Cellular and Molecular Immunology

Cellular and Molecular Immunology

Fifth Edition

Abul K. Abbas, MBBS

Professor and Chair
Department of Pathology
University of California-San Francisco School of Medicine
San Francisco, California

Andrew H. Lichtman, MD, PhD

Associate Professor of Pathology
Harvard Medical School
Brigham and Women's Hospital
Boston, Massachusetts

Illustrations by
David L. Baker, MA
Alexandra Baker, MS, CMI
DNA Illustrations, Inc.

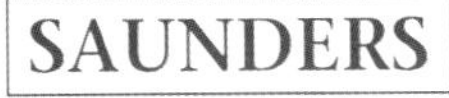

An Imprint of Elsevier Science

SAUNDERS
An Imprint of Elsevier Science

The Curtis Center
Independence Square West
Philadelphia, PA 19106

CELLULAR AND MOLECULAR IMMUNOLOGY ISBN 0-7216-0008-5
Copyright 2003, Elsevier Science (USA). All rights reserved.

No part of this publication may be reproduced, stored in a retrieval system, or transmitted in any form or by any means, electronic, mechanical, photocopying, recording or otherwise, without prior permission of the publisher (Saunders, The Curtis Center, Independence Square West, Philadelphia, PA 19106-3399).

NOTICE

Medicine is an ever-changing field. Standard safety precautions must be followed, but as new research and clinical experience broaden our knowledge, changes in treatment and drug therapy may become necessary or appropriate. Readers are advised to check the most current product information provided by the manufacturer of each drug to be administered to verify the recommended dose, the method and duration of administration, and contraindications. It is the responsibility of the treating physician, relying on experience and knowledge of the patient, to determine dosages and the best treatment for each individual patient. Neither the Publisher nor the editor assumes any liability for any injury and/or damage to persons or property arising from this publication.

The Publisher

First Edition 1991. Second Edition 1994. Third Edition 1997. Fourth Edition 2000.

Library of Congress Cataloging-in-Publication Data

Abbas, Abul K.
Cellular and molecular immunology / Abul K. Abbas, Andrew H. Lichtman; illustrations by David L. Baker, Alexandra Baker.–5th ed.
p. ; cm.
Includes bibliographical references and index.
ISBN 0-7216-0008-5
1. Cellular immunity. 2. Molecular immunology. I. Title.
[DNLM: 1. Immunity, Cellular. 2. Antibody Formation–immunology.
3. Antigens–immunology. 4. Immunologic Diseases–immunology.
5. Lymphocytes–immunology. QW568 A122c 2003]
QR185.5 .A23 2003
616.07′9–dc21

2002075771

Acquisitions Editor: Jason Malley
Developmental Editor: Heather Krehling
Project Manager: Linda Lewis Grigg
Book Designer: Gene Harris

BS/DNP

Printed in China.

Last digit is the print number: 9 8 7 6 5 4 3 2 1

TO
Ann, Jonathan, Rehana
Sheila, Eben, Ariella, Amos, Ezra

Preface

The fifth edition of this book has been extensively revised to incorporate new discoveries in immunology and the constantly growing body of knowledge. It is remarkable to us that new paradigms continue to be established in the field and unifying principles continue to emerge from analysis of complex molecular systems. Examples of areas in which our understanding has grown impressively since the last edition of this book include innate immunity and the functions of Toll-like receptors, the role of chemokines and their receptors in maintaining the functional architecture of lymphoid tissues, the functions of adapter proteins and kinase pathways in immune cell signal transduction pathways, and the basis of natural killer cell recognition of ligands. We have added new information while striving to emphasize important principles and not increase the size of the book. We have also completely reviewed the book and updated sections and changed them when necessary for increased clarity, accuracy, and completeness.

The changes in format that have evolved through the previous editions to make the book easier to read have been retained. These include the use of bold italic text to highlight "take-home messages," presentation of experimental results in bulleted lists distinguishable from the main text, and the use of boxes (including several new ones) to present detailed information about experimental approaches, disease entities, and selected molecular or biological processes. We have also strived to further improve the clarity of illustrations by simplifying the iconography. The table format has been completely reworked to improve readability.

Many individuals have made invaluable contributions to this fifth edition. Among the colleagues who have helped us, we would like to convey special thanks to Shiv Pillai for his generous willingness to review chapter drafts. Our illustrators, David and Alexandra Baker of DNA Illustrations, remain full partners in the book and provide invaluable suggestions for clarity and accuracy. Our editors, Jason Malley and Bill Schmitt, have been a source of support and encouragement. Our Developmental Editor, Hazel Hacker, shepherded the book through its preparation and production. Many other members of the staff of Elsevier Science played critical roles at various stages of this project; these include Gene Harris, Linda Grigg, and Heather Krehling. We are also grateful to our students, from whom we continue to learn how to present the science of immunology in the clearest and most enjoyable way.

Abul K. Abbas
Andrew H. Lichtman

Contents

Section I

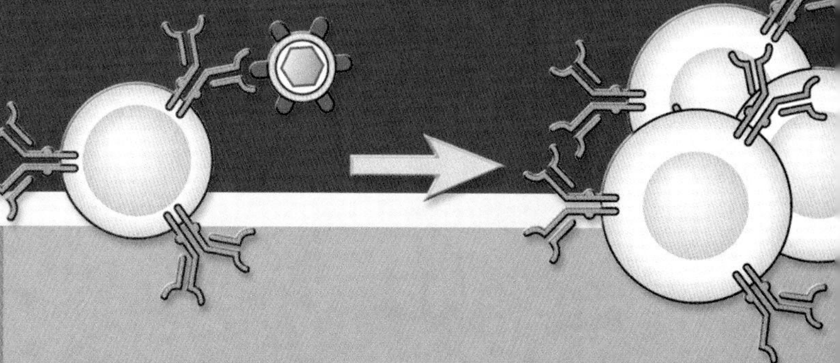

Introduction to Immunology

The first two chapters of this book introduce the nomenclature of immunology and the components of the immune system. In Chapter 1, we describe the types of immune responses and their general properties and introduce the fundamental principles that govern all immune responses. Chapter 2 is devoted to a description of the cells and tissues of the immune system, with an emphasis on their anatomic organization and structure-function relationships. This sets the stage for more thorough discussion of how the immune system recognizes and responds to antigens.

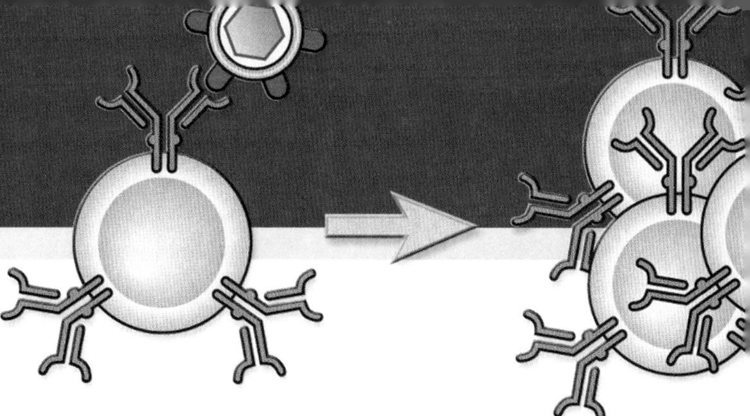

Chapter 1

General Properties of Immune Responses

The term *immunity* is derived from the Latin word *immunitas,* which referred to the protection from legal prosecution offered to Roman senators during their tenures in office. Historically, immunity meant protection from disease and, more specifically, infectious disease. The cells and molecules responsible for immunity constitute the **immune system,** and their collective and coordinated response to the introduction of foreign substances is called the **immune response.**

The physiologic function of the immune system is defense against infectious microbes. However, even noninfectious foreign substances can elicit immune responses. Furthermore, mechanisms that normally protect individuals from infection and eliminate foreign substances are themselves capable of causing tissue injury and disease in some situations. Therefore, a more inclusive definition of immunity is a reaction to foreign substances, including microbes, as well as to macromolecules such as proteins and polysaccharides, regardless of the physiologic or pathologic consequence of such a reaction. Immunology is the study of immunity in this broader sense and of the cellular and molecular events that occur after an organism encounters microbes and other foreign macromolecules.

Historians often credit Thucydides, in Athens during the fifth century BC, as having first mentioned immunity to an infection that he called "plague" (but that was probably not the bubonic plague we recognize today). The concept of immunity may have existed long before, as suggested by the ancient Chinese custom of making children resistant to smallpox by having them inhale powders made from the skin lesions of patients recovering from the disease. Immunology, in its modern form, is an experimental science, in which explanations of immunologic phenomena are based on experimental observations and the conclusions drawn from them. The evolution of immunology as an experimental discipline has depended on our ability to manipulate the function of the immune system under controlled conditions. Historically, the first clear example of this manipulation, and one that remains among the most dramatic ever recorded, was Edward Jenner's successful vaccination against smallpox. Jenner, an English physician, noticed that milkmaids who had recovered from cowpox never contracted the more serious smallpox. On the basis of this observation, he injected the material from a cowpox pustule into the arm of an 8-year-old boy. When this boy was later intentionally inoculated with smallpox, the disease did not develop. Jenner's landmark treatise on **vaccination** (Latin *vaccinus*, of or from cows) was published in 1798. It led to the widespread acceptance of this method for inducing immunity to infectious diseases, and vaccination remains the most effective method for preventing infections (Table 1–1). An eloquent testament to the importance of immunology was the announcement by the World Health Organization in 1980 that smallpox was the first disease that had been eradicated worldwide by a program of vaccination.

Since the 1960s, there has been a remarkable transformation in our understanding of the immune system and its functions. Advances in cell culture techniques (including monoclonal antibody production), immunochemistry, recombinant DNA methodology, x-ray crystallography, and creation of genetically altered animals (especially transgenic and knockout mice) have changed immunology from a largely descriptive science into one in which diverse immune phenomena can be explained in structural and biochemical terms. In this chapter, we outline the general features of immune responses and introduce the concepts that form the cornerstones of modern immunology and that recur throughout this book.

Innate and Adaptive Immunity

Defense against microbes is mediated by the early reactions of innate immunity and the later responses of adaptive immunity (Fig. 1–1 and Table 1–2). **Innate immunity** (also called natural or native immunity) consists of cellular and biochemical defense mechanisms that are in place even before infection and poised to respond rapidly to infections. These mechanisms react only to microbes and not to noninfectious substances, and they respond in essentially the same way to repeated infections. The principal components of innate immunity are (1) physical and chemical barriers, such as epithelia and antimicrobial substances produced at epithelial surfaces; (2) phagocytic cells (neutrophils, macrophages) and NK (natural killer) cells; (3) blood proteins, including members of the complement system and other mediators of inflammation; and (4) proteins called cytokines that regulate and coordinate many of the activities of the cells of innate immunity. The mechanisms of innate immunity are specific for structures that are common to groups of related microbes and may not distinguish fine differences between foreign substances. Innate immunity provides the early lines of defense against microbes.

In contrast to innate immunity, there are other immune responses that are stimulated by exposure to infectious agents and increase in magnitude and defensive capabilities with each successive exposure to a particular microbe. Because this form of immunity

Table 1–1. Effectiveness of Vaccines for Some Common Infectious Diseases

Disease	Max. number of cases	Number of cases in 2000	Percent change
Diphtheria	206,939 (1921)	2	-99.99
Measles	894,134 (1941)	63	-99.99
Mumps	152,209 (1968)	315	-99.80
Pertussis	265,269 (1934)	6,755	-97.73
Polio (paralytic)	21,269 (1952)	0	-100.0
Rubella	57,686 (1969)	152	-99.84
Tetanus	1,560 (1923)	26	-98.44
Haemophilus influenzae type B	~20,000 (1984)	1,212	-93.14
Hepatitis B	26,611 (1985)	6,646	-75.03

This table illustrates the striking decrease in the incidence of selected infectious diseases for which effective vaccines have been developed. In some cases, such as with hepatitis B, a vaccine has become available recently, and the incidence of the disease is continuing to decrease.

Adapted from Orenstein WA, AR Hinman, KJ Bart, and SC Hadler. Immunization. *In* Mandell GL, JE Bennett, and R Dolin (eds). Principles and Practices of Infectious Diseases, 4th ed. Churchill Livingstone, New York, 1995, and Morbidity and Mortality Weekly Report 49:1159–1201, 2001.

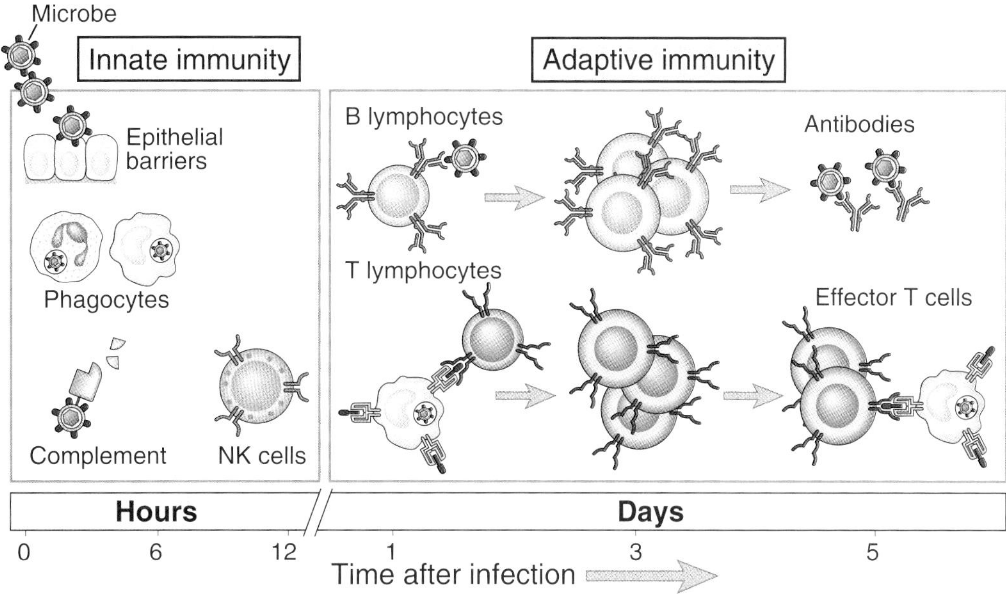

Figure 1–1 Innate and adaptive immunity.
The mechanisms of innate immunity provide the initial defense against infections. Adaptive immune responses develop later and consist of activation of lymphocytes. The kinetics of the innate and adaptive immune responses are approximations and may vary in different infections.

develops as a response to infection and adapts to the infection, it is called **adaptive immunity.** The defining characteristics of adaptive immunity are exquisite specificity for distinct molecules and an ability to "remember" and respond more vigorously to repeated exposures to the same microbe. The adaptive immune system is able to recognize and react to a large number of microbial and nonmicrobial substances. In addition, it has an extraordinary capacity to distinguish among different, even closely related, microbes and molecules, and for this reason it is also called **specific immunity.** It is also sometimes called acquired immunity, to emphasize that potent protective responses are "acquired" by experience. The components of adaptive immunity are

Table 1–2. Features of Innate and Adaptive Immunity

	Innate	Adaptive
Characteristics		
Specificity	For structures shared by groups of related microbes	For antigens of microbes and for nonmicrobial antigens
Diversity	Limited; germline-encoded	Very large; receptors are produced by somatic recombination of gene segments
Memory	None	Yes
Nonreactivity to self	Yes	Yes
Components		
Physical and chemical barriers	Skin, mucosal epithelia; antimicrobial chemicals	Lymphocytes in epithelia; antibodies secreted at epithelial surfaces
Blood proteins	Complement	Antibodies
Cells	Phagocytes (macrophages, neutrophils), natural killer cells	Lymphocytes

This table lists the major characteristics and components of innate and adaptive immune responses. Innate immunity is discussed in much more detail in Chapter 12.

lymphocytes and their products. Foreign substances that induce specific immune responses or are the targets of such responses are called **antigens.** By convention, the terms *immune responses* and *immune system* refer to adaptive immunity, unless stated otherwise.

Innate and adaptive immune responses are components of an integrated system of host defense in which numerous cells and molecules function cooperatively. The mechanisms of innate immunity provide effective defense against infections. However, many pathogenic microbes have evolved to resist innate immunity, and their elimination requires the powerful mechanisms of adaptive immunity. There are two important links between innate immunity and adaptive immunity. First, the innate immune response to microbes stimulates adaptive immune responses and influences the nature of the adaptive responses. Second, adaptive immune responses use many of the effector mechanisms of innate immunity to eliminate microbes, and they often function by enhancing the antimicrobial activities of the defense mechanisms of innate immunity. We will return to a more detailed discussion of the mechanisms and physiologic functions of innate immunity in Chapter 12.

Innate immunity is phylogenetically the oldest system of host defense, and the adaptive immune system evolved later (Box 1–1). In invertebrates, host defense against foreign invaders is mediated largely by the mechanisms of innate immunity, including phagocytes and circulating molecules that resemble the plasma proteins of innate immunity in vertebrates. Adaptive immunity, consisting of lymphocytes and antibodies, first appeared in jawed vertebrates and became increasingly specialized with further evolution.

Types of Adaptive Immune Responses

There are two types of adaptive immune responses, called humoral immunity and cell-mediated immunity, that are mediated by different components of the immune system and function to eliminate different types of microbes (Fig. 1–2). **Humoral immunity** is mediated by molecules in the blood and mucosal secretions, called **antibodies,** that are produced by cells called **B lymphocytes** (also called B cells). Antibodies recognize microbial antigens, neutralize the infectivity of the microbes, and target microbes for elimination by various effector mechanisms. Humoral immunity is the principal defense mechanism against extracellular microbes and their toxins because secreted antibodies can bind to these microbes and toxins and assist in their elimination. Antibodies themselves are specialized, and different types of antibodies may activate different effector mechanisms. For example, some types of antibodies promote phagocytosis, and others trigger the release of inflammatory mediators from leukocytes such as mast cells. **Cell-mediated immunity,** also called cellular immunity, is mediated by **T lymphocytes** (also called T cells). Intracellular microbes, such as viruses and some bacteria, survive and proliferate inside phagocytes and other host cells, where they are inac-

BOX 1–1

Evolution of the Immune System

Mechanisms for defending the host against microbes are present in some form in all multicellular organisms. These mechanisms constitute innate immunity. The more specialized defense mechanisms that constitute adaptive immunity are found in vertebrates only.

Various cells in invertebrates respond to microbes by surrounding these infectious agents and destroying them. These responding cells resemble phagocytes and have been called phagocytic amebocytes in acelomates, hemocytes in molluscs and arthropods, coelomocytes in annelids, and blood leukocytes in tunicates. Invertebrates do not contain antigen-specific lymphocytes and do not produce immunoglobulin (Ig) molecules or complement proteins. However, they contain a number of soluble molecules that bind to and lyse microbes. These molecules include lectin-like proteins, which bind to carbohydrates on microbial cell walls and agglutinate the microbes, and numerous lytic and antimicrobial factors such as lysozyme, which is also produced by neutrophils in higher organisms. Phagocytes in some invertebrates may be capable of secreting cytokines that resemble macrophage-derived cytokines in the vertebrates. Thus, host defense in invertebrates is mediated by the cells and molecules that resemble the effector mechanisms of innate immunity in higher organisms.

Many studies have shown that invertebrates are capable of rejecting foreign tissue transplants, or allografts. (In vertebrates, this process of graft rejection is dependent on adaptive immune responses.) If sponges (Porifera) from two different colonies are parabiosed by being mechanically held together, they become necrotic in 1 to 2 weeks, whereas sponges from the same colony become fused and continue to grow. Earthworms (annelids) and starfish (echinoderms) also reject tissue grafts from other species of the phyla. These rejection reactions are mediated mainly by phagocyte-like cells. They differ from graft rejection in vertebrates in that specific memory for the grafted tissue either is not generated or is difficult to demonstrate. Nevertheless, such results indicate that even invertebrates must express cell surface molecules that distinguish self from nonself, and such molecules may be the precursors of histocompatibility molecules in vertebrates.

The various components of the mammalian immune system appear to have arisen together in phylogeny and have become increasingly specialized with evolution (see Table). Thus, of the cardinal features of adaptive immune responses, specificity, memory, self/nonself discrimination, and a capacity for self-limitation are present in the lowest vertebrates, and diversity of antigen recognition

Continued on following page

	Innate immunity			Adaptive immunity	
	Phagocytes	NK cells	Antibodies	T and B lymphocytes	Lymph nodes
Invertebrates					
Protozoa	+	−	−	−	−
Sponges	+	−	−	−	−
Annelids	+	+	−	−	−
Arthropods	+	−	−	−	−
Vertebrates					
Elasmobranchs (sharks, skates, rays)	+	+	+ (IgM only)	+	−
Teleosts (common fish)	+	+	+ (IgM, others?)	+	−
Amphibians	+	+	+ (2 or 3 classes)	+	−
Reptiles	+	+	+ (3 classes)	+	−
Birds	+	+	+ (3 classes)	+	+ (some species)
Mammals	+	+	+ (7 or 8 classes)	+	+

Key: +, present; −, absent.

increases progressively in the higher species. All jawed vertebrates contain antibody molecules. The appearance of antibodies coincides with the development of specialized genetic mechanisms for generating a diverse repertoire. Fishes have only one type of antibody, called IgM; this number increases to two types in amphibians such as *Xenopus* and to seven or eight types in mammals. The diversity of antibodies is much lower in *Xenopus* than in mammals, even though the genes coding for antibodies are structurally similar. Lymphocytes that have some characteristics of both B and T cells are probably present in the earliest vertebrates, such as lampreys, and become specialized into functionally and phenotypically distinct subsets in amphibians and most clearly in birds and mammals. The major histocompatibility complex, which is the genetic locus that controls T lymphocyte antigen recognition, is present in some of the more advanced species of amphibians and fishes and in all birds and mammals. The earliest organized lymphoid tissues detected during evolution are the gut-associated lymphoid tissues; spleen, thymus, and lymph nodes are found in higher vertebrates.

cessible to circulating antibodies. Defense against such infections is a function of cell-mediated immunity, which promotes the destruction of microbes residing in phagocytes or the killing of infected cells to eliminate reservoirs of infection.

Protective immunity against a microbe may be induced by the host's response to the microbe or by the transfer of antibodies or lymphocytes specific for the microbe (Fig. 1–3). The form of immunity that is induced by exposure to a foreign antigen is called **active immunity** because the immunized individual plays an active role in responding to the antigen. Individuals and lymphocytes that have not encountered a particular antigen are said to be **naive.** Individuals who have responded to a microbial antigen and are protected from subsequent exposures to that microbe are said to be **immune.**

Immunity can also be conferred on an individual by transferring serum or lymphocytes from a specifically immunized individual, a process known as adoptive transfer in experimental situations. The recipient of such a transfer becomes immune to the particular antigen without ever having been exposed to or having responded to that antigen. Therefore, this form of immunity is called **passive immunity.** Passive immunization is a useful method for conferring resistance rapidly, without having to wait for an active immune response to develop. An example of passive immunity is the transfer of maternal antibodies to the fetus, which enables newborns to combat infections before they acquire the ability to produce antibodies themselves. Passive immunization against bacterial toxins by the administration of antibodies from immunized animals is a lifesaving treatment of potentially lethal infections, such as tetanus. The technique of adoptive transfer has also made it possible to define the various cells and molecules that are responsible for mediating specific immunity. In fact, humoral immunity was originally defined as the type of immunity that could be transferred to unimmunized, or naive, individuals by antibody-

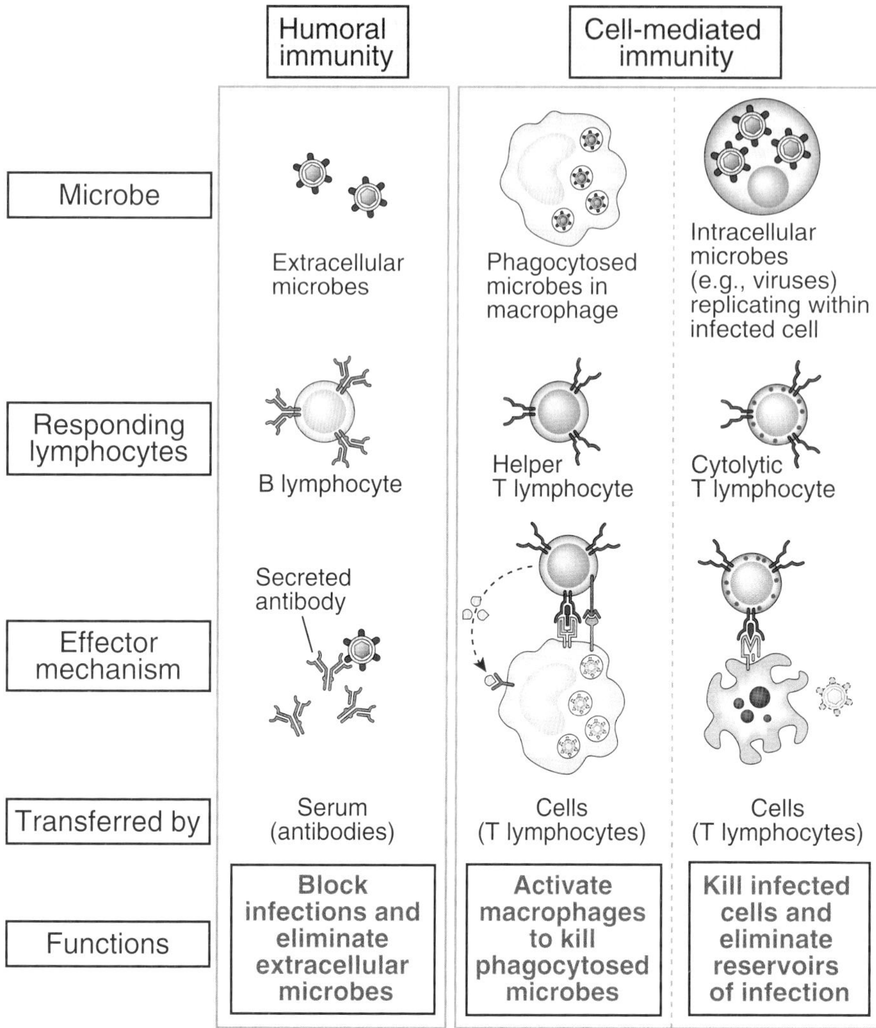

Figure 1–2 Types of adaptive immunity.
In humoral immunity, B lymphocytes secrete antibodies that prevent infections by and eliminate extracellular microbes. In cell-mediated immunity, T lymphocytes either activate macrophages to kill phagocytosed microbes or cytolytic T lymphocytes directly destroy infected cells.

containing cell-free portions of the blood (i.e., plasma or serum [once called humors]) obtained from previously immunized individuals. Similarly, cell-mediated immunity was defined as the form of immunity that can be transferred to naive individuals with cells (T lymphocytes) from immunized individuals but not with plasma or serum.

The first experimental demonstration of humoral immunity was provided by Emil von Behring and Shibasaburo Kitasato in 1890. They showed that if serum from animals who had recovered from diphtheria infection was transferred to naive animals, the recipients became specifically resistant to diphtheria infection. The active components of the serum were called antitoxins because they neutralized the pathologic effects of the diphtheria toxin. In the early 1900s, Karl Landsteiner and other investigators showed that not only toxins but also nonmicrobial substances could induce humoral immune responses. From such studies arose the more general term **antibodies** for the serum proteins that mediate humoral immunity. Substances that bound antibodies and generated the production of antibodies were then called **antigens.** (The properties of antibodies and antigens are described in Chapter 3.) In 1900, Paul Ehrlich provided a theoretical framework for the specificity of antigen-antibody reactions, the experimental proof for which came during the next 50 years from the work of Landsteiner and others using simple chemicals as antigens. Ehrlich's theories of the physicochemical complementarity of antigens and antibodies are remarkable for their prescience. This early emphasis on antibodies led to the general acceptance of the humoral theory of immunity, according to which immunity is mediated by substances present in body fluids.

The cellular theory of immunity, which stated that host cells were the principal mediators of immunity, was championed initially by Elie Metchnikoff. His demonstration of phagocytes surrounding a thorn stuck into a translucent starfish larva, published in 1893, was perhaps the first experimental evidence that cells respond to foreign invaders. Sir Almroth Wright's observation in the early 1900s that factors in immune serum enhanced the phagocytosis of bacteria by coating the bacteria, a process known as opsonization, lent support to the belief that antibodies prepared microbes

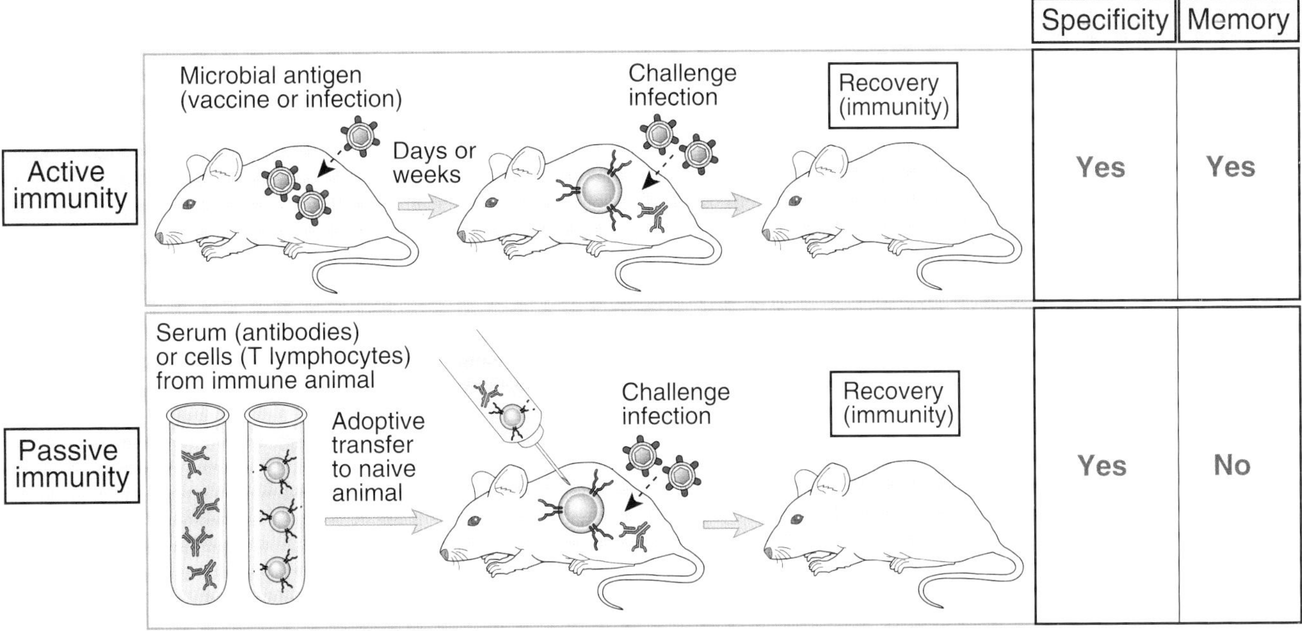

Figure 1–3 Active and passive immunity.
Active immunity is conferred by a host response to a microbe or microbial antigen, whereas passive immunity is conferred by adoptive transfer of antibodies or T lymphocytes specific for the microbe. Both forms of immunity provide resistance to infection (immunity) and are specific for microbial antigens, but only active immune responses generate immunologic memory.

for ingestion by phagocytes. These early "cellularists" were unable to prove that specific immunity to microbes could be mediated by cells. The cellular theory of immunity became firmly established in the 1950s, when George Mackaness showed that resistance to an intracellular bacterium, *Listeria monocytogenes*, could be adoptively transferred with cells but not with serum. We now know that the specificity of cell-mediated immunity is due to lymphocytes, which often function in concert with other cells, such as phagocytes, to eliminate microbes.

In the clinical setting, immunity to a previously encountered microbe is measured indirectly, either by assaying for the presence of products of immune responses (such as serum antibodies specific for microbial antigens) or by administering substances purified from the microbe and measuring reactions to these substances. A reaction to a microbial antigen is detectable only in individuals who have previously encountered the antigen; these individuals are said to be "sensitized" to the antigen, and the reaction is an indication of "sensitivity." Although the reaction to the purified antigen has no protective function, it implies that the sensitized individual is capable of mounting a protective immune response to the microbe.

Cardinal Features of Adaptive Immune Responses

All humoral and cell-mediated immune responses to foreign antigens have a number of fundamental properties that reflect the properties of the lymphocytes that mediate these responses (Table 1–3).

- ***Specificity and diversity.*** Immune responses are specific for distinct antigens and, in fact, for different portions of a single complex protein, polysaccharide, or other macromolecule (Fig. 1–4). The

Table 1–3. Cardinal Features of Adaptive Immune Responses

Feature	Functional significance
Specificity	Ensures that distinct antigens elicit specific responses
Diversity	Enables immune system to respond to a large variety of antigens
Memory	Leads to enhanced responses to repeated exposures to the same antigens
Specialization	Generates responses that are optimal for defense against different types of microbes
Self-limitation	Allows immune system to respond to newly encountered antigens
Nonreactivity to self	Prevents injury to the host during responses to foreign antigens

The features of adaptive immune responses are essential for the functions of the immune system.

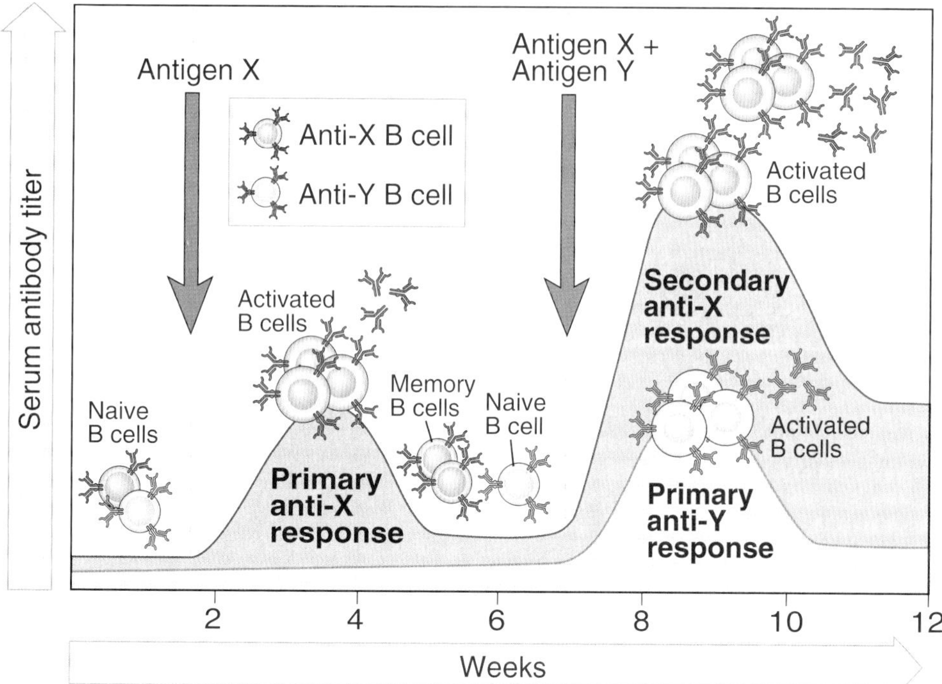

Figure 1–4 Specificity, memory, and self-limitation of immune responses. Antigens X and Y induce the production of different antibodies (specificity). The secondary response to antigen X is more rapid and larger than the primary response (memory). Antibody levels decline with time after each immunization (self-limitation).The same features are seen in cell-mediated immune responses.

parts of such antigens that are specifically recognized by individual lymphocytes are called determinants or epitopes. This fine specificity exists because individual lymphocytes express membrane receptors that are able to distinguish subtle differences in structure between distinct antigens. Clones of lymphocytes with different specificities are present in unimmunized individuals and are able to recognize and respond to foreign antigens. This concept is the basic tenet of the clonal selection hypothesis, which is discussed in more detail later in this chapter.

The total number of antigenic specificities of the lymphocytes in an individual, called the **lymphocyte repertoire,** is extremely large. It is estimated that the immune system of an individual can discriminate 10^7 to 10^9 distinct antigenic determinants. This property of the lymphocyte repertoire is called **diversity**. It is the result of variability in the structures of the antigen-binding sites of lymphocyte receptors for antigens. In other words, there are many different clones of lymphocytes that differ in the structures of their antigen receptors and therefore in their specificity for antigens, creating a total repertoire that is extremely diverse. The molecular mechanisms that generate such diverse antigen receptors are discussed in Chapter 7.

- ***Memory.*** Exposure of the immune system to a foreign antigen enhances its ability to respond again to that antigen. Responses to second and subsequent exposures to the same antigen, called secondary immune responses, are usually more rapid, larger, and often qualitatively different from the first, or primary, immune response to that antigen (see Fig. 1–4). Immunologic memory occurs partly because each exposure to an antigen expands the clone of lymphocytes specific for that antigen. In addition, stimulation of naive lymphocytes by antigens generates long-lived memory cells (discussed in detail in Chapter 2). These memory cells have special characteristics that make them more efficient at eliminating the antigen than are naive lymphocytes that have not previously been exposed to the antigen. For instance, memory B lymphocytes produce antibodies that bind antigens with higher affinities than do previously unstimulated B cells, and memory T cells are better able to home to sites of infection than are naive T cells.
- ***Specialization.*** As we have already noted, the immune system responds in distinct and special ways to different microbes, maximizing the efficiency of antimicrobial defense mechanisms. Thus, humoral immunity and cell-mediated immunity are elicited by different classes of microbes or by the same microbe at different stages of infection (extracellular and intracellular), and each type of immune response protects the host against that class of microbe. Even within humoral or cell-mediated immune responses, the nature of the antibodies or T lymphocytes that are generated may vary from one class of microbe to another. We will return to the mechanisms and functional significance of such specialization in Sections III and IV of this book.
- ***Self-limitation.*** All normal immune responses wane with time after antigen stimulation, thus returning the immune system to its resting basal state, a process called **homeostasis** (see Fig. 1–4). Homeostasis is

maintained largely because immune responses are triggered by antigens and function to eliminate antigens, thus eliminating the essential stimulus for lymphocyte activation. In addition, antigens and the immune responses to them stimulate regulatory mechanisms that inhibit the response itself. These homeostatic mechanisms are discussed in Chapter 10.

- ***Nonreactivity to self.*** One of the most remarkable properties of every normal individual's immune system is its ability to recognize, respond to, and eliminate many foreign (nonself) antigens while not reacting harmfully to that individual's own (self) antigenic substances. Im-munologic unresponsiveness is also called **tolerance.** Tolerance to self antigens, or self-tolerance, is maintained by several mechanisms. These include eliminating lymphocytes that express receptors specific for some self antigens and allowing lymphocytes to encounter other self antigens in settings that either fail to stimulate or lead to functional inactivation of the self-reactive lymphocytes. The mechanisms of self-tolerance and discrimination between self and foreign antigens are discussed in Chapter 10. Abnormalities in the induction or maintenance of self-tolerance lead to immune responses against self antigens (autologous antigens), often resulting in disorders called **autoimmune diseases.** The development and pathologic consequences of autoimmunity are described in Chapter 18.

These features of adaptive immunity are necessary if the immune system is to perform its normal function of host defense (see Table 1–3). Specificity and memory enable the immune system to mount heightened responses to persistent or recurring stimulation with the same antigen and thus to combat infections that are prolonged or occur repeatedly. Diversity is essential if the immune system is to defend individuals against the many potential pathogens in the environment. Specialization enables the host to "custom design" responses to best combat many different types of microbes. Self-limitation allows the system to return to a state of rest after it eliminates each foreign antigen and to be prepared to respond to other antigens. Self-tolerance is vital for preventing reactions against one's own cells and tissues while maintaining a diverse repertoire of lymphocytes specific for foreign antigens.

Cellular Components of the Adaptive Immune System

The principal cells of the immune system are lymphocytes, antigen-presenting cells, and effector cells. Lymphocytes are the cells that specifically recognize and respond to foreign antigens and are therefore the mediators of humoral and cellular immunity. There are distinct subpopulations of lymphocytes that differ in how they recognize antigens and in their functions (Fig. 1–5). **B lymphocytes** are the only cells capable of producing antibodies. They recognize extracellular (including cell surface) antigens and differentiate into antibody-secreting cells, thus functioning as the mediators of humoral immunity. **T lymphocytes,** the cells of cell-mediated immunity, recognize the antigens of intracellular microbes and function to destroy these microbes or the infected cells. T cells do not produce antibody molecules. Their antigen receptors are membrane molecules distinct from but structurally related to antibodies (see Chapter 6). T lymphocytes have a restricted specificity for antigens; they recognize only peptide antigens attached to host proteins that are encoded by genes in the major histocompatibility complex (MHC) and that are expressed on the surfaces of other cells. As a result, these T cells recognize and respond to cell surface–associated but not soluble antigens (see Chapter 5). T lymphocytes consist of functionally distinct populations, the best defined of which are **helper T cells** and **cytolytic,** or **cytotoxic, T lymphocytes** (CTLs). In response to antigenic stimulation, helper T cells secrete proteins called cytokines, whose function is to stimulate the proliferation and differentiation of the T cells as well as other cells, including B cells, macrophages, and other leukocytes. CTLs kill cells that produce foreign antigens, such as cells infected by viruses and other intracellular microbes. Some T lymphocytes, which are called regulatory T cells, may function mainly to inhibit immune responses. The nature and physiologic roles of these regulatory T cells are incompletely understood (see Chapter 10). A third class of lymphocytes, natural killer (NK) cells, is involved in innate immunity against viruses and other intracellular microbes. We will return to a more detailed discussion of the properties of lymphocytes in Chapter 2.

The initiation and development of adaptive immune responses require that antigens be captured and displayed to specific lymphocytes. The cells that serve this role are called **antigen-presenting cells** (APCs). The most highly specialized APCs are dendritic cells, which capture microbial antigens that enter from the external environment, transport these antigens to lymphoid organs, and present the antigens to naive T lymphocytes to initiate immune responses. Other cell types function as APCs at different stages of cell-mediated and humoral immune responses. We will describe the functions of APCs in Chapter 5.

The activation of lymphocytes by antigen leads to the generation of numerous mechanisms that function to eliminate the antigen. Antigen elimination often requires the participation of cells called **effector cells.** Activated T lymphocytes, mononuclear phagocytes, and other leukocytes function as effector cells in different immune responses.

Lymphocytes and accessory cells are concentrated in anatomically discrete lymphoid organs, where they interact with one another to initiate immune responses. Lymphocytes are also present in the blood; from the blood, they can recirculate to lymphoid tissues and to

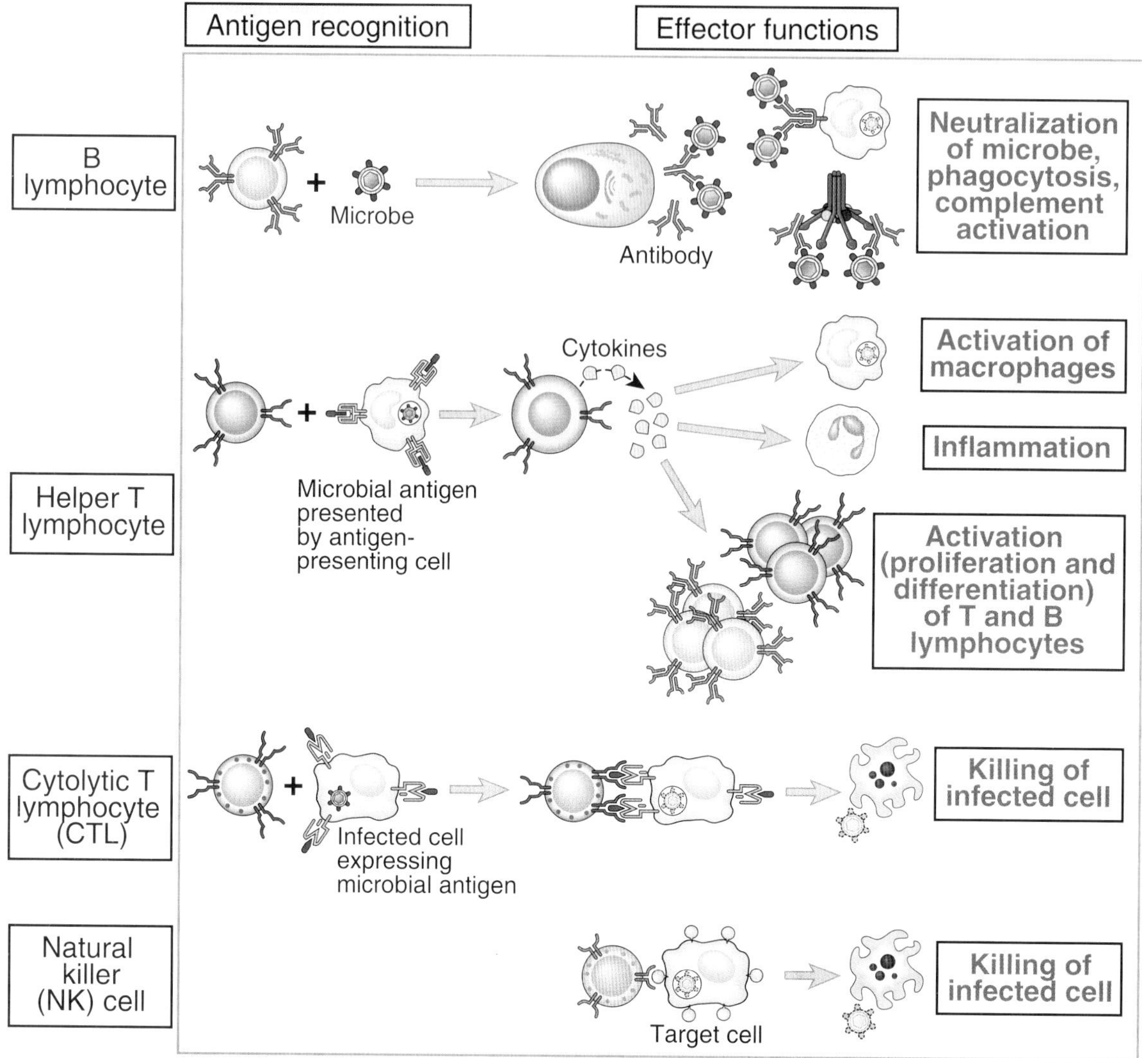

Figure 1–5 Classes of lymphocytes.
B lymphocytes recognize soluble antigens and develop into antibody-secreting cells. Helper T lymphocytes recognize antigens on the surfaces of antigen-presenting cells and secrete cytokines, which stimulate different mechanisms of immunity and inflammation. Cytolytic T lymphocytes recognize antigens on infected cells and kill these cells. Natural killer cells use receptors that are not fully identified to recognize and kill their targets, such as infected cells.

peripheral sites of antigen exposure to eliminate the antigen (see Chapter 2).

Phases of Adaptive Immune Responses

Adaptive immune responses may be divided into distinct phases—the recognition of antigen, the activation of lymphocytes, and the effector phase of antigen elimination—followed by the return to homeostasis and the maintenance of memory (Fig. 1–6). All immune responses are initiated by the specific recognition of antigens. This recognition leads to the activation of the lymphocytes that recognize the antigen and culminates in the development of effector mechanisms that mediate the physiologic function of the response, namely, the elimination of the antigen. After the antigen is eliminated, the immune response abates and homeostasis is restored. We summarize the important features of each phase in the following section, and we will discuss the mechanisms of adaptive immunity in the context of these phases throughout the book.

Recognition of Antigens

Every individual possesses numerous clonally derived lymphocytes, each clone having arisen from a single precursor and being capable of recognizing and responding to a distinct antigenic determinant, and when an antigen enters, it selects a specific preexisting clone and activates it (Fig. 1–7). This fundamental concept is called the **clonal selection hypothesis.** It was first suggested by Niels Jerne in 1955, and most clearly enunciated by Macfarlane Burnet in 1957, as a hypo-

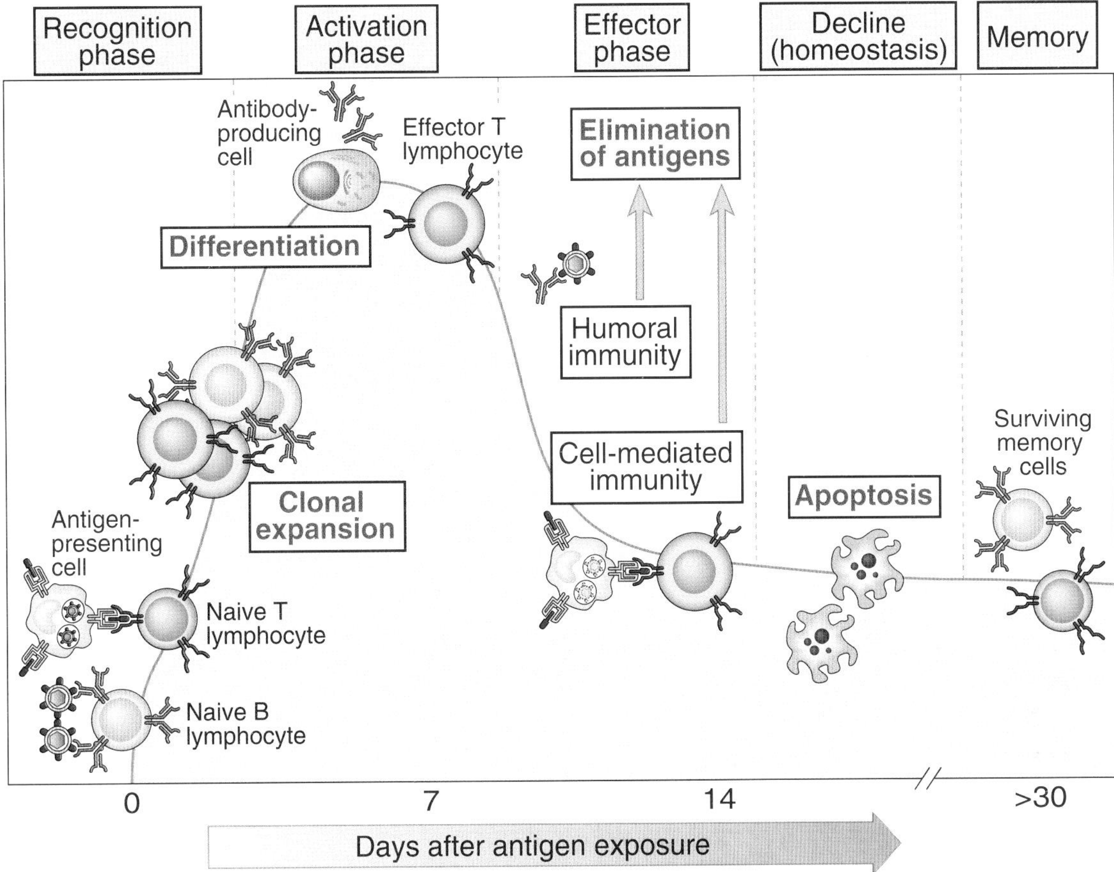

Figure 1–6 Phases of adaptive immune responses. Adaptive immune responses consist of distinct phases, the first three being the recognition of antigen, the activation of lymphocytes, and the effector phase (elimination of antigen). The response declines as antigen-stimulated lymphocytes die by apoptosis, and the antigen-specific cells that survive are responsible for memory. The duration of each phase may vary in different immune responses. The y-axis represents an arbitrary measure of the magnitude of the response. These principles apply to humoral immunity (mediated by B lymphocytes) and cell-mediated immunity (mediated by T lymphocytes).

thesis to explain how the immune system could respond to a large number and variety of antigens. According to this hypothesis, antigen-specific clones of lymphocytes develop before and independent of exposure to antigen. The cells constituting each clone have identical antigen receptors, which are different from the receptors on the cells of all other clones. Although it is difficult to place an upper limit on the number of antigenic determinants that can be recognized by the mammalian immune system, a frequently used estimate is on the order of 10^7 to 10^9. This is a reasonable approximation of the number of different antigen receptor proteins that are produced and therefore reflects the number of distinct clones of lymphocytes present in each individual. Foreign antigens interact with preexisting clones of antigen-specific lymphocytes in the specialized lymphoid tissues where immune responses are initiated.

The key postulates of the clonal selection hypothesis have been convincingly proved by a variety of experiments and form the cornerstone of the current concepts of lymphocyte specificity and antigen recognition.

- Definitive proof that antigen-specific clones of lymphocytes exist before antigen exposure came when the structure of antigen receptors and the molecular basis of receptor expression were defined. All the lymphocytes of a particular clone express receptors of one specificity, and these receptors are expressed at a stage and site of maturation where the lymphocytes have not encountered antigens (see Chapter 7).

- The fact that an individual clone of lymphocytes can recognize and respond to only one antigen was established by limiting dilution culture experiments. In this type of experiment, lymphocytes are distributed in culture wells in such a way that each well contains cells from a single clone. When mixtures of antigens are added to these wells, the cells in each well respond to only one of the antigens (e.g., by producing antibodies specific for that antigen).

- More recently, methods for assaying the expansion of antigen-specific lymphocyte populations *in vivo* have shown that administration of an antigen stimulates expansion of specific lymphocyte populations and no detectable response of other, "bystander," lymphocyte populations that are not specific for that antigen (see Chapters 8 and 9).

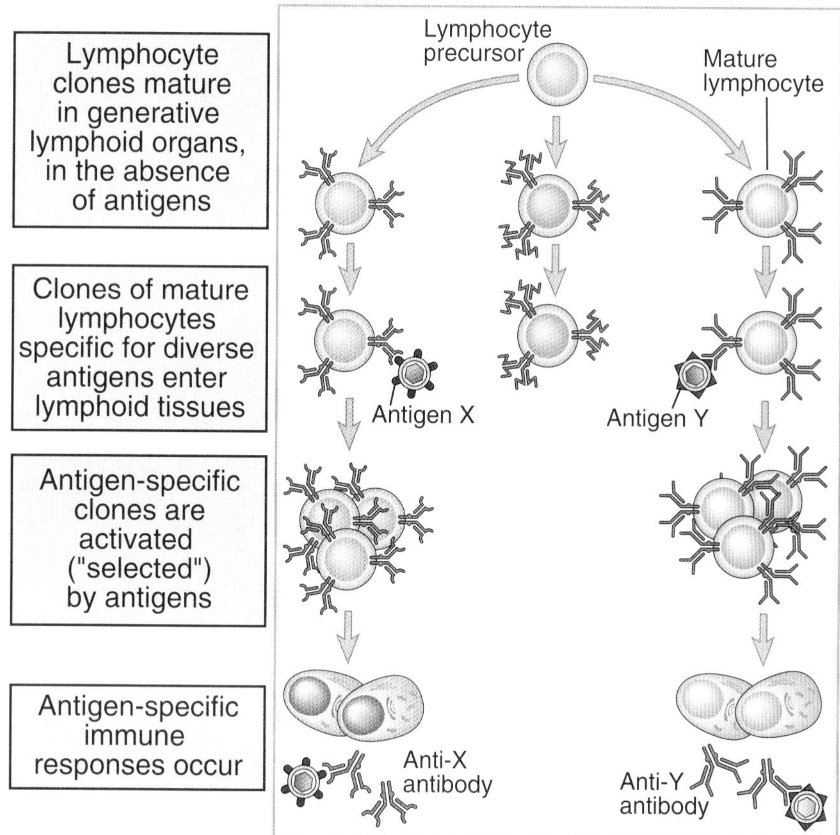

Figure 1–7 The clonal selection hypothesis.

Each antigen (X or Y) selects a preexisting clone of specific lymphocytes and stimulates the proliferation and differentiation of that clone. The diagram shows only B lymphocytes giving rise to antibody-secreting effector cells, but the same principle applies to T lymphocytes.

Activation of Lymphocytes

The activation of lymphocytes requires two distinct signals, the first being antigen and the second being either microbial products or components of innate immune responses to microbes (Fig. 1–8). This idea is called the **two-signal hypothesis** for lymphocyte activation. The requirement for antigen (so-called signal 1) ensures that the ensuing immune response is specific. The requirement for additional stimuli triggered by microbes or innate immune reactions to microbes (signal 2) ensures that immune responses are induced when they are needed (i.e., against microbes and other noxious substances) and not against harmless substances, including self antigens. We will return to the nature of second signals for lymphocyte activation in Chapters 8 and 9.

The responses of lymphocytes to antigens and second signals consist of the synthesis of new proteins, cellular proliferation, and differentiation into effector and memory cells. We will discuss these events in more detail in Chapter 2 and later chapters, after we describe the properties of lymphocytes.

Effector Phase of Immune Responses: Elimination of Antigens

During the effector phase of immune responses, lymphocytes that have been specifically activated by antigens perform the effector functions that lead to the elimination of the antigens. Antibodies and T lymphocytes eliminate extracellular and intracellular microbes, respectively. These functions of antibodies and T cells often require the participation of other, nonlymphoid effector cells and defense mechanisms that also operate in innate immunity. Thus, the same innate immune mechanisms that provide the early lines of defense against infectious agents may be used by the subsequent adaptive response to eliminate microbes. In fact, as we mentioned earlier, an important general function of adaptive immune responses is to enhance the effector mechanisms of innate immunity and to focus these effector mechanisms on those tissues and cells that contain foreign antigen.

Homeostasis: Decline of Immune Responses

At the end of an immune response, the immune system returns to its basal resting state, in large part because most of the progeny of antigen-stimulated lymphocytes die by apoptosis. Apoptosis is a form of regulated, physiologic cell death in which the nucleus undergoes condensation and fragmentation, the plasma membrane shows blebbing and vesiculation, the internal sequestration of some membrane lipids is lost, and the dead cells are rapidly phagocytosed without their contents being released. (This process contrasts with necrosis, a type of cell death in which the nuclear and plasma membranes break down and cellular contents often spill out, inducing a local inflammatory reaction.) A large fraction of antigen-stimulated lymphocytes undergoes apoptosis, probably because the survival of lym-

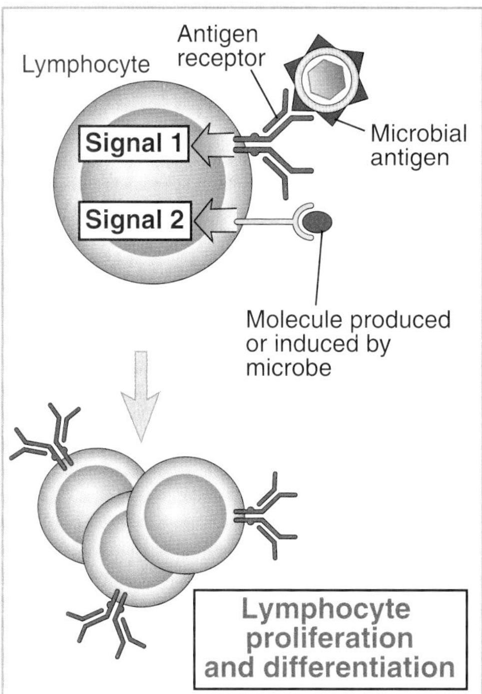

Figure 1–8 The two-signal requirement for lymphocyte activation.

Antigen recognition by lymphocytes provides signal 1 for the activation of the lymphocytes, and components of microbes or substances produced during innate immune responses to microbes provide signal 2. In this illustration, the lymphocytes are B cells, but the same principles apply to T lymphocytes. The nature of second signals differs for B and T cells and is described in later chapters.

phocytes is dependent on antigen and antigen-induced growth factors, and as the immune response eliminates the antigen that initiated it, the lymphocytes become deprived of essential survival stimuli. A considerable amount of information has accumulated about the mechanisms of apoptosis, and its regulation, in lymphoid cells (see Box 10–2, Chapter 10).

In Sections II, III, and IV, we describe in detail the recognition, activation, effector phases, and regulation of adaptive immune responses. The principles introduced in this chapter recur throughout the book.

Summary

- Protective immunity against microbes is mediated by the early reactions of innate immunity and the later responses of adaptive immunity. Innate immunity is stimulated by structures shared by groups of microbes. Adaptive immunity is specific for different microbial and nonmicrobial antigens and is increased by repeated exposures to antigen (immunologic memory).
- Humoral immunity is mediated by B lymphocytes and their secreted products, antibodies, and functions in defense against extracellular microbes. Cell-mediated immunity is mediated by T lymphocytes and their products, such as cytokines, and is important for defense against intracellular microbes.
- Immunity may be acquired by a response to antigen (active immunity) or conferred by transfer of antibodies or cells from an immunized individual (passive immunity).
- The immune system possesses several properties that are of fundamental importance for its normal functions. These include specificity for different antigens, a diverse repertoire capable of recognizing a wide variety of antigens, memory for antigen exposure, specialized responses to different microbes, self-limitation, and the ability to discriminate between foreign antigens and self antigens.
- Lymphocytes are the only cells capable of specifically recognizing antigens and are thus the principal cells of adaptive immunity. The two major subpopulations of lymphocytes are B cells and T cells, and they differ in their antigen receptors and functions. Specialized antigen-presenting cells capture microbial antigens and display these antigens for recognition by lymphocytes. The elimination of antigens often requires the participation of various effector cells.
- The adaptive immune response is initiated by the recognition of foreign antigens by specific lymphocytes. Lymphocytes respond by proliferating and by differentiating into effector cells, whose function is to eliminate the antigen, and into memory cells, which show enhanced responses on subsequent encounters with the antigen. The activation of lymphocytes requires antigen and additional signals that may be provided by microbes or by innate immune responses to microbes.
- The effector phase of adaptive immunity requires the participation of various defense mechanisms, including the complement system and phagocytes, that also operate in innate immunity. The adaptive immune response enhances the defense mechanisms of innate immunity.

Selected Readings

Burnet FM. A modification of Jerne's theory of antibody production using the concept of clonal selection. Australian Journal of Science 20:67–69, 1957.

du Pasquier L. The immune system of invertebrates and vertebrates. Comparative Biochemistry and Physiology Part B: Biochemistry and Molecular Biology 129:1–15, 2001.

Jerne NK. The natural-selection theory of antibody formation. Proceedings of the National Academy of Sciences USA 41:849–857, 1955.

Silverstein AM. A History of Immunology. Academic Press, San Diego, 1989.

Silverstein AM. Paul Ehrlich's Receptor Immunology: The Magnificent Obsession. Academic Press, New York, 2001.

Chapter 2

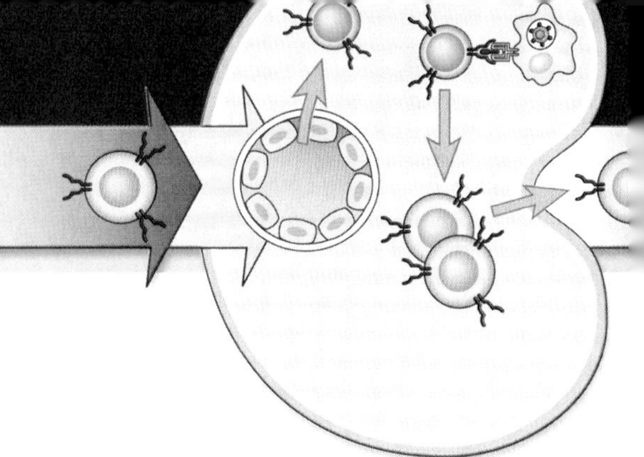

Cells and Tissues of the Immune System

The cells of the adaptive immune system are normally present as circulating cells in the blood and lymph, as anatomically defined collections in lymphoid organs, and as scattered cells in virtually all tissues. The anatomic organization of these cells and their ability to circulate and exchange among blood, lymph, and tissues are of critical importance for the generation of immune responses. The immune system faces numerous challenges to generate effective protective responses against infectious pathogens. First, the system must be able to respond to small numbers of many different microbes that may be introduced at any site in the body. Second, very few naive lymphocytes specifically recognize and respond to any one antigen. Third, the effector mechanisms of the immune system (antibodies and effector T cells) may have to locate and destroy microbes at sites that are distant from the site of initial infection. The ability of the immune system to meet these challenges and to perform its protective functions optimally is dependent on several properties of its cells and tissues.

- ***Specialized tissues, called peripheral lymphoid organs, function to concentrate antigens that are introduced through the common portals of entry (skin and gastrointestinal and respiratory tracts).*** The capture of antigen and its transport to lymphoid organs are the first steps in adaptive immune responses.

- ***Naive lymphocytes (i.e., lymphocytes that have not previously encountered antigens) migrate through these peripheral lymphoid organs, where they recognize antigens and initiate immune responses.*** Effector and memory lymphocytes develop from the progeny of antigen-stimulated naive cells.

- ***Effector and memory lymphocytes circulate in the blood, home to peripheral sites of antigen entry, and are efficiently retained at these sites.*** This ensures that immunity is systemic (i.e., that protective mechanisms can act anywhere in the body).

Adaptive immune responses develop through a series of steps, in each of which the special properties of immune cells and tissues play critical roles. The key phases of these responses and the roles of different cells and tissues are illustrated schematically in Figure 2–1. This chapter describes the cells and organs of the immune system and concludes with a discussion of the circulation of lymphocytes.

Cells of the Immune System

The cells that are involved in adaptive immune responses are antigen-specific lymphocytes, specialized antigen-presenting cells (APCs) that display antigens and activate lymphocytes, and effector cells that function to eliminate antigens. These cell types were introduced in Chapter 1. Here we describe the morphology and functional characteristics of lymphocytes and APCs and then explain how these cells are organized in lymphoid tissues. The numbers of some of these cell types in the blood are listed in Table 2–1. Although these cells are found in the blood, their responses to antigens are localized to lymphoid and other tissues and are generally not reflected in changes in the total numbers of circulating leukocytes.

Lymphocytes

Lymphocytes are the only cells in the body capable of specifically recognizing and distinguishing different antigenic determinants and are therefore responsible for the two defining characteristics of the adaptive immune response, specificity and memory. Several lines of evidence have established the role of lymphocytes as the cells that mediate adaptive immunity.

- Protective immunity to microbes can be adoptively transferred from immunized to naive individuals only by lymphocytes or their secreted products.
- Some congenital and acquired immunodeficiencies are associated with reduction of lymphocytes in the peripheral circulation and in lymphoid tissues. Furthermore, depletion of lymphocytes with drugs, irradiation, or cell type–specific antibodies, and more recently by targeted gene disruptions in mice, leads to impaired immune responses.
- Stimulation of lymphocytes by antigens in culture leads to responses *in vitro* that show many of the characteristics of immune responses induced under more physiologic conditions *in vivo.*
- Most important, specific high-affinity receptors for antigens are produced by lymphocytes but not by any other cells.

Table 2–1. Normal Blood Cell Counts

	Mean number per microliter	Normal range
White blood cells (leukocytes)	7,400	4,500–11,000
Neutrophils	4,400	1,800–7,700
Eosinophils	200	0–450
Basophils	40	0–200
Lymphocytes	2,500	1,000–4,800
Monocytes	300	200–800

Morphology

Naive lymphocytes, which are cells that have not previously been stimulated by antigens, are called small lymphocytes by morphologists. The small lymphocyte is 8 to 10 µm in diameter. It has a large nucleus with dense heterochromatin and a thin rim of cytoplasm that contains a few mitochondria, ribosomes, and lysosomes but no specialized organelles (Fig. 2–2). Before antigenic stimulation, small lymphocytes are in a state of rest, or in the G_0 stage of the cell cycle. In response to stimulation, resting small lymphocytes enter the G_1 stage of the cell cycle. They become larger (10 to 12 µm in diameter), have more cytoplasm and organelles and increased amounts of cytoplasmic RNA, and are called large lymphocytes, or lymphoblasts (see Fig. 2–2).

Classes of Lymphocytes

Lymphocytes consist of distinct subsets that are different in their functions and protein products but are morphologically indistinguishable (Table 2–2). This heterogeneity of lymphocytes was introduced in Chapter 1 (see Fig. 1–5). **B lymphocytes,** the cells that produce antibodies, were so called because in birds they were found to mature in an organ called the bursa of Fabricius. In mammals, no anatomic equivalent of the bursa exists, and the early stages of B cell maturation occur in the bone marrow. Thus, "B" lymphocytes refer to bursa-derived lymphocytes or bone marrow–derived lymphocytes. **T lymphocytes,** the mediators of cellular immunity, were named because their precursors arise in the bone marrow but then migrate to and mature in the thymus; "T" lymphocyte refers to thymus derived. T lymphocytes consist of two subsets, helper T lymphocytes and cytolytic (or cytotoxic) T lymphocytes (CTLs). Both B and T lymphocytes have clonally distributed antigen receptors, meaning that there are many clones of these cells with different antigen specificities, and all the members of each clone express antigen receptors of the same specificity that are different from the receptors of other clones. The genes encoding the antigen receptors of B and T lymphocytes are formed by recombinations of DNA segments during the development of these cells. The somatic recombinations generate millions of different receptor genes that result in a highly diverse repertoire of lymphocytes (see Chapter 7). **NK (natural killer) cells** are a third population of lymphocytes whose receptors are different from those of B and T cells and whose major function is in innate immunity.

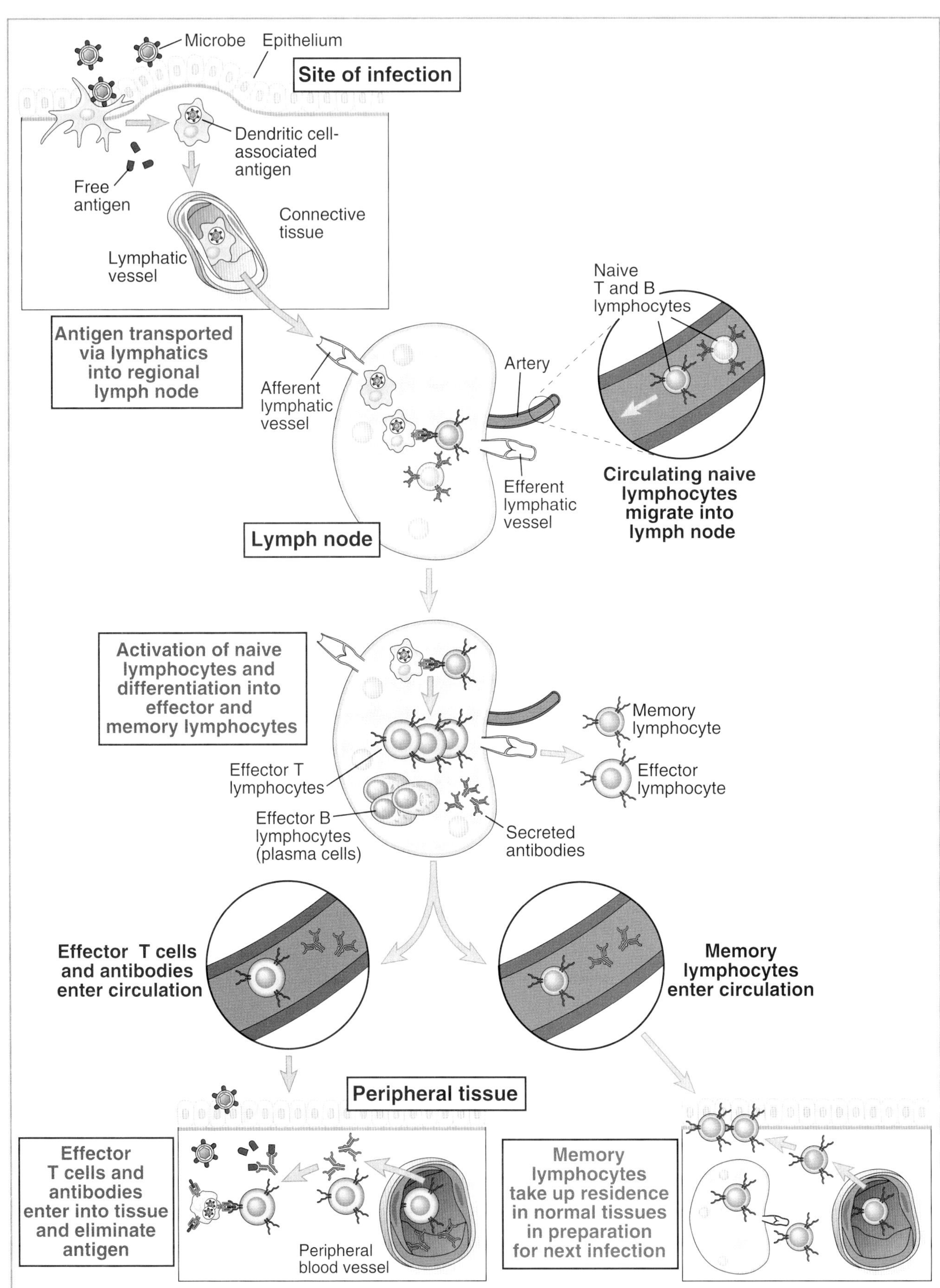

Figure 2–1 *See legend on opposite page.*

Figure 2–1 Overview of immune responses *in vivo*.
Antigens are captured from their site of entry by dendritic cells and concentrated in lymph nodes, where they activate naive lymphocytes that migrate to the nodes through blood vessels. Effector and memory T cells develop in the nodes and enter the circulation, from which they may migrate to peripheral tissues. Antibodies are produced in lymphoid organs and enter the circulation, from which they may locate antigens at any site. Memory cells also enter the circulation and may reside in lymphoid organs and other tissues. This illustration depicts the key events in an immune response to a protein antigen in a lymph node; responses in other peripheral lymphoid organs are similar.

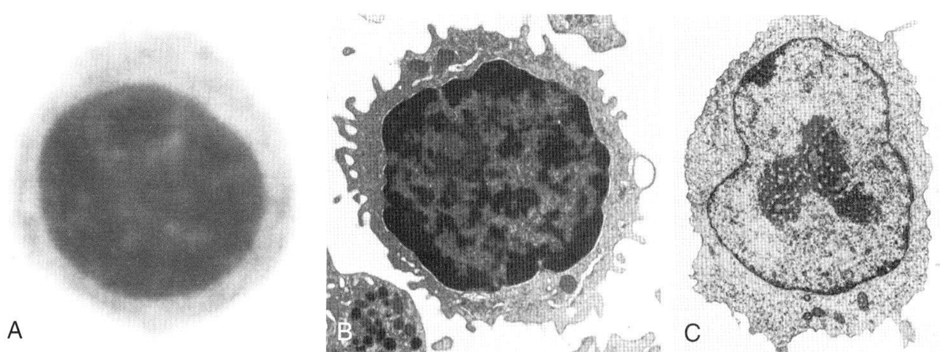

Figure 2–2 Morphology of lymphocytes.
A. Light micrograph of a lymphocyte in a peripheral blood smear.
B. Electron micrograph of a small lymphocyte. (Courtesy of Dr. Noel Weidner, Department of Pathology, University of California, San Diego.)
C. Electron micrograph of a large lymphocyte (lymphoblast). (From Fawcett DW. Bloom & Fawcett Textbook of Histology, 12th ed. WB Saunders, Philadelphia, 1994.)

Table 2–2. Lymphocyte Classes

Class	Functions	Antigen receptor	Selected phenotype markers	Percent of total lymphocytes		
				Blood	Lymph node	Spleen
T lymphocytes						
Helper T lymphocytes	Stimuli for B cell growth and differentiation (humoral immunity) Macrophage activation by secreted cytokines (cell-mediated immunity)	αβ heterodimers	$CD3^+$, $CD4^+$, $CD8^-$	50–60*	50–60	50–60
Cytolytic T lymphocytes	Killing of virus-infected cells, tumor cells; rejection of allografts (cell-mediated immunity)	αβ heterodimers	$CD3^+$, $CD4^-$, $CD8^+$	20–25	15–20	10–15
B lymphocytes	Antibody production (humoral immunity)	Surface antibody (immunoglobulin)	Fc receptors; class II MHC; CD19; CD21	10–15	20–25	40–45
Natural killer cells	Killing of virus-infected cells, tumor cells; antibody-dependent cellular toxicity	Killer cell Ig-like receptor	Fc receptor for IgG (CD16)	~10	Rare	~10

*In most tissues, the ratio of $CD4^+$ $CD8^-$ to $CD8^+$ $CD4^-$ cells is about 2:1.

The major classes of lymphocytes, their functions and selected surface molecules, and numbers in different tissues are shown. Some T lymphocytes, called regulatory cells (not included), function to inhibit immune responses and differ in phenotype and function from helper and cytolytic T cells. Smaller populations of lymphocytes, such as NK-T cells and γδ T cells, are also not listed.

Membrane proteins may be used as phenotypic markers to distinguish functionally distinct populations of lymphocytes (see Table 2–2). For instance, most helper T cells express a surface protein called CD4, and most CTLs express a different surface protein called CD8. Antibodies that are specific for such markers, labeled with probes that can be detected by various methods, are often used to identify and isolate various lymphocyte populations. (Techniques for detecting labeled antibodies are described in Appendix III.) Many of the surface proteins that were initially recognized as phenotypic markers for various lymphocyte subpopulations have turned out, on further analysis, to play important roles in the activation and functions of these cells. The accepted nomenclature for lymphocyte markers uses the CD number designation. CD stands for "cluster of differentiation," a historical term referring to a cluster (or collection) of monoclonal antibodies that are specific for various markers of lymphocyte differentiation. The CD system provides a uniform way to identify cell surface molecules on lymphocytes, APCs, and many other cell types in the immune system (Box 2–1). Examples of some CD proteins are mentioned in Table 2–2, and the biochemistry and functions of the most important ones are described in later chapters. A current list of known CD markers for leukocytes is provided in Appendix II.

Development of Lymphocytes

Like all blood cells, lymphocytes arise from stem cells in the bone marrow.

The origin of lymphocytes from bone marrow progenitors was first demonstrated by experiments with radiation-induced bone marrow chimeras. Lympho-

BOX 2–1

Lymphocyte Markers and the CD Nomenclature System

From the time that functionally distinct classes of lymphocytes were recognized, immunologists have attempted to develop methods for distinguishing them. The basic approach was to produce antibodies that would selectively recognize different subpopulations. This was initially done by raising alloantibodies (i.e., antibodies that might recognize allelic forms of cell surface proteins) by immunizing inbred strains of mice with lymphocytes from other strains. Such techniques were successful and led to the development of antibodies that reacted with murine T cells (anti–Thy-1 antibodies) and even against functionally different subsets of T lymphocytes (anti–Lyt-1 and anti–Lyt-2 antibodies). The limitations of this approach are obvious, however, because it is useful only for cell surface proteins that exist in allelic forms. The advent of hybridoma technology gave such analyses a tremendous boost, with the production of monoclonal antibodies that reacted specifically and selectively with defined populations of lymphocytes, first in humans and subsequently in many other species. (Alloantibodies and monoclonal antibodies are described in Chapter 3.)

Functionally distinct classes of lymphocytes express distinct types of cell surface proteins. Immunologists often rely on monoclonal antibody probes to detect these surface molecules. The cell surface molecules recognized by monoclonal antibodies are called antigens, because antibodies can be raised against them, or markers, because they identify and discriminate between ("mark") different cell populations. These markers can be grouped into several categories; some are specific for cells of a particular lineage or maturational pathway, and the expression of others varies according to the state of activation or differentiation of the same cells. Biochemical analyses of cell surface proteins recognized by different monoclonal antibodies demonstrated that these antibodies, in many instances, recognized the equivalent protein in different species. Considerable confusion was created because these surface markers were initially named according to the antibodies that reacted with them. To resolve this, a uniform nomenclature system was adopted, initially for human leukocytes. According to this system, a surface marker that identifies a particular lineage or differentiation stage, that has a defined structure, and that is recognized by a group ("cluster") of monoclonal antibodies is called a member of a cluster of differentiation. Thus, all leukocyte surface antigens whose structures are defined are given a CD designation (e.g., CD1, CD2). Although this nomenclature was originally used for human leukocyte antigens, it is now common practice to refer to homologous markers in other species and on cells other than leukocytes by the same CD designation. Newly developed monoclonal antibodies are periodically exchanged among laboratories, and the antigens recognized are assigned to existing CD structures or introduced as new "workshop" candidates (CDw).

The classification of lymphocytes by CD antigen expression is now widely used in clinical medicine and experimental immunology. For instance, most helper T lymphocytes are $CD3^+CD4^+CD8^-$, and most CTLs are $CD3^+CD4^-CD8^+$. This has allowed immunologists to identify the cells participating in various immune responses, isolate them, and individually analyze their specificities, response patterns, and effector functions. Such antibodies have also been used to define specific alterations in particular subsets of lymphocytes that might be occurring in various diseases. For example, the declining number of blood $CD4^+$ T cells is often used to follow the progression of disease and response to treatment in human immunodeficiency virus (HIV)–infected patients. Further investigations of the effects of monoclonal antibodies on lymphocyte function have shown that these surface proteins are not merely phenotypic markers but are themselves involved in a variety of lymphocyte responses. The two most frequent functions attributed to various CD molecules are (1) promotion of cell-cell interactions and adhesion, and (2) transduction of signals that lead to lymphocyte activation. Examples of both types of functions are described in Chapters 6 and 8.

cytes and their precursors are radiosensitive and are killed by high doses of γ-irradiation. If a mouse of one inbred strain is irradiated and then injected with bone marrow cells of another strain that can be distinguished from the host, all the lymphocytes that develop subsequently are derived from the bone marrow cells of the donor. Such approaches have proved useful for examining the maturation of lymphocytes and other blood cells (see Chapter 7).

All lymphocytes go through complex maturation stages during which they express antigen receptors and acquire the functional and phenotypic characteristics of mature cells (Fig. 2–3). B lymphocytes attain full maturity in the bone marrow, and T lymphocytes mature in the thymus. We will discuss these processes of B and T lymphocyte maturation in much more detail in Chapter 7. After the cells have matured, they leave the marrow or thymus, enter the circulation, and populate the peripheral lymphoid organs. These mature cells are called naive lymphocytes.

The population of naive lymphocytes is maintained at a steady state by the generation of new cells from bone marrow progenitors and the death of cells that do not encounter antigens. The function of naive lymphocytes is to recognize antigens and initiate adaptive immune responses. If they do not encounter antigen, the cells eventually die by a process of apoptosis (see Chapter 10, Box 10–2). The half-life of a naive lymphocyte is estimated to be 3 to 6 months in mice and a few years in humans. It is believed that the survival of naive lymphocytes is maintained by weak recognition of self antigens, so that the cells receive signals that are enough to keep them alive but not enough to activate them to differentiate into effector cells. The nature of the self antigens involved in lymphocyte survival is not known. It is known that the antigen receptor on naive lymphocytes is required not only for recognition of foreign antigens leading to effector cell differentiation but also for survival of the cells in the naive state. In addition, secreted proteins called cytokines are also essential for the survival of naive lymphocytes.

- The need for antigen receptor expression to maintain the pool of naive lymphocytes in peripheral lymphoid organs has been demonstrated by studies in which the immunoglobulin (Ig) gene that encodes the antigen receptors of B cells was knocked out after the B cells had matured, or the antigen receptors of T cells were knocked out in mature T cells. (The method used is called the cre-lox technique and is described in Appendix III.) Mature naive lymphocytes that lost their antigen receptors died within 2 or 3 weeks.
- Among T cells, there is evidence that survival of particular clones of naive cells in peripheral lymphoid organs depends on recognition of the same ligands that the clones saw during their maturation in the thymus. In Chapter 7, we will discuss the process of T cell maturation and the selection of T cells by recognition of self antigens in the thymus. This selection process ensures that the cells that mature are capable of surviving in peripheral tissues by recognizing the selecting self antigens.
- If naive lymphocytes are transferred into a mouse that does not have any lymphocytes of its own, the transferred lymphocytes begin to proliferate and increase in number until they reach roughly the numbers of lymphocytes in normal mice. This process is called **homeostatic proliferation** because it serves to maintain homeostasis (a steady state of cell numbers) in the immune system. The proliferation of naive lymphocytes in the absence of overt exposure to antigen is triggered by the recognition of self antigens. In addition, a cytokine called interleukin (IL)–7 is also essential for proliferation of the naive cells. These results imply that IL-7 may be a survival factor for naive cells in normal

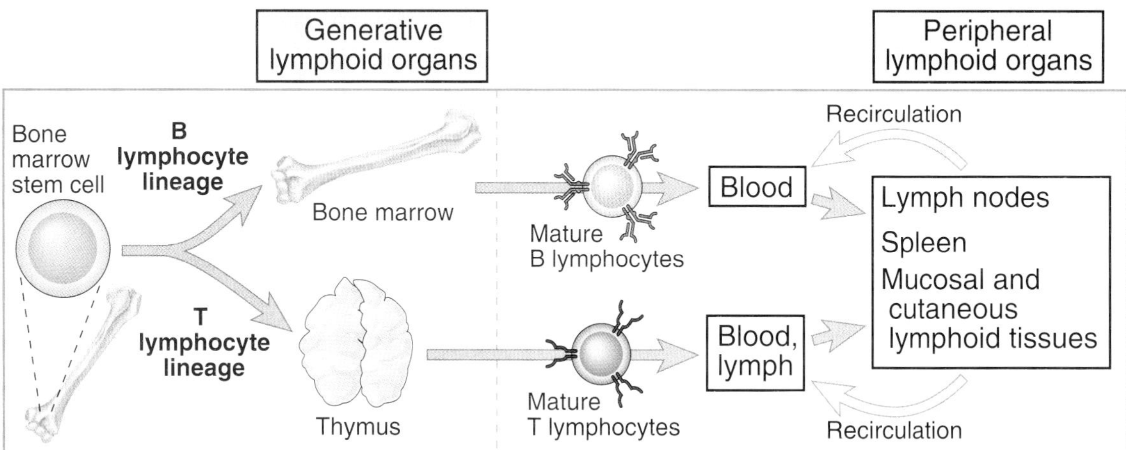

Figure 2–3 Maturation of lymphocytes.
Mature lymphocytes develop from bone marrow stem cells in the generative lymphoid organs, and immune responses to foreign antigens occur in the peripheral lymphoid tissues.

mice (i.e., not just in the experimental system of transfer into lymphocyte-deficient recipients). As we shall see in Chapter 7, the same cytokine, IL-7, is also essential for the survival and proliferation of immature lymphocytes in the generative lymphoid organs.

Activation of Lymphocytes

In adaptive immune responses, naive lymphocytes are activated by antigens and other stimuli to differentiate into effector and memory cells (Fig. 2–4). The activation of lymphocytes follows a series of sequential steps.

SYNTHESIS OF NEW PROTEINS

Early after stimulation, lymphocytes begin to transcribe genes that were previously silent and to synthesize a variety of new proteins. These proteins include secreted cytokines (in T cells), which stimulate the growth and differentiation of the lymphocytes themselves and of other effector cells; cytokine receptors, which make lymphocytes more responsive to cytokines; and many other proteins involved in gene transcription and cell division.

CELLULAR PROLIFERATION

In response to antigen and growth factors made by the antigen-stimulated lymphocytes and by other cells, the antigen-specific lymphocytes undergo mitotic division. This results in proliferation and increased size of the antigen-specific clone, so-called clonal expansion. In some acute viral infections, the numbers of virus-specific T cells may increase 50,000-fold, from a basal (unstimulated) level of about 1 in 1 million lymphocytes to 1 in 10 at the peak of the infection!

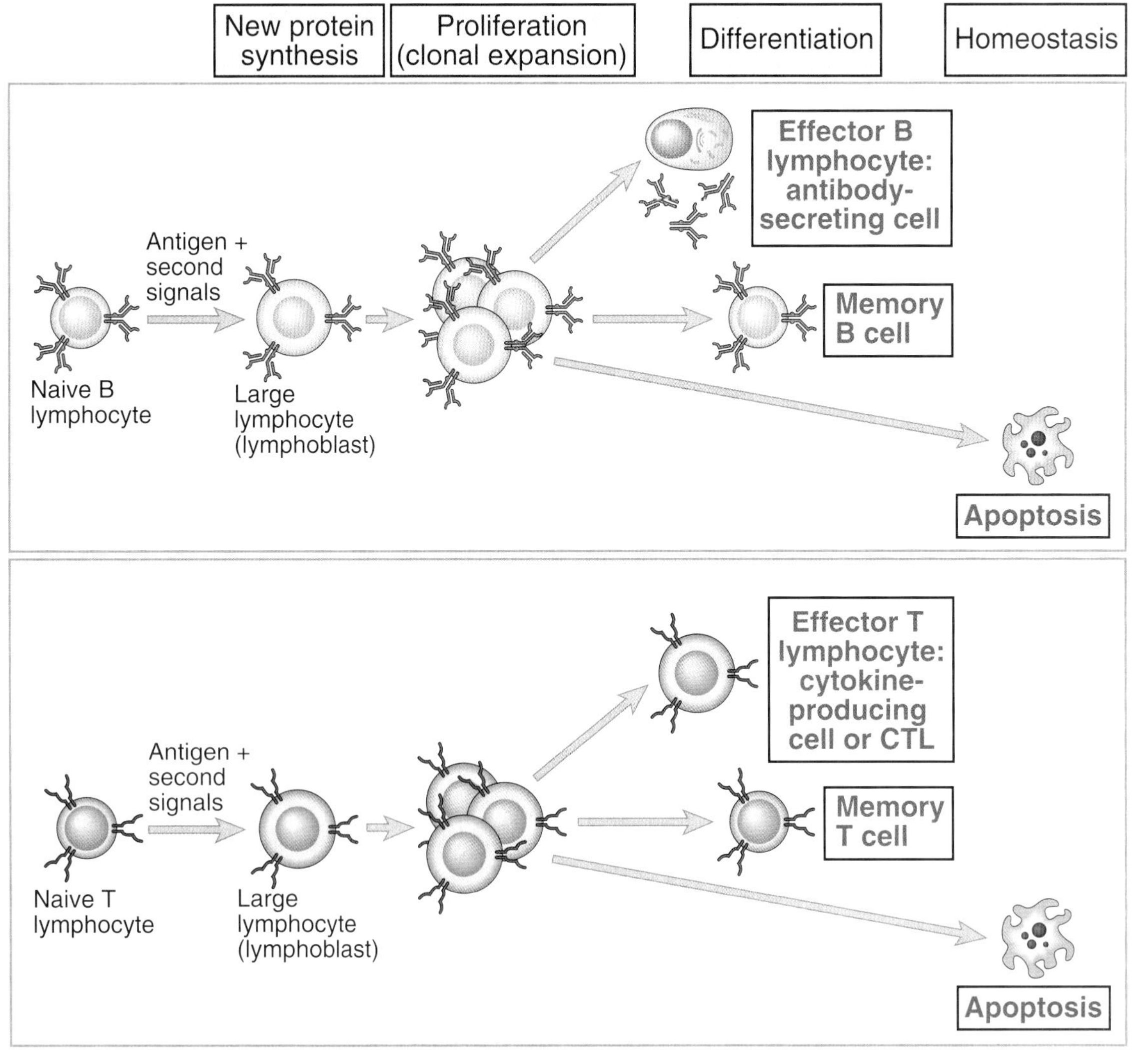

Figure 2–4 Phases of lymphocyte activation.
Naive B lymphocytes *(top panel)* and T lymphocytes *(bottom panel)* respond to antigens and second signals by protein synthesis, cellular proliferation, and differentiation into effector and memory cells. Homeostasis is restored as many of the antigen-activated lymphocytes die by apoptosis. Note that these phases of lymphocyte responses correspond to the phases of adaptive immunity illustrated in Figure 1–6, Chapter 1.

These are remarkable examples of the magnitude of clonal expansion during immune responses to microbes.

DIFFERENTIATION INTO EFFECTOR CELLS

Some of the progeny of the antigen-stimulated lymphocytes differentiate into effector cells, whose function is to eliminate the antigen. Effector lymphocytes include helper T cells, CTLs, and antibody-secreting B cells. Differentiated helper T cells express surface proteins that interact with ligands on other cells, such as macrophages and B lymphocytes, and they secrete cytokines that activate other cells. Differentiated CTLs develop granules containing proteins that kill virus-infected and tumor cells. B lymphocytes differentiate into cells that actively synthesize and secrete antibodies. Some of these antibody-producing cells are identifiable as **plasma cells.** They have characteristic nuclei, abundant cytoplasm containing dense, rough endoplasmic reticulum that is the site where antibodies (and other secreted and membrane proteins) are synthesized, and distinct perinuclear Golgi complexes where antibody molecules are converted to their final forms and packaged for secretion (Fig. 2–5). It is estimated that half or more of the messenger RNA in plasma cells codes for antibody proteins. Plasma cells develop in lymphoid organs and at sites of immune responses and often migrate to the bone marrow, where some of them may survive for long periods after the immune response is induced and even after the antigen is eliminated. The majority of differentiated effector lymphocytes are short-lived and not self-renewing.

DIFFERENTIATION INTO MEMORY CELLS

Some of the progeny of antigen-stimulated B and T lymphocytes differentiate into **memory cells,** whose function is to mediate rapid and enhanced (i.e., secondary or recall) responses to second and subsequent exposures to antigens. Memory cells may survive in a functionally quiescent or slowly cycling state for many years after the antigen is eliminated. Several lines of evidence indicate that memory cells do not require antigen recognition for their prolonged survival *in vivo.*

- If memory $CD8^+$ or $CD4^+$ T cells are transferred into mice that lack major histocompatibility complex (MHC) molecules, the memory cells survive almost as well as they do in normal mice. Since MHC-deficient mice cannot display antigens that are recognizable by T cells, the survival of the memory cells must be antigen independent.
- If the antigen receptors of T cells are knocked out after cells have matured (as in the experiment described in our discussion of naive cells), memory cells that were generated by previous antigen exposure continue to survive even without antigen receptors.

Memory cells express surface proteins that distinguish them from naive and recently activated effector lymphocytes, although it is still not clear which of these surface proteins are definitive markers of memory populations (Table 2–3). Memory B lymphocytes express certain classes (isotypes) of membrane Ig, such as IgG, IgE, or IgA, as a result of isotype switching, whereas naive B cells express only IgM and IgD (see Chapters 3 and 9). Compared with naive T cells, memory T lymphocytes express higher levels of adhesion molecules, such as integrins and CD44 (see Chapter 6), which promote the migration of the memory cells to sites of infection anywhere in the body. In humans, most naive T cells express a 200-kD isoform of a surface molecule called CD45 that contains a segment encoded by an exon designated A. This CD45 isoform can be recognized by antibodies specific for the A-encoded segment and is therefore called CD45RA (for "restricted A"). In contrast, most activated and memory T cells express a 180-kD isoform of CD45 in which the A exon RNA has been spliced out; this isoform is called CD45RO. However, this way of distinguishing between naive and memory T cells is not

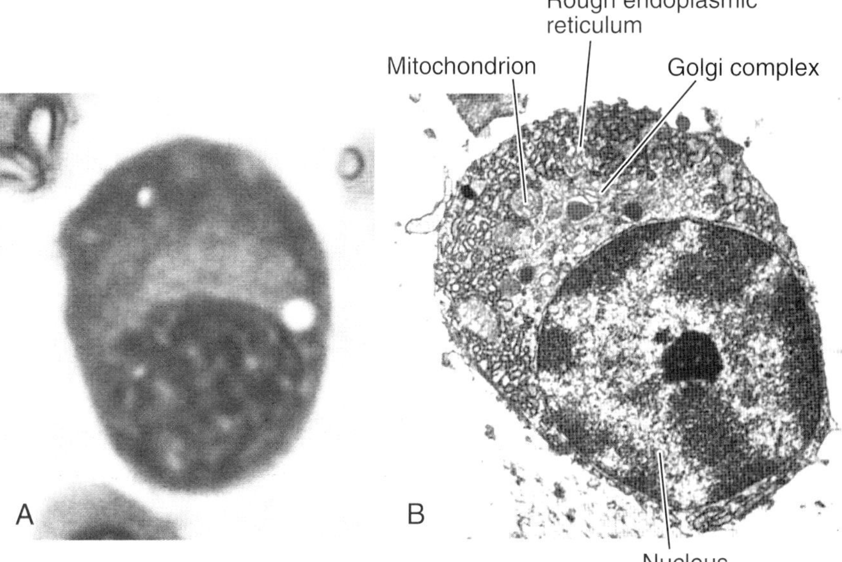

Figure 2–5 Morphology of plasma cells.
A. Light micrograph of a plasma cell in tissue.
B. Electron micrograph of a plasma cell. (Courtesy of Dr. Noel Weidner, Department of Pathology, University of California, San Diego.)

Table 2–3. Characteristics of Naive, Effector, and Memory Lymphocytes

	Naive lymphocytes	Activated or effector lymphocytes	Memory lymphocytes
T lymphocytes			
Migration	Preferentially to peripheral lymph nodes	Preferentially to inflamed tissues	Preferentially to inflamed tissues, mucosal tissues
Frequency of cells responsive to particular antigen	Very low	High	Low
Effector functions	None	Cytokine secretion; cytolytic activity	None
Cell cycling	No	Yes	+/−
Surface protein expression			
High-affinity IL-2 receptor	Low	High	Low
Peripheral lymph node homing receptor (L-selectin, CD62L)	High	Low	Low or variable
Adhesion molecules: integrins, CD44	Low	High	High
Chemokine receptor: CCR7	High	Low	Variable
Major CD45 isoform (humans only)	CD45RA	CD45RO	CD45RO; variable
Morphology	Small; scant cytoplasm	Large; more cytoplasm	Small
B lymphocytes			
Membrane immunoglobulin (Ig) isotype	IgM and IgD	Frequently IgG, IgA, IgE	Frequently IgG, IgA, IgE
Affinity of Ig produced	Relatively low	Increases during immune response	Relatively high
Effector function	None	Antibody secretion	None
Morphology	Small; scant cytoplasm	Large; more cytoplasm; plasma cell	Small
Chemokine receptor: CXCR5	High	Low	?

perfect, and interconversion between $CD45RA^+$ and $CD45RO^+$ populations has been documented.

Memory cells appear to be heterogeneous in many respects. Some migrate preferentially to lymph nodes, where they provide a pool of antigen-specific lymphocytes that can rapidly be activated to proliferate and differentiate into effector cells if the antigen is reintroduced. Other memory cells reside in mucosal tissues or circulate in the blood, from which they may be recruited to any site of infection and mount rapid effector responses that serve to eliminate the antigen.

Several key questions about memory cells remain unanswered. We do not know what stimuli induce a small fraction of the progeny of antigen-stimulated lymphocytes to differentiate into memory cells. It is also not known how memory cells are able to survive *in vivo* apparently without antigen, given that both naive and recently activated lymphocytes die by apoptosis unless they are constantly exposed to survival stimuli, including antigen and growth factors.

Antigen-Presenting Cells

Antigen-presenting cells (APCs) are cell populations that are specialized to capture microbial and other antigens, display them to lymphocytes, and provide signals that stimulate the proliferation and differen-

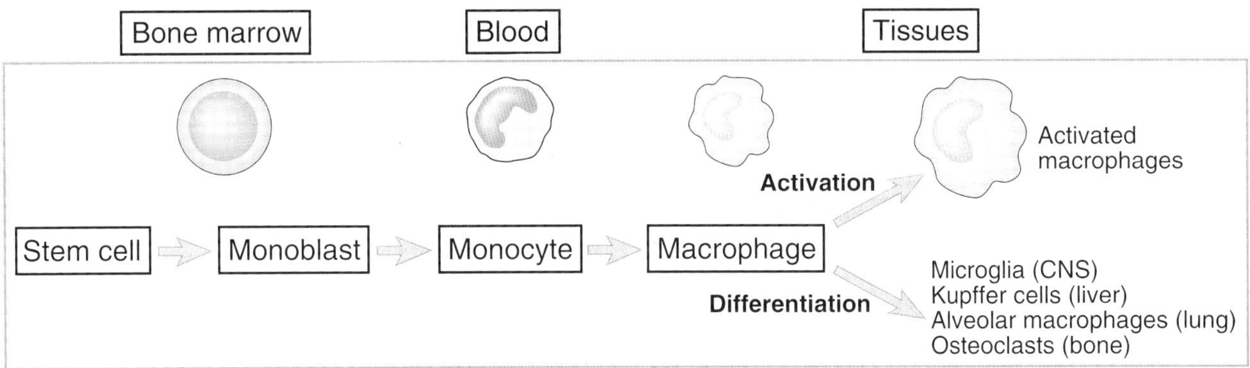

Figure 2–6 Maturation of mononuclear phagocytes.
Mononuclear phagocytes develop in the bone marrow, circulate in the blood as monocytes, and are resident in all tissues of the body as macrophages. They may differentiate into specialized forms in particular tissues. CNS, central nervous system.

tiation of the lymphocytes. By convention, APC usually refers to a cell that displays antigens to T lymphocytes. The major type of APC that is involved in initiating T cell responses is the dendritic cell. Macrophages present antigens to T cells during cell-mediated immune responses, and B lymphocytes function as APCs for helper T cells during humoral immune responses. A specialized cell type called the follicular dendritic cell displays antigens to B lymphocytes during particular phases of humoral immune responses.

Dendritic Cells

Dendritic cells play important roles in antigen capture and the induction of T lymphocyte responses to protein antigens. Dendritic cells are found under epithelia and in most organs, where they are poised to capture foreign antigens and transport these antigens to peripheral lymphoid organs. Most of these dendritic cells are derived from the monocyte lineage and are called myeloid dendritic cells. We will return to the biology and function of dendritic cells in antigen presentation in Chapter 5.

Mononuclear Phagocytes

The **mononuclear phagocyte system** consists of cells that have a common lineage whose primary function is phagocytosis. The cells of the mononuclear phagocyte system originate in the bone marrow, circulate in the blood, and mature and become activated in various tissues (Fig. 2–6). The first cell type that enters the peripheral blood after leaving the marrow is incompletely differentiated and is called the **monocyte.** Monocytes are 10 to 15 µm in diameter, and they have bean-shaped nuclei and finely granular cytoplasm containing lysosomes, phagocytic vacuoles, and cytoskeletal filaments (Fig. 2–7). Once they settle in tissues, these cells mature and become **macrophages.** Macrophages

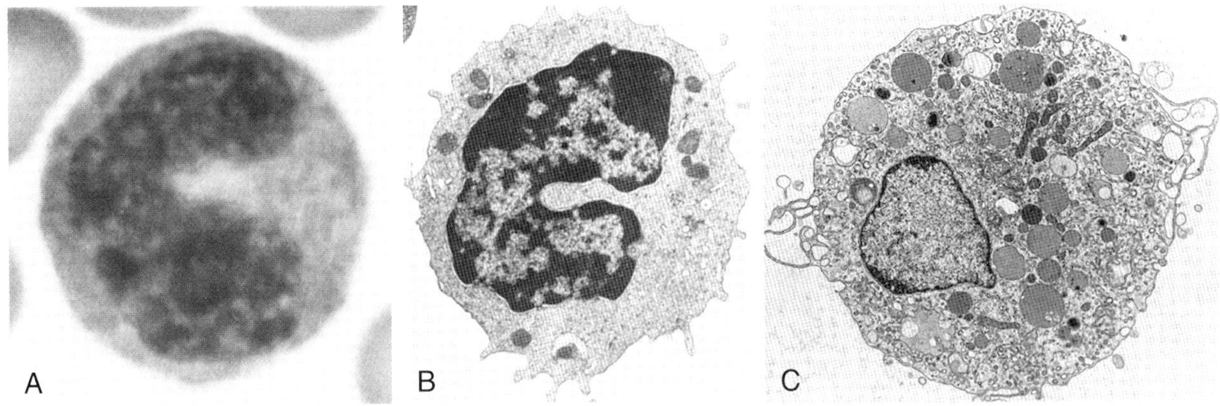

Figure 2–7 Morphology of mononuclear phagocytes.
A. Light micrograph of a monocyte in a peripheral blood smear.
B. Electron micrograph of a peripheral blood monocyte. (Courtesy of Dr. Noel Weidner, Department of Pathology, University of California, San Diego.)
C. Electron micrograph of an activated tissue macrophage showing numerous phagocytic vacuoles and cytoplasmic organelles. (From Fawcett DW. Bloom & Fawcett Textbook of Histology, 12th ed. WB Saunders, Philadelphia, 1994.)

may assume different morphologic forms after activation by external stimuli, such as microbes. Some develop abundant cytoplasm and are called epithelioid cells because of their resemblance to epithelial cells of the skin. Activated macrophages can fuse to form multinucleate giant cells. Macrophages are found in all organs and connective tissues and have been given special names to designate specific locations. For instance, in the central nervous system, they are called microglial cells; when lining the vascular sinusoids of the liver, they are called Kupffer cells; in pulmonary airways, they are called alveolar macrophages; and multinucleate phagocytes in bone are called osteoclasts.

Mononuclear phagocytes function as APCs in T cell–mediated adaptive immune responses. Macrophages containing ingested microbes display microbial antigens to differentiated effector T cells. The effector T cells then activate the macrophages to kill the microbes. This process is a major mechanism of cell-mediated immunity against intracellular microbes (see Chapter 13). Macrophages that have ingested microbes may also play a role in activating naive T cells to induce primary responses to microbial antigens, although it is likely that dendritic cells are more effective inducers of primary responses.

Mononuclear phagocytes are also important effector cells in both innate and adaptive immunity. Their effector functions in innate immunity are to phagocytose microbes and to produce cytokines that recruit and activate other inflammatory cells (see Chapter 12). Macrophages serve numerous roles in the effector phases of adaptive immune responses. As mentioned above, in cell-mediated immunity, antigen-stimulated T cells activate macrophages to destroy phagocytosed microbes. In humoral immunity, antibodies coat, or opsonize, microbes and promote the phagocytosis of the microbes through macrophage surface receptors for antibodies (see Chapter 14).

Follicular Dendritic Cells

Follicular dendritic cells (FDCs) are cells with membranous projections present in the germinal centers of lymphoid follicles in the lymph nodes, spleen, and mucosal lymphoid tissues. Most FDCs are not derived from precursors in the bone marrow and are unrelated to the dendritic cells that present antigens to T lymphocytes. FDCs trap antigens complexed to antibodies or complement products and display these antigens on their surfaces for recognition by B lymphocytes. This is important for the selection of activated B lymphocytes whose antigen receptors bind the displayed antigens with high affinity (see Chapter 9).

Anatomy and Functions of Lymphoid Tissues

To optimize the cellular interactions necessary for the recognition and activation phases of specific immune responses, lymphocytes and accessory cells are localized and concentrated in anatomically defined tissues or organs, which are also the sites where foreign antigens are transported and concentrated. Such anatomic compartmentalization is not fixed because, as we will discuss later in this chapter, many lymphocytes recirculate and constantly exchange between the circulation and the tissues.

Lymphoid tissues are classified as generative organs, also called primary lymphoid organs, where lymphocytes first express antigen receptors and attain phenotypic and functional maturity, and as peripheral organs, also called secondary lymphoid organs, where lymphocyte responses to foreign antigens are initiated and develop (see Fig. 2–3). Included in the generative lymphoid organs of mammals are the bone marrow, where all the lymphocytes arise, and the thymus, where T cells mature and reach a stage of functional competence. The peripheral lymphoid organs and tissues include the lymph nodes, spleen, cutaneous immune system, and mucosal immune system. In addition, poorly defined aggregates of lymphocytes are found in connective tissue and in virtually all organs except those in the central nervous system.

Bone Marrow

The bone marrow is the site of generation of all circulating blood cells in the adult, including immature lymphocytes, and is the site of B cell maturation. During fetal development, the generation of all blood cells, called **hematopoiesis,** occurs initially in blood islands of the yolk sac and the para-aortic mesenchyme and later in the liver and spleen. This function is taken over gradually by the bone marrow and increasingly by the marrow of the flat bones so that by puberty, hematopoiesis occurs mostly in the sternum, vertebrae, iliac bones, and ribs. The red marrow that is found in these bones consists of a spongelike reticular framework located between long trabeculae. The spaces in this framework are filled with fat cells, stromal fibroblasts, and precursors of blood cells. These precursors mature and exit through the dense network of vascular sinuses to enter the vascular circulation. When the bone marrow is injured or when an exceptional demand for production of new blood cells occurs, the liver and spleen can be recruited as sites of extramedullary hematopoiesis.

All the blood cells originate from a common **stem cell** that becomes committed to differentiate along particular lineages (i.e., erythroid, megakaryocytic, granulocytic, monocytic, and lymphocytic) (Fig. 2–8). Stem cells lack the markers of differentiated blood cells and instead express two proteins called CD34 and stem cell antigen-1 (Sca-1). These markers are used to identify and enrich stem cells from suspensions of bone marrow or peripheral blood cells for use in bone marrow transplantation. The proliferation and maturation of precursor cells in the bone marrow are stimulated by cytokines. Many of these cytokines are called colony-stimulating factors because they were originally assayed by their ability to stimulate the growth and development of various leukocytic

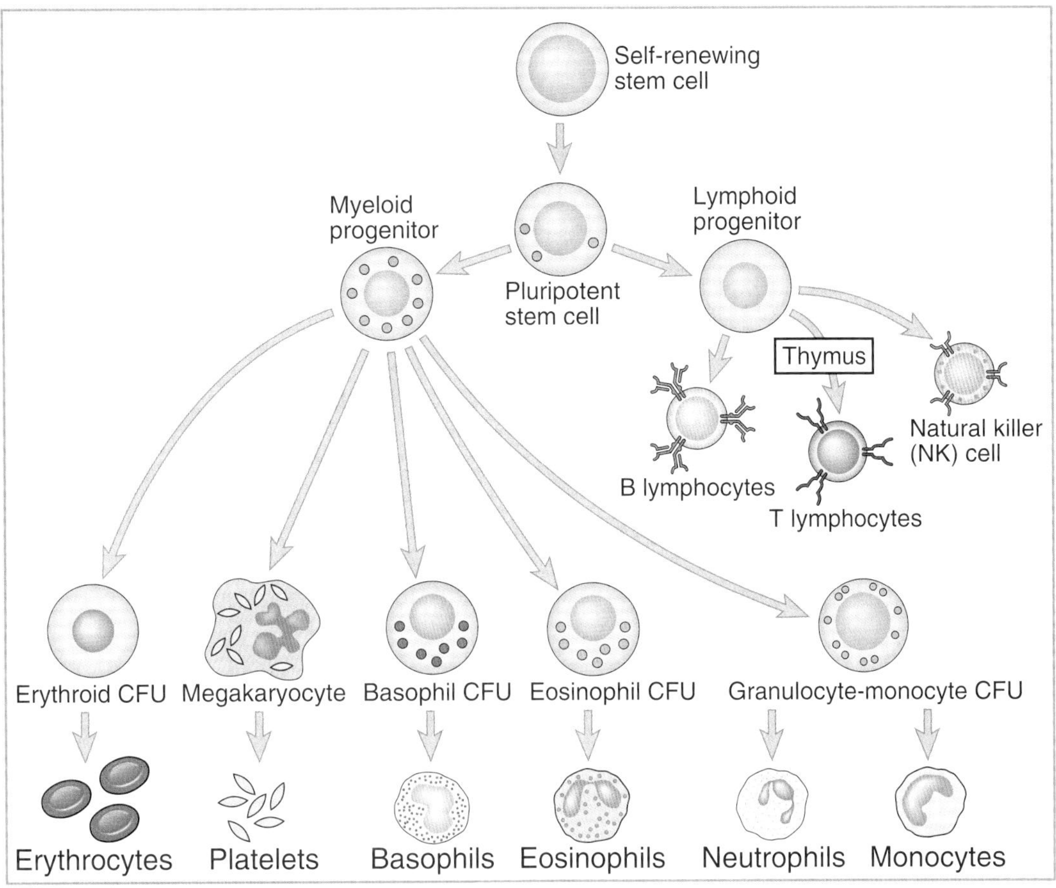

Figure 2–8 Hematopoiesis.
The development of the different lineages of blood cells is depicted in this "hematopoietic tree." The roles of cytokines in hematopoiesis are illustrated in Chapter 11, Figure 11–15. CFU, colony-forming unit.

or erythroid colonies from marrow cells. These molecules are discussed in Chapter 11 (see Fig. 11–15). Hematopoietic cytokines are produced by stromal cells and macrophages in the bone marrow, thus providing the local environment for hematopoiesis. They are also produced by antigen-stimulated T lymphocytes and cytokine-activated or microbe-activated macrophages, providing a mechanism for replenishing leukocytes that may be consumed during immune and inflammatory reactions.

In addition to self-renewing stem cells and their differentiating progeny, the marrow contains numerous antibody-secreting plasma cells. These plasma cells are generated in peripheral lymphoid tissues as a consequence of antigenic stimulation of B cells and then migrate to the marrow, where they may live and continue to produce antibodies for many years.

Thymus

The thymus is the site of T cell maturation. The thymus is a bilobed organ situated in the anterior mediastinum. Each lobe is divided into multiple lobules by fibrous septa, and each lobule consists of an outer cortex and an inner medulla (Fig. 2–9). The cortex contains a dense collection of T lymphocytes, and the lighter staining medulla is more sparsely populated with lymphocytes. Scattered throughout the thymus are nonlymphoid epithelial cells, which have abundant cytoplasm, as well as bone marrow–derived macrophages and dendritic cells. Some of these thymic dendritic cells express markers, such as CD8α, that are typically found on T lymphocytes and are called lymphoid dendritic cells to distinguish them from the myeloid dendritic cells described earlier. In the medulla are structures called Hassall's corpuscles, which are composed of tightly packed whorls of epithelial cells that may be remnants of degenerating cells. The thymus has a rich vascular supply and efferent lymphatic vessels that drain into mediastinal lymph nodes. The thymus is derived from invaginations of the ectoderm in the developing neck and chest of the embryo, forming structures called branchial clefts. In the "nude" mouse strain, a mutation in the gene encoding a transcription factor causes a failure of differentiation of certain types of epithelial cells that are required for normal development of the thymus and hair follicles. Consequently, these mice lack T cells and hair (see Chapter 20). Humans with DiGeorge syndrome also suffer from T cell deficiency because of mutations in genes required for thymus development.

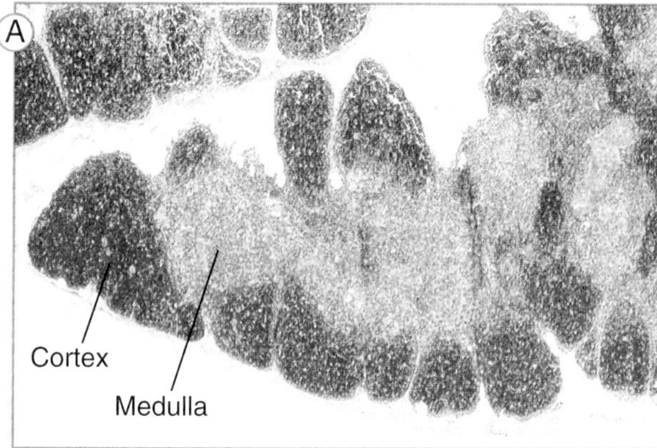

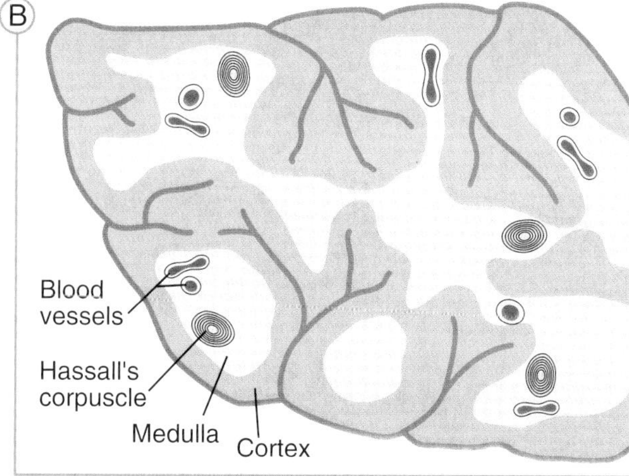

Figure 2–9 Morphology of the thymus.
A. Light micrograph of a lobe of the thymus showing the cortex and medulla. The blue-stained cells are developing T cells called thymocytes. (Courtesy of Dr. James Gulizia, Department of Pathology, Brigham and Women's Hospital, Boston.)
B. Schematic diagram of the thymus illustrating a portion of a lobe divided into multiple lobules by fibrous trabeculae.

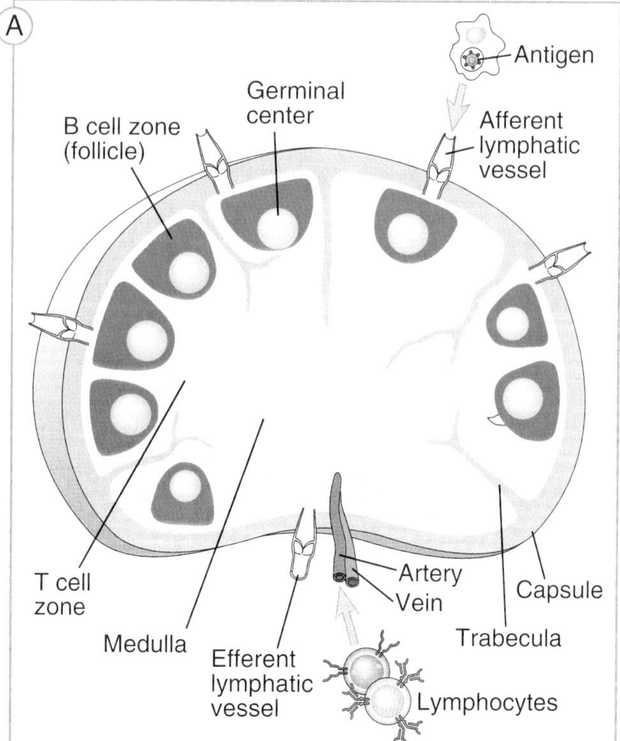

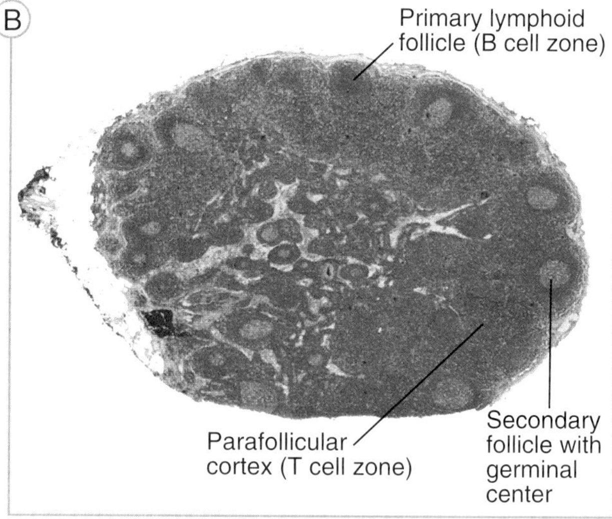

Figure 2–10 Morphology of a lymph node.
A. Schematic diagram of a lymph node illustrating the T cell–rich and B cell–rich zones and the routes of entry of lymphocytes and antigen (shown captured by a dendritic cell).
B. Light micrograph of a lymph node illustrating the T cell and B cell zones. (Courtesy of Dr. James Gulizia, Department of Pathology, Brigham and Women's Hospital, Boston.)

The lymphocytes in the thymus, also called **thymocytes,** are T lymphocytes at various stages of maturation. In general, the most immature cells of the T cell lineage enter the thymic cortex through the blood vessels. Maturation begins in the cortex, and as thymocytes mature, they migrate toward the medulla, so that the medulla contains mostly mature T cells. Only mature T cells exit the thymus and enter the blood and peripheral lymphoid tissues. The details of thymocyte maturation are described in Chapter 7.

Lymph Nodes and the Lymphatic System

Lymph nodes are the organs in which adaptive immune responses to lymph-borne antigens are initiated. Lymph nodes are small nodular aggregates of lymphocyte-rich tissue situated along lymphatic channels throughout the body. A lymph node consists of an outer cortex and an inner medulla. Each lymph node is surrounded by a fibrous capsule that is pierced by numerous afferent lymphatics, which empty the lymph into a subcapsular or marginal sinus (Fig. 2–10). The lymph percolates through the cortex into the medullary sinus and leaves the node through the efferent lymphatic vessel in the hilum. Beneath the subcapsular sinus, the outer cortex contains aggregates of cells called **follicles.** Some follicles contain central areas called germinal centers, which stain lightly with commonly used histologic stains. Follicles without germinal centers are called primary follicles, and those with germinal centers are secondary follicles. The cortex around the follicles is organized into cords, which are spaces containing lymphocytes as well as dendritic cells and mononuclear phagocytes, arranged around lymphatic and vascular sinusoids. Lymphocytes and APCs in these cords are often found near one another, but they do not form intercellular junctions, which is important for maintaining the ability of the lymphocytes to migrate and recirculate among lymph, blood, and tissues. Beneath the cortex is the medulla, consisting of medullary cords that lead to the medullary sinus. These cords are populated by macrophages and plasma cells. Blood is delivered to a lymph node by an artery that enters through the hilum and branches into capillaries in the outer cortex, and it leaves the node by a single vein that exits through the hilum.

Different classes of lymphocytes are sequestered in distinct regions of lymph nodes (Fig. 2–11). Follicles are the B cell zones of lymph nodes. Primary follicles contain mostly mature, naive B lymphocytes. Germinal centers develop in response to antigenic stimulation. They are sites of remarkable B cell proliferation, selection of B cells producing high-affinity antibodies, and generation of memory B cells. The processes of FDCs interdigitate to form a dense reticular network in the germinal centers. The T lymphocytes are located mainly beneath and between the follicles, in the cortex. Most (~70%) of these T cells are $CD4^+$ helper T cells, intermingled with relatively sparse $CD8^+$ cells. Dendritic cells are also concentrated in the T cell zones of the lymph nodes.

The anatomic segregation of different classes of lymphocytes in distinct areas of the node is dependent on cytokines (see Fig. 2–11). Naive T and B lymphocytes enter the node through an artery. These cells leave the circulation and enter the stroma of the node through specialized vessels called high endothelial venules in the cortex (described in more detail later). The naive T cells express a receptor for a chemoattractant cytokine, or chemokine; this receptor is called CCR7. (Chemokines and other cytokines will be described in Chapter 11.) CCR7 recognizes chemokines that are produced only in the T cell zone of the node, and these chemokines attract the naive T

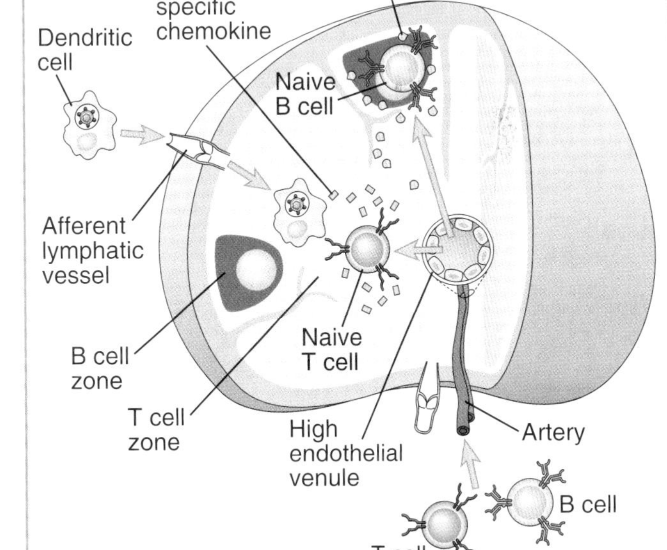

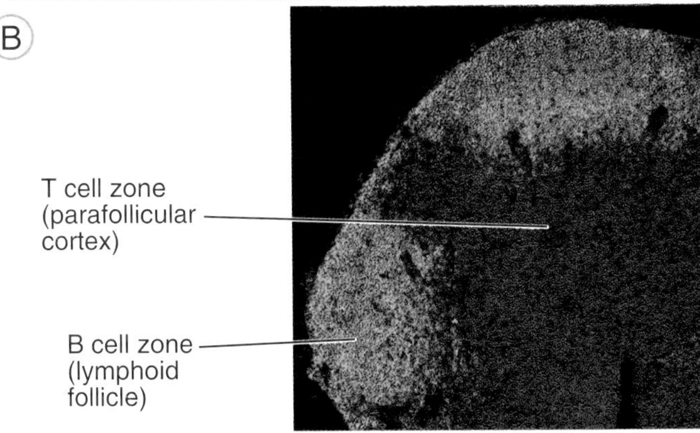

Figure 2–11 Segregation of B cells and T cells in a lymph node.

A. The schematic diagram illustrates the path by which naive T and B lymphocytes migrate to different areas of a lymph node. The lymphocytes enter through a high endothelial venule, shown in cross-section, and are drawn to different areas of the node by chemokines that are produced in these areas and bind selectively to either cell type. Also shown is the migration of dendritic cells, which pick up antigens from the sites of antigen entry, enter through afferent lymphatic vessels, and migrate to the T cell–rich areas of the node.

B. In this section of a lymph node, the B lymphocytes, located in the follicles, are stained green; the T cells, in the parafollicular cortex, are red. The method used to stain these cells is called immunofluorescence (see Appendix III for details). (Courtesy of Drs. Kathryn Pape and Jennifer Walter, University of Minnesota School of Medicine, Minneapolis.)

The anatomic segregation of T and B cells is also seen in the spleen (not shown).

cells into the T cell zone. Dendritic cells also express CCR7, and this is why they migrate to the same area of the node as do naive T cells (see Chapter 5). Naive B cells express another chemokine receptor, CXCR5, that recognizes a chemokine produced only in follicles. Thus, B cells are attracted into the follicles, which are the B cell zones of lymph nodes. Another cytokine, called lymphotoxin, may play a role in stimulating chemokine production in different regions of the lymph node, especially in the follicles. The functions of various cytokines in directing the movement of lymphocytes in lymphoid organs and in the formation of these organs have been established by numerous studies in mice.

- Knockout mice lacking the membrane form of the cytokine lymphotoxin (LTβ) or the LTβ receptor show absence of peripheral lymph nodes and a marked disorganization of the architecture of the spleen, with loss of the segregation of B and T cells.
- Overexpression of lymphotoxin or tumor necrosis factor in an organ, either as a transgene in experimental animals or in response to chronic inflammation in humans, can lead to the formation in that organ of lymph node–like structures that contain B cell follicles with FDCs and interfollicular T cell–rich areas containing mature dendritic cells.
- Knockout mice lacking CXCR5 show absent B cell zones in lymph nodes and spleen. Similarly, knockout mice lacking CCR7 show absent T cell zones.

The anatomic segregation of T and B cells ensures that each lymphocyte population is in close contact with the appropriate APCs (i.e., T cells with dendritic cells and B cells with FDCs). Furthermore, because of this precise segregation, B and T lymphocyte populations are kept apart until it is time for them to interact in a functional way. As we will see in Chapter 9, after stimulation by antigens, T and B cells lose their anatomic constraints and begin to migrate toward one another. Activated T cells may ultimately exit the node and enter the circulation, whereas activated B cells migrate into germinal centers or the medulla, from which they secrete antibodies.

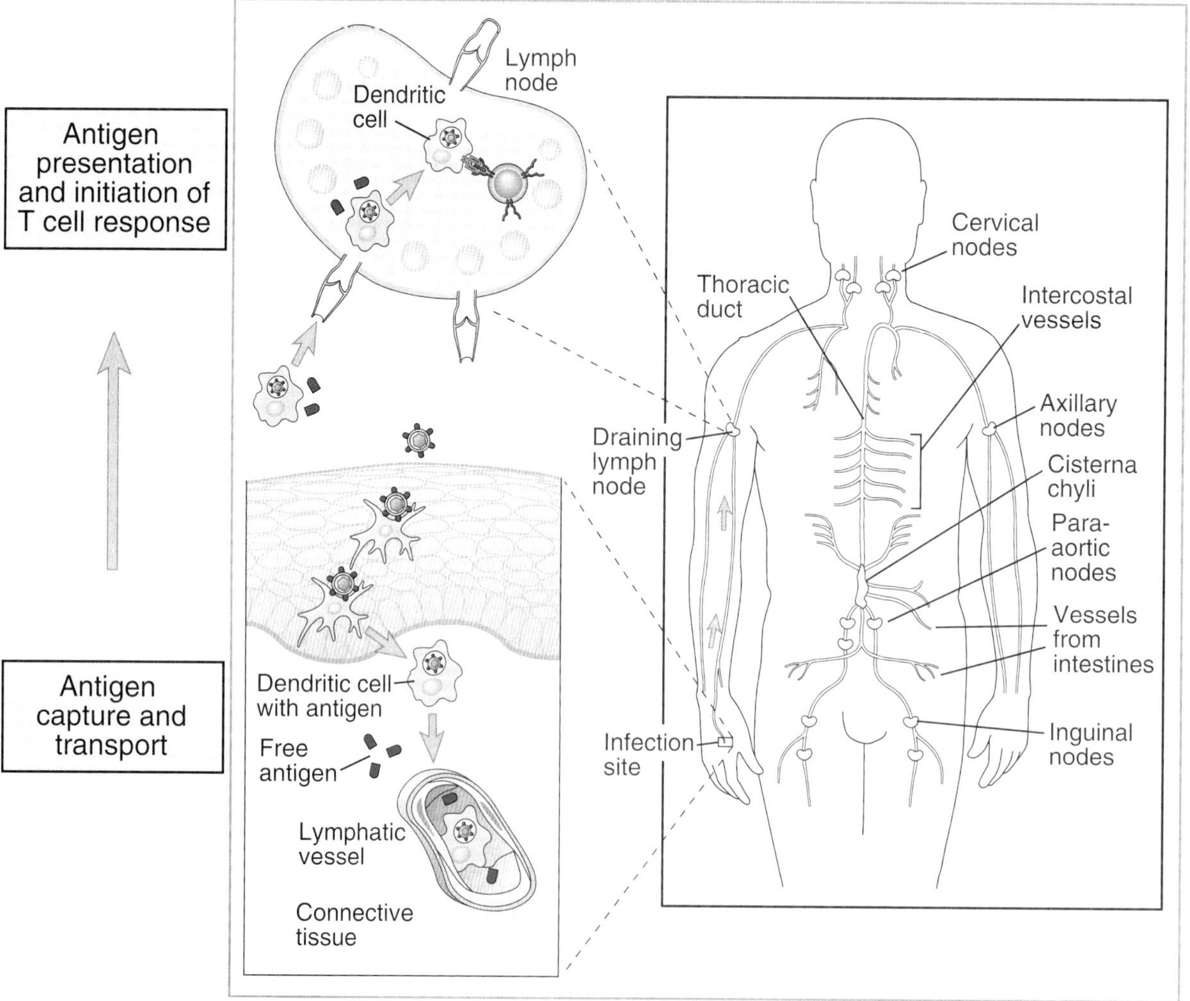

Figure 2–12 The lymphatic system.
The major lymphatic vessels and collections of lymph nodes are illustrated on the right. The left panels show where antigens are captured from a site of infection, and the draining lymph node to which these antigens are transported, and where the immune response is initiated.

Antigens are transported to lymph nodes mainly in lymphatic vessels. The functions of collecting antigens from their portals of entry and delivering them to lymph nodes are performed largely by the lymphatic system (Fig. 2–12). The skin, epithelia, and parenchymal organs contain numerous lymphatic capillaries that absorb and drain interstitial fluid (made of plasma filtrate) from these sites. The absorbed interstitial fluid, called **lymph,** flows through the lymphatic capillaries into convergent, ever larger lymphatic vessels, eventually culminating in one large lymphatic vessel called the thoracic duct. Lymph from the thoracic duct is emptied into the superior vena cava, thus returning the fluid to the blood stream. Liters of lymph are normally returned to the circulation each day, and disruption of the lymphatic system may lead to rapid tissue swelling.

Microbes enter the body most often through the skin and the gastrointestinal and respiratory tracts. All these tissues are lined by epithelia that contain dendritic cells. The dendritic cells capture microbial antigens and enter lymphatic vessels. Lymph nodes are interposed along lymphatic vessels and act as filters that sample the lymph at numerous points before it reaches the blood. In this way, antigens captured from the portals of entry are transported to lymph nodes. Cell-free antigens may also be transported in the lymph. Lymphatic vessels that carry lymph into a lymph node are referred to as afferent, and vessels that drain the lymph from the node are called efferent. Because lymph nodes are connected in series along the lymphatics, an efferent lymphatic exiting one node may serve as the afferent vessel for another.

When lymph enters a lymph node through an afferent lymphatic vessel, it percolates through the nodal stroma. Antigen-bearing dendritic cells enter the T cell zone and settle in this region. Lymph-borne soluble antigens can be extracted from the fluid by cells, such as dendritic cells and macrophages, that are resident in the stroma of the nodes (see Chapter 5). The net result of antigen uptake by these various cell types is accumulation and concentration of the antigen in the lymph node and display of the antigen in a form that can be recognized by specific T lymphocytes.

Spleen

The spleen is the major site of immune responses to blood-borne antigens. The spleen, an organ weighing about 150 g in adults, is located in the left upper quadrant of the abdomen. It is supplied by a single splenic artery, which pierces the capsule at the hilum and divides into progressively smaller branches that remain surrounded by protective and supporting fibrous trabeculae (Fig. 2–13). Small arterioles are surrounded by cuffs of lymphocytes, which are the T cell zone of the spleen. Because of their anatomic location, morphologists call these areas periarteriolar lymphoid sheaths. Lymphoid follicles, some of which contain germinal centers, are attached to the T cell zones; as in the lymph nodes, the follicles are the B cell zones. The follicles are surrounded by a rim of lymphocytes and macrophages,

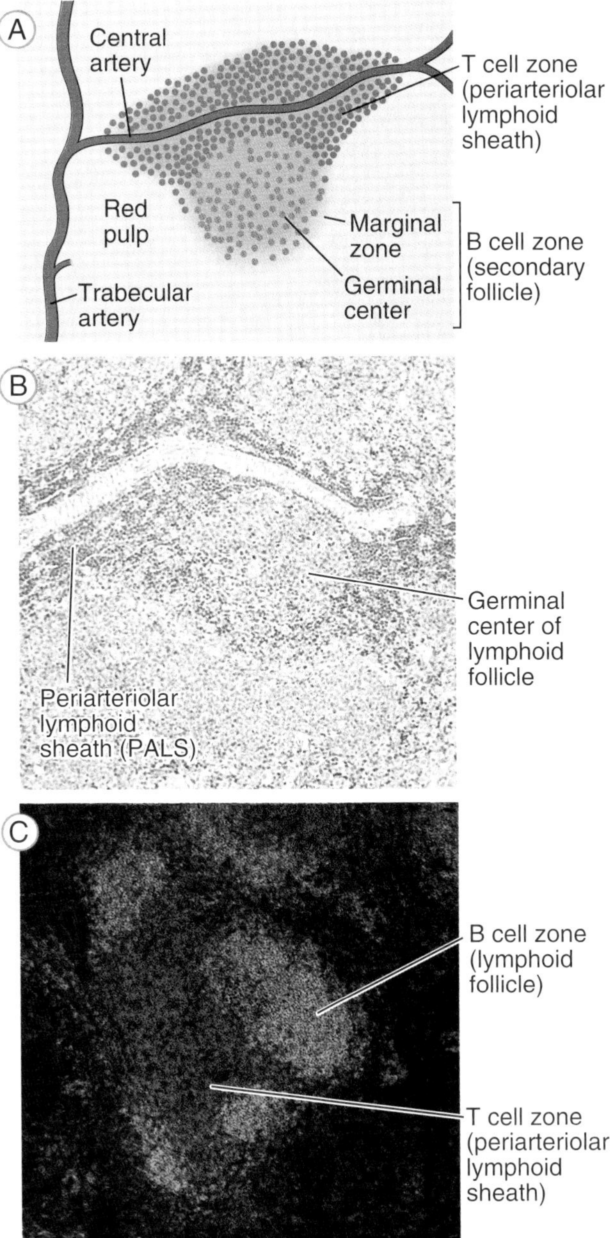

Figure 2–13 Morphology of the spleen.

A. Schematic diagram of the spleen illustrating T cell and B cell zones, which make up the white pulp.

B. Photomicrograph of a section of human spleen showing a trabecular artery with adjacent periarteriolar lymphoid sheath and a lymphoid follicle with a germinal center. Surrounding these areas is the red pulp, rich in vascular sinusoids.

C. Immunohistochemical demonstration of T cell and B cell zones in the spleen, shown in a cross-section of the region around an arteriole. T cells in the periarteriolar lymphoid sheath are stained red, and B cells in the follicle are stained green. (Courtesy of Drs. Kathryn Pape and Jennifer Walter, University of Minnesota School of Medicine, Minneapolis.)

called the marginal zone. These dense lymphoid tissues constitute the white pulp of the spleen. The arterioles ultimately end in vascular sinusoids, scattered among which are large numbers of erythrocytes, macrophages, dendritic cells, sparse lymphocytes, and plasma cells; these constitute the red pulp. The sinusoids end in venules that drain into the splenic vein, which carries blood out of the spleen and into the portal circulation.

Different classes of lymphocytes are segregated in the spleen as they are in lymph nodes, and the mechanisms of this segregation are similar in both organs (see Fig. 2–11). Antigens and lymphocytes enter the spleen through the vascular sinusoids. In response to chemokines, T cells are attracted to the T cell zones adjacent to arterioles, and B cells enter the follicles.

The spleen is also an important filter for the blood. Its red pulp macrophages clear the blood of microbes and other particles, and the spleen is the major site for the phagocytosis of antibody-coated (opsonized) microbes. Individuals lacking a spleen are extremely susceptible to infections with encapsulated bacteria such as pneumococci and meningococci because such organisms are normally cleared by opsonization and phagocytosis, and this function is defective in the absence of the spleen.

Cutaneous Immune System

The skin contains a specialized cutaneous immune system consisting of lymphocytes and APCs. The skin is the largest organ in the body and is an important physical barrier between an organism and its external environment. In addition, the skin is an active participant in host defense, with the ability to generate and support local immune and inflammatory reactions. Many foreign antigens gain entry into the body through the skin, so that many immune responses are initiated in this tissue.

The principal cell populations within the epidermis are keratinocytes, melanocytes, epidermal Langerhans cells, and intraepithelial T cells (Fig. 2–14). The keratinocytes and melanocytes do not appear to be important mediators of adaptive immunity, although keratinocytes do produce several cytokines that may contribute to innate immune reactions and cutaneous inflammation. Langerhans cells, located in the suprabasal portion of the epidermis, are the immature dendritic cells of the cutaneous immune system. Langerhans cells form an almost continuous meshwork that enables them to capture antigens that enter through the skin. On stimulation by proinflammatory cytokines, Langerhans cells retract their processes, lose their adhesiveness for epidermal cells, and migrate into the dermis. They subsequently home to lymph nodes through lymphatic vessels, and this process may be stimulated by chemokines that act specifically on Langerhans cells.

Intraepidermal lymphocytes constitute only about 2% of skin-associated lymphocytes (the rest reside in the dermis), and the majority are $CD8^+$ T cells. Intraepidermal T cells may express a more restricted set of antigen receptors than do T lymphocytes in most extracutaneous tissues. In mice (and some other species), many intraepidermal lymphocytes are T cells that express an uncommon type of antigen receptor formed by γ and δ chains instead of the usual α and β chains of the antigen receptors of $CD4^+$ and $CD8^+$ T cells (see Chapter 6). As we shall discuss shortly, this is also true of intraepithelial lymphocytes in the intestine, raising the possibility that $\gamma\delta$ T cells, at least in some species, may be uniquely committed to recognizing microbes that are commonly encountered at epithelial surfaces. However, neither the specificity nor the function of this T cell subpopulation is clearly defined.

The dermis contains T lymphocytes (both $CD4^+$ and $CD8^+$ cells), predominantly in a perivascular location, and scattered macrophages. This is essentially similar to connective tissues in other organs. The T cells usually express phenotypic markers typical of activated or memory cells. It is not clear whether these cells reside permanently within the dermis or are merely in transit between blood and lymphatic capillaries as part of memory T cell recirculation (described later). Many dermal T cells also express a carbohydrate epitope, called the cutaneous lymphocyte antigen-1, that may play a role in specific homing of the cells to the skin. This is discussed further at the end of the chapter.

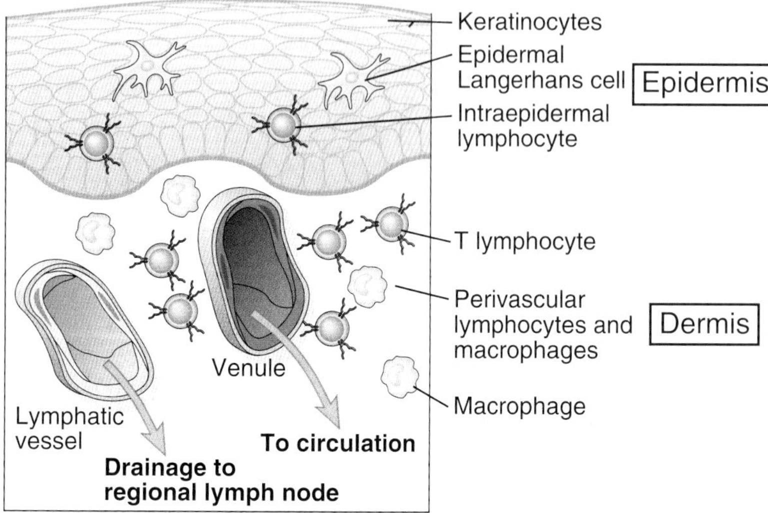

Figure 2–14 Cellular components of the cutaneous immune system.
The major components of the cutaneous immune system shown in this schematic diagram include keratinocytes, Langerhans cells, and intraepidermal lymphocytes, all located in the epidermis, and T lymphocytes and macrophages, located in the dermis.

Mucosal Immune System

The mucosal surfaces of the gastrointestinal and respiratory tracts, like the skin, are colonized by lymphocytes and APCs that initiate immune responses to ingested and inhaled antigens. Like the skin, these mucosal epithelia are barriers between the internal and external environments and are therefore an important site of entry of microbes. Much of our knowledge of mucosal immunity is based on studies of the gastrointestinal tract, and this is emphasized in the discussion that follows. In comparison, little is known about immune responses in the respiratory mucosa, even though the airways are a major portal of antigen entry. It is likely, however, that the features of immune responses are similar in all mucosal lymphoid tissues.

In the mucosa of the gastrointestinal tract, lymphocytes are found in large numbers in three main regions—within the epithelial layer, scattered throughout the lamina propria, and in organized collections in the lamina propria such as **Peyer's patches** (Fig. 2–15). Cells at each site have distinct phenotypic and functional characteristics. The majority of intraepithelial lymphocytes are T cells. In humans, most of these are $CD8^+$ cells. In mice, about 50% of intraepithelial lymphocytes express the $\gamma\delta$ form of the T cell receptor (TCR), similar to intraepidermal lymphocytes in the skin. In humans, only about 10% of intraepithelial lymphocytes are $\gamma\delta$ cells, but this proportion is still higher than the proportions of $\gamma\delta$ cells found among T cells in other tissues. Both the $\alpha\beta$ and the $\gamma\delta$ TCR-expressing intraepithelial lymphocytes show limited diversity of antigen receptors. All these findings support the idea that intraepithelial lymphocytes have a limited range of specificity, distinct from that of most T cells, which may have evolved to recognize commonly encountered intraluminal antigens.

The intestinal lamina propria contains a mixed population of cells. These include T lymphocytes, most of which are $CD4^+$ and have the phenotype of activated cells. It is likely that T cells initially recognize and respond to antigens in mesenteric lymph nodes draining the intestine and migrate back to the intestine to populate the lamina propria. This is similar to the postulated origin of T cells in the dermis of the skin. The lamina propria also contains large numbers of activated B lymphocytes and plasma cells as well as macrophages, dendritic cells, eosinophils, and mast cells.

In addition to scattered lymphocytes, the mucosal immune system contains organized lymphoid tissues, the most prominent of which are the Peyer's patches of the small intestine. Like lymphoid follicles in the spleen

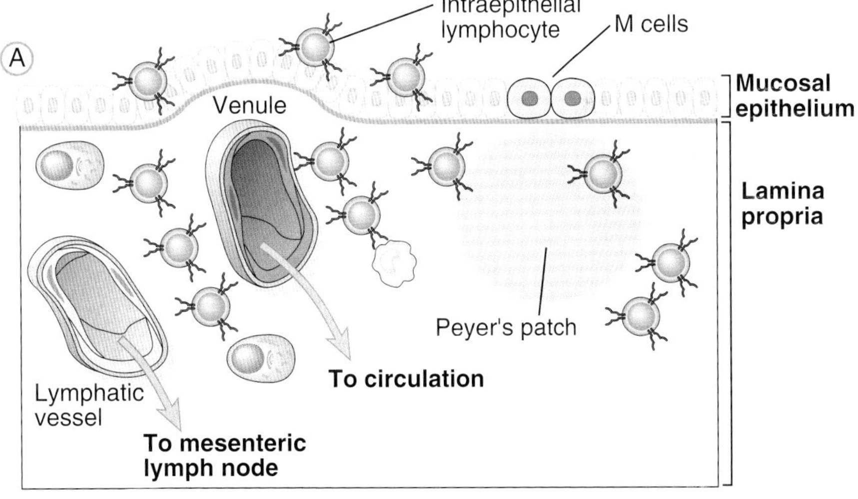

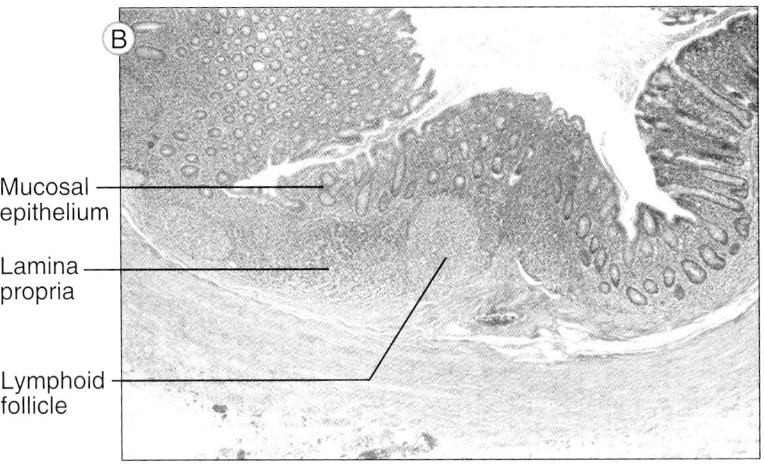

Figure 2–15 The mucosal immune system.

A. Schematic diagram of the cellular components of the mucosal immune system.

B. Photomicrograph of mucosal lymphoid tissue in the human appendix. Similar aggregates of lymphoid tissue are found throughout the gastrointestinal tract and the respiratory tract.

and lymph nodes, the central regions of these mucosal follicles are B cell–rich areas that often contain germinal centers. Peyer's patches also contain small numbers of $CD4^+$ T cells, mainly in the interfollicular regions. In adult mice, 50% to 70% of Peyer's patch lymphocytes are B cells, and 10% to 30% are T cells. Some of the epithelial cells overlying Peyer's patches are specialized M (membranous) cells. M cells lack microvilli, are actively pinocytic, and transport macromolecules from the intestinal lumen into subepithelial tissues. They are thought to play an important role in delivering antigens to Peyer's patches. (Note, however, that M cells do not function as APCs.) Follicles similar to Peyer's patches are abundant in the appendix and are found in smaller numbers in much of the gastrointestinal and respiratory tracts. Pharyngeal tonsils are also mucosal lymphoid follicles analogous to Peyer's patches.

Immune responses to oral antigens differ in some fundamental respects from responses to antigens encountered at other sites. The two most striking differences are the high levels of IgA antibody production associated with mucosal tissues (see Chapter 14) and the tendency of oral immunization with protein antigens to induce T cell tolerance rather than activation (see Chapter 10).

Pathways and Mechanisms of Lymphocyte Recirculation and Homing

Lymphocytes continuously move through the blood stream and lymphatics, from one peripheral (secondary) lymphoid tissue to another, and then to peripheral inflammatory sites (Fig. 2–16). The movement of lymphocytes between these various locations is called **lymphocyte recirculation,** and the process by which particular subsets of lymphocytes selectively enter some tissues but not others is called **lymphocyte homing.** Recirculation of lymphocytes serves critical functions in adaptive immune responses. First, it enables the limited number of lymphocytes in an individual that are specific for a particular foreign antigen to search for that antigen throughout the body. Second, it ensures that particular subsets of lymphocytes are delivered to the particular tissue microenvironments where they are required for adaptive immune responses and not, wastefully, to places where they would serve no purpose. For instance, the recirculation pathways of naive lymphocytes differ from those of effector and memory lymphocytes, and these differences are fundamental to the way immune responses develop (see Fig. 2–16). Specifically, naive lymphocytes recirculate through peripheral lymphoid organs and effector lymphocytes migrate to peripheral tissues at sites of infection and inflammation. In the following section, we describe the mechanisms and pathways of lymphocyte recirculation. Our discussion emphasizes T cells because much more is known about their movement through tissues than is known about B cell recirculation.

Lymphocyte recirculation and migration to particular tissues are mediated by adhesion molecules on lymphocytes, endothelial cells and extracellular matrix, and chemokines produced in the endothelium and in tissues. Adhesion of lymphocytes to the endothelial cells lining postcapillary venules in particular tissues determines which tissues the lymphocytes will enter. Adhesion to and detachment from extracellular matrix components within tissues determine how long lymphocytes are retained at a particular extravascular site before they return through the lymphatics to the blood. The adhesion molecules expressed by the lymphocytes are called homing receptors, and their ligands expressed on vascular endothelium are called addressins. The homing receptors on lymphocytes include members of three families of molecules, the selectins, the integrins, and the Ig superfamily. These homing receptors are distinct from antigen receptors, and the normal patterns of recirculation are independent of antigen. The only role of antigen recognition in lymphocyte recirculation may be to increase the affinity of lymphocyte integrins for their ligands, leading to retention of those cells that encounter their antigen at the anatomic site where the antigen is present.

Recirculation of Naive T Lymphocytes Through Lymphoid Organs

Naive T cells preferentially home to and recirculate through peripheral lymphoid organs, where they recognize and respond to foreign antigens. The net flux of lymphocytes through lymph nodes is very high, and it has been estimated that approximately 25×10^9 cells pass through lymph nodes each day (i.e., each lymphocyte goes through a node once a day on the average). Antigens are concentrated in the lymph nodes and spleen, where they are presented by mature dendritic cells, the APCs that are best able to initiate responses of naive T cells. Thus, movement of naive T cells through the lymph nodes and spleen maximizes the chances of specific encounter with antigen and initiation of an adaptive immune response.

Naive lymphocytes that enter lymph nodes in the blood leave the circulation and migrate into the stroma of lymph nodes selectively through modified postcapillary venules that are lined by plump endothelial cells, which are therefore called **high endothelial venules** (HEVs) (Fig. 2–17). HEVs are also present in mucosal lymphoid tissues, such as Peyer's patches in the gut, but not in the spleen. Naive T cell migration from the circulation into the stroma of a lymph node involves a multistep sequence of interactions between lymphocytes and endothelial cells in HEVs. This sequence, which is similar for migration of leukocytes into peripheral tissues, includes initial low-affinity interactions mediated by selectins, followed by chemokine-mediated up-regulation of T cell integrin affinity, and then integrin-mediated firm adhesion of the T cell to the HEV. Naive lymphocytes express on their surface a homing receptor that belongs to the selectin family and is called **L-selectin** (CD62L) (Fig. 2–18). HEVs express

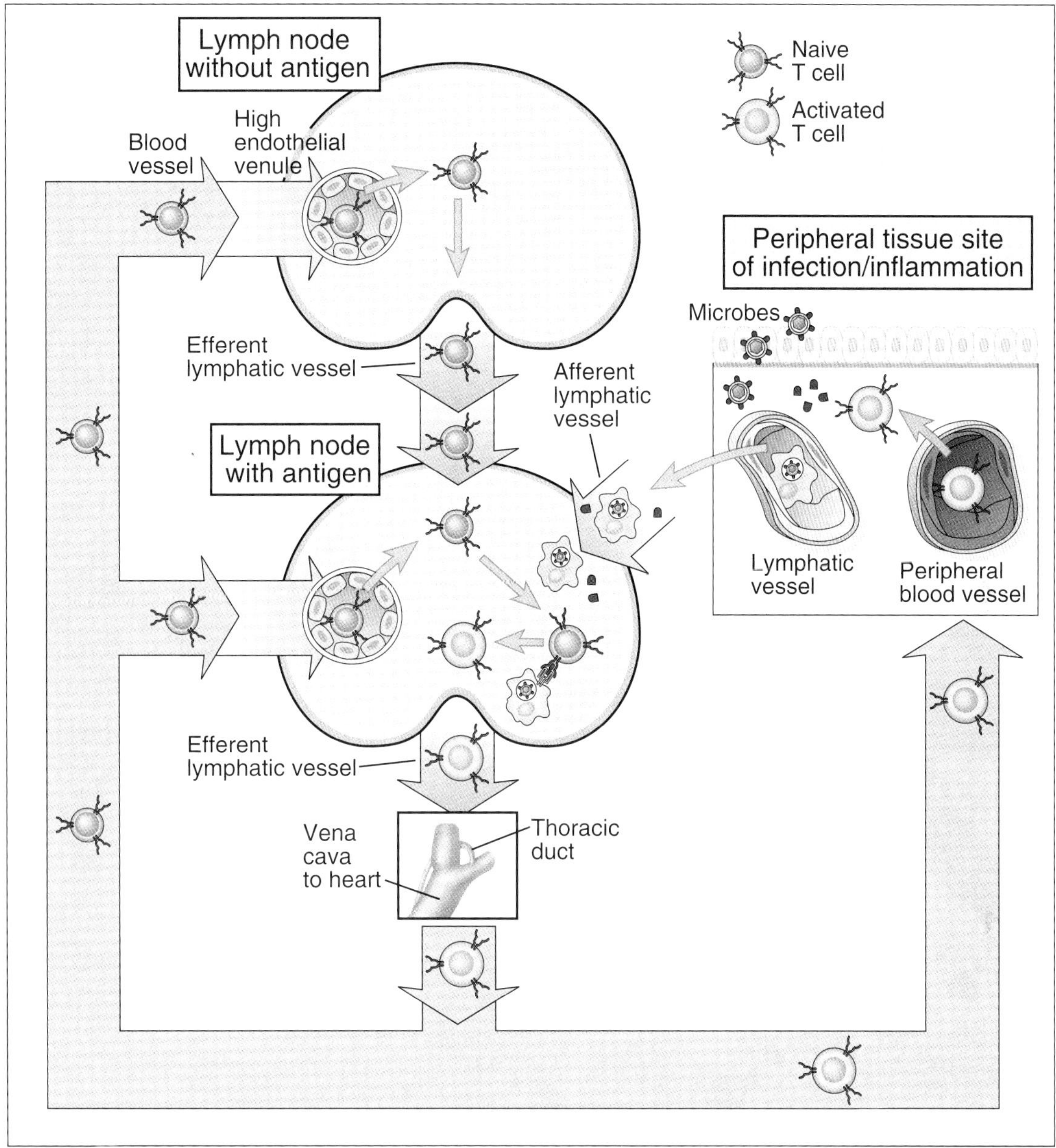

Figure 2–16 Pathways of T lymphocyte recirculation.
Naive T cells preferentially leave the blood and enter lymph nodes across the high endothelial venules. Dendritic cells bearing antigen enter the lymph node through lymphatic vessels. If the T cells recognize antigen, they are activated, and they return to the circulation through the efferent lymphatics and the thoracic duct, which empties into the superior vena cava, then into the heart, and ultimately into the arterial circulation. Effector and memory T cells preferentially leave the blood and enter peripheral tissues through venules at sites of inflammation. Recirculation through peripheral lymphoid organs other than lymph nodes is not shown.

sulfated glycosaminoglycans, collectively called peripheral node addressin (PNAd), that are ligands for L-selectin. The carbohydrate groups that bind L-selectin may be attached to different sialomucins on the endothelium in different tissues. For example, on lymph node HEVs, the PNAd is displayed by two sialomucins, called GlyCAM-1 (glycan-bearing cell adhesion molecule-1) and CD34. In Peyer's patches in the intestinal wall, the L-selectin ligand is a molecule called MadCAM-1 (mucosal addressin cell adhesion molecule-1). Thus, different molecules bearing carbohydrate ligands for L-selectin may be important for recruitment of naive T cells to endothelium in different tissues. The binding of L-selectin to its ligand is a low-affinity interaction that is readily broken by the shear force of the flowing blood. As a result, naive T cells that attach to HEVs remain loosely attached only for a few seconds, detach, bind again, and thus begin to roll on the endothelial surface. Meanwhile, chemokines that are produced in the lymph node may be displayed on the surface of the endothelial cells bound to glycosaminoglycans. Rolling T cells that encounter these chemokines are able to increase their strength of attachment further, to spread out into motile forms,

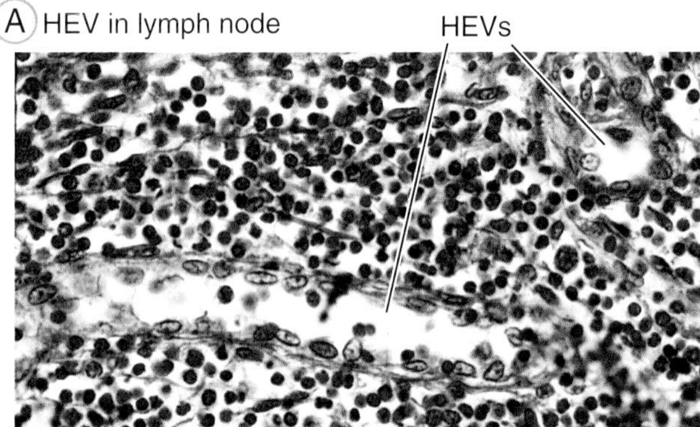

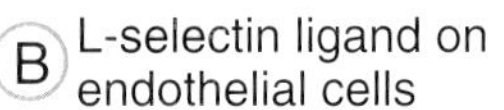

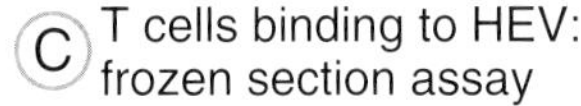

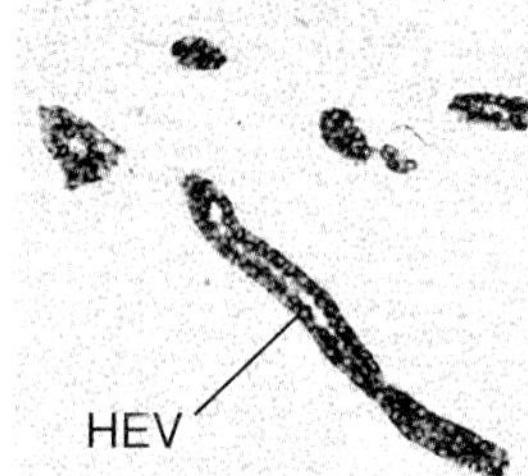

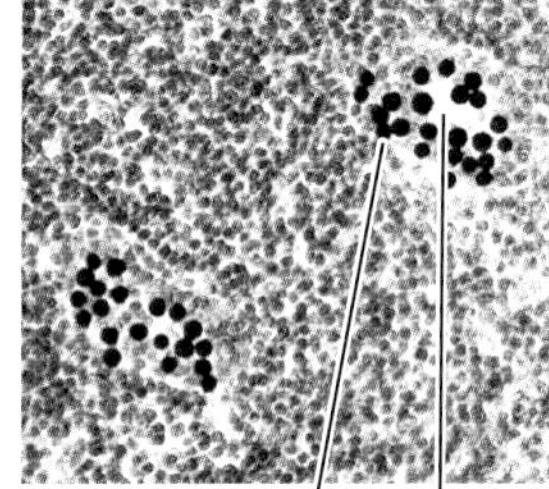

D T cells binding to HEV: electron micrograph

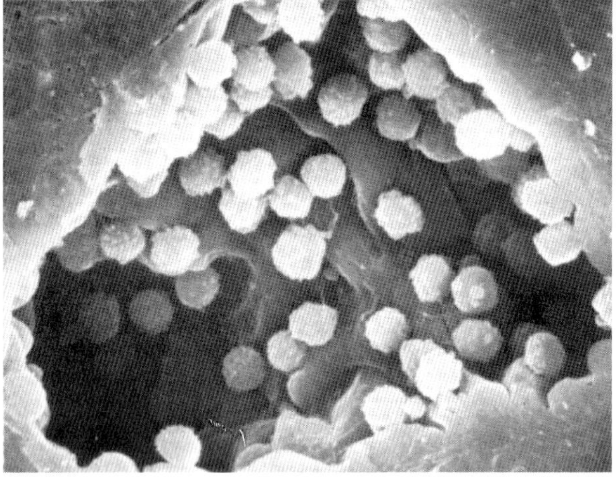

Figure 2–17 High endothelial venules (HEVs).
A. Light micrograph of an HEV in a lymph node illustrating the tall endothelial cells. (Courtesy of Dr. Steve Rosen, Department of Anatomy, University of California San Francisco.)
B. Expression of L-selectin ligand on HEVs, stained with a specific antibody by the immunoperoxidase technique. (The location of the antibody is revealed by a brown reaction product of peroxidase, which is coupled to the antibody; see Appendix III for details.) The HEVs are abundant in the T cell zone of the lymph node. (Courtesy of Drs. Steve Rosen and Akio Kikuta, Department of Anatomy, University of California San Francisco.)
C. A binding assay in which lymphocytes are incubated with frozen sections of a lymph node. The lymphocytes (stained dark blue) bind selectively to HEVs. (Courtesy of Dr. Steve Rosen, Department of Anatomy, University of California San Francisco.)
D. Scanning electron micrograph of an HEV with lymphocytes attached to the luminal surface of the endothelial cells. (Courtesy of J. Emerson and T. Yednock, University of California San Francisco School of Medicine, San Francisco. From Rosen SD, and LM Stoolman. Potential role of cell surface lectin in lymphocyte recirculation. *In* Olden K, and J Parent. Vertebrate Lectins. Van Nostrand Reinhold, New York, 1987.)

and to crawl between the endothelial cells into the stroma of the lymph node. Once the lymphocytes exit the HEVs, the cells migrate toward the chemokine gradient. As mentioned previously, naive T cells express the chemokine receptor CCR7 and migrate into the T cell zones, where the chemokines that bind to CCR7 are produced, and naive B cells express CXCR5 and migrate into lymphoid follicles under the influence of chemokines that bind to CXCR5. The important role for L-selectin and chemokines in lymphocyte homing to secondary lymphoid tissues is supported by many different experimental observations.

- Lymphocytes from L-selectin knockout mice do not bind to peripheral lymph node HEVs, and the mice have a marked reduction in the number of lymphocytes in peripheral lymph nodes.
- Immunohistochemical and *in situ* hybridization studies indicate that SLC and ELC, two chemokines that bind to CCR7 on T cells, are produced in T cell zones of lymph nodes, whereas BCA-1, a chemokine that attracts B cells, is produced in follicles.

Less is known about the nature of homing receptors or addressins involved in lymphocyte recirculation through the spleen, even though the rate of lymphocyte passage through the spleen is about half the total lymphocyte population every 24 hours. MadCAM-1 is expressed on the endothelial cells of the marginal sinus in the T cell zones of the spleen and is likely to play a role in naive T cell homing. The spleen does not contain morphologically identifiable HEVs, and it is possible that homing of lymphocytes to the spleen does not show the same degree of selectivity for naive cells as do lymph nodes.

Naive T cells that enter a lymph node may be activated by antigens that are transported to that node (see Fig. 2–1). Within a few hours after antigen exposure at a peripheral site, blood flow through a draining lymph node may increase by more than 20-fold, allowing an increased number of naive lymphocytes access to the site where antigens are concentrated. Efflux of cells from the node may decrease at the same time. These changes are probably due to an inflammatory reaction to microbes or adjuvants associated with the antigen. Naive T cells that enter the T cell zones of a lymph node scan dendritic cells in these areas for the presence of antigens that the T cells may recognize. If naive T cells do recognize antigen, they undergo clonal expansion, differentiate into effector or memory T cells, and enter a distinct recirculation pattern, as described next. If the naive T cells do not encounter antigen, they exit through an efferent lymphatic vessel, re-enter the circulation, and home to other lymph nodes.

Migration of Effector and Memory T Lymphocytes to Sites of Inflammation

Effector and memory T cells exit lymph nodes and preferentially home to peripheral tissues at sites of infection, where they are needed to eliminate microbes in the effector phase of adaptive immune responses.

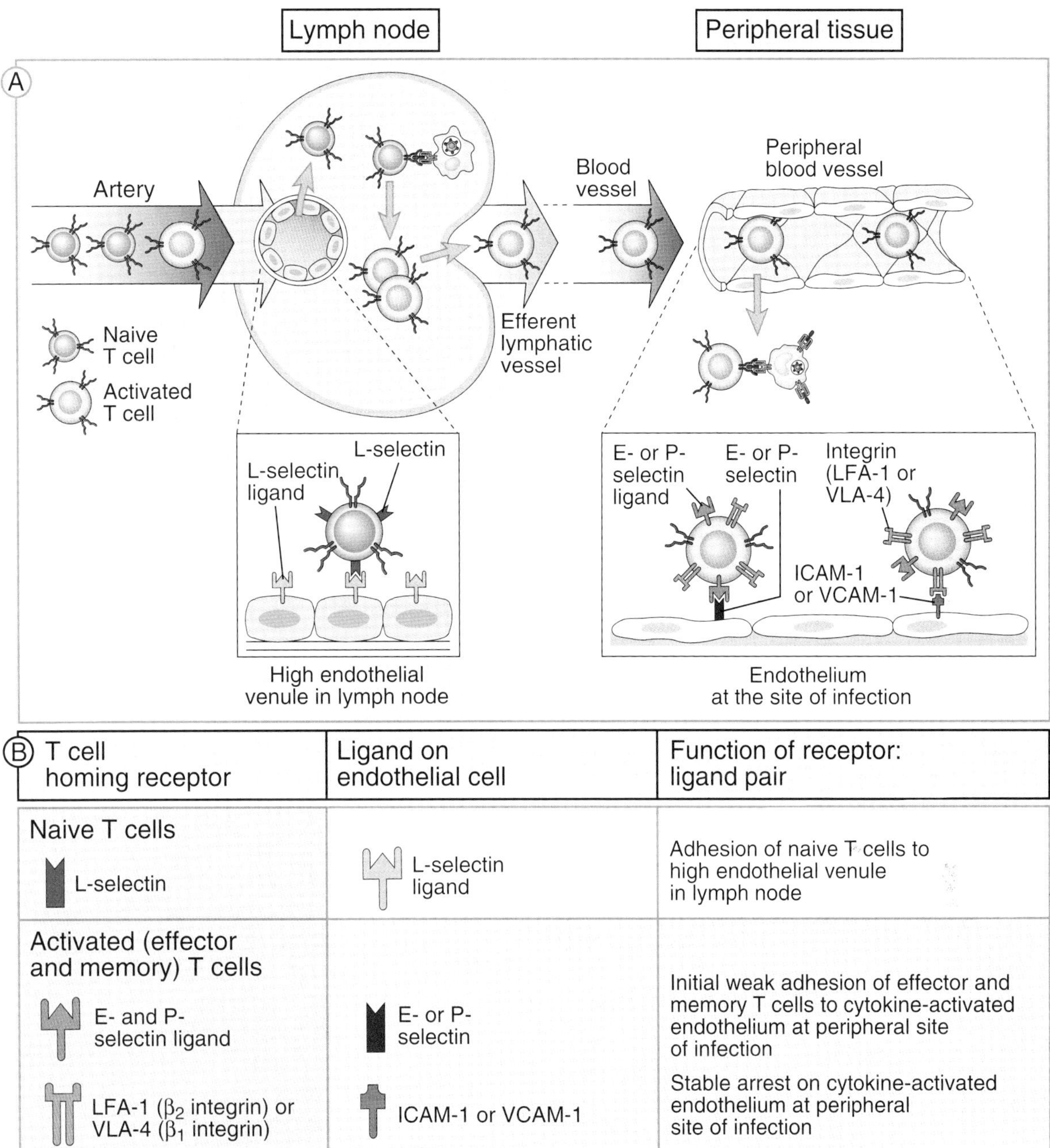

T cell homing receptor	Ligand on endothelial cell	Function of receptor: ligand pair
Naive T cells		
L-selectin	L-selectin ligand	Adhesion of naive T cells to high endothelial venule in lymph node
Activated (effector and memory) T cells		
E- and P-selectin ligand	E- or P-selectin	Initial weak adhesion of effector and memory T cells to cytokine-activated endothelium at peripheral site of infection
LFA-1 (β_2 integrin) or VLA-4 (β_1 integrin)	ICAM-1 or VCAM-1	Stable arrest on cytokine-activated endothelium at peripheral site of infection

Figure 2–18 Migration of naive and effector T lymphocytes.
A. Naive T lymphocytes home to lymph nodes as a result of L-selectin binding to its ligand on high endothelial venules, which are present only in lymph nodes. Activated T lymphocytes, including effector cells, home to sites of infection in peripheral tissues, and this migration is mediated by E- and P-selectins and integrins. In addition, different chemokines that are produced in lymph nodes and sites of infection also participate in the recruitment of T cells to these sites (not shown).
B. The ligands for the principal T cell homing receptors, and the functions of these receptors and ligands, are shown.

The differentiation of naive T cells into effector cells, which occurs in the peripheral lymphoid organs, is accompanied by changes in several adhesion molecules. The expression of L-selectin decreases, and the levels of several integrins, ligands for E- and P-selectins, and CD44 increase (see Fig. 2–18). (We will describe selectins and integrins in more detail in Chapter 6.) Differentiated effector T cells also lose expression of the CCR7 chemokine receptor. As a result, effector cells are no longer constrained to stay in the node, and they leave through efferent lymphatics and enter the circulation. At sites of infection, there is an innate immune response during which several cytokines are produced. Some of these cytokines act on the vascular endothelium at the site and stimulate expression of ligands for the integrins as well as E- and P-selectins and secretion of chemokines that act on T cells. In response to these chemokines, the T cells increase the binding avidity of their integrins for the ligands. As a result, the T cells bind firmly to the endothelium and migrate out of the vessel into the area of infection. Because integrins and CD44 also bind to extracellular matrix proteins, effector T cells are retained at these sites. Thus, the effector cells are able to perform their function of eradicating the infection. We will describe this process in more detail in Chapter 13, when we consider cell-mediated immunity.

Memory T cells are heterogeneous in their patterns of expression of adhesion molecules and in their propensity to migrate to different tissues. Some memory cells migrate to mucosal tissues and skin, and special adhesion molecules may be involved in these processes. For instance, some memory cells express an integrin ($\alpha_4\beta_6$) that interacts with the mucosal endothelial addressin MadCAM-1 and thus mediates homing of memory T cells to mucosal lymphoid tissues. T cells within the intestinal epithelium express a different integrin ($\alpha_E\beta_7$) that can bind to E-cadherin molecules on epithelial cells, allowing T cells to maintain residence as intraepithelial lymphocytes. Other memory T cells that preferentially home to skin express a carbohydrate ligand called CLA-1 (for cutaneous lymphocyte antigen-1) that binds to E-selectin. Yet other memory cells express L-selectin and CCR7, and these preferentially migrate to lymph nodes, where they can expand rapidly if they encounter the antigen that activated them initially.

Recirculation of B Lymphocytes

In principle, the migration of B lymphocytes to different tissues is similar to that of T lymphocytes and is regulated by the same molecular mechanisms. Naive B cells migrate to lymph nodes, and specifically to follicles, using L-selectin and the CXCR5 chemokine receptor to do so. On activation, the B cells lose expression of CXCR5 and exit the follicles into the T cell zones of the lymphoid organ. Activated B cells express integrins and use these to migrate to peripheral tissues. Some antibody-producing plasma cells migrate to the bone marrow; the molecules involved in this process are not identified. Other antibody-secreting cells remain in the lymphoid organs, and the antibodies they produce enter the circulation and find antigens throughout the body.

Summary

- The anatomic organization of the cells and tissues of the immune system is of critical importance for the generation of immune responses. This organization permits the small number of lymphocytes specific for any one antigen to locate and respond effectively to that antigen regardless of where in the body the antigen is introduced.
- The adaptive immune response depends on antigen-specific lymphocytes, antigen-presenting cells required for lymphocyte activation, and effector cells that eliminate antigens.
- B and T lymphocytes express highly diverse and specific antigen receptors and are the cells responsible for the specificity and memory of adaptive immune responses. NK cells are a distinct class of lymphocytes that do not express highly diverse antigen receptors and whose functions are largely in innate immunity. Many surface molecules are differentially expressed on different subsets of lymphocytes, as well as on other leukocytes, and these are named according to the CD nomenclature.
- Both B and T lymphocytes arise from a common precursor in the bone marrow. B cell development proceeds in the bone marrow, whereas T cell precursors migrate to and mature in the thymus. After maturing, B and T cells leave the bone marrow and thymus, enter the circulation, and populate peripheral lymphoid organs.
- Naive B and T cells are mature lymphocytes that have not been stimulated by antigen to become differentiated lymphocytes. When they encounter antigen, they differentiate into effector lymphocytes that have functions in protective immune responses. Effector B lymphocytes are antibody-secreting plasma cells. Effector T cells include cytokine-secreting $CD4^+$ helper T cells and $CD8^+$ CTLs.
- Some of the progeny of antigen-activated B and T lymphocytes differentiate into memory cells that survive for long periods in a quiescent state. These memory cells are responsible for the rapid and enhanced responses to subsequent exposures to antigen.
- Antigen-presenting cells (APCs) function to display antigens for recognition by lymphocytes and to promote the activation of lymphocytes. APCs include dendritic cells, mononuclear phagocytes, and follicular dendritic cells (FDCs).
- The organs of the immune system may be divided into the generative organs (bone marrow and thymus), where lymphocytes mature, and the peripheral organs (lymph nodes and spleen), where naive lymphocytes are activated by antigens.
- Bone marrow contains the stem cells for all blood cells, including lymphocytes, and is the site of maturation of all of these cell types except T cells, which mature in the thymus.
- The lymph nodes are the sites where B and T cells respond to antigens that are collected by the lymph draining peripheral tissues. The spleen is the organ in which lymphocytes respond to blood-borne antigens. Both lymph nodes and spleen are organized into B cell zones (the follicles) and T cell zones. The T cell areas are also the sites of residence of mature dendritic cells, which are APCs specialized for the activation of naive T cells. FDCs reside in the B cell areas and serve to activate B cells during humoral immune responses to protein antigens. The devel-

opment of secondary lymphoid tissue architecture depends on cytokines.

- The cutaneous immune system consists of specialized collections of APCs and lymphocytes adapted to respond to environmental antigens encountered in the skin. A network of immature dendritic cells called Langerhans cells, present in the epidermis of the skin, serves to trap antigens and then transport them to draining lymph nodes. The mucosal immune system includes specialized collections of lymphocytes and APCs organized to optimize encounters with environmental antigens introduced through the respiratory and gastrointestinal tracts.
- Lymphocyte recirculation is the process by which lymphocytes continuously move between sites throughout the body through blood and lymphatic vessels, and it is critical for the initiation and effector phases of immune responses.
- Naive T cells normally recirculate among the various peripheral lymphoid organs, increasing the likelihood of encounter with antigen displayed by APCs such as mature dendritic cells. Effector T cells more typically are recruited to peripheral sites of inflammation where microbial antigens are located. Memory T cells may enter either lymphoid organs or peripheral tissues.
- The process of lymphocyte recirculation is regulated by adhesion molecules on lymphocytes, called homing receptors, and their ligands on vascular endothelial cells, called addressins. Endothelial cells in different tissues may express different ligands for homing receptors that promote tissue-specific lymphocyte homing.
- Different populations of lymphocytes exhibit distinct patterns of homing. Naive T cells migrate preferentially to lymph nodes; this process is largely mediated by binding of L-selectin on the T cells to peripheral lymph node addressin on high endothelial venules in lymph nodes. The effector and memory T cells that are generated by antigen stimulation of naive T cells exit the lymph node. They have decreased L-selectin expression but increased expression of integrins and E-selectin and P-selectin ligands, and these molecules mediate binding to endothelium at peripheral inflammatory sites.

Selected Readings

Cyster JG. Chemokines and cell migration in secondary lymphoid organs. Science 286:2098–2102, 1999.

Dutton RW, LM Bradley, and SL Swain. T cell memory. Annual Review of Immunology 16:201–223, 1998.

Fu YX, and DD Chaplin. Development and maturation of secondary lymphoid tissues. Annual Review of Immunology 17:399–433, 1999.

Kraal G, and RE Mebius. High endothelial venules: lymphocyte traffic control and controlled traffic. Advances in Immunology 65:347–395, 1997.

Kunkel EJ, and EC Butcher. Chemokines and the tissue-specific migration of lymphocytes. Immunity 16:1–4, 2002.

Kupper TS. T cells, immunosurveillance, and cutaneous immunity. Journal of Dermatologic Science 24 Supplement 1:S41–45, 2000.

Nagler-Anderson C. Man the barrier! Strategic defences in the intestinal mucosa. Nature Reviews Immunology 1:59–67, 2001.

Neutra MR, NJ Mantis, and J-P Kraehenbuhl. Collaboration of epithelial cells with organized mucosal lymphoid tissue. Nature Immunology 2:1004–1009, 2001.

Salmi M, and D Jalkanen. How do lymphocytes know where to go: current concepts and enigmas of lymphocyte homing. Advances in Immunology 64:139–218, 1997.

Von Andrian UH, and CR Mackay. T cell function and migration: two sides of the same coin. New England Journal of Medicine 343:1020–1034, 2000.

Section II

Recognition of Antigens

Adaptive immune responses are initiated by the specific recognition of antigens by lymphocytes. This section is devoted to a discussion of the cellular and molecular basis of antigen recognition and the specificities of B and T lymphocytes.

We begin with antibodies, which are the antigen receptors and effector molecules of B lymphocytes, because our understanding of the structural basis of antigen recognition has evolved from studies of these molecules. Chapter 3 describes the structure of antibodies and how these proteins recognize antigens.

The next three chapters consider antigen recognition by T lymphocytes, which play a central role in all immune responses to protein antigens. In Chapter 4, we describe the genetics and biochemistry of the major histocompatibility complex (MHC), whose products are integral components of the ligands that T cells specifically recognize. Chapter 5 discusses the association of foreign peptide antigens with MHC molecules and the cell biology and physiologic significance of antigen presentation. Chapter 6 deals with the T cell antigen receptor and the other T cell membrane molecules that are involved in the recognition of antigens and the responses of the T cells.

Chapter 3

Antibodies and Antigens

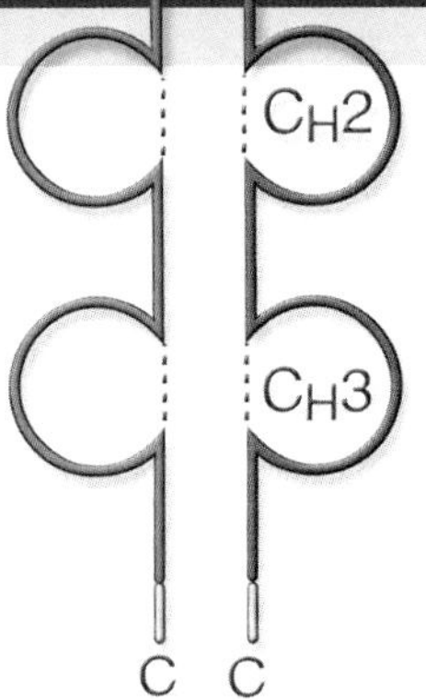

One of the earliest experimental demonstrations of adaptive immunity was the induction of humoral immunity against microbial toxins. In the early 1900s, patients with life-threatening diphtheria infection were successfully treated by the administration of serum from horses immunized with diphtheria toxin. This form of immunity, called humoral immunity, is mediated by a family of glycoproteins called **antibodies**. Antibodies, major histocompatibility complex (MHC) molecules (see Chapter 4), and T cell antigen receptors (see Chapter 6) are the three classes of molecules used in adaptive immunity to recognize antigens (Table 3–1). Of these three, antibodies bind the widest range of antigenic structures, show the greatest ability to discriminate among different antigens, and bind antigens with the greatest strength. Antibodies are also the best studied of the three types of antigen-binding molecules. Therefore, we begin our discussion of how the immune system specifically recognizes antigens by describing the structure and the antigen-binding properties of antibodies.

Antibodies specifically bind antigens in both the recognition phase and the effector phase of humoral immunity. Antibodies are produced in a membrane-bound form by B lymphocytes, and these membrane molecules function as B cell receptors for antigens. The interaction of antigen with membrane antibodies on naive B cells initiates B cell responses and thus constitutes the recognition phase of humoral immune responses. Antibodies are also produced in a secreted form by antigen-stimulated B cells. In the effector phase of humoral immunity, these secreted antibodies bind to antigens and trigger several effector mechanisms that eliminate the antigens. The elimination of antigen often requires interaction of antibody with components of the innate immune system, including molecules such as complement proteins and cells such as phagocytes and eosinophils. Antibody-mediated effector functions include neutralization of microbes or toxic microbial products; activation of the complement system; opsonization of antigens for enhanced phagocytosis; antibody-dependent cell-mediated cytotoxicity

Table 3–1. Features of Antigen Binding by the Antigen-Recognizing Molecules of the Immune System

Feature	Antigen-binding molecule		
	Immunoglobulin (Ig)	T cell receptor (TCR)	MHC molecules*
Antigen-binding site	Made up of three CDRs in V_H and three CDRs in V_L	Made up of three CDRs in V_α and three CDRs in V_β	Peptide-binding cleft made of $\alpha1$ and $\alpha2$ (class I) or $\alpha1$ and $\beta1$ (class II)
Nature of antigen that may be bound	Macromolecules (proteins, lipids, polysaccharides) and small chemicals	Peptide-MHC complexes	Peptides
Nature of antigenic determinants recognized	Linear and conformational determinants of various macromolecules and chemicals	Linear determinants of peptides; only 2 or 3 amino acid residues of a peptide bound to an MHC molecule	Linear determinants of peptides; only some amino acid residues of a peptide
Affinity of antigen binding	K_d $10^{-7}-10^{-11}$ M; average affinity of Igs increases during immune response	K_d $10^{-5}-10^{-7}$ M	K_d 10^{-6} M
On-rate and off-rate	Rapid on-rate, variable off-rate	Slow on-rate, slow off-rate	Slow on-rate, very slow off-rate

*The structures and functions of MHC and TCR molecules are discussed in Chapters 4 and 6, respectively.
Abbreviations: CDR, complementarity-determining region; K_d, dissociation constant; MHC, major histocompatibility complex; V_H, variable domain of heavy chain Ig; V_L, variable domain of light chain Ig.

(ADCC), by which antibodies target microbes for lysis by cells of the innate immune system; and immediate hypersensitivity, in which antibodies trigger mast cell activation. These effector functions of antibodies are described in detail in Chapter 14. In this chapter, we discuss the structural features of antibodies that underlie their antigen recognition and effector functions.

Natural Distribution and Production of Antibodies

Antibodies are distributed in biologic fluids throughout the body and are found on the surface of a limited number of cell types. B lymphocytes are the only cells that synthesize antibody molecules. Within B cells, antibodies are present in cytoplasmic membrane-bound compartments (endoplasmic reticulum and Golgi complex) and on the surface, where they are expressed as integral membrane proteins. Secreted forms of antibodies are present in the plasma (fluid portion of the blood), in mucosal secretions, and in the interstitial fluid of the tissues. Antibodies synthesized and secreted by B cells often attach to the surface of certain other immune effector cells, such as mononuclear phagocytes, NK (natural killer) cells, and mast cells, which have specific receptors for binding antibody molecules (see Chapter 14).

When blood or plasma forms a clot, antibodies remain in the residual fluid, called **serum.** Serum that contains a detectable number of antibody molecules that bind to a particular antigen is commonly called **antiserum**. (The study of antibodies and their reactions with antigens is therefore classically called **serology**.) The concentration of serum antibody molecules specific for a particular antigen is often estimated by determining how many serial dilutions of the serum can be made before binding can no longer be observed; sera with a high concentration of antibody molecules specific for a particular antigen are said to have a "high titer."

A healthy 70-kg adult human produces about 3 g of antibodies every day. Almost two thirds of this is an antibody called IgA, which is produced by B cells in the walls of the gastrointestinal and respiratory tracts and actively transported into the lumens. The large amount of IgA produced reflects the large surface areas of these organs. After exposure to an antigen, much of the initial antibody response occurs in lymphoid tissues, mainly the spleen, lymph nodes, and mucosal lymphoid tissues, but long-lived antibody-producing cells may persist in other tissues, especially in the bone marrow (see Chapter 9). Antibodies that enter the circulation have limited half-lives. The most common type of antibody found in the serum, called IgG, has a half-life of about 3 weeks.

Molecular Structure of Antibodies

Early studies of antibody structure relied on antibodies purified from the blood of individuals immunized with various antigens. It was not possible, by use of this approach, to define antibody structure precisely because serum contains mixtures of different antibodies produced by many clones of B lymphocytes that may respond to different portions (epitopes) of an antigen (so-called polyclonal antibodies). Two breakthroughs were critical for providing antibodies whose structures could be elucidated. The first was the discovery that patients with multiple myeloma, a monoclonal tumor of antibody-producing plasma cells, often have large amounts of biochemically identical antibody molecules (produced by the neoplastic clone) in their blood and urine. Immunologists found that these antibodies can be purified to homogeneity and analyzed. The second, and more important, breakthrough was the technique for producing monoclonal antibodies, described by Georges Köhler and Cesar Milstein in 1975. They developed a method for immortalizing individual antibody-secreting cells from an immunized animal by producing "hybridomas," enabling them to isolate individual **monoclonal antibodies** of predetermined specificity (Box 3–1). The availability of homo-

BOX 3–1

Monoclonal Antibodies

The ability to produce virtually unlimited quantities of identical antibody molecules specific for a particular antigenic determinant has revolutionized immunology and has had a far-reaching impact on research in diverse fields as well as in clinical medicine. The first and now generally used method for producing homogeneous or monoclonal antibodies of known specificity was described by Georges Köhler and Cesar Milstein in 1975. This technique is based on the fact that each B lymphocyte produces antibody of a single specificity. Because normal B lymphocytes cannot grow indefinitely, it is necessary to immortalize B cells that produce a specific antibody. This is achieved by cell fusion, or somatic cell hybridization, between a normal antibody-producing B cell and a myeloma cell, followed by selection of fused cells that secrete antibody of the desired specificity derived from the normal B cell. Such fusion-derived immortalized antibody-producing cell lines are called **hybridomas,** and the antibodies they produce are **monoclonal antibodies.**

The technique of producing hybridomas requires cultured myeloma cell lines that will grow in normal culture medium but not in a defined "selection" medium because they lack functional genes required for DNA synthesis in this selection medium. Fusing normal cells to these defective myeloma fusion partners provides the necessary genes from the normal cells, so that only the somatic cell hybrids will grow in the selection medium. Moreover, the uncontrolled growth property of the myeloma cell makes such hybrids immortal. Myeloma cell lines that can be used as fusion partners are created by inducing defects in nucleotide synthesis pathways. Normal animal cells synthesize purine nucleotides and thymidylate, both precursors of DNA, by a *de novo* pathway requiring tetrahydrofolate. Antifolate drugs, such as aminopterin, block activation of tetrahydrofolate, thereby inhibiting the synthesis of purines and therefore preventing DNA synthesis by the *de novo* pathway. Aminopterin-treated cells can use a salvage pathway in which purine is synthesized from exogenously supplied hypoxanthine by the enzyme hypoxanthine-guanine phosphoribosyltransferase (HGPRT), and thymidylate is synthesized from thymidine by the enzyme thymidine kinase (TK). Therefore, cells grow normally in the presence of aminopterin if the culture medium is also supplemented with hypoxanthine and thymidine (called HAT medium). Myeloma cell lines can be made defective in HGPRT or TK by mutagenesis followed by selection in media containing substrates for these enzymes that yield lethal products. Only HGPRT- or TK-deficient cells will survive under these selection conditions. Such HGPRT- or TK-negative myeloma cells cannot use the salvage pathway and will therefore die in HAT medium. If normal B cells are fused to HGPRT- or TK-negative cells, the B cells provide the necessary enzymes so that the hybrids synthesize DNA and grow in HAT medium.

To produce a monoclonal antibody specific for a defined antigen, a mouse or rat is immunized with that antigen, and B cells are isolated from the spleen or lymph nodes of the animal. These B cells are then fused with an appropriate immortalized cell line. Myeloma lines are the best fusion partners for B cells because like cells tend to fuse and give rise to stable hybrids more efficiently than unlike cells. In current practice, the myeloma lines that are used do not produce their own immunoglobulin, and cell fusion is achieved with polyethylene glycol. Hybrids are selected for growth in HAT medium; under these conditions, unfused HGPRT- or TK-negative myeloma cells die because they cannot use the salvage pathway, and unfused B cells cannot survive for more than 1 to 2 weeks because they are not immortalized, so that only hybrids will grow (see Figure). The fused cells are cultured at a concentration at which each culture well is expected initially to contain only one hybridoma cell. The culture supernatant from each well in which growing cells are detected is then tested for the presence of antibody reactive with the antigen used for immunization. The screening method depends on the antigen being used. For soluble antigens, the usual technique is radioimmunoassay (RIA) or enzyme-linked immunosorbent assay (ELISA); for cell surface antigens, a variety of assays for antibody binding to viable cells can be used (see Appendix III: Laboratory Methods Using Antibodies). Once positive wells (i.e., wells containing hybridomas producing the desired antibody) are identified, the cells are cloned in semisolid agar or by limiting dilution, and clones producing the antibody are isolated by another round of screening. These cloned hybridomas produce monoclonal antibodies of a desired specificity. Hybridomas can be grown in large volumes or

Continued on following page

BOX 3–1

Monoclonal Antibodies (*Continued*)

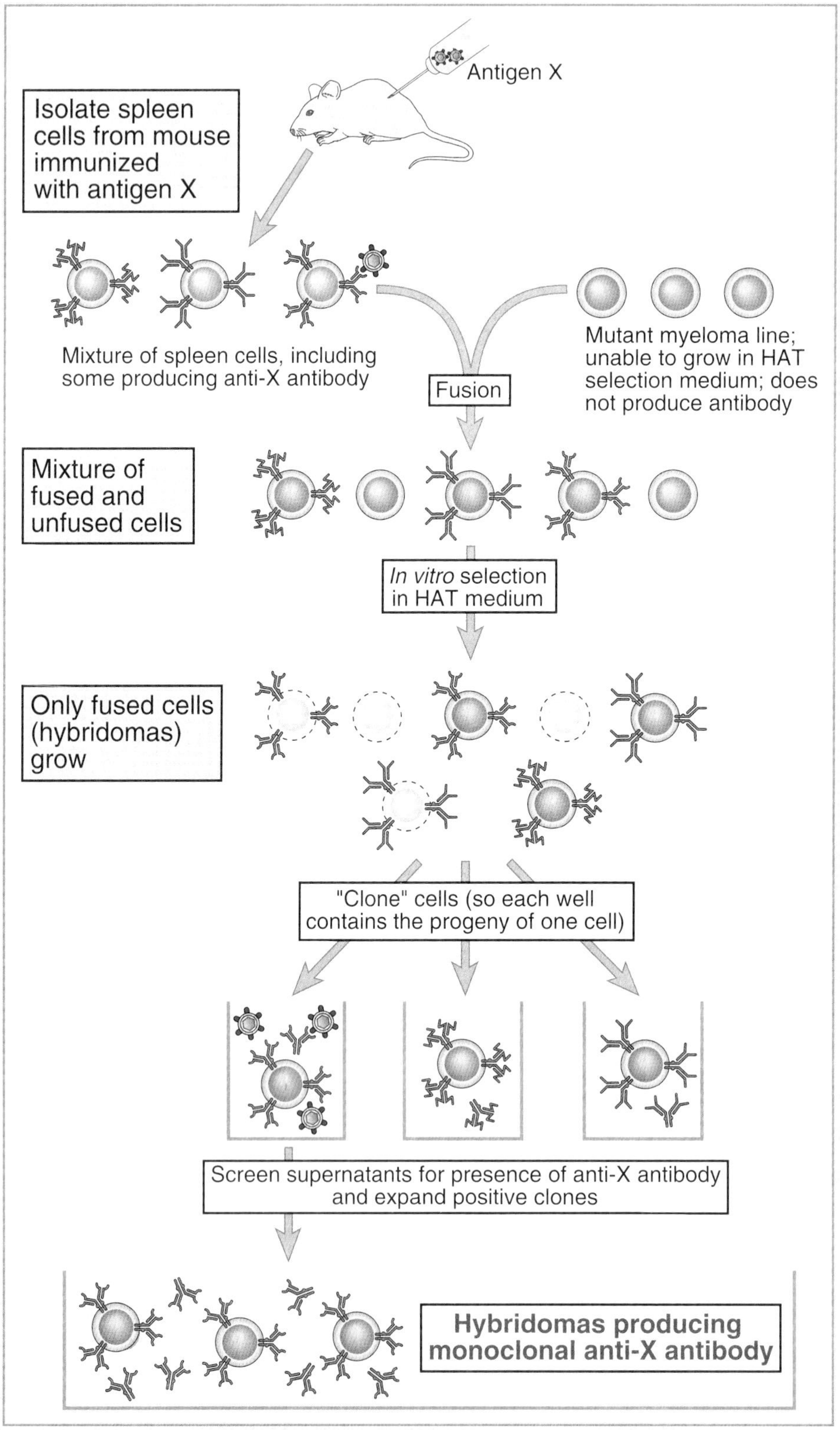

Antigen X

Isolate spleen cells from mouse immunized with antigen X

Mixture of spleen cells, including some producing anti-X antibody

Mutant myeloma line; unable to grow in HAT selection medium; does not produce antibody

Fusion

Mixture of fused and unfused cells

In vitro selection in HAT medium

Only fused cells (hybridomas) grow

"Clone" cells (so each well contains the progeny of one cell)

Screen supernatants for presence of anti-X antibody and expand positive clones

Hybridomas producing monoclonal anti-X antibody

Continued on following page

as ascitic tumors in syngeneic mice to produce large quantities of monoclonal antibodies.

Some of the common applications of hybridomas and monoclonal antibodies include the following:

- Identification of phenotypic markers unique to particular cell types. The basis for the modern classification of lymphocytes and other leukocytes is the binding of population-specific monoclonal antibodies. These have been used to define clusters of differentiation (CD markers) for various cell types (see Chapter 2).
- Immunodiagnosis. The diagnosis of many infectious and systemic diseases relies on the detection of particular antigens or antibodies in the circulation or in tissues by use of monoclonal antibodies in immunoassays.
- Tumor diagnosis and therapy. Tumor-specific monoclonal antibodies are used for detection of tumors by imaging techniques and for immunotherapy of tumors *in vivo.*
- Functional analysis of cell surface and secreted molecules. In immunologic research, monoclonal antibodies that bind to cell surface molecules and either stimulate or inhibit particular cellular functions are invaluable tools for defining the functions of surface molecules, including receptors for antigens. Antibodies that bind and neutralize cytokines are routinely used for detecting the presence and functional roles of these protein hormones *in vitro* and *in vivo.*

At present, hybridomas are most often produced by fusing HAT-sensitive mouse myelomas with B cells from immunized mice, rats, or hamsters. The same principle is used to generate mouse T cell hybridomas, by fusing T cells with a HAT-sensitive, T cell–derived tumor line. Attempts are being made to generate human monoclonal antibodies, primarily for administration to patients, by developing human myeloma lines as fusion partners. (It is a general rule that the stability of hybrids is low if cells from species that are far apart in evolution are fused, and this is presumably why human B cells do not form hybridomas with mouse myeloma lines at high efficiency.)

Genetic engineering techniques are used to expand the usefulness of monoclonal antibodies. The complementary DNAs (cDNAs) that encode the polypeptide chains of a monoclonal antibody can be isolated from a hybridoma, and these genes can be manipulated *in vitro.* As we shall discuss later in the chapter, only small portions of the antibody molecule are responsible for binding to antigen; the remainder of the antibody molecule can be thought of as a "framework." This structural organization allows the DNA segments encoding the antigen-binding sites from a murine monoclonal antibody to be "stitched" into a cDNA encoding a human myeloma protein, creating a hybrid gene. When expressed, the resultant hybrid protein, which retains antigen specificity, is referred to as a humanized antibody. Humanized antibodies are far less likely to appear "foreign" in humans and to induce anti-antibody responses (see Box 3–3) that limit the usefulness of murine monoclonal antibodies when they are administered to patients.

Genetic engineering is also being used to create monoclonal antibody–like molecules of defined specificity without the need for producing hybridomas. One approach uses random collections of cDNAs encoding just the antigen-binding regions of antibodies. These cDNAs are generated from RNA, isolated from the spleens of immunized mice, by polymerase chain reaction (PCR) technology. The cDNAs are then put into bacteriophages to form phage display libraries. Although the antigen-binding regions of antibodies are formed from two different polypeptide chains, synthetic antigen-binding sites can be created by expressing fusion proteins in which sequences from the two chains are covalently joined in a tandem array. Such fusion proteins can be expressed on the surfaces of the bacteriophages, and pools of phage can be tested for their ability to bind to a particular antigen. The virus that binds to the antigen presumably contains cDNA encoding the desired synthetic antigen-binding site. The cDNA is isolated from that virus and linked with DNA encoding the non–antigen-binding parts of a generic antibody molecule. The final construct can then be transfected into a suitable cell type, expressed in soluble form, purified, and used. The advantage of phage display technology lies in the fact that the number of binding sites that can be screened for the desired specificity is three to four orders of magnitude greater than the practical limit of hybridomas that can be screened!

geneous populations of antibodies and antibody-producing cells permitted complete amino acid sequence determination and molecular cloning of individual antibody molecules. These studies culminated in the x-ray crystallographic determinations of the three-dimensional structure of several antibody molecules and of antibodies with bound antigens.

General Features of Antibody Structure

Plasma or serum glycoproteins are traditionally separated by solubility characteristics into albumins and globulins and may be further separated by migration in an electric field, a process called electrophoresis. Most antibodies are found in the third-fastest migrating group of globulins, named **gamma globulins** for the third letter of the Greek alphabet. Another common name for antibody is **immunoglobulin (Ig)**, referring to the immunity-conferring portion of the gamma globulin fraction. The terms *immunoglobulin* and *antibody* are used interchangeably throughout this book.

All antibody molecules share the same basic structural characteristics but display remarkable variability in the regions that bind antigens. This variability of the antigen-binding regions accounts for the capacity of different antibodies to bind a tremendous number of structurally diverse antigens. There are more than 10^7, and perhaps as many as 10^9, different antibody molecules in every individual, each with unique amino acid sequences in their antigen-combining sites. The effector functions and common physicochemical properties of antibodies are associated with the non–antigen-

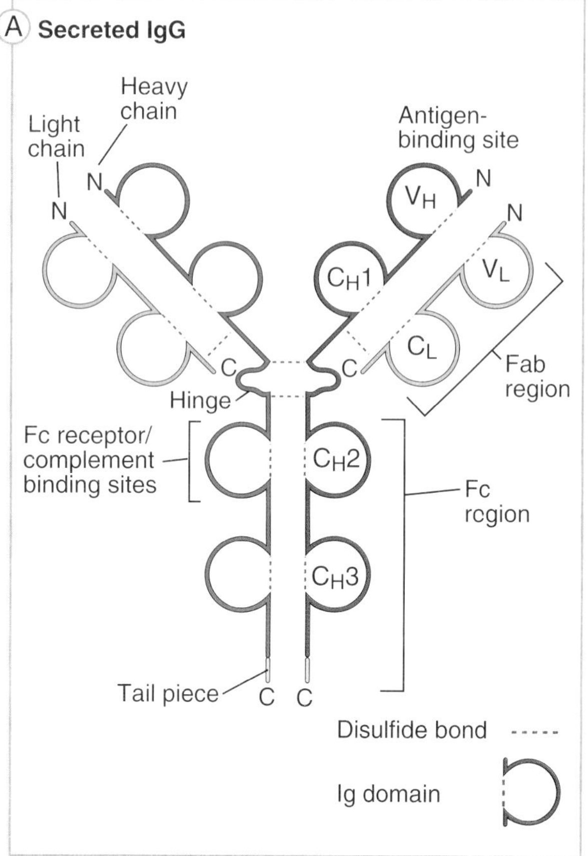

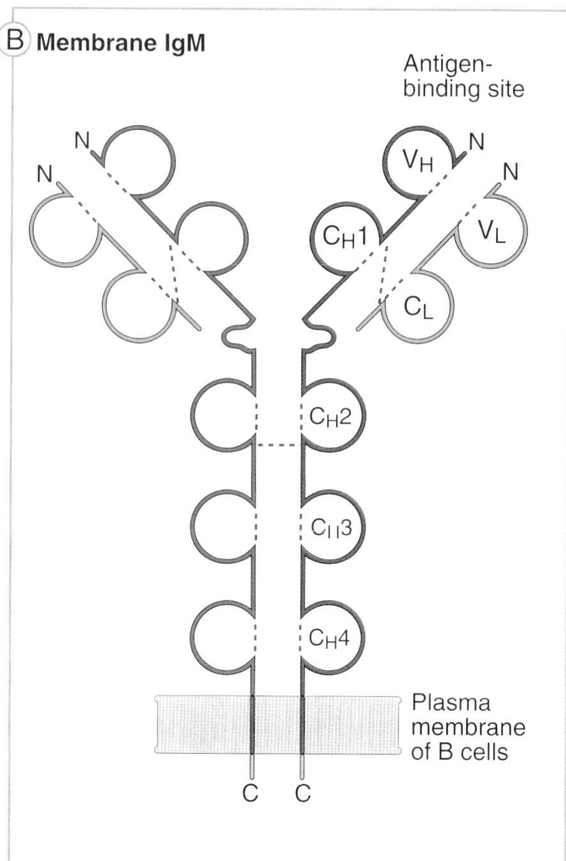

Crystal structure of secreted IgG

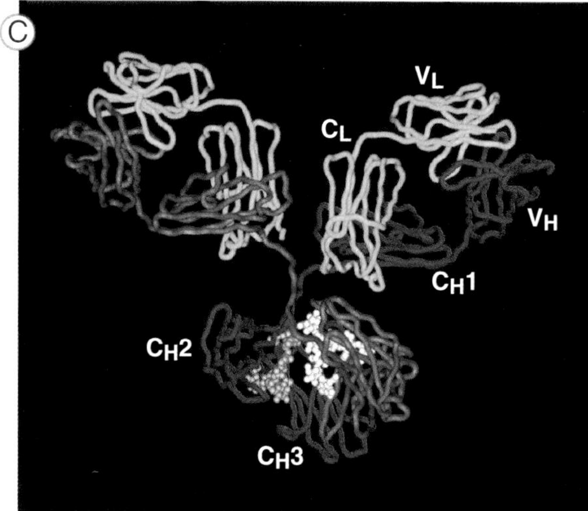

Figure 3–1 Structure of an antibody molecule.
A. Schematic diagram of a secreted IgG molecule. The antigen-binding sites are formed by the juxtaposition of variable light chain (V_L) and variable heavy chain (V_H) domains. The heavy chain C regions end in tail pieces. The locations of complement- and Fc receptor–binding sites within the heavy chain constant regions are approximations.
B. Schematic diagram of a membrane-bound IgM molecule on the surface of a B lymphocyte. The IgM molecule has one more heavy chain C region (C_H) domain than IgG, and the membrane form of the antibody has C-terminal transmembrane and cytoplasmic portions that anchor the molecule in the plasma membrane.
C. Structure of a human IgG molecule as revealed by x-ray crystallography. In this ribbon diagram of a secreted IgG molecule, the heavy chains are colored blue and red, and the light chains are colored green; carbohydrates are shown in gray. (Courtesy of Dr. Alex McPherson, University of California, Irvine.)

binding portions, which exhibit relatively few variations among different antibodies.

An antibody molecule has a symmetric core structure composed of two identical light chains and two identical heavy chains (Fig. 3–1). Each light chain is about 24 kD, and each heavy chain is 55 to 70 kD. One light chain is covalently attached to one heavy chain by a disulfide bond, and the two heavy chains are attached to each other by disulfide bonds. Both the light chains and the heavy chains contain a series of repeating, homologous units, each about 110 amino acid residues in length, that fold independently in a globular motif that is called an **Ig domain**. An Ig domain contains two layers of β-pleated sheet, each layer composed of three to five strands of antiparallel polypeptide chain (Fig. 3–2). Many other proteins of importance in the immune system contain domains that use the same folding motif and have amino acid sequences that are similar to Ig amino acid sequences. All molecules that contain this motif are said to belong to the **Ig super-**

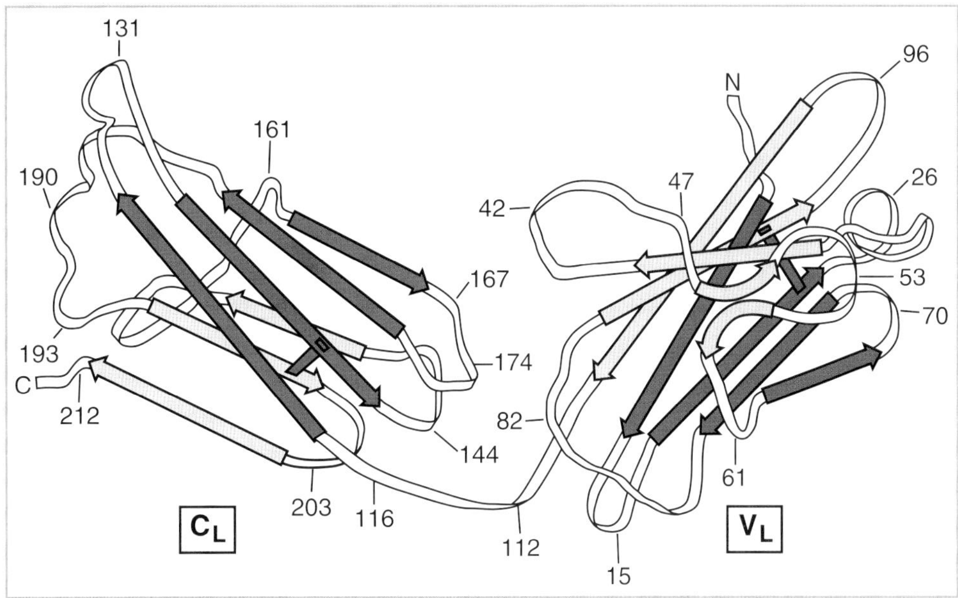

Figure 3–2 Structure of an antibody light chain.

The secondary and tertiary structures of a human Ig light chain are shown schematically. The variable (V) and constant (C) regions each independently fold into Ig domains. Each domain is composed of two antiparallel arrays of β-strands represented by the flat arrows, colored yellow and red, respectively, to form two β-pleated sheets. In the C domain, there are three and four β-strands in the two sheets. In the V domain, which is about 16 amino acid residues longer than the C domain, the two sheets are composed of five and four strands. The dark blue bars are intrachain disulfide bonds, and the numbers indicate the positions of amino acid residues counting from the amino (N) terminus. These Ig C and V domain structures are found in the extracellular portions of many other membrane proteins in the immune system, as discussed in Box 3–2. (Adapted from Edmundson AB, KR Ely, EE Abola, M Schiffer, and N Panagiotopoulos. Rotational allostery and divergent evolution of domains in immunoglobulin light chains. Biochemistry 14:3953–3961, 1975. Copyright 1975 American Chemical Society.)

family, and all the gene segments encoding the Ig domains of these molecules are believed to have evolved from one ancestral gene (Box 3–2).

Both heavy chains and light chains consist of amino terminal variable (V) regions that participate in antigen recognition and carboxyl terminal constant (C) regions; the C regions of the heavy chains mediate effector functions. In the heavy chains, the V region is composed of one Ig domain and the C region is composed of three or four Ig domains. Each light chain is made up of one V region Ig domain and one C region Ig domain. Variable regions are so named because they contain regions of variability in amino acid sequence that distinguish the antibodies made by one clone of B cells from the antibodies made by other clones. The V region of one heavy chain (V_H) is juxtaposed with the V region of one light chain (V_L) to form an antigen-binding site (see Fig. 3–1). Because the core structural unit of each antibody molecule contains two heavy chains and two light chains, it has two antigen-binding sites. The C region domains are separate from the antigen-binding site and do not participate in antigen recognition. The heavy chain C regions interact with other effector molecules and cells of the immune system and therefore mediate most of the biologic functions of antibodies. In addition, the carboxyl terminal ends of the heavy chains anchor membrane-bound antibodies in the plasma membranes of B lymphocytes. The C regions of light chains do not participate in effector functions and are not attached to cell membranes.

Structural Features of Variable Regions and Their Relationship to Antigen Binding

Most of the sequence differences among different antibodies are confined to three short stretches in the V regions of heavy and light chains called the hypervariable segments. These hypervariable regions are each about 10 amino acid residues long, and they are held in place by more conserved framework sequences that make up the Ig domain of the V region (Fig. 3–3; see also Fig. 3–2). The genetic mechanisms leading to the amino acid variability are discussed in Chapter 7. In an antibody molecule, the three hypervariable regions of a V_L domain and the three hypervariable regions of a V_H domain are brought together in three-dimensional space to form an antigen-binding surface. Because these sequences form a surface that is complementary to the three-dimensional structure of the bound antigen, the hypervariable regions are also called **complementarity-determining regions (CDRs)** (see Fig. 3–3). Proceeding from either the V_L or the V_H amino terminus, these regions are called CDR1, CDR2, and CDR3, respectively. The CDR3s of both the V_H segment and the V_L segment are the most variable of the CDRs. As we will discuss in Chapter 7, there are special genetic

BOX 3–2

The Ig Superfamily

Many of the cell surface and soluble molecules that mediate recognition, adhesion, or binding functions in the vertebrate immune system share partial amino acid sequence homology and tertiary structural features that were originally identified in Ig heavy and light chains. In addition, the same features are found in many molecules outside the immune system that also perform similar functions. These diverse proteins are members of the **Ig superfamily** (sometimes called the Ig supergene family). A superfamily is broadly defined as a group of proteins that share a certain degree of sequence homology, usually at least 15%. The conserved sequences shared by superfamily members often contribute to the formation of compact tertiary structures referred to as domains, and most often

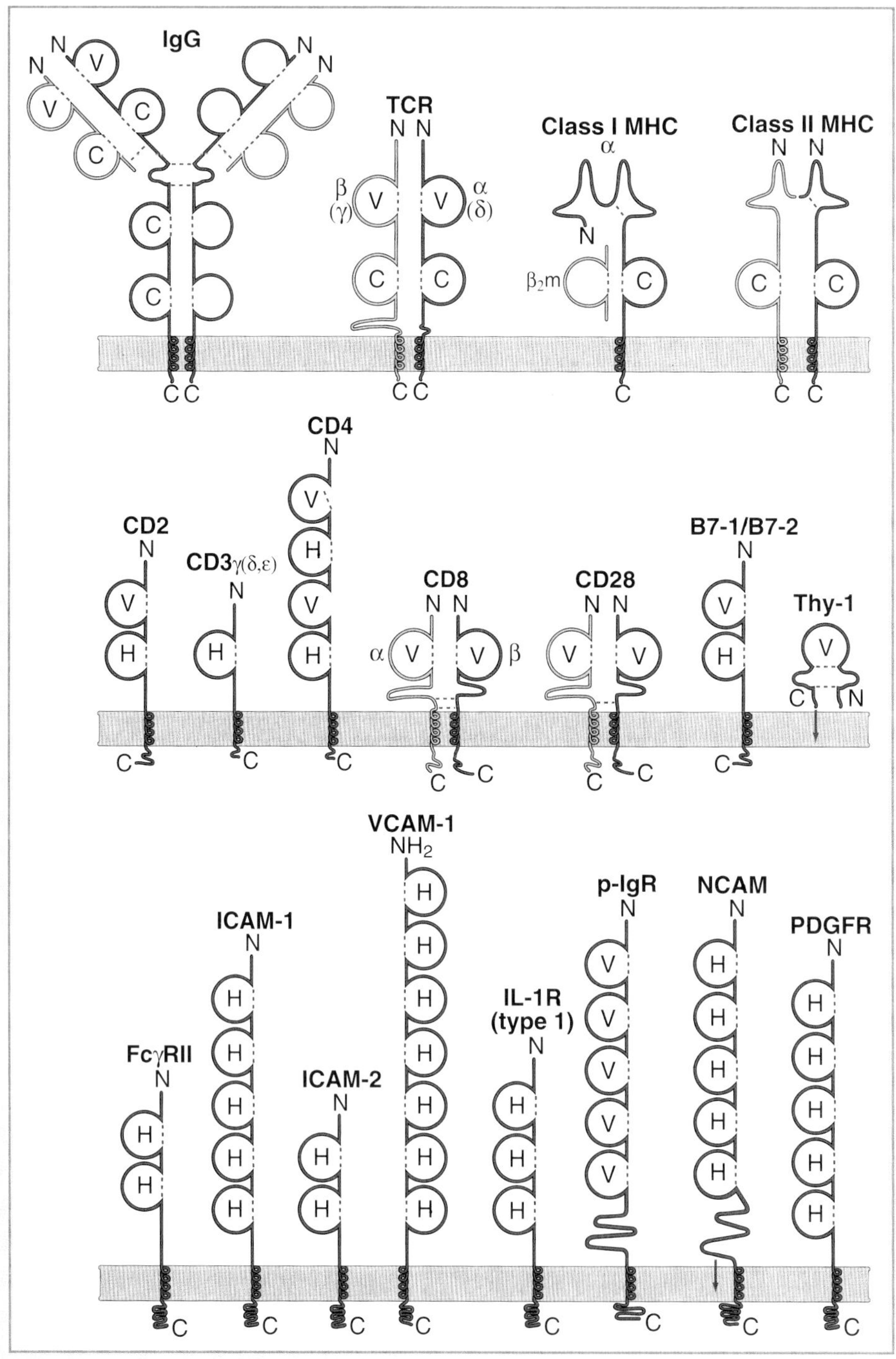

Continued on following page

the entire sequence of a domain characteristic of a particular superfamily is encoded by a single exon. Members of a superfamily are likely to be derived from a common precursor gene by divergent evolution, and multidomain proteins may belong to more than one superfamily. The criterion for inclusion of a protein in the Ig superfamily is the presence of one or more Ig domains (also called Ig homology units), which are regions of 70 to 110 amino acid residues homologous to either Ig variable (V) or Ig constant (C) domains. The Ig domain contains conserved residues that permit the polypeptide to assume a globular tertiary structure called an antibody (or Ig) fold, composed of a sandwich arrangement of two β-sheets, each made up of three to five antiparallel β-strands of five to ten amino acid residues. This sandwich-like structure is stabilized by hydrophobic amino acid residues on the β-strands pointing inward, which alternate with hydrophilic residues pointing out. Because the inward-pointing residues are essential for the stability of the tertiary structure, they are the major contributors to the regions that are conserved between Ig superfamily members. In addition, there are usually conserved cysteine residues that contribute to the formation of an intrachain disulfide-bonded loop of 55 to 75 amino acids (approximately 90 kD). Ig domains are classified as V-like or C-like on the basis of closest homology to either Ig V or Ig C domains. V domains are formed from a longer polypeptide than are C domains and contain two extra β-strands within the β-sheet sandwich. A third type of Ig domain, called C2 or H, has a length similar to C domains but has sequences typical of both V and C domains.

Using several criteria of evolutionary relatedness, such as primary sequence, intron-exon structure, and ability to undergo DNA rearrangements, molecular biologists have postulated a scheme, or family tree, depicting the evolution of members of the Ig superfamily. In this scheme, an early event was the duplication of a gene for a primordial surface receptor followed by divergence of V and C exons. Modern members of the superfamily contain different numbers of V or C domains. The early divergence is reflected by the lack of significant sequence homology in Ig and TCR V and C units, although they share similar tertiary structures. A second early event in the evolution of this family was the acquisition of the ability to undergo DNA recombination, which has remained a unique feature of the antigen receptor gene members of the family.

Most identified members of the Ig superfamily (see Figure) are integral plasma membrane proteins with Ig domains in the extracellular portions, transmembrane domains composed of hydrophobic amino acids, and widely divergent cytoplasmic tails, usually with no intrinsic enzymatic activity. There are exceptions to these generalizations. For example, the platelet-derived growth factor receptors have cytoplasmic tails with tyrosine kinase activity, and the Thy-1 molecule has no cytoplasmic tail but, rather, is anchored to the membrane by a phosphatidylinositol linkage.

One recurrent characteristic of the Ig superfamily members is that interactions between Ig domains on different polypeptide chains are essential for the functions of the molecules. These interactions can be homophilic, occurring between identical domains on opposing polypeptide chains of a multimeric protein, as in the case of C_H:C_H pairing to form functional Fc regions of Ig molecules. Alternatively, they can be heterophilic, as occurs in the case of V_H:V_L or V_β:V_α pairing to form the antigen-binding sites of Ig or TCR molecules, respectively. Heterophilic interactions can also occur between Ig domains on entirely distinct molecules expressed on the surfaces of different cells. Such interactions provide adhesive forces that stabilize immunologically significant cell-cell interactions. For example, the presentation of an antigen to a helper T cell by an antigen-presenting cell probably involves heterophilic intercellular Ig domain interactions between at least three pairs of Ig superfamily molecules, including CD4:class II MHC, CD2:LFA-3, and CD28:B7 (see Chapter 6). Several Ig superfamily members have been identified on cells of the developing and mature nervous system, consistent with the functional importance of highly regulated cell-cell interactions in these sites.

mechanisms for generating more sequence diversity in CDR3 than in CDR1 and CDR2. Crystallographic analyses of antibodies reveal that the CDRs form extended loops that are exposed on the surface of the antibody and are thus available to interact with antigen (see Fig. 3–3). Sequence differences among the CDRs of different antibody molecules result in unique chemical structures being displayed at the surfaces of the projecting loops and therefore in different specificities for antigens. The ability of a V region to fold into an Ig domain is mostly determined by the conserved sequences of the framework regions adjacent to the CDRs. Confining the sequence variability to three short stretches allows the basic structure of all antibodies to be maintained despite the variability among different antibodies.

Antigen binding by antibody molecules is primarily a function of the hypervariable regions of V_H and V_L. Crystallographic analyses of antigen-antibody complexes show that the amino acid residues of the hypervariable regions form multiple contacts with bound antigen (Fig. 3–4). The most extensive contact is with the third hypervariable region (CDR3), which is also the most variable of the three. However, antigen binding is not solely a function of the CDRs, and some framework residues may also contact the antigen. Moreover, in the binding of some antigens, one or more of the CDRs may be outside the region of contact with antigen, thus not participating in antigen binding.

Structural Features of Constant Regions and Their Relationship to Effector Functions

Antibody molecules can be divided into distinct classes and subclasses on the basis of differences in the structure of their heavy chain C regions. The classes of antibody molecules are also called isotypes and are named IgA, IgD, IgE, IgG, and IgM (Table 3–2). In humans, IgA and IgG isotypes can be further subdivided into closely related subclasses, or subtypes, called IgA1 and IgA2, and IgG1, IgG2, IgG3, and IgG4. (Mice,

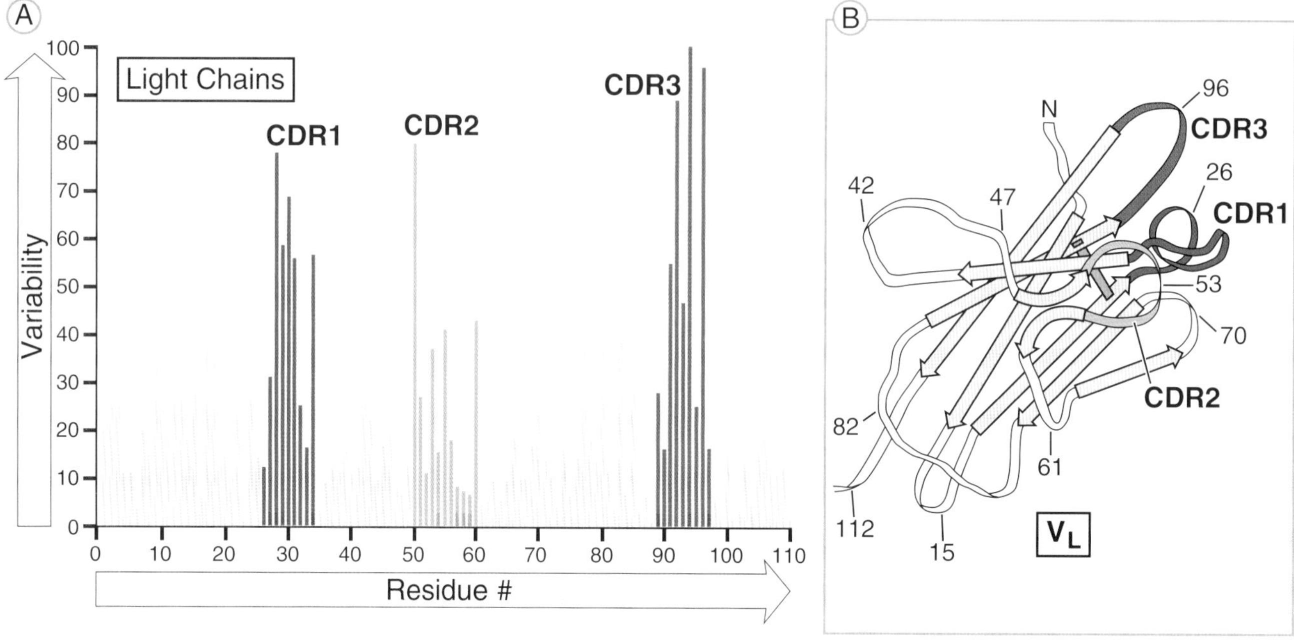

Figure 3–3 Hypervariable regions in Ig molecules.

A. Kabat-Wu plot of amino acid variability in Ig molecules. The histograms depict the extent of variability defined as the number of differences in each amino acid residue among various independently sequenced Ig light chains, plotted against amino acid residue number, measured from the amino terminus. This method of analysis, developed by Elvin Kabat and Tai Te Wu, indicates that the most variable residues are clustered in three "hypervariable" regions, colored in blue, yellow, and red corresponding to CDR1, CDR2, and CDR3, respectively. Three hypervariable regions are also present in heavy chains. (Courtesy of Dr. E. A. Kabat, Department of Microbiology, Columbia University College of Physicians and Surgeons, New York.)

B. Three-dimensional view of the hypervariable CDR loops in a light chain variable (V) domain. The V region of a light chain is shown with CDR1, CDR2, and CDR3 loops, colored in blue, yellow, and red, respectively. These loops correspond to the hypervariable regions in the variability plot in A. Heavy chain hypervariable regions (not shown) are also located in three loops, and all six loops are juxtaposed in the antibody molecule to form the antigen-binding surface (see Fig. 3–4).

which are often used in the study of immune responses, differ in that the IgG isotype is divided into the IgG1, IgG2a, IgG2b, and IgG3 subclasses.) The heavy chain C regions of all antibody molecules of one isotype or subtype have essentially the same amino acid sequence. This sequence is different in antibodies of other isotypes or subtypes. Heavy chains are designated by the letter of the Greek alphabet corresponding to the isotype of the antibody: IgA1 contains α1 heavy chains; IgA2, α2; IgD, δ; IgE, ε; IgG1, γ1; IgG2, γ2; IgG3, γ3; IgG4, γ4; and IgM, μ. In human IgM and IgE antibodies, the C regions contain four tandem Ig domains. The

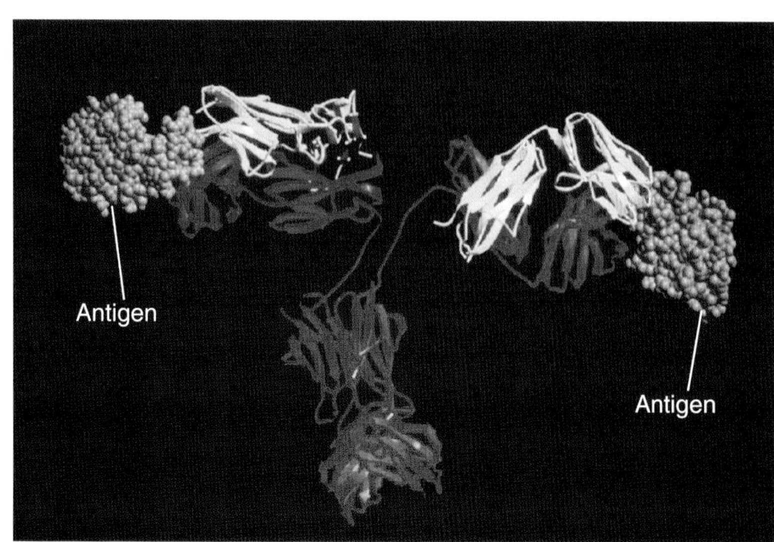

Figure 3–4 Binding of an antigen by an antibody.

This model of a globular protein antigen (chicken lysozyme) bound to an antibody molecule shows how the antigen-binding site can accommodate soluble macromolecules in their native (folded) conformation. The heavy chains of the antibody are colored red and the light chains are yellow, and the antigen is colored blue. (Courtesy of Dr. Dan Vaughn, Cold Spring Harbor Laboratory.)

Table 3–2. Human Antibody Isotypes

Isotype of antibody	Subtypes	H chain	Serum concentr. (mg/mL)	Serum half-life (days)	Secreted form	Functions
IgA	IgA1, 2	α (1 or 2)	3.5	6	**IgA (dimer)** Monomer, dimer, trimer Cα1 Cα2 Cα3 J chain	Mucosal immunity
IgD	None	δ	Trace	3	None	Naive B cell antigen receptor
IgE	None	ε	0.05	2	**IgE** Monomer Cε1 Cε2 Cε3 Cε4	Immediate hypersensitivity
IgG	IgG1–4	γ (1, 2, 3, or 4)	13.5	23	**IgG1** Monomer V_H Cγ1 V_L C_L Cγ2 Cγ3	Opsonization, complement activation, antibody-dependent cell-mediated cytotoxicity, neonatal immunity, feedback inhibition of B cells
IgM	None	μ	1.5	5	**IgM** Pentamer Cμ1 Cμ2 Cμ3 Cμ4 J chain	Naive B cell antigen receptor, complement activation

The effector functions of antibodies are discussed in detail in Chapter 14.

C regions of IgG, IgA, and IgD contain only three Ig domains. These domains are designated C_H and numbered sequentially from amino terminus to carboxyl terminus (e.g., C_H1, C_H2, and so on). In each isotype, these regions may be designated more specifically (e.g., $C_\gamma1$, $C_\gamma2$ in IgG). Antibodies can act as antigens when introduced into foreign hosts, eliciting the production of anti-antibodies (Box 3–3). By immunizing an animal of one species with Ig of another species, it is possible to produce anti-antibodies specific for one Ig class or subclass, and such antibodies are routinely used in the clinical and experimental analyses of humoral immune responses.

Different isotypes and subtypes of antibodies perform different effector functions. The reason for this is that most of the effector functions of antibodies are mediated by the binding of heavy chain C regions to receptors on different cells, such as phagocytes, NK cells, and mast cells, and to plasma proteins, such as complement proteins. Antibody isotypes and subtypes differ in their C regions and therefore in what they bind to and what effector functions they perform. The effec-

BOX 3–3

Anti-Ig Antibodies: Allotypes and Idiotypes

Antibody molecules are proteins and can therefore be immunogenic. Immunologists have exploited this fact to produce antibodies specific for Ig molecules that can be used as reagents to analyze the structure and function of the Ig molecules. To obtain an anti-antibody response, it is necessary that the Ig molecules used to immunize an animal be recognized in whole or in part as foreign. The simplest approach is to immunize an animal of one species (e.g., rabbit) with Ig molecules of a second species (e.g., mouse). Populations of antibodies generated by such cross-species immunizations are largely specific for epitopes present in the constant (C) regions of light or heavy chains. Antisera generated in this way can be used to define the isotype of an antibody.

When an animal is immunized with Ig molecules derived from another animal of the same species, the immune response is confined to epitopes of the immunizing Ig that are absent or uncommon on the Ig molecules of the responder animal. Two types of determinants have been defined by this approach. First, determinants may be formed by minor structural differences (polymorphisms) in amino acid sequences located in the conserved portions of Ig molecules, called **allotopes.** All antibody molecules that share a particular allotope are said to belong to the same **allotype.** Most allotopes are located in the C regions of light or heavy chains, but some are found in the framework portions of variable (V) regions. Allotypic differences have been important in the study of Ig genetics. For example, allotypes detected by anti-Ig antibodies were initially used to locate the position of Ig genes by linkage analysis. In addition, the remarkable observation that, in homozygous animals, all the heavy chains of a particular isotype (e.g., IgM) share the same allotype even though the V regions of these antibodies have different amino acid sequences provided the first evidence that the C regions of all Ig molecules of a particular isotype are encoded by a single gene segment that is separate from the gene segments encoding V regions. As is discussed in Chapter 7, we now know that this surprising conclusion is correct.

The second type of determinant on antibody molecules that can be recognized as foreign by other animals of the same species is that formed by the hypervariable regions of the Ig variable domains. When a homogeneous population of antibody molecules (e.g., a myeloma protein, or a monoclonal antibody) is used as an immunogen, antibodies are produced that react with the unique hypervariable loops of that antibody. These determinants are recognized as foreign because they are usually present in very small quantities in any given animal (i.e., at too low a level to induce self-tolerance). The unique determinants of individual antibody molecules are called **idiotopes,** and all antibody molecules that share an idiotope are said to belong to the same **idiotype.** As is discussed in Chapter 7, hypervariable sequences that form idiotopes arise both from inherited germline diversity and from somatic events. Idiotopes may be involved in regulation of B cell functions. The theory of lymphocyte regulation through idiotopes of antigen receptors called the network hypothesis, is mentioned in Chapter 10.

In addition to experimentally elicited anti-Ig antibodies, immunologists have been interested in naturally occurring antibodies reactive with self Ig molecules. Anti-Ig antibodies are particularly prevalent in an autoimmune disease called rheumatoid arthritis (see Chapter 18), in which setting they are known as rheumatoid factor. Rheumatoid factor is usually an IgM antibody that reacts with the constant regions of self IgG. The significance of rheumatoid factor in the pathogenesis of rheumatoid arthritis is unknown.

Patients treated with mouse monoclonal antibodies may make antibodies against the mouse Ig, called a human anti-mouse antibody (HAMA) response. These anti-Ig antibodies eliminate the injected monoclonal. Humanized antibodies have been developed to circumvent this problem, but even humanized antibodies contain hypervariable regions derived from the original monoclonal, and these can elicit a response in treated patients.

tor functions mediated by each antibody isotype are listed in Table 3–2 and are discussed in more detail later in this chapter and in Chapter 14.

Antibody molecules are flexible, permitting them to bind to different arrays of antigens. Every antibody contains at least two antigen-binding sites, each formed by a pair of V_H and V_L domains. Many Ig molecules can orient these binding sites so that two antigen molecules on a planar (e.g., cell) surface may be engaged at once (Fig. 3–5). This flexibility is conferred, in large part, by a **hinge region** located between C_H1 and C_H2 in certain isotypes. The hinge region varies from 10 to more than 60 amino acid residues in different isotypes. Portions of this sequence assume a random and flexible conformation, permitting molecular motion between C_H1 and C_H2. Some of the greatest differences between the constant regions of the IgG subclasses are concentrated in the hinge. This leads to different overall shapes of the IgG subtypes. In addition, some flexibility of antibody molecules is due to the ability of each V_H domain to rotate with respect to the adjacent C_H1 domain.

There are two classes or isotypes of light chains, called κ and λ, which are distinguished by their carboxyl terminal constant (C) regions. An antibody molecule has either two κ light chains or two λ light chains, but never one of each. The amino acid sequences of the κ light chain C regions (C_κ) differ from the sequences of the λ chain C regions (C_λ), but all C_κ sequences of different antibody molecules are identical, as are all C_λ sequences. Despite the sequence differences, C_κ and C_λ are structurally homologous to each other, and each folds into one Ig domain. In humans, about 60% of antibody molecules have κ light chains, and about 40% have λ light chains. Marked changes in this ratio can occur in patients with monoclonal B cell tumors because the neoplastic clone produces antibody molecules with

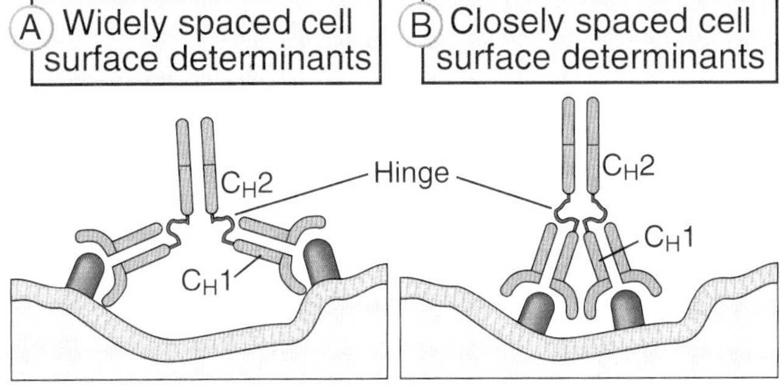

Figure 3–5 Flexibility of antibody molecules.
The two antigen-binding sites of an Ig monomer can simultaneously bind to two determinants separated by varying distances. In A, an Ig molecule is depicted binding to two widely spaced determinants on a cell surface, and in B, the same antibody is binding to two determinants that are close together. This flexibility is mainly due to the hinge regions located between the first constant heavy chain (C_H1) and the second constant heavy chain (C_H2) domains, which permit independent movement of antigen-binding sites relative to the rest of the molecule.

the same light chain. In fact, the ratio of κ-bearing cells to λ-bearing cells is often used clinically in the diagnosis of B cell lymphomas. In mice, κ-containing antibodies are about 10 times more abundant than λ-containing antibodies. Unlike in heavy chain isotypes, there are no known differences in function between κ-containing antibodies and λ-containing antibodies.

Antibodies may be expressed in secreted or membrane-associated forms, which differ in the amino acid sequence of the carboxyl terminal end of the heavy chain C region. In the secreted form, found in blood and other extracellular fluids, the sequence of the last C_H region terminates with charged and hydrophilic amino acid residues. In the membrane form of antibody, found only on the plasma membrane of the B lymphocytes that synthesize the antibody, the last C_H region is followed by 26 amino acids with hydrophobic side chains and variable numbers of basic amino acid residues (Fig. 3–6). This structural motif is characteristic of integral membrane proteins. The hydrophobic residues form an α-helix that extends across the lipid bilayer of the plasma membrane, and the basic terminal (cytoplasmic) amino acids are located in the cytoplasm, where their side chains interact with the phospholipid head groups on the cytoplasmic surface of the membrane and anchor the protein to the membrane. In membrane IgM and IgD molecules, the cytoplasmic portion of the heavy chain is short, only 3 amino acid residues in length; in membrane IgG and IgE molecules, it is somewhat longer, up to 30 amino acid residues in length.

Secreted IgG and IgE, and all membrane Ig molecules, regardless of isotype, are monomeric with respect to the basic antibody structural unit (i.e., they contain two heavy chains and two light chains). In contrast, the secreted forms of IgM and IgA form multimeric complexes in which two or more of the four-chain core antibody structural units are covalently joined. These complexes are formed by interactions between regions, called tail pieces, that are located at the carboxyl terminal ends of μ and α heavy chains (see Table 3–2). Multimeric IgM and IgA molecules also contain an additional 15-kD polypeptide called the joining (J) chain, which is disulfide bonded to the tail pieces and serves to stabilize the multimeric complexes.

Associations Between Heavy and Light Chains

Heavy chains and light chains are covalently linked in such a way that the V_H and V_L domains are juxtaposed to form the antigen-binding sites and the C_H domains form the sites that interact with cell surface receptors or effector molecules (see Fig. 3–1). The covalent interactions that link the heavy and light chains are disulfide bonds formed between cysteine residues in the carboxyl terminus of the light chain and the C_H1 domain of the heavy chain. Noncovalent interactions between the V_L and V_H domains and between the C_L and C_H1 domains may also contribute to the association of heavy and light chains.

The two heavy chains of each antibody molecule are also covalently linked by disulfide bonds. In IgG antibodies, these bonds are formed between cysteine residues in the C_H2 regions, close to the hinge. In other isotypes, the disulfide bonds may be in different locations. Noncovalent interactions (e.g., between the third C_H domains [$C_\gamma3$]) may also contribute to heavy chain pairing.

- The associations between the chains of antibody molecules and the functions of different regions of antibodies were first deduced from experiments done by Rodney Porter in which rabbit IgG was cleaved by proteolytic enzymes into fragments with distinct structural and functional properties. In IgG molecules, the hinge between $C_\gamma1$ and $C_\gamma2$ of the heavy chain is the region most susceptible to proteolytic cleavage. If rabbit IgG is treated with the enzyme papain under conditions of limited proteolysis, the enzyme acts on the hinge region and cleaves the IgG into three separate pieces (Fig. 3–7). Two of the pieces are identical to each other and consist of the complete light chain (V_L and C_L) associated with a V_H-$C_\gamma1$ fragment of the heavy chain. These fragments retain the ability to bind antigen because each contains paired V_L and V_H domains, and they are called **Fab** (fragment, antigen binding). The third piece is composed of two identical, disulfide-linked peptides containing the heavy chain $C_\gamma2$ and $C_\gamma3$ domains. This piece of IgG has a propensity to self-associate and to crystallize into a lattice and is therefore called **Fc** (fragment, crystallizable).

- When pepsin (instead of papain) is used to cleave rabbit IgG under limiting conditions, proteolysis is restricted to the carboxyl terminus of the hinge region, generating an antigen-binding fragment of IgG with the hinge and the interchain disulfide bonds intact (see Fig. 3–7). Fab fragments retaining the heavy chain hinge are called Fab′; when the interchain disulfide bonds are preserved, the two Fab′ fragments remain associated in a form called **F(ab′)₂**. Fab and F(ab′)₂ are

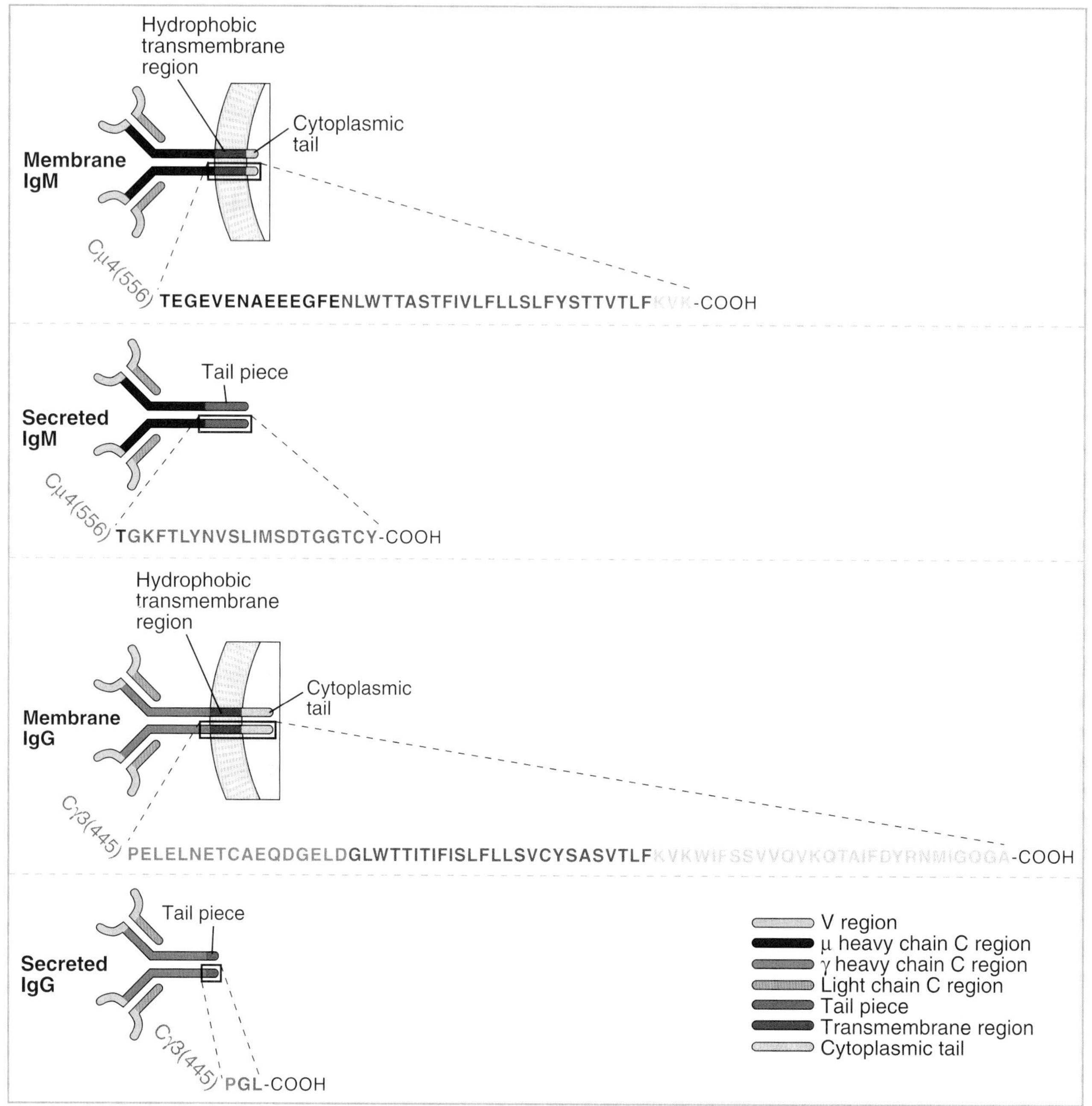

Figure 3–6 Membrane and secreted forms of Ig heavy chains.
The membrane forms of the Ig heavy chains, but not the secreted forms, contain transmembrane regions made up of hydrophobic amino acid residues and cytoplasmic domains that differ significantly among the different isotypes. The cytoplasmic portion of the membrane form of the μ chain contains only 3 residues, whereas the γ3 cytoplasmic region contains 28 residues. The secreted forms of the antibodies end in C-terminal tail pieces, which also differ among isotypes: μ has a long tail piece (21 residues) that is involved in pentamer formation, whereas γ3 has only a short tail piece (3 residues). In this figure, the μ and γ3 chains are compared, but other γ isotype heavy chains have structures similar to γ3. Amino acids are shown in the letter code, and the last amino acid of the terminal C region domain (i.e., $C_{\mu}4$ or $C_{\gamma}3$) is indicated.

useful experimental tools because they can bind to antigens without activating Fc-dependent effector mechanisms.

The results of limited papain or pepsin proteolysis of other isotypes besides IgG, or of IgGs of species other than the rabbit, do not always recapitulate the studies with rabbit IgG. However, the basic organization of the Ig molecule that Porter deduced from his experiments is common to all Ig molecules of all isotypes and of all species. In fact, these proteolysis experiments provided the first evidence that the antigen recognition functions and the effector functions of Ig molecules are spatially segregated.

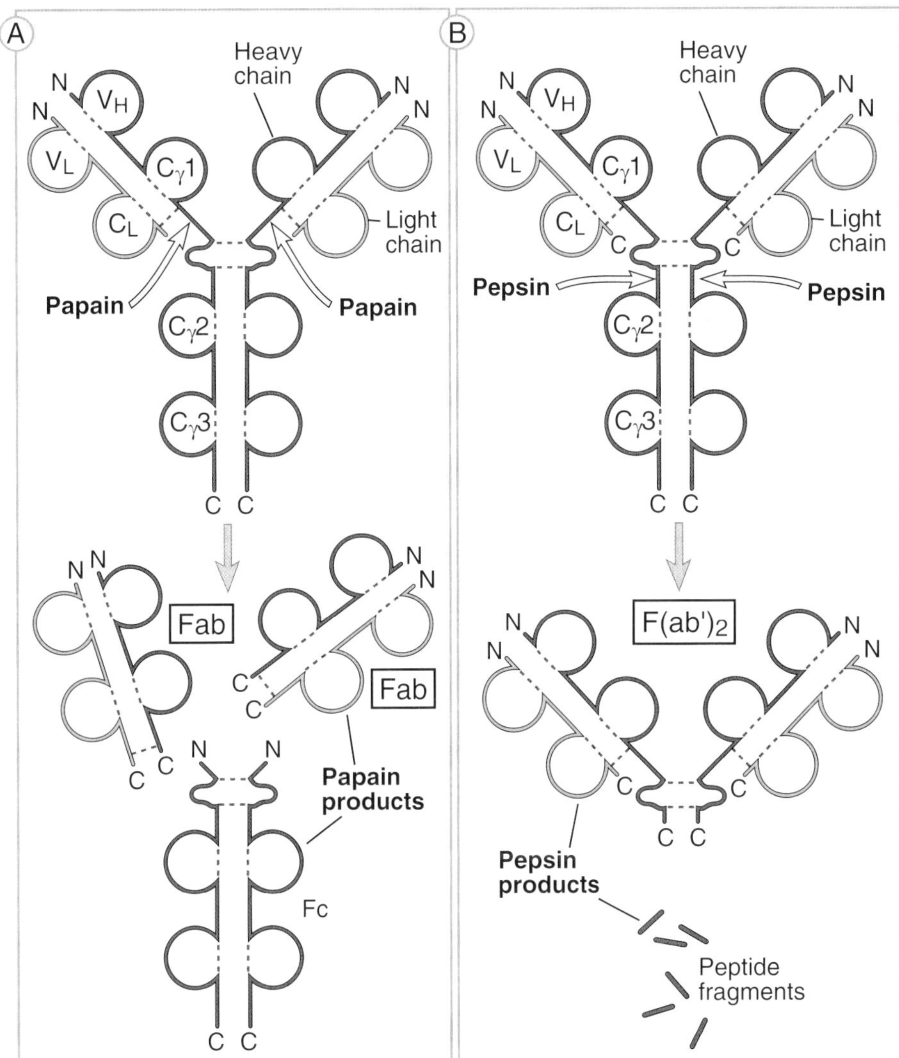

Figure 3–7 Proteolytic fragments of an IgG molecule.
IgG molecules are cleaved by the enzymes papain (A) and pepsin (B) at the sites indicated by arrows. Papain digestion allows separation of two antigen-binding regions (the Fab fragments) from the portion of the IgG molecule that binds to complement and Fc receptors (the Fc fragment). Pepsin generates a single bivalent antigen-binding fragment, $F(ab')_2$.

Synthesis, Assembly, and Expression of Ig Molecules

Ig heavy and light chains, like most secreted and membrane proteins, are synthesized on membrane-bound ribosomes in the rough endoplasmic reticulum. The proper folding of Ig heavy chains and their assembly with light chains are regulated by proteins resident in the endoplasmic reticulum called chaperones. These proteins, which include calnexin and a molecule called BiP (binding protein), bind to newly synthesized Ig polypeptides and ensure that they are retained or targeted for degradation unless they become properly folded and assembled into Ig molecules. The covalent association of heavy and light chains, created by the formation of disulfide bonds, and N-linked glycosylation also occur in the endoplasmic reticulum. After assembly, the Ig molecules are released from the chaperones and directed into the cisternae of the Golgi complex, where carbohydrates are modified, and the antibodies are then transported to the plasma membrane in vesicles, where they become anchored into the cell membrane or are secreted by a process of exocytosis. Other proteins that bind to Ig are coordinately regulated. For instance, secreted IgA and IgM antibodies are maintained as multimers by the attached J chains. In cells producing such antibodies, transcription of Ig heavy and light chain genes is accompanied by coordinate J chain gene transcription and biosynthesis.

The maturation of B cells from bone marrow progenitors is accompanied by specific changes in Ig gene expression, resulting in the production of Ig molecules in different forms (Fig. 3–8). The earliest cell in the B lymphocyte lineage that produces Ig polypeptides, called the pre-B cell, synthesizes the membrane form of the μ heavy chain, but most of the protein remains in the cytoplasm. This is because chaperone proteins associated with newly synthesized μ heavy chains restrict their movement out of the cell. Most of the cytoplasmic μ heavy chains in pre-B cells are degraded intracellularly. A small amount of these μ chains is expressed on the cell surface in association with proteins called surrogate light chains to form the pre-B cell receptor. Immature and mature B cells produce κ or λ light chains (see Fig. 3–8), which associate with μ proteins to form IgM molecules. This assembly protects the heavy

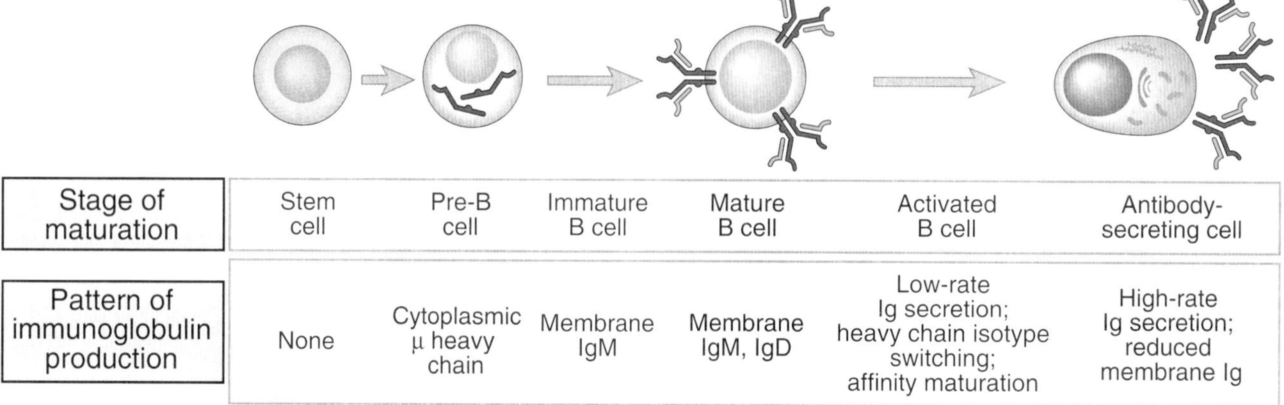

Stage of maturation	Stem cell	Pre-B cell	Immature B cell	Mature B cell	Activated B cell	Antibody-secreting cell
Pattern of immunoglobulin production	None	Cytoplasmic μ heavy chain	Membrane IgM	Membrane IgM, IgD	Low-rate Ig secretion; heavy chain isotype switching; affinity maturation	High-rate Ig secretion; reduced membrane Ig

Figure 3–8 Immunoglobulin expression during B lymphocyte maturation. Stages in B lymphocyte maturation are shown with associated changes in the production of Ig heavy and light chains. The molecular events accompanying these changes are discussed in Chapters 7 and 9.

chains from intracellular degradation and allows the IgM to be expressed on the cell surface. Mature B cells express membrane forms of IgM and IgD (the μ and δ heavy chains associated with κ or λ light chains). These membrane Ig receptors serve as cell surface receptors that recognize antigens and initiate the process of B cell activation. B cell antigen receptors are noncovalently associated with two other membrane proteins, Igα and Igβ, which serve signaling functions and are essential for surface expression of IgM and IgD. The molecular and cellular events in B cell maturation underlying these changes in antibody expression are discussed in detail in Chapters 7 and 9.

When mature B lymphocytes are activated by antigens and other stimuli, the cells differentiate into antibody-secreting cells. This process is also accompanied by changes in the pattern of Ig production. One such change is the conversion of membrane Ig to secreted Ig; the structural basis of this conversion has been discussed previously (see Fig. 3–6). The second change is the expression of Ig heavy chain isotypes other than IgM and IgD. This process, called heavy chain isotype (or class) switching, is described later in this chapter and in more detail in Chapter 9, when we discuss B cell activation.

Antibody Binding of Antigens

Features of Biologic Antigens

An **antigen** is any substance that may be specifically bound by an antibody molecule or T cell receptor. Antibodies can recognize as antigens almost every kind of biologic molecule, including simple intermediary metabolites, sugars, lipids, autacoids, and hormones, as well as macromolecules such as complex carbohydrates, phospholipids, nucleic acids, and proteins. This is in contrast to T cells, which recognize only peptides (see Chapter 5). Only macromolecules are capable of stimulating B lymphocytes to initiate humoral immune responses. Molecules that stimulate immune responses are called **immunogens**. Small chemicals, such as dinitrophenol, may bind to antibodies but cannot activate B cells on their own (i.e., they are not immunogenic). To generate antibodies specific for such small chemicals, immunologists commonly attach them to macromolecules before immunization. In these cases, the small chemical is called a **hapten,** and the macromolecule is called a **carrier**. The hapten-carrier complex, unlike free hapten, can act as an immunogen.

Macromolecules are usually much bigger than the antigen-binding region of an antibody molecule (see Fig. 3–4). Therefore, any antibody binds to only a portion of the macromolecule, which is called a **determinant** or an **epitope.** These two words are synonymous and are used interchangeably throughout the book. Macromolecules typically contain multiple determinants, some of which may be repeated, and each of which, by definition, can be bound by an antibody. The presence of multiple identical determinants in an antigen is referred to as **polyvalency** or **multivalency.** Most globular proteins do not contain multiple identical epitopes and are not polyvalent, unless they are in aggregates. In the case of polysaccharides and nucleic acids, many identical epitopes may be regularly spaced, and the molecules are said to be polyvalent. Cell surfaces, including microbes, often display polyvalent arrays of protein or carbohydrate antigenic determinants.

The spatial arrangement of different epitopes on a single protein molecule may influence the binding of antibodies in several ways. When determinants are well separated, two or more antibody molecules can be bound to the same protein antigen without influencing each other; such determinants are said to be nonoverlapping. When two determinants are close to one another, the binding of antibody to the first determinant may cause steric interference with the binding of antibody to the second; such determinants are said to be overlapping. In rarer cases, binding of the first antibody may cause a conformational change in the struc-

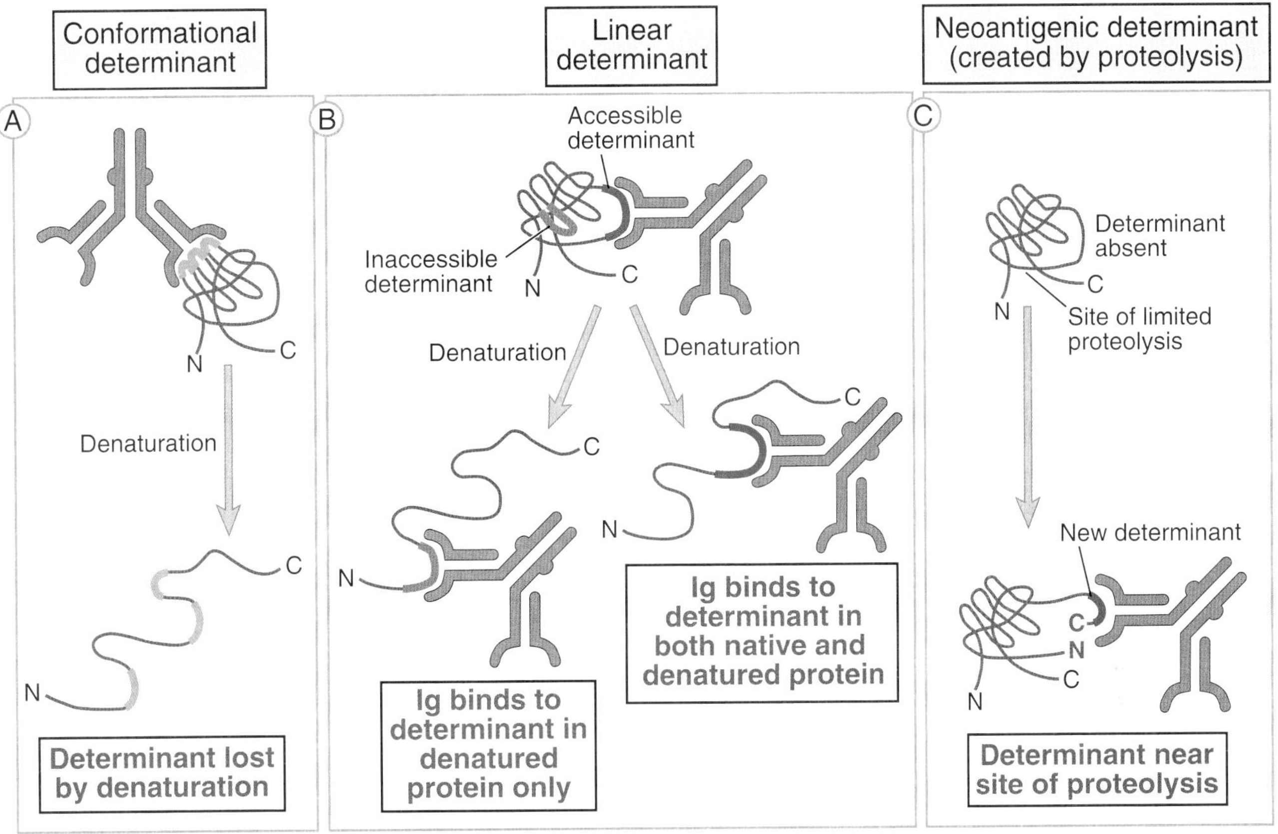

Figure 3–9 The nature of antigenic determinants.
Antigenic determinants (shown in orange, red, and blue) may depend on protein folding (conformation) as well as on covalent structure. Some determinants are accessible in native proteins and are lost on denaturation (A), whereas others are exposed only on protein unfolding (B). Neodeterminants arise from covalent modifications such as peptide bond cleavage (C).

ture of the antigen, influencing the binding of the second antibody by means other than steric hindrance. Such interactions are called allosteric effects.

Antigenic determinants may be formed by the covalent structure of a molecule or, in the case of proteins and nucleic acids, by the noncovalent folding of the molecule (Fig. 3–9). The antigenic determinants of complex carbohydrates and phospholipids are usually formed by the covalent structure. In the case of proteins, the formation of some determinants depends only on covalent structure, and formation of other determinants reflects tertiary structure. Epitopes formed by several adjacent amino acid residues are called **linear determinants.** The antigen-binding site of an antibody can usually accommodate a linear determinant made up of about six amino acids. If linear determinants appear on the external surface or in a region of extended conformation in the native folded protein, they may be accessible to antibodies. More often, linear determinants may be inaccessible in the native conformation and appear only when the protein is denatured. In contrast, **conformational determinants** are formed by amino acid residues that are not in a sequence but become spatially juxtaposed in the folded protein. Antibodies specific for certain linear determinants and antibodies specific for conformational determinants can be used to ascertain whether a protein is denatured or in its native conformation, respectively. Proteins may be subjected to modifications such as phosphorylation or proteolysis. These modifications, by altering the covalent structure, can produce new epitopes. Such epitopes are called **neoantigenic determinants,** and they too may be recognized by specific antibodies.

Structural and Chemical Basis of Antigen Binding

The antigen-binding sites of most antibodies are planar surfaces that can accommodate conformational epitopes of macromolecules, allowing the antibodies to bind large macromolecules. As is discussed in Chapter 4, this is a key difference between the antigen-binding sites of antibody molecules and those of certain other antigen-binding molecules of the immune system, namely, MHC molecules, which contain antigen-binding clefts that bind small peptides but not native globular proteins (see Table 3–1). In some instances, such as antibodies specific for small carbohydrates, the antigen is bound in a cleft between V_L and V_H domains.

The recognition of antigen by antibody involves noncovalent, reversible binding. Various types of noncovalent interactions may contribute to antibody

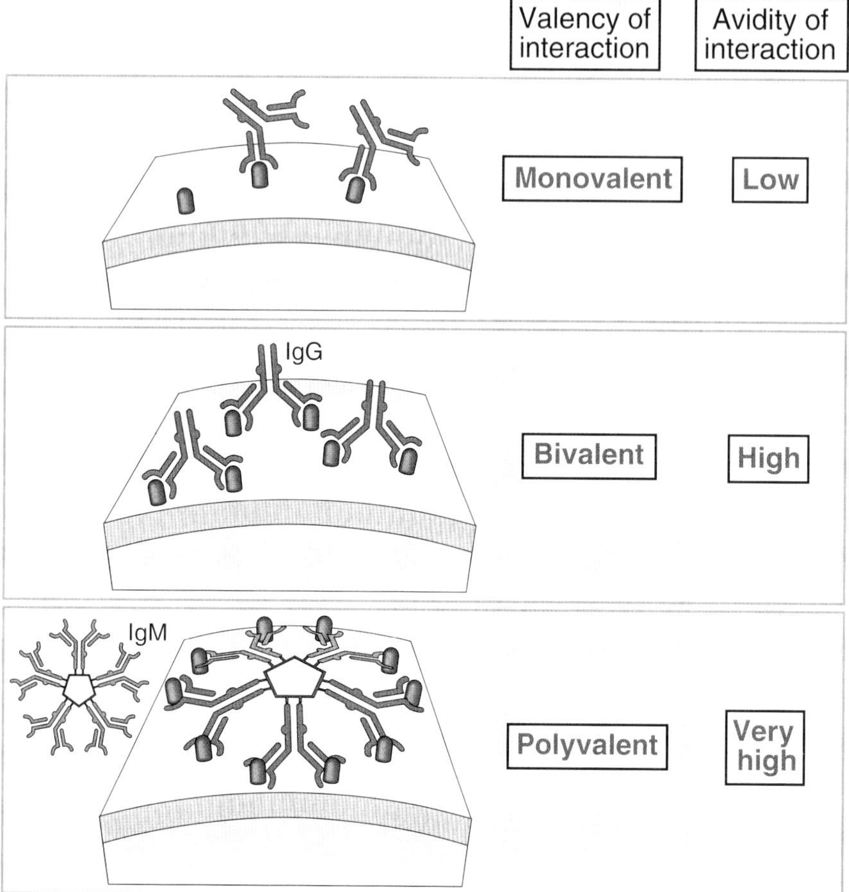

Figure 3–10 Valency and avidity of antibody-antigen interactions. Monovalent antigens, or epitopes spaced far apart on cell surfaces, will interact with a single binding site of one antibody molecule. Although the affinity of this interaction may be high, the overall avidity is relatively low. When repeated determinants on a cell surface are close enough, both the antigen-binding sites of a single IgG molecule can bind, leading to a higher avidity bivalent interaction. The hinge region of the IgG molecule accommodates the shape change needed for simultaneous engagement of both binding sites. IgM molecules have 10 identical antigen-binding sites that can theoretically bind simultaneously with 10 repeating determinants on a cell surface, resulting in a polyvalent, very high avidity interaction.

binding of antigen, including electrostatic forces, hydrogen bonds, van der Waals forces, and hydrophobic interactions. The relative importance of each of these depends on the structures of the binding site of the individual antibody and of the antigenic determinant. The strength of the binding between a single combining site of an antibody and an epitope of an antigen, which can be determined experimentally by equilibrium dialysis (see Appendix III), is called the **affinity** of the antibody. The affinity is commonly represented by a dissociation constant (K_d), which indicates the concentration of antigen that is required to occupy the combining sites of half the antibody molecules present in a solution of antibody. A smaller K_d indicates a stronger or higher affinity interaction because a lower concentration of antigen is needed to occupy the sites. The K_d of antibodies produced in typical humoral immune responses usually varies from about 10^{-7} M to 10^{-11} M. Serum from an immunized individual will contain a mixture of antibodies with different affinities for the antigen, depending primarily on the amino acid sequences of the CDRs.

Because the hinge region of antibodies gives them flexibility, a single antibody may attach to a single multivalent antigen by more than one binding site. For IgG or IgE, this attachment can involve, at most, two binding sites, one on each Fab. For pentameric IgM, however, a single antibody may bind at up to 10 different sites (Fig. 3–10). Polyvalent antigens will have more than one copy of a particular determinant. Although the affinity of any one antigen-binding site will be the same for each epitope of a polyvalent antigen, the strength of attachment of the antibody to the antigen must take into account binding of all the sites to all the available epitopes. This overall strength of attachment is called the **avidity** and is much greater than the affinity of any one antigen-binding site. Mathematically, the avidity increases almost geometrically (rather than additively) for each occupied site. Thus, a low-affinity IgM molecule can still bind tightly to a polyvalent antigen because many low-affinity interactions (up to 10 per IgM molecule) can produce a single high-avidity interaction.

Polyvalent interactions between antigen and antibody are of biologic significance because many effector functions of antibodies are triggered optimally when two or more antibody molecules are brought close together by binding to a polyvalent antigen. If a polyvalent antigen is mixed with a specific antibody in a test tube, the two interact to form immune complexes (Fig. 3–11). At the correct concentration, called a zone of equivalence, antibody and antigen form an extensively cross-linked network of attached molecules such that most or all of the antigen and antibody molecules are complexed into large masses. Immune complexes may be dissociated into smaller aggregates either by increasing the concentration of antigen so that free

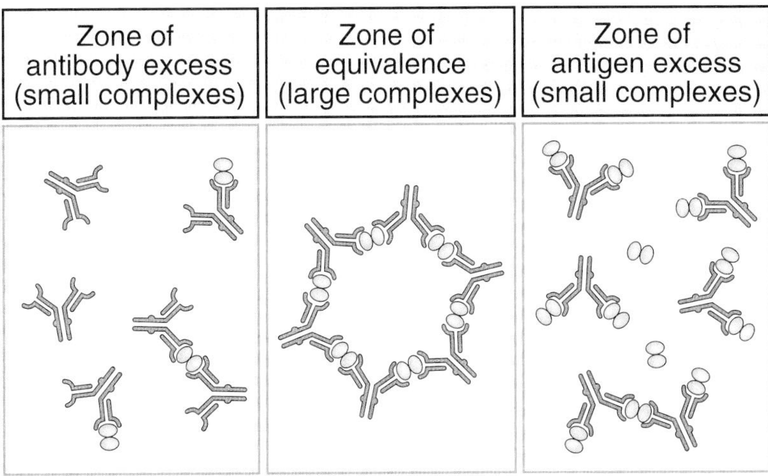

Figure 3–11 Antigen-antibody complexes. The sizes of antigen-antibody (immune) complexes are a function of relative concentrations of antigen and antibody. Large complexes are formed at concentrations of multivalent antigens and antibodies that are termed the zone of equivalence; the complexes are smaller in relative antigen or antibody excess.

antigen molecules will displace antigen bound to the antibody (zone of antigen excess) or by increasing antibody so that free antibody molecules will displace bound antibody from antigen determinants (zone of antibody excess). If a zone of equivalence is reached *in vivo*, large immune complexes can form in the circulation. Immune complexes that are trapped or formed in tissues can initiate an inflammatory reaction, resulting in immune complex diseases (see Chapter 18).

Structure-Function Relationships in Antibody Molecules

Many structural features of antibodies are critical for their ability to recognize antigens and for their effector functions. In the following section, we summarize how the structure of antibodies contributes to their functions.

Features Related to Antigen Recognition

Antibodies are able to specifically recognize a wide variety of antigens with varying affinities. All the features of antigen recognition reflect the properties of antibody V regions.

Specificity

Antibodies can be remarkably specific for antigens, distinguishing between small differences in chemical structure.

- Classic experiments performed by Karl Landsteiner in the 1930s demonstrated that antibodies made in response to an aminobenzene hapten with a meta-substituted sulfonate group would bind strongly to this hapten but weakly or not at all to ortho- or para-substituted isomers. These antigens are structurally similar and differ only in the location of the sulfonate group on the benzene ring.

The fine specificity of antibodies applies to the recognition of all classes of molecules. For example, antibodies can distinguish between two linear protein determinants differing by only a single conservative amino acid substitution that has little effect on secondary structure. Because the biochemical constituents of all living organisms are fundamentally similar, this high degree of specificity is necessary so that antibodies generated in response to the antigens of one microbe usually do not react with structurally similar self molecules or the antigens of other microbes. However, some antibodies produced against one antigen may bind to a different but structurally related antigen. This is referred to as a **cross-reaction**. Antibodies that are produced in response to a microbial antigen sometimes cross-react with self antigens, and this may be the basis for certain immunologic diseases (see Chapter 18).

Diversity

As we discussed earlier in this chapter, an individual is capable of making a tremendous number of structurally distinct antibodies, perhaps up to 10^9, each with a distinct specificity. The presence of a large number of antibodies that bind different antigens is called **diversity,** and the total collection of antibodies with different specificities is called the **antibody repertoire.** The genetic mechanisms that can generate such a large antibody repertoire occur exclusively in lymphocytes. They are based on the random recombination of a limited set of inherited germline DNA sequences into functional genes that encode the V regions of heavy and light chains as well as on the random addition of nontemplate nucleotide sequences to these V segment genes. These mechanisms are discussed in detail in Chapter 7. The millions of resulting variations in structure are concentrated in the hypervariable regions of both heavy and light chains and thereby determine specificity for antigens.

Affinity and Avidity

The ability of antibodies to neutralize toxins and infectious microbes is dependent on tight binding of the

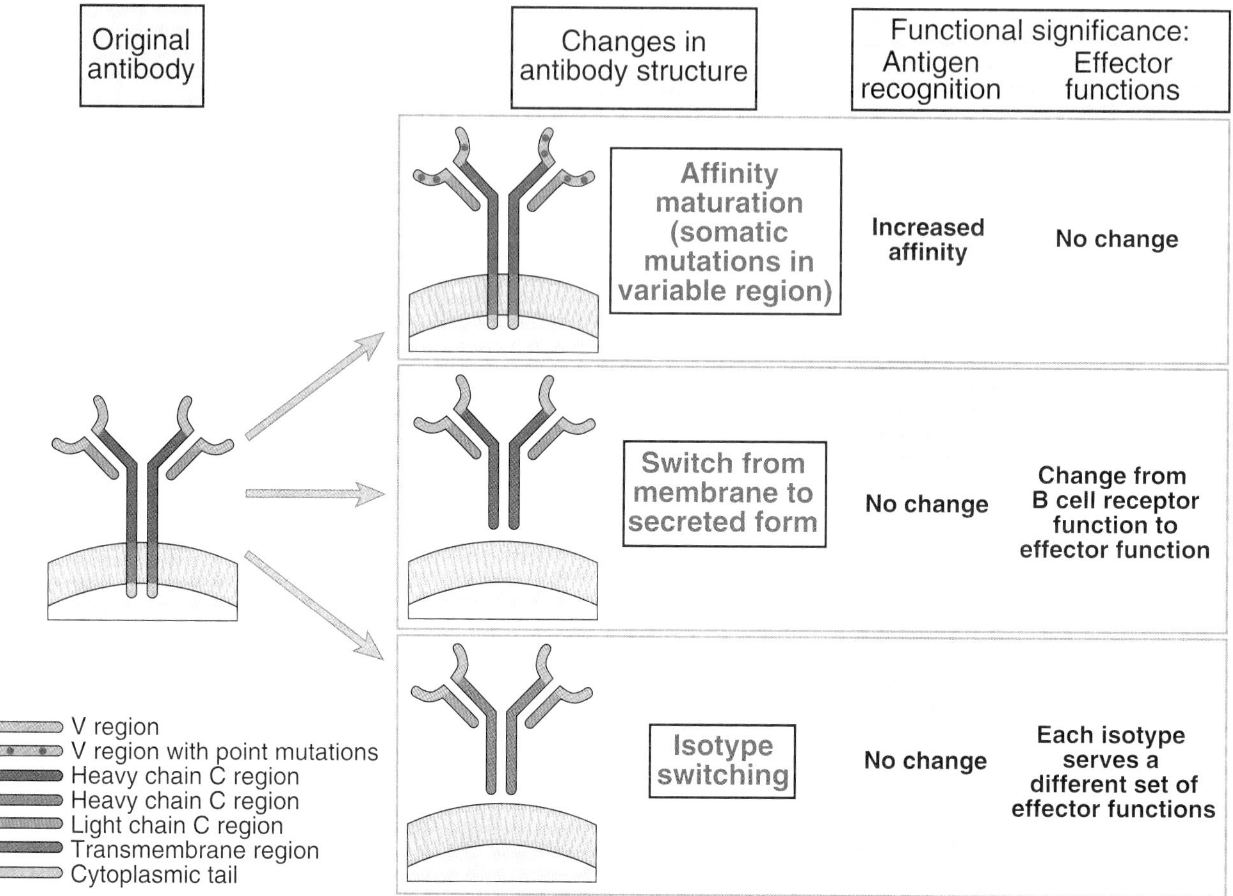

Figure 3–12 Changes in antibody structure during humoral immune responses. The illustration depicts the changes in the structure of antibodies that may be produced by the progeny of activated B cells (one clone) and the related changes in function. During affinity maturation, mutations in the variable (V) region (indicated by red dots) lead to changes in fine specificity without changes in constant (C) region–dependent effector functions. Activated B cells may shift production from largely membrane-bound antibodies containing transmembrane and cytoplasmic regions to secreted antibodies. Secreted antibodies may or may not show V gene mutations (i.e., secretion of antibodies occurs before and after affinity maturation). In isotype switching, the C regions change (indicated by color change from blue to orange) without changes in the antigen-binding V region. Isotype switching is seen in membrane-bound and secreted antibodies. The molecular basis for these changes is discussed in Chapter 9.

antibodies. As we have discussed, tight binding is achieved by high-affinity and high-avidity interactions. A mechanism for the generation of high-affinity antibodies involves subtle changes in the structure of the V regions of antibodies during the humoral responses. These changes come about by a process of somatic mutation in antigen-stimulated B lymphocytes that generates new V domain structures, some of which bind the antigen with greater affinity than did the original V domains (Fig. 3–12). Those B cells producing the higher affinity antibodies are preferentially stimulated by antigen and become the dominant B cells with each subsequent exposure to the antigen. This process, called **affinity maturation,** results in an increase in the average binding affinity of antibodies for an antigen as a humoral response develops. Thus, an antibody produced during a primary immune response to a protein antigen often has a K_d in the range of 10^{-7} to 10^{-9} M; in secondary responses, the affinity increases, with a K_d of 10^{-11} M or even less. The mechanisms of affinity maturation are discussed in Chapter 9.

Features Related to Effector Functions

Many of the effector functions of immunoglobulins are mediated by the Fc portions of the molecules, and antibody isotypes that differ in these Fc regions perform distinct functions. We have mentioned previously that the effector functions of antibodies require the binding of heavy chain C regions, which make up the Fc portions, to other cells and plasma proteins. For example, IgG coats microbes and targets them for phagocytosis by neutrophils and macrophages. This occurs because the antigen-complexed IgG molecule is able to bind, through its Fc region, to γ heavy chain–specific Fc receptors (FcRs) that are expressed on neutrophils and macrophages. In contrast, IgE coats helminths and targets them for destruction by eosinophils because eosinophils express IgE-specific FcRs. Another Fc-dependent effector mechanism of humoral immunity is activation of the classical pathway of the complement system. The system generates inflammatory mediators and promotes microbial phagocytosis and lysis. It is initiated by the binding of a complement protein called C1q to the Fc portions of antigen-complexed IgG or IgM. The FcR- and complement-binding sites of antibodies are found within the heavy chain C domains of the different isotypes (see Fig. 3–1). The structure and functions of FcRs and complement proteins are discussed in more detail in Chapter 14.

The effector functions of antibodies are initiated only by antibodies that have bound antigens and not by free Ig. The reason that only antibodies with bound antigens activate effector mechanisms is that two or more adjacent antibody Fc portions are needed to bind to and trigger various effector systems, such as complement proteins and FcRs of phagocytes (see Chapter 14). This requirement for adjacent antibody molecules ensures that the effector functions are targeted specifically toward eliminating antigens that are recognized by the antibody and that circulating free antibodies do not wastefully trigger effector responses.

Changes in the isotypes of antibodies during humoral immune responses influence how and where the responses work to eradicate antigen. After stimulation by an antigen, a single clone of B cells may produce antibodies with different isotypes yet identical V domains, and therefore identical antigen specificity. Naive B cells, for example, simultaneously produce IgM and IgD that function as membrane receptors for antigens. When these B cells are activated by an antigen such as a microbe, they may undergo a process called **isotype switching** in which the type of C_H region, and therefore the antibody isotype, produced by the B cell changes, but the V regions and the specificity do not (see Fig. 3–12). As a result of isotype switching, different progeny of the original IgM- and IgD-expressing B cell may produce isotypes and subtypes that are best able to eliminate the antigen. For example, the antibody response to many bacteria and viruses is dominated by IgG antibodies, which promote phagocytosis of the microbes, and the response to helminths consists mainly of IgE, which aids in the destruction of the parasites. The mechanisms and functional significance of isotype switching are discussed in Chapter 9.

The heavy chain C regions of antibodies also determine the tissue distribution of antibody molecules. IgA is the only isotype that can be secreted efficiently through mucosal epithelia, and therefore it is the major class of antibody in mucosal secretions and milk. Neonates are protected from infections by IgG antibodies they acquire from their mothers during gestation and early after birth. This transfer of maternal IgG is mediated by a special type of Fc receptor that is expressed in the placenta (through which antibodies enter the fetal circulation) and in the intestine of the neonate (through which antibodies are absorbed from ingested milk).

Summary

- Antibodies, or immunoglobulins, are a family of structurally related glycoproteins produced in membrane-bound or secreted form by B lymphocytes. Membrane-bound antibodies serve as receptors that mediate the antigen-triggered activation of B cells. Secreted antibodies function as mediators of specific humoral immunity by engaging various effector mechanisms that serve to eliminate the bound antigens.

- The antigen-binding regions of antibody molecules are highly variable, and any one individual produces up to 10^9 different antibodies, each with distinct antigen specificity.

- All antibodies have a common symmetric core structure of two identical covalently linked heavy chains and two identical light chains, each linked to one of the heavy chains. Each chain consists of two or more independently folded Ig domains of about 110 amino acids containing conserved sequences and intrachain disulfide bonds.

- The N-terminal domains of heavy and light chains form the V regions of antibody molecules, which differ among antibodies of different specificities. The V regions of heavy and light chains each contain three separate hypervariable regions of about 10 amino acids that are spatially assembled to form the antigen-combining site of the antibody molecule.

- Antibodies are classified into different isotypes and subtypes on the basis of differences in the heavy chain C regions, which consist of three or four Ig C domains, and these classes and subclasses have different functional properties. The antibody classes are called IgM, IgD, IgG, IgE, and IgA. Both light chains of a single Ig molecule are of the same light chain isotype, either κ or λ, that differ in their single C domains.

- Most of the effector functions of antibodies are mediated by the C regions of the heavy chains, but these functions are triggered by binding of antigens to the spatially distant combining site in the V region.

- Antigens are substances specifically bound by antibodies or T lymphocyte antigen receptors. Antigens that bind to antibodies are a wide variety of biologic molecules, including sugars, lipids, carbohydrates, proteins, and nucleic acids. This is in contrast to T cell antigen receptors, which recognize only peptide antigens.

- Macromolecular antigens contain multiple epitopes, or determinants, each of which may be recognized by an antibody. Linear epitopes of protein antigens may be formed by a sequence of adjacent amino acids, and conformational determinants may be formed by folding of a polypeptide chain.

- The affinity of the interaction between the combining site of a single antibody molecule and a single epitope is measured as a dissociation constant (K_d).

Polyvalent antigens contain multiple identical epitopes to which identical antibody molecules can bind. Antibodies can bind to two or, in the case of IgM, up to 10 identical epitopes simultaneously, leading to enhanced avidity of the antibody-antigen interaction. The relative concentrations of polyvalent antigens and antibodies may favor the formation of immune complexes that may deposit in tissues and cause damage.

- Antibody binding to antigen can be highly specific, distinguishing small differences in chemical structures, but cross-reactions may also occur in which two or more antigens may be bound by the same antibody.
- Several changes in the structure of antibodies made by one clone of B cells may occur in the course of an immune response. B cells initially produce only membrane-bound Ig, but changes in the carboxyl terminal end of the antibody lead to secretion of soluble Ig with the same specificity as the original membrane-bound Ig receptor. Changes in the use of C region gene segments without changes in V regions are the basis of isotype switching, which leads to changes in effector function without a change in specificity. Point mutations in the V regions of an antibody specific for an antigen lead to increased affinity for that antigen (affinity maturation).

Selected Readings

Harris LJ, SB Larsen, and A McPherson. Comparison of intact antibody structures and the implications for effector functions. Advances in Immunology 72:191–208, 1999.

Huston JS, and AJ George. Engineered antibodies take center stage. Human Antibodies 10:127–142, 2001.

Köhler G, and C Milstein. Continuous cultures of fused cells secreting antibody of predefined specificity. Nature 256:495–497, 1975.

Ravetch JV, and S Bolland. IgG Fc receptors. Annual Review of Immunology 19:275–290, 2001.

Wilson IA, and RL Stanford. Antibody-antigen interactions: new structures and new conformational changes. Current Opinions in Structural Biology 4:857–867, 1994.

Chapter 4

The Major Histocompatibility Complex

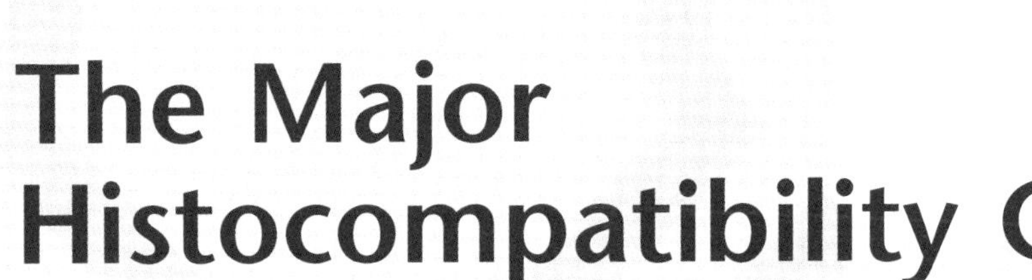

The principal functions of T lymphocytes are defense against intracellular microbes and activation of other cells, such as macrophages and B lymphocytes. All these functions require that T lymphocytes interact with other cells, which may be infected host cells, dendritic cells, macrophages, and B lymphocytes. T lymphocytes are able to interact with other cells because the antigen receptors of T cells can only recognize antigens that are displayed on other cells. This specificity of T lymphocytes is in contrast to that of B lymphocytes and their secreted products, antibodies, which can recognize soluble antigens as well as cell-associated antigens. The task of displaying cell-associated antigens for recognition by T cells is performed by specialized proteins that are encoded by genes in a locus called the **major histocompatibility complex** (MHC). The MHC was discovered as an extended locus containing highly polymorphic genes that determined the outcome of tissue transplants exchanged between individuals. We now know that the physiologic function of MHC molecules is the presentation of peptides to T cells. In fact, MHC molecules are integral components of the ligands that most T cells recognize because the antigen receptors of T cells are actually specific for complexes of foreign peptide antigens and self MHC molecules (schematically illustrated in Figure 4–1). There are two main types of MHC gene products, called **class I MHC molecules** and **class II MHC molecules,** which sample different pools of protein antigens, cytosolic (intracellular) antigens and extracellular antigens that have been endocytosed, respectively. Class I molecules present peptides to $CD8^+$ cytolytic T lymphocytes (CTLs), and class II molecules to $CD4^+$ helper T cells. Thus, knowledge of the structure and biosynthesis of MHC molecules and the association of peptide antigens with MHC molecules is fundamental to understanding how T cells recognize foreign antigens.

We begin our discussion of antigen recognition by T cells with a description of the structure of MHC molecules, the biochemistry of peptide binding to MHC molecules, and the genetics of the MHC. In Chapter 5, we will discuss in more detail the presentation of anti-

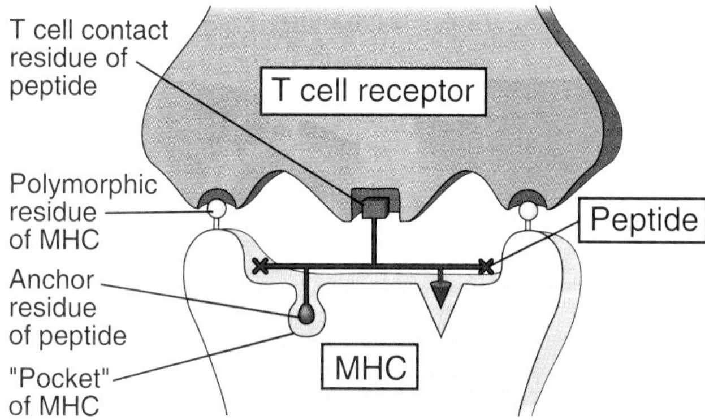

Figure 4–1 T cell recognition of a peptide-MHC complex. This schematic illustration shows an MHC molecule binding and displaying a peptide and a T cell receptor recognizing two polymorphic residues of the MHC molecule and one residue of the peptide. Details of the interactions among peptides, MHC molecules, and T cell receptors are described in Chapters 4, 5, and 6.

gens to T lymphocytes, the roles of class I and class II MHC molecules in this process, and the physiologic significance of MHC-associated antigen presentation. The structure of T cell antigen receptors is described in Chapter 6. The role of MHC molecules in graft rejection is described in Chapter 16. The terminology and genetics of the MHC are best understood from a historical perspective, and we begin with a description of how the MHC was discovered.

Discovery of the MHC and Its Role in Immune Responses

Discovery of the Mouse MHC

The MHC was discovered as the genetic locus whose products were responsible for rapid rejection of tissue grafts exchanged between inbred strains of mice. Key to understanding this discovery is the concept of genetic polymorphism. Some genes are represented by only one normal nucleic acid sequence in all the members of a species (except for relatively rare mutations); such genes are said to be nonpolymorphic, and the normal, or wild-type, gene sequence is usually present on both chromosomes of a pair in every member of the species. In the case of other genes, alternative forms, or variants, are present at stable frequencies in different members of the population. Such genes are said to be **polymorphic,** and each common variant of a polymorphic gene is called an **allele.** For polymorphic genes, an individual can have the same allele at that genetic locus on both chromosomes of the pair and is said to be homozygous, or an individual can have two different alleles, one on each chromosome, and is termed heterozygous.

In the 1940s, George Snell and his colleagues used genetic techniques to analyze the rejection of transplanted tumors and other tissues grafted between strains of laboratory mice. To do this, it was necessary first to produce inbred mouse strains by repetitive mating of siblings. After about 20 generations, every member of an inbred strain has identical nucleic acid sequences at all locations on all chromosomes. In other words, inbred mice are homozygous at every genetic locus, and every mouse of an inbred strain is genetically identical (**syngeneic**) to every other mouse of the same strain. In the case of polymorphic genes, each inbred strain, because it is homozygous, expresses a single allele from the original population. Different strains may express different alleles and are said to be **allogeneic** to one another.

When a tissue or an organ, such as a patch of skin, is grafted from one animal to another, two possible outcomes may ensue. In some cases, the grafted skin survives and functions as normal skin. In other cases, the immune system destroys the graft, a process called **rejection.** Skin grafting experiments showed that grafts exchanged between animals of one inbred strain are accepted, whereas grafts exchanged between animals of different inbred strains (or between outbred animals) are rejected (Fig. 4–2). Therefore, the recognition of a graft as self or foreign is an inherited trait. The genes responsible for causing a grafted tissue to be perceived as similar to or different from one's own tissues were called **histocompatibility genes** (for genes that determine tissue compatibility between individuals), and the differences between self and foreign were attributed to genetic polymorphisms among different histocompatibility gene alleles.

The tools of genetics, namely, breeding and analysis of the offspring, were then applied to identify the relevant genes (Box 4–1). The critical strategy in this effort was the breeding of congenic mouse strains; in two congenic strains, the mice are identical at all loci except the one at which they are selected to be different. Analyses of congenic mice that were selected for their ability to reject grafts from one another indicated that a single genetic region is primarily responsible for rapid graft rejection, and this region was called the major histocompatibility locus. The particular locus that was identified in mice by Snell's group was linked to a gene on chromosome 17 encoding a polymorphic blood group antigen called antigen II, and therefore this region was named histocompatibility-2 or, simply, H-2. Initially, this locus was thought to contain a single gene that controlled tissue compatibility. However, occasional recombination events occurred within the H-2 locus during interbreeding of different strains, indicating that it actually contained several different but closely linked genes, each involved in graft rejection. The genetic region that controlled graft rejection and contained several linked genes was named the major histocompatibility complex, or MHC. Genes that determine the fate of grafted tissues are present in all mammalian species, are homologous to the *H-2* genes first identified in mice, and are all called MHC genes (Fig. 4–3). Other genes that contribute to graft rejection to a lesser degree are called minor histocompatibility genes; we will return to these in Chapter 16, when we discuss transplantation immunology. The

Transplantation

A

MHC^a MHC^b

Donor Donor

Skin graft

Recipient (MHC^a) Recipient (MHC^a)

Graft rejection No Yes

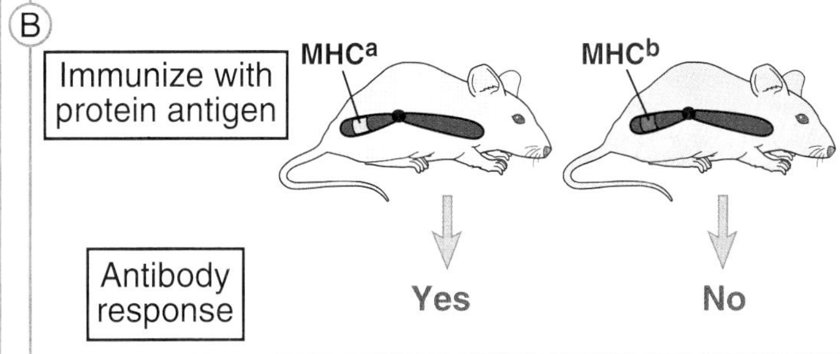

Figure 4–2 MHC genes control graft rejection and immune responses.

The two strains of mice shown are identical except for their MHC alleles (referred to as a and b). These strains reject skin grafts from each other (A) and respond differently to immunization with a model protein antigen (usually a simple polypeptide) (B).

BOX 4–1

Identification and Nomenclature of MHC Genes in Mice

Our knowledge of the organization of the MHC locus is in large part the result of mouse breeding studies. A key development in these studies was the creation of congenic mouse strains that differ only in the genes responsible for graft rejection. Mice of a congenic strain are identical to one another at every genetic locus except the one for which they are selected to differ. The strategy for deriving congenic mice is based on breeding and selection for a particular trait. In their original experiments, Snell and colleagues used acceptance or rejection of transplantable tumors as their assay for histocompatibility, but this is more easily done with skin grafts. For instance, a cross between inbred strains A and B generates $(A \times B)F_1$ offspring (F_1 for first filial generation). The offspring are repeatedly backcrossed to parental strain A, and at each stage the mice that are selected for breeding are those that accept a skin graft from strain B. By this method, one can generate mice that are genetically identical to strain A except that they have the MHC locus of strain B. In other words, mice with the strain B MHC do not recognize strain B tissues as foreign and will accept strain B grafts, even though all other genetic loci are from strain A. Such mice are said to be congenic to strain A and to have the "B MHC on an A background." Such congenic strains have been used to study the function of the MHC genes and to produce antibodies against MHC-encoded proteins.

In mice, the MHC alleles of particular inbred strains are designated by lowercase letters (e.g., *a, b, c*). The individual genes within the MHC are named for the MHC type of mouse strain in which they were first identified. The two independent MHC loci known to be most important for graft rejection in mice are called *H-2K* and *H-2D*. The *K* gene was first discovered in a strain whose MHC had been designated k, and the *D* gene was first discovered in a strain whose MHC had been designated d. In the parlance of mouse geneticists, the allele of the *H-2K* gene in a strain with the k-type MHC is called K^k (pronounced K of k), whereas the allele of the *H-2K* gene in a strain of MHC d is called K^d (K of d). A third locus similar to K and D was discovered later and called L.

Several other genes were subsequently mapped to the region between the *K* and *D* genes responsible for skin rejection. For example, *S* genes were found that coded for polymorphic serum proteins, now known to be components of the complement system. Most important, the polymorphic immune response (Ir) genes described in the text were assigned to a region within the MHC called I (the letter, not the Roman numeral). The I region, in turn, was further subdivided into I-*A* and I-*E* subregions on the basis of recombination events during breeding between congenic strains. The *I* region was also found to code for certain cell surface antigens against which antibodies

Continued on following page

BOX 4–1

Identification and Nomenclature of MHC Genes in Mice *(Continued)*

could be produced by interstrain immunizations. These antigens were called I region–associated molecules, or Ia molecules. The genes of the *I-A* and *I-E* loci, which were discovered as Ir genes, code for Ia antigens, which are called I-A and I-E molecules, respectively. The I-A molecule found in the inbred mouse strain with the K^k and D^k alleles is called $I\text{-}A^k$ (pronounced I A of k). Similar terminology is used for I-E molecules. The elucidation of the molecular structure of the mouse class II region revealed some surprises that were not anticipated by classical genetics. For instance, the *I-A* subregion, originally defined by recombinations during interbreeding of inbred strains, codes for the α and β chains of the I-A molecule as well as for the highly polymorphic β chain of the I-E molecule. The *I-E* subregion identified from breeding codes for only the less polymorphic α chain of the I-E molecule.

nomenclature of mouse MHC genes is described in Box 4–1.

MHC genes control immune responsiveness to protein antigens. For almost 20 years after the MHC was discovered, its only documented role was in graft rejection. This was a puzzle to immunologists because transplantation is not a normal phenomenon, and there was no obvious reason why a set of genes should be preserved through evolution if the only function of the genes was to control the rejection of foreign tissue grafts. In the 1960s and 1970s, it was discovered that MHC genes are of fundamental importance for all immune responses to protein antigens. Baruj Benacerraf, Hugh McDevitt, and their colleagues found that inbred strains of guinea pigs and mice differed in their ability to make antibodies against simple synthetic polypeptides, and responsiveness was inherited as a dominant mendelian trait (see Fig. 4–2). The relevant genes were called **immune response (Ir) genes,** and they were all found to map to the MHC. We now know that Ir genes are, in fact, MHC genes that encode MHC molecules that differ in their ability to bind and display peptides derived from various protein antigens. Responder strains inherit MHC alleles whose products do bind such peptides, forming peptide-MHC complexes that can be recognized by helper T cells. These T cells then help B cells to produce antibodies. Nonresponder strains express MHC molecules that are not capable of binding peptides derived from the polypeptide antigen, and therefore these strains cannot generate helper T cells or antibodies specific for the antigen.

Definitive proof of the importance of MHC molecules in T cell antigen recognition came with the discovery of the phenomenon of **MHC restriction** of T cells, which we will describe in Chapter 5 when we consider the characteristics of the ligands that T cells recognize.

Discovery of the Human MHC

Human MHC molecules are called human leukocyte antigens (HLA) and are equivalent to the H-2 molecules of mice. The kinds of experiments used to discover and define MHC genes in mice, requiring inbreeding, obviously cannot be performed in humans. However, the development of blood transfusion and especially organ transplantation as methods of treatment in clinical medicine provided a strong impetus to detect and define genes that control rejection reactions in humans. Jean Dausset, Jan van Rood, and their colleagues first showed that patients who reject kidneys or have transfusion reactions to white blood cells often contain circulating antibodies reactive with antigens on the white blood cells of the blood or organ donor. Sera

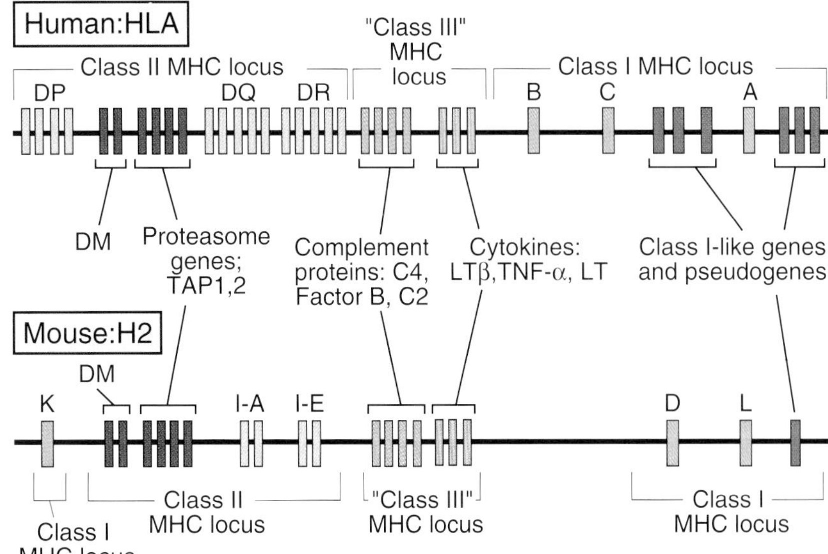

Figure 4–3 Schematic maps of human and mouse MHC loci.

Sizes of genes and intervening DNA segments are not shown to scale. A more detailed map of the human MHC is in Figure 4–10. Class III MHC locus refers to genes that encode molecules other than peptide-display molecules; this term is not used commonly.

that react against the cells of other, allogeneic individuals are called **alloantisera** and are said to contain **alloantibodies,** whose molecular targets are called **alloantigens.** It was presumed that these alloantigens are the products of polymorphic genes that distinguish foreign tissues from self tissues. Panels of alloantisera were collected from alloantigen-immunized donors, including multiparous women (who are immunized by paternal alloantigens expressed by the fetus during pregnancy), actively immunized volunteers, and transfusion or transplant recipients. These sera were compared for their ability to bind to and lyse lymphocytes from different donors. Efforts at several international workshops, involving exchanges of reagents among laboratories, led to the identification of several polymorphic genetic loci, clustered together in a single locus on chromosome 6, whose products are recognized by alloantibodies. Because these alloantigens are expressed on human leukocytes, they were called **human leukocyte antigens** (HLAs). Family studies were then used to construct the map of the HLA locus (see Fig. 4–3). The first three genes defined by purely serologic approaches were called *HLA-A, HLA-B,* and *HLA-C.*

The use of antibodies to study alloantigenic differences between donors and recipients was complemented by the mixed leukocyte reaction (MLR), a test for T cell recognition of allogeneic cells. The MLR is also an *in vitro* model for allograft rejection and will be discussed more fully in the context of transplantation (see Chapter 16). It was found that T lymphocytes from one individual would proliferate in response to leukocytes of another individual, and this assay was used to map the genes that elicited allogeneic T cell reactions. The first gene to be identified from these studies of cellular responses mapped to a region adjacent to the serologically defined HLA locus and was therefore called *HLA-D.* The protein encoded by the *HLA-D* locus was later detected by alloantibodies and was called the HLA-D–related, or HLA-DR, molecule. Two additional genes that mapped adjacent to *HLA-D* were found to encode proteins structurally similar to HLA-DR and also were found to contribute to MLRs; these genes were called *HLA-DQ* and *HLA-DP,* with Q and P chosen for their proximity in the alphabet to R.

We now know that differences in HLA alleles between individuals are important determinants of the rejection of grafts from one individual to another (see Chapter 16). Thus, the HLA locus of humans is functionally equivalent to the H-2 locus of mice defined by transplantation experiments. As we shall see later, MHC molecules in all mammals have essentially the same structure and function.

The accepted nomenclature of MHC genes and their encoded proteins is based on sequence and structural homologies and is applicable to all vertebrate species (see Fig. 4–3). The genes identified as determinants of graft rejection in mice (*H-2K, H-2D,* and *H-2L*) are homologous to the serologically defined human HLA genes (*HLA-A, HLA-B,* and *HLA-C*), and all of these are grouped as **class I MHC genes.** The Ir genes of mice (*I-A* and *I-E*) are homologous to the human genes identified by lymphocyte responses in the MLR (*HLA-DR, HLA-DP,* and *HLA-DQ*) and are grouped as **class II MHC genes.** There are many other genes contained within the MHC; we will return to these later in the chapter.

Properties of MHC Genes

Several important characteristics of MHC genes and their products were deduced from the classical genetic analyses done in mice and humans.

- ***The two types of polymorphic MHC genes, namely, the class I and class II MHC genes, encode two groups of structurally distinct but homologous proteins.*** Class I MHC molecules present peptides to and are recognized by $CD8^+$ T cells, and class II MHC molecules present peptides to $CD4^+$ T cells.
- ***MHC genes are the most polymorphic genes present in the genome.*** The studies of the mouse MHC were accomplished with a limited number of inbred and congenic strains. Although it was appreciated that mouse MHC genes were polymorphic, only about 20 alleles of each MHC gene were identified in the available inbred strains of mice. The human serologic studies were conducted on outbred human populations. A remarkable feature to emerge from the studies of the human MHC genes is the unprecedented and unanticipated extent of their polymorphism. For some HLA loci, more than 250 alleles have been identified by serologic assays. Molecular sequencing has shown that a single serologically defined HLA allele may actually consist of multiple variants that differ slightly. Therefore, the polymorphism is even greater than that predicted from serologic studies.
- ***MHC genes are codominantly expressed in each individual.*** In other words, each individual expresses both the MHC alleles that are inherited from the two parents. For the individual, this maximizes the number of MHC molecules available to bind peptides for presentation to T cells.

The set of MHC alleles present on each chromosome is called an **MHC haplotype.** In humans, each HLA allele is given a numerical designation. For instance, an HLA haplotype of an individual could be HLA-A2, HLA-B5, HLA-DR3, and so on. All heterozygous individuals, of course, have two HLA haplotypes. In mice, each H-2 allele is given a letter designation. Inbred mice, being homozygous, have a single haplotype. Thus, the haplotype of an $H\text{-}2^d$ mouse is $H\text{-}2K^d$ $I\text{-}A^d$ $I\text{-}E^d$ D^d L^d. In humans, certain HLA alleles at different loci are inherited together more frequently than would be predicted by random assortment, a phenomenon called linkage disequilibrium.

The discoveries of the phenomena of MHC-linked immune responsiveness and MHC restriction (see Chapter 5) led to the conclusion that MHC genes control not only graft rejection but also immune responses to all protein antigens. These breakthroughs moved the study of the MHC to the forefront of immunology research.

Structure of MHC Molecules

The elucidation of the biochemistry of MHC molecules has been one of the most important accomplishments of modern immunology. The key advance in this field was the solution of the crystal structures for the extracellular portions of human class I and class II molecules by Don Wiley, Jack Strominger, and their colleagues. Subsequently, many MHC molecules with bound peptides have been crystallized and analyzed in detail. On the basis of this knowledge, we now understand how MHC molecules function to display peptides.

In this section of the chapter, we first summarize the biochemical features that are common to class I and class II MHC molecules and that are most important for the function of these molecules. We then describe the structures of class I and class II proteins, pointing out their important similarities and differences (Table 4–1).

Properties of MHC Molecules

All MHC molecules share certain structural characteristics that are critical for their role in peptide display and antigen recognition by T lymphocytes.

- ***Each MHC molecule consists of an extracellular peptide-binding cleft, or groove, followed by a pair of immunoglobulin (Ig)–like domains and is anchored to the cell by transmembrane and cytoplasmic domains.*** As we shall see later, class I molecules are composed of one polypeptide chain encoded in the MHC and a second, non–MHC-encoded chain, whereas class II molecules are made up of two MHC-encoded polypeptide chains. Despite this difference, the overall three-dimensional structures of class I and class II molecules are similar.
- ***The polymorphic amino acid residues of MHC molecules are located in and adjacent to the peptide-binding cleft.*** This cleft is formed by the folding of the amino termini of the MHC-encoded proteins and is composed of paired α-helices resting on a floor made up of an eight-stranded β-pleated sheet. The polymorphic residues, which are the amino acids that vary among different MHC alleles, are located in and around this cleft. This portion of the MHC molecule binds peptides for display to T cells, and the antigen receptors of T cells interact with the displayed peptide and with the α-helices of the MHC molecules (see Fig. 4–1). Because of amino acid variability in this region, different MHC molecules bind and display different peptides and are recognized specifically by the antigen receptors of different T cells. We will return to a discussion of peptide binding by MHC molecules later in this chapter.
- ***The nonpolymorphic Ig-like domains of MHC molecules contain binding sites for the T cell molecules CD4 and CD8.*** CD4 and CD8 are expressed on distinct subpopulations of mature T lymphocytes and participate, together with antigen receptors, in the recognition of antigen; that is, CD4 and CD8 are T cell "coreceptors" (see Chapter 6). CD4 binds selectively to class II MHC molecules, and CD8 binds to class I molecules. This is why $CD4^+$ T cells recognize only peptides displayed by class II molecules, and $CD8^+$ T cells recognize peptides presented by class I molecules. Most $CD4^+$ T cells function as helper cells, and most $CD8^+$ cells are CTLs.

Class I MHC Molecules

Class I molecules consist of two noncovalently linked polypeptide chains: an MHC-encoded **α chain** (or heavy chain) of 44 to 47 kD and a non–MHC-encoded 12-kD subunit called **β_2-microglobulin** (Fig. 4–4). Each α

Table 4–1. Features of Class I and Class II MHC Molecules

Feature	Class I MHC	Class II MHC
Polypeptide chains	α (44-47 kD) β_2-Microglobulin (12 kD)	α (32-34 kD) β (29-32 kD)
Locations of polymorphic residues	α1 and α2 domains	α1 and β1 domains
Binding site for T cell coreceptor	α3 region binds CD8	β2 region binds CD4
Size of peptide-binding cleft	Accommodates peptides of 8-11 residues	Accommodates peptides of 10-30 residues or more
Nomenclature		
Human	HLA-A, HLA-B, HLA-C	HLA-DR, HLA-DQ, HLA-DP
Mouse	H-2K, H-2D, H-2L	I-A, I-E

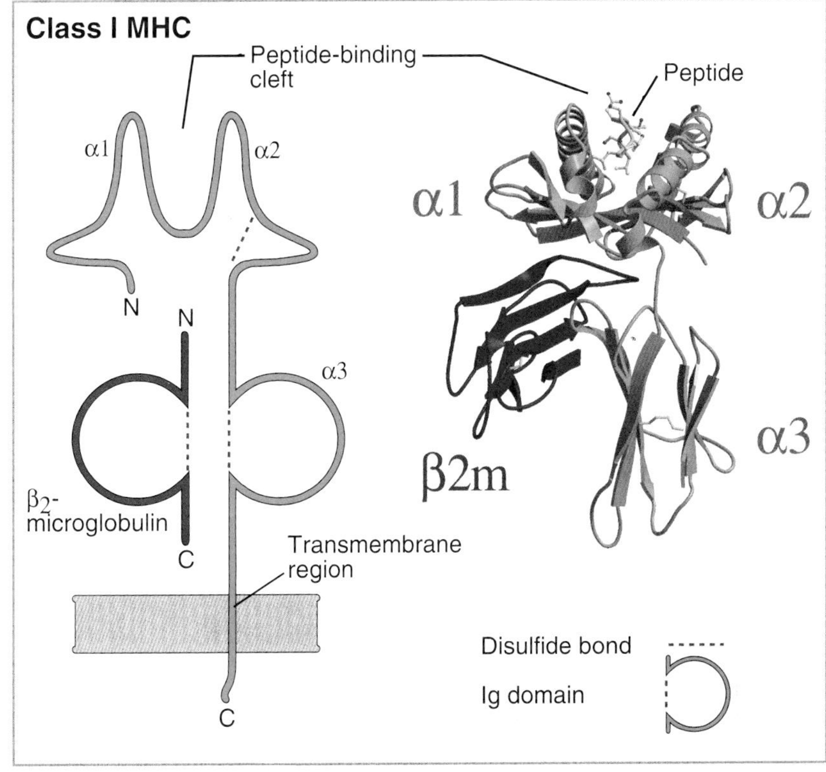

Figure 4–4 Structure of a class I MHC molecule.

The schematic diagram *(left)* illustrates the different regions of the MHC molecule (not drawn to scale). Class I molecules are composed of a polymorphic α chain noncovalently attached to the nonpolymorphic β_2-microglobulin (β2m). The α chain is glycosylated; carbohydrate residues are not shown. The ribbon diagram *(right)* shows the structure of the extracellular portion of the HLA-B27 molecule with a bound peptide, resolved by x-ray crystallography. (Courtesy of Dr. P. Bjorkman, California Institute of Technology, Pasadena.)

chain is oriented so that about three quarters of the complete polypeptide extends into the extracellular milieu, a short hydrophobic segment spans the cell membrane, and the carboxy terminal residues are located in the cytoplasm. The amino terminal (N-terminal) α1 and α2 segments of the α chain, each approximately 90 residues long, interact to form a platform of an eight-stranded, antiparallel β-pleated sheet supporting two parallel strands of α-helix. This forms the peptide-binding cleft of class I molecules. Its size is large enough (~25 Å × 10 Å × 11 Å) to bind peptides of 8 to 11 amino acids in a flexible, extended conformation. The ends of the class I peptide-binding cleft are closed so that larger peptides cannot be accommodated. Therefore, native globular proteins have to be "processed" to generate fragments that are small enough to bind to MHC molecules and to be recognized by T cells (see Chapter 5). The polymorphic residues of class I molecules are confined to the α1 and α2 domains, where they contribute to variations among different class I alleles in peptide binding and T cell recognition (Fig. 4–5). The α3 segment of the α chain folds into an Ig domain whose amino acid sequence is conserved among all class I molecules. This segment contains a loop that serves as the binding site for CD8. At the carboxy terminal end of the α3 segment is a stretch of approximately 25 hydrophobic amino acids that traverses the lipid bilayer of the plasma membrane. Immediately following this are approximately 30 residues located in the cytoplasm, included in which is a cluster of basic amino acids that interact with phospholipid head groups of the inner leaflet of the lipid bilayer and anchor the MHC molecule in the plasma membrane.

The light chain of class I molecules, which is encoded by a gene outside the MHC, is identical to a protein previously identified in human urine and is called β_2-microglobulin for its electrophoretic mobility (β_2), size (micro), and solubility (globulin). β_2-microglobulin interacts noncovalently with the α3 domain of the α chain. Like the α3 segment, β_2-microglobulin is structurally homologous to an Ig domain and is invariant among all class I molecules.

The fully assembled class I molecule is a heterotrimer consisting of an α chain, β_2-microglobulin, and a bound antigenic peptide, and stable expression of class I molecules on cell surfaces requires the presence of all three components of the heterotrimer. The reason for this is that the interaction of the α chain with β_2-microglobulin is stabilized by binding of peptide antigens to the cleft formed by α1 and α2, and conversely, the binding of peptide is strengthened by the interaction of β_2-microglobulin with the α chain. Because antigenic peptides are needed to stabilize the MHC molecules, only useful peptide-loaded MHC molecules are expressed on cell surfaces. The process of assembly of stable peptide-loaded class I molecules will be detailed in Chapter 5.

Every normal (heterozygous) individual expresses six different class I molecules on every cell, containing α chains derived from the two alleles of *HLA-A*, *HLA-B*, and *HLA-C* genes that are inherited from the parents.

Class II MHC Molecules

Class II MHC molecules are composed of two noncovalently associated polypeptide chains, an α chain of 32

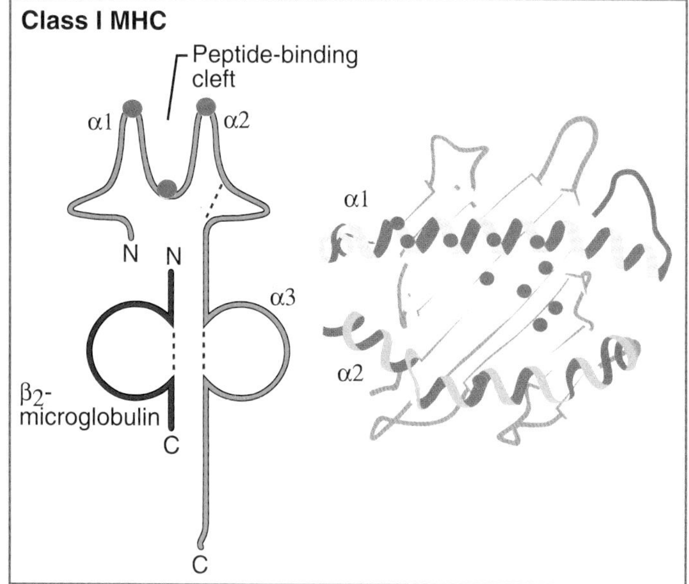

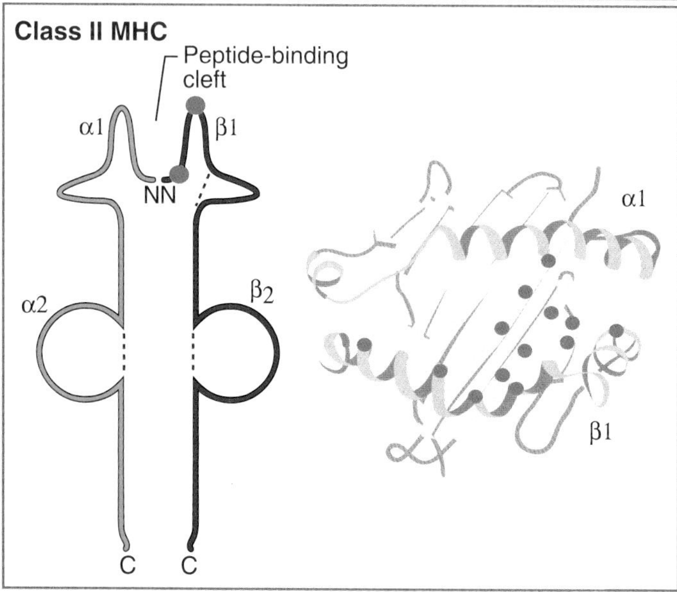

Figure 4–5 Polymorphic residues of a class I MHC molecule.

The polymorphic residues of class I and class II MHC molecules (shown as red circles) are located in the peptide-binding clefts and the α-helices around the clefts. In the class II molecule shown (HLA-DR), essentially all the polymorphism is in the β chain. However, other class II molecules in humans and mice show varying degrees of polymorphism in the α chain and usually much more in the β chain. (Courtesy of Dr. J. McCluskey, University of Melbourne, Parkville, Australia.)

to 34 kD and a β chain of 29 to 32 kD (Fig. 4–6). Unlike class I molecules, both chains of class II molecules are encoded by polymorphic MHC genes.

The amino terminal α1 and β1 segments of the class II chains interact to form the peptide-binding cleft, which is structurally similar to the cleft of class I molecules. Four strands of the floor of the cleft and one of the helices are formed by α1, and the other four strands of the floor and the second helix are formed by β1. The polymorphic residues are located in α1 and β1, in and around the peptide-binding cleft, as in class I molecules. In human class II molecules, most of the polymorphism is in the β chain. In class II molecules, the ends of the peptide-binding cleft are open, so that peptides of 30 residues or more can fit.

The α2 and β2 segments of class II molecules, like class I α3 and $β_2$-microglobulin, are folded into Ig domains and are nonpolymorphic among various alleles of a particular class II gene. A loop in the β2 segment of class II molecules is the binding site for CD4, similar to the binding site for CD8 in α3 of the class I heavy chain. In general, α chains of one class II MHC locus (e.g., DR) most often pair with β chains of the same locus and less commonly with β chains of other loci (e.g., DQ, DP).

The carboxy terminal ends of the α2 and β2 segments continue into short connecting regions followed by approximately 25–amino acid stretches of hydrophobic transmembrane residues. In both chains, the transmembrane regions end with clusters of basic amino acid residues, followed by short, hydrophilic cytoplasmic tails.

A nonpolymorphic polypeptide called the **invariant chain** (I_i) is associated with newly synthesized class II molecules. The I_i plays important roles in the traffic of class II molecules and in the determination of where in the cell peptides bind to class II molecules (see Chapter 5).

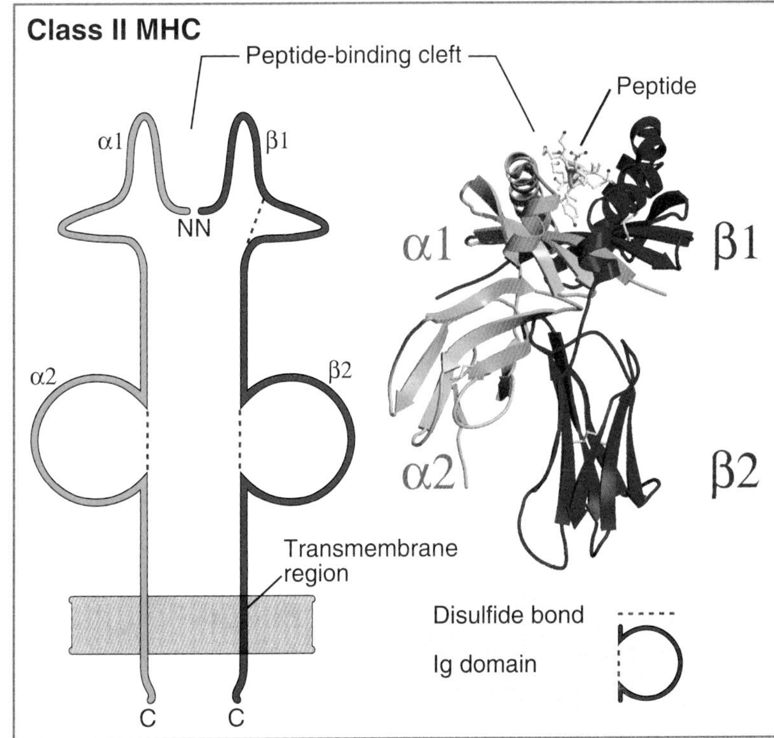

Figure 4–6 Structure of a class II MHC molecule.
The schematic diagram *(left)* illustrates the different regions of the MHC molecule (not drawn to scale). Class II molecules are composed of a polymorphic α chain noncovalently attached to a polymorphic β chain. Both chains are glycosylated; carbohydrate residues are not shown. The ribbon diagram *(right)* shows the structure of the extracellular portion of the HLA-DR1 molecule with a bound peptide, resolved by x-ray crystallography. (Courtesy of Dr. P. Bjorkman, California Institute of Technology, Pasadena.)

The fully assembled class II molecule is a heterotrimer consisting of an α chain, a β chain, and a bound antigenic peptide, and stable expression of class II molecules on cell surfaces requires the presence of all three components of the heterotrimer. As in class I molecules, this ensures that the MHC molecules that end up on the cell surface are the molecules that are serving their normal function of peptide display.

Six class II MHC alleles are inherited, three from each parent (one set of DP, DQ, and DR). However, there may be some heterologous pairing (e.g., DQα from one chromosome with DQβ from another). Therefore, the total number of class II molecules in a heterozygous individual is about 10 to 20, more than the 6 class II alleles that are inherited from both parents.

Binding of Peptides to MHC Molecules

With the realization that MHC molecules are the peptide display molecules of the adaptive immune system, considerable effort has been devoted to elucidating the molecular basis of peptide-MHC interactions and the characteristics of peptides that allow them to bind to MHC molecules. These issues are important not only for understanding the biology of T cell antigen recognition but also for defining the properties of a protein that make it immunogenic. For a protein to be immunogenic in an individual, it must contain peptides that can bind to the MHC molecules of that individual. Such information may be used to design vaccines, by inserting MHC-binding amino acid sequences into antigens used for immunization. In the following section of this chapter, we summarize the key features of the interactions between peptides and class I or class II MHC molecules.

Several analytical methods have been used to study peptide-MHC interactions.

- The earliest studies relied on functional assays of helper T cells and CTLs responding to antigen-presenting cells that were incubated with different peptides. By determining which types of peptides derived from complex protein antigens could activate T cells from animals immunized with these antigens, it was possible to define the features of peptides that allowed them to be presented by antigen-presenting cells.
- After MHC molecules were purified, it was possible to study their interactions with radioactively or fluorescently labeled peptides in solution by methods such as equilibrium dialysis and gel filtration to quantitate bound and free peptides.
- The nature of MHC-binding peptides generated *in vivo* from intact proteins has been analyzed by exposing antigen-presenting cells to a protein antigen for various times, purifying the MHC molecules from these cells by affinity chromatography, and eluting the bound peptides for mass spectroscopy or amino acid sequencing. The same approach may be used to define the endogenous peptides that are displayed by antigen-presenting cells isolated from animals or humans.
- X-ray crystallographic analysis of peptide-MHC complexes has provided valuable information about how peptides sit in the clefts of MHC molecules and about the residues of each that participate in this binding.

On the basis of such studies, we now understand the physicochemical characteristics of peptide-MHC interactions in considerable detail. It has also become apparent that the binding of peptides to MHC molecules is fundamentally different from the binding of antigens to the antigen receptors of B and T lymphocytes (see Chapter 3, Table 3–1).

Characteristics of Peptide-MHC Interactions

MHC molecules show a broad specificity for peptide binding, and the fine specificity of antigen recognition resides largely in the antigen receptors of T lymphocytes. Every peptide against which an immune response can be generated must contain some residues that contribute to binding to the clefts of MHC molecules and must also contain other residues that project from the clefts, where they are recognized by T cells. There are several important features of the interactions of MHC molecules and antigenic peptides.

- ***Each class I or class II MHC molecule has a single peptide-binding cleft that can accommodate many different peptides.*** The ability of one MHC molecule to bind many different peptides was established by several lines of experimental evidence.
  - If a T cell specific for one peptide is stimulated by antigen-presenting cells presenting that peptide, the response is inhibited by the addition of an excess of other, structurally similar peptides (Fig. 4–7). In these experiments, the MHC molecule bound different peptides, but the T cell recognized only one of these peptides presented by the MHC molecule.
  - Direct binding studies with purified MHC molecules in solution definitively established that a single MHC molecule can bind multiple different peptides (albeit only one at a time) and that multiple peptides compete with one another for binding to the single binding site of each MHC molecule.
  - The analyses of peptides eluted from MHC molecules purified from antigen-presenting cells showed that many different peptides can be eluted from any one type of MHC molecule.

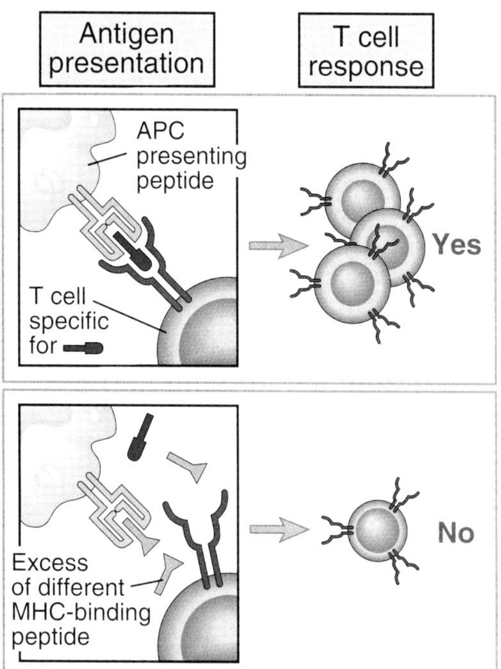

Figure 4–7 Antigen competition for T cells. A T cell recognizes a peptide presented by one MHC molecule. An excess of a different peptide that binds to the same MHC molecule competitively inhibits presentation of the peptide that the T cell recognizes. APC, antigen-presenting cell.

The solution of the crystal structures of class I and class II MHC molecules confirmed the presence of a single peptide-binding cleft in these molecules (see Figs. 4–4 and 4–6). It is not surprising that a single MHC molecule can bind multiple peptides because each individual contains only a few different MHC molecules (6 class I and 10 to 20 class II molecules in a heterozygous individual), and these must be able to present peptides from the enormous number of protein antigens that one is likely to encounter.

- ***The peptides that bind to MHC molecules share structural features that promote this interaction.*** One of these features is the size of the peptide—class I molecules can accommodate peptides that are 8 to 11 residues long, and class II molecules bind peptides that may be 10 to 30 residues long or longer, the optimal length being 12 to 16 residues. In addition, peptides that bind to a particular allelic form of an MHC molecule contain amino acid residues that allow complementary interactions between the peptide and that allelic MHC molecule (Table 4–2). The residues of a peptide that bind to MHC molecules are distinct from those that are recognized by T cells.
- ***The association of antigenic peptides and MHC molecules is a saturable, low-affinity interaction (dissociation constant [K_d] ~10^{-6} M) with a slow on-rate and a very slow off-rate.*** The affinity of peptide-MHC interactions is much lower than that of antigen-antibody binding, which usually has a K_d of 10^{-7} to 10^{-11} M (see Chapter 3, Table 3–1). Because the K_d is equal to the ratio of the rate constants for dissociation (K_{off}) and association (K_{on}), a low-affinity interaction can be stable (i.e., have a slow K_{off}) as long as the K_{on} is also slow. In a solution, saturation of peptide binding to class II MHC molecules takes 15 to 30 minutes. Once bound, peptides may stay associated for hours to many days! The extraordinarily slow off-rate of peptide dissociation from MHC molecules allows peptide-MHC complexes to persist long enough on the surfaces of antigen-presenting cells to ensure productive interactions with antigen-specific T cells.
- ***The MHC molecules of an individual do not discriminate between foreign peptides (e.g., those derived from microbial antigens) and peptides derived from the antigens of that individual (self***

Table 4–2. Peptide Binding to MHC Molecules

HLA molecule (allele)	HLA-binding residues required in peptides at position #		
	#2	#5	#8/9
HLA-A2	Leucine/isoleucine	Variable	Variable; usually valine/ leucine/isoleucine
HLA-B27	Arginine	Variable	Arginine/lysine
HLA-B8	Lysine/arginine	Lysine/arginine	Valine/leucine/isoleucine
HLA-B35	Proline	Variable	Tyrosine/phenylalanine/ tryptophan

Different MHC alleles bind different peptides, which often share conserved features. The table lists some examples of class I human MHC alleles, each of which binds peptides with particular residues at certain positions.

antigens). Thus, MHC molecules display both self peptides and foreign peptides, and T cells survey these displayed peptides for the presence of foreign antigens. This process is central to the surveillance function of T cells. However, the inability of MHC molecules to discriminate between self antigens and foreign antigens raises two questions. First, because MHC molecules are continuously exposed to, and presumably occupied by, abundant self peptides, how can they bind and display foreign peptides, which are likely to be relatively rare? Second, if self peptides are constantly being presented, why do individuals not develop autoimmune reactions? The answer to these questions lies in the cell biology of MHC biosynthesis and assembly, in the specificity of T cells, and in the exquisite sensitivity of these cells to small amounts of peptide-MHC complexes. We will return to these questions in more detail in Chapter 5.

Structural Basis of Peptide Binding to MHC Molecules

The binding of peptides to MHC molecules is a noncovalent interaction mediated by residues both in the peptides and in the clefts of the MHC molecules. Protein antigens are proteolytically cleaved in antigen-presenting cells to generate the peptides that will be bound and displayed by MHC molecules (see Chapter 5). These peptides bind to the clefts of MHC molecules in an extended conformation. Once bound, the peptides and their associated water molecules fill the clefts, making extensive contacts with the amino acid residues that form the β-strands of the floor and the α-helices of the sides of the cleft (Fig. 4–8). In most MHC molecules, the β-strands in the floor of the cleft contain "pockets." The amino acid residues of a peptide may contain side chains that fit into these pockets and bind to complementary amino acids in the MHC molecule, often through hydrophobic interactions (see Table 4–2). Such residues of the peptide are called **anchor residues** because they contribute most of the favorable interactions of the binding (i.e., they anchor the peptide in the cleft of the MHC molecule). The anchor residues of peptides may be located in the middle or at the ends of the peptide. Each MHC-binding peptide usually contains only one or two anchor residues, and this presumably allows greater variability in the other residues of the peptide, which are the residues that are recognized by specific T cells. Not all peptides use anchor residues to bind to MHC molecules, especially to class II molecules. Specific interactions of peptides with the α-helical sides of the MHC cleft also contribute to peptide binding by forming hydrogen bonds or charge interactions (salt bridges). Class I–binding peptides usually contain hydrophobic or basic amino acids at their carboxyl termini that also contribute to the interaction.

Because many of the residues in and around the peptide-binding cleft of MHC molecules are polymorphic (i.e., they differ among various MHC alleles), different alleles favor the binding of different peptides. This is the structural basis of the function of MHC genes as "immune response genes"; only animals that express MHC alleles that can bind a particular peptide and display it to T cells can respond to that peptide.

A portion of the bound peptide is exposed from the open top of the cleft of the MHC molecule, and the amino acid side chains of this portion of the peptide are recognized by the antigen receptors of specific T cells. The same T cell receptor also interacts with polymorphic residues of the α-helices of the MHC molecule itself (see Fig. 4–1). Thus, amino acids from both the antigenic peptide and the MHC molecules contribute to T cell antigen recognition, with the peptide being responsible for the fine specificity of antigen recognition and the MHC residues accounting for the MHC restriction of the T cells. Predictably, variations either in the peptide antigen or in the peptide-binding cleft of the MHC molecule will alter presentation of that peptide or its recognition by T cells. In fact, one can enhance the immunogenicity of a peptide by incorporating into it a residue that strengthens its binding to commonly inherited MHC molecules in a population.

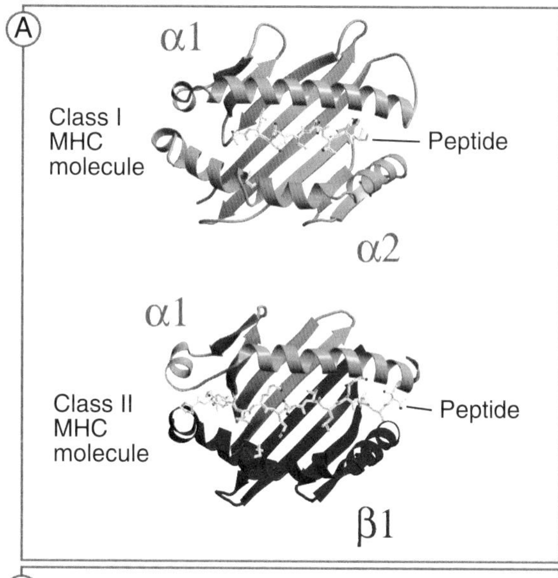

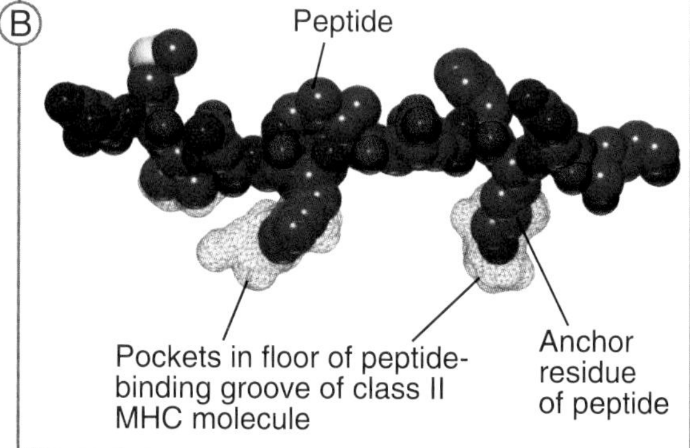

Figure 4–8 Peptide binding to MHC molecules.

A. These top views of the crystal structures of MHC molecules show how peptides (in yellow) lie on the floors of the peptide-binding clefts and are available for recognition by T cells. The class I molecule shown is HLA-A2, and the class II molecule is HLA-DR1. Note that the cleft of the class I molecule is closed, whereas that of the class II molecule is open. As a result, class II molecules accommodate longer peptides than do class I molecules. (Courtesy of Dr. P. Bjorkman, California Institute of Technology, Pasadena.)

B. The side view of a cut-out of a peptide bound to a class II MHC molecule shows how anchor residues of the peptide hold it in the pockets in the cleft of the MHC molecule. (From Scott CA, PA Peterson, L Teyton, and IA Wilson. Crystal structures of two I-A^d–peptide complexes reveal that high affinity can be achieved without large anchor residues. Immunity 8:319–329, 1998. Copyright 1998, with permission from Elsevier Science.)

This approach is being tried for the synthesis of custom-designed vaccines.

- By introducing mutations in an immunogenic peptide, it is possible to identify residues involved in binding to MHC molecules and those that are critical for T cell recognition. This approach has been applied to many peptide antigens, using T cells to measure responses to these peptides (Fig. 4–9).

The realization that the polymorphic residues of MHC molecules determine the specificity of peptide binding and T cell antigen recognition has led to the question of why MHC genes are polymorphic. One possibility is that the presence of multiple MHC alleles in a population will ensure that virtually all peptides derived from microbial antigens will be recognized by the immune system of at least some individuals. At the population level, this will increase the range of microbial peptides that may be presented to T cells and reduce the likelihood of a microbe's evading the immune systems of all individuals by mutating its antigenic proteins.

Genomic Organization of the MHC

In humans, the MHC is located on the short arm of chromosome 6 and β_2-microglobulin is encoded by a gene on chromosome 15. The human MHC occupies a large segment of DNA, extending about 3500 kilobases (kb). (For comparison, a large human gene may extend up to 50 to 100 kb, and the size of the entire *Escherichia coli* genome is approximately 4500 kb.) In classical genetic terms, the MHC extends about 4 centimorgans, meaning that crossovers within the MHC occur with a frequency of about 4% at each meiosis. A molecular map of the human MHC is shown in Figure 4–10.

Many of the proteins involved in the processing of protein antigens and the presentation of peptides to T cells are encoded by genes located within the MHC. In other words, this genetic locus contains much of the information needed for the machinery of antigen presentation. The class I genes, *HLA-A, HLA-B,* and *HLA-C,* are in the most telomeric portion of the HLA locus, and the class II genes are the most centromeric in the HLA locus. Within the class II locus are genes that encode several proteins that play critical roles in antigen processing. One of these proteins, called the **transporter associated with antigen processing** (TAP), is a heterodimer that transports peptides from the cytosol into the endoplasmic reticulum, where the peptides can associate with newly synthesized class I molecules. The two subunits of the TAP dimer are encoded by two genes within the class II region. Other genes in this cluster encode subunits of a cytosolic protease complex, called the **proteasome,** that degrades cytosolic proteins into peptides that are subsequently presented by class I MHC molecules. Another pair of genes, called *HLA-DMA* and *HLA-DMB,* encodes a nonpolymorphic heterodimeric class II–like molecule, called **HLA-DM** (or H-2M in mice), that is involved in peptide binding to class II molecules. The functions of these proteins in antigen presentation are discussed in Chapter 5.

Between the class I and class II gene clusters are genes that code for several components of the com-plement system; for three structurally related cytokines, tumor necrosis factor, lymphotoxin, and lymphotoxin-β; and for some heat shock proteins. The genes within the MHC that encode these diverse proteins have been called class III MHC genes. Between HLA-C and HLA-A, and telomeric to HLA-A, are many genes that are called class I–like because they resemble class I genes but exhibit little or no polymorphism. Some of these encode proteins that are expressed in association

Figure 4–9 MHC-binding residues and T cell receptor contact residues of a model peptide antigen.

The immunodominant epitope of the protein hen egg lysozyme (HEL) in H-2[k] mice is a peptide composed of residues 52–62. The ribbon diagrams modeled after crystal structures show the surface of the peptide-binding cleft of the I-A[k] class II molecule and the bound HEL peptide with amino acid residues (P1–P9) indicated as spheres (A) and with side chains (B). Mutational analysis of the peptide has shown that the residues involved in binding to MHC molecules are P1 (Asp52), P4 (Ile55), P6 (Gln57), P7 (Ile 58), and P9 (Ser60); these are the residues that project down and fit into the peptide-binding cleft. The residues involved in recognition by T cells are P2 (Tyr53), P5 (Leu56), P8 (Asn59), P10 (Arg61), and P11 (Trp62); these residues project upward and are available to T cells. (From Fremont DH, D Monnale, CA Nelson, WA Hendrickson, and ER Unanue. Crystal structure of I-A in complex with a dominant epitope of lysozyme. Immunity 8:305–317, 1998. Copyright 1998, with permission from Elsevier Science.)

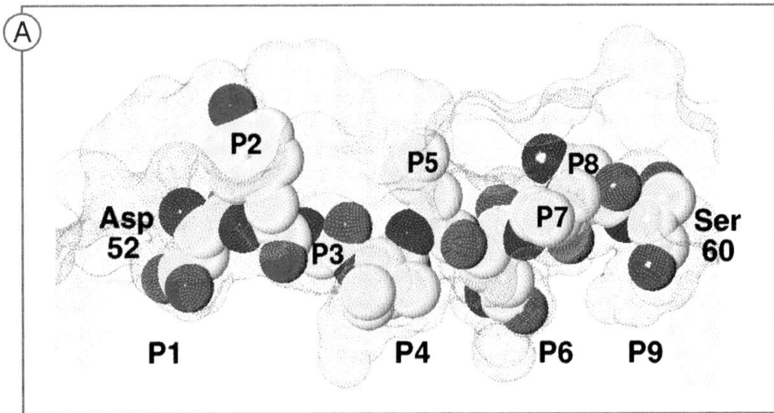

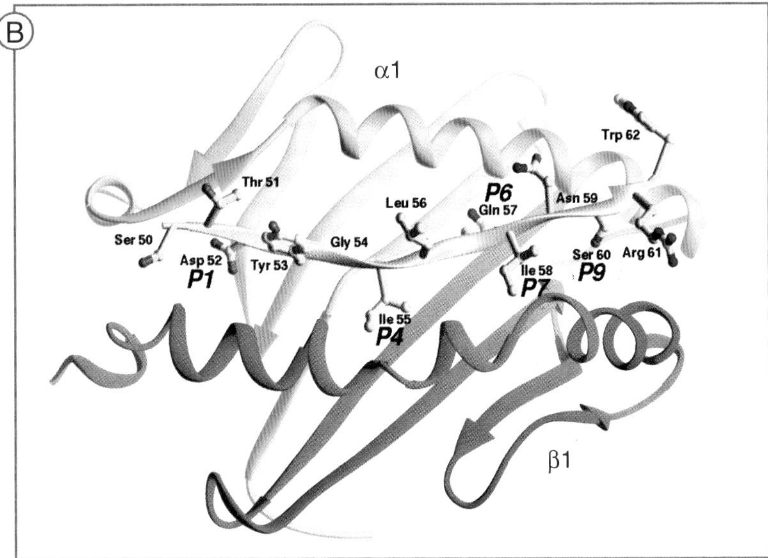

with β_2-microglobulin and are called class IB molecules, to distinguish them from the classical polymorphic class I molecules. Among the class IB molecules is HLA-G, which may play a role in antigen recognition by NK (natural killer) cells, and HLA-H, which appears to be involved in iron metabolism and has no known function in the immune system. Many of the class I–like sequences are pseudogenes. The functions of most of these class I–like genes and pseudogenes are not known. One function may be that these DNA sequences serve as a repository of coding sequences to be used for generating polymorphic sequences in conventional class I and class II MHC molecules by the process of gene conversion. In this process, a portion of the sequence of one gene is replaced with a portion of another gene without a reciprocal recombination event. Gene conversion is a more efficient mechanism than point mutation for producing genetic variation without loss of function because several changes can be introduced at once, and amino acids necessary for maintaining protein structure can remain unchanged if identical amino acids at those positions are encoded by both of the genes involved in the conversion event. It is clear from population studies that the extraordinary polymorphism of MHC molecules has been generated by gene conversion and not by point mutations.

The mouse MHC, located on chromosome 17, occupies about 2000 kb of DNA, and the genes are organized in an order slightly different from the human MHC gene. One of the mouse class I genes (*H-2K*) is centromeric to the class II region, but the other class I genes and the nonpolymorphic class IB genes are telomeric to the class II region. As in the human, β_2-microglobulin is encoded not by the MHC but by a gene located on a separate chromosome (chromosome 2).

There are β_2-microglobulin–associated proteins other than class I MHC molecules that may serve important functions in the immune system. These include the neonatal Fc receptor (see Chapter 14) and the CD1 molecules, which may be involved in presenting nonpeptidic antigens to unusual populations of T cells. These proteins are homologous to the class I MHC α chain but are encoded outside the MHC, on different chromosomes.

Individual class I and class II MHC genes have the same pattern of intron-exon organization. The first exon encodes the signal sequence, and each of the approximately 90–amino acid residue extracellular segments (e.g., class I α1, α2, and α3 or class II α1, α2, β1,

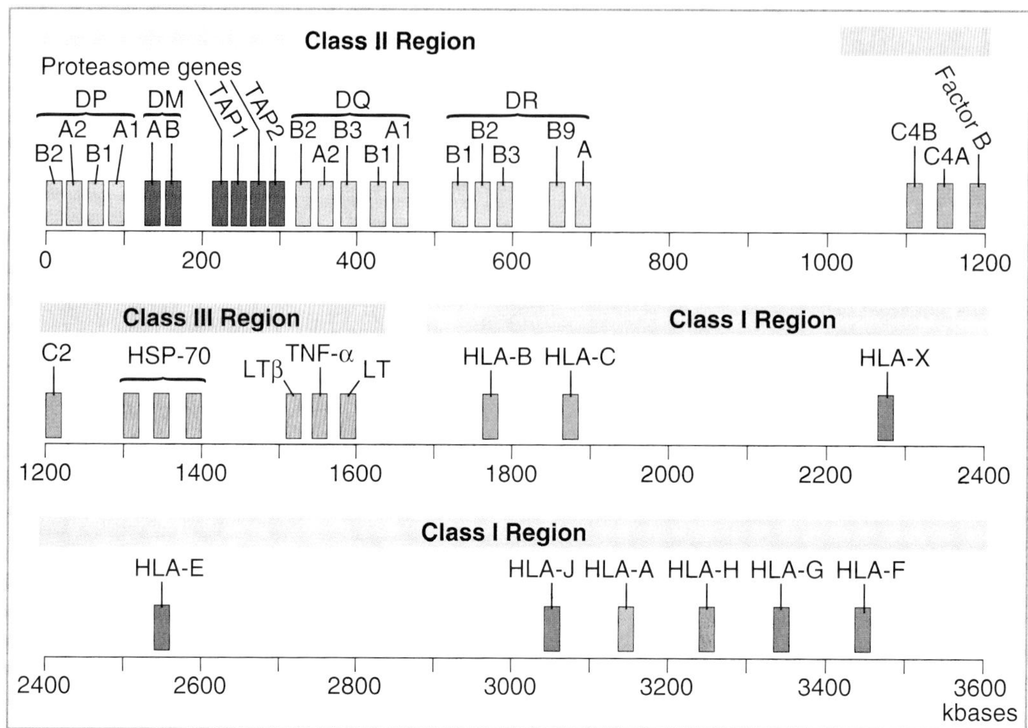

Figure 4–10 Map of the human MHC.
This map is simplified to exclude many genes that are of unknown function. HLA-E, HLA-F, HLA-G, HLA-J, and HLA-X are class I–like molecules; HLA-H does not appear to be involved in the immune system. C4, C2, B, complement proteins; DM, TAP, proteasomes, proteins involved in antigen processing; HLA, human leukocyte antigen; HSP, heat shock protein; LT, TNF, cytokines.

and β2) is encoded by a separate exon. The transmembrane and cytoplasmic regions are encoded by several small exons.

Expression of MHC Molecules

Because MHC molecules are required to present antigens to T lymphocytes, the expression of MHC genes in a cell determines whether foreign (e.g., microbial) antigens in that cell will be recognized by T cells. There are several important features of the expression of MHC molecules.

- ***Class I molecules are constitutively expressed on virtually all nucleated cells, whereas class II molecules are normally expressed on only dendritic cells, B lymphocytes, macrophages, and a few other cell types.*** This pattern of MHC expression is intimately linked to the functions of class I–restricted and class II–restricted T cells. The effector function of class I–restricted CD8$^+$ T cells is to kill cells infected with intracellular microbes, such as viruses. Because viruses can infect virtually any nucleated cell, the ligands that CD8$^+$ T cells recognize need to be displayed on all nucleated cells. The expression of class I MHC molecules on nucleated cells serves precisely this purpose, providing a display system for viral antigens. In contrast, class II–restricted CD4$^+$ helper T lymphocytes have a set of functions that require recognizing antigen presented by a more limited number of cell types. In particular, naive CD4$^+$ T cells need to recognize antigens that are presented by dendritic cells in peripheral lymphoid organs. Differentiated CD4$^+$ helper T lymphocytes function mainly to activate (or help) macrophages to eliminate extracellular microbes that have been phagocytosed and to activate B lymphocytes to make antibodies that also eliminate extracellular microbes. Class II molecules are expressed mainly on these cell types and provide a system for displaying peptides derived from extracellular microbes and proteins.
- ***The expression of MHC molecules is increased by cytokines produced during both innate and adaptive immune responses*** (Fig. 4–11). On most cell types, the interferons IFN-α, IFN-β, and IFN-γ increase the level of expression of class I molecules, and tumor necrosis factor (TNF) and lymphotoxin (LT) can have the same effect. (The properties and biologic activities of cytokines are discussed in Chapter 11.) The interferons are produced during the early innate immune response to many viruses, and TNF and LT are produced in response to many microbial infections. Thus, innate immune responses to microbes increase the expression of the MHC molecules that display microbial antigens to microbe-specific T cells. This is one of the mechanisms by which innate immunity stimulates adaptive immune responses.

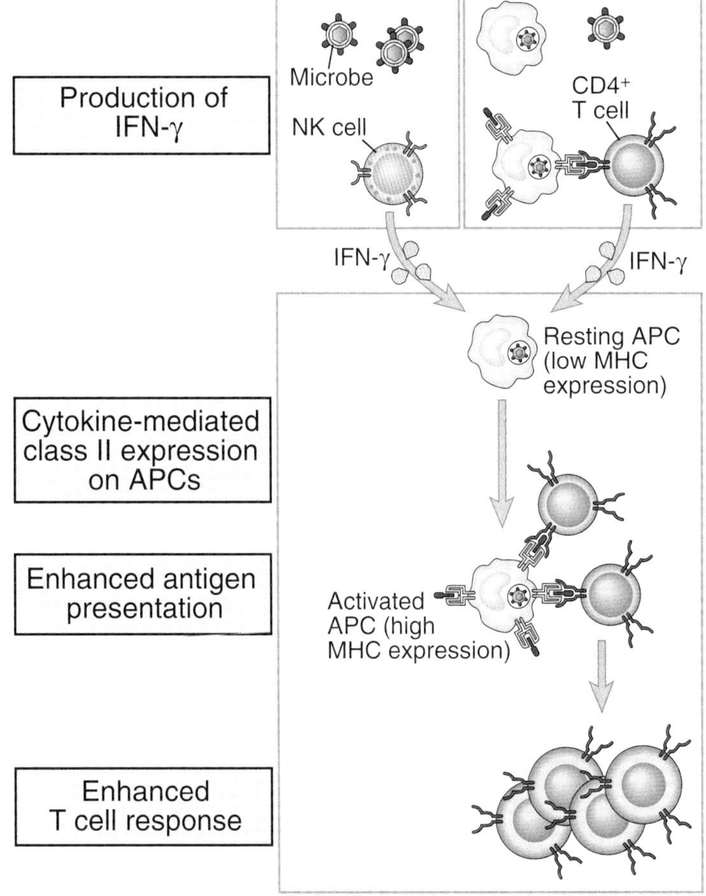

Figure 4–11 Enhancement of class II MHC expression by IFN-γ.

IFN-γ, produced by NK cells during innate immune reactions to microbes or by T cells during adaptive immune reactions, stimulates class II MHC expression on antigen-presenting cells (APCs) and thus enhances the activation of $CD4^+$ T cells. IFN-γ has a similar effect on the expression of class I MHC molecules and the activation of $CD8^+$ T cells.

The expression of class II molecules is also regulated by different cytokines in different cells. IFN-γ is the principal cytokine involved in stimulating expression of class II molecules, in antigen-presenting cells such as macrophages. These cells express low levels of class II molecules until stimulated to do so by IFN-γ (see Fig. 4–11). The IFN-γ may be produced by NK cells during innate immune reactions; this is one mechanism by which innate immunity stimulates adaptive immunity. IFN-γ is also produced by antigen-activated T cells during adaptive immune reactions, and its ability to increase class II expression on antigen-presenting cells is an amplification mechanism in adaptive immunity. In dendritic cells, the expression of class II molecules increases as these cells mature, often under the influence of cytokines such as TNF. B lymphocytes constitutively express class II molecules and can increase expression in response to interleukin-4. Vascular endothelial cells, like macrophages, increase class II expression in response to IFN-γ. Most nonimmune cell types express few, if any, class II MHC molecules unless exposed to high levels of IFN-γ. These cells are unlikely to present antigens to $CD4^+$ T cells except in unusual circumstances. Some cells, such as neurons, never appear to express class II molecules. Human, but not mouse, T cells express class II molecules after activation; however, no cytokine has been identified in this response, and its functional significance is unknown.

The rate of transcription is the major determinant of the level of MHC molecule synthesis and expression on the cell surface. Cytokines enhance MHC expression by stimulating the rate of transcription of class I and class II genes in a wide variety of cell types. These effects are mediated by the binding of cytokine-activated transcription factors to regulatory DNA sequences in the promoter regions of MHC genes. Several transcription factors may be assembled and bind a protein called the class II transcription activator (CIITA), and the entire complex binds to the class II promoter and promotes efficient transcription. By keeping the complex of transcription factors together, CIITA functions as a master regulator of class II gene expression. CIITA is synthesized in response to IFN-γ, explaining how this cytokine can increase expression of class II MHC molecules. Mutations in several of these transcription factors have been identified as the cause of human immunodeficiency diseases associated with defective expression of MHC molecules. The best studied of these disorders is the **bare lymphocyte syndrome** (see Chapter 20). Knockout mice lacking CIITA also show an absence of class II expression on dendritic cells and B lymphocytes and an inability of IFN-γ to induce class II on macrophages.

The expression of many of the proteins involved in antigen processing and presentation is coordinately regulated. For instance, IFN-γ increases the transcription not only of class I and class II genes but also of β_2-microglobulin, of the genes that encode two of the subunits of the proteasome, and of the genes encoding the subunits of the TAP heterodimer.

Summary

- The MHC is a large genetic region coding for class I and class II MHC molecules as well as for other proteins. MHC genes are highly polymorphic, with more than 250 alleles for some of these genes in the population.
- MHC molecules were originally recognized for their role in triggering T cell responses that caused the rejection of transplanted tissue. It is now known that MHC-encoded class I and class II molecules bind peptide antigens and display them for recognition by antigen-specific T lymphocytes. Peptide antigens associated with class I molecules are recognized by $CD8^+$ CTLs, whereas class II–associated peptide antigens are recognized by $CD4^+$ (mostly helper) T cells.
- Class I MHC molecules are composed of an α (or heavy) chain in a noncovalent complex with a nonpolymorphic polypeptide called β_2-microglobulin. The class II molecules contain two MHC-encoded polymorphic chains, an α chain and a β chain. Both classes of MHC molecules are structurally similar and consist of an extracellular peptide-binding cleft, a nonpolymorphic Ig-like region, a transmembrane region, and a cytoplasmic region. The peptide-binding cleft of MHC molecules has α-helical sides and an eight-stranded antiparallel β-pleated sheet floor. The peptide-binding cleft of class I molecules is formed by the α1 and α2 segments of the α chain, and that of class II molecules by the α1 and β1 segments of the two chains. The Ig-like domains of class I and class II molecules contain the binding sites for the T cell coreceptors CD8 and CD4, respectively.
- MHC molecules bind only one peptide at a time, and all the peptides that bind to a particular MHC molecule share common structural motifs. Peptide binding is of low affinity (K_d ~10^{-6}M), and the off-rate is very slow, so that complexes, once formed, persist for a sufficiently long time to be recognized by T cells. The peptide-binding cleft of class I molecules can accommodate peptides that are 8 to 11 amino acid residues long, whereas the cleft of class II molecules allows larger peptides (up to 30 amino acid residues in length or more) to bind. The polymorphic residues of MHC molecules are localized to the peptide-binding domain. Some polymorphic MHC residues determine the binding specificities for peptides by forming structures, called pockets, that interact with complementary residues of the bound peptide, called anchor residues. Other polymorphic MHC residues and some residues of the peptide are not involved in binding to MHC molecules but instead form the structure recognized by T cells. Every MHC molecule has a broad specificity for peptides and can bind multiple peptides that have common structural features, such as anchor residues.
- In addition to the polymorphic class I and class II genes, the MHC contains genes encoding complement proteins, cytokines, nonpolymorphic class I–like molecules, and several proteins involved in antigen processing.
- Class I molecules are expressed on all nucleated cells, whereas class II molecules are expressed mainly on specialized antigen-presenting cells, such as dendritic cells, macrophages, and B lymphocytes, and a few other cell types, including endothelial cells and thymic epithelial cells. The expression of MHC gene products is enhanced by inflammatory and immune stimuli, particularly cytokines like IFN-γ, which stimulate the transcription of MHC genes.

Selected Readings

Bjorkman PJ, MA Saper, B Samraoui, WS Bennett, JL Strominger, and DC Wiley. Structure of the human class I histocompatibility antigen HLA-A2. Nature 329:506–512, 1987.

Campbell RD, and J Trowsdale. Map of the human MHC. Immunology Today 14:349–352, 1993.

Engelhard VH. Structure of peptides associated with class I and class II MHC molecules. Annual Review of Immunology 12:181–207, 1994.

Hammer J, T Sturniolo, and F Sinigaglia. HLA class II binding specificity and autoimmunity. Advances in Immunology 66:67–100, 1997.

Klein J, and A Sato. The HLA system. New England Journal of Medicine 343:702–709 and 782–786, 2000.

Mach B, V Steimle, E Martinez-Soria, and W Reith. Regulation of MHC class II genes: lessons from a disease. Annual Review of Immunology 14:301–331, 1996.

Madden DR. The three dimensional structure of peptide-MHC complexes. Annual Review of Immunology 13:587–622, 1995.

Parham P, and T Ohta. Population biology of antigen presentation by class I MHC molecules. Science 272:67–74, 1996.

Chapter 5

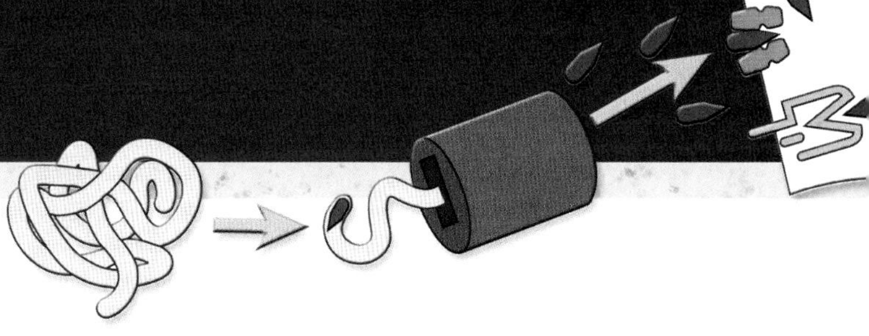

Antigen Processing and Presentation to T Lymphocytes

T lymphocytes play central roles in all adaptive immune responses against protein antigens. In cell-mediated immunity, $CD4^+$ T cells activate macrophages to destroy phagocytosed microbes, and $CD8^+$ T cells kill cells infected with intracellular microbes. In humoral immunity, $CD4^+$ helper T cells interact with B lymphocytes and stimulate the proliferation and differentiation of these B cells. Both the induction phase and the effector phase of T cell responses are triggered by the specific recognition of antigen. In Chapter 4, we introduced the concept that T cells recognize peptide fragments that are derived from protein antigens and are bound to cell surface molecules encoded by genes of the major histocompatibility complex (MHC) (see Fig. 4–1). The cells that display MHC-associated peptides are called **antigen-presenting cells** (APCs). Certain APCs present antigens to naive T cells during the recognition phase of immune responses to initiate these responses, and some APCs present antigens to differentiated T cells during the effector phase to trigger the mechanisms that eliminate the antigens. In Chapter 4, we focused on the structures and functions of MHC molecules. In this chapter, we continue the discussion of the ligands that T cells recognize by focusing on the generation of peptide-MHC complexes on APCs. Specifically, we describe the characteristics of the APCs that form and display these peptide-MHC complexes and how protein antigens are converted by APCs to peptides that associate with MHC molecules. We conclude with a discussion of the importance of MHC-restricted antigen presentation in immune responses.

Properties of Antigens Recognized by T Lymphocytes

Our current understanding of T cell antigen recognition is the culmination of a vast amount of research that began with studies of the nature of antigens that stimulate cell-mediated immunity. The early studies showed that the physicochemical forms of antigens that are recognized by T cells are different from those recognized by B lymphocytes and antibodies, and this knowledge led to the discovery of the role of the MHC in T cell antigen recognition. Several features of antigen recognition are unique to T lymphocytes (Table 5–1).

- ***Most T lymphocytes recognize only peptides,*** whereas B cells can recognize peptides, proteins, nucleic acids, polysaccharides, lipids, and small chemicals. As a result, T cell–mediated immune responses are induced only by protein antigens (the natural source of foreign peptides), whereas humoral immune responses are seen with protein and nonprotein antigens. Some T cells are specific for small chemical haptens such as dinitrophenol, urushiol of poison ivy, and β lactams of penicillin antibiotics. In these situations, it is likely that the haptens bind to self proteins and that hapten-conjugated peptides are recognized by T cells. Rare populations of T cells have been described that recognize nonpeptide antigens; these include so-called γδ T cells (see Chapter 6).
- ***T cells are specific for amino acid sequences of peptides.*** In contrast, B cells may recognize conformational determinants that exist when antigens, such as globular proteins, are in their native tertiary (folded) configuration.

  When an animal is immunized with a native protein, the antigen-specific T cells that are stimulated will respond to denatured or even proteolytically digested forms of that protein. In contrast, after immunization with a native protein, B cells produce antibodies that react with only the native protein (Table 5–2).

  The antigen receptors of T cells recognize very few residues even within a single peptide, and different T cells can distinguish peptides that differ even at single amino acid residues. We will return to the structural basis of this remarkable fine specificity of T cells in Chapter 6.
- ***T cells recognize and respond to foreign peptide antigens only when the antigens are attached to the surfaces of APCs,*** whereas B cells and secreted antibodies bind soluble antigens in body fluids as well as exposed cell surface antigens. This is because T cells can recognize only peptides bound to and displayed by MHC molecules, and MHC molecules are integral membrane proteins expressed on APCs. The properties and functions of APCs are discussed later in this chapter.
- ***T cells from any one individual recognize foreign peptide antigens only when these peptides are bound to and displayed by the MHC molecules of that individual.*** This feature of antigen recognition by T cells, called **self MHC restriction,** can be demonstrated in experimental situations in which T lymphocytes from one individual are mixed with APCs from another individual.

  The first demonstration of MHC restriction came from the studies of Rolf Zinkernagel and Peter Doherty that examined the recognition of virus-infected cells by virus-specific cytolytic T lymphocytes (CTLs) in inbred mice. If a mouse is infected with a virus, $CD8^+$ CTLs specific for the virus develop in the animal. These

Table 5–1. Features of T Cell Antigen Recognition

Features of antigens recognized by T cells	Explanation
Most T cells recognize peptides and no other molecules	Only peptides bind to MHC molecules
T cells recognize linear and not conformational determinants of peptide antigens	Peptides bind to clefts of MHC molecules in linear (extended) conformation, and extended peptides cannot form conformational determinants
T cells recognize cell-associated and not soluble antigens	MHC molecules are membrane proteins that display stably bound peptides on cell surfaces
$CD4^+$ and $CD8^+$ T cells preferentially recognize antigens sampled from the extracellular and cytosolic pools, respectively	Pathways of assembly of MHC molecules ensure that class II molecules preferentially display peptides that are derived from extracellular proteins and taken up into vesicles in APCs, and class I molecules present peptides from cytosolic proteins; CD4 and CD8 bind to nonpolymorphic regions of class II and class I, respectively

Abbreviations: APC, antigen-presenting cell; MHC, major histocompatibility complex.

Table 5–2. Differences in Antigen Recognition by T and B Lymphocytes

Primary immunization	Secondary antigen challenge	Secondary immune response	
		B cell response (Antibody production)	T cell response (Delayed-type hypersensitivity)
Native protein	Native protein	+	+
Denatured protein	Native protein	−	+
Native protein	Denatured protein	−	+
Denatured protein	Denatured protein	+	+

In an animal immunized with a protein antigen, B cells are specific for conformational determinants of the antigen and therefore distinguish between native and denatured antigens. In contrast, T cells do not distinguish between native and denatured antigens because T cells recognize linear epitopes on peptides derived from the native antigens.

CTLs recognize and lyse virus-infected cells only if the infected cells express alleles of MHC molecules that are expressed in the animal in which the CTLs were generated (Fig. 5–1). By use of MHC congenic strains of mice, it was shown that the CTLs and the infected target cell must be derived from mice that share a class I MHC allele. Thus, the recognition of antigens by $CD8^+$ CTLs is restricted by self class I MHC alleles. Essentially similar experiments demonstrated that responses of $CD4^+$ helper T lymphocytes to antigens are self class II MHC restricted.

The self MHC restriction of T cells is a consequence of selection processes during T cell maturation in the thymus, and it ensures that each individual's T cells are able to recognize foreign antigens displayed by that individual's APCs. During the maturation of T cells, the cells that express antigen receptors specific for self MHC–associated peptides are selected to survive, and the cells that do not "see" self MHC are allowed to die (see Chapter 7). This process ensures that the T cells that attain maturity are the useful ones because they will be able to recognize antigens displayed by the individual's MHC molecules. The discovery of self MHC restriction provided the definitive evidence that T cells see not only protein antigens but also polymorphic residues of MHC molecules, which are the residues that distinguish self from foreign MHC. Thus, MHC molecules display peptides for recognition by T lymphocytes and are also integral components of the ligands that T cells recognize. Although T cells are self MHC restricted, they recognize foreign MHC molecules present in tissue grafts and reject these grafts. The basis of this cross-reaction against foreign MHC molecules will be described in Chapter 16.

- ***$CD4^+$ helper T cells recognize peptides bound to class II MHC molecules, whereas $CD8^+$ CTLs recognize peptides bound to class I MHC molecules.*** Stated differently, $CD4^+$ T cells are class II MHC restricted, and $CD8^+$ T cells are class I MHC restricted. In Chapter 6, we will return to the roles of CD4 and CD8 in determining the MHC restriction patterns of T cells.

- ***$CD4^+$ class II–restricted T cells recognize peptides derived mainly from extracellular proteins that are internalized into the vesicles of APCs, whereas $CD8^+$ T cells recognize peptides derived from cytosolic, usually endogenously synthesized, proteins.*** The reason for this is that vesicular proteins enter the class II peptide loading and presentation pathway, and cytosolic proteins enter the class I pathway. The mechanisms and physiologic significance of this segregation are major themes of this chapter.

- In addition to MHC-associated presentation of peptides, there is another antigen presentation system that is specialized to present lipid antigens. The class I–like nonpolymorphic molecule CD1 is expressed on a variety of APCs and epithelia, and it presents lipid antigens to unusual populations of non–MHC-restricted T cells. Studies with culture-derived cloned lines of T cells indicate that a variety of cells can recognize lipid antigens presented by CD1; these include $CD4^+$, $CD8^+$, and $CD4^-CD8^-$ T cells expressing the αβ TCR as well as γδ T cells. There has been much interest in a small subset of T cells that express markers of NK (natural killer) cells. These are called NK-T cells, and they recognize CD1-associated lipids. However, it is not known whether CD1-restricted responses to lipid antigens are important components of host defense against microbes. In this chapter, we focus on the presentation of peptide antigens by class I and class II MHC molecules to $CD8^+$ and $CD4^+$ T lymphocytes.

Presentation of Protein Antigens to $CD4^+$ T Lymphocytes

$CD4^+$ helper T lymphocytes control virtually all immune responses to protein antigens. $CD4^+$ T cells are effector cells of cell-mediated immunity and provide stimuli that are important for the proliferation and differentiation of B lymphocytes and CTLs (see Chapters 9 and 13). Therefore, a great deal of effort has been devoted to

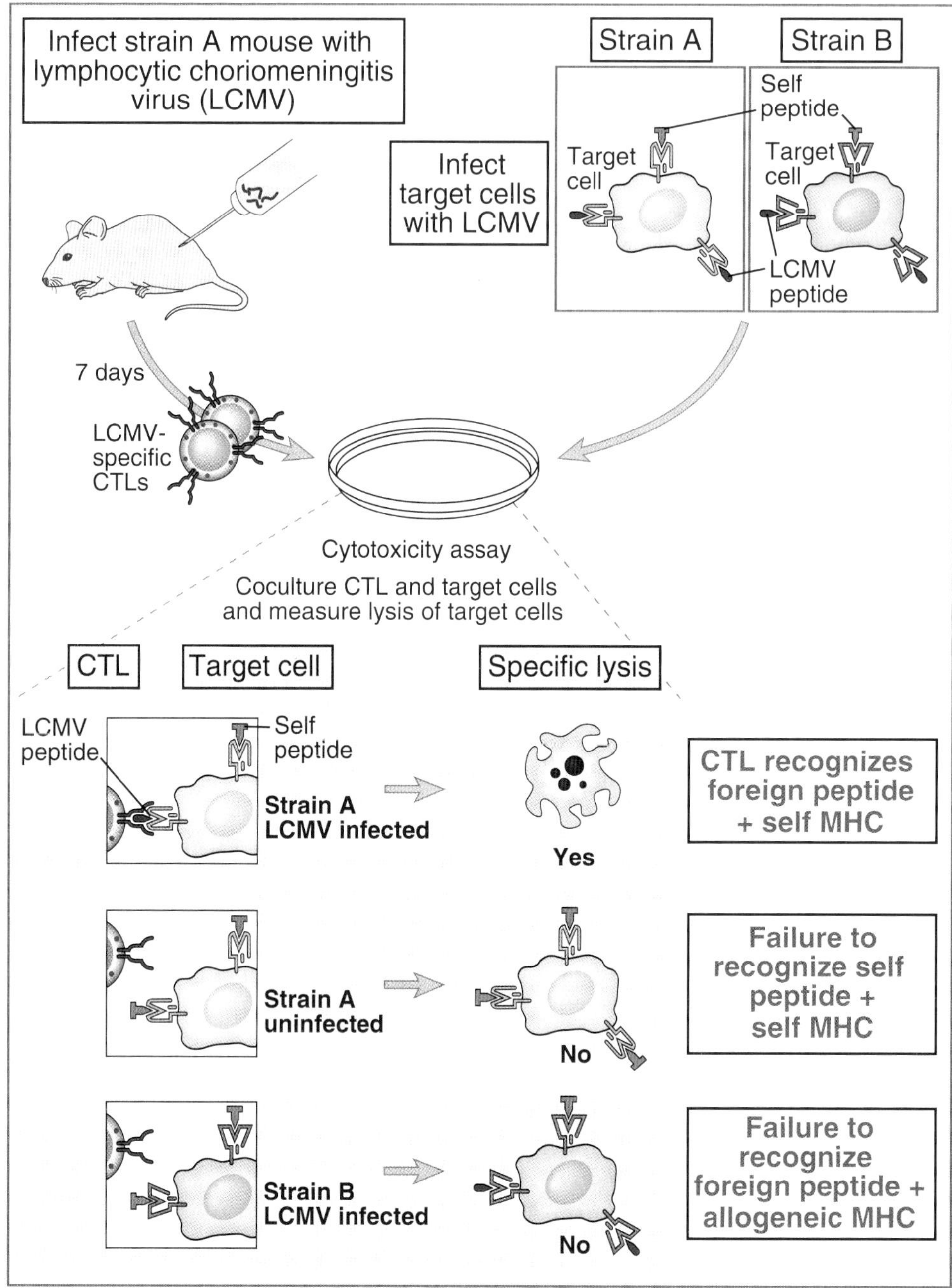

Figure 5–1 MHC restriction of cytolytic T lymphocytes.
Virus-specific cytolytic T lymphocytes (CTLs) generated from virus-infected strain A mice kill only syngeneic (strain A) target cells infected with that virus. The CTLs do not kill uninfected strain A targets (which express self peptides but not viral peptides) or infected strain B targets (which express different MHC alleles than does strain A). By use of congenic mouse strains that differ only at class I MHC loci, it has been proved that recognition of antigen by $CD8^+$ CTLs is self class I MHC restricted.

defining how antigens are presented to helper T cells to initiate immune responses. From these studies, it has become apparent that only a few cell types that express class II MHC molecules can function as APCs for $CD4^+$ T lymphocytes. In this section of the chapter, we describe the APCs that are involved in activating $CD4^+$ T cells and the functions of these APCs in immune responses to protein antigens.

Discovery of Antigen-Presenting Cells and Their Role in Immune Responses

The responses of antigen-specific T lymphocytes to protein antigens require the participation of antigen-presenting cells (APCs), which capture and display the antigens to T cells. This conclusion is based on several lines of experimental evidence.

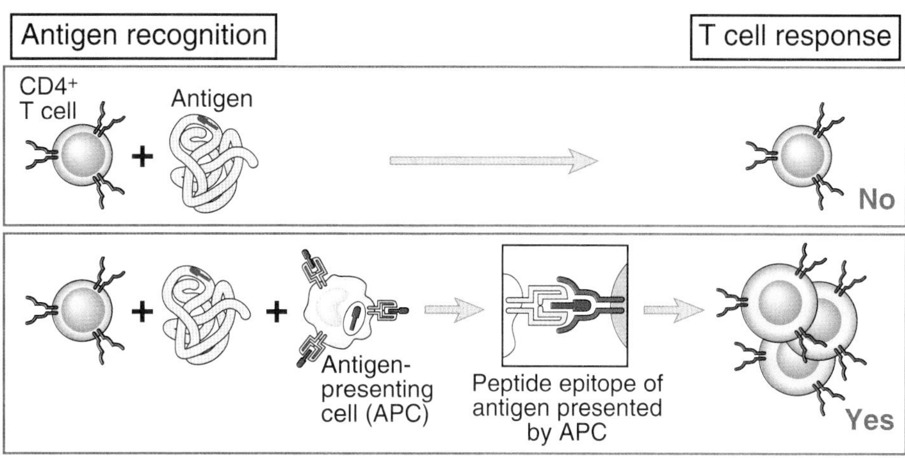

Figure 5–2 Antigen-presenting cells are required for T cell activation.
Purified $CD4^+$ T cells do not respond to a protein antigen by itself but do respond to the antigen in the presence of an antigen-presenting cell (APC). The function of the APCs is to present a peptide derived from the antigen to the T cell. APCs also express costimulators that are important for T cell activation; these are not shown.

- T cells present in the blood, spleen, or lymph nodes of individuals immunized with a protein antigen can be activated by exposure to that antigen in tissue culture. If contaminating dendritic cells, macrophages, and B cells are removed from the cultures, the purified T lymphocytes do not respond to the antigen, and responsiveness can be restored by adding back dendritic cells, macrophages, or B lymphocytes (Fig. 5–2). Such experimental approaches are commonly used to determine which cell types are able to function as APCs for the activation of T lymphocytes.
- If an antigen is taken up by macrophages or other APCs *in vitro* and then injected into mice, the amount of cell-associated antigen required to induce a response is 1000 times less than the amount of the same antigen required when administered by itself in a cell-free form. In other words, cell-associated proteins are much more immunogenic than are soluble proteins on a molar basis. The explanation for this finding is that the immunogenic form of the antigen is the APC-associated form, and only a small fraction of injected free antigen ends up associated with APCs *in vivo*. This concept is now being exploited to immunize patients with cancer against their tumors by growing APCs (specifically, dendritic cells) from these patients, incubating the APCs with tumor antigens, and injecting them back into the patients as a cell-based vaccine.

APCs serve two important functions in the activation of $CD4^+$ T cells. First, APCs convert protein antigens to peptides, and they display peptide-MHC complexes for recognition by the T cells. The conversion of native proteins to MHC-associated peptide fragments by APCs is called **antigen processing** and is discussed later in the chapter. Second, some APCs provide stimuli to the T cell beyond those initiated by recognition of peptide-MHC complexes by the T cell antigen receptor. These stimuli, referred to as **costimulators,** are required for the full responses of the T cells. The nature and mode of action of costimulators are discussed further in Chapters 6 and 8.

To induce a T cell response to a protein antigen in a vaccine or experimentally, the antigen must be administered with substances called adjuvants. Adjuvants promote T cell activation by several mechanisms. Adjuvants induce local inflammation and thus stimulate the influx of APCs to sites of antigen exposure. Adjuvants activate APCs to increase the expression of costimulators and to produce soluble proteins, called cytokines, that stimulate T cell responses. Some adjuvants may also act on APCs to prolong the persistence of peptide-MHC complexes on the cell surface. Protein antigens administered in aqueous form, without adjuvants, either fail to induce T cell responses or induce a state of unresponsiveness, called tolerance (see Chapter 10). Microbes produce substances that, like adjuvants, elicit innate immune reactions that stimulate T cell responses (see Chapter 12). In fact, many potent adjuvants are products of microbes, such as killed mycobacteria. It is not possible to use most of these microbial adjuvants in humans because of the pathologic inflammation that microbial products elicit. Attempts are ongoing to develop adjuvants for clinical use, mainly to maximize the immunogenicity of vaccines.

Types of Antigen-Presenting Cells for $CD4^+$ Helper T Lymphocytes

The two requisite properties that allow a cell to function as an APC for class II MHC–restricted helper T lymphocytes are the ability to process endocytosed antigens and the expression of class II MHC gene products. Most mammalian cells are capable of endocytosing and proteolytically digesting protein antigens, but only specialized cell populations normally express class II MHC molecules.

The best defined APCs for helper T lymphocytes are dendritic cells, mononuclear phagocytes, and B lymphocytes, and they play different roles in T cell responses (Fig. 5–3 and Table 5–3). Dendritic cells are the most effective APCs for initiating T cell responses, macrophages present antigens to differentiated (effector) $CD4^+$ T cells in the effector phase of cell-mediated immunity, and B lymphocytes present antigens to helper T cells during humoral immune responses. Dendritic cells, macrophages, and B lymphocytes have also been called professional APCs; however, this term is sometimes used to refer only to dendritic cells because this is the only cell type specialized to serve the sole function of antigen capture and presentation.

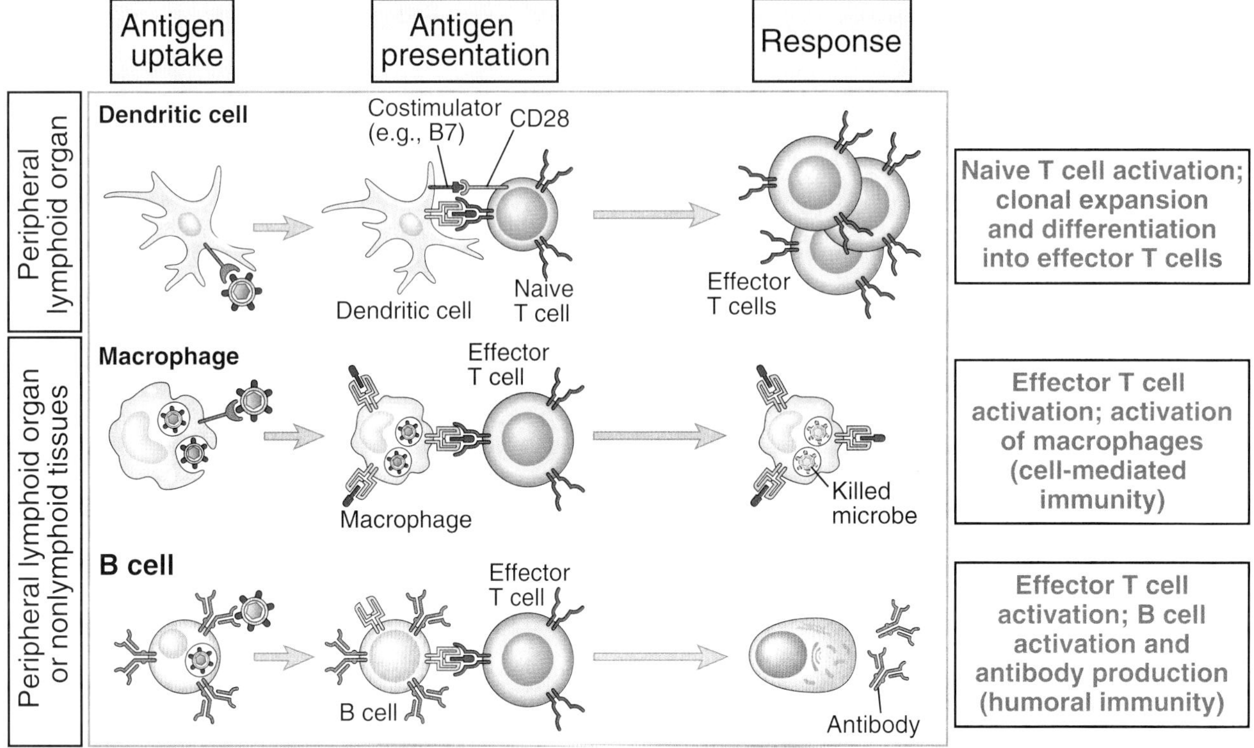

Figure 5–3 Functions of different antigen-presenting cells.
The three major types of antigen-presenting cells for $CD4^+$ T cells function to display antigens at different stages and in different types of immune responses. Note that effector T cells activate macrophages and B lymphocytes by production of cytokines and by expressing surface molecules; these will be described in later chapters.

Table 5–3. Properties and Functions of Antigen-Presenting Cells

Cell type	Expression of		Principal function
	Class II MHC	Costimulators	
Dendritic cells	Constitutive; increases with maturation; increased by IFN-γ	Constitutive; increases with maturation; inducible by IFN-γ, CD40-CD40L interactions	Initiation of T cell responses to protein antigens (priming)
Macrophages	Low or negative; inducible by IFN-γ	Inducible by LPS, IFN-γ, CD40-CD40L interactions	Effector phase of cell-mediated immune responses
B lymphocytes	Constitutive; increased by IL-4	Induced by T cells (CD40-CD40L interactions), antigen receptor cross-linking	Antigen presentation to $CD4^+$ helper T cells in humoral immune responses (cognate T cell–B cell interactions)
Vascular endothelial cells	Inducible by IFN-γ; constitutive in humans	Constitutive (inducible in mice)	May promote activation of antigen-specific T cells at site of antigen exposure
Various epithelial and mesenchymal cells	Inducible by IFN-γ	Probably none	No known physiologic function

Dendritic cells are present in lymphoid organs, in the epithelia of the skin and gastrointestinal and respiratory tracts, and in most parenchymal organs. These cells are identified morphologically by their membranous or spinelike projections (Fig. 5–4). All dendritic cells are thought to arise from bone marrow precursors, and most, called myeloid dendritic cells, are related in lineage to mononuclear phagocytes. Immature dendritic cells are located in the epithelia of the skin and gastrointestinal and respiratory systems, which are the main portals through which microbes can enter. The prototypes of immature dendritic cells are the Langerhans cells of the epidermis. Because of their long cytoplasmic processes, Langerhans cells occupy as much as 25% of the surface area of the epidermis, even though they constitute less than 1% of the cell population. The function

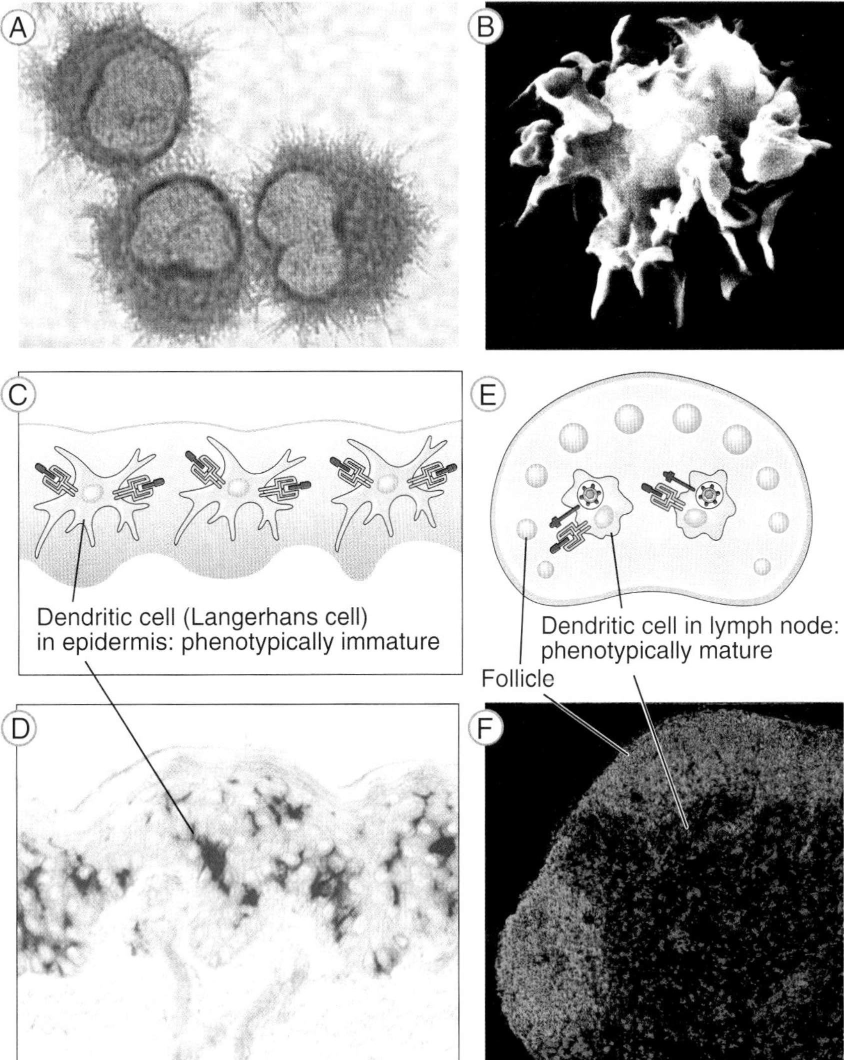

Figure 5–4 Dendritic cells.
A. Light micrograph of cultured dendritic cells derived from bone marrow precursors. (Courtesy of Dr. Y-J. Liu, DNAX, Palo Alto, Calif.)
B. A scanning electron micrograph of a dendritic cell, showing the extensive membrane projections. (Courtesy of Dr. Y-J. Liu, DNAX, Palo Alto, Calif.)
C, D. Dendritic cells in the skin, illustrated schematically (C) and in a section of the skin stained with an antibody specific for Langerhans cells (which appear blue in this immunoenzyme stain) (D). (The micrograph of the skin is courtesy of Dr. Y-J. Liu, DNAX, Palo Alto, Calif.)
E, F. Dendritic cells in a lymph node, illustrated schematically (E) and in a section of a mouse lymph node stained with fluorescently labeled antibodies against B cells in follicles (green) and dendritic cells in the T cell zone (red) (F). (The micrograph is courtesy of Drs. Kathryn Pape and Jennifer Walter, University of Minnesota School of Medicine, Minneapolis.)

of epithelial dendritic cells is to capture microbial protein antigens and to transport the antigens to draining lymph nodes. During their migration to the lymph nodes, the dendritic cells mature to become extremely efficient at presenting antigens and stimulating naive T cells. Mature dendritic cells reside in the T cell zones of the lymph nodes, and in this location they display antigens to the T cells. These lymph node dendritic cells are called interdigitating dendritic cells or, simply, dendritic cells. There are subsets of dendritic cells that may be distinguished by the expression of various cell surface markers. Studies are ongoing to determine whether these subsets are important in initiating different types of T cell responses. The process of antigen capture by dendritic cells is described more fully later.

Macrophages are APCs that actively phagocytose large particles. Therefore, they play an important role in presenting antigens derived from phagocytosed infectious organisms such as bacteria and parasites. In the effector phase of cell-mediated immunity, differentiated effector T cells recognize microbial antigens on phagocytes and activate the macrophages to destroy the phagocytosed microbes (see Chapter 13). Most macrophages express low levels of class II MHC molecules, and much higher levels are induced by the cytokine interferon-γ (IFN-γ). This is a mechanism by which IFN-γ enhances antigen presentation and T cell activation (see Chapter 4, Fig. 4–11).

B lymphocytes use their antigen receptors to bind and internalize soluble protein antigens and present processed peptides derived from these proteins to helper T cells. The antigen-presenting function of B cells is essential for helper T cell–dependent antibody production (see Chapter 9).

Vascular endothelial cells in humans express class II MHC molecules and may present antigens to blood T cells that have become adherent to the vessel wall. This may contribute to the recruitment and activation of T cells in cell-mediated immune reactions (see Chapter 13). Endothelial cells in grafts are also targets of T cells reacting against graft antigens (see Chapter 16). Various epithelial and mesenchymal cells may express class II MHC molecules in response to IFN-γ. The physiologic significance of antigen presentation by these cell populations is unclear. Because they generally do not express costimulators, it is unlikely that they play an important role in most T cell responses. Thymic epithelial cells constitutively express class II MHC molecules and play a specialized role in presenting peptide-MHC complexes to maturing T cells in the thymus as part of the selection processes that shape the repertoire of T cell specificities (see Chapter 7).

Capture and Presentation of Protein Antigens *in Vivo*

The responses of CD4⁺ T cells are initiated in the peripheral lymphoid organs, to which protein antigens are transported after being collected from their portal of entry (Fig. 5–5). The common routes through which foreign antigens, such as microbes, enter a host are the skin and the epithelia of the gastrointestinal and respiratory systems. In addition, microbial antigens may be produced in any tissue that has been infected. The skin, mucosal epithelia, and parenchymal organs contain numerous lymphatic capillaries that drain lymph from these sites and into the regional lymph nodes. The lymph drained from the skin, mucosa, and other sites contains a sampling of all the soluble and particulate antigens present in these tissues. Lymph nodes that are interposed along lymphatic vessels act as filters that sample the lymph at numerous points before it reaches the blood (see Fig. 2–12, Chapter 2). Antigens that enter the blood stream may be similarly sampled by the spleen.

Immature dendritic cells that are resident in epithelia and tissues capture protein antigens and transport the antigens to draining lymph nodes (Fig. 5–6). Immature dendritic cells express membrane receptors that bind microbes, such as receptors for mannose and Toll-like receptors (see Chapter 12). Dendritic cells use these receptors to capture microbial antigens, to endocytose the antigens, and to begin to process the proteins into peptides capable of binding to MHC molecules. Microbes also stimulate innate immune reactions, during which inflammatory cytokines are produced. The combination of microbes and cytokines activates the dendritic cells. The cells lose their adhesiveness for epithelia and begin to express a chemokine receptor

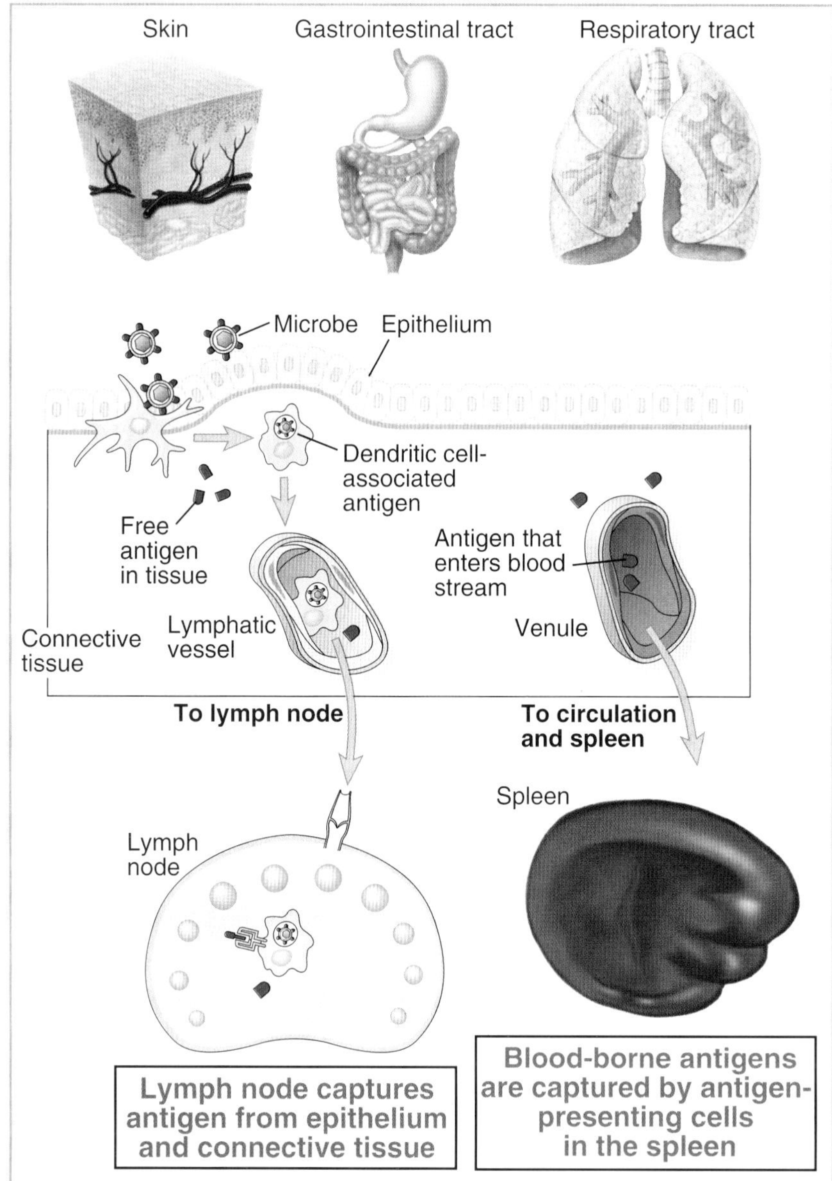

Figure 5–5 Routes of antigen entry. Microbial antigens commonly enter through the skin and gastrointestinal and respiratory tracts, where they are captured by dendritic cells and transported to regional lymph nodes. Antigens that enter the blood stream are captured by antigen-presenting cells in the spleen.

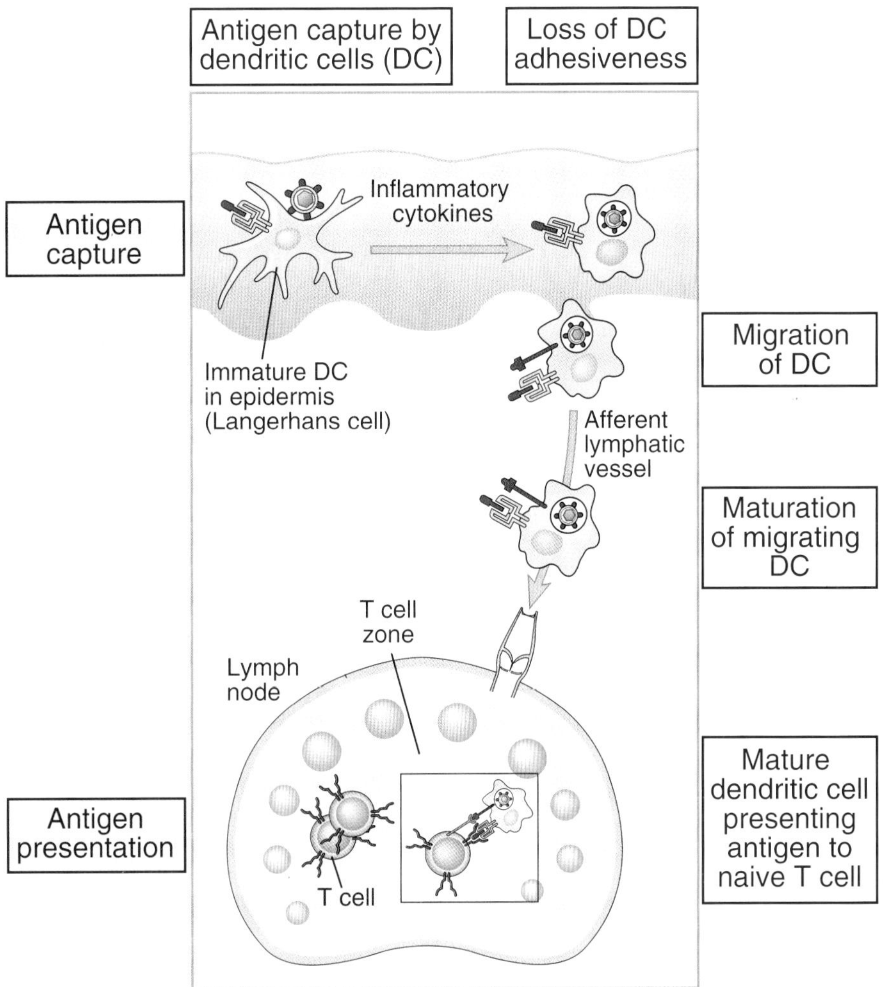

	Immature dendritic cell	Mature dendritic cell
Principal function	Antigen capture	Antigen presentation to T cells
Expression of Fc receptors, mannose receptors	++	–
Expression of molecules involved in T cell activation: B7, ICAM-1, IL-12	– or low	++
Class II MHC molecules		
Half-life on surface	~10 hr	>100 hr
Number of surface molecules	~10^6	~7×10^6

Figure 5–6 Role of dendritic cells in antigen capture and presentation. Immature dendritic cells in the skin (Langerhans cells) capture antigens that enter through the epidermis and transport the antigens to regional lymph nodes. During this migration, the dendritic cells mature and become efficient antigen-presenting cells. The table summarizes some of the changes during dendritic cell maturation that are important in the functions of these cells.

called CCR7 that is specific for chemokines produced in the T cell zones of lymph nodes. The chemokines attract the dendritic cells bearing microbial antigens into the T cell zones of the regional lymph nodes. (Recall that in Chapter 2 we mentioned that naive T cells also express CCR7, and this is why naive T cells migrate to the same regions of lymph nodes where antigen-bearing dendritic cells are concentrated.) Immature dendritic cells that have encountered microbes and are transporting microbial antigens to lymph nodes mature during this migration from cells whose function is to capture antigen into cells that are able to display antigens to naive T cells and activate the cells. Mature dendritic cells express high levels of class II MHC molecules with bound peptides as well as costimulators required for T cell activation. This process of maturation can be reproduced *in vitro* by culturing bone marrow–derived immature dendritic cells with cytokines (such as tumor necrosis factor and granulocyte-macrophage colony-stimulating factor) and microbial products (such as endotoxin). Thus, by the time these cells become resident in lymph nodes, they have developed into potent APCs. Naive T lymphocytes that recirculate through lymph nodes encounter these APCs. T cells that are specific for the displayed peptide-MHC complexes are activated, and an immune response is initiated.

Dendritic cells are the most effective APCs for initiating primary T cell responses, for several reasons. First, dendritic cells are strategically located at the common sites of entry of microbes and foreign antigens and in organs that may be colonized by microbes. Second, dendritic cells express receptors that enable them to capture microbes. Third, these cells migrate preferentially to the T cell zones of lymph nodes, through which naive T lymphocytes circulate searching for foreign antigens. Fourth, mature dendritic cells express costimulators, which are needed to activate naive T cells.

Antigens may also be transported to lymph nodes in soluble form. When lymph enters a lymph node through an afferent lymphatic vessel, it percolates through the node. Here, the lymph-borne soluble antigens can be extracted from the fluid by APCs, such as dendritic cells and macrophages. Macrophages, through phagocytosis, are particularly adept at extracting particulate and opsonized antigens. B cells in the node may also recognize and internalize soluble antigens. Dendritic cells, macrophages, and B cells that have taken up protein antigens can then process and present these antigens to naive T cells and to effector T cells that have been generated by previous antigen stimulation. Thus, APC populations in lymph nodes accumulate and concentrate antigens and display them in a form that can be recognized by antigen-specific $CD4^+$ T lymphocytes.

The collection and concentration of foreign antigens in lymph nodes are supplemented by two other anatomic adaptations that serve similar functions. First, the mucosal surfaces of the gastrointestinal and respiratory systems, in addition to being drained by lymphatic capillaries, contain specialized collections of secondary lymphoid tissue that can directly sample the luminal contents of these organs for the presence of antigenic material. The best characterized of these mucosal lymphoid organs are Peyer's patches of the ileum and the pharyngeal tonsils. Second, the blood stream is monitored by APCs in the spleen for any antigens that reach the circulation. Such antigens may reach the blood either directly from the tissues or by way of the lymph from the thoracic duct.

In the effector phase of $CD4^+$ T cell responses, previously activated effector or memory cells may recognize and respond to antigens in nonlymphoid tissues. Foreign antigens can, of course, be produced in any tissue that is infected or into which an antigen is introduced. The effector phase of the immune response is designed to eliminate the antigen in any tissue. Previously activated T cells migrate to peripheral sites of inflammation or infection, where antigens are presented by macrophages and other APCs. This process will be described in more detail when we discuss cell-mediated immunity (see Chapter 13). In humoral immune responses, B lymphocytes that recognize antigens internalize and process these antigens and present peptides to differentiated helper T cells. This process occurs mostly in lymphoid organs and is described in Chapter 9.

Presentation of Protein Antigens to $CD8^+$ T Lymphocytes

All nucleated cells can present class I MHC–associated peptides, derived from cytosolic protein antigens, to $CD8^+$ T lymphocytes because all nucleated cells express class I MHC molecules. Most foreign protein antigens that are present in the cytosol are endogenously synthesized, such as viral proteins in virus-infected cells and mutated proteins in tumor cells. All nucleated cells are susceptible to viral infections and cancer-causing mutations. Therefore, it is important that the immune system be able to recognize cytosolic antigens harbored in any cell type. Differentiated $CD8^+$ T cells, which function as CTLs, are able to recognize class I–associated peptides and to kill any antigen-expressing cell. The ubiquitous expression of class I molecules allows class I–restricted CTLs to recognize and eliminate any type of virus-infected or tumor cell. Phagocytosed particulate antigens may also be recognized by $CD8^+$ CTLs because some proteins may be transported from phagocytic vesicles into the cytosol.

The induction of a primary CTL response poses a special problem because the antigen may be produced by a cell type, such as a virus-infected or tumor cell, that is not an APC. To be activated to proliferate and differentiate into effector CTLs, naive $CD8^+$ T cells must recognize class I–associated peptide antigens and also encounter costimulators on APCs or signals provided by helper T cells. It is likely that virus-infected or tumor cells are captured by APCs, such as dendritic cells, and that the viral or tumor antigens are presented to naive $CD8^+$ T cells by the APCs to initiate a primary response (Fig. 5–7). This process is called cross-presentation, or cross-priming, to indicate that one cell type (the APC) can present antigens from another cell (the virus-infected or tumor cell) and prime, or activate, T cells specific for these antigens. We will return to a discussion of CTL responses in Chapter 13.

Cell Biology of Antigen Processing

The pathways of antigen processing convert protein antigens derived from the extracellular space or the cytosol into peptides and load these peptides onto MHC molecules for display to T lymphocytes (Fig. 5–8). Our understanding of the cell biology of antigen

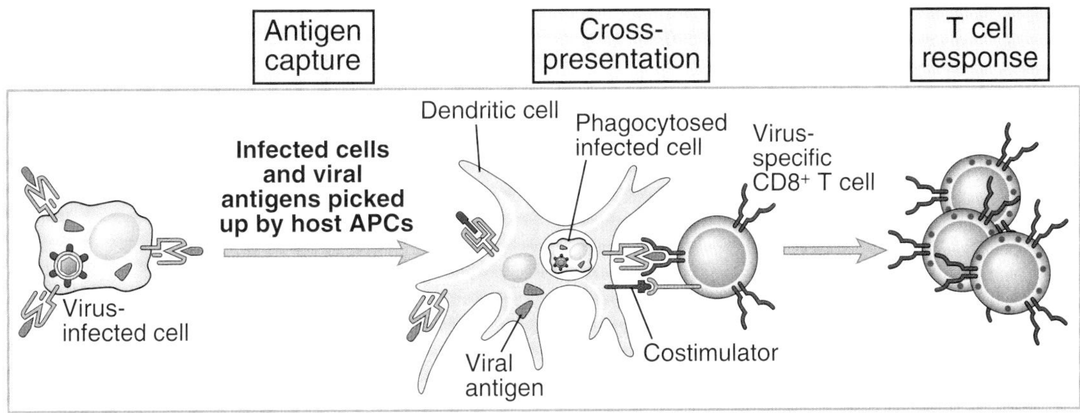

Figure 5–7 Cross-presentation of antigens to CD8$^+$ T cells.
Cells infected with intracellular microbes, such as viruses, are captured by professional antigen-presenting cells (APCs), particularly dendritic cells, and the antigens of the infectious microbes are broken down and presented in association with the MHC molecules of the APCs. T cells recognize the microbial antigens and costimulators expressed on the APCs, and the T cells are activated. This example shows CD8$^+$ T cells recognizing class I MHC–associated antigens; the same cross-presenting APC may display class II MHC–associated antigens from the microbe for recognition by CD4$^+$ helper T cells.

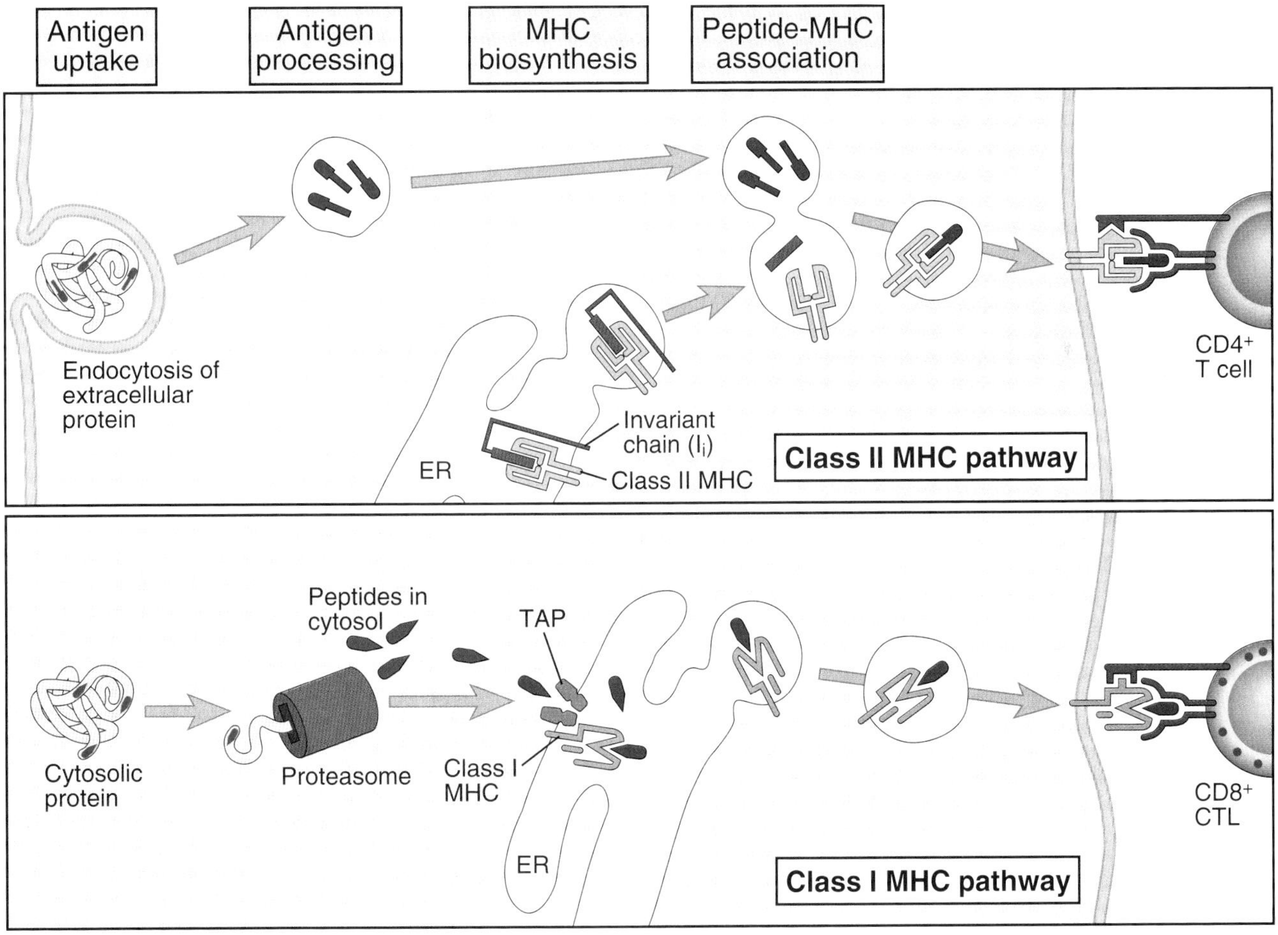

Figure 5–8 Pathways of antigen processing and presentation.
In the class II MHC pathway *(top panel),* extracellular protein antigens are endocytosed into vesicles, where the antigens are processed and the peptides bind to class II MHC molecules. In the class I MHC pathway *(bottom panel),* protein antigens in the cytosol are processed by proteasomes, and peptides are transported into the endoplasmic reticulum (ER), where they bind to class I MHC molecules. Details of these processing pathways are in Figures 5–10 and 5–14. TAP, transporter associated with antigen processing.

processing has increased greatly since the 1980s with the discovery and characterization of the molecules and organelles that generate peptides from intact proteins and promote the assembly and peptide loading of MHC molecules. Both class I and class II MHC pathways of antigen processing and presentation use subcellular organelles and enzymes that have generalized protein degradation and recycling functions that are not exclusively used for antigen display to the immune system. In other words, both class I and class II MHC antigen presentation pathways have evolved as adaptations of basic cellular functions. The cellular pathways of antigen processing are designed to generate peptides that have the structural characteristics required for associating with MHC molecules and to place these peptides in the same cellular location as the appropriate MHC molecules with available peptide-binding clefts. Peptide binding to MHC molecules occurs before cell surface expression and is an integral component of the biosynthesis and assembly of MHC molecules. In fact, peptide association is required for the stable assembly and surface expression of both class I and class II MHC molecules.

Protein antigens present in acidic vesicular compartments of APCs generate class II–associated peptides, whereas antigens present in the cytosol generate class I–associated peptides. The different fates of vesicular and cytosolic antigens are due to the segregated pathways of biosynthesis and assembly of class I and class II MHC molecules (see Fig. 5–8).

This fundamental difference between vesicular and cytosolic antigens was demonstrated experimentally by analyzing the presentation of the same antigen introduced into APCs in different ways (Fig. 5–9). If a globular protein is added in soluble form to APCs and endocytosed into the vesicles of the APCs, it is subsequently presented as class II–associated peptides and is recognized by antigen-specific $CD4^+$ T cells. In contrast, the same protein antigen produced in the cyto-

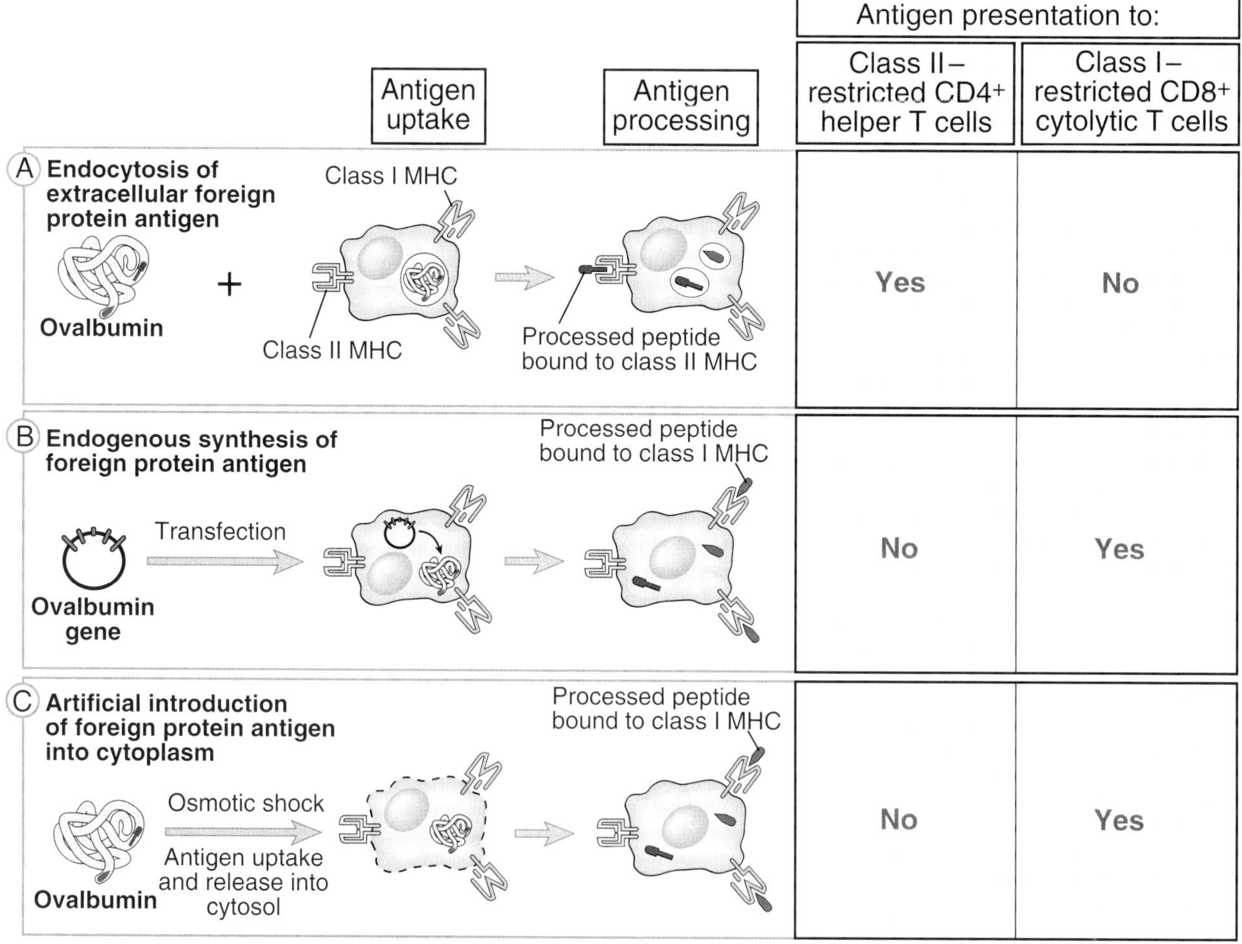

Figure 5–9 Presentation of extracellular and cytosolic antigens.
When a model protein ovalbumin is added as an extracellular antigen to an antigen-presenting cell that expresses both class I and class II MHC molecules, ovalbumin-derived peptides are presented only in association with class II molecules (A). When ovalbumin is synthesized intracellularly as a result of transfection of its gene (B), or when it is introduced into the cytoplasm through membranes made leaky by osmotic shock (C), ovalbumin-derived peptides are presented in association with class I MHC molecules. The measured response of class II–restricted helper T cells is cytokine secretion, and the measured response of class I–restricted CTLs is killing of the antigen-presenting cells.

plasm of APCs as the product of a transfected gene, or introduced directly into the cytoplasm of the APCs by osmotic shock, is presented in the form of class I–associated peptides that are recognized by $CD8^+$ T cells.

The major comparative features of the class I and class II MHC pathways of antigen presentation are summarized in Table 5–4. In the following sections, we describe these pathways individually in more detail.

Processing of Endocytosed Antigens for Class II MHC–Associated Presentation

The generation of class II MHC–associated peptides from endocytosed antigens involves the proteolytic degradation of internalized proteins in endocytic vesicles and the binding of peptides to class II MHC molecules in these vesicles. This sequence of events is illustrated in Figure 5–10, and the individual steps are described here.

1. UPTAKE OF EXTRACELLULAR PROTEINS INTO VESICULAR COMPARTMENTS OF APCS

Most class II–associated peptides are derived from protein antigens that are captured and internalized into endosomes by specialized APCs. The initial steps in the presentation of an extracellular protein antigen are the binding of the native antigen to an APC and the internalization of the antigen. Different APCs can bind protein antigens in several ways and with varying efficiencies and specificities. Dendritic cells and macrophages express a variety of surface receptors that recognize structures shared by many microbes (see Chapter 12). Thus, these APCs bind and internalize microbes efficiently. Macrophages also express receptors for the Fc portions of antibodies and receptors for the complement protein C3b, which bind antigens with attached antibodies or complement proteins and enhance their internalization. Another example of specific receptors on APCs is the surface immunoglobulin on B cells, which, because of its high affinity for antigens, can effectively mediate the internalization of proteins present at very low concentrations in the extracellular fluid (see Chapter 9).

After their internalization, protein antigens become localized in intracellular membrane-bound vesicles called **endosomes.** Endosomes are vesicles with acidic pH that contain proteolytic enzymes. The endosomal pathway of intracellular protein traffic communicates with lysosomes, which are more dense membrane-bound enzyme-containing vesicles. A subset of class II

Table 5–4. Comparative Features of Class II and Class I MHC Pathways of Antigen Processing and Presentation

Feature	Class II MHC pathway	Class I MHC pathway
Composition of stable peptide-MHC complex	Polymorphic α and β chains, peptide 	Polymorphic α chain, β_2-microglobulin, peptide
Types of APCs	Dendritic cells, mononuclear phagocytes, B lymphocytes; endothelial cells, thymic epithelium	All nucleated cells
Responsive T cells	$CD4^+$ T cells	$CD8^+$ T cells
Source of protein antigens	Endosomal/lysosomal proteins (mostly internalized from extracellular environment)	Cytosolic proteins (mostly synthesized in the cell; may enter cytosol from phagosomes)
Enzymes responsible for peptide generation	Endosomal and lysosomal proteases (e.g., cathepsins)	Cytosolic proteasome
Site of peptide loading of MHC	Specialized vesicular compartment	Endoplasmic reticulum
Molecules involved in transport of peptides and loading of MHC molecules	Calnexin in ER; invariant chain in ER, Golgi and MIIC/CIIV; DM	Calnexin, calreticulin, TAP in ER

Abbreviations: APC, antigen-presenting cell; CIIV, class II vesicle ; ER, endoplasmic reticulum; MHC, major histocompatibility complex; MIIC, MHC class II compartment; TAP, transporter associated with antigen processing.

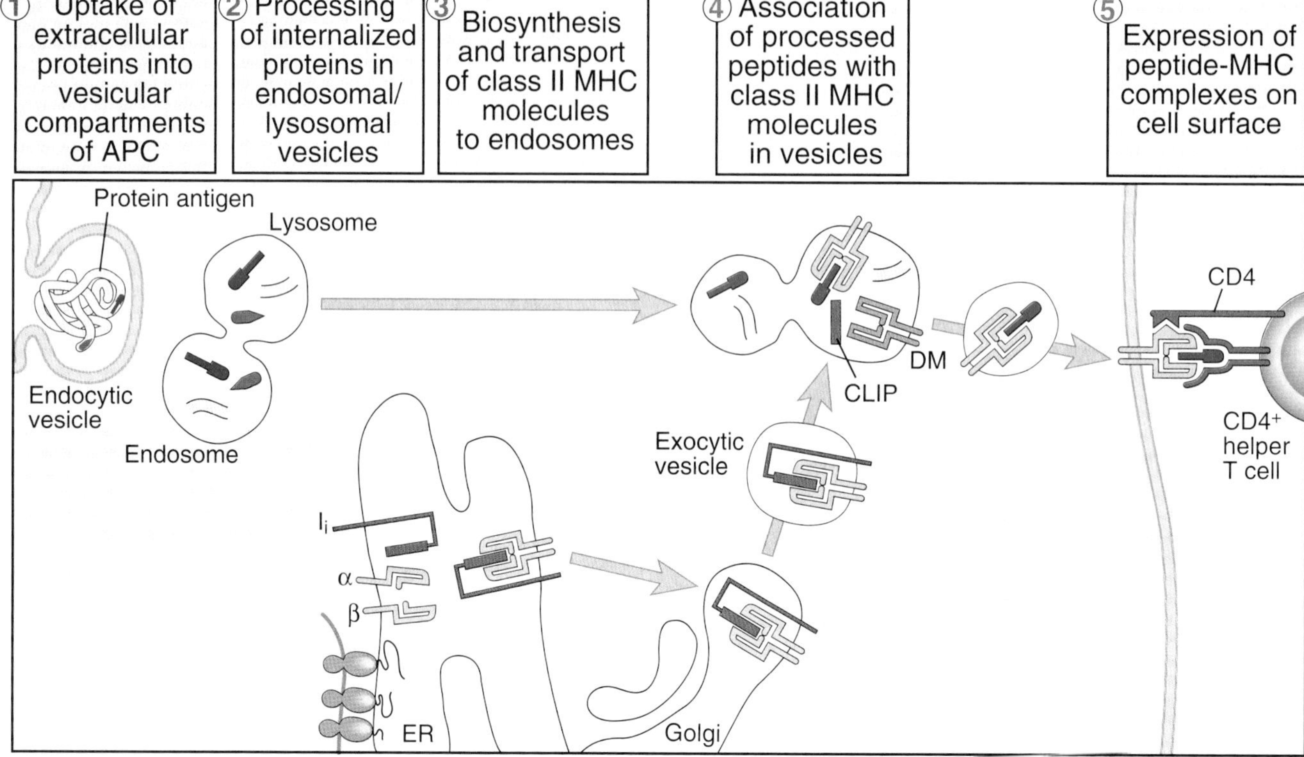

Figure 5–10 The class II MHC pathway of antigen presentation.
The numbered stages in processing of extracellular antigens correspond to the stages described in the text. APC, antigen-presenting cell; CLIP, class II–associated invariant chain peptide; ER, endoplasmic reticulum; I_i, invariant chain.

MHC–rich endosomes plays a special role in antigen processing and presentation by the class II pathway; this is described next. Particulate microbes are internalized into vesicles called **phagosomes,** which may fuse with lysosomes, producing vesicles called phagolysosomes or secondary lysosomes. Some microbes, such as mycobacteria and *Leishmania,* may survive and even replicate within phagosomes or endosomes, providing a persistent source of antigens in vesicular compartments.

2. PROCESSING OF INTERNALIZED PROTEINS IN ENDOSOMAL AND LYSOSOMAL VESICLES

Internalized proteins are degraded enzymatically in endosomes and lysosomes to generate peptides, many of which have the structural properties that enable them to bind to the peptide-binding clefts of class II MHC molecules. The degradation of protein antigens in vesicles is an active process mediated by proteases that have acidic pH optima.

- The processing of soluble proteins by macrophages (and other APCs) is inhibited by rendering the APCs metabolically inert by chemical fixation (Fig. 5–11) or by increasing the pH of intracellular acid vesicles with agents such as chloroquine.
- Several types of proteases, notably cathepsins (see following), are present in endosomes and lysosomes, and specific inhibitors of these enzymes block the presentation of protein antigens by APCs.
- The processed forms of most protein antigens that T cells recognize can be artificially generated by proteolysis in the test tube. Macrophages that are chemically fixed or treated with chloroquine before they have processed a protein antigen can effectively present predigested peptide fragments of that antigen, but not the intact protein, to specific T cells (see Fig. 5–11).

The enzymes that degrade protein antigens in the endosomes are not fully defined. The most abundant proteases of endosomes are cathepsins, which are thiol and aspartyl proteases with broad substrate specificities. Cathepsins may play an important role in generating peptides for the class II pathway. Knockout mice lacking cathepsin S show defects in class II–associated antigen presentation.

Although most class II MHC–binding peptides are derived from proteins internalized from the extracellular milieu, cytoplasmic and membrane proteins may also occasionally enter the class II pathway. In some cases, this may result from the normal cellular pathway for the turnover of cytoplasmic contents, referred to as autophagy. In this pathway, cytoplasmic proteins are trapped within endoplasmic reticulum (ER)–derived vesicles called autophagosomes; these vesicles fuse with lysosomes, and the cytoplasmic proteins are proteolytically degraded. The peptides generated by this route may be delivered to the same class II–bearing vesicular compartment as are peptides derived from extracellular antigens. Some peptides that associate with class II

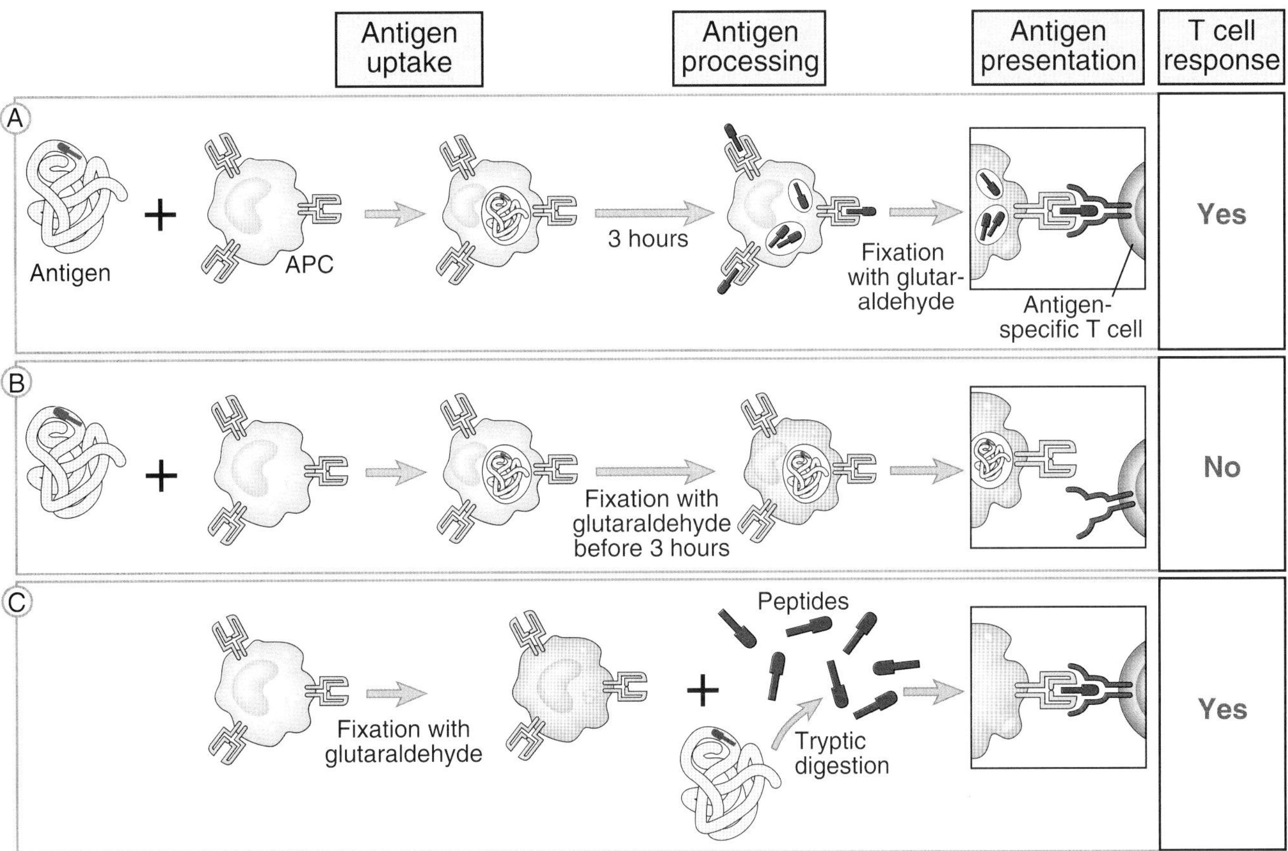

Figure 5–11 Antigen processing requires time and cellular metabolism and can be mimicked by *in vitro* proteolysis.

If an antigen-presenting cell (APC) is allowed to process antigen and is then chemically fixed (rendered metabolically inert) 3 hours or more after antigen internalization, it is capable of presenting antigen to T cells (A). Antigen is not processed or presented if APCs are fixed less than 3 hours after antigen uptake (B). Fixed APCs bind and present proteolytic fragments of antigens to specific T cells (C). The artificial proteolysis therefore mimics physiologic antigen processing by APCs. Effective antigen presentation is assayed by measuring a T cell response, such as cytokine secretion. (Note that this type of experiment is done with populations of antigen-specific T cells, such as T cell hybridomas, which respond to processed antigens on fixed APCs, but that normal T cells require costimulators that may be destroyed by fixation. Also, the time required for antigen processing is 3 hours in this experiment, but it may be different with other antigens and APCs.)

molecules are derived from membrane proteins. Before they are expressed on the surface, these proteins may have ready access to class II MHC molecules because they would be synthesized and transported through the same ER-Golgi compartments as the class II molecules. It is also possible that after cell surface expression, some membrane proteins reenter the cell by the same endocytic pathway as extracellular proteins. Thus, even viruses, which replicate in the cytoplasm of infected cells, may produce cytoplasmic and membrane proteins that are degraded into peptides that enter the class II MHC pathway of antigen presentation. This may be a mechanism for the activation of viral antigen–specific CD4$^+$ helper T cells.

3. BIOSYNTHESIS AND TRANSPORT OF CLASS II MHC MOLECULES TO ENDOSOMES

Class II MHC molecules are synthesized in the ER and transported to endosomes with an associated protein called the invariant chain (I_i), which occupies the peptide-binding clefts of the newly synthesized class II molecules. The α and β chains of class II MHC molecules are coordinately synthesized and associate with each other in the ER. Nascent class II dimers are structurally unstable, and their folding and assembly are aided by ER-resident chaperones, such as calnexin. The nonpolymorphic I_i also associates with the class II MHC αβ heterodimers in the ER. The I_i is a trimer composed of three 30-kD subunits, each of which binds one newly synthesized class II αβ heterodimer in a way that interferes with peptide loading of the cleft formed by the α and β chains (Fig. 5–12). As a result, class II MHC molecules cannot bind and present peptides they encounter in the ER, leaving such peptides to associate with class I molecules. The I_i may also promote folding and assembly of class II molecules and direct newly formed class II molecules to the specialized endosomal vesicles where internalized proteins have been proteolytically degraded into peptides. During their passage toward the cell surface, the exocytic vesicles transporting class II molecules out of the ER meet and fuse with the endocytic vesicles containing internalized and processed antigens. The net

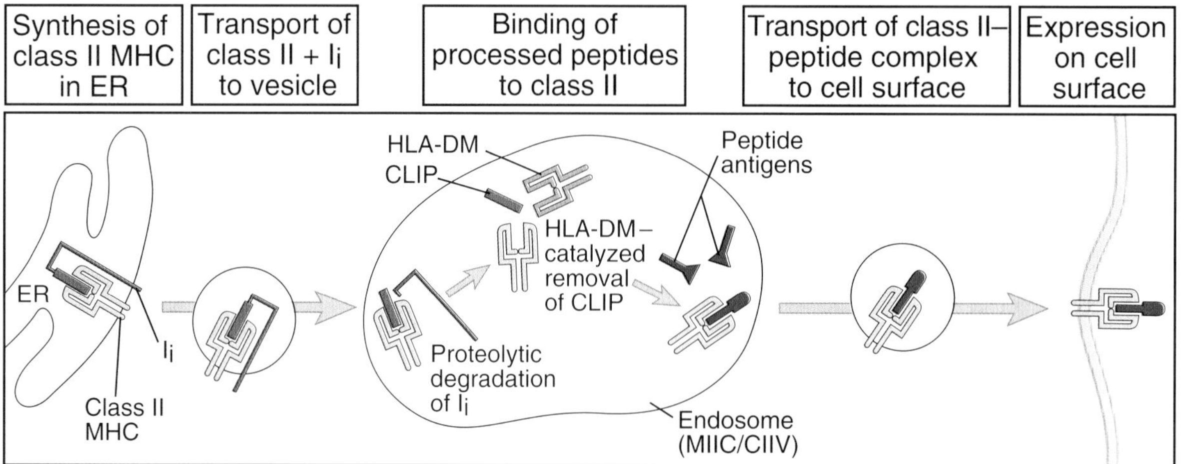

Figure 5–12 The functions of class II MHC–associated invariant chains and HLA-DM. Class II molecules with bound invariant chain, or CLIP, are transported into vesicles (the MIIC/CIIV), where the CLIP is removed by the action of DM. Antigenic peptides generated in the vesicles are then able to bind to the class II molecules. Another class II–like protein, called HLA-DO, may regulate the DM-catalyzed removal of CLIP. CIIV, class II vesicle; CLIP, class II–associated invariant chain peptide; ER, endoplasmic reticulum; I_i, invariant chain; MIIC, MHC class II compartment.

result of this sequence of events is that class II molecules enter the vesicles that also contain peptides generated by proteolysis of endocytosed proteins.

Immunoelectron microscopy and subcellular fractionation studies have defined a class II–rich subset of endosomes that plays an important role in antigen presentation (Fig. 5–13). In macrophages and human B cells, it is called the MHC class II compartment, or MIIC. (In some mouse B cells, a similar organelle containing class II molecules has been identified and named the class II vesicle [CIIV].) The MIIC has a characteristic multilamellar appearance. Importantly, it contains all the components required for peptide–class II association, including the enzymes that degrade protein antigens, the class II molecules, the I_i (or invariant chain–derived peptides), and a molecule called human leukocyte antigen DM (HLA-DM) whose function is described next.

APCs from knockout mice lacking the I_i show defective presentation of some protein antigens but are still able to present class II–associated peptides derived from a wide variety of proteins. This suggests that the importance of the I_i may vary according to the antigen being presented.

4. ASSOCIATION OF PROCESSED PEPTIDES WITH CLASS II MHC MOLECULES IN VESICLES

Within the MIIC, the I_i is removed from class II MHC molecules by the combined action of proteolytic enzymes and the HLA-DM molecule, and antigenic peptides are then able to bind to the available peptide-binding clefts of the class II molecules. Because the I_i blocks access to the peptide-binding cleft of a class II MHC molecule, it must be removed before complexes of peptide and class II molecules can form. The same proteolytic enzymes, such as cathepsin S, that generate peptides from internalized proteins also act on the I_i, degrading it and leaving only a 24–amino acid remnant

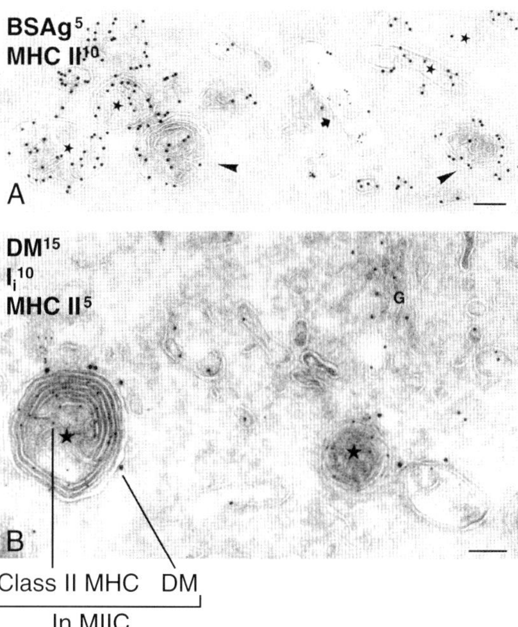

Figure 5–13 Morphology of class II MHC–rich endosomal vesicles.

A. Immunoelectron micrograph of a B lymphocyte that has internalized bovine serum albumin into early endosomes (labeled with 5-nm gold particles, *arrow*) and contains class II MHC molecules (labeled with 10-nm gold particles) in MIICs *(arrowheads)*. The internalized albumin will reach the MIICs ultimately. (From Kleijmeer MJ, S Morkowski, JM Griffith, AY Rudensky, and HJ Geuze. Major histocompatibility complex class II compartments in human and mouse B lymphoblasts represent conventional endocytic compartments. The Journal of Cell Biology 139:639–649, 1997, by copyright permission of The Rockefeller University Press.)

B. Immunoelectron micrograph of a B cell showing location of class II MHC molecules and DM in MIICs *(stars)* and invariant chain concentrated in the Golgi (G) complex. In this example, there is virtually no invariant chain detected in the MIIC, presumably because it has been cleaved to generate CLIP. (Photographs courtesy of Drs. H. J. Geuze and M. Kleijmeer, Department of Cell Biology, Utrecht University, The Netherlands.)

called class II–associated invariant chain peptide (CLIP). X-ray crystallographic analysis has shown that the CLIP sits in the peptide-binding cleft in the same way that other peptides bind to class II MHC molecules. Therefore, removal of CLIP is required before the cleft becomes accessible to peptides produced from extracellular proteins. This is accomplished by the action of a molecule called HLA-DM (or H-2M in the mouse), which is encoded within the MHC, has a structure similar to that of class II MHC molecules, and colocalizes with class II molecules in the MIIC compartment. HLA-DM molecules differ from class II MHC molecules in several respects: they are not polymorphic, they do not associate with the I_i, and they are not expressed on the cell surface. HLA-DM acts as a peptide exchanger, facilitating the removal of CLIP and the addition of other peptides to class II MHC molecules (see Fig. 5–12).

The critical role of HLA-DM is demonstrated by the finding that mutant cell lines that lack DM, and knockout mice that lack the homologous mouse protein H-2M, are defective in presenting peptides derived from extracellular proteins. When class II MHC molecules are isolated from these DM-mutant cell lines or from APCs from H-2M knockout mice, they are found to have CLIP almost exclusively in their peptide-binding clefts, consistent with a role for DM in removing CLIP. Transfection of the gene encoding DM into these mutant cell lines restores normal class II–associated antigen presentation.

Once CLIP is removed, peptides generated by proteolysis of internalized protein antigens are able to bind to class II MHC molecules. The HLA-DM molecule may accelerate the rate of peptide binding to class II molecules. Because the ends of the class II MHC peptide-binding cleft are open, large peptides or even unfolded whole proteins may bind, yet the size of peptides eluted from cell surface class II MHC molecules is usually restricted to 10 to 30 amino acids. It is possible that larger polypeptides initially bind to class II MHC molecules and are then "trimmed" by proteolytic enzymes to the appropriate size for T cell recognition.

B lymphocytes, but not other APCs, express another nonpolymorphic class II–like heterodimer called HLA-DO. Much of the DO in the cell is found in association with DM, suggesting that the DO molecule may regulate the efficiency of antigen presentation or the types of peptides that are generated in B cells. However, DO is clearly not required for antigen processing, and its function remains poorly defined.

5. EXPRESSION OF PEPTIDE–CLASS II COMPLEXES ON THE APC SURFACE

Class II MHC molecules are stabilized by the bound peptides, and the stable peptide–class II complexes are delivered to the surface of the APC, where they are displayed for recognition by CD4⁺ T cells. The requirement for bound peptide to stabilize class II MHC molecules ensures that only properly loaded peptide-MHC complexes will survive long enough to get displayed on the cell surface. A similar phenomenon occurs in class I MHC assembly. Once expressed on the APC surface, the peptide–class II complexes are recognized by specific $CD4^+$ T cells, with the CD4 coreceptor playing an essential role by binding to nonpolymorphic regions of the class II molecule. The slow off-rate and therefore long half-life of peptide-MHC complexes increase the chance that a T cell specific for such a complex will make contact, bind, and be activated by that complex. Interestingly, while peptide-loaded class II molecules traffic from the MIIC vesicular compartment to the cell surface, other molecules involved in antigen presentation, such as DM, stay in the vesicle and are not expressed as membrane proteins. The mechanism of this selective traffic is unknown.

Very small numbers of peptide-MHC complexes are capable of activating specific T lymphocytes. Because APCs continuously present peptides derived from all the proteins they encounter, only a very small fraction of cell surface peptide-MHC complexes will contain the same peptide. Furthermore, most of the bound peptides will be derived from normal self proteins because there is no mechanism to distinguish self proteins from foreign proteins in the process that generates the peptide-MHC complexes. This is borne out by studies in which class II MHC molecules are purified from APCs from normal individuals and the bound peptides are eluted and sequenced; it is seen that most of these peptides are derived from self proteins. These findings raise two important questions that were introduced in Chapter 4. First, how can a T cell recognize and be activated by any foreign antigen when it encounters only APCs that are predominantly displaying self peptide–MHC complexes? The answer is that T cells are remarkably sensitive and need to specifically recognize very few peptide-MHC complexes to be activated. It has been estimated that as few as 100 complexes of a particular peptide with a class II MHC molecule on the surface of an APC can initiate a specific T cell response. This represents less than 0.1% of the total number of class II molecules likely to be present on the surface of the APC. Thus, a newly introduced antigen may be processed into peptides that load enough MHC molecules of APCs to activate T cells specific for that antigen, even though most of the MHC molecules are occupied with self peptides. In fact, the ability of APCs to internalize, process, and present the heterogeneous mix of self proteins and foreign proteins ensures that the immune system will not miss transient or quantitatively small exposures to foreign antigens. Second, if individuals process their own proteins and present them in association with their own class II MHC molecules, why do we normally not develop immune responses against self proteins? The answer is that self peptide–MHC complexes are formed but do not induce autoimmunity because T cells specific for such complexes are deleted or inactivated. In other words, T cells are tolerant to self antigens (see Chapter 10).

Processing of Cytosolic Antigens for Class I MHC–Associated Presentation

Class I MHC–associated peptides are produced by the proteolytic degradation of cytosolic proteins, the transport of the generated peptides into the ER, and the binding to newly synthesized class I molecules. This sequence of events is illustrated in Figure 5–14, and the individual steps are described here.

1. PRODUCTION OF PROTEINS IN THE CYTOSOL

The peptides that are presented bound to class I MHC molecules are derived from cytosolic proteins, most of which are endogenously synthesized in nucleated cells. Foreign antigens in the cytosol may be the products of viruses or other intracellular microbes that infect such cells and synthesize their own proteins during their life cycle. (Many normal self proteins are also present in the cytosol, from which they may enter the class I pathway.) In tumor cells, mutated self genes or oncogenes often produce protein antigens that are recognized by class I–restricted CTLs (see Chapter 17). Peptides that are presented in association with class I molecules may also be derived from microbes and other particulate antigens that are phagocytosed into phagosomes. Some microbes are able to damage cellular membranes and create pores through which the microbes and their antigens may exit phagosomes and enter the cytosol. For instance, pathogenic strains of *Listeria monocytogenes* produce a protein, called listeriolysin, that enables bacteria to escape from vesicles into the cytosol. (This escape is a mechanism that the bacteria have evolved to resist killing by the microbicidal mechanisms of phagocytes, most of which are limited to phagolysosomes; see Chapter 12.) Once the antigens of the phagocytosed microbes are in the cytosol, they are processed like other cytosolic antigens.

2. PROTEOLYTIC DEGRADATION OF CYTOSOLIC PROTEINS

The major mechanism for the generation of peptides from cytosolic protein antigens is proteolysis by the proteasome. The proteasome is a large multiprotein enzyme complex with a broad range of proteolytic activity that is found in the cytoplasm of most cells. A 700-kD form of proteasome appears as a cylinder composed of a stacked array of two inner and two outer rings, each ring being composed of seven subunits. Three of the seven subunits are the catalytic sites for proteolysis. A larger, 1500-kD proteasome is likely to be most important for generating class I–binding peptides and is composed of the 700-kD structure plus several additional subunits that regulate proteolytic activity. Two catalytic subunits present in many 1500-kD proteasomes, called LMP-2 and LMP-7, are encoded by genes in the MHC and are particularly important for generating class I–binding peptides.

The proteasome performs a basic housekeeping function in cells by degrading many different cytoplasmic proteins. These proteins are targeted for proteasomal degradation by covalent linkage of several copies of a small polypeptide called ubiquitin. After ubiquitination, the proteins are unfolded, the ubiquitin is removed, and the proteins are "threaded" through proteasomes. The proteasome has broad substrate specificity and can generate a wide variety of peptides from cytosolic proteins (but usually does not degrade proteins completely into single amino acids). Interestingly, in cells treated with the cytokine IFN-γ, there is

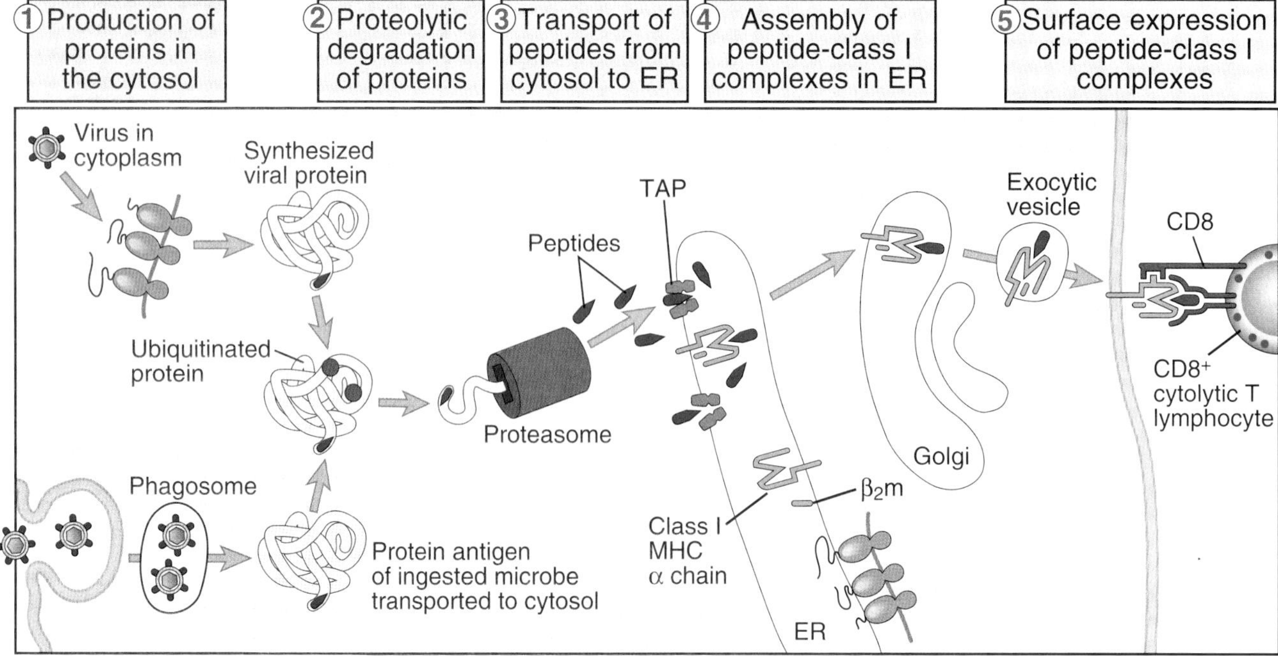

Figure 5–14 The class I MHC pathway of antigen presentation.
The numbered stages in the processing of cytosolic proteins correspond to the stages described in the text. β_2m, β_2-microglobulin; ER, endoplasmic reticulum; TAP, transporter associated with antigen processing.

increased transcription and synthesis of LMP-2 and LMP-7, and these proteins replace two of the subunits of the proteasome. This results in a change in the substrate specificity of the proteasome so that the peptides produced are 6 to 30 residues long and usually contain carboxyl terminal basic or hydrophobic amino acids. Both features are typical of peptides that are transported into the class I pathway and that bind to class I molecules (often after further trimming). This is one mechanism by which IFN-γ enhances antigen presentation. Thus, proteasomes are excellent examples of organelles whose basic cellular function has been adapted for a specialized role in antigen presentation.

Many lines of evidence have conclusively established that proteasomal degradation of cytosolic proteins is required for entry into the class I antigen-processing pathway.

- Specific inhibitors of proteasomal function block presentation of a cytoplasmic protein to class I MHC–restricted T cells specific for a peptide epitope of that protein. However, if the peptide that is recognized by the CTLs is synthesized directly in the cytoplasm of a cell as the product of a transfected minigene, the peptide is presented and the cell can be killed by the CTLs. In this situation, presentation of the peptide is not blocked by inhibitors of proteasomal enzymes, indicating that once antigens are converted to cytosolic peptides, they no longer need proteasomal degradation.
- In some cell lines, inhibition of ubiquitination also inhibits the presentation of cytoplasmic proteins to class I MHC–restricted T cells specific for a peptide epitope of that protein. Conversely, modification of proteins by attachment of an N-terminal sequence that is recognized by ubiquitin-conjugating enzymes leads to enhanced ubiquitination and more rapid class I MHC–associated presentation of peptides derived from those proteins.
- Mice in which the genes encoding selected subunits of proteasomes (LMP-2 or LMP-7) are deleted show defects in the generation of CTLs against some viruses, presumably because of defective class I–associated presentation of viral antigens.

Thus, the proteolytic mechanisms that generate antigenic peptides that bind to class I MHC molecules are different from the mechanisms described earlier for peptide–class II MHC molecule associations. This is also evident from the observation that agents that raise endosomal and lysosomal pH, or directly inhibit endosomal proteases, block class II–restricted but not class I–restricted antigen presentation, whereas inhibitors of ubiquitination or proteasomes selectively block class I–restricted antigen presentation.

Some protein antigens apparently do not require ubiquitination or proteasomes to be presented by the class I MHC pathway. This may be because other, less well defined mechanisms of cytoplasmic proteolysis exist. In addition, some class I MHC molecules bind peptides that may be generated by proteolytic enzymes resident in the ER. For example, the signal sequences of membrane and secreted proteins are usually degraded proteolytically in the ER during translation of these proteins. This ER degradation generates class I–binding peptides without a need for proteolysis in the cytosol.

3. TRANSPORT OF PEPTIDES FROM THE CYTOSOL TO THE ER

Peptides generated in the cytosol are translocated by a specialized transporter into the ER, where newly synthesized class I MHC molecules are available to bind the peptides. Because antigenic peptides for the class I pathway are generated in the cytosol, but class I MHC molecules are synthesized in the ER, a mechanism must exist for delivery of cytosolic peptides into the ER. The initial insights into this mechanism came from studies of cell lines that are defective in assembling and displaying peptide–class I MHC complexes on their surfaces. The mutations responsible for this defect turned out to involve two genes located within the MHC that are homologous to the ABC transporter family of genes, which encode proteins that mediate adenosine triphosphate (ATP)–dependent transport of low molecular weight compounds across cellular membranes. The genes in the MHC that belong to this family encode the two chains of a heterodimer called the **transporter associated with antigen processing** (TAP). (Interestingly, the *TAP1* and *TAP2* genes are next to the genes encoding LMP-2 and LMP-7 in the MHC, and the synthesis of the TAP protein is also stimulated by IFN-γ.) The TAP protein is located mainly in the ER, where it mediates the active, ATP-dependent transport of peptides from the cytosol into the ER lumen (Fig. 5–15). Although the TAP heterodimer has a broad range of specificities, it optimally transports peptides ranging from 6 to 30 amino acids long and containing carboxyl termini that are basic (in humans) or hydrophobic (in humans and mice). As mentioned before, the proteasome generates peptides with these features. Therefore, the TAP dimer delivers to the ER peptides of the right size and characteristics for binding to class I MHC molecules.

- TAP-deficient cell lines, and mice in which the *TAP1* gene is deleted, show defects in class I MHC expression and cannot effectively present class I–associated antigens to T cells. The class I MHC molecules that do get expressed in TAP-deficient cells have bound peptides that are mostly derived from signal sequences of proteins destined for secretion or membrane expression. As mentioned before, these signal sequences may be degraded to peptides within the ER, without a requirement for TAP.
- Rare examples of human *TAP1* and *TAP2* gene mutations have been identified, and the patients carrying these mutant genes also show defective class I MHC–associated antigen presentation and increased susceptibility to infections with some bacteria.

On the luminal side of the ER membrane, the TAP protein is noncovalently attached to newly

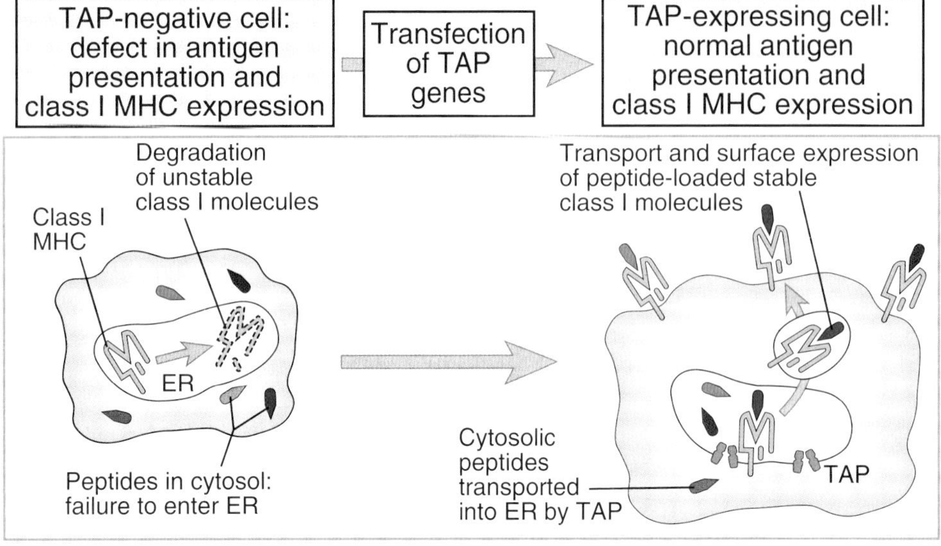

Figure 5–15 Role of TAP in class I MHC–associated antigen presentation. In a cell line lacking functional TAP, class I molecules are not efficiently loaded with peptides and are degraded, mostly in the endoplasmic reticulum (ER). When a functional TAP gene is transfected into the cell line, normal assembly and expression of peptide-associated class I MHC molecules are restored. Note that the TAP dimer may be attached to class I molecules by a linker protein called tapasin, which is not shown in this and other illustrations. TAP, transporter associated with antigen processing.

synthesized class I MHC molecules by a linker protein called tapasin. Thus, the class I molecule is strategically located at the site where it can receive peptides.

4. ASSEMBLY OF PEPTIDE–CLASS I MHC COMPLEXES IN THE ER

Peptides translocated into the ER bind to class I MHC molecules that are attached to the TAP dimer. The synthesis and assembly of class I molecules involve a multistep process in which peptide binding plays a key role. Class I α chains and β_2-microglobulin are synthesized in the ER. Appropriate folding of the nascent α chains is assisted by various ER chaperone proteins, such as calnexin and calreticulin. Within the ER, the newly formed "empty" class I dimers remain attached to the TAP complex by tapasin. When peptide enters the ER via TAP, the peptide binds to the cleft of the associated class I molecule. The peptide–class I complex is then released from tapasin, and it is able to exit the ER and be transported to the cell surface. In the absence of bound peptide, many of the newly formed α chain–β_2-microglobulin dimers are unstable, cannot be transported out of the ER efficiently, and are presumably degraded in the ER (see Fig. 5–15).

Peptides transported into the ER preferentially bind to class I, but not class II, MHC molecules, for two reasons. First, newly synthesized class I molecules are attached to the luminal aspect of the TAP complex, ready to receive peptides. Second, as mentioned previously, in the ER the peptide-binding clefts of newly synthesized class II molecules are blocked by the associated I_i.

5. SURFACE EXPRESSION OF PEPTIDE–CLASS I COMPLEXES

Class I MHC molecules with bound peptides are structurally stable and are expressed on the cell surface. Stable peptide–class I MHC complexes that were produced in the ER move through the Golgi complex and are transported to the cell surface by exocytic vesicles. Once expressed on the cell surface, the peptide–class I complexes may be recognized by peptide antigen–specific $CD8^+$ T cells, with the CD8 coreceptor playing an essential role by binding to nonpolymorphic regions of the class I molecule. In later chapters, we will return to a discussion of the role of class I–restricted CTLs in protective immunity. Several viruses have evolved mechanisms that interfere with class I assembly and peptide loading, emphasizing the importance of this pathway for antiviral immunity (see Chapter 15).

Physiologic Significance of MHC-Associated Antigen Presentation

So far, we have discussed the specificity of $CD4^+$ and $CD8^+$ T lymphocytes for MHC-associated foreign protein antigens and the mechanisms by which complexes of peptides and MHC molecules are produced. In this section, we consider the impact of MHC-associated antigen presentation on the role that T cells play in protective immunity, the nature of T cell responses to different antigens, and the types of antigens that T cells recognize.

T Cell Surveillance for Foreign Antigens

The class I and class II pathways of antigen presentation sample available proteins for display to T cells. Most of these proteins are self proteins. Foreign proteins are relatively rare; these may be derived from infectious microbes, other foreign antigens that are introduced, and tumors. T cells survey all the displayed peptides for the presence of these rare foreign peptides and respond to the foreign antigens (Fig. 5–16). MHC molecules sample both the extracellular space and the cytosol of nucleated cells, and this is important because microbes may reside in both locations. Even though peptides derived from foreign (e.g., microbial) anti-

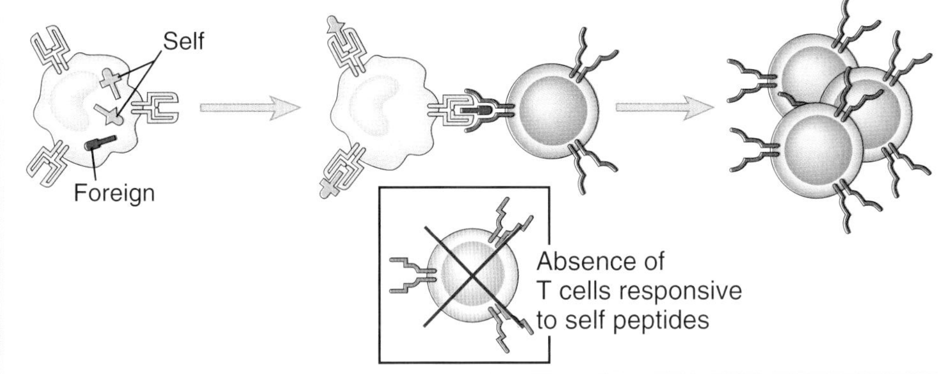

Figure 5–16 T cells survey APCs for foreign peptides. Antigen-presenting cells (APCs) present self peptides and foreign peptides associated with MHC molecules, and T cells respond to the foreign peptides. In response to infections, APCs also express costimulators (not shown) that activate T cells specific for the microbial antigens.

gens may not be abundant, these foreign antigens are recognized by the immune system because of the exquisite sensitivity of T cells. In addition, infectious agents stimulate the expression of costimulators on APCs that enhance T cell responses, thus ensuring that T cells will be activated when microbes are present.

Nature of T Cell Responses

The expression and functions of MHC molecules determine how T cells respond to different types of antigens and mediate their effector functions.

- ***The presentation of endosomal versus cytosolic proteins by the class II or class I MHC pathways, respectively, determines which subsets of T cells will respond to antigens found in these two pools of proteins*** (Fig. 5–17). Extracellular antigens usually end up in the endosomal pool and activate class II–restricted CD4$^+$ T cells because the pathways by which extracellular proteins are internalized converge with the pathway of class II expression. These CD4$^+$ T cells function as helpers to stimulate effector mechanisms, such as antibodies and phagocytes, that serve to eliminate extracellular antigens. Conversely, endogenously synthesized antigens are present in the cytoplasmic pool of proteins, where they are inaccessible to antibodies and phagocytes. These cytosolic antigens enter the pathway for loading class I molecules and activate class I–restricted CD8$^+$ CTLs, which kill the cells producing the intracellular antigens. The expression of class I molecules in all nucleated cells ensures that peptides from virtually any intracellular protein may be displayed for recognition by CD8$^+$ T cells. Thus, antigens from microbes that reside in different cellular locations selectively stimulate the T cell responses that are most effective at eliminating that type of microbe. This is especially important because the antigen receptors of helper T cells and CTLs cannot distinguish between extracellular and intracellular microbes. By segregating peptides derived from these types of microbes, the MHC molecules guide these subsets of T cells to respond to the microbes that each subset can best combat.

- ***The unique specificity of T cells for cell-bound antigens is essential for the functions of T lymphocytes, which are largely mediated by interactions requiring direct cell-cell contact and by cytokines that act at short distances.*** APCs not only present antigens to T lymphocytes but also are the targets of T cell effector functions (see Fig. 5–17). For instance, macrophages with phagocytosed microbes present microbial antigens to CD4$^+$ T cells, and the T cells respond by activating the macrophages to destroy the microbes. B lymphocytes that have specifically bound and endocytosed a protein antigen present peptides derived from that antigen to helper T cells, and the T cells then stimulate the B lymphocytes to produce antibodies against the protein. B lymphocytes and macrophages are two of the principal cell types that express class II MHC genes, function as APCs for CD4$^+$ helper T cells, and focus helper T cell effects to their immediate vicinity. Similarly, the presentation of class I–associated peptides allows CD8$^+$ CTLs to detect and respond to antigens produced in any nucleated cell and to destroy these cells. We will return to a fuller discussion of these interactions of T cells with APCs when we discuss the effector functions of T cells in later chapters.

Immunogenicity of Protein Antigens

MHC molecules determine the immunogenicity of protein antigens in two related ways.

- ***The epitopes of complex proteins that are most likely to elicit T cell responses are often the peptides that are generated by proteolysis in APCs and bind most avidly to MHC molecules.*** If an individual is immunized with a multideterminant protein antigen, in many instances the majority of the

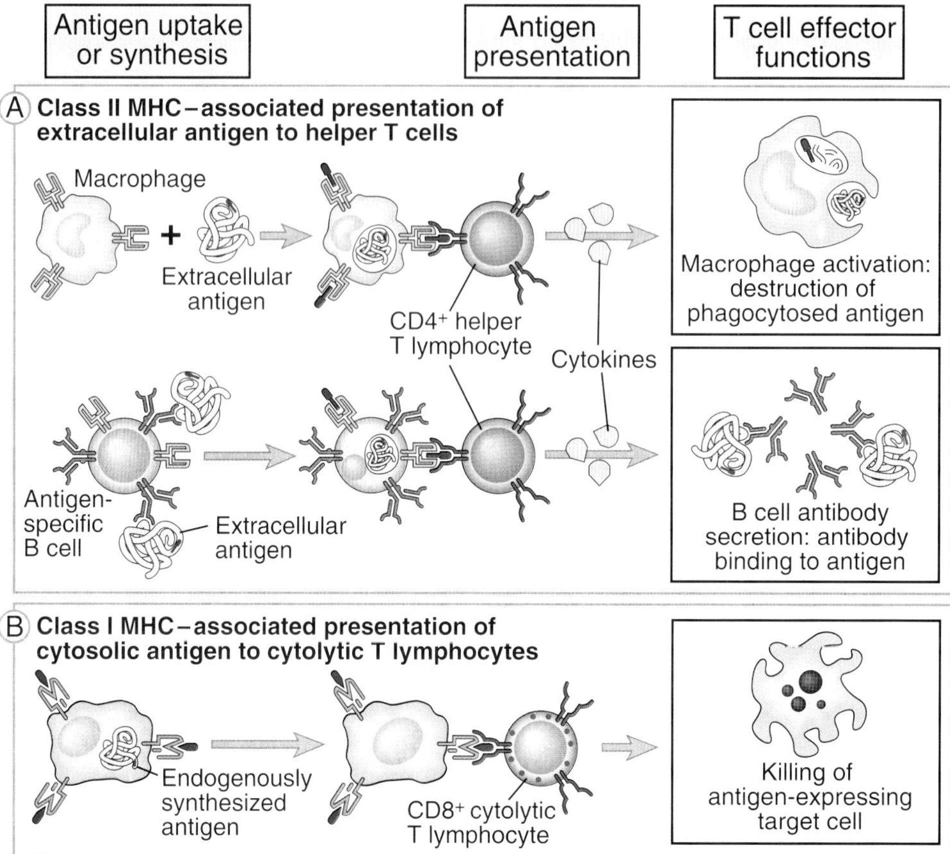

Figure 5–17 Presentation of extracellular and cytosolic antigens to different subsets of T cells.

A. Extracellular antigens are presented by macrophages or B lymphocytes to $CD4^+$ helper T lymphocytes, which activate the macrophages or B cells and eliminate the extracellular antigens.

B. Cytosolic antigens are presented by nucleated cells to $CD8^+$ CTLs, which kill (lyse) the antigen-expressing cells.

responding T cells are specific for one or a few linear amino acid sequences of the antigen. These are called the **immunodominant epitopes** or determinants. The proteases involved in antigen processing produce a variety of peptides from natural proteins, and only some of these peptides possess the characteristics that enable them to bind to the MHC molecules present in each individual (Fig. 5–18).

In H-2^k mice immunized with the antigen hen egg lysozyme (HEL), a large proportion of the HEL-specific T cells are specific for one epitope formed by residues 52–62 of HEL in association with the I-A^k class II molecule. This is because the HEL(52–62) peptide binds to I-A^k better than do other HEL peptides. *In vitro*, if I-A^k–expressing APCs are incubated with HEL, up to 20% of the I-A^k molecules may get loaded with this one peptide. Thus, the 52–62 peptide is the immunodominant epitope of HEL in H-2^k mice. This approach has been used to identify immunodominant epitopes of many other protein antigens. In inbred mice infected with a virus, such as the lymphocytic choriomeningitis virus, all the virus-specific T cells that are activated may be specific for as few as two or three viral peptides recognized in association with one of the inherited class I alleles. Similarly, in humans infected with the human immunodeficiency virus, individual patients contain T cells that recognize a small number of viral epitopes. The same phenomenon has been seen with many viruses and intracellular bacteria. These results imply that even complex microbes produce very few peptides capable of binding to any one allelic MHC molecule.

It is important to define the structural basis of immunodominance because this may permit the efficient manipulation of the immune system with synthetic peptides. An application of such knowledge is the design of vaccines. For example, a viral protein could be analyzed for the presence of amino acid sequences that would form typical immunodominant epitopes capable of binding to MHC molecules with high affinity. Synthetic peptides containing these epitopes may be effective vaccines for eliciting T cell responses against the viral peptide expressed on an infected cell.

The expression of particular class II MHC alleles in an individual determines the ability of that individual to respond to particular antigens. The phenomenon of genetically controlled immune responsiveness was introduced in Chapter 4. We now

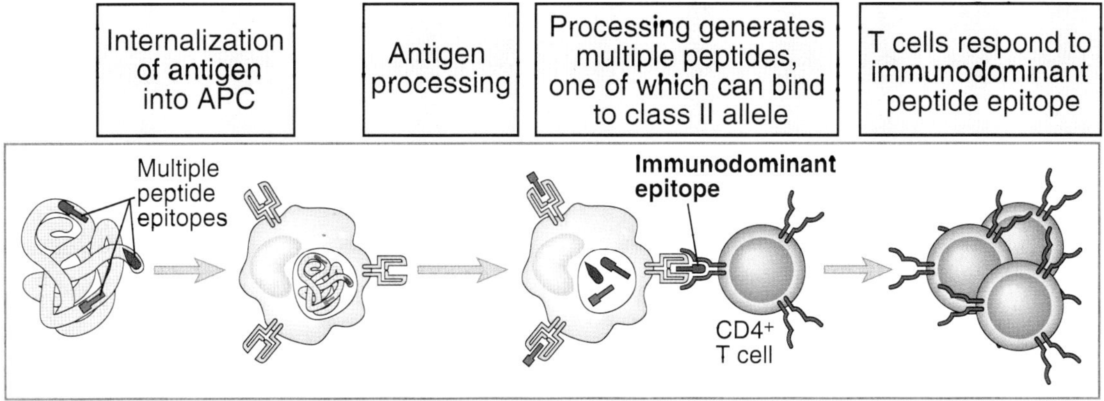

Figure 5–18 Immunodominance of peptides.
Protein antigens are processed to generate multiple peptides; immunodominant peptides are the ones that bind best to the available class I and class II MHC molecules. The illustration shows an extracellular antigen generating a class II–binding peptide, but this also applies to peptides of cytosolic antigens that are presented by class I MHC molecules. APC, antigen-presenting cell.

know that the immune response (Ir) genes that control antibody responses are the class II MHC structural genes. They influence immune responsiveness because various allelic class II MHC molecules differ in their ability to bind different antigenic peptides and therefore to stimulate specific helper T cells.

H-2^k mice are responders to HEL(52–62), but H-2^d mice are nonresponders to this epitope. Equilibrium dialysis experiments have shown that HEL(52–62) binds to I-A^k but not to I-A^d molecules. X-ray crystallographic analysis of peptide-MHC complexes shows that the HEL(52–62) peptide binds tightly to the peptide-binding cleft of the I-A^k molecule (see Chapter 4, Fig. 4–9). Modeling studies indicate that the HEL(52–62) peptide cannot bind tightly to the cleft of the I-A^d molecule (which has different amino acids in the binding cleft than does I-A^k). This explains why the H-2^d mouse is a nonresponder to this peptide. Similar results have been obtained with numerous other peptides.

These findings support the **determinant selection model** of MHC-linked immune responses. This model, which was proposed many years before the demonstration of peptide-MHC binding, states that the products of MHC genes in each individual select which determinants of protein antigens will be immunogenic in that individual. We now realize that the structural basis of determinant selection and Ir gene function is simply the ability of individual MHC molecules to bind some but not all peptides. Most Ir gene phenomena have been studied by measuring helper T cell–dependent responses, but the same principles apply to CTLs. Individuals with certain MHC alleles may be incapable of generating CTLs against some viruses. In this situation, of course, the Ir genes will map to one of the class I MHC loci.

These concepts of immunodominance and genetically controlled immune responsiveness are based largely on studies with simple peptide antigens and inbred homozygous strains of mice because in these cases, limited numbers of epitopes are presented by few MHC molecules, making the analyses simple. However, the same principles are also relevant to the understanding of responses to complex multideterminant protein antigens in outbred species. It is likely that most individuals will express at least one MHC molecule capable of binding at least one determinant of a complex protein, so that all individuals will be responders to such complex antigens. As we mentioned in Chapter 4, the need for every species to produce MHC molecules capable of binding many different peptides may be the evolutionary pressure for maintaining MHC polymorphism.

Summary

- T cells recognize antigens only in the form of peptides displayed by the products of self MHC genes on the surface of APCs. CD4$^+$ helper T lymphocytes recognize antigens in association with class II MHC gene products (class II MHC–restricted recognition), and CD8$^+$ CTLs recognize antigens in association with class I gene products (class I MHC–restricted recognition).
- Specialized APCs, such as dendritic cells, macrophages, and B lymphocytes, capture extracellular protein antigens, internalize and process them, and display class II–associated peptides to CD4$^+$ T cells. Dendritic cells are the most efficient APCs for initiating primary responses by activating naive T cells, and macrophages and B lymphocytes present antigens to differentiated helper T cells in the effector phase of cell-mediated immunity and in humoral immune responses, respectively. All nucleated cells can present class I–associated peptides,

derived from cytosolic proteins such as viral and tumor antigens, to $CD8^+$ T cells.

- Antigen processing is the conversion of native proteins into MHC-associated peptides. This process consists of the introduction of exogenous protein antigens into APCs or the synthesis of antigens in the cytosol, the proteolytic degradation of these proteins into peptides, the binding of peptides to MHC molecules, and the display of the peptide-MHC complexes on the APC surface for recognition by T cells. Antigen-processing pathways in APCs use basic cellular proteolytic mechanisms that also operate independently of the immune system. Both extracellular and intracellular proteins are sampled by these antigen-processing pathways, and peptides derived from both normal self proteins and foreign proteins are displayed by MHC molecules for surveillance by T lymphocytes.
- For class II–associated antigen presentation, extracellular proteins are internalized into endosomes, where these proteins are proteolytically cleaved by enzymes that function at acidic pH. Newly synthesized class II MHC molecules associated with the I_i are transported from the ER to the endosomal vesicles. Here the I_i is proteolytically cleaved, and a small peptide remnant of the I_i, called CLIP, is removed from the peptide-binding cleft of the MHC molecule by the DM molecules. The peptides that were generated from extracellular proteins then bind to the available cleft of the class II MHC molecule, and the trimeric complex (class II MHC α and β chains and peptide) moves to and is displayed on the surface of the cell.
- For class I–associated antigen presentation, cytosolic proteins are proteolytically degraded in the proteasome, generating peptides with features that enable them to bind to class I molecules. These peptides are delivered from the cytoplasm to the ER by an ATP-dependent transporter called TAP. Newly synthesized class I MHC–β_2-microglobulin dimers in the ER are attached to the TAP complex and receive peptides transported into the ER. Stable complexes of class I MHC molecules with bound peptides move out of the ER, through the Golgi complex, to the cell surface.
- These pathways of MHC-restricted antigen presentation ensure that most of the body's cells are screened for the possible presence of foreign antigens. The pathways also ensure that proteins from extracellular microbes preferentially generate peptides bound to class II MHC molecules for recognition by $CD4^+$ helper T cells, which activate effector mechanisms that eliminate extracellular antigens. Conversely, proteins synthesized by intracellular (cytosolic) microbes generate peptides bound to class I MHC molecules for recognition by $CD8^+$ CTLs, which function to eradicate cells harboring intracellular infections. The immunogenicity of foreign protein antigens depends on the ability of antigen-processing pathways to generate peptides from these proteins that bind to self MHC molecules.

Selected Readings

Alfonso C, and L Karlsson. Nonclassical MHC class II molecules. Annual Review of Immunology 18:113–142, 2000.

Chapman HA. Endosomal proteolysis and class II MHC function. Current Opinion in Immunology 10:93–102, 1998.

Elliott T. Transporter associated with antigen processing. Advances in Immunology 65:47–109, 1997.

Germain RN. MHC-dependent antigen processing and peptide presentation: providing ligands for T lymphocyte activation. Cell 76:287–299, 1994.

Geuze HJ. The role of endosomes and lysosomes in MHC class II functioning. Immunology Today 19:282–287, 1998.

Hart DNJ. Dendritic cells: unique leukocyte populations which control the primary immune response. Blood 90:3245–3287, 1997.

Pamer E, and P Cresswell. Mechanisms of MHC class I–restricted antigen processing. Annual Review of Immunology 16:323–358, 1998.

Porcelli SA, and RL Modlin. The CD1 system: antigen-presenting molecules for T cell recognition of lipids and glycolipids. Annual Review of Immunology 17:297–329, 1999.

Rock KL, and AL Goldberg. Degradation of cell proteins and generation of MHC class I–presented peptides. Annual Review of Immunology 17:739–779, 1999.

Tanaka K, N Tanahashi, C Tsurumi, K Yokota, and N Shimbara. Proteasomes and antigen processing. Advances in Immunology 64:1–38, 1997.

Villadangos JA, and HL Ploegh. Proteolysis in MHC class II antigen presentation: who's in charge? Immunity 12:233–239, 2000.

Wolf PR, and HL Ploegh. How MHC class II molecules acquire peptide cargo: biosynthesis and trafficking through the endocytic pathway. Annual Review of Developmental and Cell Biology 11:267–306, 1995.

Yewdell JW, CC Norbury, and JR Bennink. Mechanisms of exogenous antigen presentation by MHC class I molecules *in vitro* and *in vivo*: implications for generating $CD8^+$ T cell responses to infectious agents, tumors, transplants, and vaccines. Advances in Immunology 73:1–77, 1999.

Yewdell JW, and JR Bennink. Immunodominance in major histocompatibility class I–restricted T lymphocyte responses. Annual Review of Immunology 17:51–88, 1999.

A series of brief reviews on dendritic cells was published in Cell 106:255–274, 2001.

Chapter 6

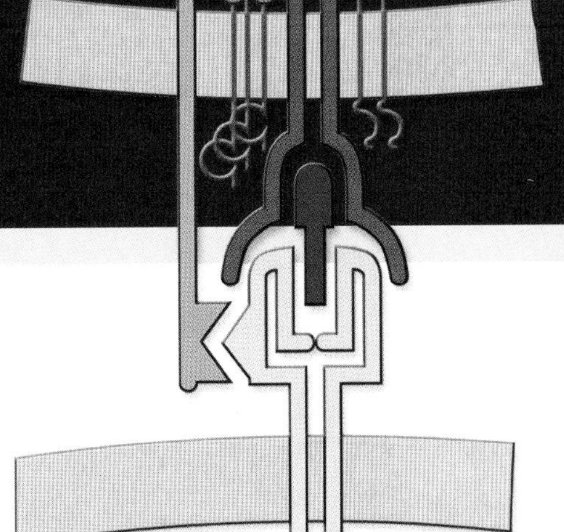

Antigen Receptors and Accessory Molecules of T Lymphocytes

T lymphocytes respond to peptide fragments of protein antigens that are displayed by antigen-presenting cells (APCs). The initiation of these responses requires specific antigen recognition by the T cells, stable adhesion of the T cells to the APCs, and transduction of activating signals to the T cells. Each of these events is mediated by distinct sets of molecules on the T cells (Fig. 6–1). In this chapter, we describe the molecules involved in T cell antigen recognition, adhesion, and signaling.

T lymphocytes have a dual specificity: they recognize polymorphic residues of self major histocompatibility complex (MHC) molecules, which accounts for their MHC restriction, and they also recognize residues of peptide antigens displayed by these MHC molecules, which is responsible for their specificity. As we discussed in Chapters 4 and 5, MHC molecules and peptides form complexes on the surface of APCs. The receptor that recognizes these peptide-MHC complexes is called the **T cell receptor** (TCR). The TCR is a clonally distributed receptor, meaning that clones of T cells with different specificities express different TCRs. The biochemical signals that are triggered in T cells by antigen recognition are transduced not by the TCR itself but by invariant proteins called CD3 and ζ, which are noncovalently linked to the antigen receptor to form the **TCR complex.** Thus, in T cells, and as we shall see in Chapter 9 in B cells as well, antigen recognition and signaling are segregated among two sets of molecules—a highly variable antigen receptor (the TCR in T cells and membrane immunoglobulin [Ig] in B cells) and invariant signaling proteins (CD3 and ζ chains in T cells and Igα and Igβ in B cells) (Fig. 6–2). T cells also express other membrane receptors that do not recognize antigen but participate in responses to antigens; these are collectively called **accessory molecules.** The physiologic role of some accessory molecules is to deliver signals to the T cell that function in concert with signals from the TCR complex to fully activate the cells. Other accessory molecules function as adhesion molecules to stabilize the binding of T cells to APCs, thus allowing the TCR to be engaged by antigen long enough to transduce the necessary signals. Adhesion molecules also regulate the migration of T cells to the sites where they locate and respond to antigens. Activated T cells express some membrane and secreted molecules that mediate the various effector functions of the cells; these are mentioned at the end of the chapter.

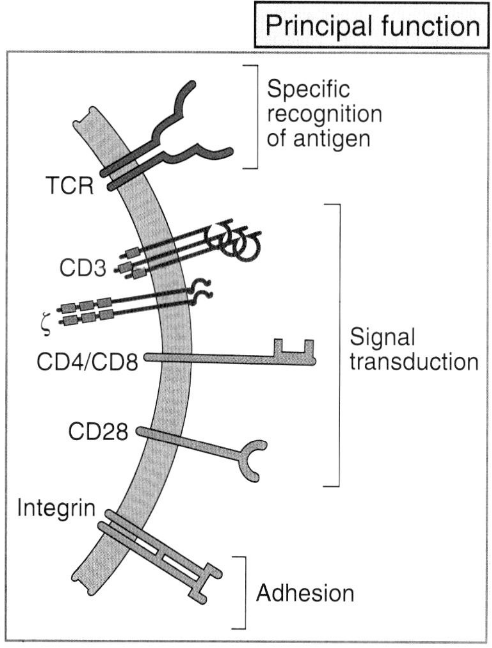

Figure 6–1 T cell receptors and accessory molecules. The principal T cell membrane proteins involved in antigen recognition and in responses to antigens are shown. The functions of these proteins fall into three groups: antigen recognition, signal transduction, and adhesion.

With this background, we proceed with a description of the T cell membrane molecules that are required for antigen recognition and the initiation of functional responses. The maturation of T cells is discussed in Chapter 7, and the biology and biochemistry of T cell responses to antigen are discussed in Chapter 8.

αβ TCR for MHC-Associated Peptide Antigen

The TCR responsible for MHC-restricted antigen recognition was identified at the same time as the structure of MHC-associated peptides was being defined. The key technological advances that led to the discovery of the TCR and the elucidation of its structure were the development of monoclonal T cell populations and the cloning of T cell–specific genes that rearrange during T cell development and are homologous to Ig genes (Box 6–1). These studies have culminated in the x-ray crystallographic analysis of TCRs and, most impressively, of trimolecular complexes of MHC molecules, bound peptides, and specific TCRs. As we shall see in the following section, on the basis of these analyses, we now understand the structural features of antigen recognition by the TCR precisely. The components of the TCR complex, in addition to the TCR itself, have been identified by biochemical analyses and molecular cloning (Table 6–1).

Structure of the αβ TCR

The antigen receptor of MHC-restricted CD4⁺ helper T cells and CD8⁺ cytolytic T lymphocytes (CTLs) is a heterodimer consisting of two transmembrane polypeptide chains, designated α and β, covalently linked to each other by disulfide bonds (Fig. 6–3). (Another less common type of TCR, found on a small subset of T cells, is composed of γ and δ chains and is

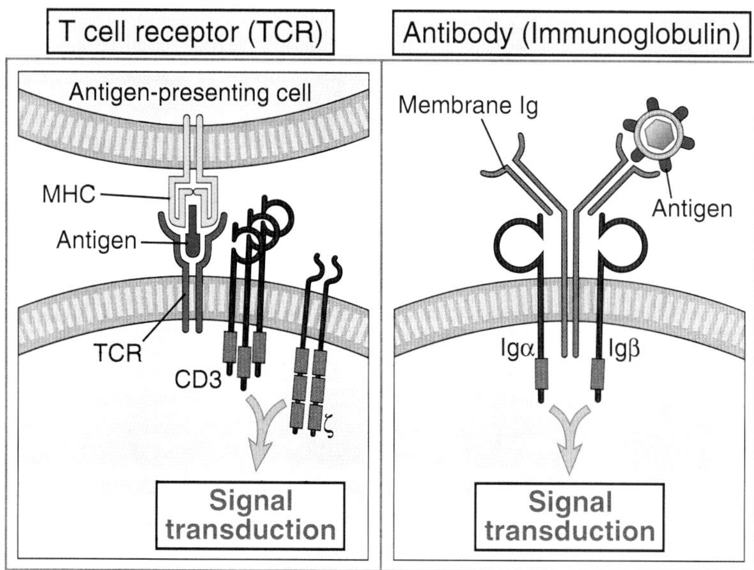

Figure 6–2 Antigen recognition and signaling functions of lymphocyte antigen receptors. The antigen recognition and signaling functions of antigen receptors are mediated by distinct proteins of the antigen receptor complex. When TCR or Ig molecules recognize antigens, signals are delivered to the lymphocytes by proteins associated with the antigen receptors. The antigen receptors and attached signaling proteins form the T and B cell receptor complexes. Note that single antigen receptors are shown recognizing antigens, but signaling requires the cross-linking of two or more receptors by binding to adjacent antigen molecules.

BOX 6–1

Identification of the TCR

To identify TCRs for MHC-associated peptide antigens, it was necessary to develop monoclonal T cell populations in which all the cells express the same TCR. The first such populations to be used for studying TCR proteins were tumors derived from T lymphocytes. Subsequently, methods were developed for propagating monoclonal T cell populations *in vitro,* including T-T hybridomas and antigen-specific T cell clones (see Chapter 8, Box 8–1). The earliest techniques for purifying TCR molecules for biochemical studies relied on producing antibodies specific for unique (idiotypic) determinants of the antigen receptors of a clonal T cell population. Antigen receptors were isolated by use of such antibodies, and limited amino acid sequencing of these receptor proteins suggested that the TCRs were structurally homologous to Ig molecules and contained highly variable regions that differed from one clone to another. However, the protein sequencing studies did not reveal the structure of the complete TCR.

The breakthrough came from attempts to clone the genes encoding TCRs, and this was accomplished before the structure of the proteins was fully defined. The strategy for the identification of TCR genes was based on the knowledge of Ig genes. Three criteria were chosen that needed to be fulfilled for genes to be considered TCR genes: (1) these genes would be uniquely expressed in T cells, (2) they would undergo somatic rearrangements during T cell development (as Ig genes do during B cell development; see Chapter 7), and (3) they would be homologous to Ig genes. One method that was used to identify TCR genes was subtractive hybridization, aimed at identifying T cell–specific genes. In this method, complementary DNA (cDNA) is prepared from T cell mRNA and hybridized to B cell mRNA. All the cDNAs that are common to T and B cells hybridize to the mRNA and can be removed by various separation techniques. The cDNAs that are left behind are unique to T cells. Some of the genes contained in this library of T cell–specific cDNAs were found to be homologous in sequence to Ig genes, and Southern blot hybridization showed that these genes had a different structure in non-T cells than in T cells. This was a known characteristic of Ig genes (see Chapter 7) and suggested that the T cell genes that had been found encoded clonally distributed antigen receptors of T cells that underwent somatic rearrangement only in cells of the T lymphocyte lineage. Furthermore, the predicted amino acid sequences of the proteins encoded by these genes agreed with the partial sequences obtained from putative TCR proteins purified with TCR-specific anti-idiotypic antibodies. Other investigators discovered TCR genes among a library of T cell genes (without subtractive hybridization) based solely on the criteria mentioned before.

The molecular cloning of the TCR was a landmark achievement that came soon after the detailed structural analysis of MHC molecules and provided the structural basis for understanding how T cells recognize peptide-MHC complexes. The ability to express TCRs in ways that allowed them to be cleaved from cell membranes and solubilized was key to the crystallization of TCRs bound to peptide-MHC complexes. These advances have revolutionized our understanding of T cell antigen recognition and paved the way for many important techniques, including the expression of single TCRs of known specificities in transgenic animals. We will refer to such approaches for analyzing immune responses in many later chapters.

Table 6–1. Components of the TCR Complex

Protein	Size (kD)		Function(s)
	Human	Mouse	
TCRα	40-60	44-55	One chain of αβ TCR for peptide-MHC complexes
TCRβ	40-50	40-55	One chain of αβ TCR for peptide-MHC complexes
TCRγ	45-60	45-60	One chain of γδ TCR on subset of T cells
TCRδ	40-60	40-60	One chain of γδ TCR on subset of T cells
CD3γ	25-28	21	Signal transduction; surface expression of TCR
CD3δ	20	28	Signal transduction; surface expression of TCR
CD3ε	20	25	Signal transduction; surface expression of TCR
ζ	16	16	Signal transduction; surface expression of TCR

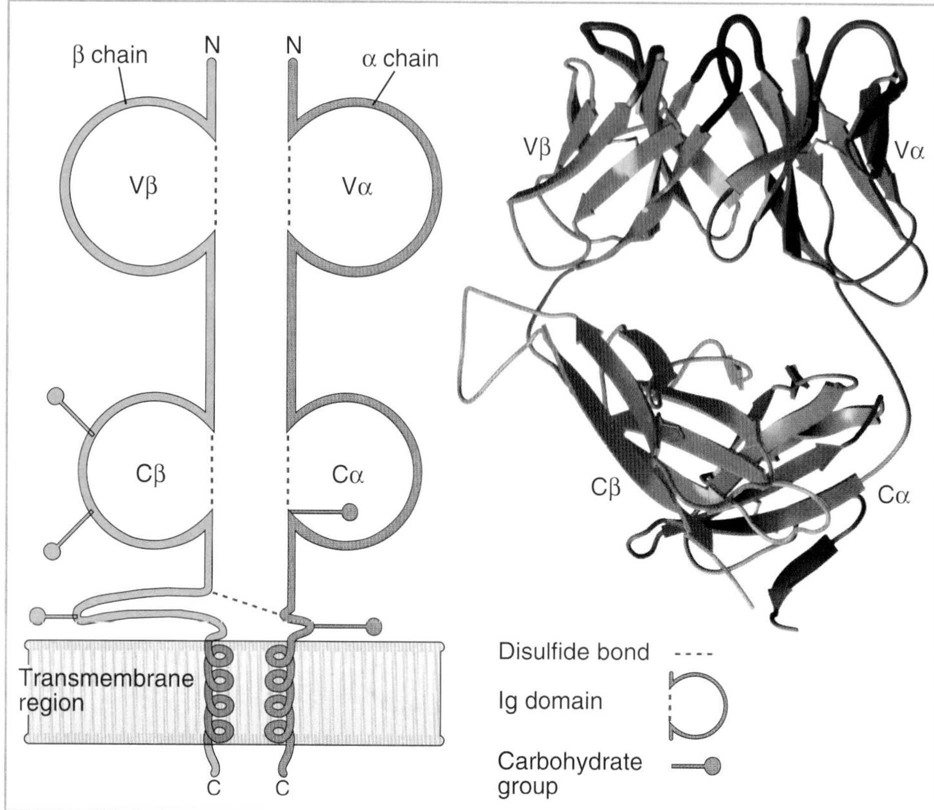

Figure 6–3 Structure of the T cell receptor.
The schematic diagram of the αβ TCR *(left)* shows the domains of a typical TCR specific for a peptide-MHC complex. The antigen-binding portion of the TCR is formed by the V_α and V_β domains. The ribbon diagram *(right)* shows the structure of the extracellular portion of a TCR as revealed by x-ray crystallography. The hypervariable segment loops that form the peptide-MHC binding site are at the top. (Adapted from Bjorkman PJ. MHC restriction in three dimensions: a view of T cell receptor/ligand interactions. Cell 89:167–170, 1997. Copyright Cell Press.)

discussed later.) Each α chain and β chain consists of one Ig-like N-terminal variable (V) domain, one Ig-like constant (C) domain, a hydrophobic transmembrane region, and a short cytoplasmic region. Thus, the extracellular portion of the αβ heterodimer is structurally similar to the antigen-binding fragment (Fab) of an Ig molecule, which is made up of the V and C regions of a light chain and the V region and one C region of a heavy chain (see Chapter 3).

The V regions of the TCR α and β chains contain short stretches of amino acids where the variability between different TCRs is concentrated, and these form the hypervariable or complementarity-determining regions (CDRs). Three CDRs in the α chain are juxtaposed to three similar regions in the β chain to form the part of the TCR that specifically recognizes peptide-MHC complexes (described in the following section). The β chain V domain contains a fourth hypervariable region, which does not appear to participate in antigen recognition but is the binding site for microbial products called superantigens (see Chapter 15, Box 15–1). Each TCR chain, like Ig heavy and light chains, is encoded by multiple gene segments that undergo somatic rearrangements during the maturation of the T lymphocytes (see Chapter 7). In the α and β chains of the TCR, the third hypervariable regions (which form CDR3) are composed of sequences encoded by V and J (joining) gene segments (in the α chain) or V, D (diversity), and J segments (in the β chain). The CDR3 regions also contain sequences that are not present in the genome but are encoded by different types of nucleotide additions, so-called N regions and P nucleotides (see Chapter 7, Fig. 7–11). Therefore, most of the sequence variability in TCRs is concentrated in CDR3.

The C regions of both α and β chains continue into short hinge regions, which contain cysteine residues that contribute to a disulfide bond linking the two chains. The hinge is followed by the hydrophobic transmembrane portions, an unusual feature of which is the presence of positively charged amino acid residues, including a lysine residue (in the α chain) or a lysine and an arginine residue (in the β chain). These residues interact with negatively charged residues present in the transmembrane portions of other polypeptides (CD3 and ζ) that form the TCR complex. Both α and β chains have carboxyl terminal cytoplasmic tails that are 5 to 12 amino acids long. Like membrane Ig on B cells, these cytoplasmic regions are too small to transduce signals, and the molecules physically associated with the TCR serve the signal-transducing functions.

TCRs and Ig molecules are structurally similar, but there are also several significant differences between these two types of antigen receptors (Table 6–2). The TCR is not produced in a secreted form, and it does not perform effector functions on its own. Instead, on binding peptide-MHC complexes, the TCR complex initiates signals that activate the effector functions of T cells. Also, unlike Ig, the TCR chains do not undergo changes in C region expression (i.e., isotype switching) or affinity maturation during T cell differentiation.

Table 6–2. Properties of Lymphocyte Antigen Receptors: T Cell Receptors and Immunoglobulins

	T cell receptor (TCR)	Immunoglobulin (Ig)
Components	α and β chains	Heavy and light chains
Number of Ig domains	One V domain and one C domain in each chain	Heavy chain: one V domain, three or four C domains Light chain: one V domain and one C domain
Number of CDRs	Three in each chain for antigen binding; fourth hypervariable region in β chain (of unknown function)	Three in each chain
Associated signaling molecules	CD3 and ζ	Igα and Igβ
Affinity for antigen (K_d)	10^{-5}–10^{-7} M	10^{-7}–10^{-11} M (secreted Ig)
Changes after cellular activation		
Production of secreted form	No	Yes
Isotype switching	No	Yes
Somatic mutations	No	Yes

Role of the αβ TCR in the Recognition of MHC-Associated Peptide Antigen

The recognition of peptide-MHC complexes is mediated by the CDRs formed by both the α and β chains of the TCR. Several types of experiments have definitively established that both the α and β chains form a single heterodimeric receptor that is responsible for both the antigen (peptide) specificity and the MHC restriction of a T cell.

- Cloned lines of T cells with different peptide specificities and MHC restrictions differ in the sequences of the V regions of both α and β chains.
- TCR α and β genes can be isolated from a T cell clone of defined peptide and MHC specificity. When both these genes are expressed in other T cells by transfection, they confer on the recipient cell both the peptide specificity and the MHC restriction of the original clone from which they were isolated (Fig. 6–4). Neither TCR chain alone is adequate for providing specific recognition of peptide-MHC complexes.
- To create transgenic mice expressing a TCR of a particular antigen specificity and MHC restriction, it is necessary to express both the α and β chains of the TCR as transgenes.

The antigen-binding site of the TCR is a flat surface formed by the CDRs of the α and β chains (Fig. 6–5). This resembles the antigen-binding surface of antibody molecules, which is formed by the V regions of the heavy and light chains (see Chapter 3, Fig. 3–4). In the TCR structures that have been analyzed in detail, the TCR contacts the peptide-MHC complex in a diagonal orientation, fitting between the high points of the MHC α-helices. In general, the CDR1 loops of the TCR α and β chains are positioned over the ends of the bound peptide, the CDR2 loops are over the helices of the MHC molecule, and the CDR3 loop is positioned over the center of the MHC-associated peptide. One surprising result of these structural analyses is that the side chains of only one or two amino acid residues of the MHC-bound peptide make contact with the TCR. This is structural proof for the remarkable ability of T cells to distinguish among diverse antigens on the basis of very few amino acid differences. Recall that mutational analyses of peptides described in Chapter 4 also showed that very few residues of the peptide are responsible for the specificity of T cell antigen recognition (see Fig. 4–9).

The affinity of the TCR for peptide-MHC complexes is low, much lower than that of most antibodies (see Chapter 3, Table 3–1). In the few T cells that have been analyzed in detail, the dissociation constant (K_d) of TCR interactions with peptide-MHC complexes varies from ~10^{-5} to ~10^{-7}M. This low affinity of specific antigen binding is the likely reason that accessory molecules are needed to stabilize the adhesion of T cells to APCs, thus allowing biologic responses to be initiated. Signaling by the TCR complex appears to require prolonged or repeated engagement of peptide-MHC complexes, which is also promoted by stable adhesion between T cells and APCs. The TCR and accessory molecules in the T cell plasma membrane move coordinately with their ligands in the APC membrane to form a transient supramolecular structure that has been called the **immunological synapse.** The formation of this synapse regulates TCR-mediated signal transduction. We will return to a discussion of signal transduction by the TCR complex and the role of the synapse in Chapter 8.

Virtually all αβ TCR–expressing cells are MHC restricted and express either the CD4 or the CD8

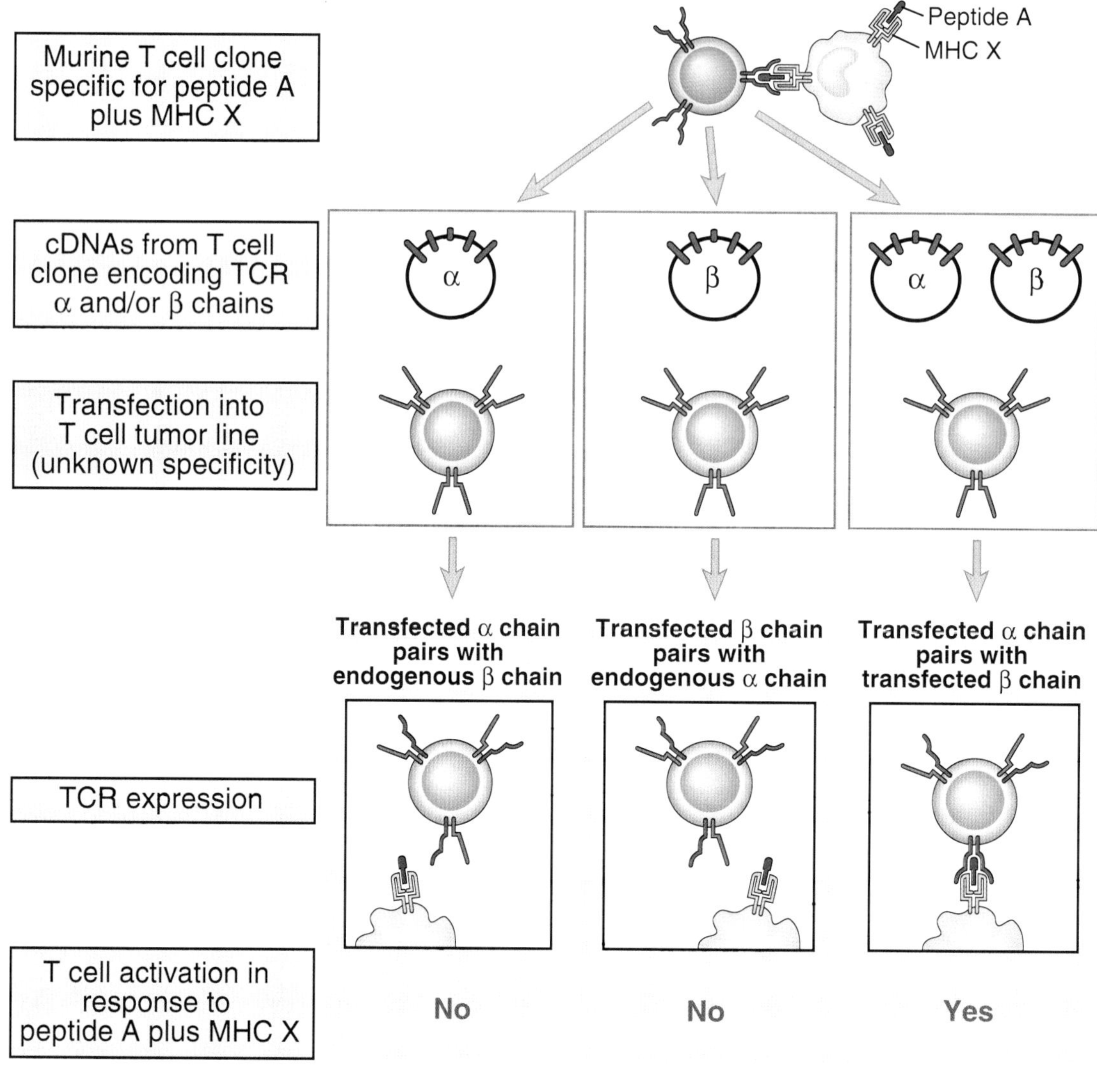

Figure 6–4 Role of the αβ TCR in MHC-restricted antigen recognition. The TCR α and β genes from a T cell clone of known specificity are expressed in a T cell tumor line. Transfection of both α and β genes is required to give the tumor line the antigen specificity and MHC restriction of the original T cell clone.

coreceptor. The functions of these coreceptors are described later in the chapter. A small population of T cells also expresses markers that are found on NK (natural killer) cells; these are called **NK-T cells**. The TCR α chains expressed by NK-T cells have limited diversity, and the TCRs recognize lipids that are bound to class I MHC–like molecules called CD1 molecules. Other cloned lines of T cells that recognize CD1-associated lipid antigens may be $CD4^+$, $CD8^+$, or $CD4^-CD8^-$ αβ T cells. These lipid antigen–specific T cells are capable of rapidly producing cytokines such as interleukin (IL)-4 and interferon (IFN)-γ. Their physiologic function is not known.

CD3 and ζ Proteins of the TCR Complex

The CD3 and ζ proteins are noncovalently associated with the TCR αβ heterodimer, and when the TCR recognizes antigen, these associated proteins transduce the signals that lead to T cell activation. The components of the TCR complex are illustrated in Figure 6–6 and listed in Table 6–1. The CD3 molecule actually consists of three proteins that are designated CD3 γ, δ, and ε. The TCR complexes also contain a disulfide-linked homodimer of the ζ chain. The CD3 proteins and the ζ chain are identical in all T cells regardless of specificity, which is consistent with their role in signaling and not in antigen recognition.

Structure and Association of CD3 and ζ Proteins

The CD3 proteins were identified before the αβ heterodimer by the use of monoclonal antibodies raised against T cells, and the ζ chain was identified later by co-immunoprecipitation with αβ and CD3 proteins. The physical association of the αβ heterodimer, CD3, and ζ chains has been demonstrated in two ways.

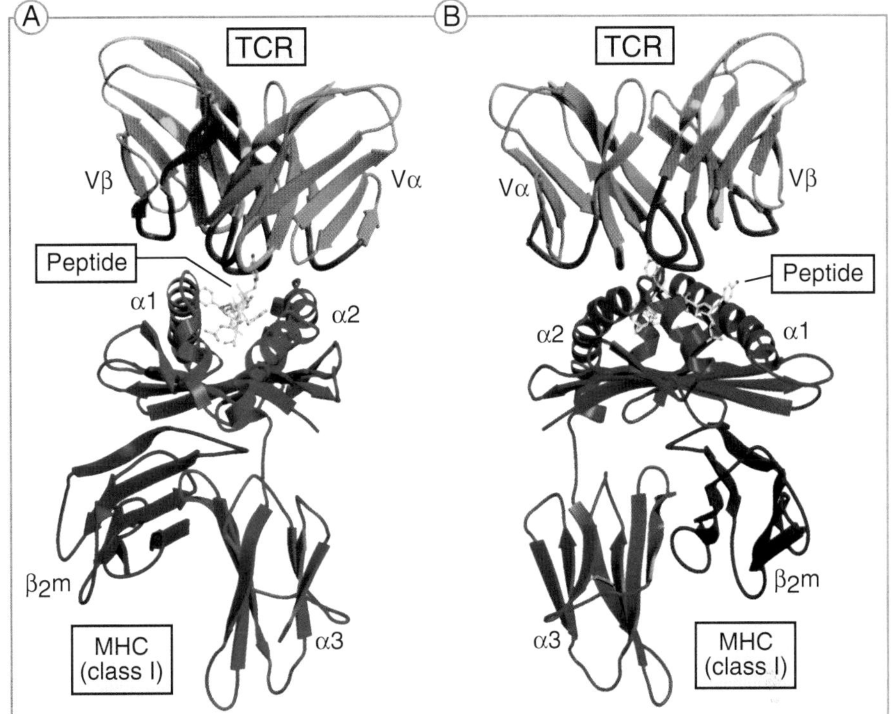

Figure 6–5 Binding of a TCR to a peptide-MHC complex. The V domains of a TCR are shown interacting with a human class I MHC molecule, HLA-A2, presenting a viral peptide (in yellow). A is a front view and B is a side view of the x-ray crystal structure of the trimolecular MHC-peptide-TCR complex. (From Bjorkman PJ. MHC restriction in three dimensions: a view of T cell receptor/ligand interactions. Cell 89:167–170, 1997. Copyright Cell Press.)

- Antibodies against the TCR αβ heterodimer or any of the CD3 proteins coprecipitate the heterodimer and all the associated proteins from solubilized plasma membranes of T cells.
- When intact T cells are treated with either anti-CD3 or anti-TCR αβ antibodies, the entire TCR complex is endocytosed and disappears from the cell surface (i.e., all the proteins are comodulated).

The CD3 γ, δ, and ε proteins are homologous to each other. The N-terminal extracellular regions of γ, δ, and ε chains each contains a single Ig-like domain, and therefore these three proteins are members of the Ig

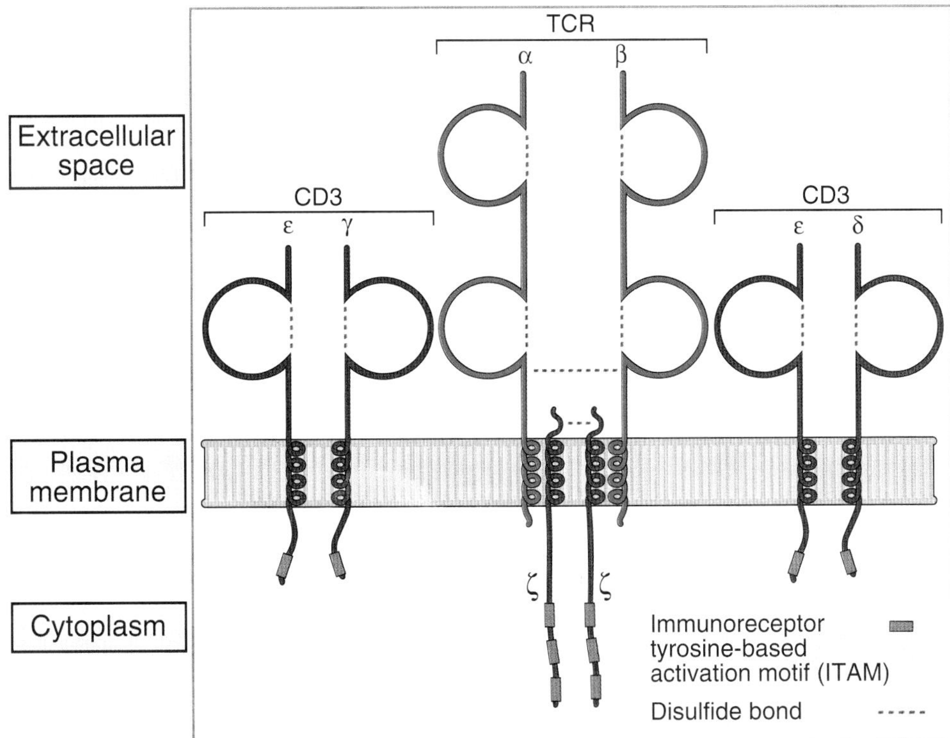

Figure 6–6 Components of the TCR complex. The TCR complex of MHC-restricted T cells consists of the αβ TCR noncovalently linked to the CD3 and ζ proteins. One possible stoichiometric combination is shown, but this may vary. The associations of these proteins are mediated by charged residues in their transmembrane regions, which are not shown.

superfamily. The transmembrane segments of all three CD3 chains contain a negatively charged aspartic acid residue, which binds to positively charged residues in the transmembrane domains of the TCR α and β chains, thus keeping the complex intact. The cytoplasmic domains of the CD3 γ, δ, and ε proteins range from 44 to 81 amino acid residues long, and each of these domains contains one copy of a conserved sequence motif important for signaling functions that is called the **immunoreceptor tyrosine-based activation motif** (ITAM). An ITAM contains two copies of the sequence tyrosine-X-X-leucine (in which X is an unspecified amino acid), separated by six to eight residues. ITAMs play a central role in signaling by the TCR complex. They are also found in the cytoplasmic tails of several other lymphocyte membrane proteins that are involved in signal transduction, including the ζ chain of the TCR complex, Igα and Igβ proteins associated with membrane Ig molecules of B cells (see Chapter 9, Fig. 9–3), and components of several Fc receptors (see Chapter 14, Box 14–1).

The ζ chain has a short extracellular region of nine amino acids, a transmembrane region containing a negatively charged aspartic acid residue (similar to the CD3 chains), and a long cytoplasmic region (113 amino acids) that contains three ITAMs. It is normally expressed as a homodimer. In mice, about 10% of T cells express a heterodimer composed of one ζ chain and an alternative splice product of the ζ gene called the η chain. There is no known functional correlate of these minor differences in the composition of the TCR complex. The ζ chain is also associated with signaling receptors on lymphocytes other than T cells, such as the Fcγ receptor (FcγRIII) of NK cells.

The expression of the TCR complex requires synthesis of all its components. The need for all components of the complex to be present for expression was first established in cell lines (Fig. 6–7). During the maturation of T cells in the thymus, CD3 and ζ proteins are synthesized before the TCR α and β genes are expressed (see Chapter 7). The CD3 γ, δ, and ε chains form core structures, but neither these nor the ζ proteins make their way to the plasma membrane, and they are apparently proteolytically degraded in the endoplasmic reticulum (ER). Chaperones, such as calnexin, may retain individual members of the TCR complex in the ER before the complex is fully assembled. As T cell maturation proceeds, the TCR αβ dimer is synthesized, and the entire TCR complex is assembled in the ER, transported to the Golgi complex where carbohydrates are added and modified, and expressed on the cell surface. This sequence of events is essentially similar to the events that lead to expression of the B cell antigen receptor complex in B lymphocytes.

Functions of CD3 and ζ Proteins

The CD3 and ζ chains link antigen recognition by the TCR to the biochemical events that lead to functional activation of the T cells. Several lines of evidence support the critical role of these components of the TCR complex in signal transduction in T cells.

- Antibodies against CD3 proteins often stimulate T cell functional responses that are identical to antigen-induced responses. Unlike antigens, which stimulate only specific T cells, anti-CD3 antibodies bind to and stimulate all T cells, regardless of antigen specificity. Thus, anti-CD3 antibodies are polyclonal activators of T cells.
- The cytoplasmic tail of either the CD3ε or the ζ protein is sufficient to transduce the signals necessary for T cell activation in the absence of the other components of the TCR complex. This was shown by expressing in

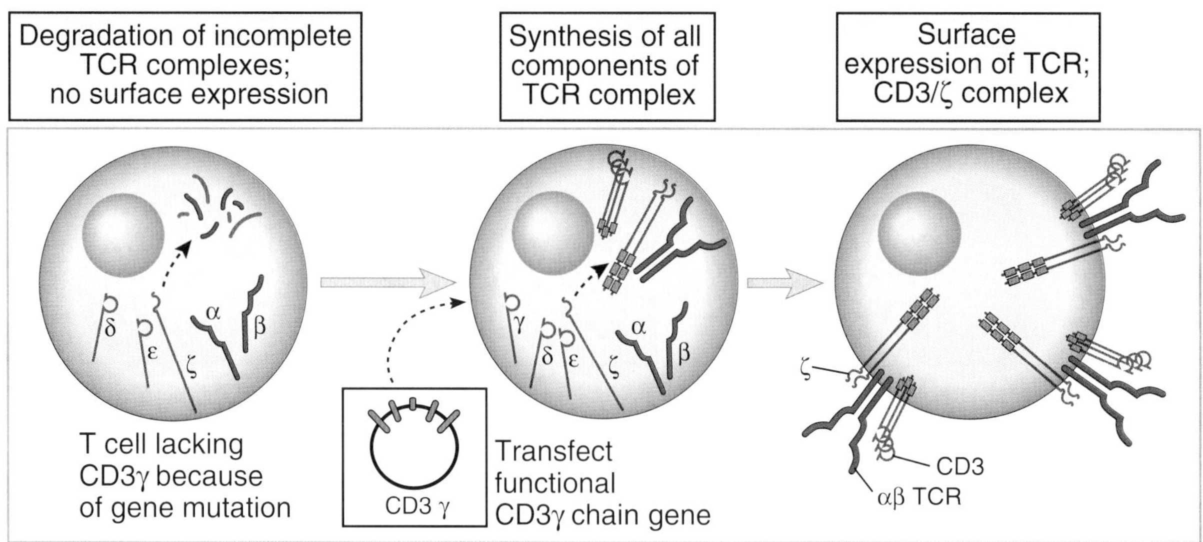

Figure 6–7 Assembly and surface expression of the TCR complex. In the absence of any one component (in this case, the CD3γ protein), the TCR complex is not assembled and all its proteins are degraded within the cell, probably in the endoplasmic reticulum. Introduction of the missing component by gene transfection allows the complex to be assembled and transported to the cell surface.

certain T cell lines genetically engineered chimeric molecules containing the cytoplasmic portion of CD3ε or the ζ chain fused to the extracellular and transmembrane domains of other cell surface receptors for soluble ligands, such as the IL-2 receptor. Binding of the ligand (e.g., IL-2) to the chimeric receptors results in activation responses identical to those induced by stimulation through the normal TCR complex on the same T cells.

The earliest intracellular event that occurs in T cells after antigen recognition is the phosphorylation of tyrosine residues within the ITAMs in the cytoplasmic tails of the CD3 and ζ proteins. The phosphotyrosines become docking sites for adapter proteins and for tyrosine kinases with Src homology 2 (SH2) domains, including a kinase called ZAP-70 (70-kD ζ-associated protein) that binds to the ζ chain and another kinase called Fyn that binds to CD3. Subsequent activation of these kinases triggers signal transduction pathways that ultimately lead to changes in gene expression in the T cells. The process of T cell activation is described in Chapter 8.

γδ TCR

The γδ TCR is a second type of diverse, disulfide-linked heterodimer that is expressed on a small subset of αβ-negative T cells associated with CD3 and ζ proteins. (The γδ TCR should not be confused with the γ and δ components of the CD3 complex.) The TCR γ and δ chains consist of extracellular Ig-like V and C regions, short connecting or hinge regions, hydrophobic transmembrane segments, and short cytoplasmic tails, similar to the α and β chains. The hinge regions contain cysteine residues involved in interchain disulfide linkages. The transmembrane regions of γ and δ chains, similar to α and β chains, contain positively charged amino acid residues that interact with the negatively charged residues in the transmembrane regions of the CD3 polypeptides. The γδ heterodimer associates with the same CD3 and ζ proteins as do αβ receptors. Furthermore, TCR-induced signaling events typical of αβ-expressing T cells are also observed in γδ T cells. The majority of γδ T cells do not express CD4 or CD8. A number of biologic activities have been ascribed to γδ T cells that are also characteristic of αβ T cells, including secretion of cytokines and lysis of target cells.

T cells expressing the γδ TCR are a lineage distinct from the more numerous αβ-expressing, MHC-restricted T lymphocytes. The percentages of γδ T cells vary widely in different tissues and species, but overall, less than 5% of all T cells express this form of TCR. Different subsets of γδ T cells may develop at different times during ontogeny, contain different V regions, and populate different tissues. For example, in mice, many skin γδ T cells develop in neonatal life and express one particular TCR with essentially no variability in the V region, whereas many of the γδ T cells in the vagina, uterus, and tongue appear later and express another TCR with a different V region. It is not known whether these subsets perform different functions, but the distinct V regions suggest that the subsets may be specific for different ligands. One intriguing feature of γδ T cells is their abundance in epithelial tissues of certain species. For example, more than 50% of lymphocytes in the small bowel mucosa of mice and chickens, called **intraepithelial lymphocytes,** are γδ-expressing T cells. In mouse skin, most of the intraepidermal T cells express the γδ receptor. Equivalent cell populations are not as abundant in humans; only about 10% of human intestinal intraepithelial T cells express the γδ receptor.

The functions of γδ T cells remain largely unresolved. γδ T cells do not recognize MHC-associated peptide antigens and are not MHC restricted. Some γδ T cell clones recognize small phosphorylated molecules, alkyl amines or lipids that may be presented by "nonclassical" class I MHC–like molecules and that are commonly found in mycobacteria and other microbes. Other γδ T cells recognize protein or nonprotein antigens that do not require processing or any particular type of APCs for their presentation. The limited diversity of the γδ TCRs in many tissues suggests that the ligands for these receptors are invariant and conserved. A working hypothesis for the specificity of γδ T cells is that they may recognize antigens that are frequently encountered at epithelial boundaries between the host and the external environment. Thus, they may initiate immune responses to a small number of common microbes at these sites, before the recruitment of antigen-specific αβ T cells. However, mice lacking γδ T cells, created by targeted disruption of the γ or δ TCR gene, have little or no immunodeficiency and only a modest increase in susceptibility to infections by some intracellular bacteria.

Accessory Molecules of T Cells

T cells express several integral membrane proteins, other than the members of the TCR complex, that play crucial roles in the responses of these cells to antigen recognition. These proteins, often collectively called **accessory molecules,** were discovered and initially characterized by the use of monoclonal antibodies raised against T cells. Some of these antibodies were shown to block or trigger functional responses of T cells and thus served as probes for studying the physiologic roles of accessory molecules. Subsequently, the antibodies were used to identify and characterize the T cell surface molecules by immunofluorescence and immunoprecipitation techniques.

These accessory molecules share several common properties that determine their roles in immune responses.

- ***Accessory molecules on T lymphocytes specifically bind other molecules (ligands) that are present on the surfaces of other cells, such as APCs and vascular endothelial cells, and in the extracellular matrix.*** Several different accessory molecules and their ligands on APCs or CTL target cells are known, and their principal functions are established (Fig. 6–8 and Table 6–3). The central role of accessory

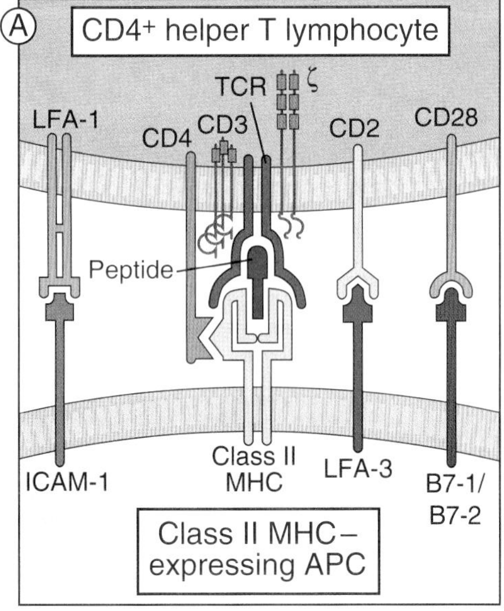

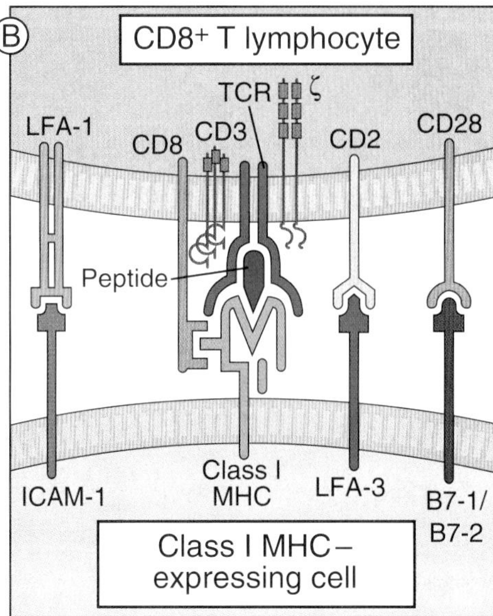

Figure 6–8 Accessory molecules of T lymphocytes. The interaction of a CD4⁺ helper T cell with an APC (A), or of a CD8⁺ CTL with a target cell (B), involves multiple T cell membrane proteins that recognize different ligands on the APC or target cell. Only selected accessory molecules and their ligands are illustrated. APC, antigen-presenting cell; CTL, cytolytic T lymphocyte.

molecules in T cell responses to antigens is illustrated by the finding that when T cells recognize antigens on APCs, accessory molecules are redistributed in an ordered way at the site of T cell–APC contact to form the immunological synapse (see Chapter 8).

- ***Accessory molecules are nonpolymorphic and invariant.*** Unlike the TCR, each accessory molecule is identical on all the T cells in all individuals of a species. Therefore, these molecules have no capacity to specifically recognize different, variable ligands, such as antigens. As we shall see later, many of the accessory molecules of T lymphocytes and their ligands are members of the Ig, integrin, and selectin families of proteins.
- ***Many accessory molecules transduce biochemical signals to the interior of the T cell that are important in regulating functional responses.*** Signal transduction occurs as a consequence of ligand binding and may act in concert with signals generated by the TCR complex. This signaling function is best defined for the coreceptors CD4 and CD8 and for T cell receptors for costimulators.
- ***The binding of some accessory molecules to their ligands on the surfaces of APCs increases the strength of adhesion between T cells and APCs.*** This property helps to ensure that the T cells and APCs remain attached to one another long enough to allow antigen-specific TCRs the opportunity to locate, recognize, and respond to peptide-MHC complexes displayed by the APCs. Multiple adhesive interactions between T cells and APCs may be needed to compensate for the low affinity of TCRs for their peptide-MHC ligands. As we shall see later, regulated adhesion mediated by accessory molecules is critical for the functional responses of T cells.
- ***The binding of accessory molecules to endothelial cells and extracellular matrix proteins is responsible for the homing of T cells to tissues and the retention of T cells in tissues.*** The affinity and expression of some accessory molecules on T lymphocytes increase on encountering antigen and inflammatory stimuli. The ligands for these molecules may be differentially expressed on endothelium in different tissues, and expression of the ligands also increases in response to local inflammation. Thus, the regulated expression of both accessory molecules and their ligands influences the way T cells migrate from blood to sites of antigen in lymphoid organs and nonlymphoid peripheral tissues.
- T cell accessory molecules are useful cell surface "markers" that facilitate the identification of T cells in normal tissues and in pathologic lesions, such as T cell tumors and inflammatory diseases. In addition, antibodies against these markers can be used to physically isolate T cells for experimental or diagnostic procedures.

In the following sections, we discuss selected T cell accessory molecules whose structures, functions, and importance in T cell activation are well understood. We begin with molecules whose principal role is to transduce signals that are involved in T cell activation and then discuss accessory molecules that function mainly to strengthen adhesions between T cells and other cells. Many other T cell surface molecules have been identified that may contribute to T cell responses, but their roles in physiologic immune responses are less well defined, and they are not discussed individually. Information about these accessory molecules is summarized in Table 6–3 and in Appendix II.

CD4 and CD8: Coreceptors Involved in MHC-Restricted T Cell Activation

CD4 and CD8 are T cell proteins that bind to nonpolymorphic regions of MHC molecules and transduce signals that together with signals delivered by the TCR complex initiate T cell activation. Mature αβ T

Table 6–3. The Principal Accessory Molecules of T Lymphocytes

Name of molecule	Synonyms	Biochemical features	Gene family	Cellular expression	Ligand	Affinity ($K_d \times 10^{-6}$ M)	Role in T cell activation	
							Adhesion	Signaling
CD4	T4 (human) L3T4 (mouse)	55-kD monomer	Ig	Class II–restricted T cells	Class II MHC		±	+
CD8	T8 (human) Lyt2 (mouse)	αβ or αα dimer; 78-kD α chain; 32- to 34-kD β chain	Ig	Class I–restricted T cells	Class I MHC	200	±	+
CD28	Tp44	Homodimer of ~44-kD chains	Ig	>90% CD4+ T cells, ~50% CD8+ T cells	B7-1 (CD80), B7-2 (CD86)	4	–	+
CTLA-4 (CD152)		Homodimer of 33- to 34-kD chains; may be monomer; >90% is intracellular	Ig	Activated T cells	B7-1, B7-2	0.4	–	+
CD45R	T200; leukocyte common antigen	180–220-kD monomer; cytoplasmic phosphatase		Leukocytes	Unknown		–	+
CD2	T11, LFA-2	50-kD monomer	Ig	>90% T cells (human), NK cells	LFA-3	10-20	+	+
LFA-1	CD11aCD18	Dimer of 180-kD α chain, 95-kD β chain	Integrin	Leukocytes, platelets	ICAM-1, ICAM-2, ICAM-3	0.1	+	±
L-selectin	CD62L, Mel-14	150-kD monomer	Selectin	Leukocytes	Carbohydrate ligands on HEV	105	+	–
CD44	Pgp-1	80–200-kD monomer		Lymphocytes, granulocytes	Matrix proteins		+	±

Abbreviations: HEV, high endothelial venule; ICAM, intercellular adhesion molecule; LFA, leukocyte function–associated antigen.

cells express either CD4 or CD8, but not both. CD4 and CD8 interact with class II and class I MHC molecules, respectively, when the antigen receptors of T cells specifically recognize peptide-MHC complexes on APCs (see Fig. 6–8). The major function of CD4 and CD8 is in signal transduction at the time of antigen recognition; they may also strengthen the binding of T cells to APCs. Because CD4 and CD8 operate together with the TCR in recognition of MHC molecules and in T cell activation, they are often called **coreceptors.** About 65% of mature αβ-positive T cells in the blood and lymphoid tissues express CD4, and 35% express CD8.

Structure of CD4 and CD8

CD4 and CD8 are transmembrane glycoprotein members of the Ig superfamily, with similar functions but different structures. CD4 is expressed as a monomer on the surface of peripheral T cells and thymocytes and is also present on mononuclear phagocytes and some dendritic cells. CD4 has four extracellular Ig-like domains, a hydrophobic transmembrane region, and a highly basic cytoplasmic tail 38 amino acids long (Fig. 6–9). The CD4 protein binds through its two N-terminal Ig-like domains to the nonpolymorphic β2 domain of the class II MHC molecule.

Most CD8 molecules exist as disulfide-linked heterodimers composed of two related chains called CD8α and CD8β. Both the α chain and the β chain have a single extracellular Ig domain, a hydrophobic transmembrane region, and a highly basic cytoplasmic tail about 25 amino acids long. The Ig domain of CD8 binds to the nonpolymorphic α3 domain of class I MHC molecules (Fig. 6–9). Some T cells express CD8 αα homo-

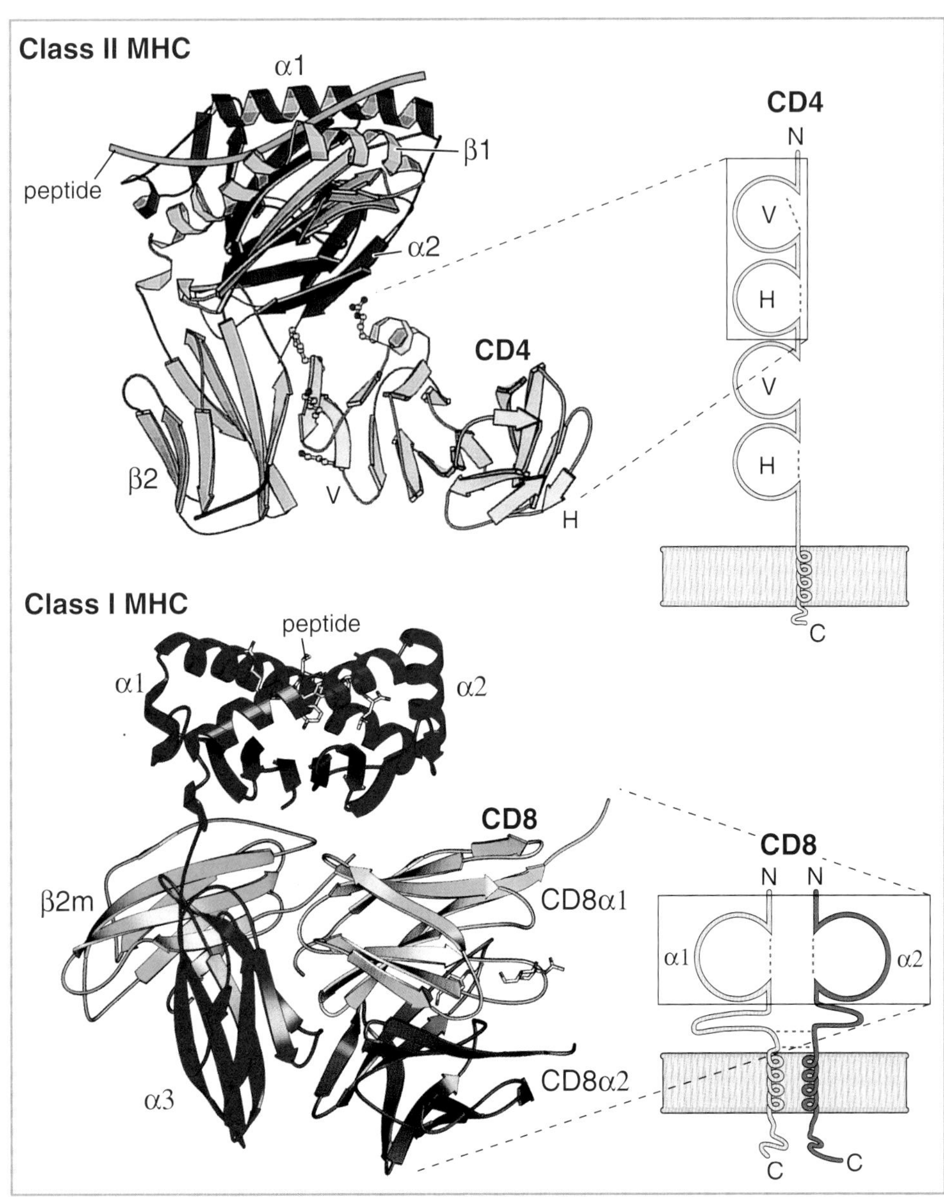

Figure 6–9 Structure of CD4 and CD8.

The models of CD4 and CD8 binding to class II MHC and class I MHC molecules, respectively, are based on the structures defined by x-ray crystallography. Both CD4 and CD8 bind to nonpolymorphic regions of MHC molecules (CD4 to the class II β2 domain and CD8 to the class I α3 domain) away from the peptide-binding clefts. (From Kern PS, M-K Teng, A Smolyar, et al. Structural basis of CD8 coreceptor function revealed by crystallographic analysis of a marine CD8αα ectodomain fragment in complex with H-2k. Immunity 9:519–530, 1998. Copyright 1998, with permission from Elsevier Science.)

dimers, but this different form appears to function like the more common CD8 αβ heterodimers.

Functions of CD4 and CD8

The selective binding of CD4 to class II MHC molecules and of CD8 to class I MHC molecules ensures that CD4⁺ T cells respond to class II–associated peptide antigens and that CD8⁺ T cells respond to class I–associated peptides. In Chapter 5, we described the processes by which class I and class II MHC molecules present peptides derived from intracellular (cytosolic) and extracellular (endocytosed) protein antigens, respectively. The segregation of $CD4^+$ and $CD8^+$ T cell responses to these different pools of antigens is because of the specificities of CD4 and CD8 for different classes of MHC molecules. CD4 binds to class II MHC molecules and is expressed on T cells whose TCRs recognize complexes of peptide and class II MHC molecules. Most $CD4^+$ class II–restricted T cells are cytokine-producing helper cells and function in host defense against extracellular microbes. CD8 binds to class I MHC molecules and is expressed on T cells whose TCRs recognize complexes of peptide and class I MHC molecules. Most $CD8^+$ class I–restricted T cells are CTLs, which serve to eradicate infections by intracellular microbes. Some $CD4^+$ T cells, especially in humans, function as CTLs, but even these are class II restricted. Thus, the expression of CD4 or CD8 determines the MHC restriction of the T cells and not necessarily their functional capabilities. The physiologic importance of this segregation was discussed in Chapter 5 (see Fig. 5–17).

The essential roles of CD4 and CD8 in the functional responses of T cells have been demonstrated by many types of experiments (Fig. 6–10).

- Antibodies specific for CD4 selectively block the stimulation of class II MHC–restricted T cells by antigen and APCs, and antibodies to CD8 selectively block killing of target cells by class I MHC–restricted CTLs.

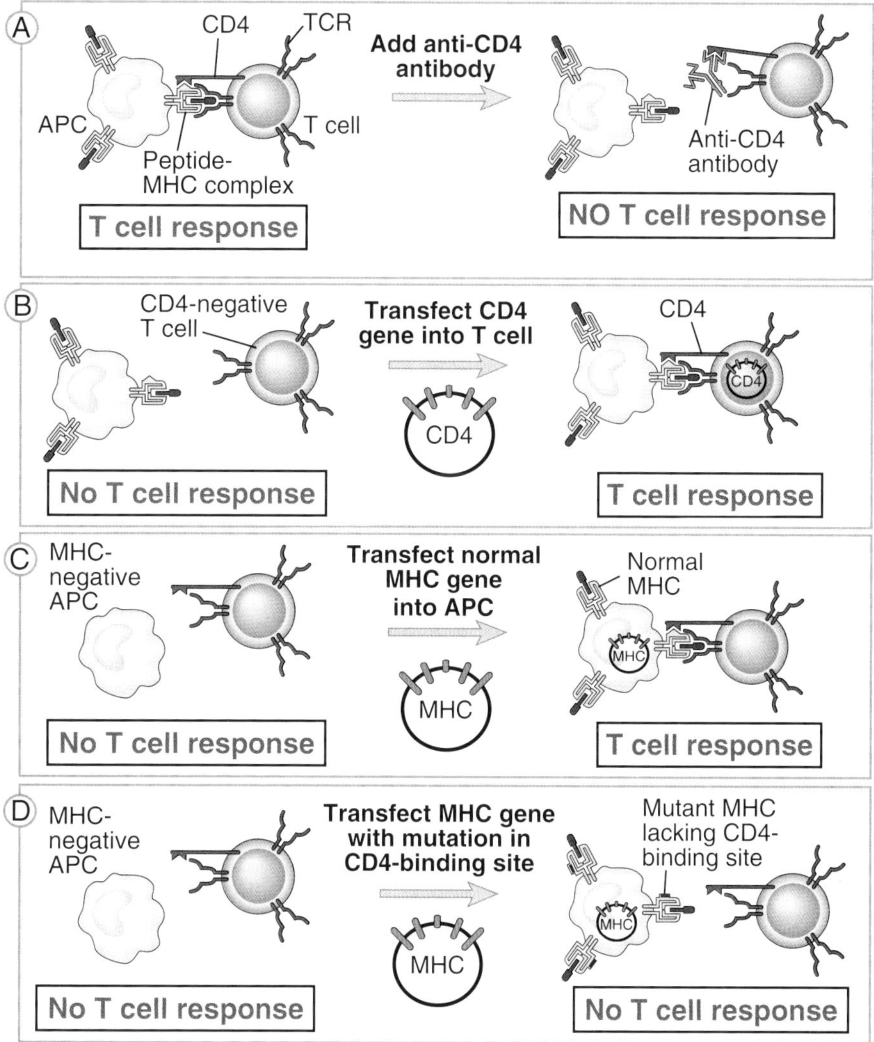

Figure 6–10 Role of the CD4 coreceptor in T cell responses to antigens.
During a T cell response to an MHC-associated peptide, CD4 binds to the MHC molecule. An antibody against CD4 blocks its binding to the MHC molecule and prevents T cell activation (A). A CD4-negative T cell does not respond to antigen, and introduction of CD4 into the T cell restores responsiveness (B). An MHC-negative antigen-presenting cell (APC) fails to activate T cells. Antigen-presenting function is restored by expressing normal MHC molecules in the APC (C) but not by expressing mutant MHC molecules that cannot bind CD4 (D).

- Formal proof of the obligatory function of these molecules came from gene transfection experiments. For example, if the TCR α and β genes are isolated from a CD4$^+$ T cell clone and transfected into another T cell line that does not express CD4, the TCR-expressing transfected line will not respond to APCs bearing the relevant class II MHC–associated antigen. Responsiveness is restored if the CD4 gene is cotransfected along with the TCR genes. The same type of experiment has established the importance of CD8 in the responses of class I–restricted T cells.

- An APC lacking MHC molecules cannot present antigen to or activate T cells. The ability to activate T cells is restored by transfecting into the APC normal MHC molecules but not by transfecting MHC molecules in which the CD4-binding or CD8-binding nonpolymorphic domain is mutated.

- Knockout mice lacking CD4 or CD8 do not contain mature class II–restricted or class I–restricted T cells, respectively, because these coreceptors play essential roles in the maturation of T cells in the thymus (see Chapter 7).

CD4 and CD8 serve two important functions in the activation of T cells.

- ***CD4 and CD8 participate in the early signal transduction events that occur after T cell recognition of peptide-MHC complexes on APCs.*** These signal-transducing functions are mediated by a T cell–specific Src family tyrosine kinase called **Lck** that is noncovalently but tightly associated with the cytoplasmic tails of both CD4 and CD8. CD4/CD8-associated Lck is required for the maturation and activation of T cells, as demonstrated by studies with knockout mice and mutant cell lines.
  - Disruption of the *lck* gene in mice leads to a block in T cell maturation, like the maturational arrest caused by deletion of CD4 and CD8 (see Chapter 7).
  - In T cell lines or in knockout mice lacking CD4, normal T cell responses or maturation can be restored by reintroducing and expressing a wild-type CD4 gene but not by expressing a mutant form of CD4 that does not bind Lck.

When a T cell recognizes peptide-MHC complexes by its antigen receptor, simultaneous interaction of

CD4 or CD8 with the MHC molecule brings the coreceptor and its associated Lck close to the TCR complex. Lck then phosphorylates tyrosine residues in the ITAMs of CD3 and ζ chains, thus initiating the T cell activation cascade (see Chapter 8).

- ***CD4 and CD8 promote the adhesion of MHC-restricted T cells to APCs or target cells expressing peptide-MHC complexes.*** The adhesive function of CD4 and CD8 has been demonstrated in several ways.
  - $CD4^+$ T cells adhere more firmly to class II MHC–expressing cellular monolayers than to cells lacking class II, and this adhesion is blocked by anti-CD4 antibodies.
  - The formation of conjugates between $CD4^+$ T cells and APCs, or between $CD8^+$ CTLs and their targets, is inhibited by antibodies against CD4 or CD8, respectively.

The affinities of CD4 and CD8 for MHC molecules are very low (see Table 6–3), and therefore these coreceptors probably play a minor role in T cell–APC adhesion. Also, it is likely that if these coreceptors strengthen the adhesion of T cells to APCs, they do so only with other accessory molecules.

In addition to its physiologic roles, CD4 is a receptor for the human immunodeficiency virus (see Chapter 20).

CD28 and CTLA-4: Receptors That Regulate T Cell Activation

CD28 is a membrane protein that transduces signals that function together with signals delivered by the TCR complex to activate naive T cells. A general property of naive T and B lymphocytes is that they need two distinct extracellular signals to initiate their proliferation and differentiation into effector cells. This two-signal concept was introduced in Chapter 1. The first signal is provided by antigen binding to the antigen receptor and is responsible for ensuring the specificity of the subsequent immune response. In the case of T cells, binding of peptide-MHC complexes to the TCR (and to the CD4 or CD8 coreceptor) provides signal 1. The second signal for T cell activation is provided by molecules that are collectively called **costimulators.** The best defined costimulators for T lymphocytes are a pair of related proteins, called B7-1 (CD80) and B7-2 (CD86), that are expressed on professional APCs. These B7 costimulators on APCs are recognized by specific receptors on T cells. The first of these receptors for B7 to be discovered was the **CD28** molecule, which is expressed on more than 90% of $CD4^+$ T cells and on 50% of $CD8^+$ T cells in humans (and on all naive T cells in mice). CD28 is a homodimer of two chains with Ig domains. Binding of B7 molecules on APCs to CD28 delivers signals to the T cells that induce the expression of anti-apoptotic proteins, stimulate production of growth factors and other cytokines, and promote T cell proliferation and differentiation. Thus, CD28 is the principal receptor for delivering second signals for T cell activation. A second receptor for B7 molecules was discovered later and called **CTLA-4** (CD152). CTLA-4 is structurally homologous to CD28, but CTLA-4 is expressed on recently activated $CD4^+$ and $CD8^+$ T cells, and its function is to inhibit T cell activation by counteracting signals delivered by CD28. Thus, CTLA-4 is involved in terminating T cell responses. How two TCRs deliver opposing signals even though they recognize the same B7 molecules on APCs is an intriguing question and an issue of active research. Several other T cell receptors have recently been discovered that are homologous to CD28 and bind to ligands that are homologous to B7 molecules (see Chapter 8, Box 8–2). These costimulatory signals may serve different roles in various types of immune responses. We will discuss the mechanisms and biologic significance of costimulation in more detail in Chapter 8, when we describe the activation of T lymphocytes.

Other Accessory Molecules with Signaling Functions: CD45, CD2

CD45 (originally called leukocyte common antigen), a cell surface glycoprotein with a cytoplasmic tyrosine phosphatase domain, is believed to play a role in T cell activation. Various forms of CD45 are expressed on immature and mature leukocytes, including T and B cells, thymocytes, mononuclear phagocytes, and polymorphonuclear leukocytes. The CD45 family consists of multiple members that are all products of a single complex gene. This gene contains 34 exons, and the primary RNA transcripts of three of the exons (called A, B, and C) are alternatively spliced to generate up to eight different messenger RNAs (mRNAs) and eight different protein products. The predicted amino acid sequences of the protein products include external domains of varying lengths, a transmembrane region, and a 705–amino acid cytoplasmic domain that is one of the largest identified among membrane proteins. Isoforms of CD45 proteins that are expressed on a restricted group of cell types are designated CD45R. Most naive human T cells express a form of CD45R that is called CD45RA, whereas memory T cells express a different isoform called CD45RO (see Chapter 2). However, these expression patterns are not fixed. There is no evidence that the distinct isoforms of CD45R perform different functions.

The cytoplasmic domain of CD45 contains a region with intrinsic protein tyrosine phosphatase activity, which catalyzes the removal of phosphates from tyrosine residues in several substrates. One such substrate is Lck, the tyrosine kinase that is associated with the cytoplasmic tails of CD4 and CD8. Some studies with T cell lines suggest that CD45-mediated dephosphorylation may allow Lck to become active, but it is not clear whether this is an essential step in the activation of normal T cells by antigens. CD45 gene knockout mice show a block in T cell maturation and defects in B cell and mast cell activation, the mechanisms of which are not defined. The physiologic ligand for CD45 is not known.

CD2 is a glycoprotein present on more than 90% of mature T cells, on 50% to 70% of thymocytes, and on

NK cells. The molecule contains two extracellular Ig domains, a hydrophobic transmembrane region, and a long (116 amino acid residues) cytoplasmic tail. The principal ligand for CD2 in humans is a molecule called leukocyte function–associated antigen-3 (LFA-3, or CD58), also an Ig superfamily member. LFA-3 is expressed on a wide variety of hematopoietic and nonhematopoietic cells, either as an integral membrane protein or as a phosphatidyl inositol–anchored membrane molecule. In mice, the principal ligand for CD2 is CD48, which is distinct from but structurally similar to LFA-3.

CD2 is an example of an accessory molecule that functions both as an intercellular adhesion molecule and as a signal transducer.

- Some anti-CD2 antibodies increase cytokine secretion by and proliferation of human T cells cultured with anti-TCR/CD3 antibodies, indicating that CD2 signals can enhance TCR-triggered T cell responses.
- Some anti-CD2 antibodies block conjugate formation between T cells and other LFA-3–expressing cells, indicating that CD2 binding to LFA-3 also promotes cell-cell adhesion. Such antibodies inhibit both CTL activity and antigen-dependent helper T cell responses.
- Knockout mice lacking both CD28 and CD2 have more profound defects in T cell responses than do mice lacking either molecule alone. This indicates that CD28 and CD2 may compensate for each other, an example of the redundancy of accessory molecules of T cells.

On the basis of such findings, anti-CD2 antibodies are now in clinical trials for blocking the rejection of transplants.

Adhesion Molecules of T Cells: Integrins, Selectins, CD44

Some accessory molecules of T cells function as intercellular adhesion molecules and play important roles in the interactions of T cells with APCs and in the migration of T cells to sites of infection and inflammation. The major adhesion molecules of T cells are members of the integrin and selectin families and CD44.

Integrins

The integrins are heterodimeric proteins, expressed on leukocytes, whose cytoplasmic domains bind to the cytoskeleton (Box 6–2). There are two subfamilies of

BOX 6–2

Integrins

The specific (nonrandom) adhesion of cells to other cells or to extracellular matrices is a basic component of cell migration and recognition and underlies many biologic processes, including embryogenesis, tissue repair, and immune and inflammatory responses. It is therefore not surprising that many different genes have evolved that encode proteins with specific adhesive functions. The integrin superfamily consists of about 30 structurally homologous proteins that promote cell-cell or cell-matrix interactions. The name of this family of proteins derives from the hypothesis that they coordinate (i.e., "integrate") signals generated when they bind extracellular ligands with cytoskeleton-dependent motility, shape change, and phagocytic responses. The Ig superfamily, which was described in Box 3–2, is another set of homologous proteins with adhesive and recognition functions.

All integrins are heterodimeric cell surface proteins composed of two noncovalently linked polypeptide chains, α and β. The α chain varies in size from 120 to 200 kD, and the β chain varies from 90 to 110 kD. The amino terminus of each chain forms a globular head that contributes to interchain linking and to ligand binding. These globular heads contain divalent cation-binding domains. Divalent cations are essential for integrin receptor function and may interact directly with integrin ligands. Stalks extend from the globular heads to the plasma membrane, followed by transmembrane segments and cytoplasmic tails, which are usually less than 50 amino acid residues long. The extracellular domains of the two chains bind to various ligands, including extracellular matrix glycoproteins, activated complement components, and proteins on the surfaces of other cells. Several integrins bind to Arg-Gly-Asp (RGD) sequences in fibronectin and vitronectin molecules. The cytoplasmic domains of the integrins interact with cytoskeletal components (including vinculin, talin, actin, α-actinin, and tropomyosin).

Three integrin subfamilies were originally defined on the basis of which of three β subunits were used to form the heterodimers. This led to a simplified organizational scheme because it was thought that each of these β chains could pair with a distinct and nonoverlapping set of α chains. More recently, five additional β chains have been identified, and many examples have been found of a single α chain pairing with more than one kind of β chain. Nonetheless, the subfamily designation is still useful for consideration of integrins relevant to the immune system; the major members of these subfamilies are listed in the table.

The β_1-containing integrins are also called VLA molecules, referring to "very late activation" molecules, because $\alpha_1\beta_1$ and $\alpha_2\beta_1$ were first shown to be expressed on T cells 2 to 4 weeks after repetitive stimulation *in vitro*. In fact, other VLA integrins, including VLA-4, are constitutively expressed on some T cells or rapidly induced on others. The β_1 integrins are also called CD49a–fCD29, CD49a–f referring to different α chains (α_1 to α_6) and CD29 referring to the common β_1 subunit. Most of the β_1 integrins are widely expressed on leukocytes and non-blood cells and mediate attachment of cells to extracellular matrices. VLA-4 ($\alpha_4\beta_1$ or CD49dCD29) is expressed only on leukocytes and can mediate attachment of these cells to endothelium by interacting with vascular cell adhesion molecule-1 (VCAM-1). VLA-4 is one of the principal surface proteins that mediate homing of lymphocytes to endothelium at peripheral sites of inflammation.

Continued on following page

BOX 6–2

Integrins (*Continued*)

Subunits		Name	Ligands/counterreceptors	Functions
β_1	α_1	VLA-1 (CD49aCD29)	Collagens, laminin	Cell-matrix adhesion
	α_2	VLA-2 (CD49bCD29)	Collagens, laminin	Cell-matrix adhesion
	α_3	VLA-3 (CD49cCD29)	Fibronectin, collagens, laminin	Cell-matrix adhesion
	α_4	VLA-4 (CD49dCD29)	Fibronectin, VCAM-1, MadCAM-1	Cell-matrix adhesion; homing; T cell costimulation?
	α_5	VLA-5 (CD49eCD29)	Fibronectin	Cell-matrix adhesion
	α_6	VLA-6 (CD49fCD29)	Laminin	Cell-matrix adhesion
	α_7	CD49gCD29	Laminin	Cell-matrix adhesion
	α_8	CD49hCD29	?	?
	α_v	CD51CD29	Vitronectin, fibronectin	Cell-matrix adhesion
β_2	α_L	CD11aCD18 (LFA-1)	ICAM-1, ICAM-2, ICAM-3	Leukocyte adhesion to endothelium; T cell–APC adhesion; T cell costimulation?
	α_M	CD11bCD18 (MAC-1, CR3)	iC3b, fibrinogen, factor X, ICAM-1	Leukocyte adhesion and phagocytosis; cell-matrix adhesion
	α_X	CD11cCD18 (p150,95; CR4)	iC3b; fibrinogen	Leukocyte adhesion and phagocytosis; cell-matrix adhesion
β_3	α_{IIb}	GPIIb/IIIa (CD41CD61)	Fibrinogen, fibronectin, von Willebrand factor, vitronectin, thrombospondin	Platelet adhesion and aggregation
	α_V	Vitronectin receptor (CD51CD61)	Fibrinogen, fibronectin, von Willebrand factor, thrombospondin, fibronectin, osteopontin, collagen	Cell-matrix adhesion
β_4	α_6	CD49fCD104	Laminin	Cell-matrix adhesion
β_5	α_v		Vitronectin	Cell-matrix adhesion
β_6	α_v		Fibronectin	Cell-matrix adhesion
β_7	α_4	LPAM-1	Fibronectin, VCAM-1, MadCAM-1	Lymphocyte homing ot mucosal lymphoid tissues
	α_E	HML-1	E-cadherin	Retention of intraepithelial T cells

Abbreviations: APC, antigen-presenting cell; iC3b, C3b inactivated; ICAM, intercellular adhesion molecule; LFA, leukocyte function–associated antigen; MadCAM-1, mucosal addressin cell adhesion molecule-1; VCAM-1, vascular cell adhesion molecule-1. Adapted from Hynes RO. Integrins: versatility, modulation, and signaling in cell adhesion. Cell 69:11–25, 1992. © Cell Press.

The β_2 integrins, also known as the leukocyte function–associated antigen-1 (LFA-1) family, were identified by monoclonal antibodies that blocked adhesion-dependent lymphocyte functions such as killing of target cells by CTLs. LFA-1 plays an important role in the adhesion of lymphocytes with other cells, such as APCs and vascular endothelium. This family is also called CD11a–cCD18, CD11 referring to different α chains and CD18 to the common β_2 subunit. LFA-1 itself is termed CD11aCD18. Other members of the family include CD11bCD18 (Mac-1 or CR3) and CD11cCD18 (p150,95 or CR4), both of which have the same β subunit as LFA-1. CD11bCD18 and CD11cCD18 both mediate leukocyte attachment to endothelial cells and subsequent extravasation. CD11bCD18 also functions as a fibrinogen receptor and as a complement receptor on phagocytic cells, binding particles opsonized with a by-product of complement activation called the inactivated C3b (iC3b) fragment. An autosomal recessive inherited deficiency in LFA-1, Mac-1, and p150,95 proteins, called type 1 leukocyte adhesion deficiency (LAD-1), has been identified in a few families and is characterized by recurrent bacterial and fungal

Continued on following page

infections, lack of polymorphonuclear leukocyte accumulations at sites of infection, and profound defects in adherence-dependent lymphocyte functions. The disease is a result of mutations in the CD18 gene, which encodes the β chain of LFA-1 subfamily molecules, and it demonstrates the physiologic importance of the LFA-1–related proteins. In knockout mice, deficiency of either LFA-1 or Mac-1 causes less severe immunologic defects than does the loss of all β_2 integrins.

In addition to adhesion, integrins may deliver stimulatory signals to cells on ligand binding. The mechanism of signaling involves tyrosine phosphorylation of different substrates, inositol lipid turnover, and elevated cytoplasmic calcium. The functional consequences of these integrin-mediated signals vary with cell type; in T lymphocytes, ICAM-1 binding to the β_2 integrins can provide costimulatory signals that enhance cytokine gene expression. However, the signaling role of integrins has been demonstrated mostly in nonphysiologic *in vitro* experimental systems, and its importance in conventional immune responses is not known.

integrins, and the members of each family express a conserved β chain (β_1, or CD18, and β_2, or CD29) associated with different α chains. The major integrin adhesion molecules on T cells are β_1 integrins, also known as VLA (very late activation) antigens, and the β_2 integrin commonly called leukocyte function–associated antigen-1 (LFA-1, also known as CD11aCD18). LFA-1 is expressed on more than 90% of thymocytes and mature T cells, B cells, granulocytes, and monocytes. One specific ligand for LFA-1 is intercellular adhesion molecule-1 (ICAM-1, or CD54), a membrane glycoprotein that is expressed on a variety of hematopoietic and nonhematopoietic cells, including B and T cells, dendritic cells, macrophages, fibroblasts, keratinocytes, and endothelial cells. Two other ligands for LFA-1 are ICAM-2, which is expressed on endothelial cells, and ICAM-3, which is expressed on lymphocytes. The β_1 integrin (VLA) subfamily consists of six members with different α chains. VLA-4 (CD49dCD29) binds to a protein called vascular cell adhesion molecule-1 (VCAM-1) that is expressed on cytokine-activated endothelial cells. T cell VLA molecules also bind to extracellular matrix ligands, such as fibronectin (VLA-4 and VLA-5) and laminin (VLA-6).

The major functions of T cell integrins are to mediate adhesion to APCs, endothelial cells, and extracellular matrix proteins. When the integrins bind their specific ligands, the T cell reorganizes its cytoskeleton, and this change leads to firm adhesion of the T cell. These adhesion functions of integrins are regulated by changes in the avidity of the integrins for their ligands, changes in the level of expression of the integrins, and changes in the expression of their ligands.

The avidity of integrins for their ligands is increased rapidly on exposure of the T cells to cytokines called chemokines and after stimulation of T cells through the TCR (Fig. 6–11). This rapid increase in binding avidity allows integrins to respond quickly when there is local inflammation (which is associated

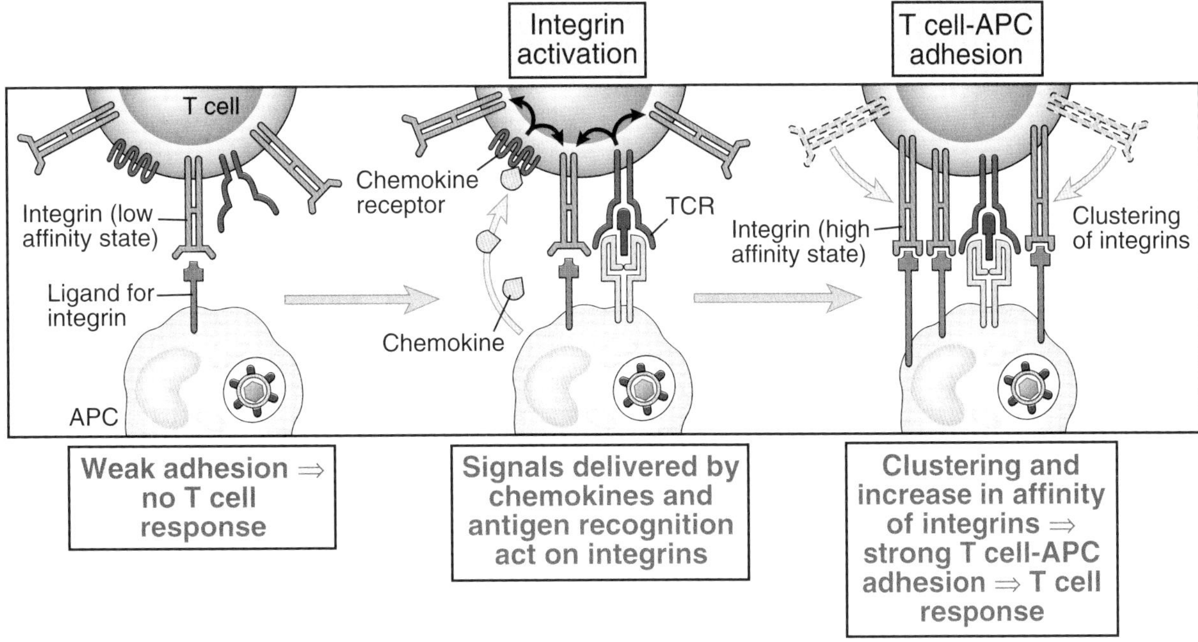

Figure 6–11 Regulation of integrin avidity.
Integrins are present in a low-affinity state in resting T cells. Chemokines produced by the antigen-presenting cell (APC) and signals induced by the TCR when it recognizes antigen both act on integrins and lead to their clustering and to conformational changes that increase the affinity of the integrins for their ligands. As a result, the integrins bind with high avidity to their ligands on APCs and thus promote T cell activation.

with the production of chemokines) and when T cells recognize antigens (leading to TCR-mediated signaling). The increase in integrin avidity in these situations ensures that integrin-mediated intercellular adhesion functions together with antigen recognition, especially at sites of inflammation, to optimize T cell–APC and T cell–endothelium interactions. This type of signaling, in which a stimulus (antigen or cytokine) changes the ability of a membrane protein to interact with the external environment, has been called inside-out signaling. The increase in integrin avidity is likely to involve changes in cytoskeletal organization, leading to clustering of integrins at the site of contact, and perhaps conformational changes in the extracellular regions of the integrins, leading to increased affinity of binding to ligands.

The expression of integrins on T cells is increased after activation, and the expression of the ligands for integrins on APCs and endothelial cells is increased by exposure to inflammatory cytokines. For these reasons, effector and memory T cells that have previously been stimulated by antigens bind more strongly than do naive T cells to APCs and to endothelium at sites of infection and inflammation. The tendency of antigen-stimulated T cells to home to sites of infection or inflammation is largely due to integrin-mediated binding of the T cells to ligands on the endothelium at these sites (see Chapters 2 and 13).

Integrins, particularly LFA-1, are essential for most adhesion-dependent lymphocyte functions, including antigen- and APC-induced helper T cell stimulation, CTL-mediated killing of target cells, and lymphocyte adhesion to endothelium. Antibodies against integrins or their ligands block all these interactions. Integrin-mediated adhesion may play a key role in the induction of antigen-specific T cell responses. T cells may first bind transiently to APCs through integrins and scan the APC surface for the presence of peptide-MHC complexes. If the APC expresses complexes that a T cell recognizes by its antigen receptors, the T cell is activated, the binding avidity of its integrins is increased, and the T cell remains attached for long enough to result in a productive response. Integrins also play critical roles in the interaction of nonlymphoid cells (granulocytes, macrophages) with other cells, such as endothelial cells. Some *in vitro* experiments suggest that integrins deliver activating signals to T cells, but it is unclear whether the signaling function of these molecules is critical for T cell activation.

The ability of integrins (and CD44) to bind to matrix molecules is responsible for the retention of antigen-stimulated T cells in lymphoid organs and at peripheral sites of infection and antigen persistence. Thus, in response to antigen and associated inflammation, effector and memory T cells leave the circulation and migrate into tissues. Those cells that specifically recognize the antigen increase the avidity of their integrins and, therefore, their ability to bind to matrix molecules. As a result, antigen-specific T cells are preferentially retained in the tissues, where they are needed to respond to and eliminate the antigen. We will return to a more detailed discussion of this sequence of events in Chapter 13, when we discuss cell-mediated immune reactions.

Selectins and Selectin Ligands

Selectins are carbohydrate-binding proteins present on leukocytes, endothelial cells, and platelets; their principal function is to regulate the migration of leukocytes to various tissues (Box 6–3). The leukocyte selectin, called L-selectin, is expressed at high levels on naive T

BOX 6–3

Selectins and Selectin Ligands

The selectins are a family of three separate but closely related proteins that mediate adhesion of leukocytes to endothelial cells (see Table). One member of this family of adhesion molecules is expressed on leukocytes, and two other members are expressed on endothelial cells, but all three participate in the process of leukocyte-endothelium attachment. Each of the selectin molecules is a single-chain transmembrane glycoprotein with a similar modular structure. The amino terminus, expressed extracellularly, is related to the family of mammalian carbohydrate-binding proteins known as C-type lectins. Like other C-type lectins, ligand binding by selectins is calcium dependent (hence the name C-type). The lectin domain is followed by a domain homologous to part of the epidermal growth factor, which in turn is followed by a number of tandemly repeated domains related to structures previously identified in complement regulatory proteins as short consensus repeats. These short consensus repeats are followed by a hydrophobic transmembrane region and a short cytoplasmic carboxyl terminal region.

L-selectin, or CD62L, is expressed on lymphocytes and other leukocytes. It serves as a homing receptor for lymphocytes to lymph node high endothelial venules and is also expressed on other leukocytes. On neutrophils, it serves to bind these cells to endothelial cells that are activated by cytokines (TNF-α, IL-1, and IFN-γ) found at sites of inflammation. L-selectin binding to its ligand has a fast on-rate but also has a fast off-rate and is of low affinity; this property allows L-selectin to mediate initial attachment and subsequent rolling of leukocytes on endothelium in the face of flowing blood. L-selectin is located on the tips of microvillus projections of leukocytes, facilitating its interaction with ligands on endothelium. The rolling is followed by more stable integrin-mediated attachment of the neutrophils to ICAM-1, spreading, and LFA-1–mediated transmigration. At least three endothelial cell ligands can bind L-selectin: glycan-bearing cell adhesion molecule-1 (GlyCAM-1), a secreted proteoglycan found on high endothelial venules of lymph node; mucosal addressin cell adhesion molecule-1 (MadCAM-1), expressed on endothe-

Continued on following page

Selectin	Size	Distribution	Ligand
L-selectin (CD62L)	90–110 kD (variation due to glycosylation)	Lymphocytes (high expression on naive T cells, low expression on activated effector and memory cells)	Sulfated glycosamino-glycans on GlyCAM-1, CD34, MadCAM-1, others
E-selectin (CD62E)	110 kD	Endothelium activated by cytokines (TNF, IL-1)	Sialylated Lewis X and related glycans (e.g., CLA-1) on various glycoproteins
P-selectin (CD62P)	140 kD	Storage granules and surface of endothelium and platelets	Sialylated Lewis X and related glycans on PSGL-1 and other glycoproteins

Abbreviations: CLA-1, cutaneous lymphocyte antigen-1; GlyCAM-1, glycan-bearing cell adhesion molecule-1; IL-1, interleukin-1; MadCAM-1, mucosal addressin cell adhesion molecule-1; PSGL-1, P-selectin glycoprotein ligand-1; TNF, tumor necrosis factor.

lial cells in gut-associated lymphoid tissues; and CD34, a proteoglycan on endothelial cells (and bone marrow cells).

E-selectin, also known as endothelial leukocyte adhesion molecule-1 (ELAM-1) or CD62E, is exclusively expressed by cytokine-activated endothelial cells, hence the designation E. E-selectin recognizes complex sialylated carbohydrate groups related to the Lewis X or Lewis A family found on various surface proteins of granulocytes, monocytes, and certain previously activated effector and memory T cells. E-selectin is important in the homing of effector and memory T cells to some peripheral sites of inflammation, particularly in the skin. On a subset of T cells, the carbohydrate ligand for E-selectin is called cutaneous lymphocyte antigen-1 (CLA-1) and is implicated in homing of these T cells to the skin. Endothelial cell expression of E-selectin is a hallmark of acute cytokine-mediated inflammation, and antibodies to E-selectin can block leukocyte accumulation *in vivo.*

P-selectin (CD62P) was first identified in the secretory granules of platelets, hence the designation P. It has since been found in secretory granules of endothelial cells, which are called Weibel-Palade bodies. When endothelial cells or platelets are stimulated, P-selectin is translocated within minutes to the cell surface as part of the exocytic secretory process. On reaching the cell surface, P-selectin mediates binding of neutrophils, T lymphocytes, and monocytes. In mice, P-selectin expression is regulated by cytokines, similar to the regulation of E-selectin. The complex carbohydrate ligands recognized by P-selectin appear similar to those recognized by E-selectin. A protein called P-selectin glycoprotein ligand-1 (PSGL-1) is post-translationally modified in leukocytes to express functional ligands for P-selectin. This involves both sulfation and fucosylation.

The synthesis of selectin ligands is differentially regulated in subsets of T cells, and this reflects differential expression of glycosyl transferase enzymes that attach carbohydrates to the protein backbone of the ligands. For example, naive T cells express virtually no E- and P-selectin ligands, and T_H1 cells express significantly more than do T_H2 cells. The genes for the three selectins are located in tandem on chromosome 1 in both mice and humans. The selectin structural motif clearly arose from duplication of an ancestral selectin gene. The differences among the three selectins serve to confer both differences in binding specificity and differences in tissue expression. However, it is thought that all three selectins mediate rapid low-affinity attachment of leukocytes to endothelium, an early and important step in leukocyte homing, although E-selectin may mediate high-affinity attachment as well.

The physiologic roles of selectins have been reinforced by studies of gene knockout mice. L-selectin–deficient mice have small, poorly formed lymph nodes and defective induction of T cell–dependent immune responses and inflammatory reactions. Mice lacking either E-selectin or P-selectin have only mild defects in leukocyte recruitment, suggesting that these two molecules are functionally redundant in this species. Double knockout mice lacking both E-selectin and P-selectin have significantly impaired leukocyte recruitment and increased susceptibility to infections. Humans who lack one of the enzymes needed to express the carbohydrate ligands for E-selectin and P-selectin on neutrophils have similar problems, resulting in a syndrome called type 2 leukocyte adhesion deficiency (LAD-2) (see Chapter 20).

lymphocytes, and its expression is reduced on activated T cells. It specifically binds carbohydrate moieties found on glycoproteins on the specialized endothelial cells of high endothelial venules in lymph nodes. Therefore, L-selectin mediates the migration of naive T cells into lymph nodes, where antigens are concentrated and immune responses are initiated (see Chapter 2). Two other selectins are called E-selectin (for endothelial selectin) and P-selectin (for platelet selectin, also found in endothelial cells). Both are rapidly expressed on endothelial cells that are activated by cytokines during inflammatory reactions. Activated T cells express ligands for E- and P-selectins. These ligands are heavily glycosylated membrane proteins, and their interactions with the selectins are also important for the migration of effector and memory T cells to sites of inflammation.

CD44

CD44 is an acidic sulfated membrane glycoprotein expressed in several alternatively spliced and variably glycosylated forms on a variety of cell types, including mature T cells, thymocytes, B cells, granulocytes, macrophages, erythrocytes, and fibroblasts. Recently activated and memory T cells express higher levels of CD44 than do naive T cells. CD44 binds hyaluronate, and this property is responsible for the retention of T cells in extravascular tissues at sites of infection and for the binding of activated and memory T cells to endothelium at sites of inflammation and in mucosal tissues (see Chapters 2 and 13).

Effector Molecules of T Lymphocytes

T lymphocytes express many other molecules that are involved in their effector functions and their regulation. Activated $CD4^+$ T cells express a surface protein called CD40 ligand (CD40L or CD154), which binds to CD40 on B lymphocytes, macrophages, dendritic cells, and endothelial cells and activates these cells. Thus, CD40L is an important mediator of many of the effector functions of helper T cells, such as the stimulation of B cells to produce antibodies and the activation of macrophages to destroy phagocytosed microbes. The role of CD40:CD40L interactions in humoral immune responses is discussed in Chapter 9 and in cell-mediated immunity in Chapter 13.

Activated T cells also express a ligand for the death receptor Fas (CD95). Engagement of Fas by Fas ligand on T cells results in apoptosis and is important for eliminating T cells that are repeatedly stimulated by antigens (see Chapter 10, Box 10–2). Fas ligand also provides one of the mechanisms by which CTLs kill their targets (see Chapter 13).

Activated T cells secrete cytokines, which function as growth and differentiation factors of the T cells and act on many other cell populations. Activated T cells also express receptors for many of these cytokines. We will discuss these effector molecules in later sections of the book when we describe the biologic responses and effector functions of T lymphocytes.

Summary

- The functional responses of T cells are initiated by the recognition of peptide-MHC complexes on the surfaces of APCs. These responses require specific antigen recognition, stable adhesion between the T cells and APCs, and delivery of activating signals to the T cells. The various components of T cell responses to antigens are mediated by distinct sets of molecules expressed on the T cells.
- MHC-restricted T cells recognize peptide-MHC complexes on APCs by clonally distributed TCRs. These TCRs are composed of two disulfide-linked polypeptide chains, called α and β, that are homologous to the heavy and light chains of Ig molecules. Each chain of the αβ TCR consists of a V region and a C region.
- The V segment of each TCR chain contains three hypervariable (complementarity-determining) regions, which form the portions of the receptor that recognize complexes of processed peptide antigens and MHC molecules. During T cell antigen recognition, the TCR makes contact with amino acid residues of the peptide as well as with polymorphic residues of the presenting self MHC molecules, accounting for the dual recognition of peptide and self MHC molecules.
- The γδ TCR is another clonally distributed heterodimer that is expressed on a small subset of αβ-negative T cells. These γδ T cells are not MHC restricted, and they recognize different forms of antigen than αβ T cells do, including lipids and some small molecules presented by nonpolymorphic MHC-like molecules.
- The αβ (and γδ) heterodimers are noncovalently associated with four invariant membrane proteins, three of which are components of CD3; the fourth is the ζ chain. The assembly of the TCR, CD3, and ζ chain is called the TCR complex. When the αβ TCR binds peptide-MHC complexes, the CD3 and ζ proteins transduce signals that initiate the process of T cell activation.
- In addition to expressing the TCR complex, T cells express several accessory molecules that are important in antigen-induced activation. Some of these molecules bind ligands on APCs or target cells and thereby provide stabilizing adhesive forces, and others transduce activating signals to the T cells.
- CD4 and CD8 are coreceptors expressed on mutually exclusive subsets of mature T cells that bind nonpolymorphic regions of class II and class I MHC molecules, respectively. CD4 is expressed on class II–restricted helper T cells, and CD8 is expressed on class I–restricted CTLs. When T cells recognize peptide-MHC complexes, CD4 and CD8 deliver signals that are critical for initiating T cell responses.
- CD28 is a receptor on T cells that binds to B7 costimulatory molecules expressed on professional APCs. CD28 delivers signals, often called signal 2, that are required in addition to TCR complex–generated signals (signal 1) for full T cell activation. A second receptor for B7, called CTLA-4, is induced after T cell activation and functions to inhibit responses.
- CD45 is a protein tyrosine phosphatase that plays a role in regulating tyrosine kinases during early T cell activation. CD2 is a T cell molecule that serves both adhesive and signaling functions.
- The T cell integrins LFA-1 and VLA-4 bind ICAMs and VCAM-1, respectively, on the surfaces of other cells. These adhesive interactions are important for stable conjugation of T cells and APCs and for T cell migration from blood into tissues. The binding of integrins to their ligands is regulated by changes in the avidity and expression of the integrins and by changes in the expression of their ligands.

- CD40 ligand and Fas ligand are T cell surface molecules whose expression is induced by T cell activation and that perform specialized effector functions.

Selected Readings

Bjorkman PJ. MHC restriction in three dimensions: a view of T cell receptor/ligand interactions. Cell 89:167–170, 1997.

Davis MM, JJ Boniface, Z Reich, D Lyons, J Hampl, B Arden, and YH Chien. Ligand recognition by γδ T cell receptors. Annual Review of Immunology 16:523–544, 1998.

Garcia KC, L Teyton, and IA Wilson. Structural basis of T cell recognition. Annual Review of Immunology 17:369-397, 1999.

Hayday AC. γδ T cells: a right time and a right place for a conserved third way of protection. Annual Review of Immunology 18:975–1026, 2000.

Hemler ME. VLA proteins in the integrin family: structure, functions, and their role on leukocytes. Annual Review of Immunology 8:365–400, 1990.

Hennecke J, and DC Wiley. T cell receptor–MHC interactions up close. Cell 104:1–4, 2001.

Hynes RO. Integrins: Bidirectional, allosteric signaling machines. Cell 110:673–687, 2002.

Miceli MC, and JR Parnes. The role of CD4 and CD8 in T cell activation and differentiation. Advances in Immunology 53:59–122, 1993.

Section III

Maturation, Activation, and Regulation of Lymphocytes

The activation of lymphocytes by foreign antigens is the central event in adaptive immune responses. Much of the science of immunology is devoted to studying the biology of B and T lymphocytes. In this section of the book, we focus on the generation of mature lymphocytes and the responses of these lymphocytes to antigen recognition.

Chapter 7 describes the development of B and T lymphocytes from uncommitted progenitors, with an emphasis on the molecular basis of the expression of antigen receptors and the generation of diverse lymphocyte repertoires. In Chapter 8, we discuss the biology and biochemistry of T lymphocyte activation. Chapter 9 deals with the activation of B lymphocytes and the mechanisms that lead to the production of antibodies against different types of antigens. In Chapter 10, we discuss the phenomenon of immunologic tolerance and the mechanisms that control immune responses and maintain homeostasis in the immune system.

Chapter 7

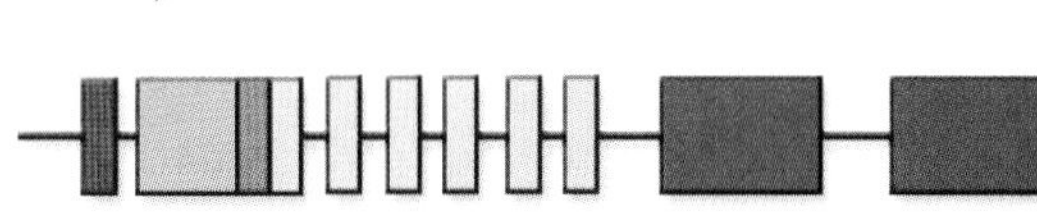

Lymphocyte Maturation and Expression of Antigen Receptor Genes

Lymphocytes are the only cells in the body to express highly diverse antigen receptors that recognize a wide variety of foreign substances. This diversity is generated during the development of mature B and T lymphocytes from precursor cells that do not express antigen receptors and cannot recognize and respond to antigens. The process by which bone marrow–derived lymphocyte progenitors are converted to mature lymphocytes that populate peripheral lymphoid tissues is called **lymphocyte maturation.** The collection of antigen receptors, and therefore specificities, expressed in B and T lymphocytes is called the **lymphocyte repertoire.** During maturation, a program of sequential gene expression leads to proliferation of the developing cells, generation of a diverse repertoire, changes in the phenotypes, acquisition of functional competence, and selection events to ensure that most of the lymphocytes entering peripheral tissues are useful in that they respond to foreign antigens but not to many self antigens. The expression of antigen receptor genes is the central feature of lymphocyte maturation, and there are many fundamental similarities in the processes by which B cells acquire the ability to express immunoglobulin (Ig) genes and T cells acquire the ability to express T cell receptor (TCR) genes. We begin this chapter with a discussion of the common cellular and genetic features of B and T lymphocyte maturation. This is followed by a description of the processes that are unique to B cell development and then of those unique to T cell development.

General Features of Lymphocyte Maturation

The maturation of B and T lymphocytes consists of sequential stages—early maturation involving lineage commitment and proliferation, expression of antigen receptor genes, and selection of the mature

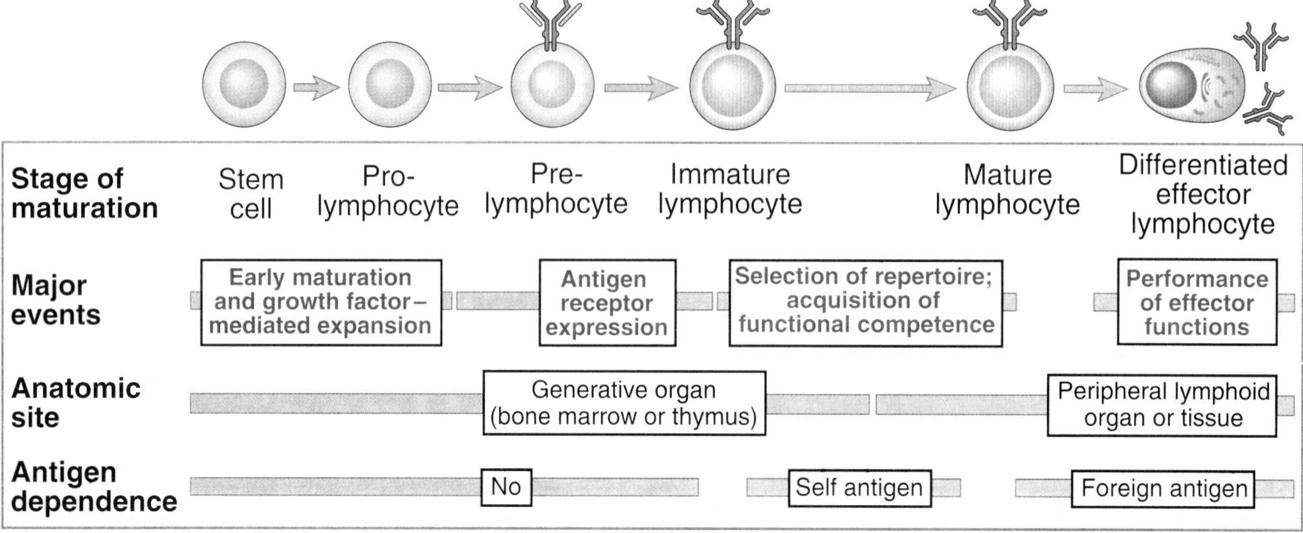

Figure 7–1 Stages of lymphocyte maturation. Development of both B and T lymphocytes involves the sequence of maturational stages shown. B cell maturation is illustrated, but the basic stages of T cell maturation are similar.

repertoires. During each of these stages, the cells undergo distinct cellular and genetic changes (Fig. 7–1).

Early Maturation

Pluripotent stem cells in the bone marrow (and fetal liver) give rise to all lineages of blood cells, including the lymphocyte lineage. It has been difficult to precisely define the mechanisms by which stem cells become committed to the lymphoid lineage or the phenotypic characteristics of these lymphoid progenitors. The existence of lymphoid progenitors is indicated by gene mutations in experimental animals or human patients that result in a block in development of lymphocytes but not other bone marrow–derived cells (Box 7–1). Some of these genes involved in lymphocyte maturation encode transcription factors, and others encode growth factors or growth factor receptors. The lymphoid progenitors give rise to B and T lymphocytes and NK (natural killer) cells. B and T lymphocytes develop from precursors that are not well defined by unique phenotypic markers, but their existence is convincingly demonstrated by genetic abnormalities in either early B cell development or early T cell development, but not both (see Box 7–1). The maturation of B cells from progenitors committed to this lineage proceeds in the bone marrow. In contrast, precursors of T lymphocytes leave the bone marrow and circulate to the thymus, where they complete their maturation. Despite their different anatomic locations, the early maturation events of both B and T lymphocytes are fundamentally similar.

Early B and T cell maturation is characterized by high mitotic activity, stimulated mainly by the cytokine interleukin (IL)-7, resulting in marked increases in cell numbers. The mitotic activity ensures that a large enough pool of cells will be generated to provide a highly diverse repertoire of antigen-specific lymphocytes. IL-7 is produced by stromal cells in the bone marrow and thymus. Mice with targeted mutations in either the IL-7 gene or the IL-7 receptor gene have profound deficiencies in mature T and B cells and little maturation of lymphocyte precursors beyond the earliest stages (see Box 7–1). Mutations in a chain of the IL-7 receptor, called the common γ chain because it is shared by several cytokine receptors, give rise to an immunodeficiency disease in humans called **X-linked severe combined immunodeficiency disease.** This disease is characterized by a block mainly in T cell development, perhaps because human B cell progenitors are able to proliferate in the absence of IL-7 signals (see Chapter 20). The proliferative activity in early lymphocyte development, driven mainly by IL-7, ceases before the cells express their antigen receptor genes. After the developing lymphocytes express antigen receptors, these molecules take over the function of stimulating proliferation.

Antigen Receptor Gene Recombination and Expression

The expression of antigen receptor genes is the key event in lymphocyte maturation required for the generation of a diverse repertoire and for the processes that ensure selective survival of lymphocytes with useful specificities. As we discussed in Chapters 3 and 6, each clone of B or T lymphocytes produces an antigen receptor with a unique antigen-binding structure, and in any individual, there may be 10^7 or more different B and T lymphocyte clones. The ability of each individual to generate these enormously diverse lymphocyte repertoires has evolved in a way that does not require an equally large number of distinct antigen receptor genes;

otherwise, a large proportion of the mammalian genome would be devoted to encoding Ig and TCR molecules. Functional antigen receptor genes are produced in immature B cells in the bone marrow and in immature T cells in the thymus by a process of **somatic recombination,** in which a set of inherited, or germline, DNA sequences that are initially separated from one another are brought together by enzymatic deletion of intervening DNA and religation. The diversity of the lymphocyte repertoire is generated during the joining of different gene segments. The DNA recombination events that lead to production of antigen receptors are not dependent on or influenced by the presence of antigens. In other words, as the clonal selection hypothesis had proposed, antigen receptors are expressed before encounter with antigens. We will discuss the molecular details of antigen receptor gene recombination later in the chapter.

Antigen receptors deliver signals to developing lymphocytes that are required for the survival of these cells and for their proliferation and continued maturation (Fig. 7–2). In the absence of antigen receptor expression, developing lymphocytes enter a default pathway of death by apoptosis. This requirement for antigen receptor expression in lymphocyte maturation is a quality control mechanism to ensure that only useful lymphocytes with functional antigen receptors are generated. During an intermediate stage of matu-

BOX 7–1

Genetic Blocks in Lymphocyte Maturation

Studies of natural and targeted gene mutations in mice, as well as identification of the affected genes in several inherited human immunodeficiency diseases, have contributed to our understanding of the role of individual molecules in the development of mature B and T lymphocytes. The genes identified by these approaches encode transcription factors, components of the pre-T and pre-B antigen receptor complexes, enzymes and adapter proteins involved in signal transduction in lymphocyte precursors, and proteins required for the formation of ligands involved in positive selection of lymphocytes. Some of these genetic blocks, especially mutations in transcription factors, have helped establish the existence of stem cells and early precursors committed to differentiate into either B or T lineages. Other mutations have contributed to our understanding of different stages of B or T lineage maturations, often referred to as checkpoints because these mutations block development of cells that are not able to express useful antigen receptors. Not surprisingly, many of these checkpoint mutations are found in genes encoding the structural or signaling components of the pre-B or pre-T receptors. Analyses of mutations in transcription factors and signaling molecules are also beginning to reveal the essential signaling pathways involved in lymphocyte maturation. In several cases, the mutations in homologous genes in mice and humans result in different degrees of developmental blockade. For example, mutations in the IL-2 receptor common γ chain, the cause of X-linked severe combined immunodeficiency disease in humans, result in a block only in T cell development in humans, but knockout of the same gene in mice results in failure of both T cell and B cell maturation. Mutations in the Btk kinase, the cause of X-linked agammaglobulinemia, result in a complete absence of mature B cells in humans but only a partial failure of B cell development in mice. Such observations suggest that maturation of lymphocytes is dependent on distinct sets of stimuli to different extents in different species. Thus, for maturation of B cells, signals from the pre-B cell receptor, which involve the Btk kinase, may be more important in humans, and signals delivered by cytokines, such as IL-7, which uses the IL-2R γ chain, may be critical in mice.

The following table includes a summary of many of the identified genetic blocks in lymphocyte maturation.

Maturation block	Defective *gene*/product	Function of encoded protein	Experimental model or human disease
Stem cell committed B or T lineage precursor	Ikaros	Transcription factor	Mouse gene knockout
	PU-1	Transcription factor	Mouse gene knockout
	IL-7	Cytokine: growth factor for immature lymphocytes	Mouse gene knockout
	IL-7 receptor α chain	IL-7–induced signaling	Mouse gene knockout
	Common cytokine receptor γ chain	IL-7– and other cytokine-induced signaling	Mouse gene knockout, human X-linked SCID (no B cell maturation defect in humans)
	Jak 3	IL-7 receptor–associated tyrosine kinase	Mouse gene knockout, human autosomal SCID
Stem cell committed B precursor, pro-B cell	Pax-5	Transcription factor	Mouse gene knockout
	E2A	Transcription factor	Mouse gene knockout
	EBF	Transcription factor	Mouse gene knockout
	Sox-4	Transcription factor	Mouse gene knockout

Continued on following page

BOX 7–1

Genetic Blocks in Lymphocyte Maturation (*Continued*)

Maturation block	Defective *gene*/product	Function of encoded protein	Experimental model or human disease
Pro-B cell pre-B cell	Igα	Pre-B receptor complex signaling	Rare human agammaglobulinemia
	RAG-1,RAG-2	Lymphocyte-specific components of V(D)J recombinase	Mouse gene knockout, human autosomal SCID
	Scid (DNA-protein kinase)	V(D)J recombinase component	Natural mouse mutation
	Ku80	V(D)J recombinase component	Mouse gene knockout
	μ heavy chain	Ig heavy chain component of pre-B receptor	Mouse gene knockout, rare human agammaglobulinemia
	λ5	Surrogate light chain component of pre-B receptor	Mouse gene knockout, rare human agammaglobulinemia
	Syk	Protein tyrosine kinase involved in pre-B cell receptor signaling	Mouse gene knockout
	B cell tyrosine kinase (Btk)	Tyrosine kinase	Human X-linked agammaglobulinemia, mouse gene knockout
	B cell linker protein (BLNK)/SLP-65	Adapter protein	Mouse gene knockout, rare human agammaglobulinemia
	Phospholipase Cγ2	Enzyme involved in B cell receptor signaling	Mouse gene knockout
Pre-B cell immature B cell	κ light chain gene	Component of Ig B cell antigen receptor	Mouse gene knockout
Immature B cell mature B cell	Igβ	B cell receptor complex signaling	Mouse gene knockout
Stem cell committed T lineage precursor	Winged helix nude	Transcription factor (expressed in thymic epithelium)	Natural mouse mutation
Committed T lineage precursor early double-negative thymocyte	GATA-3	Transcription factor	Mouse gene knockout
Early pre-T to double-positive thymocyte	RAG-1 or RAG-2	Lymphocyte-specific component of V(D)J recombinase	Mouse gene knockout, rare human immunodeficiency
	Scid (mouse)	DNA-dependent kinase	Natural mouse mutant
	Pre-Tα	Component of pre-T cell receptor	Mouse gene knockout
	TCRβ	Component of pre-T receptor and mature T cell antigen receptor	Mouse gene knockout
	CD3ε	Signaling chain of the pre-T and mature T cell antigen receptor complex	Mouse gene knockout
	CD3γ	Signaling chain of the pre-T and mature T cell antigen receptor complex	Mouse gene knockout
	Lck	CD4- and CD8-associated protein tyrosine kinase	Mouse gene knockout
	Itk	Protein tyrosine kinase involved in pre-T and mature TCR signaling	Mouse gene knockout
Double-positive thymocyte to single-positive thymocyte	TCRα enhancer	Regulates expression of α chain of TCR	Mouse gene knockout
	CD3γ	Signaling component of TCR	Mouse gene knockout
	ZAP-70	Protein tyrosine kinase involved in pre-T and mature TCR signaling	Mouse gene knockout, rare human immunodeficiency
	MHC class I or II	Component of TCR ligand required for positive selection	Mouse gene knockout
	CIITA and RFX genes	Required for class II MHC gene transcription	Mouse gene knockouts, human bare lymphocyte syndrome
	TAP-1 or TAP-2	Peptide transporter required for class I MHC assembly	Mouse gene knockout, rare human immunodeficiency
	CD4 or CD8	Component of TCR ligand required for positive selection	Mouse gene knockout, rare human immunodeficiency (CD8)

Abbreviation: SCID, severe combined immunodeficiency.

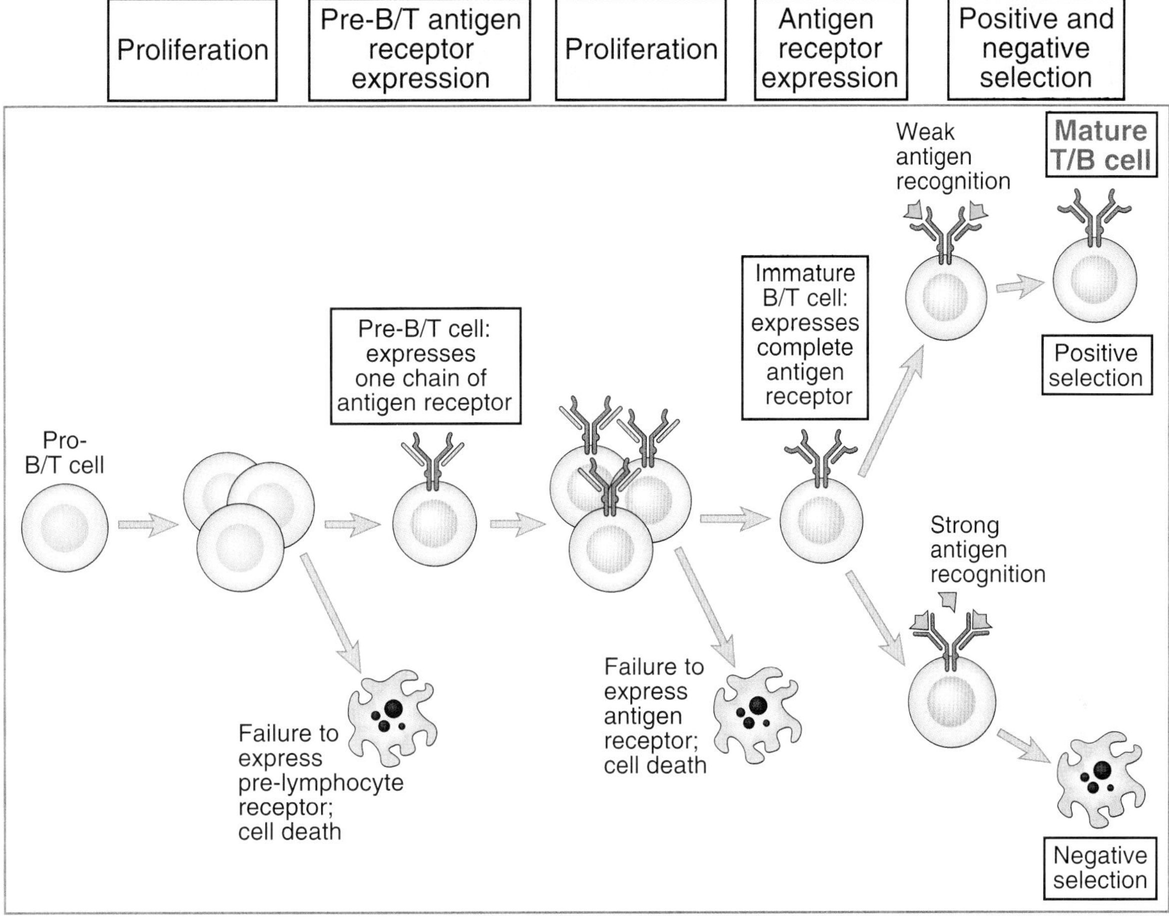

Figure 7–2 Checkpoints in lymphocyte maturation.
During development, the lymphocytes that express receptors required for continued proliferation and maturation are selected to survive, and cells that do not express functional receptors die by apoptosis. Positive and negative selection further preserve cells with useful specificities. The presence of multiple checkpoints ensures that only cells with useful receptors complete their maturation.

ration, called the pre-B cell or pre-T cell stage, an immature form of antigen receptor is formed. This pre-B or pre-T cell receptor is composed of one of the chains of the mature antigen receptor (the Ig heavy chain in pre-B cells and the TCR β chain in pre-T cells) attached to an additional invariant protein (which differs between B and T cell lineages). Although it is not clear what, if any, ligands these immature receptors bind, it is known they transduce signals that induce further maturation steps. Importantly, the signals also rescue the developing pre-lymphocytes from programmed cell death, also called death by neglect. Thus, the receptor of the pre-lymphocytes provides an intermediate checkpoint to ensure that the first somatic recombination was successful. In more mature lymphocytes, the complete antigen receptor is expressed (Ig heavy chains + light chains in B cells, TCR α chains + β chains in T cells), and signals from this receptor promote cell survival, proliferation, and continued maturation, providing the next checkpoint during maturation. The process of somatic recombination of antigen receptor genes often fails to produce functional Ig or TCR genes. As a result, many developing B and T cells, estimated to be 90% to 95% of the immature cells, fail to express these antigen receptors and die by apoptosis.

Selection Processes That Shape the B and T Lymphocyte Repertoires

After immature lymphocytes express antigen receptors, the cells with useful receptors are preserved, and many potentially harmful, self antigen–reactive cells are eliminated by processes of selection induced by antigen receptor engagement (Fig. 7–3). Because the expression of antigen receptors results from gene recombinations that are not influenced by the specificities of the receptors that will be produced, many immature lymphocytes may express antigen receptors that are of no use. The preservation of useful specificities is called **positive selection,** and it is best understood in T lymphocytes. Positive selection ensures maturation of T cells whose receptors bind with low avidity (weakly) to self major histocompatibility complex (MHC) molecules. Mature T cells whose precursors were positively selected by self MHC molecules in the thymus are able to recognize foreign peptide antigens displayed by the

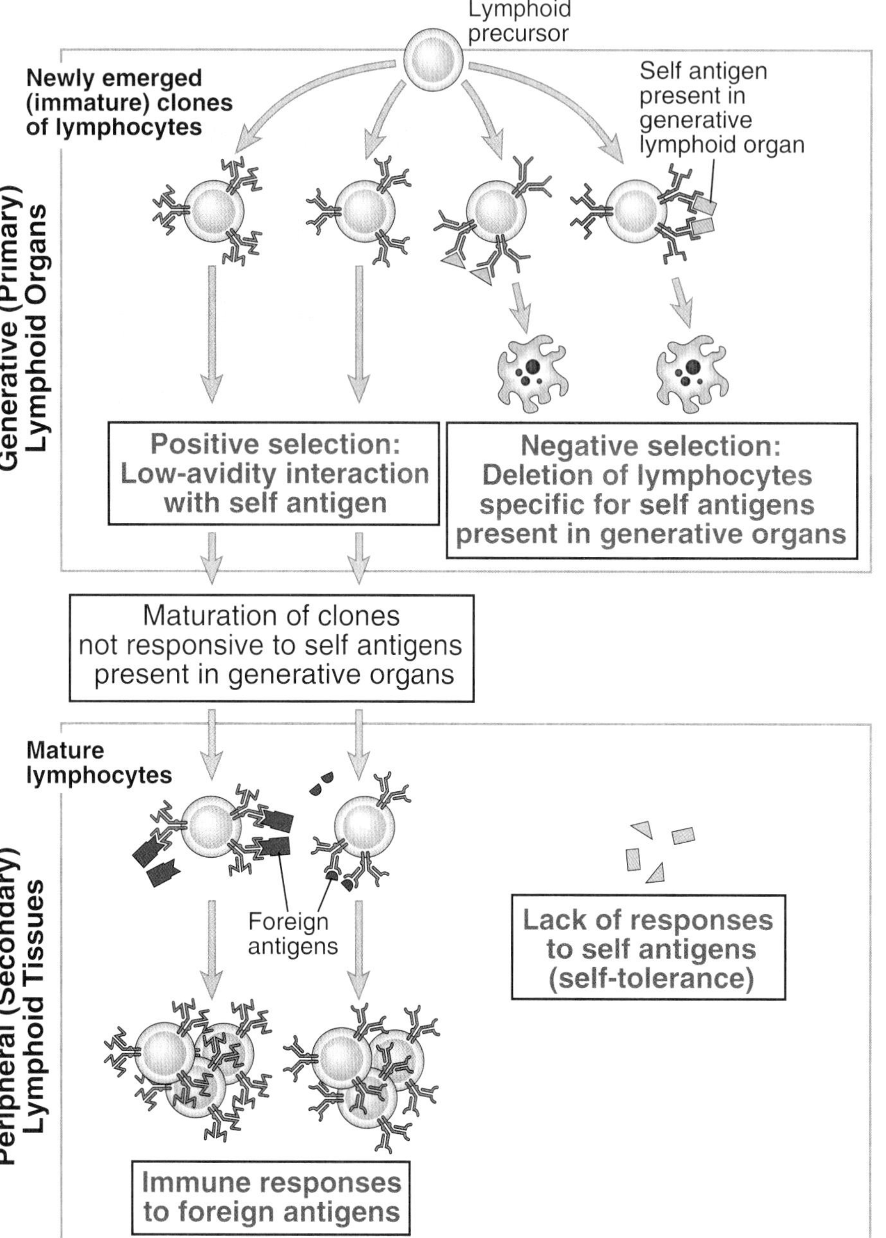

Figure 7–3 Selection processes in lymphocyte maturation. After immature clones of lymphocytes in generative lymphoid organs express antigen receptors, they are subject to both positive and negative selection processes. In positive selection, lymphocyte precursors with antigen receptors that bind some self ligand, probably with low avidity, are selected to survive and mature further. These positively selected lymphocytes enter peripheral lymphoid tissues, where they respond to foreign antigens. In negative selection, cells that bind ubiquitous antigens present within the generative organs, with high avidity, receive signals that lead to cell death. As a result, the repertoire of mature lymphocytes lacks cells capable of responding to these self antigens. The diagram illustrates selection of B cells; the principles are the same for T lymphocytes.

same self MHC molecules on antigen-presenting cells in peripheral tissues. If the TCR on a developing T cell cannot recognize any MHC molecules in the thymus, the cell dies by apoptosis; such a cell would not be able to recognize MHC-associated antigens in that individual. Thus, positive selection serves to generate a self MHC–restricted T cell repertoire. Pre-B cells and immature B cells may be positively selected by weak recognition of some self antigens or simply by virtue of antigen receptor expression, ensuring that all the B cells that mature express functional antigen receptors. The ligands that may trigger receptor-mediated signals in maturing B cells are not known.

Negative selection is the process that eliminates developing lymphocytes whose antigen receptors bind strongly to self antigens present in the generative lymphoid organs. Both developing B cells and developing T cells are susceptible to negative selection during a short period after antigen receptors are expressed. The mechanism of negative selection is apoptosis that is actively induced by antigen receptor–generated signals in immature lymphocytes. Negative selection of developing lymphocytes is an important mechanism for maintaining so-called tolerance to ubiquitous self antigens; this is called central tolerance (see Chapter 10).

Acquisition of Functional Competence

During the late stages of maturation, lymphocytes acquire the ability to respond to antigens and generate the effector mechanisms that serve to eliminate antigens. Functional maturation involves the expression of a variety of cell surface and intracellular molecules that participate in lymphocyte activation and effector functions. B cells acquire the ability to secrete antibodies in response to antigens and other signals. Distinct subsets of T cells with different functions develop within the thymus. The clearest example of functional heterogeneity acquired during T cell development is the maturation of precursors that express both CD4 and CD8 into either $CD4^+$ class II MHC–restricted T cells or $CD8^+$ class I MHC–restricted T cells. The $CD4^+$ cells that leave the thymus can be activated by antigens to differentiate into helper T cells whose effector functions are mediated by particular membrane molecules and the production of cytokines. The $CD8^+$ cells can differentiate into cytolytic T lymphocytes whose major effector function is to kill infected target cells.

With this introduction, we proceed to a more detailed discussion of lymphocyte maturation, starting with the key event in maturation, the expression of antigen receptors.

Formation of Functional Antigen Receptor Genes in B and T Lymphocytes

The diverse antigen receptors of B and T lymphocytes are produced in immature cells from genes that are formed by somatic recombination of a limited number of inherited gene segments. Elucidation of the mechanisms of antigen receptor gene expression is one of the landmark achievements of modern immunology and has provided a basis for understanding the specificity and diversity of antigen receptors.

The first insights into how millions of different antigen receptors could be generated from a small number of genes came from analyses of the amino acid sequences of Ig molecules. These analyses showed that the polypeptide chains of many different antibodies of the same isotype share identical sequences at one end of the chains (the constant regions) but differ considerably in the sequences at the other end (the variable regions) (see Chapter 3). Contrary to the general assumption of the time that single polypeptide chains are encoded by single genes, Dreyer and Bennett postulated in 1965 that each antibody chain is actually encoded by at least two genes, one variable and the other constant, and that the two become joined at the level of the DNA or the messenger RNA (mRNA) to give rise to functional Ig proteins. (The evidence for this conclusion is described later in the chapter.)

Formal proof of this hypothesis came more than a decade later when Susumu Tonegawa demonstrated that the structure of Ig genes in the cells of an antibody-producing tumor, called a myeloma or plasmacytoma, is different from that in embryonic tissues or in non-lymphoid tissues not committed to Ig production. These differences arise because during B cell development, there is a recombination of DNA sequences within the loci encoding Ig heavy and light chains. Furthermore, similar rearrangements occur during T cell development in the loci encoding the polypeptide chains of TCRs. Antigen receptor gene recombination is best understood by first describing the unrearranged, or germline, organization of Ig and TCR genes and then describing their rearrangement during lymphocyte maturation.

Organization of Ig and TCR Genes in the Germline

The germline organizations of Ig and TCR genetic loci are fundamentally similar and are characterized by spatial segregation of sequences that must be joined together to produce functional genes coding for antigen receptor proteins. We first describe the Ig loci and then discuss the TCR loci in comparison.

Organization of Ig Gene Loci

Three separate loci encode, respectively, all the Ig heavy chains, the Ig κ light chain, and the Ig λ light chain. Each locus is on a different chromosome. The organization of human Ig genes* is illustrated in Figure 7–4, and the relationship of gene segments to the domains of the Ig heavy and light chain proteins is shown in Figure 7–5A. Ig genes are organized in essentially the same way in all mammals, although their chromosomal locations and the number and sequence of different gene segments in each locus may vary. Each germline Ig locus is made up of multiple copies of at least three different types of gene segments, the V, C, and joining (J) segments. In addition, the Ig heavy chain locus has diversity (D) segments. Within each locus, the sets of each type of gene segment are separated from one another by stretches of noncoding DNA.

At the 5′ end of each of the Ig loci, there is a cluster of **V gene segments,** each about 300 base pairs long, separated from one another by noncoding DNA of varying lengths. The numbers of V genes (used here synonymously with V region exons) vary considerably among the different Ig loci and among different species. For example, there are about 35 V genes in the human κ

*In Ig and TCR loci, the term *gene* usually refers to the DNA encoding the complete polypeptide chain (e.g., an Ig heavy or light chain) or a TCR α or β chain. As we shall discuss presently, each complete gene consists of multiple "gene segments" that code for V, C, and other regions and are separated from one another in the genome by large stretches of DNA that are never transcribed. Each V and C gene segment is further composed of coding sequences that are present in the mature mRNA; these are called **exons.** For instance, each C_H gene segment that gives rise to a heavy chain C region is composed of five or six exons. Exons are separated by pieces of DNA, called **introns,** that are transcribed and present in the primary (nuclear) RNA but absent from the mRNA. The removal of introns from the primary transcript is the process of RNA **splicing.** Sometimes, the terms *gene, gene segment,* and *exon* are used interchangeably. For instance, "V gene" might refer to the gene segment coding for the complete V region of an Ig heavy or light chain, which actually consists of a V region exon and additional segments (J and D, as we shall see later), or "V gene" might refer to a V region exon only (as in "V gene families," discussed in this chapter).

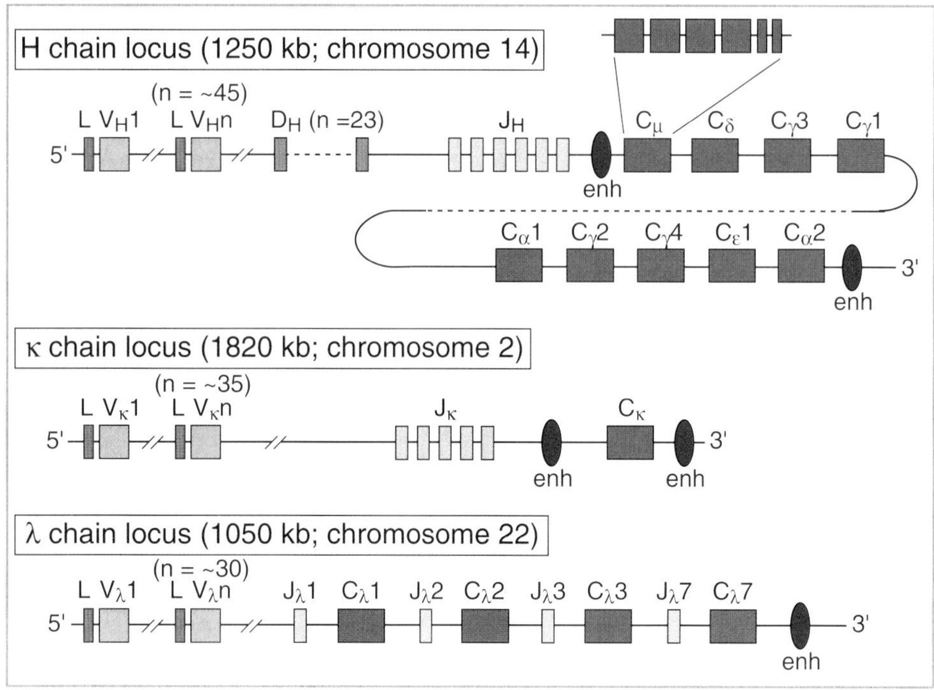

Figure 7–4 Germline organization of human Ig loci.
The human heavy chain, κ light chain, and λ light chain loci are shown. Only functional genes are shown; pseudogenes have been omitted for simplicity. Exons and introns are not drawn to scale. Each C_H gene is shown as a single box but is composed of several exons, as illustrated for C_μ. Gene segments are indicated as follows: L, leader (usually called signal sequence); V, variable; D, diversity; J, joining; C, constant; enh, enhancer.

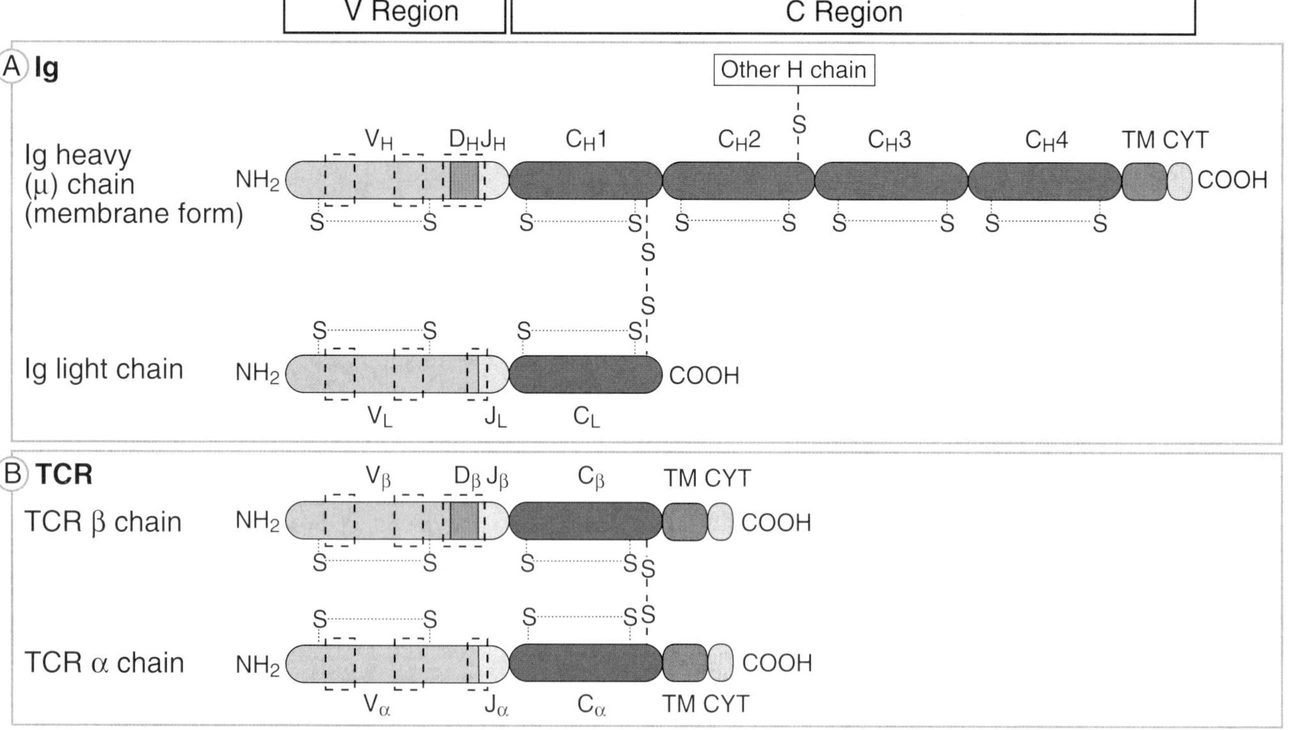

Figure 7–5 Domains of Ig and TCR proteins.
The domains of Ig heavy and light chains are shown in A, and the domains of TCR α and β chains are shown in B. The relationships between the Ig and TCR gene segments and the domain structure of the antigen receptor polypeptide chains are indicated. The variable (V) and constant (C) regions of each polypeptide are encoded by different gene segments. The locations of intrachain and interchain disulfide bonds (S-S) are approximate. Areas in the dashed boxes are the hypervariable (complementarity-determining) regions. In the Ig μ chain and the TCR α and β chains, transmembrane (TM) and cytoplasmic (CYT) domains are encoded by separate exons.

light chain locus and about 45 in the human heavy chain locus, whereas the mouse λ light chain locus has only 2V genes and the mouse heavy chain locus has more than 1000V genes. The V gene segments for each locus are spaced over large stretches of DNA, up to 2000 kilobases long. Although each V gene segment differs in sequence from every other one, the V genes of each locus can be grouped into multiple families on the basis of sequence homology. The members of each family are identical to one another at 70% to 80% of their nucleotide sequences, and they probably arose during evolution by duplication of a single V gene exon. The physiologic significance of these V gene families remains uncertain; members of each family do not appear to encode antigen receptor V regions with a similar specificity. At the 5′ end of each V region exon is a nucleotide sequence that encodes the 20 to 30 N-terminal residues of the translated protein. These terminal residues are moderately hydrophobic and make up the leader (or signal) peptide. Signal sequences are found in all newly synthesized secreted and transmembrane proteins and are involved in guiding the emerging polypeptides during their synthesis on ribosomes into the lumen of the endoplasmic reticulum. Here, the signal sequences are rapidly cleaved, probably before translation is complete, and they are not present in the mature proteins.

At varying distances 3′ of the V genes are the **C gene segments.** Again, each Ig locus has a distinct arrangement and number of C genes. In humans, the Ig κ light chain locus has a single C gene (C_κ) and the λ light chain locus has four functional C genes (C_λ). The Ig heavy chain locus has nine C genes (C_H), arranged in a tandem array, that encode the C regions of the nine different Ig isotypes and subtypes (see Chapter 3). The C_κ and C_λ genes are each composed of a single exon that encodes the entire extracellular C region of the light chains. In contrast, each C_H gene is composed of five or six exons. Three or four exons (each similar in size to a V region exon) encode the complete C region of each heavy chain isotype, and two smaller exons code for the carboxyl terminal ends, including the transmembrane and cytoplasmic domains of the heavy chains (Fig. 7–5A).

Between the V and C genes in each Ig locus, and separated by introns of varying lengths, are additional coding sequences, 30 to 50 base pairs long, that make up the **J segments** and, in the Ig heavy chain locus, the **D segments.** In the human Ig heavy chain locus, 5′ of the entire array of C_H gene segments, there is one cluster of 6 functional J segments and one cluster of more than 20 D segments. In the human κ chain locus, there is a cluster of five J segments 5′ of C_κ, and in the human λ locus, there is one J segment 5′ of each of the four functional C_λ genes. The D and J gene segments code for the carboxyl terminal ends of the V regions, including the third hypervariable (complementarity-determining) regions of antibody molecules. Thus, in an Ig light chain protein (κ or λ), the V region is encoded by the V and J gene segments. In the Ig heavy chain protein, the V region is encoded by the V, D, and J gene segments (Fig. 7–5A).

The V and C domains of Ig (and TCR) molecules share structural features, including a tertiary structure called the Ig fold. As we discussed in Chapters 3 and 6, proteins that include this structure are members of the **Ig superfamily** (see Chapter 3, Box 3–2). On the basis of tandem organization of V and C genes in each Ig or TCR locus and the structural homologies between them, it is believed that these genes evolved from repeated duplication of a primordial gene. Each Ig domain of heavy and light chains is encoded by one exon.

Although the introns between exons are not expressed in mature mRNA, they play an important role in the production of antigen receptors. As we shall see later, recognition sequences that dictate recombination of different gene segments are present in the introns between these gene segments. In addition, the introns contain nucleotide sequences, such as promoters, enhancers, and silencers, that regulate transcription and gene expression.

Organization of TCR Gene Loci

The genes encoding the TCR α chain, the TCR β chain, and the TCR γ chain are in three separate loci, and the TCR δ chain locus is contained within the TCR α locus (Fig. 7–6). Each germline TCR locus includes V, J, and C gene segments. In addition, TCR β and TCR δ loci also have D segments, like the Ig heavy chain locus. At the 5′ end of each of the TCR loci, there is a cluster of several **V gene segments,** arranged similarly to the Ig V genes. Like Ig V genes, TCR V gene segments can also be grouped into multiple families on the basis of sequence homology. Some microbial products called superantigens can bind to TCR β chain V regions encoded by any member of a particular V_β family. In this way, superantigens can activate large numbers of T cells and cause considerable disease (see Chapter 15, Box 15–1). At the 5′ end of each TCR V region exon is a signal sequence.

At varying distances 3′ of the TCR V genes are the **C gene segments.** There are two C genes in each of the human TCR β (C_β) and TCR γ (C_γ) loci and only one C gene in each of the TCR α (C_α) and TCR δ (C_δ) loci. Each TCR C region gene is composed of four exons encoding the extracellular C region, a short hinge region, the transmembrane segment, and the cytoplasmic tail.

There are J segments between the V and C genes in all the TCR loci, and there are D segments in the TCR β and TCR δ chain loci. Each human TCR C gene segment has its own associated 5′ cluster of J (and D) segments. In a TCR α or γ chain, the V region is encoded by the V and J exons, and in the TCR β and δ proteins, the V region is encoded by the V, D, and J gene segments.

The relationship of the TCR gene segments and the corresponding portions of TCR proteins that they encode is shown in Figure 7–5B. As in Ig molecules, the TCR V and C domains assume an Ig-fold tertiary structure, and thus the TCR is a member of the Ig superfamily of proteins.

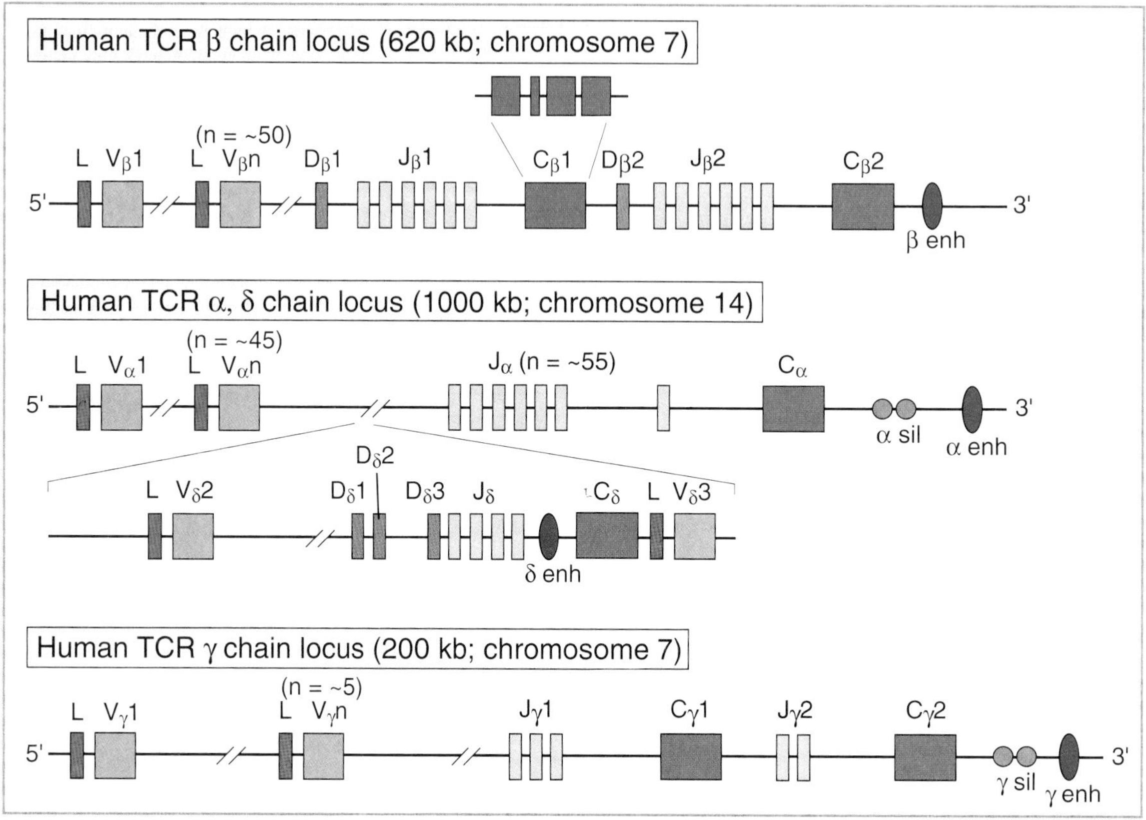

Figure 7–6 Germline organization of human TCR loci.
The human TCR β, α, γ, and δ chain loci are shown, as indicated. Exons and introns are not drawn to scale, and nonfunctional pseudogenes are not shown. Each constant (C) gene is shown as a single box but is composed of several exons, as illustrated for C_β. Gene segments are indicated as follows: L, leader (usually called signal sequence); V, variable; D, diversity; J, joining; C, constant; enh, enhancer; sil, silencer (sequences that regulate TCR gene transcription).

Antigen Receptor Gene Recombination

The germline organization of Ig and TCR loci described in the preceding section exists in all cell types in the body. Germline genes cannot be transcribed into mRNA that gives rise to antigen receptor proteins. Functional antigen receptor genes are created only in developing B and T lymphocytes by rearrangements of DNA that make the V, D, and J gene segments contiguous. This somatic recombination involves bringing together the appropriate gene segments, introducing double-strand breaks at the ends of these segments, and ligating them to produce genes that can be transcribed.

The recombination of antigen receptor genes can be demonstrated by a technique called Southern blot hybridization, which is used to examine the sizes of DNA fragments produced by restriction enzyme digestion of genomic DNA (see Appendix III for a description of the technique). By this method, it can be shown that the enzyme-generated DNA fragments containing Ig or TCR gene segments are a different size when the DNA is from cells that make antibodies or TCRs, respectively, than when the DNA is from cells that do not make these antigen receptors (Fig. 7–7). The explanation for these different sizes is that V and C regions of antigen receptor chains are encoded by different gene segments that are located far apart in embryonic and nonlymphoid cells and brought close together in cells committed to antibody or TCR synthesis (i.e., in B or T lymphocytes).

The process of somatic recombination involves selecting one V gene, one J gene, and one D gene (when present) in each developing lymphocyte and bringing these gene segments together to form a single V(D)J gene that will code for the variable region of an antigen receptor protein (Fig. 7–8). The C gene remains separate from the V(D)J gene in the DNA and in the primary RNA transcript. The primary RNA is then processed so that the V(D)J segment becomes contiguous with the C gene, forming an mRNA that is translated to produce one of the chains of the antigen receptor protein. Different clones of lymphocytes use different combinations of V, D, and J genes. In addition, during V(D)J recombination, nucleotides are added to or removed from the joints. As we will discuss in more detail later, these processes generate the diversity characteristic of lymphocyte antigen receptors. The details and unique features of recombination of Ig and TCR genes will be described when we consider the maturation of B and T lymphocytes, respectively.

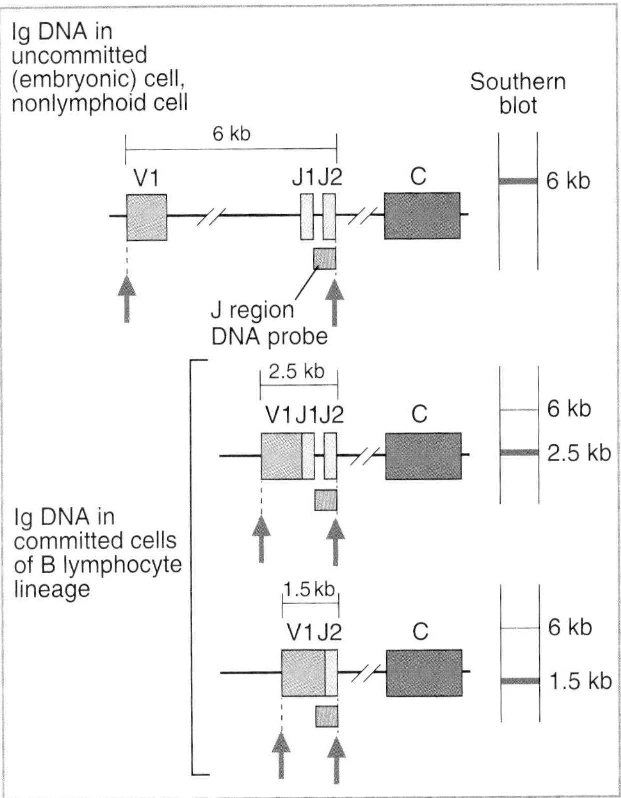

Figure 7–7 Antigen receptor gene rearrangements. Southern blot analysis (see Appendix III) of DNA from nonlymphoid cells and from two monoclonal populations of B lymphocyte lineage (e.g., B cell tumors) is shown. The DNA is digested with a restriction enzyme, different-sized fragments are separated by electrophoresis, and the fragments are blotted onto a filter. The sites at which the restriction enzyme cleaves the DNA are indicated by arrows. The size of the fragments containing the joining (J) segment of the Ig κ light chain gene is determined by use of a radioactive probe that specifically binds to J segment DNA. In the hypothetical example shown, the size of the J segment containing DNA fragments from each of two B cells is smaller than that from non-B cell DNA. This indicates that the specific sites where the restriction enzyme cuts the DNA are in a different position in the genome of the B cells compared with the non-B cells. Thus, a rearrangement of the germline DNA sequence in the Ig κ locus has occurred in the B cells. Note that the fragment from the rearranged DNA may be larger or smaller than the fragment from the germline DNA, depending on the location of the sites where the restriction enzyme cuts the DNA.

Mechanisms of Somatic Recombination of Antigen Receptor Genes

Rearrangement of Ig and TCR genes is a special kind of DNA recombination involving nonhomologous gene segments, mediated by the coordinated activities of several enzymes, some of which are found only in developing lymphocytes and others of which are ubiquitous DNA repair enzymes. Together, these enzymes are called the **V(D)J recombinase.** The lymphocyte-specific components of the V(D)J recombinase recognize certain DNA sequences called **recombination signal sequences,** located 3′ of each V gene segment, 5′ of each J segment, and flanking both sides of each D segment (Fig. 7–9). The recombination signal sequences consist of a highly conserved stretch of 7 nucleotides, called the heptamer, located adjacent to the coding sequence, followed by a spacer of exactly 12 or 23 nonconserved nucleotides, followed by a highly conserved stretch of 9 nucleotides, called the nonamer. The 12- and 23-nucleotide spacers roughly correspond to one or two turns of a DNA helix, and they presumably bring the heptamer and nonamer into positions that can be simultaneously accessible to the recombinase enzymes. The V(D)J recombinase introduces double-stranded breaks in the DNA between the recombination signal sequence and the adjacent V, D, or J coding sequence. In Ig light chain V-to-J recombination, for example, breaks will be made 3′ of a V segment and 5′ of a J segment. Temporary hairpin loop structures are formed connecting the parallel strands of DNA on either side of the breaks. The intervening double-stranded DNA is removed in the form of a circle. This is followed by joining of the two broken ends and therefore joining of the V and J coding sequences. Some V genes, especially in the Ig κ locus, are in the opposite orientation, such that the recognition sequences 5′ of these V segments and 3′ of the J segments face the same direction. In these cases, the intervening DNA is inverted and the V and J exons fuse at one end. Most Ig and TCR gene rearrangements occur by deletion; rearrangement by inversion occurs in up to 50% of rearrangements in the Ig κ locus. Recombination occurs between two segments only if

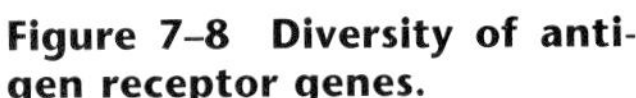

Figure 7–8 Diversity of antigen receptor genes. From the same germline DNA, it is possible to generate recombined DNA sequences and mRNAs that differ in their V-D-J junctions. In the example shown, three distinct antigen receptor mRNAs are produced from the same germline DNA by the use of different gene segments and the addition of nucleotides to the junctions.

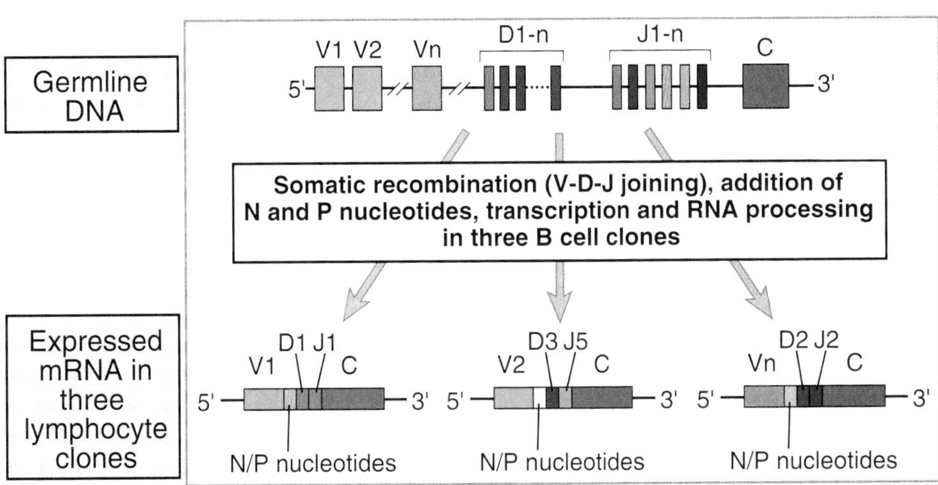

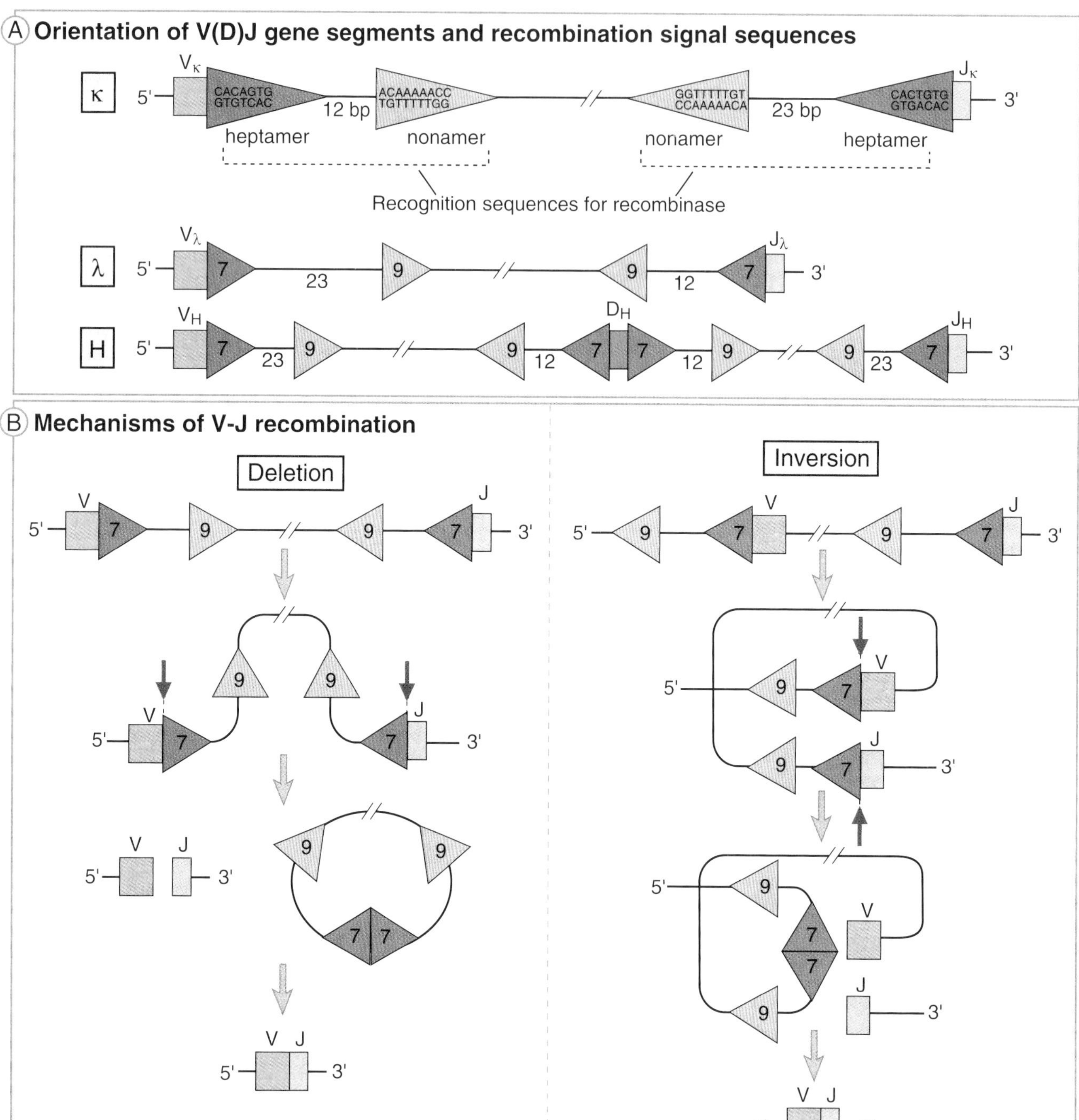

Figure 7–9 V(D)J recombination.

The DNA sequences and mechanisms involved in recombination in the Ig gene loci are depicted. The same sequences and mechanisms apply to recombinations in the TCR loci.

A. Conserved heptamer (7 bp) and nonamer (9 bp) sequences, separated by 12- or 23-bp spacers, are located adjacent to V and J exons (for κ and λ loci) or to V, D, and J exons (in the H chain locus). The V(D)J recombinase recognizes these recombination signal sequences and brings the exons together.

B. Recombination of V and J exons may occur by deletion of intervening DNA and ligation of the V and J segments *(left panel)* or, if the V gene is in the opposite orientation, by inversion of the DNA followed by ligation of adjacent gene segments *(right panel)*. Red arrows indicate the sites where germline sequences are cleaved and later rejoined.

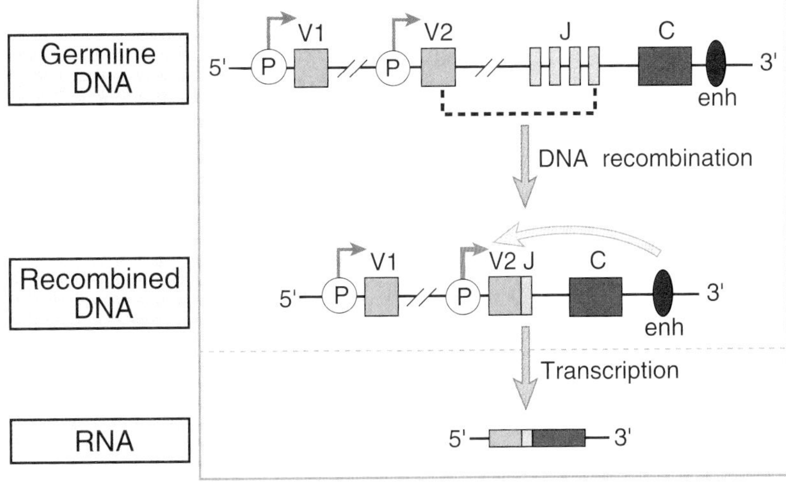

Figure 7–10 Transcriptional regulation of Ig genes.
V-D-J recombination brings promoter sequences (shown as P) close to the enhancer (enh) located between the J and C loci. The enhancer promotes transcription of the rearranged V gene (V2, whose active promoter is indicated by a bold green arrow).

one of the segments is flanked by a 12-nucleotide spacer and the other is flanked by a 23-nucleotide spacer; this is called the 12/23 rule. The location of the spacers and signal sequences ensures that the appropriate gene segments will recombine. For example, in the Ig heavy chain locus, both V and J segments have 23-nucleotide spacers and therefore cannot join directly; D-to-J recombination is required first, followed by V-to-DJ recombination, and this is possible because the D segments are flanked on both sides by 12-nucleotide spacers, allowing V-D and D-J joining. Also, these recombination signal sequences are unique to Ig and TCR genes. Therefore, the V(D)J recombinase can act on antigen receptor genes but on no other genes.

The lymphocyte-specific component of the V(D)J recombinase, which binds to and cleaves DNA at the recombination signal sequences, is a complex of two proteins encoded by genes called ***recombination-activating gene 1*** and ***recombination-activating gene 2*** (*RAG1* and *RAG2*). The RAG-1 protein is a dimer that is thought to bind to and cleave the DNA (i.e., it functions as a specific endonuclease), but it is enzymatically active only when complexed with the RAG-2 protein. The importance of this enzyme is illustrated by the finding that knockout mice lacking either *RAG1* or *RAG2* genes fail to produce Ig and TCR proteins and lack mature B and T lymphocytes. The RAG-1 and RAG-2 components of the V(D)J recombinase have several important properties. First, RAG-1 and RAG-2 are cell type specific, being produced only in cells of the B and T lymphocyte lineages. Second, the *RAG* genes are expressed only in immature lymphocytes. Therefore, the V(D)J recombinase is active in immature B and T lymphocytes but not in mature cells, explaining why Ig and TCR gene rearrangements do not continue in cells that express functional antigen receptors. Third, *RAG* genes are expressed mainly in the G_0 and G_1 stages of the cell cycle and are silenced in proliferating cells. It is thought that limiting DNA cleavage and recombination to nondividing cells minimizes the risk of inappropriate DNA breaks during DNA replication in mitosis. The same recombinase mediates recombination at both Ig and TCR loci. Because complete functional rearrangement of Ig genes normally occurs only in B cells and rearrangement of TCR genes normally occurs only in T cells, some other mechanism must control the cell type specificity of recombination. It is likely that the accessibility of the Ig and TCR loci to the recombinase is differentially regulated in developing B and T cells by several mechanisms, including alterations in chromatin structure, DNA methylation, and basal transcriptional activity in the unrearranged loci.

The other enzymes that are part of the V(D)J recombinase are expressed in many cell types and are involved mainly in DNA repair. Their role in Ig and TCR gene recombination is to repair the double-stranded breaks introduced by the recombinase. One such enzyme, called the DNA-dependent protein kinase (DNA-PK) complex, is a double-stranded DNA repair enzyme that is defective in mice carrying the severe combined immunodeficiency *(scid)* mutation (see Chapter 20). Like *RAG*-deficient mice, *scid* mice fail to produce mature lymphocytes.

One of the consequences of V-J or V-D-J recombination is that the process brings promoters located 5′ of V regions close to enhancers that are located in the introns between V and C gene segments or even 3′ of the C genes (Fig. 7–10). These enhancers maximize the transcriptional activity of the V gene promoters and are thus important for high-level transcription of the V genes in lymphocytes.

Because Ig and TCR genes are sites for multiple DNA recombinations in B and T cells, and because these sites become transcriptionally active after recombination, from other loci genes can be abnormally translocated to these loci and, as a result, may be aberrantly transcribed. In tumors of B and T lymphocytes, oncogenes are often translocated to Ig or TCR gene loci. Such chromosomal translocations are frequently accompanied by enhanced transcription of the oncogenes and are believed to be one of the factors causing the development of lymphoid tumors (Box 7–2).

BOX 7–2

Chromosomal Translocations in Tumors of Lymphocytes

Reciprocal chromosomal translocations in many tumors, including lymphomas and leukemias, were first noted by cytogeneticists in the 1960s, but their significance remained unknown until almost 20 years later. At this time, sequencing of switch regions of IgH genes in B cell tumors revealed the presence of DNA segments that were not derived from Ig genes. This was first observed in two tumors derived from B lymphocytes, human Burkitt's lymphoma and murine myelomas. The "foreign" DNA was identified as a portion of the c-*myc* proto-oncogene, which is normally present on chromosome 8 in humans. Proto-oncogenes are normal cellular genes that often code for proteins involved in the regulation of cellular proliferation, differentiation, and survival, such as growth factors, receptors for growth factors, or transcription-activating factors. In normal cells, their function is tightly regulated. When these genes are altered by mutations, inappropriately expressed, or incorporated into and reintroduced in cells by RNA retroviruses, they can exhibit either enhanced or aberrant activities and function as oncogenes. Dysfunction of oncogenes is one important mechanism leading to increased cellular growth and, ultimately, neoplastic transformation. The most common translocation in Burkitt's lymphoma is t(8;14), involving the Ig heavy chain locus on chromosome 14; less commonly, t(2;8) or t(8;22) translocations are found, involving the κ or λ light chain loci, respectively. In all cases of Burkitt's lymphoma, c-*myc* is translocated from chromosome 8 to one of the Ig loci, which explains the reciprocal 8;14, 2;8, or 8;22 translocations detectable in these tumors. The *myc* gene product is a transcription factor, and translocation of the gene leads to its dysregulated expression. Increased Myc activity is believed to lead to uncontrolled cell proliferation at the expense of differentiation, but the precise mechanism of this effect is not known. Thus, Myc is an example of a transcription factor that serves as an oncoprotein.

Because antigen receptor genes normally undergo several genetic rearrangements during lymphocyte maturation, they are likely sites for accidental translocations of distant genes. DNA sequencing of antigen receptor genes involved in chromosomal translocations has suggested that these mistakes may occur at the time of attempted V(D)J rearrangement in pre-B and pre-T cells, during switch recombination in germinal center B cells, and possibly during the process of somatic hypermutation (also in germinal center B cells). In some translocations associated with lymphoid tumors, DNA breakage near proto-oncogenes occurs at sites that resemble heptamer and nonamer sequences, suggesting that they may be caused by an aberrant V(D)J recombinase activity. However, in most instances (and, more generally, in all translocations found in nonlymphoid tumors), such sequences are

Type of tumor	Chromosomal translocation	Genes involved in translocation
B cell derived		
Burkitt's lymphoma	t(8;**14**)(q24.1;**q32.3**) most common	c-*myc*, *IgH*
Acute lymphoblastic leukemia (pre-B ALL)	t(12;**21**)(p13;q22) (25% of childhood cases)	*TEL1, AML1*
Pre-B ALL; also chronic myelogenous leukemia	t(9;**22**)(q34;**q11.2**) (25% of adult ALL, 3% of childhood ALL)	*bcr, abl* (Philadelphia chromosome)
Follicular lymphoma	t(**14**;18)(**q32.3**;q21.3)	*bcl-2, IgH*
Diffuse B cell lymphoma, large cell type	t(3;**14**)(q27;**q32.3**)	*bcl-6* (DNA-binding protein), *IgH*
Mantle cell lymphoma	t(11;**14**)(q13;**q32.3**)	*cyclin D1, IgH*
T cell derived		
Pre-T cell acute lymphoblastic leukemia	t(1;**14**)(p32;**q11.2**) (5% of cases); del(1p32) (20% of cases)	*TAL1, TCRα; TAL1, SCL*
T cell lymphoma, anaplastic large cell type	t(2;5)(p23;q35)	*ALK* (tyrosine kinase), *NPM* (unknown function)

This box was written with the assistance of Dr. Jon Aster, Department of Pathology, Brigham & Women's Hospital and Harvard Medical School, Boston.

These are some examples of chromosomal translocations that have been molecularly cloned in human lymphoid tumors. Each translocation is indicated by the letter t. The first pair of numbers refers to the chromosomes involved, for example, (8;14), and the second pair to the bands of each chromosome, for example, (q24.1; q32.3). The normal chromosomal locations of antigen receptor genes (indicated in bold) are IgH, 14q32.3; Igκ, 2p12; Igλ, 22q11.2; TCRαδ, 14q11.2; TCRβ, 7q34; and TCRγ, 7p15.

Continued on following page

lacking and the cause of DNA breakage within or adjacent to proto-oncogenes is uncertain.

Since the discovery of *myc* translocations in B cell lymphomas, the genes involved in translocations in many other lymphoid (and nonlymphoid) tumors have been identified (see Table). In most cases, these translocations result in dysregulation of transcription factors, cell survival proteins, or signal-transducing molecules such as kinases. One gene that has proved to be particularly important in acute lymphoid and myeloid leukemias is *AML1*, a gene on chromosome 21 that encodes a member of the runt family of transcription factors. About 25% of childhood acute lymphoblastic leukemias have a balanced (12;21) translocation that produces a fusion gene encoding the DNA-binding portion of AML-1 and the dimerization domain of TEL-1, a member of the Ets family of transcription factors. Similarly, about 20% of acute myelogenous leukemias have a balanced (8;21) translocation involving a different Ets-like transcription factor, ETO, and AML-1. In both instances, the oncogenic AML-1 fusion proteins appear to have "dominant negative" activity that inhibits normal AML-1 function and results in a block in differentiation. This implies that the normal role of AML-1 is to promote the terminal differentiation of blood cell progenitors, which is supported by the observation that AML-1 knockout mice die during embryogenesis because of a failure to produce blood cells. The "Philadelphia chromosome," found in chronic myelogenous leukemia and some acute lymphoblastic leukemias, is created by a balanced t(9;22) translocation. This yields a fusion gene consisting of the c-*abl* and *bcr* genes that encodes a novel tyrosine kinase. The t(14;18) translocation found in the most common B cell lymphoma, follicular lymphoma, leads to overexpression of a survival gene, *bcl-2*, and prevention of programmed cell death. In another type of B cell lymphoma, mantle cell lymphoma, the *bcl-1* gene is translocated to the IgH locus; *bcl-1* codes for cyclin D, a protein that regulates cell cycle progression. The most frequent chromosomal rearrangements in T cell acute leukemias lead to inappropriate expression of *TAL1*, a gene encoding a basic helix-loop-helix transcription factor that appears to specifically interfere with T cell differentiation.

Generation of Diversity of the B and T Cell Repertoires

The enormous diversity of the mature B and T cell repertoires is generated during somatic recombination of Ig and TCR genes. Several genetic mechanisms contribute to this diversity, and the relative importance of each mechanism varies among the different antigen receptor loci (Table 7–1).

- **Combinatorial diversity.** Somatic recombinations involve multiple germline gene segments that may combine randomly, and different combinations produce different antigen receptors. The maximum possible number of combinations of these gene segments is the product of the numbers of V, J, and (if present) D gene segments at each antigen receptor locus. Therefore, the amount of combinatorial diversity that can be generated at each locus reflects the number of germline V, J, and D gene segments at that locus. After somatic recombination and expression of antigen receptor chains, combinatorial diversity is further enhanced by the juxtaposition of two different, randomly generated V regions (i.e., V_H and V_L in Ig molecules and V_α and V_β in TCR molecules). Therefore, the total combinatorial diversity is theoretically the product of the combinatorial diversity of each of the two associating chains. The actual degree of combinatorial diversity in the expressed Ig and TCR repertoires in any individual is likely to be considerably less than the theoretical maximum. This is because not all recombinations of gene segments are equally likely to occur, and not all

Table 7–1. Contributions of Different Mechanisms to the Generation of Diversity in Ig and TCR Genes

Mechanism	Immunoglobulin		TCR αβ		TCR γδ	
	Heavy chain	κ	α	β	γ	δ
Variable (V) segments	45	35	45	50	5	2
Diversity (D) segments	23	0	0	2	0	3
D segments read in all three reading frames	Rare	--	--	Often	--	Often
N region diversification	V-D, D-J	None	V-J	V-D, D-J	V-J	V-D1, D1-D2, D1-J
Joining (J) segments	6	5	55	12	5	4
Total potential repertoire with junctional diversity	~10^{11}		~10^{16}		~10^{18}	

The potential number of antigen receptors with junctional diversity is much greater than the number that can be generated only by combinations of V, D, and J gene segments. Note that although the upper limit on the numbers of Ig and TCR proteins that may be expressed is very large, it is estimated that each individual contains on the order of 107 clones of B and T cells with distinct specificities and receptors; in other words, only a fraction of the potential repertoire may actually be expressed.

pairings of Ig heavy and light chains or TCR α and β chains may form functional antigen receptors. Importantly, since the numbers of V, J, and D segments in each locus are limited (see Figs. 7–4 and 7–6), the maximum possible numbers of combinations are on the order of thousands. This is, of course, much less than the actual diversity of antigen receptors in mature lymphocytes.

Junctional diversity. The largest contribution to the diversity of antigen receptors is made by the removal or addition of nucleotides between V and D, D and J, or V and J segments at the time of joining. These processes result in variability at the junctions of V, D, and J gene segments, called junctional diversity. One way this can occur is if endonucleases remove nucleotides from the germline sequences at the ends of the J segments (Fig. 7–11A). In addition, new nucleotide sequences, not present in the germline, may be added at junctions. Gene segments (e.g., V and J gene segments) that are cleaved by the RAG enzyme form hairpin loops whose ends are often cleaved asymmetrically, so that one DNA strand is longer than the other (see Fig. 7–11B). The shorter strand has to be extended with nucleotides complementary to the longer strand before the ligation of the two segments. The short lengths of added nucleotides are called P nucleotides, and their addition introduces new sequences at the V-D-J junctions. Another mechanism of junctional diversity is the random addition of up to 20 non–template-encoded nucleotides called N nucleotides (see Fig. 7–11B). N region diversification is more common in Ig heavy chains and in TCR β and γ chains than in Ig κ or λ chains. This addition of new nucleotides is mediated by an enzyme called terminal deoxyribonucleotidyl transferase (TdT). In mice rendered deficient in TdT by gene knockout, the diversity of B and T cell repertoires is substantially less than in normal mice. The addition of P nucleotides and N nucleotides at the recombination sites may introduce frameshifts, theoretically generating termination codons in two of every three joining events. Such inefficiency is a price that is paid for generating diversity.

Because of junctional diversity, antibody and TCR molecules show the greatest variability at the junctions of V and C regions that form the third hypervariable region, or CDR3. The CDR3 regions of Ig and TCR molecules, which are formed at the sites of V(D)J recombination (see Fig. 7–5), are also the most important portions of these molecules for determining the specificity of antigen binding (see Chapters 3 and 6). In fact, because of junctional diversity, the numbers of different amino acid sequences that are present in the CDR3 regions of Ig and TCR molecules are much greater than the numbers that can be encoded by germline gene segments. Thus, the greatest diversity in antigen receptors is concentrated in the regions of the receptors that are the most important for antigen binding.

Although the theoretical limit of the number of Ig and TCR proteins that can be produced is enormous (see Table 7–1), the actual number of Ig and TCR genes expressed in each individual is only on the order of 10^7. This probably reflects the fact that most receptors, which are generated randomly, do not pass the selection processes needed for maturation, as we shall discuss later.

A practical application of our knowledge of junctional diversity is the determination of the clonality of lymphoid tumors that have arisen from B or T cells. Because every lymphocyte clone expresses a unique

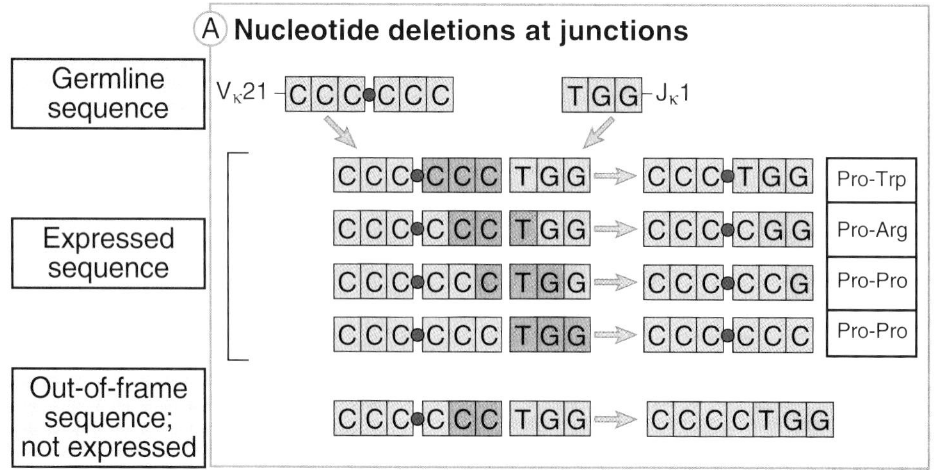

Figure 7–11 Junctional diversity.

A. During the joining of different V and J exons, removal of nucleotides (indicated as purple boxes) by nucleases may lead to the generation of novel nucleotide and amino acid sequences or to out-of-frame nonfunctional recombinations. All the indicated amino acid sequences have been detected in different $V_\kappa 21$-containing mouse antibodies. (Adapted from Nature. Weigert M, R Perry, D Kelley, T Hunkapiller, J Schilling, and L Hood. The joining of V and J gene segments creates antibody diversity. Nature 283:497–499, 1980. Copyright 1980 Macmillan Magazines Limited.)

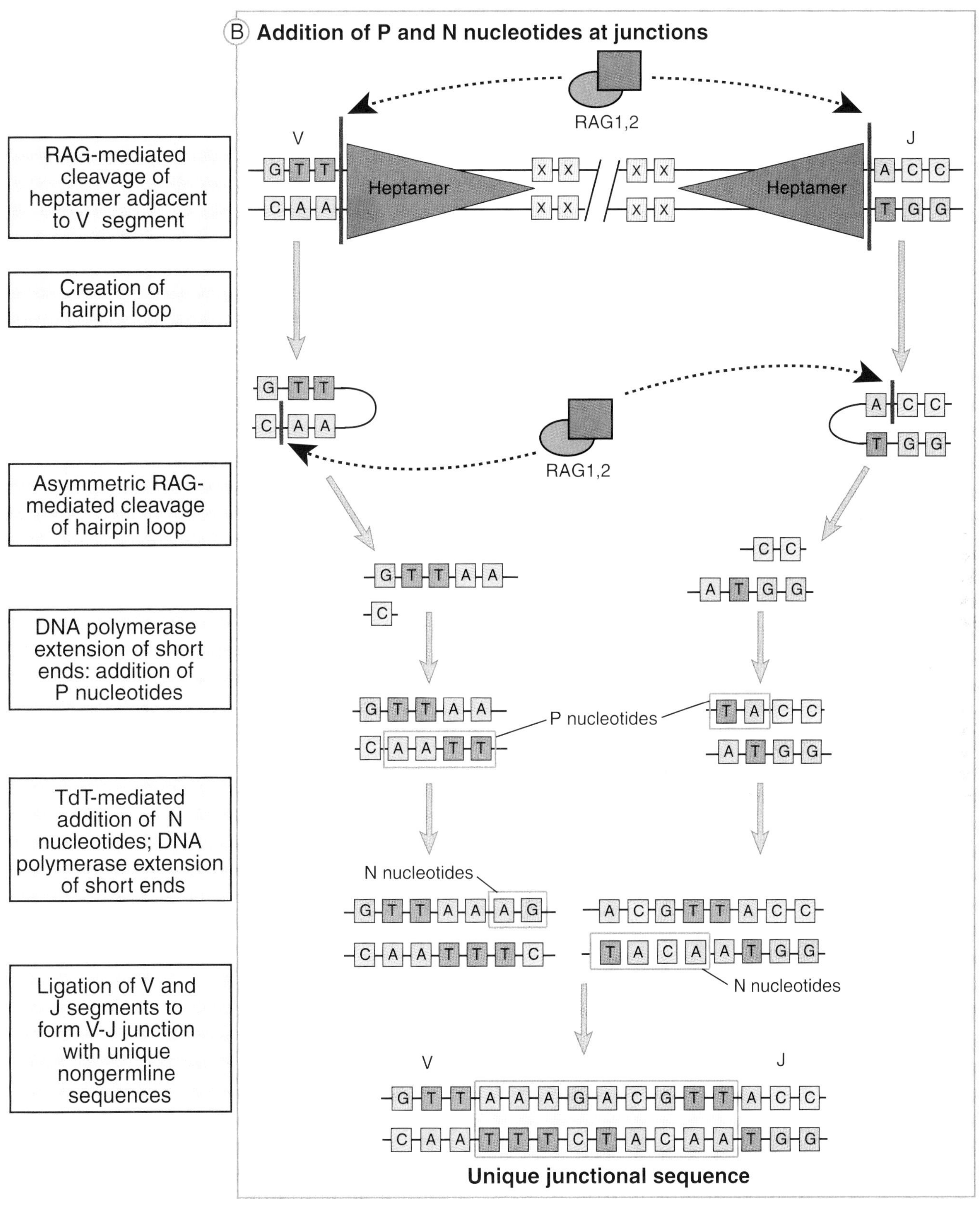

Figure 7–11 *(Continued)*
B. Nucleotides (P sequences) may be added to broken DNA ends to repair asymmetric breaks. Other nucleotides (N regions) may be added to the sites of VD, VJ, or DJ junctions by the action of the enzyme terminal deoxyribonucleotidyl transferase (TdT), generating new sequences that are not present in the germline.

antigen receptor CDR3 region, the sequence of nucleotides at the V(D)J recombination site serves as a specific marker for each clone. Thus, by sequencing the junctional regions of Ig or TCR genes in different B or T cell tumors, even from the same patient, one can establish whether these tumors arose from one clone or independently from different clones. Furthermore, polymerase chain reaction–mediated amplification of these clone-specific sequences may be used as a sensitive detection method for small numbers of tumor cells in the blood or tissues.

With this background, we will proceed to discussion of the maturation of B lymphocytes and then of T cells.

Maturation of B Lymphocytes

The principal events during the maturation of B lymphocytes are rearrangement and expression of Ig genes in a precise order, proliferation of immature cells, and selection of the mature repertoire (Fig. 7–12). The maturation of B lymphocytes from committed precursors occurs in the fetal liver and, after birth, in the bone marrow. During this process, Ig-negative B cell progenitors develop into mature B cells that express membrane-bound IgM and IgD molecules and then leave the bone marrow to populate peripheral lymphoid organs, where they use their membrane Ig to recognize and respond to foreign antigens. The development of a mature B cell from a lymphoid progenitor is estimated to take 2 to 3 days in humans.

Stages of B Lymphocyte Maturation

During their maturation, cells of the B lymphocyte lineage go through stages characterized by a specific pattern of Ig gene expression and the expression of other cell surface proteins that serve as phenotypic markers of these maturational stages (see Fig. 7–12). The earliest bone marrow cell committed to the B cell lineage is called a **pro-B cell.** Pro-B cells do not produce Ig, but they can be distinguished from other immature cells by the expression of B lineage–restricted surface molecules such as CD19 and CD10. RAG proteins are first expressed at this stage, and the first recombination of Ig genes occurs in the heavy chain locus. This recombination brings together one D and one J gene segment, with deletion of the intervening DNA (Fig. 7–13A). The D segments that are 5′ of the rearranged D segment, and the J segments that are 3′ of the rearranged J segment, are not affected by this recom-

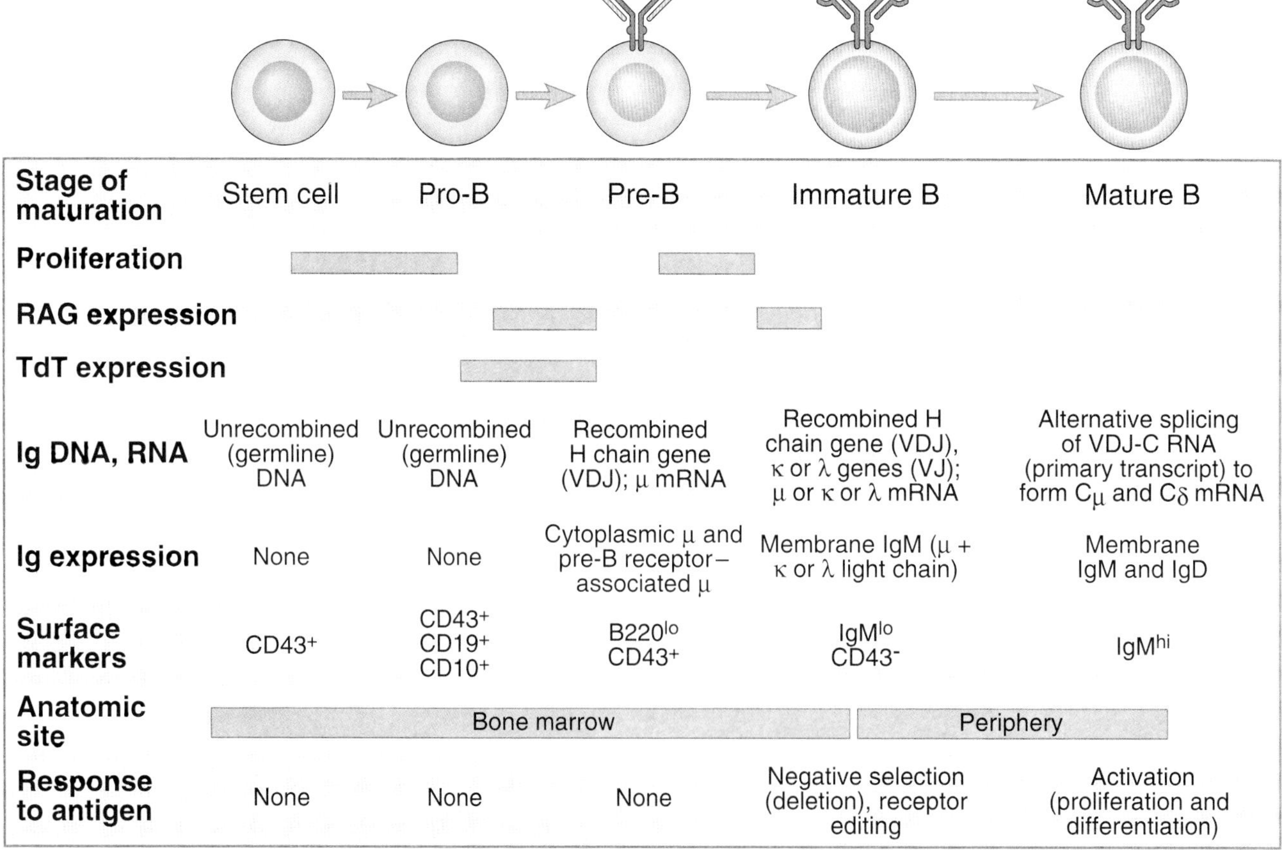

Figure 7–12 Stages of B cell maturation.
Events corresponding to each stage of B cell maturation from a bone marrow stem cell to a mature B lymphocyte are illustrated. Several surface markers in addition to those shown have been used to define distinct stages of B cell maturation. TdT, terminal deoxyribonucleotidyl transferase.

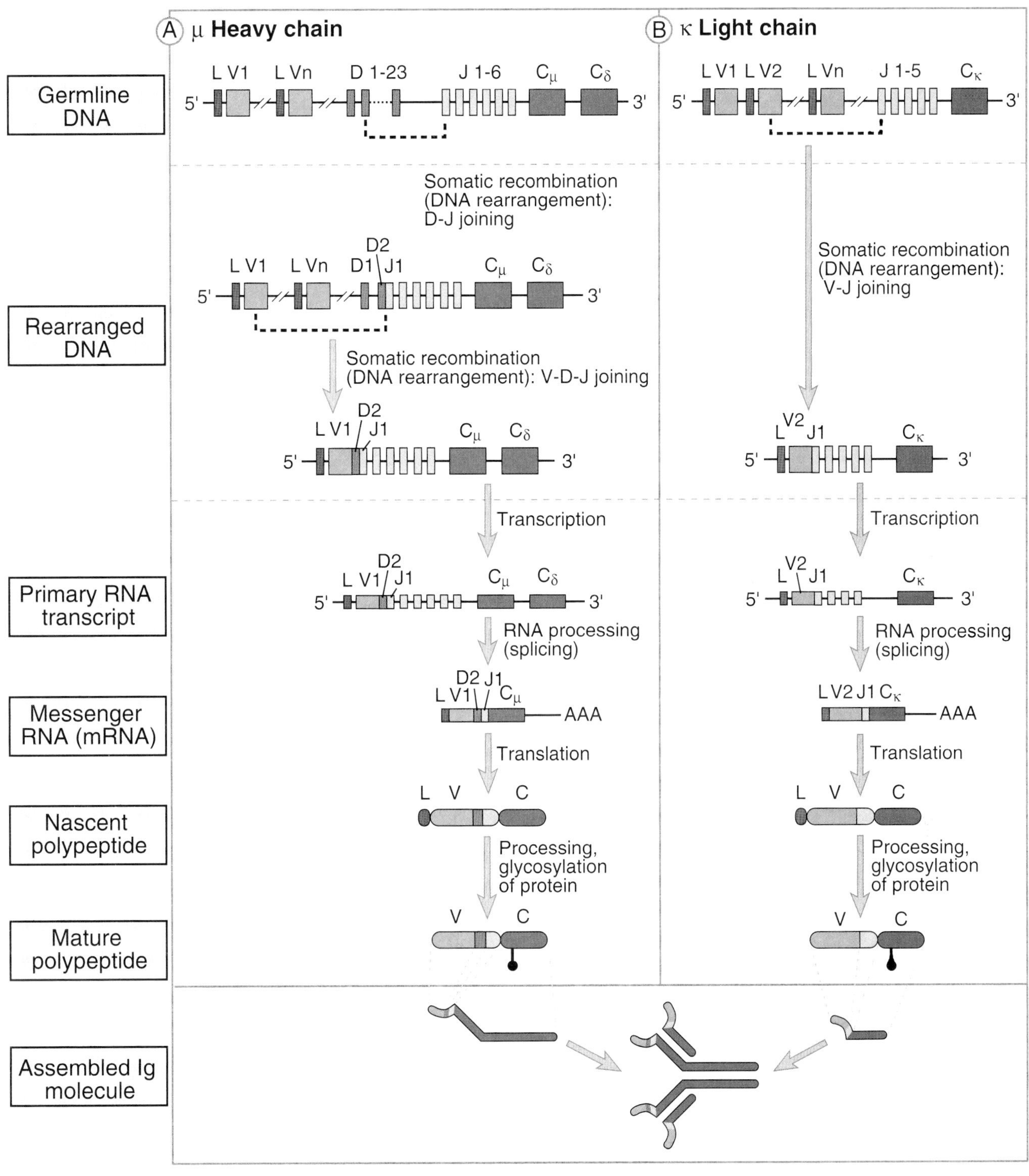

Figure 7–13 Ig heavy and light chain gene recombination and expression. The sequence of DNA recombination and gene expression events is shown for the Ig μ heavy chain (A) and the Ig κ light chain (B). In the example shown in A, the variable (V) region of the μ heavy chain is encoded by the exons V1, D2, and J1. In the example shown in B, the V region of the κ chain is encoded by the exons V1 and J1.

bination (e.g., D1 and J2 to J6 in Figure 7–13A). Ig heavy chain D-to-J rearrangements do not appear to be B lineage restricted because they are commonly found in T cells as well. After the D-J recombination, one of the many 5′ V genes is joined to the DJ complex, giving rise to a rearranged VDJ gene. At this stage, all V and D segments between the rearranged V and D genes are also deleted. V-to-DJ recombination in the Ig H chain locus occurs only in committed B lymphocyte precursors and is a critical checkpoint in Ig expression because only the rearranged V gene is subsequently transcribed. The TdT enzyme, which catalyzes the addition of junctional N nucleotides, is expressed most abundantly during the pro-B stage when heavy chain VDJ recombination occurs, and levels of TdT decrease early in the next stage before light chain V-J recombination is complete. Therefore, junctional diversity attributed to N nucleotides is more abundant in heavy chains than in light chains. The heavy chain C region genes remain separated from the VDJ complex by DNA containing the distal J segments, and Ig protein is not produced at this stage.

The **pre-B cell** represents the next stage of development and is the earliest cell type that synthesizes a detectable Ig gene product, namely, cytoplasmic μ heavy chain. Pre-B cells are found only in hematopoietic tissues. The rearranged Ig heavy chain gene is transcribed to produce a primary transcript that includes the rearranged VDJ complex and the proximal (μ and δ) C genes. Multiple adenine nucleotides, called poly-A tails, are added to one of several consensus polyadenylation sites located 3′ of the C_μ RNA. Subsequent processing of the RNA leads to splicing out of the sequences between the VDJ complex and the C_μ gene, giving rise to a functional mRNA for the μ heavy chain. Thus, the production of the mature mRNA requires both recombination of DNA segments and splicing of RNA. Translation of the μ heavy chain mRNA leads to production of the μ protein in pre-B cells.

Pre-B cells do not express membrane-bound antigen receptors because expression of complete membrane Ig molecules requires synthesis of both heavy and light chains. Therefore, these cells cannot recognize or respond to antigen. Some of the μ heavy chains in pre-B cells associate with proteins called **surrogate light chains,** which are structurally homologous to κ and λ light chains but are invariant (i.e., they are identical in all B cells). Complexes of μ and surrogate light chains, called **pre-B cell receptors** (Fig. 7–14A), are expressed on the cell surface at low levels. The pre-B cell receptor (pre-BCR) associates with other proteins, called Igα and Igβ, that function in transducing signals from the receptor; Igα and Igβ also associate with membrane Ig molecules in mature B cells (see Chapter 9). Pre-BCRs stimulate the proliferation and continued maturation of the developing B cells, and expression of these receptors is essential if the developing B cells are to complete their maturation successfully.

The importance of pre-BCRs is illustrated by studies of knockout mice and rare cases of human deficiencies of these receptors. For instance, in mice, knockout of the gene encoding the μ chain or one of the surrogate light chains, called λ5, results in markedly reduced numbers of mature B cells. This suggests that the μ-λ5 complex delivers signals required for B cell maturation and that if either gene is disrupted, maturation does not proceed.

It is not known what the pre-BCR complex recognizes or what biochemical signals it delivers. A kinase called the B cell tyrosine kinase (Btk) is associated with the pre-BCR and is required for delivering signals from this receptor that stimulate B cell maturation beyond

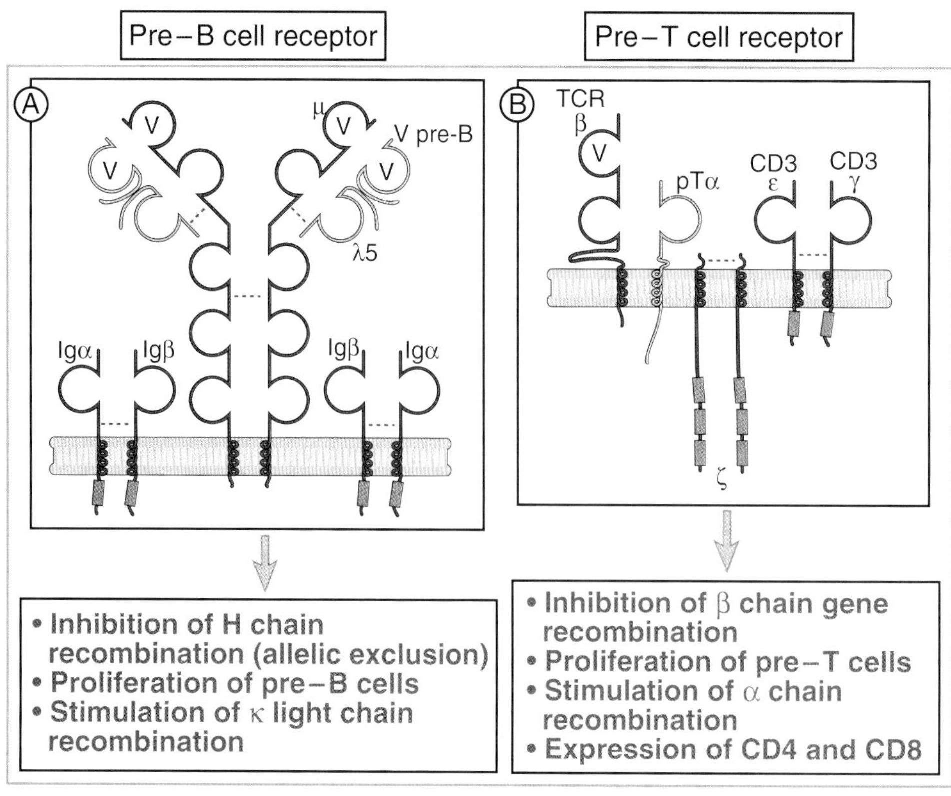

Figure 7–14 Pre-B cell and pre-T cell receptors.
The pre-B cell receptor (A) and the pre-T cell receptor (B) are expressed during the pre-B and pre-T cell stages of maturation, respectively, and both receptors share similar structures and functions. The pre-B cell receptor is composed of the μ heavy chain and an invariant surrogate light chain. The surrogate light chain is composed of two proteins, the variable (V) pre-B protein, which is homologous to a light chain V domain, and a λ5 protein that is covalently attached to the μ heavy chain by a disulfide bond. The pre-T cell receptor (B) is composed of the TCR β chain and the invariant pre-Tα chain. The pre-B cell receptor is associated with the Igα and Igβ signaling molecules that are part of the BCR complex in mature B cells (see Chapter 9), and the pre-T cell receptor associates with the CD3 and ζ proteins that are part of the TCR complex in mature T cells (see Chapter 8).

the pre-B cell stage. In humans, mutations in the *btk* gene result in the disease called **X-linked agammaglobulinemia** (XLA), which is characterized by failure of B cell maturation (see Chapter 20). In mice, mutations in *btk* result in a less severe B cell defect in a mouse strain called the Xid (for X-linked immunodeficiency) mouse.

The pre-BCR regulates further somatic recombination of Ig genes in two ways. First, if a μ protein is produced from the recombined heavy chain locus on one chromosome and forms a pre-BCR, this receptor signals to irreversibly inhibit rearrangement of the heavy chain locus on the other chromosome. If the first rearrangement is nonproductive because of deletions or frameshifts during recombination that produce stop codons, the heavy chain genes on the second allelic chromosome can recombine. Thus, in any B cell clone, one heavy chain allele is productively rearranged and expressed, and the other is in the germline configuration or is aberrantly rearranged. As a result, an individual B cell can express Ig heavy chain proteins encoded by only one of the two inherited alleles. This phenomenon is called **allelic exclusion,** and it ensures that every B cell can have only one specificity. If both alleles undergo nonproductive recombinations, the developing cell cannot produce Ig and undergoes programmed cell death. This occurs frequently and is one of the reasons that only a small fraction of the cells arising from B cell progenitors develop into mature B lymphocytes (see Fig. 7–2). Ig heavy chain allelic exclusion is likely to be due to permanent changes in chromatin structure in the heavy chain locus that limit accessibility to the V(D)J recombinase. In addition to mediating allelic exclusion, pre-BCR signaling also stimulates light chain gene rearrangement. However, μ chain expression is not absolutely required for light chain gene recombination, as shown by the finding that knockout mice lacking the μ gene do show light chain gene rearrangements in some immature B cells (which, of course, cannot express functional antigen receptors and proceed to maturity).

At the next stage in its maturation, each developing B cell also rearranges a κ or a λ light chain gene and produces the light chain, which associates with the previously synthesized μ chain to produce a complete IgM protein. The IgM-expressing B cell is called the **immature B cell.** DNA recombination in the κ or λ light chain locus occurs in a similar manner as in the Ig heavy chain locus (see Fig. 7–13B). There are no D segments in the light chain loci, and therefore recombination involves only the joining of one V segment to one J segment, forming a VJ complex. This VJ complex remains separated from the C region by an intron, and this separation is retained in the primary RNA transcript. Splicing of the primary transcript joins the C region RNA to the VJ RNA, forming an mRNA that is translated to produce the κ or λ protein. In the λ locus, alternative RNA splicing may lead to the use of any one of the four functional C_λ genes, but there is no known functional difference between the resulting types of λ light chains. During the maturation of one B cell clone, the κ locus rearranges after heavy chain rearrangement and before λ gene rearrangement. Production of κ light chains inhibits rearrangement of the λ locus, and the λ locus will undergo recombination only if a κ light chain cannot be produced. Therefore, an individual B cell clone can produce only one of the two types of light chains during its life; this is called light chain isotype exclusion. As in the heavy chain locus, production of κ or λ from one of the two parental chromosomes prevents recombination at the other allele, accounting for allelic exclusion of light chains in individual B cells. Also, as for heavy chains, if one allele undergoes nonfunctional rearrangement, DNA recombination can occur on the other allele; however, if both alleles of both κ and λ chains are nonfunctional in a developing B cell, that cell dies. The light chain that is produced complexes with the previously synthesized μ heavy chain, and the assembled IgM molecules are expressed on the cell surface in association with Igα and Igβ, where they function as specific receptors for antigens. Immature B cells do not proliferate and differentiate in response to antigens. In fact, their encounter with antigens, such as self antigens in the bone marrow, may lead to cell death or functional unresponsiveness rather than activation. This property is important for the negative selection of B cells that are specific for self antigens present in the bone marrow (discussed later). Immature B cells leave the bone marrow and complete their maturation in lymphoid organs.

The next stage of development is the **mature B cell** stage. At this stage, the cells coexpress μ and δ heavy chains in association with the κ or λ light chain and therefore produce both membrane IgM and membrane IgD. Both classes of membrane Ig have the same V region and hence the same antigen specificity. Simultaneous expression of a single rearranged VDJ gene cassette with both C_μ and C_δ to form the two heavy chains in one cell occurs by alternative RNA splicing (Fig. 7–15). A long primary RNA transcript is produced containing the rearranged VDJ complex as well as the

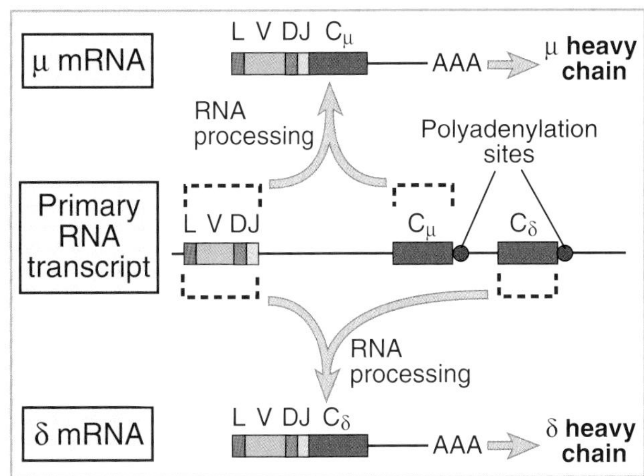

Figure 7–15 Coexpression of IgM and IgD.
Alternative processing of a primary RNA transcript results in the formation of a μ or δ mRNA. Dashed lines indicate the H chain segments that are joined by RNA splicing.

C_μ and C_δ genes. If the introns are spliced out such that the VDJ complex is attached to the C_μ gene, it gives rise to a μ mRNA. If, however, the C_μ RNA is spliced out as well so that the VDJ complex becomes contiguous with C_δ, a δ mRNA is produced. Subsequent translation results in the synthesis of a complete μ or δ heavy chain protein. Thus, alternative splicing allows a B cell to simultaneously produce mature mRNAs and proteins of two different heavy chain isotypes. The precise mechanisms that regulate the choice of polyadenylation or splice acceptor sites by which the rearranged VDJ is joined to either C_μ or C_δ are not known, nor are the signals that determine when and why a B cell expresses both IgM and IgD rather than IgM alone. The coexpression of IgM and IgD is accompanied by the acquisition of functional competence, and this is why the cells are called mature B cells. This correlation between expression of IgD and acquisition of functional competence has led to the suggestion that IgD is the essential activating receptor of mature B cells. However, as we shall discuss in Chapter 9, there is no evidence for a functional difference between membrane IgM and membrane IgD. Moreover, knockout of the δ gene in mice does not have a significant impact on the maturation or antigen-induced responses of B cells.

These mature, naive B cells are responsive to antigens, and unless the cells encounter antigen, they die in a few days or weeks. Mature B cells are found in the circulation and peripheral lymphoid organs; in the blood and lymphoid tissues of normal individuals, the majority of B cells are IgD^+IgM^+. In Chapter 9, we will discuss how these cells respond to antigens and how the pattern of Ig gene expression changes during antigen-induced B cell differentiation.

Selection of the Mature B Cell Repertoire

The repertoire of mature B cells is positively selected from the pool of immature cells before these cells leave the bone marrow. As we shall see later, positive selection is well defined in T lymphocytes and is responsible for preserving self MHC–restricted $CD4^+$ and $CD8^+$ T cells from the much larger pool of unselected, immature T cells. There is no comparable specificity or restriction for B cell antigen recognition. It is possible that only B cells that express functional membrane Ig molecules are allowed to complete their maturation, perhaps because this Ig delivers survival signals. If this is correct, positive selection in B cells may serve to preserve all the cells with the capacity to recognize antigens, regardless of specificity. However, the mechanisms of this positive selection process, and even its importance, are unknown.

Immature B cells that express high-affinity receptors for self antigens and encounter these antigens in the bone marrow may die or fail to mature further. This is the process of **negative selection,** and it is partly responsible for maintaining B cell tolerance to self antigens that are present in the bone marrow. These are the self antigens that tend to be widely distributed throughout the body, and the process of negative selection prevents potentially harmful immune responses against such self antigens (see Chapter 10). The antigens mediating negative selection–usually abundant or polyvalent (e.g., membrane-bound) self antigens–deliver strong signals to IgM-expressing immature B lymphocytes that happen to express receptors specific for these self antigens. Antigen recognition leads to apoptotic death of immature B cells. It is not clear why mature B cells proliferate in response to antigen recognition whereas immature cells die.

In addition to negative selection, some immature B cells that recognize self antigens may be induced to change their specificities by a process called **receptor editing.** In this process, antigen recognition leads to reactivation of *RAG* genes, additional light chain V-J recombinations, and production of a new Ig light chain, allowing the cell to express a different Ig receptor that is not self-reactive. Receptor editing most often involves the κ light chain locus. The VJ_κ genes encoding the autoreactive light chains are replaced by new VJ_κ rearrangements or λ light chain rearrangements. The importance of receptor editing as a mechanism for maintaining self-tolerance is not well defined.

Once the transition is made to the IgD^+IgM^+ mature B cell stage, antigen recognition leads to proliferation and differentiation, not to apoptosis or receptor editing. As a result, mature B cells that recognize antigens with high affinity in peripheral lymphoid tissues are activated, and this process leads to humoral immune responses (see Chapter 9).

B-1 Subset of B Lymphocytes

A subset of B lymphocytes, called B-1 cells, differs from the majority of B cells and has unique features of maturation and Ig gene expression. Many B-1 cells express the CD5 (Ly-1) molecule. In neonatal mice, these cells originate from the fetal liver and to a lesser extent from the bone marrow. In the adult, large numbers are found as a self-renewing population in the peritoneum. B-1 cells develop earlier during ontogeny than do conventional B cells, and they express a relatively limited repertoire of V genes with less junctional diversity than conventional B cells have. Only 5% to 10% of B cells in the blood and lymphoid tissues belong to the B-1 subset. Surprisingly, virtually all B cell–derived chronic lymphocytic leukemias are $CD5^+$ and are thought to arise from B-1 cells. Moreover, B-1 cells spontaneously secrete IgM antibodies that often react with microbial polysaccharides and some self antigens. These antibodies are sometimes called **natural antibodies** because they are present in individuals without overt immunization, although it is possible that microbial flora in the gut are the source of antigens that stimulate their production. It is not known whether B-1 cells serve a special function in immune responses. One possibility is that B-1 cells provide a source of rapid antibody production against microbes in particular sites, such as the peritoneum. These cells are also expanded in some mouse models of autoimmune disease, although their pathophysiologic role in autoimmunity is unclear. B-1 cells are analogous to γδ T cells in that they both have limited antigen receptor repertoires, and they are both presumed to respond to commonly encountered microbial antigens early in immune responses.

Marginal zone B cells in the spleen have some similarities with B-1 cells, such as limited diversity and responsiveness to polysaccharide antigens. The development of marginal zone B cells is not well understood.

Maturation of T Lymphocytes

The maturation of T lymphocytes from committed progenitors follows sequential stages consisting of somatic recombination and expression of TCR genes, cell proliferation, antigen-induced selection, and acquisition of mature phenotypes and functional capabilities (Fig. 7–16). In many ways, this is similar to B cell maturation. However, T cell maturation has some unique features that reflect the specificity of T lymphocytes for self MHC–associated peptide antigens and the need for a special microenvironment for selecting cells with this specificity.

Role of the Thymus in T Cell Maturation

The thymus is the major site of maturation of T cells. This function of the thymus was first suspected because of immunologic deficiencies associated with the lack of a thymus.

- If the thymus is removed from a neonatal mouse, this animal fails to develop mature T cells.
- The congenital absence of the thymus, as occurs in the DiGeorge syndrome in humans or in the nude mouse strain, is characterized by low numbers of mature T cells in the circulation and peripheral lymphoid tissues and severe deficiencies in T cell–mediated immunity.

The thymus involutes with age and is virtually undetectable in postpubertal humans, but some maturation of T cells continues throughout adult life, as indicated by the successful reconstitution of the immune system in adult recipients of bone marrow transplants. It may

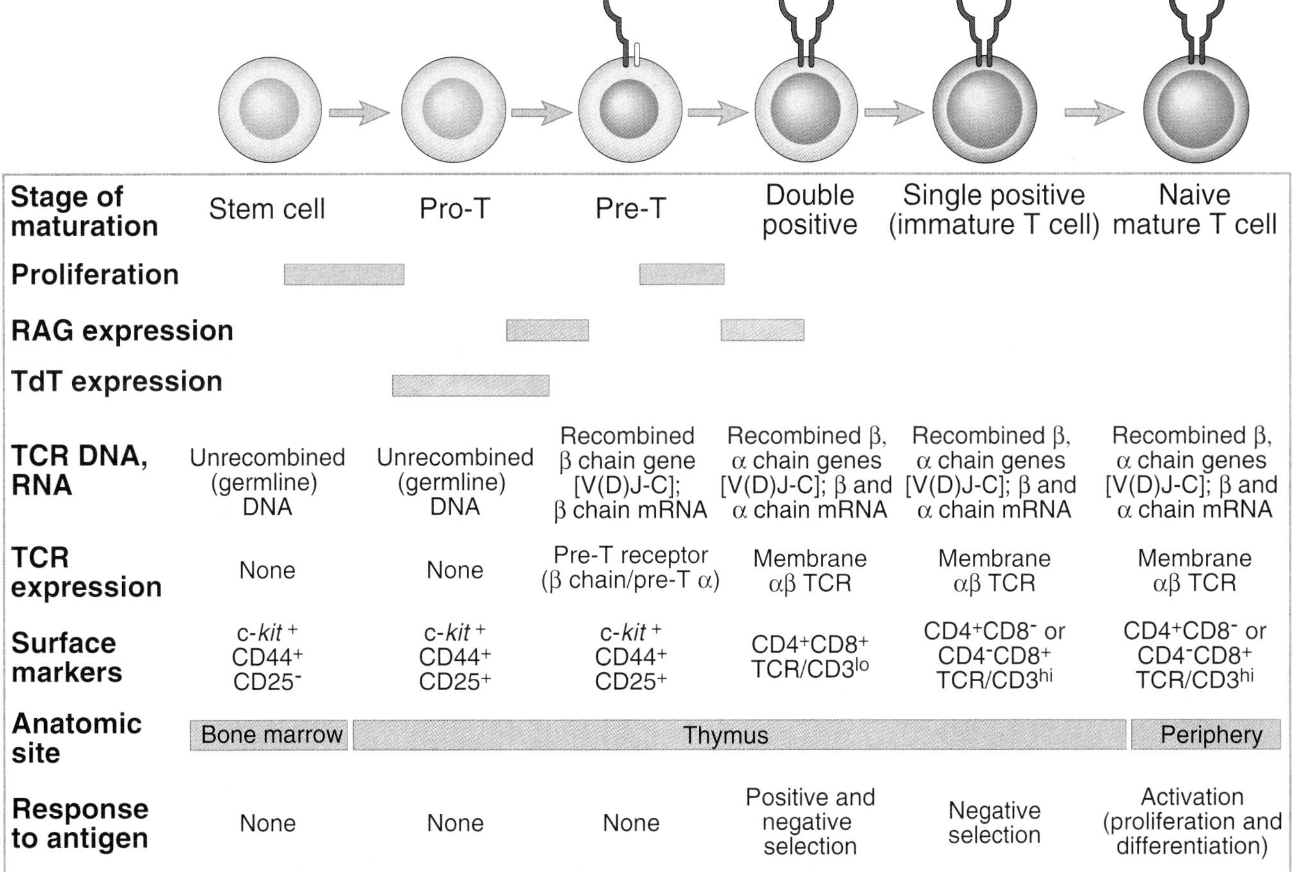

Figure 7–16 Stages of T cell maturation.
Events corresponding to each stage of T cell maturation from a bone marrow stem cell to a mature T lymphocyte are illustrated. Several surface markers in addition to those shown have been used to define distinct stages of T cell maturation. TdT, terminal deoxyribonucleotidyl transferase.

be that the remnant of the involuted thymus is adequate for some T cell maturation; extrathymic sites of T cell maturation may also exist, but none has been clearly identified. Because memory T cells have a long life span (perhaps longer than 20 years in humans) and accumulate with age, the need to generate new T cells decreases as individuals age.

T lymphocytes originate from precursors that arise in the fetal liver and adult bone marrow and seed the thymus. It is likely that progenitors of multiple lineages enter the thymus and only T cell precursors survive and mature. In mice, immature lymphocytes are first detected in the thymus on the 11th day of the normal 21-day gestation. This corresponds to about week 7 or 8 of gestation in humans. Developing T cells in the thymus are called **thymocytes.** The most immature thymocytes do not express the TCR or CD4 and CD8 coreceptors (Fig. 7–17). They are found in the subcapsular sinus and outer cortical region of the thymus. From here, the thymocytes migrate into and through the cortex, where most of the subsequent maturation events occur. It is in the cortex that the thymocytes first express TCRs and begin to mature into $CD4^+$ class II MHC–restricted or $CD8^+$ class I MHC–restricted T cells. As these thymocytes undergo the final stages of maturation, they migrate from the cortex to the medulla and then exit the thymus through the circulation.

The thymic environment provides stimuli that are required for the proliferation and maturation of thymocytes. Many of these stimuli come from cells other than the maturing T cells, which are also present within the thymus. These include thymic epithelial cells and bone marrow–derived macrophages and dendritic cells (see Chapter 2, Fig. 2–9). Within the cortex, the epithelial cells form a meshwork of long cytoplasmic processes, around which thymocytes must pass to reach the medulla. Epithelial cells are also present in the medulla. Bone marrow–derived dendritic cells are present at the corticomedullary junction and within the medulla, and macrophages are present primarily

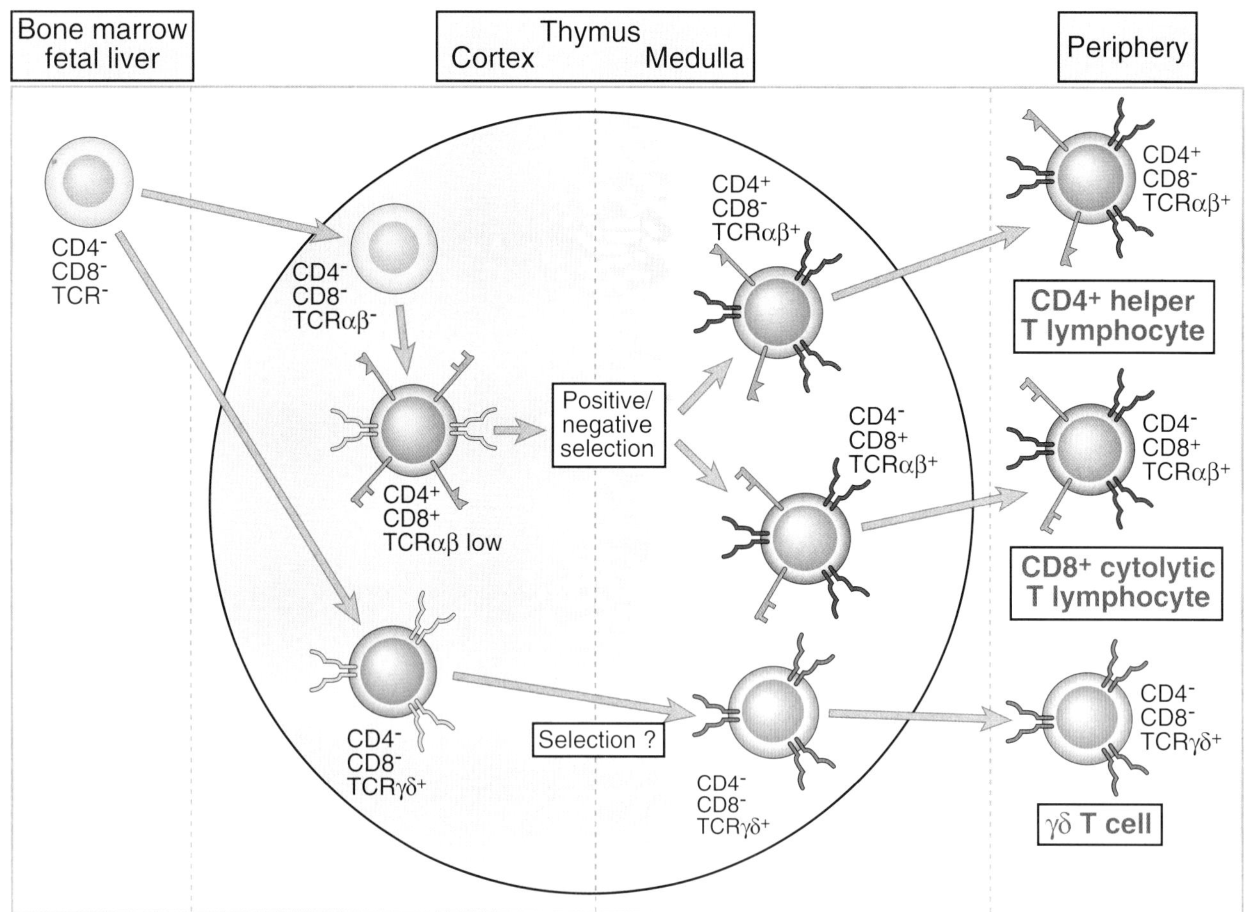

Figure 7–17 Maturation of T cells in the thymus.
Precursors of T cells travel from the bone marrow through the blood to the thymus. In the thymic cortex, progenitors of αβ T cells express TCRs and CD4 and CD8 coreceptors. Selection processes eliminate self-reactive thymocytes and promote survival of thymocytes whose TCRs bind self MHC molecules with low affinity. Functional and phenotypic differentiation into $CD4^+CD8^-$ or $CD8^+CD4^-$ T cells occurs in the medulla, and mature T cells are released into the circulation. The γδ TCR–expressing T cells are also derived from bone marrow precursors and mature in the thymus as a separate lineage.

within the medulla. The migration of thymocytes through this anatomic arrangement allows physical interactions between the thymocytes and these other cells, which are necessary for the maturation of the T lymphocytes.

Two types of molecules produced by the nonlymphoid thymic cells are important for T cell maturation. The first are MHC molecules, which are expressed by many of the nonlymphoid cells in the thymus. Epithelial cells and dendritic cells in the thymus express high levels of class I and class II MHC molecules, and macrophages express class I MHC molecules. The interactions of maturing thymocytes with these MHC molecules within the thymus are essential for the selection of the mature T cell repertoire, as we will discuss in detail later. Second, thymic stromal cells, including epithelial cells, secrete cytokines, which stimulate the proliferation of immature T cells. The best defined of these cytokines is IL-7, which was mentioned earlier as a critical lymphopoietic growth factor.

The rates of cell proliferation and apoptotic death are extremely high in cortical thymocytes. A single precursor gives rise to many progeny, and 95% of these cells die by apoptosis before reaching the medulla. The cell death is due to a combination of failure to express functional antigen receptors, failure to be positively selected by MHC molecules in the thymus, and self antigen–induced negative selection (see Figs. 7–2 and 7–3). Cortical thymocytes are also sensitive to irradiation and glucocorticoids. *In vivo*, high doses of glucocorticoids induce apoptotic death mainly in cortical thymocytes.

Stages of T Cell Maturation

During T cell maturation, there is a precise order of somatic recombination of TCR genes and expression of the TCR and CD4 and CD8 coreceptors (see Figs. 7–16 and 7–17). In the mouse, surface expression of the CD3-associated γδ TCR occurs first, 3 to 4 days after the precursor cells first arrive in the thymus, and the αβ TCR is expressed 2 or 3 days later. In human fetal thymuses, γδ receptor expression begins at about 9 weeks of gestation, followed by expression of the αβ TCR at 10 weeks. In the following section, we discuss the maturation of αβ T cells; γδ T cells are discussed later in the chapter.

The most immature cortical thymocytes, which are recent arrivals from the bone marrow, contain TCR genes in their germline configuration and do not express TCR, CD3, or ζ chains or CD4 or CD8; these cells are called **double-negative thymocytes.** This is also known as the **pro-T cell stage** of maturation. The majority (>90%) of the double-negative thymocytes will ultimately give rise to αβ TCR–expressing, MHC-restricted $CD4^+$ and $CD8^+$ T cells. RAG-1 and RAG-2 proteins are first expressed at this stage, and D_β-to-J_β rearrangements occur first and involve either joining of the $D_\beta1$ gene segment to one of the six $J_\beta1$ segments or joining of the $D_\beta2$ segment to one of the six $J_\beta2$ segments (Fig. 7–18A). D_β-to-J_β rearrangements are not lineage restricted and may occur in developing B cells, but V_β-to-DJ_β rearrangements occur only in developing T cells.

The next stage of maturation of αβ T cells is called the **pre-T cell stage.** V_β-to-DJ_β rearrangements occur at this stage. The DNA sequences between the rearranging elements, including D, J, and possibly $C_\beta1$ genes (if $D_\beta2$ and $J_\beta2$ segments are used), are deleted during this rearrangement process. The primary nuclear transcripts of the TCR β genes contain noncoding sequences between the recombined VDJ and the C genes. Poly-A tails are added to consensus polyadenylation sites located 3′ of the C_β RNA, and the sequences between the VDJ and C RNA are spliced out to form a mature mRNA in which VDJ segments are juxtaposed to either of the two C genes. Translation of this mRNA gives rise to a full-length C_β protein. The two C_β genes appear to be functionally interchangeable, and there is no evidence that an individual T cell ever switches from one C gene to another. Furthermore, the use of either C_β gene segment does not influence the function or specificity of the TCR. The β chain promoters in the 5′ flanking regions of V_β genes function together with a powerful enhancer that is located 3′ of the $C_\beta2$ gene once the two genes are brought into proximity by the V to DJ recombination. This is responsible for high-level, T cell–specific transcription of the TCR β chain. The β chain protein is expressed on the cell surface in association with an invariant protein called **pre-Tα** and with CD3 and ζ proteins to form the **pre-T cell receptor** (pre-TCR; see Fig. 7–14B). The function of the pre-TCR complex in T cell development is thought to be similar to that of the surrogate light chain–containing pre-BCR in B cell development. Signals from the pre-TCR stimulate proliferation of the pre-T cells, recombination at the α chain locus, and transition from the double-negative to the double-positive stage (see later). These signals also inhibit further rearrangements of the β chain locus on either chromosome, presumably by down-regulating expression of RAG proteins that mediate recombination and by limiting accessibility of the other allele to these enzymes. This results in β chain allelic exclusion (i.e., mature T cells express only one of the two inherited β chain alleles). As in pre-B cells, it is not known what, if any, ligand this pre-TCR recognizes. The mechanism of signaling by the pre-TCR is not well defined but probably involves the Src family tyrosine kinase Lck, which is also required for signal transduction by the TCR in mature T cells (see Chapter 8). The essential function of the pre-TCR in T cell maturation has been demonstrated by numerous studies with genetically mutated mice.

In RAG-1– or RAG-2–deficient mice, thymocytes cannot rearrange either α or β chain genes and fail to mature past the double-negative stage. If a functionally rearranged β chain gene is introduced into the RAG-deficient mice as a transgene, the expressed β chain associates with pre-Tα to form the pre-TCR, and maturation proceeds to the double-positive stage. An α chain transgene alone does not relieve the maturation block because the β chain is required for formation of the pre-TCR.

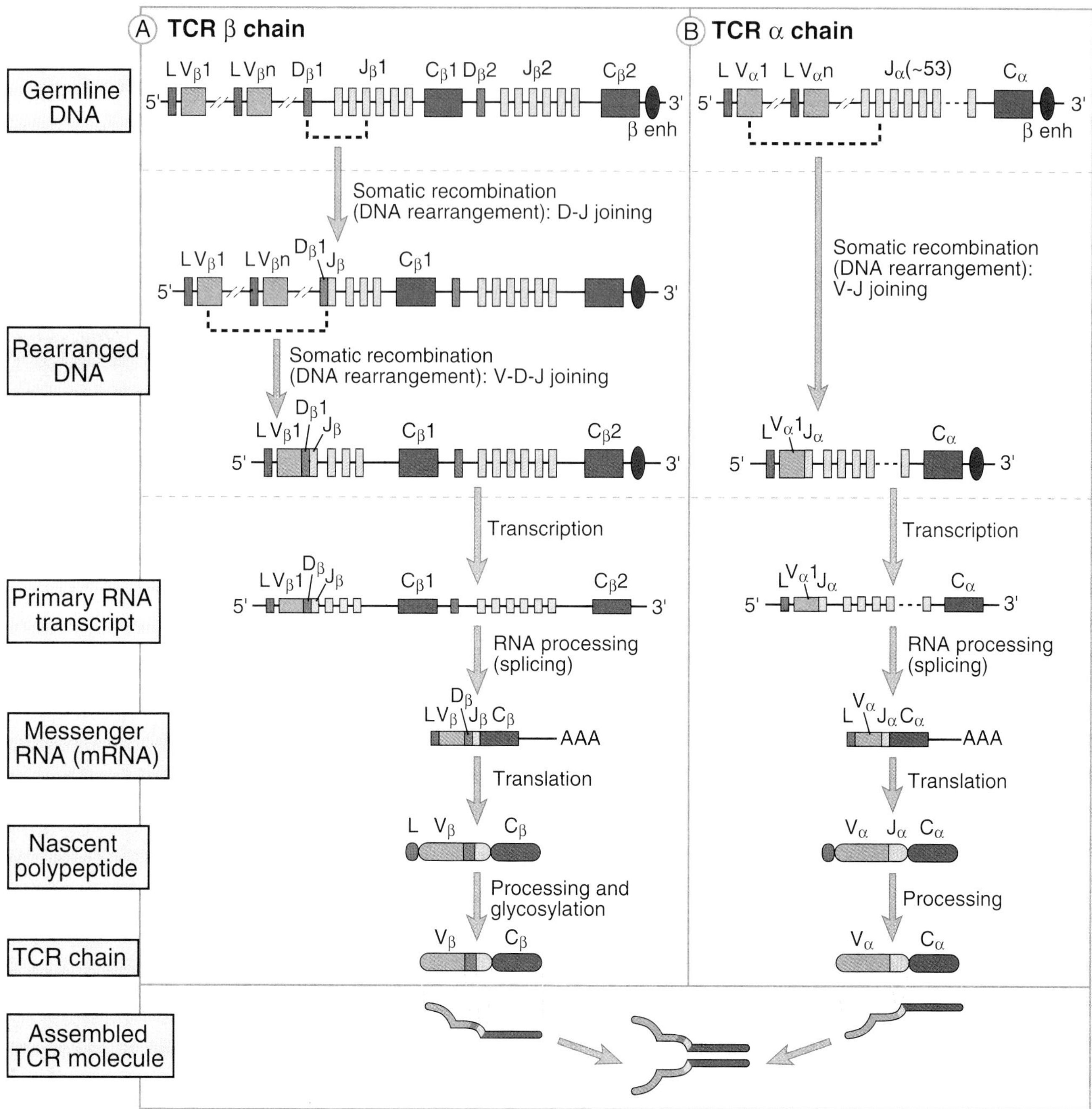

Figure 7–18 TCR α and β chain gene recombination and expression.
The sequence of recombination and gene expression events is shown for the TCR β chain (A) and the TCR α chain (B). In the example shown in A, the variable (V) region of the TCR β chain is encoded by the exons $V_{\beta}1$, $D_{\beta}1$, and the third exon in the $J_{\beta}1$ cluster, and the constant (C) region is encoded by $C_{\beta}1$. Note that in this example, the DNA recombination begins with D-to-J joining followed by V-to-DJ joining, but direct V-to-J joining may also occur in the β chain locus. In the example shown in B, the V region of the TCR α chain is encoded by $V_{\alpha}1$ and the second exon in the J_{α} cluster.

Knockout mice lacking any component of the pre-TCR complex (i.e., the TCR β chain, pre-Tα, CD3, ζ, or Lck) show a block in the maturation of T cells at the double-negative stage (see Box 7–1).

At the next stage of T cell maturation, thymocytes express both CD4 and CD8 and are called **double-positive thymocytes.** The expression of CD4 and CD8 is essential for subsequent selection events, discussed later. The rearrangement of the TCR α chain genes and the expression of TCR αβ heterodimers occur in the $CD4^+CD8^+$ double-positive population, just before or during migration of the thymocytes from the cortex to the medulla (see Figs. 7–16 and 7–17). A second wave of *RAG* gene expression late in the pre-T stage promotes TCR α gene recombinations. Once α chain rearrangement commences, it proceeds for 3 or 4 days (in mice) until the expression of the *RAG1* and *RAG2* genes is turned off by signals from the αβ TCR during positive selection (discussed later). The steps in α chain gene rearrangements are similar to those in the β chain gene (see Fig. 7–18B). Because there are no D segments in the α locus, rearrangement consists solely of the joining of V and J segments. The large number of J_α segments permits multiple attempts at productive V-J joining on each chromosome, thereby increasing the probability that a functional αβ TCR will be produced. Unlike in the β chain locus, where production of the protein and formation of the pre-TCR suppress further rearrangement, there is little or no allelic exclusion in the α chain locus. Therefore, productive TCR α rearrangements may occur on both chromosomes, and if this happens, the T cell will express two α chains. In fact, up to 30% of mature peripheral T cells do express two different TCRs, with different α chains but the same β chain. The functional consequence of this dual receptor expression is unknown. Because only one TCR is required for positive selection, it is possible that the second TCR may not have any affinity for self MHC, and therefore it would have no function. Transcriptional regulation of the α chain gene is apparently similar to that of the β chain. There are promoters 5′ of each V_α gene that have low-level activity and are responsible for high-level T cell–specific transcription when brought close to an α chain enhancer located 3′ of the C_α gene. In both the α and the β chain loci, if productive rearrangements fail to occur on either chromosome, the thymocyte will die by apoptosis.

TCRα gene expression in the double-positive stage leads to the formation of the complete αβ TCR, which is expressed on the cell surface in association with CD3 and ζ proteins. The coordinate expression of CD3 and ζ proteins and the assembly of intact TCR complexes are required for surface expression. The expression of *RAG* genes and further TCR gene recombination cease after this stage of maturation. The first cells to express TCRs are in the thymic cortex, and expression is low compared with mature T cells. By virtue of their expression of complete TCR complexes, double-positive cells become responsive to antigens and are subjected to positive and negative selection.

Cells that successfully undergo these selection processes go on to mature into $CD4^+$ or $CD8^+$ T cells, which are called **single-positive thymocytes.** Thus, the stages of T cell maturation in the thymus can readily be distinguished by the expression of CD4 and CD8 (Fig. 7–19). This phenotypic maturation is accompanied by functional maturation. $CD4^+$ cells acquire the ability to produce cytokines in response to subsequent antigen stimulation and to express effector molecules (such as CD40 ligand) that "help" B lymphocytes and macrophages, whereas $CD8^+$ cells become capable of producing molecules that kill other cells. We do not know the mechanisms by which $CD4^+$ cells become specialized to function as helper cells and $CD8^+$ cells as cytolytic T lymphocytes. Mature single-positive thymocytes enter the thymic medulla and then leave the thymus to populate peripheral lymphoid tissues.

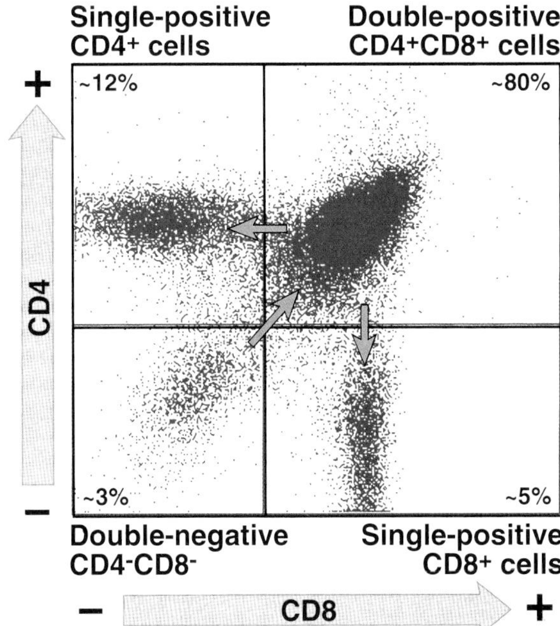

Figure 7–19 CD4 and CD8 expression on thymocytes. The maturation of thymocytes can be followed by changes in expression of the CD4 and CD8 coreceptors. A two-color flow cytometric analysis of thymocytes using anti-CD4 and anti-CD8 antibodies, each tagged with a different fluorochrome, is illustrated. The percentages of all thymocytes contributed by each major population are shown in the four quadrants. The least mature subset is the $CD4^-CD8^-$ (double-negative) cells. Arrows indicate the sequence of maturation.

Selection Processes in the Maturation of MHC-Restricted αβ T Cells

The selection of developing T cells is stimulated by recognition of antigen (peptide-MHC complexes) in the thymus and is responsible for preserving useful cells and eliminating potentially harmful ones (Fig. 7–20). The immature, or unselected, repertoire of T lymphocytes consists of cells whose receptors may recognize any peptide antigen (self or foreign) displayed by any MHC molecule (also self or foreign). In addition, receptors may be expressed that do not recognize any peptide-MHC molecule complex. In every individual, the only useful T cells are the ones specific for foreign peptides presented by that individual's MHC molecules, that is, self MHC molecules. (Recall that there are many alleles of MHC molecules in the population, and every individual inherits one allele of each MHC gene from each parent. These inherited alleles encode "self MHC" for that individual.) Also, in every individual, T cells that recognize ubiquitous self antigens with high avidity are potentially dangerous because such recognition may trigger autoimmunity.

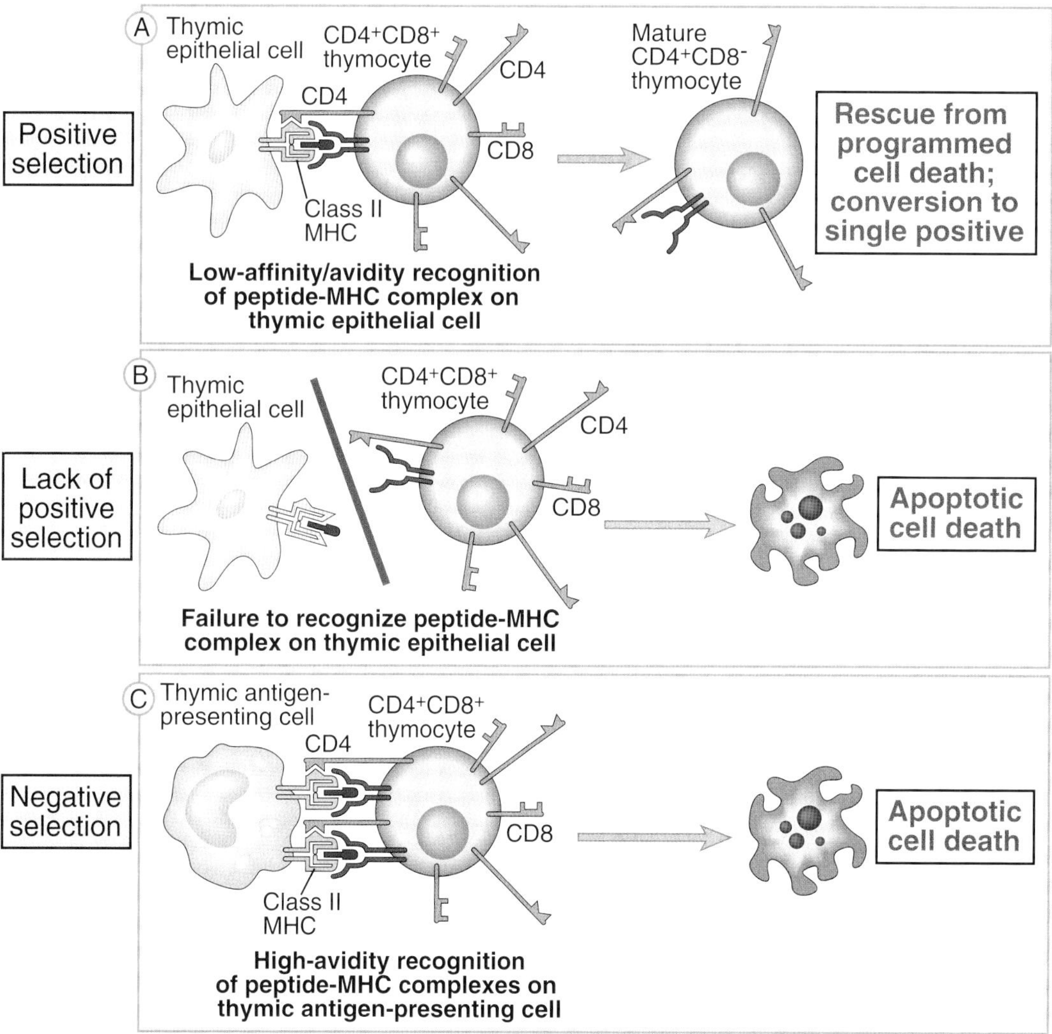

Figure 7–20 Selection processes in the thymus.
A. Positive selection. If the thymocyte TCR engages in a low-affinity interaction with a self MHC molecule on a thymic epithelial cell, it is rescued from programmed cell death and continues to mature.
B. Lack of positive selection. If the thymocyte TCR does not engage in any interactions with peptide-MHC molecule complexes on thymic epithelial cells, it will die by a default pathway of programmed cell death.
C. Negative selection. If the thymocyte TCR binds peptide-MHC complexes on a thymic antigen-presenting cell with high affinity or avidity, it is induced to undergo apoptotic cell death.

Selection processes act on the immature T cell repertoire to ensure that only the useful cells complete the process of maturation.

When double-positive thymocytes first express αβ TCRs, these receptors encounter self peptides (the only peptides normally present in the thymus) displayed by self MHC molecules (the only MHC molecules available to display peptides). **Positive selection** is the process in which thymocytes whose TCRs bind with low avidity (i.e., weakly) to self peptide–self MHC complexes are stimulated to survive (see Fig. 7–20A). Thymocytes whose receptors do not recognize self MHC molecules are permitted to die by a default pathway of apoptosis (see Fig. 7–20B). This ensures that the T cells that mature are self MHC-restricted. Positive selection also fixes the class I or class II MHC restriction of T cell subsets, ensuring that $CD8^+$ T cells are specific for peptides displayed by class I MHC molecules and $CD4^+$ T cells for class II–associated peptides. **Negative selection** is the process in which thymocytes whose TCRs bind strongly to self peptide antigens in association with self MHC molecules are deleted (see Fig. 7–20C). This eliminates developing T cells that are strongly autoreactive against ubiquitous self antigens, which are the self antigens most likely to be present in the thymus. The net result of these selection processes is that the repertoire of mature T cells that leaves the thymus is self MHC-restricted and tolerant to many self antigens. In the following sections, we discuss the details of positive and negative selection.

Positive Selection of Thymocytes: Development of the Self MHC–Restricted T Cell Repertoire

Positive selection works by promoting the selective survival and expansion of thymocytes with self MHC–restricted TCRs and by permitting thymocytes whose TCRs are not self MHC-restricted to die by apoptosis (Fig. 7–20A, B). Double-positive thymocytes are produced without antigenic stimulation and begin to express αβ TCRs with randomly generated specificities. In the thymic cortex, these immature cells encounter epithelial cells that are displaying a variety of self peptides bound to class I and class II MHC molecules. If the TCR on a cell recognizes peptide-loaded class I MHC molecules, and at the same time CD8 interacts with the class I MHC molecules, that T cell receives signals that prevent its death and promote its continued maturation. To proceed along the maturation pathway, the T cell must continue to express the TCR and CD8 but can lose expression of CD4. The result is the development of a class I MHC–restricted CD8$^+$ T cell. An entirely analogous process leads to the development of class II MHC–restricted CD4$^+$ T cells. Any T cell that expresses a TCR that does not recognize a peptide-loaded MHC molecule in the thymus will die and be lost.

Positive selection of T cells requires the recognition of self MHC molecules in the thymus by the TCRs of immature (double-positive) thymocytes. The essential roles of MHC molecules and TCR specificity have been established by a variety of experiments.

- In early studies, T cells from inbred mice of one strain were allowed to mature in the presence of a thymus of another strain, and the restriction of mature T cells to the MHC alleles of either strain was examined. If chimeric animals are created by transferring the bone marrow–derived hematopoietic stem cells from a mouse of one MHC haplotype into a lethally irradiated mouse of a partially different MHC haplotype, the mature T cells that develop in these chimeras recognize foreign antigens only in association with MHC molecules of the host strain (Table 7–2). Therefore, T cells are selected to recognize the MHC molecules of the strain in which the cells mature. The self MHC restriction of T cells refers to the MHC that the T cells encounter during their maturation and not necessarily to the MHC alleles expressed by the T cells themselves. Normally, of course, the thymus and the developing T cells express the same MHC alleles, which are "self" in each individual.
- If a thymus from one inbred strain is transplanted into chimeric animals of another strain, the T cells that mature are restricted by the MHC type of the thymus (see Table 7–2). The transplanted thymuses may be irradiated or treated with cytotoxic drugs (such as deoxyguanosine) to kill all resident bone marrow–derived macrophages, dendritic cells, and lymphoid cells, leaving only the resistant thymic epithelial cells. Again, mature T cells develop in these thymuses, and their ability to recognize antigen is restricted by MHC gene products expressed on the transplanted thymic epithelial cells and not necessarily by MHC gene products expressed on extrathymic cells. Therefore, the thymic epithelium is the critical host element for positive selection (i.e., the development of the MHC restriction patterns of T cells).
- If a transgenic αβ TCR with a known MHC restriction is expressed in a mouse strain that also expresses the MHC allele for which the TCR is specific, T cells will mature and populate peripheral lymphoid tissue. If the mouse is of another MHC haplotype and does not express the MHC molecule that the transgenic TCR recognizes, there are normal numbers of CD4$^+$CD8$^+$ thymocytes but very few mature transgenic TCR-expressing T cells (Fig. 7–21). This result demonstrates that double-positive thymocytes must express TCRs that can bind self MHC molecules to be positively selected. As we shall see later, the same experimental system has been used to study negative selection.

Table 7–2. Development of MHC Restriction in Bone Marrow plus Thymus Chimeras

Chimera			Specific killing of virus-infected targets from	
Host strain and treatment	Bone marrow donor	Thymus donor	Strain A	Strain B
(A × B)F$_1$ irradiated	(A × B)F$_1$	None	+	+
A irradiated	(A × B)F$_1$	None	+	–
A irradiated and thymectomized	(A × B)F$_1$	A	+	–
A irradiated and thymectomized	(A × B)F$_1$	B	–	+

Bone marrow chimeras are created by reconstituting an irradiated mouse of one strain with bone marrow progenitors from another strain. In this example, the strain A and B mice have different class I MHC alleles. The MHC restriction specificity of mature T cells in these mice is tested by assaying the ability of cytolytic T lymphocytes generated in response to viral infection to kill virus-infected target cells from different mouse strains *in vitro.* These experiments demonstrate that the host MHC type, and not the bone marrow donor type, determines the restriction specificity of the mature T cells and that the thymus is the site where self MHC restriction is learned.

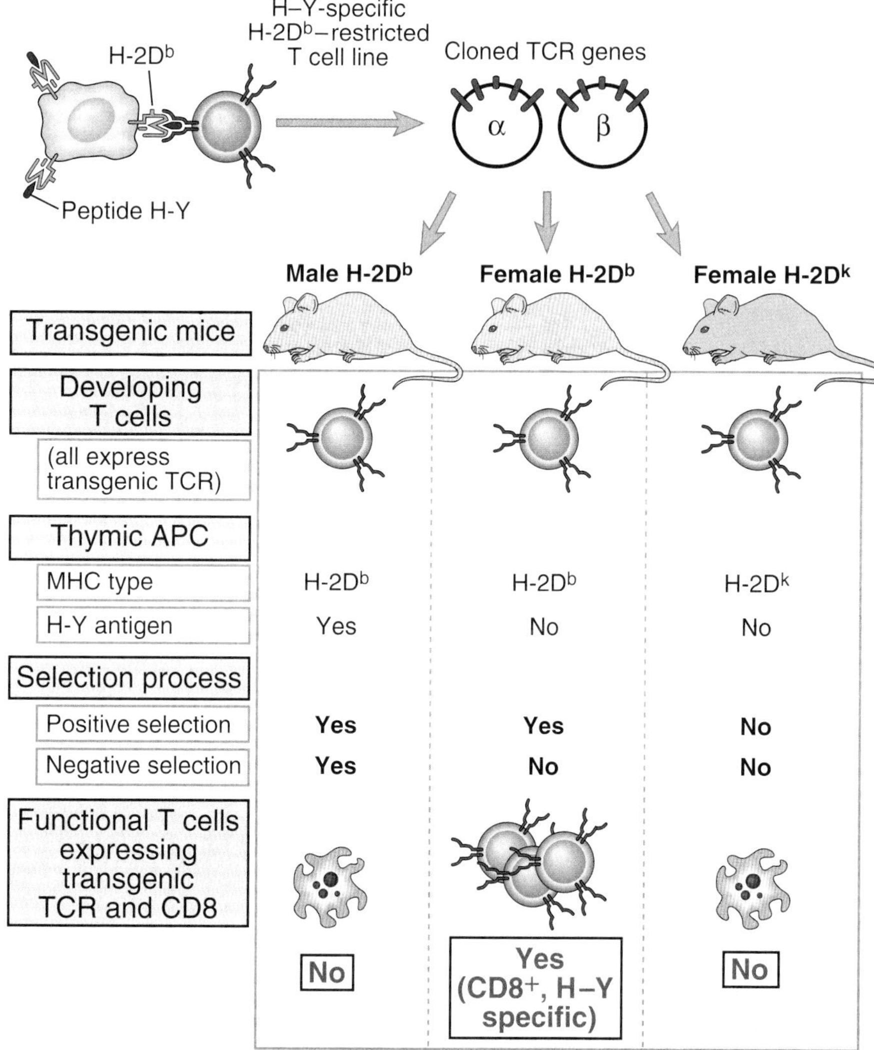

Figure 7–21 T cell maturation and selection in a TCR transgenic mouse model.

In the experiment depicted, a transgenic mouse expresses a TCR specific for an H-2D^b–associated H-Y (male-specific) antigen, which is, in effect, a foreign antigen for a female mouse. (The creation of TCR transgenic mice is described in Appendix III.) In female mice expressing the D^b MHC allele, mature T cells expressing the transgenic TCR do develop because they are positively selected by the self MHC molecules. These T cells do not mature in male H-Y–expressing mice because they are negatively selected by H-Y antigen recognition in the thymus. Furthermore, mature T cells do not develop in female mice that express D^k but do not express the D^b allele because of a lack of positive selection of the D^b-restricted TCR-expressing T cells. APC, antigen-presenting cell.

During the transition from double-positive to single-positive cells, thymocytes with class I–restricted TCRs become CD8$^+$CD4$^-$, and cells with class II–restricted TCRs become CD4$^+$CD8$^-$. CD4 and CD8 function as coreceptors with TCRs during positive selection and recognize the MHC molecules when the TCRs are recognizing peptide-MHC complexes. Signals from the TCR complex and the coreceptors function together to promote survival of thymocytes. This function of CD4 and CD8 is similar to their role in the activation of mature T cells (see Chapter 8). At this stage in maturation, there may be a random loss of either CD4 or CD8 gene, and only cells expressing the "correct" coreceptor (i.e., CD4 on a class II–restricted T cell or CD8 on a class I–restricted T cell) will continue to mature. It is also possible that the expression of the wrong coreceptor is actively suppressed, although how this is accomplished is unknown.

- Knockout mice that lack class I MHC expression in thymic epithelial cells do not develop mature CD8$^+$ T cells but do develop CD4$^+$CD8$^+$ thymocytes and mature CD4$^+$ T cells. Conversely, class II MHC–deficient mice do not develop CD4$^+$ T cells but do develop CD8$^+$ cells. These results demonstrate that thymic epithelial cells must express class I or class II MHC molecules to positively select thymocytes to become CD8$^+$ or CD4$^+$ single-positive cells, respectively.

- In transgenic mice expressing a class II MHC–restricted TCR, the mature T cells that develop are almost exclusively CD4$^+$, even though there are normal numbers of CD4$^+$CD8$^+$ thymocytes. Conversely, if the transgenic TCR is class I-restricted, the T cells that mature are CD8$^+$. Thus, the coreceptor and the MHC specificity of the TCR must match if a thymocyte is to develop into a mature T cell.

Peptides bound to MHC molecules on thymic epithelial cells play an essential role in positive selection. In Chapters 4 and 5, we described how cell surface class I and class II molecules always contain bound peptides. These MHC-associated peptides on thymic antigen-presenting cells probably serve two roles in positive selection—first, they promote stable cell surface expression of MHC molecules, and second, they may influence the specificities of the T cells that are selected. Obviously, the thymus cannot contain all the antigens to which an individual can respond. Therefore, foreign peptides cannot be involved in the positive selection of T cells that ultimately may recognize these peptides. Self peptides are required for positive selection, however, and exactly what role they are playing has been the subject of numerous studies using a variety of experimental systems.

- To address the role of peptides in T cell selection, it was necessary to develop systems in which the array of peptides presented to developing thymocytes was limited and could be manipulated experimentally. For class I MHC–dependent positive selection, this was accomplished with use of TAP-1–deficient or β_2-microglobulin–deficient mice. In these mice, the class I molecules are not loaded with cytosolic peptides and are unstable, but they can readily be loaded with exogenously added peptides. If thymuses from such mice are cultured without added peptides, few mature T cells develop (Fig. 7–22). The addition of peptides dramatically increases the development of single-positive $CD8^+$ T cells, indicating effective positive selection of thymocytes expressing class I MHC–restricted TCRs. A key finding in these experiments was that one or a few peptides induced the positive selection of a large repertoire of $CD8^+$ T cells that could potentially recognize many different unrelated peptides. However, no single peptide was sufficient to generate a normal number (or repertoire) of mature T cells. Furthermore, complex mixtures of peptides induced the maturation of more $CD8^+$ T cells than did single peptides. We do not know if the specificities of the T cells that mature are related to the peptides that induced their maturation.

The conclusion of such experiments is that peptides bound to MHC molecules are required for positive selection of T cells and that some peptides are better than others in supporting this process. It is not known what structural features may be common to positively selecting peptides. Nevertheless, the finding that peptides differ in the repertoires of T cells they select suggests that specific antigen recognition, and not just MHC recognition, has some role in positive selection. Weak, or low-avidity, recognition of peptides in the thymus protects immature T cells from a default pathway of apoptotic death and allows the cells to complete their maturation. We do not know what signals generated by weak antigen recognition protect immature T cells from death and how these signals differ from those generated by antigen recognition in mature, single-positive T cells. One consequence of self peptide–induced positive selection is that the T cells that mature have some capacity to recognize self peptides. We mentioned in Chapter 2 that the survival of naive lymphocytes before encounter with foreign antigens requires survival signals that are apparently generated by recognition of self antigens. The same self peptides that mediate positive selection of double-positive thymocytes in the thymus may be involved in keeping naive, mature (single-positive) T cells alive in peripheral lymphoid organs, such as the lymph nodes and spleen.

This model of positive selection based on weak recognition of self antigens raises a fundamental question: How does positive selection driven by self antigens produce a repertoire of mature T cells specific for foreign antigens? The likely answer is that T cells that recognize self peptides with low affinity will, after maturing, fortuitously recognize foreign peptides with a high enough affinity to be activated and to generate

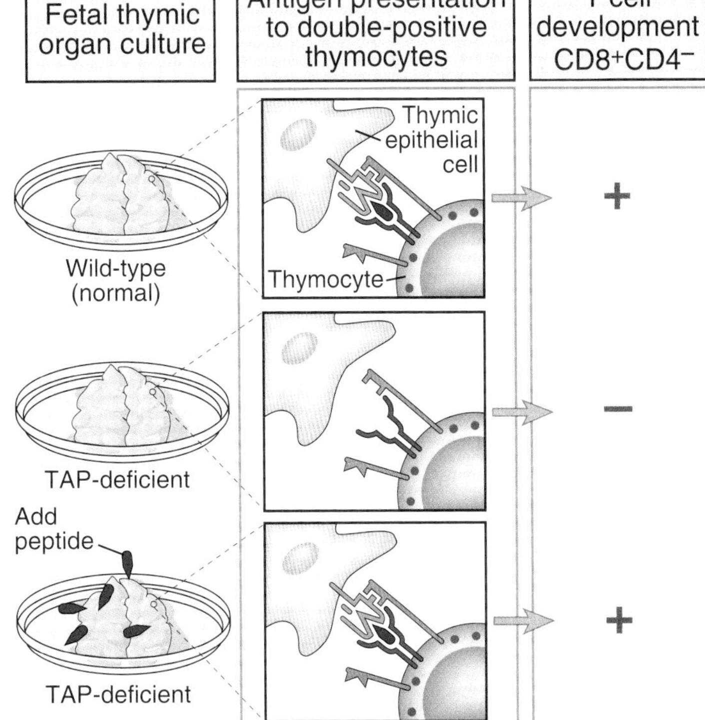

Figure 7–22 Role of peptides in positive selection. In the experiment shown, thymuses are removed from fetal mice and cultured *in vitro* (fetal thymic organ cultures). If the thymuses are removed early enough in gestation, they contain only immature thymocytes that have not yet undergone positive selection, and therefore subsequent maturation events can be followed under varying *in vitro* conditions. In thymuses from wild-type (normal) mice, both $CD4^+CD8^-$ and $CD8^+CD4^-$ T cells will develop. TAP-1–deficient mice cannot form peptide–class I MHC complexes on thymic epithelial cells (see Chapter 5), and there is little development of $CD8^+CD4^-$ T cells in the thymuses from these mice because of a lack of positive selection of class I–restricted thymocytes. However, the addition of peptides to the culture medium surrounding the TAP-1–deficient thymuses permits the formation of peptide–class I MHC complexes on the surface of thymic epithelial cells, and this restores maturation of $CD8^+CD4^-$ T cells.

immune responses. As we discuss next, strong recognition of self antigens in the thymus results in negative selection of developing T cells.

Negative Selection of Thymocytes: Development of Central Tolerance

Negative selection of thymocytes works by inducing apoptotic death of cells whose receptors recognize abundant peptide-MHC complexes in the thymus with high avidity (see Fig. 7–20C). Among the double-positive T cells that are generated in the thymus, some may express TCRs that recognize self antigens with high affinity. If these self antigens are also present at high concentrations in the thymus, the T cells will see the antigens with high avidity because the avidity of antigen recognition depends on the affinity of the TCR and the concentration of the peptide that the T cell recognizes. The peptides present at high concentration in the thymus are self peptides that are mainly derived from protein antigens widely expressed in the body (i.e., they are ubiquitous). In immature T cells, the consequence of high-avidity antigen recognition is the triggering of apoptosis, leading to death, or deletion, of the cells. Therefore, the immature thymocytes that express high-affinity receptors for ubiquitous self antigens are eliminated, resulting in negative selection of the T cell repertoire. This process eliminates the potentially most harmful self-reactive T cells and is one of the mechanisms ensuring that the immune system does not respond to many self antigens, a property called self-tolerance. Tolerance induced in immature lymphocytes by recognition of self antigens in the generative (or central) lymphoid organs is also called central tolerance, to be contrasted with peripheral tolerance induced in mature lymphocytes by self antigens in peripheral tissues. We will discuss the mechanisms and physiologic importance of immunologic tolerance in more detail in Chapter 10.

Formal proof for deletion of T cell clones reactive with antigens in the thymus (also called clonal deletion) has come from several experimental approaches that allowed investigators to observe the effects of self antigen recognition by a large number of developing T cells.

- When TCR transgenic mice are exposed to the peptide for which the TCR is specific, a large amount of cell death is induced in the thymus and a block occurs in the development of mature transgenic TCR-expressing T cells. In one such study, a transgenic mouse line was created that expressed a class I MHC–restricted TCR specific for the Y chromosome–encoded antigen H-Y, which is expressed by many cell types in male mice but not in female mice (see Fig. 7–21). Female mice with this transgenic TCR have normal numbers of thymocytes in the thymic medulla and large numbers of $CD8^+$ T cells in the periphery because they do not express the H-Y antigen that may induce negative selection. In contrast, male transgenic mice have few TCR-expressing, single-positive thymocytes in the medulla and few mature peripheral $CD8^+$ T cells because of deletion of the H-Y–specific thymocytes induced by H-Y antigen in the thymus.
- The same deletion of immature T cells is seen if transgenic mice expressing a TCR specific for a known peptide antigen are bred with mice expressing that antigen or if the mice are injected with large doses of the antigen. This can also be mimicked *in vitro* by culturing intact thymuses from TCR transgenic mice with high concentrations of the peptide for which the TCR is specific. In all these examples, there is a block of T cell maturation after the cortical double-positive stage, presumably because immature thymocytes express the transgenic TCR, recognize the antigen on thymic antigen-presenting cells, and are deleted before they can mature into single-positive cells.

The deletion of immature self-reactive T cells occurs when the TCR on a $CD4^+CD8^+$ thymocyte binds strongly to a self peptide presented by another thymic cell. Most evidence indicates that any thymic antigen-presenting cell can induce negative selection, including bone marrow–derived macrophages and dendritic cells and thymic epithelial cells, whereas epithelial cells are especially (and perhaps uniquely) effective at inducing positive selection. The key factor determining the choice between positive and negative selection is the strength of antigen recognition, with low-avidity recognition leading to positive selection and high-avidity recognition inducing negative selection. CD4 and CD8 molecules probably play a role in negative selection, as they do in positive selection, because these coreceptors participate in recognition of MHC molecules presenting self peptides. The cellular basis of negative selection in the thymus is the induction of death by apoptosis. Unlike in death by default (or neglect), which occurs in the absence of positive selection, in negative selection, active death-promoting signals are generated when the TCR of immature thymocytes binds with high affinity to antigen. The nature of these active death-inducing signals in thymocytes is not known.

Studies suggest that recognition of self antigens in the thymus can also generate a population of regulatory T cells, which function to prevent autoimmune reactions (see Chapter 10). It is not known why some self antigens cause deletion of T cells and others induce regulatory T cells.

γδ Subset of T Lymphocytes

TCR αβ- and γδ-expressing thymocytes are separate lineages with a common precursor. In fetal thymuses, the first TCR gene rearrangements involve the γ and δ loci. Recombination of TCR γ and δ loci proceeds in a fashion similar to that of other antigen receptor gene rearrangements, although the order of rearrangement appears to be less rigid than in other loci.

T cells that express functional γ and δ chains do not express αβ TCRs and vice versa. The independence of these lineages is indicated by several lines of evidence.

- Mature αβ-expressing T cells often show out-of-frame rearrangements of δ genes, indicating that these cells could never have expressed γδ receptors.

- TCR δ gene knockout mice develop normal numbers of αβ T cells, and β gene knockout mice develop normal numbers of γδ T cells.

The diversity of the γδ T cell repertoire is theoretically even greater than that of the αβ T cell repertoire, in part because the heptamer-nonamer recognition sequences adjacent to D segments permit D-to-D joining. Paradoxically, however, the actual diversity of expressed γδ TCRs is limited because only a few of the available V, D, and J segments are used in mature γδ T cells, for unknown reasons. This limited diversity is reminiscent of the limited diversity of the B-1 subset of B lymphocytes and is in keeping with the concept that γδ T cells serve as an early defense against a limited number of commonly encountered microbes at epithelial barriers.

In Chapter 6, we also mentioned another small subset of T cells, the NK-T cells, which are not MHC restricted and do not recognize peptides displayed by antigen-presenting cells. The maturation of NK-T cells is not defined.

Summary

- B and T lymphocytes arise from a common bone marrow–derived precursor that becomes committed to the lymphocyte lineage. B cell maturation proceeds in the bone marrow, whereas early T cell progenitors migrate to and complete their maturation in the thymus. Early maturation is characterized by cell proliferation induced by cytokines, mainly IL-7, leading to marked increases in the numbers of immature lymphocytes.
- B and T cell maturation involves the somatic recombination of antigen receptor gene segments and the expression of Ig molecules in B cell precursors and TCR molecules in T cell precursors. The expression of antigen receptors is essential for survival and maturation of developing lymphocytes and for selection processes that lead to a diverse repertoire of useful antigen specificities.
- The antigen receptors of B and T cells are encoded by genes formed by the somatic recombination of a limited number of gene segments that are spatially segregated in the germline antigen receptor loci. There are separate loci encoding the Ig heavy chain, Ig κ light chain, Ig λ light chain, TCR β chain, TCR α and γ chains, and TCR δ chain. These loci contain V, J, and, in the Ig heavy chain and TCR β and δ loci only, D gene segments. Somatic recombination of both Ig and TCR loci involves the joining of D and J segments in the loci that contain D segments, followed by the joining of the V segment to the recombined DJ segments in these loci, or direct V-to-J joining in the other loci. This process of somatic gene recombination is mediated by a recombinase enzyme complex that includes lymphocyte-specific components RAG-1 and RAG-2.
- The diversity of the antibody and TCR repertoires is generated by the combinatorial associations of multiple germline V, D, and J genes and junctional diversity generated by the addition of random nucleotides to the sites of recombination. These mechanisms generate the most diversity at the junction of the V and C regions that form the third hypervariable regions of both antibody and TCR polypeptides.
- B cell maturation occurs in stages characterized by different patterns of Ig gene recombination and expression. In the earliest B cell precursors, called pro-B cells, Ig genes are in the germline configuration. In the pre-B cell stage, V-D-J recombination occurs in the Ig H chain locus. A primary RNA transcript containing the VDJ complex and Ig C gene segments is produced, and the μ C region exons of the heavy chain RNA are spliced to the VDJ segment to generate a mature mRNA that is translated into μ heavy chain protein. A pre-BCR is formed by pairing of the μ chain with a nonvariable surrogate light chain and by association with the signaling molecules Igα and Igβ. This receptor mediates signals that inhibit rearrangement on the other heavy chain allele (allelic exclusion) as well as stimulate proliferation. In the immature B cell stage, V-J recombinations occur in the κ or λ loci, and light chain proteins are expressed. Heavy and light chains are then assembled into intact IgM molecules and expressed on the cell surface. Immature B cells leave the bone marrow to populate peripheral lymphoid tissues, where they complete their maturation. In the mature B cell stage, synthesis of both μ and δ heavy chains occurs in the same B cells mediated by alternative splicing of primary heavy chain RNA transcripts, and membrane IgM and IgD are expressed.
- During B lymphocyte maturation, selection processes eliminate or inactivate B cell precursors that express antigen receptors specific for ubiquitous self antigens present in the bone marrow.
- T cell maturation in the thymus also progresses in stages distinguished by expression of antigen receptor genes, CD4 and CD8 coreceptor molecules, and location in the thymus. The earliest T lineage immigrants to the thymus do not express TCRs or CD4 or CD8 molecules. The developing T cells within the thymus, called thymocytes, initially populate the outer cortex, where they undergo proliferation, rearrangement of TCR genes, and surface expression of CD3, TCR, CD4, and CD8 molecules. As the cells mature, they migrate from the cortex to the medulla.
- The least mature thymocytes, called pro-T cells, are $CD4^-CD8^-$ (double negative), and the TCR genes are in the germline configuration. In the pre-T stage, thymocytes remain double negative, but V-D-J recombination occurs in the TCR β chain locus. Primary β chain transcripts are expressed and processed to bring a C_β segment adjacent to the VDJ complex, and β chain polypeptides are produced. The β chain associates with the invariant pre-Tα protein to form a pre-TCR. The pre-TCR transduces signals that inhibit rearrangement on the other β chain allele (allelic exclusion) and promote CD4 and CD8 expression

and further proliferation of immature thymocytes. In the $CD4^+CD8^+$ (double-positive) stage of T cell development, V-J recombinations occur in the α locus, α chain polypeptides are produced, and low levels of TCRs are expressed on the cell surface.

- Selection processes drive maturation of TCR-expressing, double-positive thymocytes and shape the T cell repertoire toward self MHC restriction and self-tolerance. Positive selection of $CD4^+CD8^+$ TCRαβ thymocytes requires low-avidity recognition of peptide-MHC complexes on thymic epithelial cells, leading to a rescue of the cells from programmed death. Negative selection of $CD4^+CD8^+$ TCRαβ double-positive thymocytes occurs when these cells recognize, with high avidity, antigens that are present at high concentrations in the thymus. This process is responsible for tolerance to many self antigens. Most of the cortical thymocytes do not survive these selection processes. As the surviving TCRαβ thymocytes mature, they move into the medulla and become either $CD4^+CD8^-$ or $CD8^+CD4^-$. Medullary thymocytes acquire the ability to differentiate into either helper or cytolytic effector cells and finally emigrate to peripheral lymphoid tissues.

Selected Readings

Bevan M. In thymic selection, peptide diversity gives and takes away. Immunity 7:175–178, 1997.

Fischer A, and B Malissen. Natural and engineered disorders of lymphocyte development. Science 280:237–243, 1998.

Fugmann SD, AI Lee, PE Shockett, IJ Villey, and DG Schatz. The RAG proteins and V(D)J recombination: complexes, ends, and transposition. Annual Review of Immunology 18:495–527, 2000.

Germain RN. T cell development and the CD4–CD8 lineage decision. Nature Reviews Immunology 2:309–322, 2002.

Glimcher LH, and S Singh. Transcription factors in lymphocyte development–T and B cells get together. Cell 96:13–23, 1999.

Goldrath AW, and MJ Bevan. Selecting and maintaining a diverse T-cell repertoire. Nature 402:255–262, 1999.

Hardy RR, and K Hayakawa. B cell development pathways. Annual Review of Immunology 19:595–622, 2001.

Hogquist KA. Signal strength in thymic selection and lineage commitment. Current Opinion in Immunology 13:225–231, 2001.

Killeen N, BA Irving, S Pippig, and K Zingler. Signaling checkpoints during the development of T lymphocytes. Current Opinion in Immunology 10:360–367, 1998.

Kuppers R, and R Dalla-Favera. Mechanisms of chromosomal translocations in B cell lymphomas. Oncogene 20:5580–5594, 2001.

Matsuda F, and T Honjo. Organization of the human heavy-chain locus. Advances in Immunology 62:1–29, 1996.

Meffre E, R Casellas, and MC Nussenzweig. Antibody regulation of B cell development. Nature Immunology 1:379–385, 2000.

Muljo SA, and MS Schlissel. Pre-B and pre-T cell receptors: conservation of strategies in regulating early lymphocyte development. Immunological Reviews 175:80–93, 2000.

Nemazee D. Receptor selection in B and T lymphocytes. Annual Review of Immunology 18:19–51, 2000.

Rajewsky K. Clonal selection and learning in the antibody system. Nature 381:751–758, 1996.

Rodewald HR, and HJ Fehling. Molecular and cellular events in early thymocyte development. Advances in Immunology 69:1–112, 1998.

Rolink AG, C Schaniel, J Andersson, and F Melchers. Selection events operating at various stages in B cell development. Current Opinion in Immunology 13:202–207, 2001.

Roth DB, and SY Roth. Unequal access: regulating V(D)J recombination through chromatin remodeling. Cell 103:699–702, 2000.

Chapter 8

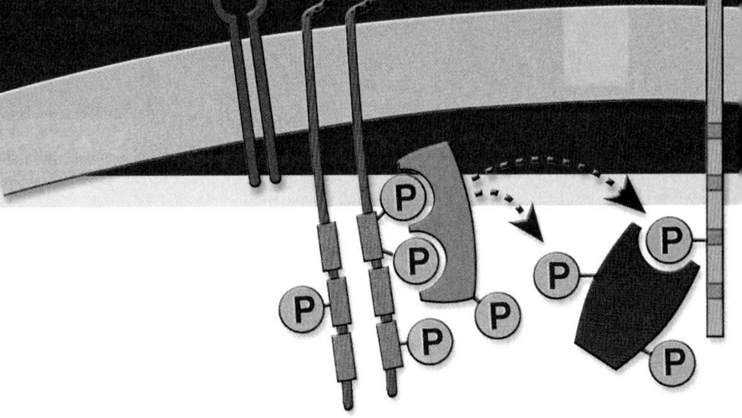

Activation of T Lymphocytes

The activation and effector phases of T cell–mediated adaptive immune responses are triggered by antigen recognition by T lymphocytes. In Chapter 5, we described the specificity of T cells for peptide fragments, derived from protein antigens, that are displayed bound to self major histocompatibility complex (MHC) molecules. In Chapter 6, we described the antigen receptors and accessory molecules of T cells that are involved in responses to antigens. In this chapter, we describe the biology and biochemistry of T cell activation by antigens and by additional signals provided by antigen-presenting cells (APCs). We start with a description of the biologic responses of T cells and proceed to a discussion of the biochemical mechanisms of T cell activation.

General Features of T Lymphocyte Activation

The expansion and differentiation of naive T cells and the effector functions of differentiated T cells are triggered by the binding of antigens to antigen receptors in combination with other stimuli. Different populations of T cells differ in their requirements for activation and in the patterns of their responses. We will summarize the general features of T cell activation before we discuss the individual responses and their functional importance.

- ***Naive T lymphocytes recognize antigens and are activated in peripheral lymphoid organs, resulting in the expansion of the antigen-specific lymphocyte pool and the differentiation of these cells into effector and memory lymphocytes*** (Fig. 8–1). Protein antigens that enter through epithelia and into the circulation are captured by "professional APCs," mainly dendritic cells, and transported to lymph nodes and spleen. Naive T cells continuously recirculate through lymph nodes. When a T cell of the correct specificity finds antigen, in the form of peptide-MHC complexes, that T cell is activated. Antigen-stimulated T cells proliferate and differentiate into effector and memory cells, some of which leave the lymphoid organs and enter the circulation.

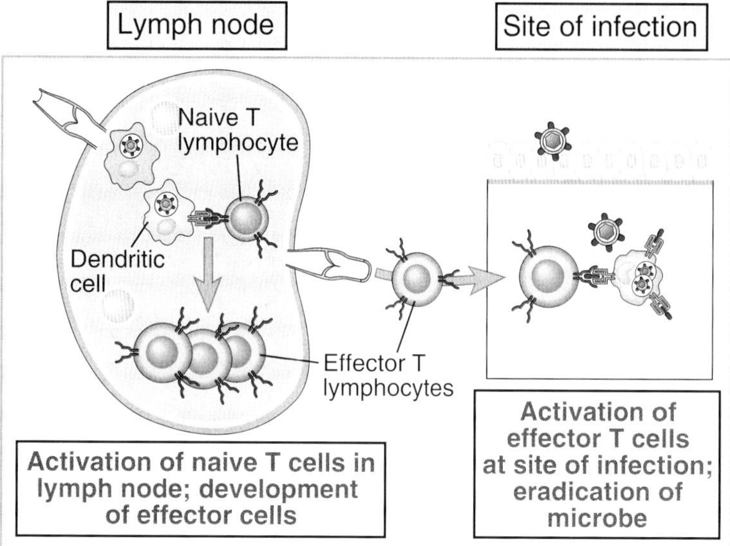

Figure 8–1 Activation of naive and effector T cells by antigen.

Antigens that are transported by dendritic cells to lymph nodes are recognized by naive T lymphocytes that recirculate through these lymph nodes. The T cells are activated to differentiate into effector and memory cells, which may remain in the lymphoid organs or migrate to nonlymphoid tissues. At sites of infection, the effector cells are again activated by antigens and perform their various functions, such as macrophage activation.

- ***Effector T cells recognize antigens in lymphoid organs or in peripheral nonlymphoid tissues and are activated to perform their effector functions*** (see Fig. 8–1). Effector T cells are able to migrate to any site of infection or inflammation. Here the cells again encounter the antigen for which they are specific and respond in ways that serve to eliminate the antigens. Effector T cells of the $CD4^+$ helper subset express membrane molecules and secrete cytokines that activate (help) macrophages to kill phagocytosed microbes and help B cells to differentiate into cells that secrete antibodies that bind to the antigens. $CD8^+$ cytolytic T lymphocytes (CTLs), the effector cells of the $CD8^+$ subset, kill infected cells and tumor cells that display class I MHC–associated antigens. We will return to the effector functions of T cells in Chapters 9 and 13. Memory T cells are an expanded population of T cells specific for antigen that can respond rapidly to subsequent encounter with the antigen and differentiate into effector cells that eliminate the antigen.

- ***The activation of T cells requires recognition of antigens displayed on APCs, costimulators ("second signals"), and cytokines produced by the APCs and by the T cells themselves.*** These stimuli work together to induce the sequential phases of T cell responses, namely, the initial activation, proliferation, and differentiation (Fig. 8–2). Recognition of peptide-MHC complexes by the T cell receptor (TCR) is the first signal for activation and provides specificity to the subsequent T cell response. The activation of the T cells is dependent on different accessory molecules that serve distinct functions (see Chapter 6). To reiterate the key points, the coreceptors CD4 and CD8 recognize class II and class I MHC molecules, respectively, and transduce activating signals to the T cells. The specificity of the coreceptors for different MHC molecules accounts for the fact that $CD4^+$ T cells are restricted to recognizing class II MHC–associated peptides (derived mainly from endocytosed proteins), and $CD8^+$ cells recognize class I MHC–associated peptides (derived from cytosolic, usually endogenously synthesized, proteins). Adhesion molecules on the T cells, primarily the integrins, stabilize the attachment of the T cells to APCs, thus ensuring that the T cells are engaged for long enough to trigger functional responses. T cell receptors for costimulators on APCs provide second signals for T cell activation; the nature and significance of these costimulatory signals are discussed later in the chapter. Cytokines drive the proliferation and differentiation of T cells and will also be discussed later and in Chapter 11.

- ***Naive T cells require activation by dendritic cells, whereas effector T cells can respond to antigens presented by a wider variety of APCs.*** Mature dendritic cells are the APCs that are most potent at activating naive T cells and initiating responses, for several reasons. Dendritic cells are strategically located to capture antigens and transport them to lymph nodes; this is why T cell responses are initiated in lymph nodes. Mature dendritic cells also express high levels of the MHC molecules that display peptides and high levels of the costimulators that provide second signals to naive T cells. Other APCs that activate T lymphocytes include macrophages and B cells, both of which are more efficient activators of differentiated effector and memory cells than of naive T cells. Thus, macrophages and B lymphocytes are important APCs in the effector phase of T cell responses. Both effector and memory T cells are less dependent on costimulators and require less antigen to be activated than do naive T cells. This is why effector and memory cells are able to react to antigens displayed by APCs other than dendritic cells in nonlymphoid organs. The nature of the APCs also influences the differentiation pathway of T cells and the choice between activation

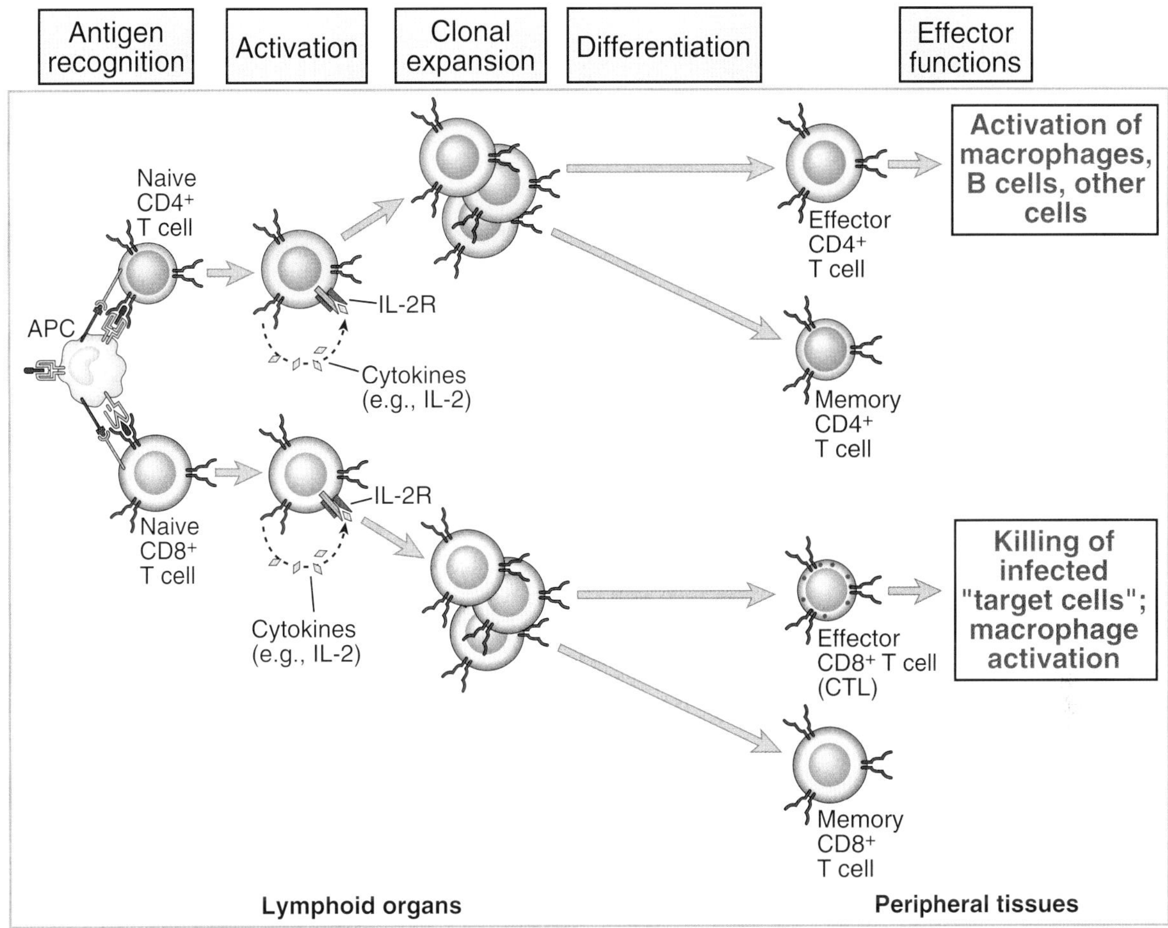

Figure 8–2 Phases of T cell responses.
Antigen recognition by T cells induces cytokine (e.g., IL-2) secretion, clonal expansion as a result of IL-2–induced autocrine cell proliferation, and differentiation of the T cells into effector cells or memory cells. In the effector phase of the response, the effector $CD4^+$ T cells respond to antigen by producing cytokines that have several actions, such as the activation of macrophages and B lymphocytes, and $CD8^+$ CTLs respond by killing other cells. APC, antigen-presenting cell; CTL, cytolytic T lymphocyte.

and tolerance. We will discuss these roles of APCs in later chapters.

Functional Responses of T Lymphocytes

The responses of T lymphocytes to antigen recognition, costimulation, and other signals consist of cytokine secretion, proliferation, and differentiation (see Fig. 8–2). Many methods have been used to analyze the activation of T cells *in vivo* and *in vitro,* and these techniques are providing a wealth of valuable information (Box 8–1). We describe the different functional responses of T cells here.

Secretion of Cytokines

Among the earliest detectable responses of T cells to antigen recognition is the secretion of proteins called cytokines. Cytokines are proteins secreted by many cells in the immune system, and they mediate many of the responses and functions of immune cells; we will discuss these proteins in more detail in Chapter 11.

In T cells, signals delivered by antigens and costimulators trigger the transcription of several cytokine genes and the synthesis of these proteins. The principal cytokine produced by naive T cells is interleukin (IL)-2, which functions as a growth factor for the T cells. Under different activation conditions, naive T cells that are stimulated by antigens may differentiate into subsets that secrete distinct sets of cytokines and perform different effector functions. The best defined of these subsets are the T_H1 and T_H2 populations of $CD4^+$ helper T cells (see Chapter 13). The cytokines produced by these differentiated effector $CD4^+$ T cells function to activate macrophages and B lymphocytes in the effector phases of cell-mediated and humoral immunity. On antigen stimulation, T cells also increase their expression of receptors for many cytokines.

BOX 8–1

Methods for Studying T Cell Activation

Our current knowledge of the cellular events in T cell activation is based on a variety of experimental techniques in which different populations of T cells are activated by defined stimuli and functional responses are measured. *In vitro* experiments have provided a great deal of information on the changes that occur in a T cell when it is stimulated by antigen. More recently, several techniques have been developed to study T cell proliferation, cytokine expression, and anatomic redistribution in response to antigen activation *in vivo.* The new experimental approaches have been particularly useful for the study of naive T cell activation and the localization of antigen-specific memory T cells after an immune response has waned.

POLYCLONAL ACTIVATION OF T CELLS ***Polyclonal activators*** of T cells bind to many or all TCR complexes regardless of specificity and activate the T cells in ways similar to peptide-MHC complexes on APCs. Polyclonal activators are mostly used *in vitro* to activate T cells isolated from human blood or the lymphoid tissues of experimental animals. Polyclonal activators can also be used to activate T cells with unknown antigen specificities, and they can evoke a detectable response from mixed populations of naive T cells, even though the frequency of cells specific for any one antigen would be too low to elicit a detectable response. The polymeric plant proteins called lectins, such as concanavalin-A (Con-A) and phytohemagglutinin (PHA), are one commonly used group of polyclonal T cell activator. Lectins bind specifically to certain sugar residues on T cell surface glycoproteins, including the TCR and CD3 proteins, and thereby stimulate the T cells. Antibodies specific for invariant framework epitopes on TCR or CD3 proteins also function as polyclonal activators of T cells. Often, these antibodies need to be immobilized on solid surfaces or beads or cross-linked with secondary anti-antibodies to induce optimal activation responses. Because soluble polyclonal activators do not provide costimulatory signals that are normally provided by APCs, they are often used together with stimulatory antibodies to receptors for costimulators, such as anti-CD28 or anti-CD2. Superantigens, another kind of polyclonal stimulus, bind to and activate all T cells that express particular types of TCR β chain (see Chapter 15, Box 15–1). T cells of any antigen specificity can also be stimulated with pharmacologic reagents, such as the combination of the phorbol ester PMA and the calcium ionophore ionomycin, that mimic signals generated by the TCR complex.

ANTIGEN-INDUCED ACTIVATION OF T CELLS ***Polyclonal populations*** of normal T cells that are enriched for T cells specific for a particular antigen can be derived from the blood and peripheral lymphoid organs of individuals after immunization with the antigen. The immunization serves to expand the number of antigen-specific T cells, which can then be restimulated *in vitro* by adding antigen and MHC-matched APCs to the T cells. This approach can be used to study antigen-induced activation of a mixed population of previously activated ("primed") T cells expressing many different TCRs, but the method does not permit analysis of responses of naive T cells.

Monoclonal populations of T cells, which express identical TCRs, have been useful for functional, biochemical, and molecular analyses. The limitation of these monoclonal populations is that they are maintained as long-term tissue culture lines and therefore may have phenotypically diverged from normal T cells *in vivo.* One type of monoclonal T cell population that is frequently used in experimental immunology is an antigen-specific T cell clone. Such clones are derived by isolating T cells from immunized individuals, as described for polyclonal T cells, followed by repetitive *in vitro* stimulation with the immunizing antigen plus MHC-matched APCs and cloning of single antigen-responsive cells in semisolid media or in liquid media by limiting dilution. Antigen-specific responses can easily be measured in these populations because all the cells in a cloned cell line have the same receptors and have been selected for growth in response to a known antigen-MHC complex. Both helper and CTL clones have been established from mice and humans. Other monoclonal T cell populations used in the study of T cell activation include antigen-specific T cell hybridomas, which are produced like B cell hybridomas (see Box 3–1, Chapter 3), and tumor lines derived from T cells have been established *in vitro* after removal of malignant T cells from animals or humans with T cell leukemias or lymphomas. Although some tumor-derived lines express functional TCR complexes, their antigen specificities are not known, and the cells are usually stimulated with polyclonal activators for experimental purposes. The Jurkat line, derived from a human T cell leukemia cell, is an example of a tumor line that is widely used as a model to study T cell signal transduction.

TCR transgenic mice are a source of homogeneous, phenotypically normal T cells with identical antigen specificities that are widely used for *in vitro* and *in vivo* experimental analyses. If the rearranged α and β chain genes of a single TCR of known specificity are expressed as a transgene in mice, a majority of the mature T cells in the mice will express that TCR. If the TCR transgene is crossed onto a RAG-1– or RAG-2–deficient background, no endogenous TCR gene expression occurs and 100% of the T cells will express only the transgenic TCR. TCR transgenic T cells can be activated *in vitro* or *in vivo* with a single peptide antigen, and they can be identified by antibodies specific for the transgenic TCR. One of the unique advantages of TCR transgenic mice is that they permit the isolation of sufficient numbers of naive T cells of defined specificity to allow one to study functional responses to the first exposure to antigen. This advantage has allowed investigators to study the *in vitro* conditions under which antigen activation of naive T cells leads to differentiation into functional subsets such as T_H1 and T_H2 cells (see Chapter 12). Naive T cells from TCR transgenic mice can also be injected into normal syngeneic recipient mice, where they home to lymphoid tissues. The recipient mouse is then exposed to the antigen for which the transgenic TCR is specific. By use of antibodies that label the TCR transgenic T cells, it is possible to follow their expansion and differentiation *in vivo* and to isolate them for analyzing recall (secondary) responses to antigen *ex vivo.*

METHODS TO ENUMERATE AND STUDY FUNCTIONAL RESPONSES OF ANTIGEN-SPECIFIC T CELLS *IN VIVO* ***Fluorescent dyes*** can be used to study prolifer-

Continued on following page

ation of T cells *in vivo*. T cells are first labeled with chemically reactive lipophilic fluorescent esters and then adoptively transferred into experimental animals. The dyes enter cells, form covalent bonds with cytoplasmic proteins, and then cannot leave the cells. One commonly used dye of this type is 5,6-carboxyfluorescein diacetate succinimidyl ester (CFSE), which can be detected in cells by standard flow cytometric techniques. Every time a T cell divides, its dye content is halved, and therefore it is possible to determine whether the adoptively transferred T cells present in lymphoid tissues of the recipient mouse have divided *in vivo* and to estimate the number of doublings each T cell has gone through.

Peptide-MHC tetramers are used to enumerate T cells with a single antigen specificity isolated from blood or lymphoid tissues of experimental animals or humans. These tetramers contain four of the peptide-MHC complexes that the T cell would normally recognize on the surface of APCs. The tetramer is made by producing a class I MHC molecule to which is attached a small molecule called biotin by use of recombinant DNA technology. Biotin binds with high affinity to a protein called avidin, and each avidin molecule binds four biotin molecules. Thus, avidin forms a substrate for assembling four biotin-conjugated MHC proteins. The MHC molecules can be loaded with a peptide of interest and thus stabilized, and the avidin molecule is labeled with a fluorochrome, such as FITC. This tetramer binds to T cells specific for the peptide-MHC complex with high enough avidity to label the T cells even in suspension. This method is the only feasible approach for identifying antigen-specific T cells in humans. For instance, it is possible to identify and enumerate circulating HLA-A2–restricted T cells specific for an HIV peptide by staining blood cells with a tetramer of HLA-A2 molecules loaded with the peptide. The same technique is being used to enumerate and isolate T cells specific for self antigens in normal individuals and in patients with autoimmune diseases. Peptide-MHC tetramers that bind to a particular transgenic TCR can also be used to quantify the transgenic T cells in different tissues after adoptive transfer and antigen stimulation. The technique is now widely used with class I MHC molecules; in class I molecules, only one polypeptide is polymorphic, and stable molecules can be produced *in vitro*. This has proved to be much more difficult for class II molecules, in which both chains are polymorphic and required for proper assembly. The use of peptide-MHC tetramers to analyze the expansion of $CD8^+$ T cells is mentioned in the text.

Cytokine secretion assays can be used to quantify cytokine-secreting effector T cells within lymphoid tissues. The most commonly used methods are cytoplasmic staining of cytokines and single-cell enzyme-linked immunosorbent assays (ELISPOT). In these types of studies, antigen-induced activation and differentiation of T cells take place *in vivo*, and then T cells are isolated and tested for cytokine expression *in vitro*. Cytoplasmic staining of cytokines requires permeabilizing the cells so that fluorochrome-labeled antibodies specific for a particular cytokine can gain entry into the cell, and the stained cells are analyzed by flow cytometry. Cytokine expression by T cells specific for a particular antigen can be determined by additionally staining T cells with peptide-MHC tetramers or, in the case of TCR-transgenic T cells, antibodies specific for the transgenic TCR. By use of a combination of CFSE and anticytokine antibodies, it is possible to examine the relationship between cell division and cytokine expression. In the ELISPOT assay, T cells freshly isolated from blood or lymphoid tissues are cultured in plastic wells coated with antibody specific for a particular cytokine. As cytokines are secreted from individual T cells, they bind to the antibodies in discrete spots corresponding to the location of individual T cells. The spots are visualized by adding secondary enzyme-linked anti-immunoglobulin, as in a standard ELISA (see Appendix III), and the number of spots is counted to determine the number of cytokine-secreting T cells.

Activated T cells are often identified by the expression of newly synthesized surface proteins, called activation markers, that are synthesized concomitantly with cytokines. One such activation marker is the α chain of the IL-2 receptor (also called CD25, see Chapter 11).

Proliferation

T cell proliferation in response to antigen recognition is mediated primarily by an autocrine growth pathway, in which the responding T cell secretes its own growth-promoting cytokines and also expresses cell surface receptors for these cytokines. The principal autocrine growth factor for most T cells is IL-2. Both the production of IL-2 and the expression of high-affinity receptors for IL-2 require antigen recognition by specific T cells. Therefore, the cells that recognize antigen bind the IL-2 they secrete and thus proliferate in response to this cytokine. IL-2 is not the only growth factor for T cells. A cytokine called IL-15, which is similar to IL-2 but produced mainly by APCs and other nonlymphoid cells, stimulates the proliferation of $CD8^+$ T cells, especially memory cells of the $CD8^+$ subset. The result of the proliferation of naive T cells is clonal expansion, which generates from a small pool of naive antigen-specific lymphocytes the large number of cells required to eliminate the antigen. Before antigen exposure, the frequency of naive T cells specific for any antigen is 1 in 10^5 to 10^6 lymphocytes. After antigen exposure, the numbers of T cells specific for that antigen may increase to about 1 in 10 for $CD8^+$ cells and 1 in 100 to 1000 for $CD4^+$ cells. These numbers rapidly decline as the antigen is eliminated, and after the immune response subsides, the surviving memory cells specific for the antigen number on the order of 1 in 10^4.

Studies in mice have revealed an unexpectedly large expansion of $CD8^+$ T cells during the acute phase of infections with intracellular microbes. In one such study, T cells specific for a dominant epitope of the lymphocytic choriomeningitis virus (LCMV) were identified by staining cell populations with a fluorescent tetramer of an appropriate MHC molecule loaded with the viral peptide (see Box 8–1). It was estimated that the frequency of LCMV-specific T cells in uninfected mice is about 1 in 10^5 $CD8^+$ cells. After infection with the virus, at the peak of the immune response, there was a twofold to threefold expansion in the total number of $CD8^+$ T cells in the spleen, and as many as one in five of these cells was specific for the viral peptide. In other words, in this infection, there was a greater than 50,000-fold expansion of antigen-specific $CD8^+$ T cells, and remarkably, this occurred within 1 week after infection. Equally remarkable was the finding that during this massive antigen-specific clonal expansion, "bystander" T cells not specific for the virus did not proliferate. The expansion of T cells specific for Epstein-Barr virus and human immunodeficiency virus (HIV) in acutely infected humans is also on this order of magnitude. Although it has been more difficult to quantitate the antigen-stimulated expansion of $CD4^+$ cells, it appears to be much less than the clonal expansion of $CD8^+$ cells. This may be expected because $CD8^+$ CTLs perform their effector functions by directly attacking infected cells, whereas a single $CD4^+$ helper cell may secrete cytokines that activate many effector cells such as macrophages, and therefore a greater number of CTLs may be needed for protective immunity.

The kinetics of T cell expansion have been determined by injecting T cells expressing a transgenic TCR specific for a known antigen into mice that produce the antigen and then identifying the specific T cells and measuring their responses. From such studies, it is estimated that T cells begin to divide within 18 hours after encountering antigen, and their doubling time is about 6 hours. This rapid proliferative capacity presumably accounts for the enormous expansion of T cells mentioned before.

Differentiation into Effector Cells

On antigen stimulation, some of the progeny of the proliferating T cells differentiate into effector cells that eliminate antigens and may activate other immune cells. This process depends both on antigen-induced activation of the T cells and on other stimuli, principally costimulators and cytokines produced at the site of antigen recognition. The progeny of antigen-stimulated $CD4^+$ T lymphocytes differentiate into effector cells whose function is to activate phagocytes and B lymphocytes. Effector $CD4^+$ cells consist of subsets that produce distinct sets of cytokines and perform different functions, such as T_H1 and T_H2 subsets (see Chapter 13). $CD8^+$ T cells differentiate into functional CTLs, with the ability to kill target cells that express the peptide-MHC complexes these T cells recognize (see Chapter 13). The differentiation of T cells is associated with the transcriptional activation of genes encoding effector molecules. Some of these effector molecules, such as cytokines and CTL granule proteins, are released from the T cell, and others, such as CD40 ligand (CD40L) and Fas ligand, are cell surface molecules that are involved in effector functions.

Differentiation into Memory Cells

Some of the progeny of antigen-stimulated T cells develop into long-lived, functionally quiescent memory cells. Although the responses of T cells to antigen stimulation last for only days or a few weeks, memory T cells survive for long periods even after the antigen is eliminated. The memory T cell population is responsible for enhanced and accelerated secondary immune responses on subsequent exposures to the same antigen. The mechanisms of memory cell generation and survival are not known. It is not even clear if memory T cells develop from differentiated effector cells or if effector and memory cells are divergent populations arising from antigen-stimulated lymphocytes. The mechanisms that determine whether the progeny of antigen-stimulated T cells will differentiate into functionally active, short-lived effector cells or functionally quiescent, long-lived memory cells are not known. The survival of memory cells does not require antigen recognition (see Chapter 2). As mentioned, the cytokine IL-15 appears to be important in maintaining the pool of memory $CD8^+$ cells, but no comparable stimulus for $CD4^+$ memory cells has been identified. Memory cells accumulate with age, having been generated by encounters with environmental microbes and other antigens. For instance, in human neonates, virtually all blood T cells are naive, whereas in the adult human, half or more of T cells appear to be memory cells. Memory cells also tend to accumulate in particular tissues, notably the mucosal immune system.

Several surface markers have been used to distinguish memory cells from naive and recently activated effector T cells (see Chapter 2). Memory T cells, like effector T cells, express high levels of some surface molecules, notably integrins and CD44, that promote their migration to peripheral sites of infection and inflammation and their retention at these sites. This property enables memory cells to rapidly locate and eliminate antigen at any site of infection or inflammation. However, memory cells do not express activation markers, such as the α chain of the IL-2 receptor, which is consistent with the fact that these cells are functionally quiescent and are neither proliferating rapidly nor performing effector functions until they are induced to do so on re-exposure to the antigen.

Memory T cells appear to be heterogeneous in their migration and functional capabilities. In humans, memory T cells consist of subsets that differ in the expression of the chemokine receptor CCR7. (Recall that CCR7 is the chemokine receptor that is also responsible for the migration of naive T cells and dendritic cells into the T cell zones of lymphoid organs; see Chapter 2.) It is believed that CCR7-high memory cells preferentially migrate to lymph nodes and proliferate rapidly on repeated encounter with antigen, providing a large pool of T cells in secondary immune responses. CCR7-low memory cells produce effector cytokines, and they may migrate preferentially to peripheral sites of infection and inflammation, where they function to eliminate antigens.

Decline of T Cell Responses

T cell responses decline after the antigen is eliminated by effector cells. This decline is important for returning the immune system to a state of rest, or homeostasis. T cell responses decline mainly because the majority of antigen-activated T cells die by apoptosis. The reason for this is that as the antigen is eliminated, lymphocytes are deprived of survival stimuli that are normally provided by the antigen and by the costimulators and cytokines produced during inflammatory reactions to the antigen. It is estimated that in the example of the viral infection mentioned earlier, more than 95% of the virus-specific $CD8^+$ T cells that arise by clonal expansion die by apoptosis as the infection is cleared. We will return to the mechanisms of homeostasis in the immune system in Chapter 10.

Role of Costimulators in T Cell Activation

The proliferation and differentiation of T cells require signals provided by molecules on APCs, called costimulators, in addition to antigen-induced signals (Fig. 8–3). In Chapter 1, we introduced the concept that naive lymphocytes, both T cells and B cells, require two distinct sets of extracellular signals to induce their proliferation and differentiation into effector cells. The first signal is provided by antigen binding to antigen receptors. In the case of T cells, binding of peptide-MHC complexes to the TCR (and to the CD4 or CD8 coreceptor) provides signal 1. The second signal for T cell activation is provided by molecules on APCs, which are called **costimulators** because they function together with antigen to stimulate T cells. In the absence of costimulation, T cells that encounter antigens either fail to respond and die by apoptosis or enter a state of unresponsiveness called anergy (see Chapter 10).

The best characterized costimulatory pathway in T cell activation involves the T cell surface molecule CD28, which binds the costimulatory molecules B7-1 (CD80) and B7-2 (CD86) expressed on activated APCs (Box 8–2). CD28 delivers signals that enhance many T cell responses to antigen, including cell survival, production of cytokines such as IL-2, and differentiation of naive T cells into effector and memory cells. The structure and expression of CD28 were described in Chapter 6. B7-1 and B7-2 are structurally similar single-chain glycoproteins, each with two extracellular Ig-like domains, a transmembrane segment, and a cytoplasmic tail. The B7 molecules are expressed mainly on APCs, including dendritic cells, macrophages, and B lymphocytes. They are absent or expressed at low levels on resting APCs and are induced by various stimuli (discussed later).

The essential role of the B7 costimulators in T cell activation has been established by several types of experiments.

- *In vitro*, purified populations of $CD4^+$ T cells respond to antigen by cytokine secretion and proliferation when the antigen is presented by APCs that express B7 molecules but not when the antigen is presented by APCs that lack B7 expression. An activating antibody that binds to CD28 can provide an artificial costimulatory signal and induce T cell responses even if the APCs lack B7 molecules (Fig. 8–4).
- If a pure population of $CD4^+$ T cells is cultured with agents that cross-link the TCR, such as anti-CD3 antibodies, the T cells produce very little cytokine and do not proliferate. Again, if an additional costimulatory signal is provided by antibodies that bind to CD28, the T cells are able to respond (see Fig. 8–4). The costimulatory signal provided by anti-CD28 antibody in the absence of the TCR signal does not by itself induce T cell responses.
- Knockout mice lacking B7-1 and B7-2 are deficient in T cell–dependent responses to immunization with protein antigens.

The expression of costimulators is regulated and ensures that T lymphocyte responses are initiated at the correct time and place. The expression of B7 costimulators is increased by microbial products, such as

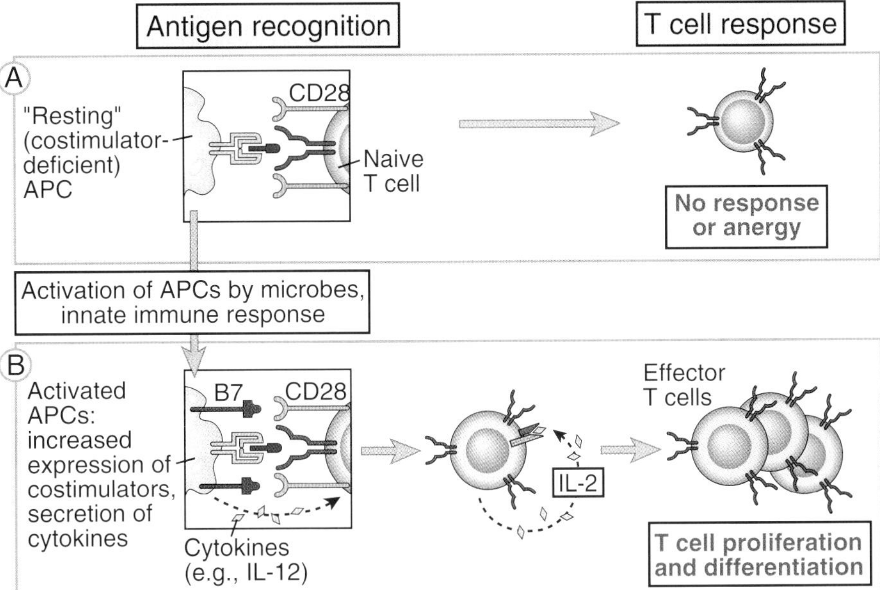

Figure 8–3 Functions of costimulators in T cell activation. The resting antigen-presenting cell (APC) expresses few or no costimulators and fails to activate naive T cells (A). (Sometimes antigen recognition without costimulation may make the T cells anergic; this phenomenon will be discussed in Chapter 10.) Microbes and cytokines produced during innate immune responses activate the APCs to express costimulators, such as B7 molecules (B). The APCs then become capable of activating naive T cells. Activated APCs also produce cytokines such as IL-12, which stimulate the differentiation of naive T cells into effector cells.

BOX 8–2

The B7 and CD28 Families of Costimulators and Receptors

The best defined costimulators for T lymphocytes are the B7 family of molecules on APCs that bind to members of the CD28 family of receptors on T cells. The first proteins to be discovered in these families were CD28 and B7-1. The existence and functions of B7-1 and CD28 were originally surmised from experiments with monoclonal antibodies specific for these molecules. The cloning of the genes encoding B7-1 and CD28 opened the way for a variety of experiments in mice that have clarified the role of these molecules and led to the identification of additional homologous proteins involved in T cell costimulation. For example, residual costimulatory activity of APCs from B7-1 knockout mice suggested the existence of additional costimulatory molecules, and homology-based cloning strategies led to the identification of the B7-2 molecule. B7-1 and B7-2 both bind to CD28 and together account for the majority of costimulatory activity provided by APCs for the activation of naive T cells. This is evident from the phenotype of B7-1/B7-2 double knockout mice, which have profound defects in adaptive immune responses to protein antigens.

Although costimulatory pathways were discovered as mediators of T cell activation, it is now clear that homologous molecules are involved in inhibiting T cell responses. The first and best defined example of an inhibitory receptor on T cells is CTLA-4, a member of the CD28 family, which was discovered and characterized by the use of monoclonal antibodies. The name CTLA-4 is based on the fact that this molecule was the fourth receptor identified in a search for molecules expressed in CTLs, but its expression and function are not restricted to CTLs. CTLA-4 is structurally homologous to CD28 and is a receptor for both B7-1 and B7-2. Unlike CD28, CTLA-4 serves as a negative regulator of T cell activation. CTLA-4 knockout mice show excessive T cell activation, proliferation, and systemic autoimmunity.

Several other proteins structurally related to B7-1 and B7-2 or to CD28 and CTLA-4 have recently been identified by homology-based cloning strategies, and their functions are now being studied. These proteins can be considered members of the B7 and CD28 families, respectively. The two recently discovered members of the family that are described here were identified first by the cloning of the receptors on T cells, and these receptors were called ICOS (inducible costimulator) and PD-1 (programmed death-1, because this molecule was thought to regulate programmed cell death of T cells). An emerging picture of T cell costimulation includes the actions of several costimulatory signals and negative regulatory signals, involving multiple members of the B7 and CD28 families whose actions are regulated with respect to location and timing of expression.

Members of the B7 family include B7-1, B7-2, ICOS-ligand (L), and PD-L1 and PD-L2 (see Figure). All these proteins are transmembrane proteins consisting of two extracellular Ig-like domains, including an N-terminal V-like domain and a membrane proximal C-like domain. Another member of the family, B7-H3, may be expressed in alternative forms, with either one pair of V and C domains like the other B7 family members or two tandem pairs of V and C domains. The main function of these molecules is to bind to CD28 family receptors on T cells, thereby stimulating signal transduction pathways in the T cells. There is no compelling evidence that the cytoplasmic tails of the B7 family members transduce activating signals in the cells on which they are expressed. B7-1 and B7-2 are mainly expressed on APCs, including dendritic cells, macrophages, and B cells. Although there is some constitutive expression on dendritic cells, expression of both molecules is strongly induced by various signals including endotoxin, inflammatory cytokines (e.g., IL-12, IFN-γ), and CD40–CD40 ligand interactions. The temporal patterns of expression of B7-1 and B7-2 differ; B7-2 is expressed constitutively at low levels and induced early after activation of APCs, whereas B7-1 is not expressed constitutively and is induced hours or days later. The other members of the B7 family, ICOS ligand and PD-L1 and PD-L2, are also expressed on APCs, but in addition, there is significant expression on a variety of nonlymphoid tissues. PD-L1 and PD-L2, for example, are expressed on endothelial cells and cardiac myocytes. The nonlymphoid expression of these molecules suggests they play a role in regulating T cell activation in peripheral tissues and perhaps in the maintenance of self-tolerance.

The CD28 family of receptors are all expressed on T cells, but PD-1 is also expressed on B cells and myeloid cells. These receptors are transmembrane proteins, all of which include a single Ig V-like domain and a cytoplasmic tail with tyrosine residues. CD28, CTLA-4, and ICOS exist as disulfide-linked homodimers; PD-1 is expressed as a monomer. Both CD28 and CTLA-4 bind both B7-1 and B7-2, with different affinities, and share a sequence motif, MYPPPY, in the V domain, which is essential for B7 binding. ICOS has an FDPPPF motif in the corresponding position, which mediates binding to ICOS-ligand but not to B7-1 or B7-2. PD-1 has neither motif and binds to PD-L1 or PD-L2 but not to B7-1, B7-2, or ICOS-ligand. The cytoplasmic tails of the CD28 family molecules contain structural motifs that mediate interaction with signaling molecules, although the signal pathways that are engaged are incompetently understood. Tyrosine residues in the tails of CD28 become phosphorylated on B7-1 or B7-2 binding, and they serve as docking sites for PI-3 kinase and Grb-2. PI-3 kinase activation is linked to the activation of the serine/threonine kinase Akt. PI-3 kinase binding and activation also occur on the cytoplasmic tail of CTLA-4, and perhaps ICOS. Consistent with their roles in negative regulation of cellular activation, both CTLA-4 and PD-1 have variations of the immunoreceptor tyrosine inhibitory motifs (ITIMs) in their cytoplasmic tails (see Box 8–3) and recruit the tyrosine phosphatase SHP-2. CD28 is constitutively expressed on $CD4^+$ and $CD8^+$ T cells. ICOS is expressed on $CD4^+$ and $CD8^+$ T cells only after TCR binding to antigen, and its induction is enhanced by CD28 signals.

X-ray crystallographic analyses of B7-1 and B7-2 interactions with CTLA-4 suggest that these molecules form a repeating lattice structure in the immunological synapse. B7-1 or B7-2 may dimerize in the APC membrane, and each monomeric subunit would bind to one chain of a different CTLA-4 dimer. This arrangement would enhance the local concentration of the ligands and receptors and

Continued on following page

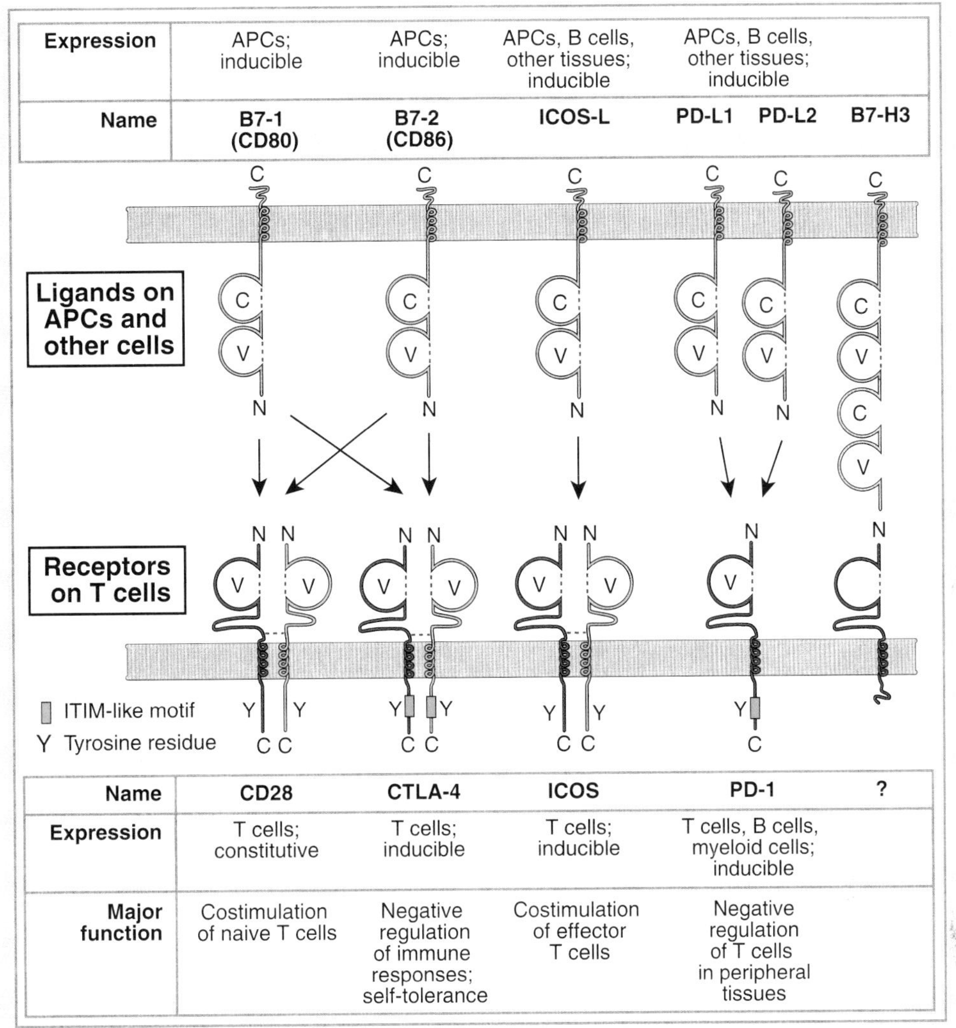

presumably enhance signaling. It is not known if such an arrangement also applies to other B7:CD28 family ligand-receptor interactions.

The functional consequences of signaling by CD28 family members differ for each molecule. CD28 signaling promotes T cell IL-2 production and clonal expansion of naive T cells and increased BCL-X_L expression resulting in enhanced T cell survival. As a built-in positive amplification mechanism, CD28 signals also up-regulate CD40 ligand expression, which leads to CD40 signaling in APCs, which in turn up-regulates the expression of the CD28 ligands B7-1 and B7-2. In contrast, ICOS signaling promotes expression of effector cytokines such as IL-10 and IL-4, but not of the T cell growth factor IL-2. It appears that ICOS is more important for costimulation of effector T cell responses, particularly T_H2 responses, than for clonal expansion of antigen-stimulated T cells. It is not known whether CTLA-4 and PD-1 play distinct or overlapping roles in inhibiting immune responses. The CTLA-4 knockout mouse develops severe enlargement of lymphoid organs and infiltration of many tissues by activated lymphocytes, whereas the PD-1 knockout develops an unusual dilated cardiomyopathy thought to be antibody mediated. These findings suggest that CTLA-4 and PD-1 do indeed inhibit different types of immune responses.

endotoxin, and by cytokines such as interferon (IFN)-γ produced during innate immune reactions to microbes. The induction of costimulators by microbes and by the cytokines of innate immunity promotes T cell responses to microbial antigens (see Chapter 12). In addition, when T cells are activated, they express a molecule called CD40 ligand (CD40L), which binds to CD40 expressed on APCs and delivers signals that enhance the expression of B7 costimulators on the APCs. In B lymphocytes, engagement of the antigen receptor stimulates B7 expression, so that B cells that encounter antigen are able to activate and be helped by $CD4^+$ helper T cells. Of all potential APCs, mature dendritic cells express the highest levels of costimulators and, as a result, are the most potent stimulators of naive T cells (which are completely dependent on costimulation for

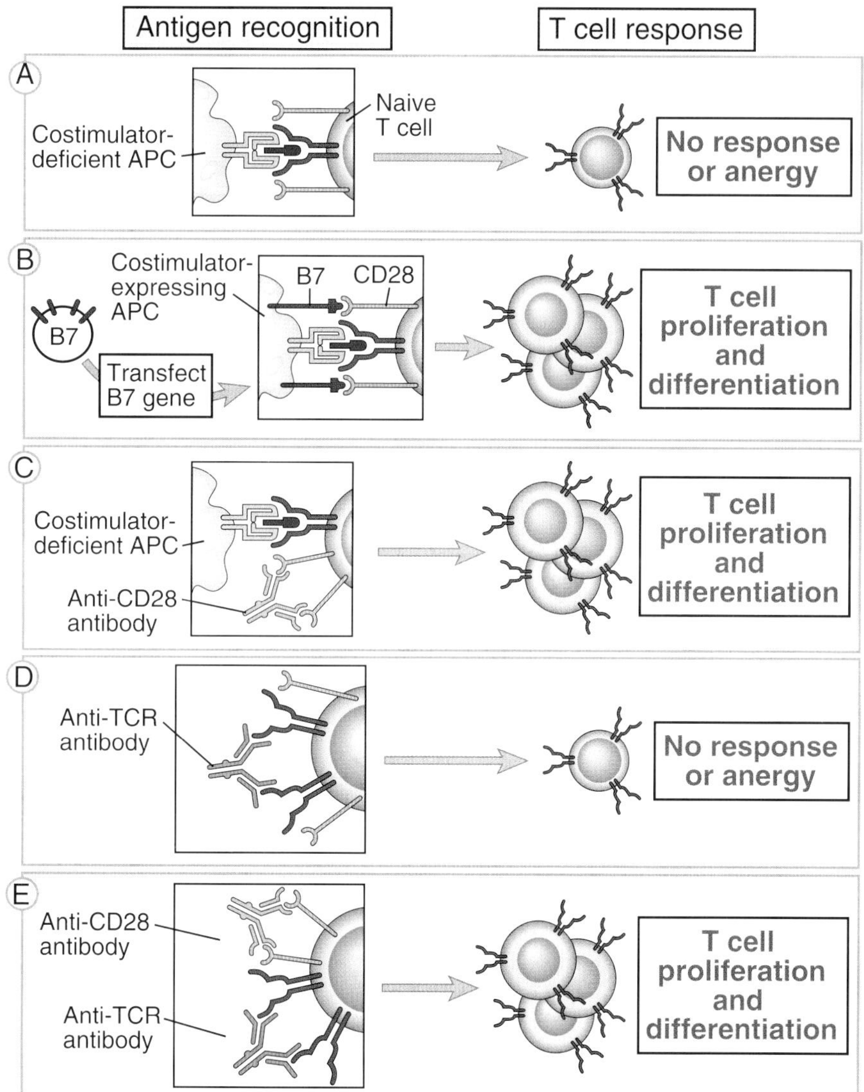

Figure 8–4 Role of B7 and CD28 in T cell activation.

A costimulator-deficient antigen-presenting cell (APC) does not stimulate responses of CD4$^+$ T cells or may induce T cell anergy (A). The expression of B7 molecules in the APCs by gene transfection (B) or the provision of a costimulatory signal with an anti-CD28 antibody (C) leads to T cell activation. Similarly, cross-linking of the TCR complex with an antibody specific for the TCR/CD3 complex does not activate the T cells (D), but the addition of an activating anti-CD28 antibody elicits T cell responses (E). Such experiments show that the B7:CD28 pathway is a costimulatory pathway for naive T cells.

activation). In Chapter 5, we mentioned the essential role of **adjuvants** in inducing primary T cell responses to protein antigens such as vaccines. Many adjuvants are products of microbes, or mimic microbes, and one of their major functions in T cell activation is to stimulate the expression of costimulators on APCs. The absence of costimulators on unactivated, or "resting," APCs in normal tissues contributes to the maintenance of tolerance to self antigens. Because such tissue APCs are capable of presenting self antigens to T cells, the lack of costimulator expression ensures that potentially self-reactive T cells are not activated and may be rendered anergic (see Chapter 10).

Previously activated effector and memory T cells are less dependent on costimulation by the B7:CD28 pathway than are naive cells. This property of effector and memory cells enables them to respond to antigens presented by various APCs that may reside in nonlymphoid tissues and may express no or low levels of B7. For instance, the differentiation of CD8$^+$ T cells into effector CTLs requires costimulation, but effector CTLs can kill other cells that do not express costimulators (see Chapter 13).

The biochemical mechanism by which CD28:B7 interactions promote T cell activation is incompletely understood. CD28-mediated signals increase the production of cytokines, especially the T cell autocrine growth factor IL-2. This may occur by a combination of enhanced transcription and stabilization of IL-2 messenger RNA. In addition, CD28 signals promote the survival of T cells, in part by increasing expression of the anti-apoptotic protein Bcl-x (see Chapter 10, Box 10–2). We will describe signaling responses to costimulators later in the chapter, after we discuss the biochemistry of T cell activation.

The CD28:B7 pathway of costimulation is the prototype of a much larger family of receptors and ligands that both stimulate and inhibit T cells (see Box 8–2). A protein called ICOS (inducible costimulator) is homologous to CD28 and is so named because it is induced on T cells after activation. The ligand for ICOS is homologous to B7-1 and B7-2. ICOS appears to be particularly important for stimulating the production of certain cytokines, notably IL-10, and for the activation of previously differentiated effector T cells. A protein called CTLA-4 (CD152) is also homologous to CD28, binds to B7-1 and B7-2, and is expressed on activated T cells. Unlike CD28, CTLA-4 functions to terminate T cell responses and plays a role in self-tolerance (Chapter 10).

The interaction of CD40L on T cells with CD40 on APCs enhances T cell activation. The likely mechanism of this effect is that the engagement of CD40 on the APCs activates the APCs to increase their expression of B7 molecules and to secrete cytokines such as IL-12 that promote T cell differentiation (Fig. 8–5). Thus, the CD40 pathway indirectly amplifies T cell responses and probably does not function as a costimulatory pathway by itself. On the basis of many experimental studies of costimulators, antagonists against B7 molecules and CD40L are in clinical trials to prevent the rejection of organ allografts and other pathologic immune responses. Many other T cell surface molecules, including CD2 and integrins, have been shown to deliver costimulatory signals *in vitro*, but their physiologic role in mice and humans is unclear.

Signal Transduction by the TCR Complex

The goal of T cell signaling pathways is to coordinately activate the transcription of genes that are silent in naive cells and whose products mediate the responses and functions of activated T cells. The recognition of antigen by the TCR initiates a sequence of biochemical signals in T cells that result in transcriptional activation of particular genes and the entry of the cells into the cell cycle. The genes that are expressed in T cells after antigen recognition encode many of the proteins that mediate the biologic responses of these cells (Fig. 8–6). The signaling cascades triggered by the TCR have been defined largely by *in vitro* analyses of various T cell populations that can be activated by the engagement of their antigen receptors (see Box 8–1). From such studies, several important general features of T cell signal transduction are now well established.

- ***Signal transduction by the TCR is triggered by ligation of multiple antigen receptors and coreceptors.*** The outcome of T cell antigen recognition is determined by the duration and affinity of the TCR-antigen interaction. The affinity of most TCRs for peptide-MHC complexes is low, with dissociation constants (K_d values) on the order of 10^{-5} to 10^{-7} M, which is much lower than the affinity of most antibodies for antigens (see Chapter 3, Table 3–1). The off-rate of the TCR-antigen interaction is rapid, and it is estimated that a single TCR engages an MHC-associated peptide for less than 10 seconds. Furthermore, on any APC, fewer than 1000 of the ~10^5 available MHC molecules are likely to be displaying any one peptide at any time. Therefore, one APC can engage a small fraction of the 10^4 to 10^5 antigen receptors on a single T cell. For all these reasons, the antigen receptors of a T cell are likely to bind to antigen-bearing APCs weakly and briefly. Activation of an individual T cell may require multiple sequential engagements of that cell's antigen receptors by peptide-MHC complexes on APCs. Thus, the T cell behaves like a signal integrator, adding up the number of times that TCR molecules bind to peptide-MHC complexes and the duration of each encounter. Full activation of the T cell, resulting in all the possible biologic responses, occurs when the TCR-induced signals reach a critical threshold. (There is, as yet, no accurate quantitative estimate of this threshold.) Incomplete signaling may result in no response; in partial activation, in which some but not all responses ensue; or even in functional inacti-

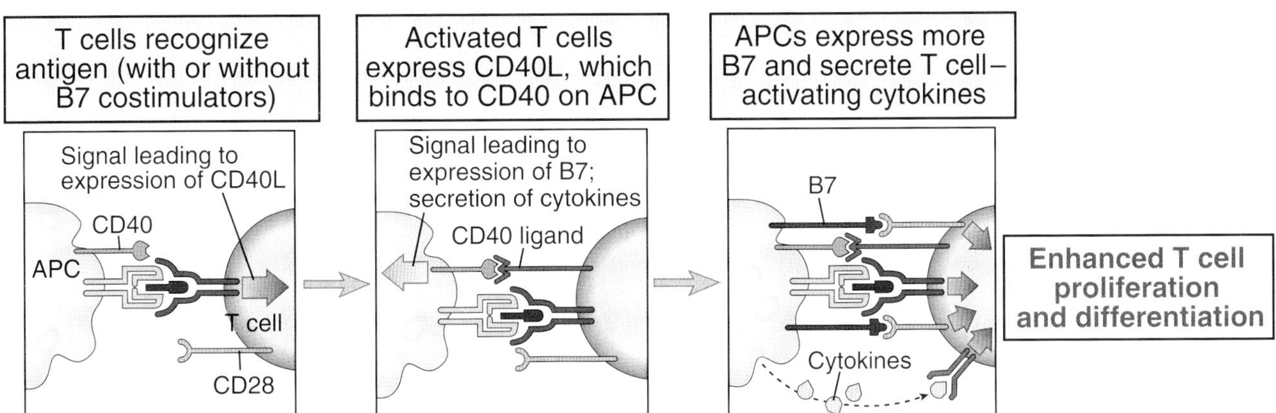

Figure 8–5 Role of CD40 in T cell activation.
Antigen recognition by T cells induces the expression of CD40 ligand (CD40L). CD40L engages CD40 on the antigen-presenting cell (APC) and stimulates the expression of B7 molecules and the secretion of cytokines that activate T cells. Thus, CD40L on the T cells makes the APCs "better" APCs. T cells can express CD40L on antigen recognition even without costimulation, but sustained expression of CD40L requires B7:CD28 costimulation as well as antigen. Thus, the B7 and CD40 pathways stimulate each other.

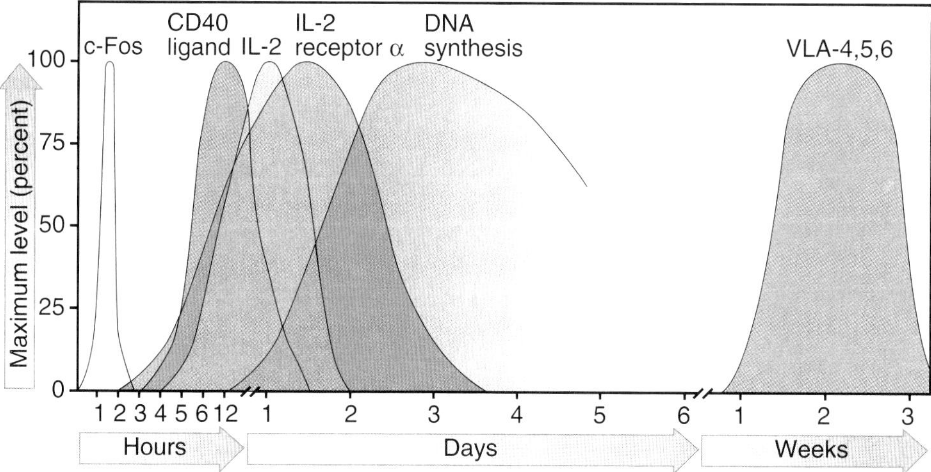

Figure 8–6 Kinetics of gene expression in antigen-stimulated T lymphocytes. T lymphocytes activated by antigens and costimulators express new genes. The approximate time course of the expression of selected genes is shown; the actual kinetics may vary in different T cell populations exposed to different stimuli.

vation of the T cells. At the end of the chapter, we will return to a discussion of how altered versions of a peptide antigen may elicit these distinct responses.

- ***The early biochemical response to antigen recognition consists of clustering of membrane receptors, tyrosine phosphorylation of several proteins, and recruitment and activation of adapter proteins*** (Fig. 8–7). The TCR does not have intrinsic enzymatic activity, but it is associated with other proteins that bind enzymes and adapter molecules that form a scaffold for the assembly of signaling intermediates. These events occur within seconds after the engagement of antigen receptors, and they result in the assembly of signaling complexes in the plasma membrane, at the site of receptor clustering. The subsequent events in signal transduction are generated from the membrane-associated complexes of receptors and adapter proteins.
- ***Signals from the antigen receptor coordinately activate a number of important biochemical pathways, the main ones being the Ras–MAP kinase pathway, the protein kinase C pathway, and the calcium-calcineurin pathway*** (see Fig. 8–7). Activation of these enzymes occurs in minutes after antigen recognition. The enzymes activated by each of these pathways induce transcription factors that stimulate the expression of various genes in the T cells, a process that takes several hours.

In the following sections, we describe the major steps in signaling by the TCR, starting with the earliest responses at the plasma membrane and culminating in the transcriptional activation of many T cell–specific genes.

Early Membrane Events: Formation of the Immunological Synapse and Recruitment and Activation of Protein Tyrosine Kinases and Adapter Proteins

The earliest events that occur after antigen recognition are designed to bring together many of the molecules that are involved in signal transduction in T cells.

Formation of the Immunological Synapse

When the TCR complex recognizes MHC-associated peptides on an APC, several T cell surface proteins and intracellular signaling molecules are rapidly mobilized to the site of T cell–APC contact (Fig. 8–8). This region of physical contact between the T cell and the APC has been called the **immunological synapse** (or the supramolecular activation cluster). The T cell molecules that are rapidly mobilized to the center of the synapse include the TCR complex (the TCR, CD3, and ζ chains), CD4 or CD8 coreceptors, receptors for costimulators (such as CD28), and enzymes and adapter proteins that associate with the cytoplasmic tails of the transmembrane receptors. Integrins remain at the periphery of the synapse, where they function to stabilize the binding of the T cell to the APC. Many signaling molecules found in synapses are localized to regions of the plasma membrane that have a lipid content different from the rest of the cell membrane and are called lipid rafts or glycolipid-enriched microdomains. The regulated movement of membrane molecules into the synapse is triggered by antigen recognition and involves signaling pathways that activate proteins of the cytoskeleton. The formation of the synapse brings signaling molecules into proximity to one another and to the receptors that activate these molecules. These molecules initiate and amplify TCR-induced signals. However, some signals may be triggered by antigen recognition before the formation of the synapse and may even be required for membrane molecules to move into the synapse. In addition, the formation of the synapse ensures that the molecules that T cells use to communicate with APCs are brought close to the target molecules on the APCs. For instance, as we shall see in Chapter 9, T cells activate B lymphocytes by using CD40L to interact with CD40, and this ligand:receptor pair is concentrated in the synapse after antigen recognition, with CD40L on the T cell side and CD40 on the B cell.

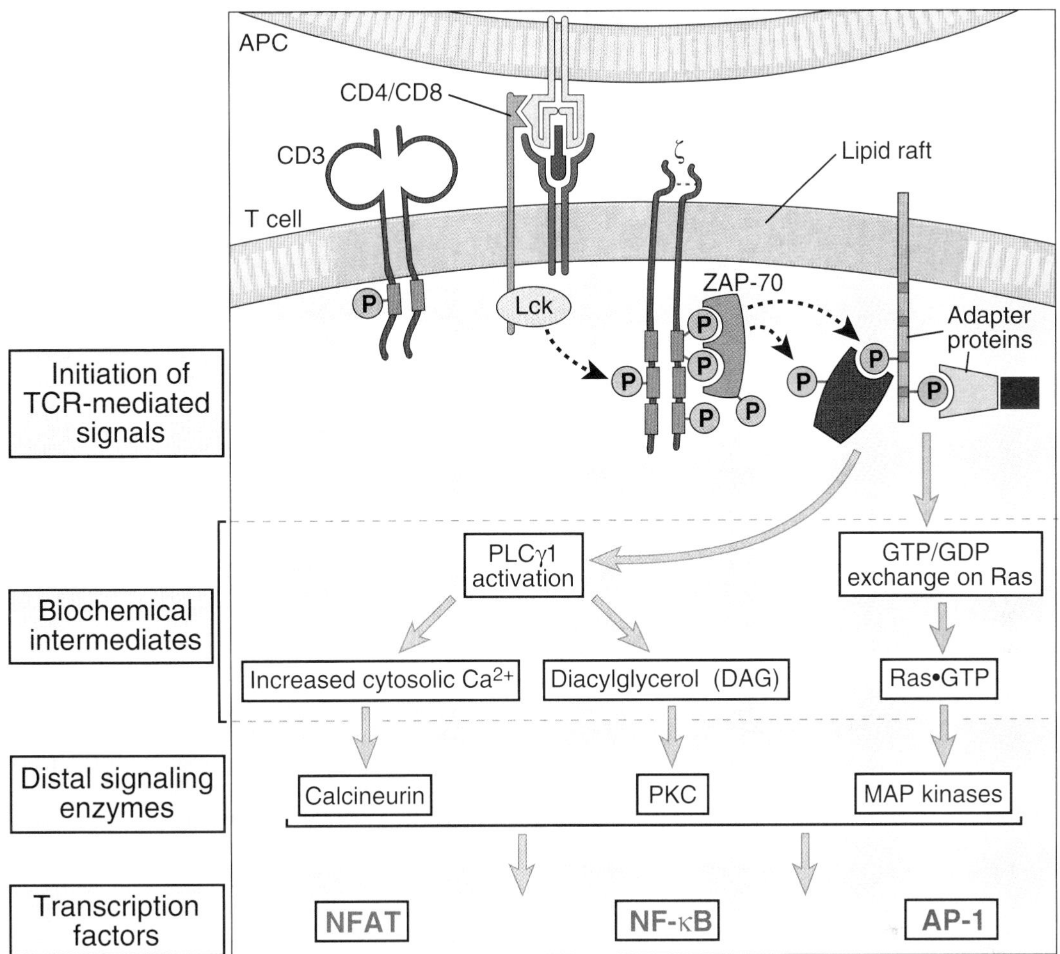

Figure 8–7 Intracellular signaling events during T cell activation.
Binding of the TCR and coreceptors to peptide-MHC complexes on the antigen-presenting cell (APC) initiates proximal signaling events, which result in phosphorylation of the ζ chain, binding and activation of ZAP-70, phosphorylation of adapter proteins, and activation of various cellular enzymes. These enzymes then activate transcription factors that stimulate the expression of various genes involved in T cell responses.

Activation of Tyrosine Kinases

The earliest biochemical events within the T cell that follow clustering of the TCR complex and coreceptor are the activation of protein tyrosine kinases associated with the cytoplasmic domains of the clustered CD3 and coreceptor proteins and phosphorylation of tyrosines in CD3 and ζ chains. Protein tyrosine kinases are enzymes that catalyze the phosphorylation of tyrosine residues in various protein substrates (Box 8–3). In T cells, several components of the TCR complex, as well as downstream intermediates, are targets of protein tyrosine kinases. The cytoplasmic portions of the CD3 chains and the ζ chains contain a total of nine conserved peptide sequences called **immunoreceptor tyrosine-based activation motifs** (ITAMs) (see Chapter 6). When TCRs bind to peptide-MHC complexes, CD4 or CD8 binds at the same time to nonpolymorphic regions of the class II or class I MHC molecule on the APC (Fig. 8–9). **Lck,** a Src family tyrosine kinase that is associated with the cytoplasmic tails of CD4 and CD8, is thus brought into proximity of the ITAMs in the CD3 and ζ chains. Lck may be activated by autophosphorylation, and the active Lck then phosphorylates the tyrosines in the ITAMs of the CD3 and ζ chains. Thus, within seconds of TCR clustering, many of the tyrosine residues within the ITAMs of the CD3 and ζ chains become phosphorylated. Another cytoplasmic tyrosine kinase that is found in physical association with the TCR complex is CD3-associated Fyn, and it may play a role similar to that of Lck. Mice lacking Lck show some defects in T cell development, and double knockout mice lacking both Lck and Fyn show even more severe defects.

The tyrosine phosphorylated ITAMs in the ζ chain become "docking sites" for the tyrosine kinase called ZAP-70 (for ζ-associated protein of 70-kD). ZAP-70 is a member of a family of tyrosine kinases distinct from the Src family. (Another member of the ZAP-70 family is Syk, which plays an important role in signal transduction in B cells and in some populations of T cells, such as γδ T cells from the intestine.) ZAP-70 contains two conserved domains called Src homology 2 (SH2) domains that can bind to phosphotyrosines (see Box

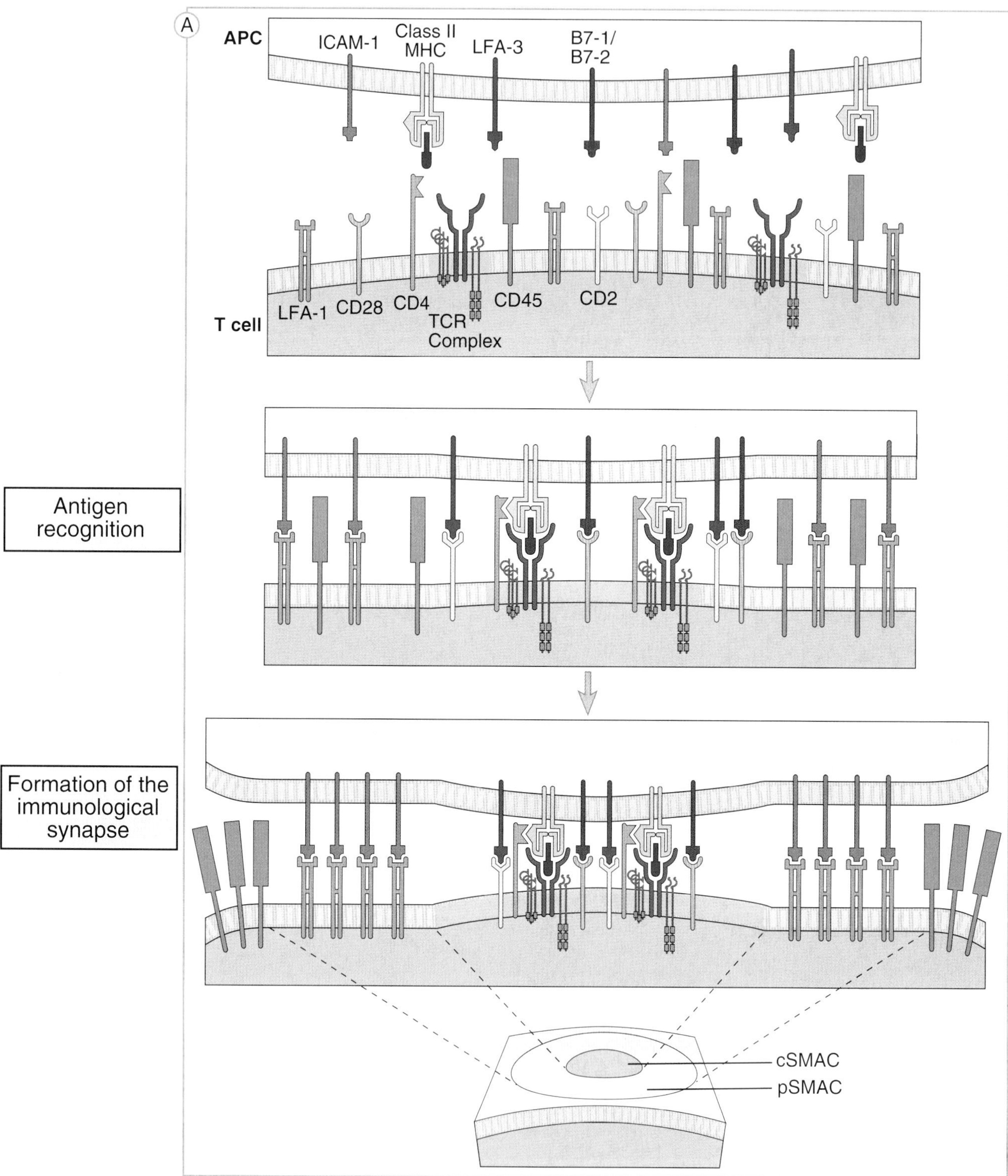

Figure 8–8 Formation of the immunological synapse.

A. This schematic diagram illustrates the steps in the formation of the immunological synapse. Before antigen recognition, various receptors on T cells and their ligands on APCs are dispersed in the plasma membranes of the two cells. When the T cell recognizes antigen presented by the antigen-presenting cell (APC), selected receptors on the T cell and their respective ligands are redistributed to a defined area of cell-cell contact, forming the synapse. The molecules in the central portion of the synapse form the central supramolecular activation cluster (cSMAC), and the molecules in the periphery form the peripheral supramolecular activation cluster (pSMAC).

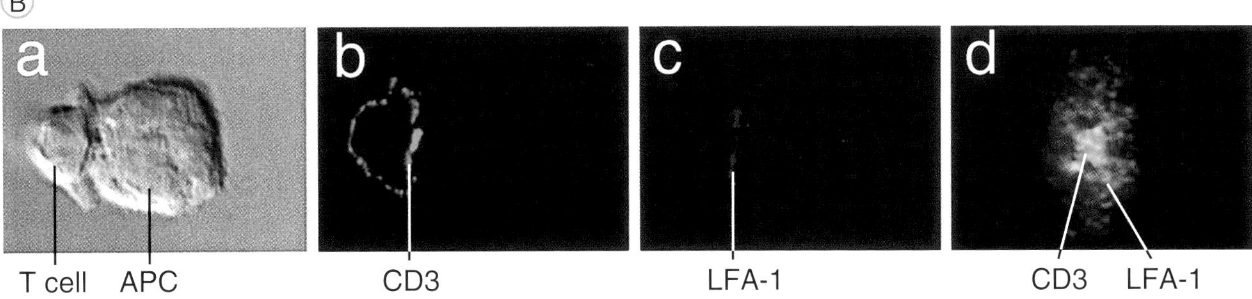

Figure 8–8 *(Continued)*
B. The formation of the synapse can be demonstrated by labeling selected molecules of T cells and APCs with fluorescent antibodies and imaging the distributions of these molecules by confocal microscopy. A T cell specific for a peptide binds to an APC presenting that peptide (a). CD3, a component of the TCR complex (b), becomes localized to the cSMAC, and leukocyte function–associated antigen (LFA-1), an accessory molecule (c), is clustered in the pSMAC. In the three-dimensional view (d), CD3 is in the center and LFA-1 is at the periphery of the T cell–APC contact site. (From Monks CRF, BA Freiberg, H Kupfer, N Sciaky, and A Kupfer. Three dimensional segregation of supramolecular activation clusters in T cells. Nature 395:82–86, 1998. Copyright 1998 Macmillan Magazines Limited.)

BOX 8–3

Protein Tyrosine Kinases and Phosphatases

Protein-protein interactions and the activities of cellular enzymes are often regulated by phosphorylation of tyrosine residues. Inducible phosphorylation of tyrosines is much less common than phosphorylation of serine or threonine residues and is usually reserved for critical regulatory steps. It is not surprising, therefore, that the kinases that catalyze tyrosine phosphorylation are essential components of many intracellular signaling cascades in lymphocytes and other cell types. These protein tyrosine kinases (PTKs) mediate the transfer of the terminal phosphate of adenosine triphosphate (ATP) to the hydroxyl group of a tyrosine residue in a substrate protein. A particular PTK will phosphorylate only a limited set of substrates, and this specificity is determined by the amino acid sequences flanking the tyrosine as well as by the tertiary structural characteristics of the substrate protein.

Some tyrosine kinases are intrinsic components of the cytoplasmic tails of cell surface receptors, such as the receptors for platelet-derived growth factor (PDGF) and epidermal growth factor (EGF). Examples of receptor tyrosine kinases that are involved in hematopoiesis include c-Kit, a receptor for stem cell factor, and the receptor for monocyte colony-stimulating factor (M-CSF). Many PTKs of importance in the immune system, however, are cytoplasmic proteins that are noncovalently associated with the cytoplasmic tails of cell surface receptors or with adapter proteins. Sometimes this association is only transiently induced in the early stages of signaling cascades. Three families of cytoplasmic PTKs that are prominent in B and T cell antigen receptor signaling cascades, as well as Fc receptor signaling, are the Src, Syk/ZAP-70, and Tec families (see Figure). The Janus kinases are another group of nonreceptor PTKs involved in many cytokine-induced signaling cascades and are discussed in Chapter 11.

Src kinases are homologous to, and named after, the transforming gene of Rous sarcoma virus, the first animal tumor virus identified. Members of this family include Src, Yes, Fgr, Fyn, Lck, Lyn, Hck, and Blk. All Src family members share tertiary structural characteristics that are distributed among four distinct domains and are critical for their function and regulation of enzymatic activity. The amino terminal end of most Src family kinases contains a consensus site for addition of a myristic acid group; this type of lipid modification serves to anchor cytoplasmic proteins to the inner side of the plasma membrane. Otherwise, the amino terminal domains of Src family PTKs

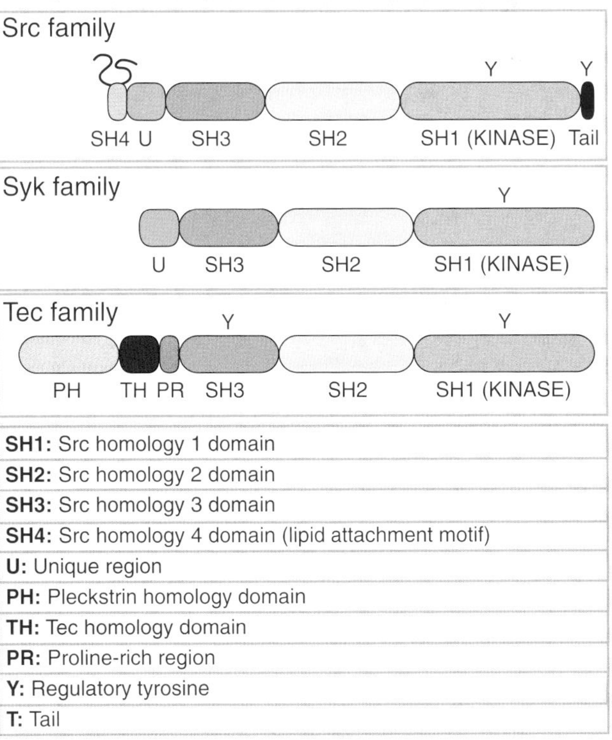

Continued on following page

BOX 8–3

Protein Tyrosine Kinases and Phosphatases (*Continued*)

are highly variable among different family members, and this region determines the ability of each member to interact specifically with different proteins. For example, the amino terminal region of the Lck protein is the contact site for interaction with the cytoplasmic tails of CD4 and CD8. The Src family PTKs have two internal domains called **Src homology 2** (SH2) and **Src homology 3** (SH3) **domains,** each of which has a distinct three-dimensional structure that permits specific noncovalent interactions with other proteins. SH2 domains are about 100 amino acids long and bind to phosphotyrosines on other proteins. Each SH2 domain has a unique binding specificity, which is determined by the three residues amino terminal to the phosphotyrosine on the target protein. SH2 domains are also found on many signaling molecules outside the Src family. SH3 domains are approximately 60 amino acids long and also mediate protein-protein binding. It is believed that SH3 domains bind to proline residues and may function cooperatively with the SH2 domains of the same protein binding to phosphotyrosines. The critical role of SH3 domains in PTK function is illustrated by mutations in the SH3 domain of Bruton's tyrosine kinase; these mutations do not alter the protein's stability or kinase activity but result in defective B cell receptor signaling and agammaglobulinemia. The carboxyl terminal SH1 domain in Src PTKs is usually the tyrosine kinase enzymatic domain. It contains binding sites for the substrate and for the ATP phosphate donor and an autophosphorylation site (a tyrosine residue) whose phosphorylation is needed for kinase activity. The carboxyl terminal domain has a second tyrosine that serves as a regulatory switch for the PTK. When it is phosphorylated, the PTK is inactive, and when the phosphate is removed by tyrosine phosphatases, the enzyme activity is turned on. The PTKs that phosphorylate Src family PTKs at this inhibitory site form yet another subfamily of PTKs, the best described member being c-Src kinase-1 (Csk-1).

The Syk/ZAP-70 family of PTKs includes only two identified members so far. Syk is abundantly expressed in B lymphocytes but is also found in lower amounts in other hematopoietic cells including some T cells. ZAP-70 is expressed in only T lymphocytes and NK (natural killer) cells. Syk and ZAP-70 play similar roles in membrane Ig and TCR signaling cascades, respectively. There are two SH2 domains in the Syk/ZAP-70 PTKs, but no SH3 domain and no inhibitory tyrosine. Syk and ZAP-70 are inactive until they bind, through their two SH2 domains, to paired phosphotyrosines within immunoreceptor tyrosine-based activation motifs (ITAMs) of antigen-receptor complex proteins (see text). Furthermore, activation of ZAP-70 probably requires Src family PTK (e.g., Lck)–mediated phosphorylation of one or more tyrosine residues.

The Tec PTKs are a third group of nonreceptor kinases that are activated by antigen receptors in B and T cells as well as by many other signals in other cell types. This family includes Btk, Tec, Itk, DSrc29, Etk, and Rlk. Btk is expressed in all hematopoietic cells, but mutations of the Btk gene primarily affect B cell development in humans, causing X-linked agammaglobulinemia. The major Tec kinases expressed by T cells are Itk, Rlk, and Tec. All the Tec family members contain a Tec homology (TH) domain, which includes sequences unique to this family (Btk homology domain) and sequences homologous with GTPase-activating protein. The TH domain mediates interactions with other signaling molecules. In addition, Tec kinases share structural similarities with the Src family kinases, including SH3 and SH2 domains that mediate interactions with other signaling molecules and a catalytic SH1 domain. Unlike the Src kinases, the Tec kinases do not have N-terminal myristoylation sites. In contrast, most Tek family kinases contain a pleckstrin homology (PH) domain, which promotes membrane localization by binding to PIP_3 generated by PI-3 kinase. The Tec kinases also do not contain a C-terminal regulatory tyrosine. Activation of a Tec kinase requires membrane localization, phosphorylation by a Src kinase, and autophosphorylation of the SH3 domain. The SH2 domains of Btk and Itk bind the phosphorylated adapter proteins BLNK/SLP-65 and SLP-76, in B and T cells, respectively, shortly after antigen recognition. Once bound to these adapter proteins, Btk and Itk can phosphorylate and activate phospholipase C.

Protein tyrosine phosphatases (PTPs) are enzymes that remove phosphate moieties from tyrosine residues, countering the actions of PTKs. PTPs may be membrane receptors or cytoplasmic proteins. One important receptor PTP, which has a role in lymphocyte activation, is CD45, a membrane-bound protein that removes autoinhibitory C-terminal phosphates from Src family kinases, such as Lck and Fyn, and is essential for T and B cell activation. The phosphatase activity of CD45 appears to require dimerization for activation, and mutations that prevent dimerization result in dysregulated activation of lymphocytes. Cytoplasmic PTPs are loosely associated with receptors or are recruited to tyrosine phosphorylated receptors through SH2 domains. These enzymes include two PTPs commonly called SH2-containing phosphatase-1 and SH2-containing phosphatase-2 (SHP-1 and SHP-2). SHP-1 is particularly abundant in hematopoietic cells. SHP-1 is a negative regulator of lymphocytes and contributes to the inhibitory signals mediated by inhibitory receptors of the immune system, such as killer inhibitory receptors of NK cells (see Chapter 12). These inhibitory receptors bind SHP-1 through special motifs called immunoreceptor tyrosine inhibitory motifs (ITIMs) by analogy to the ITAMs of the TCR and other activating receptors. The central role of SHP-1 in regulating lymphocyte function is illustrated by the "moth-eaten" mouse strain, which carries a mutation in the SHP-1 gene and is characterized by severe immunodeficiency and autoimmunity. SHP-2 plays a positive role in signaling by certain receptors, such as the EGF receptor, but may also be involved in negative regulation in CTLA-4 signaling.

Other phosphatases act on phosphorylated inositol lipids and inhibit cellular responses; an example is SHIP-1, an inositol phosphatase that is associated with an Fc receptor of B cells and serves to terminate B cell responses (see Chapter 9, Fig. 9–19).

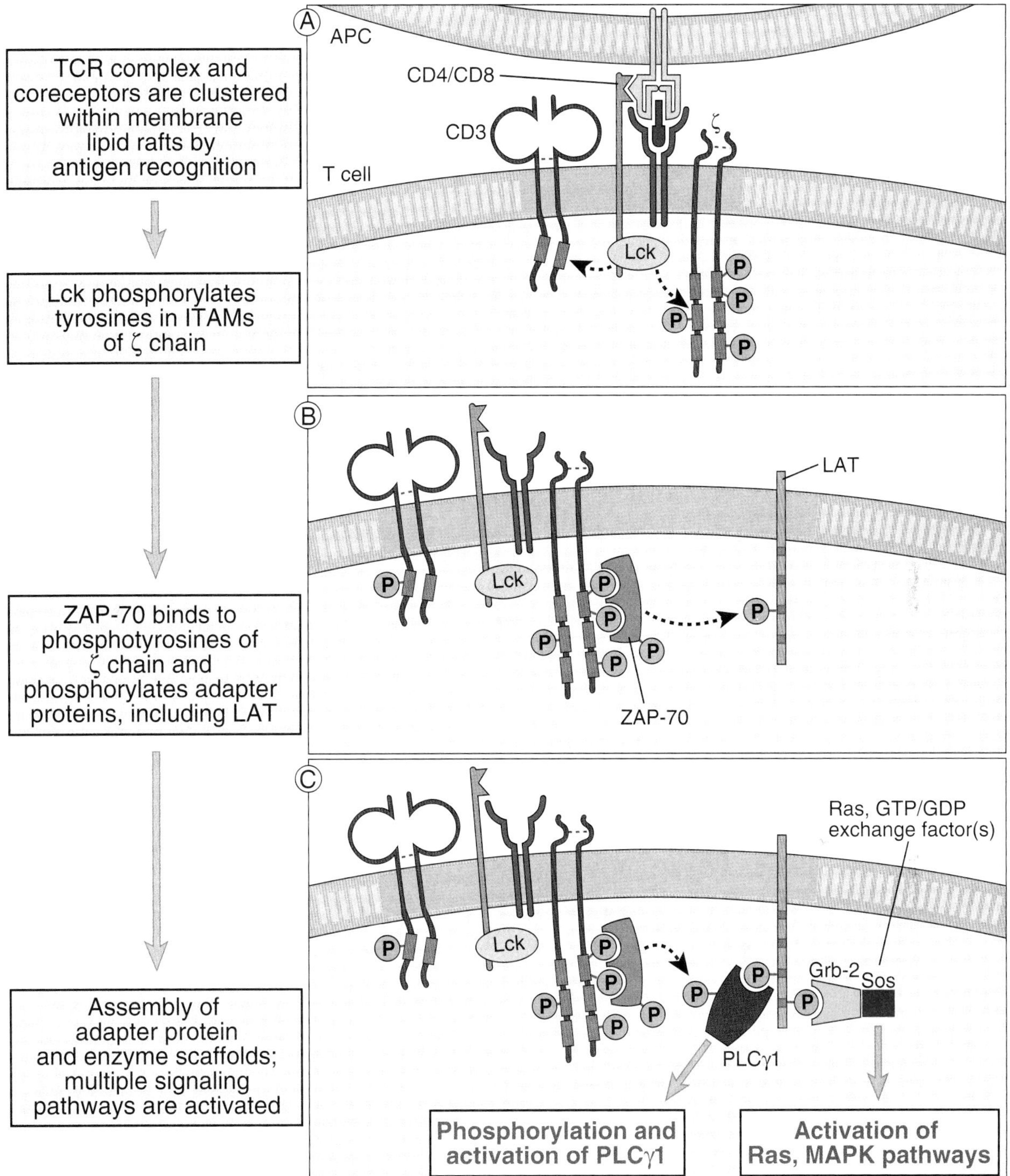

Figure 8–9 Early tyrosine phosphorylation events in T cell activation.
On antigen recognition, there is clustering of TCR complexes and coreceptors (CD4, in this case). CD4-associated Lck becomes active and phosphorylates tyrosines in the ITAMs of CD3 and ζ chains (A). ZAP-70 binds to the phosphotyrosines of the ζ chains and is itself phosphorylated and activated. (The illustration shows one ZAP-70 molecule binding to two phosphotyrosines of one ITAM in the ζ chain, but it is likely that initiation of a T cell response requires the assembly of multiple ZAP-70 molecules on each ζ chain.) Active ZAP-70 then phosphorylates tyrosines on various adapter molecules, such as LAT (B). The adapters become docking sites for cellular enzymes such as PLCγ1 and proteins that activate Ras and MAP kinases (C), and these enzymes activate various cellular responses.

8–3). Each ITAM of the ζ chain has two tyrosine residues, and both of these must become phosphorylated to form a docking site for one ZAP-70 molecule. The bound ZAP-70 becomes a substrate for the adjacent Lck, which phosphorylates the tyrosines of ZAP-70. As a result, ZAP-70 acquires its own tyrosine kinase activity and is then able to phosphorylate a number of other cytoplasmic signaling molecules. Once activated, ZAP-70 can also autophosphorylate itself. A critical threshold of ZAP-70 activity may be needed before downstream signaling events will proceed, and this threshold is achieved by the recruitment of multiple ZAP-70 molecules to the multiple phosphorylated ITAMs of the ζ chains. In fact, the need for a single T cell to bind antigen multiple times, which was mentioned earlier, may be because each binding event phosphorylates more ITAMs on the ζ chains, recruiting and activating additional ZAP-70 molecules.

The activation of ZAP-70 plays a critical role in sustaining the signaling cascade set in motion by TCR recognition of antigen.

- T cell lines and knockout mice lacking functional ZAP-70 show profound defects in TCR-induced responses. Mutations in the ZAP-70 gene are responsible for some rare immunodeficiency diseases also characterized by defective T cell maturation and activation (see Chapter 20).
- There is a strong correlation between the level of ζ chain phosphorylation and ZAP-70 activation and the subsequent T cell response. Peptides that have been mutated in their TCR contact residues often induce partial or no activation of T cells. The magnitude of T cell responses to these peptides, which are called altered peptide ligands (APLs), correlates with the extent of ζ chain phosphorylation. We will return to a discussion of APLs later in this chapter.

Another kinase pathway in T cells involves PI-3 (phosphatidylinositol-3) kinase, which phosphorylates membrane-associated inositol lipids. This enzyme is recruited to the TCR complex and associated adapter proteins and generates phosphatidylinositol triphosphate (PIP_3) from the biphosphate membrane lipid. PIP_3 is a binding site for signaling intermediates that contain pleckstrin homology domains, including phospholipase Cγ and kinases such as Itk (and Btk in B cells). PI-3 kinase is also involved in CD28 signaling, as we will discuss later.

The activity of kinases in T cell signaling pathways may be regulated by protein tyrosine phosphatases. These phosphatases can remove phosphates from tyrosine residues of the kinases, and depending on which tyrosine residue is involved, the effect may be to activate or to inhibit the enzymatic function of the kinases. Two phosphatases that are recruited to the TCR complex are SHP-1 and SHP-2 (for SH2 domain–containing phosphatases). These phosphatases serve to inhibit signal transduction by removing phosphates from key signaling molecules. Another inhibitory phosphatase is specific for inositol phospholipids and is called SHIP. In Chapter 6, we described the CD45 protein, which has an intrinsic tyrosine phosphatase in its cytoplasmic tail. CD45 may dephosphorylate inhibitory tyrosine residues in Lck that are present before antigen recognition, and this may allow Lck to become active. Mice in which CD45 is mutated so that it cannot be down-regulated develop excessive T cell activity and autoimmunity. Much of our knowledge of the function of CD45 is based on studies with T cell tumor lines. How CD45 is recruited to the TCR complex and its role in antigen-induced responses of normal T cells are not known.

Recruitment and Activation of Adapter Proteins

Activated ZAP-70 phosphorylates several adapter proteins that are able to bind signaling molecules (see Fig. 8–7). Adapter proteins serve to bring many signaling molecules into specific cellular compartments and thereby promote the activation of signal transduction pathways. Adapter proteins contain structural motifs, or domains, that bind other proteins. These domains include motifs that bind Src homology 2 and 3 (SH2 and SH3) domains, phosphotyrosine-binding (PTB) domains, and pleckstrin homology (PH) domains. Both transmembrane and cytoplasmic adapter proteins contribute to the rapid assembly of scaffolds of signaling molecules after T cells recognize antigen on APCs. A key early event in T cell activation is the ZAP-70–mediated tyrosine phosphorylation of the membrane-anchored adapter protein LAT (linker of activation of T cells). The phosphorylated tyrosines of LAT serve as docking sites for SH2 domains of other adapter proteins and enzymes involved in several signaling cascades. LAT also contains proline-rich regions that bind SH3 domains of other proteins. Activated LAT directly binds phospholipase Cγ1, a key enzyme in T cell activation (discussed later), and because it localizes within the immunological synapse, it coordinates the recruitment of several other adapter proteins, including SLP-76 (for SH2-binding leukocyte phosphoprotein of 76-kD) and Grb-2, to the synapse. Thus, LAT serves to bring a variety of downstream components of TCR signaling pathways close to their upstream activators. Because the function of many of these adapters depends on their tyrosine phosphorylation by active ZAP-70, only antigen recognition (the physiologic stimulus for ZAP-70 activation) triggers the signal transduction pathways that lead to functional T cell responses.

Ras–MAP Kinase Signaling Pathways in T Lymphocytes

The Ras pathway is activated in T cells on TCR clustering, leading to the activation of kinases called MAPkinases and eventually to the activation of transcription factors. Ras is a member of a family of 21-kD guanine nucleotide–binding proteins (small G proteins) that are involved in diverse activation responses in different cell types. Ras is loosely attached to the plasma membrane through covalently attached lipids. In its inactive form, the guanine nucleotide–binding site of Ras is occupied by guanosine diphosphate (GDP). When the bound GDP is replaced by guanosine

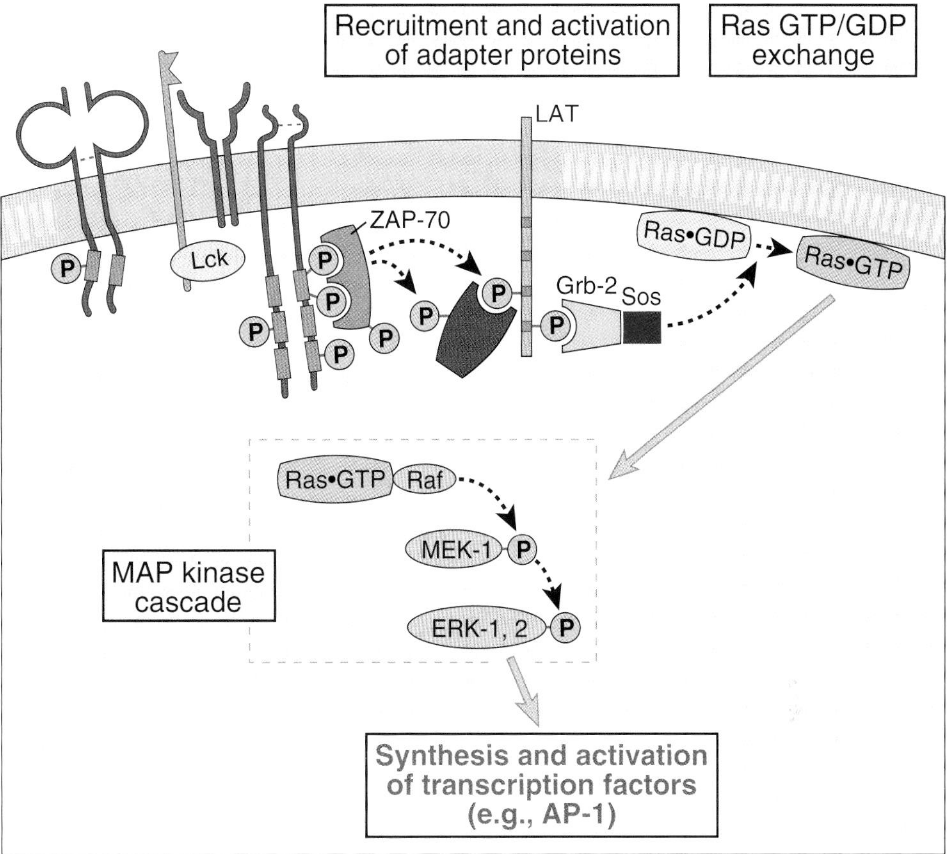

Figure 8–10 The Ras–MAP kinase pathway in T cell activation.
ZAP-70 that is activated by antigen recognition (see Fig. 8–9) phosphorylates membrane-associated adapter proteins (such as LAT), which then bind another adapter, Grb-2. ZAP-70 phosphorylates Grb-2, making it a docking site for the GTP/GDP exchange factor Sos. Sos converts Ras•GDP to Ras•GTP. Ras•GTP activates a cascade of enzymes, which culminates in the activation of the MAP kinase ERK. A parallel Rac-dependent pathway, called the stress-activated protein (SAP) kinase pathway, generates another active MAP kinase, JNK (not shown).

triphosphate (GTP), Ras undergoes a conformational change and can recruit or activate various cellular enzymes. Activation of Ras by GDP/GTP exchange is seen in response to the engagement of many types of receptors in many cell populations, including the TCR complex in T cells. Mutated Ras proteins that are constitutively active (i.e., assume the GTP-bound conformation) are associated with neoplastic transformation of many cell types.

The mechanism of Ras activation in T cells involves the adapter proteins LAT and another adapter protein, Grb-2 (Fig. 8–10). When LAT is phosphorylated by ZAP-70 at the site of TCR clustering, it serves as the docking site for the SH2 domain of Grb-2. Once attached to LAT, Grb-2 recruits to the membrane the Ras GTP/GDP exchange factor called Sos (so named because it is the mammalian homologue of a *Drosophila* protein called son of sevenless). Sos catalyzes GTP for GDP exchange on Ras. This generates the GTP-bound form of Ras (written as Ras•GTP), which then functions as an allosteric activator of enzymes called mitogen-activated protein (MAP) kinases. There are three main MAP kinases in T cells, the prototype being an enzyme called the extracellular receptor-activated kinase (ERK). ERK activation results from Ras•GTP-induced sequential activation of at least three different kinases, each of which phosphorylates (and thus activates) the next enzyme in the cascade. The activated ERK phosphorylates a protein called Elk, and phosphorylated Elk stimulates transcription of Fos, a component of the activation protein-1 (AP-1) transcription factor.

In parallel with the activation of Ras through recruitment of Grb-2 and Sos, the adapters phosphorylated by TCR-associated kinases also recruit and activate a GTP/GDP exchange protein called Vav that acts on another small 21-kD guanine nucleotide–binding protein called Rac. The Rac•GTP that is generated initiates a parallel enzyme cascade, resulting in the activation of the MAP kinase called c-Jun N-terminal kinase (JNK). JNK is sometimes called stress-activated protein (SAP) kinase because in many cells, it is activated by various forms of noxious stimuli such as ultraviolet light, osmotic stress, or proinflammatory cytokines such as tumor necrosis factor (TNF) and IL-1. Activated JNK then phosphorylates c-Jun, the second component of the AP-1 transcription factor. The third member of the MAP kinase family, in addition to ERK and JNK, is p38, and it too is activated by Rac•GTP and in turn activates various transcription factors. Rac•GTP also induces cytoskeletal reorganization and may play a role in the clustering of TCR complexes, coreceptors, and other signaling molecules into the synapse. Thus, active G proteins induced by antigen recognition stimulate at least three different MAP kinases, which in turn activate transcription factors.

The activities of ERK and JNK are eventually shut off by the action of dual-specificity protein tyrosine/threonine phosphatases. These phosphatases are induced or activated by ERK and JNK themselves, providing a negative feedback mechanism to terminate T cell activation.

Calcium- and Protein Kinase C–Mediated Signaling Pathways in T Lymphocytes

TCR signaling leads to the activation of the γ1 isoform of the enzyme phospholipase C (PLCγ1), and the products of PLCγ1-mediated hydrolysis of membrane lipids activate enzymes that generate additional active transcription factors in T cells (Fig. 8–11). PLCγ1 is a cytosolic enzyme specific for inositol phospholipids that is recruited to the plasma membrane by tyrosine phosphorylated LAT. Here the enzyme is phosphorylated by ZAP-70 and by other kinases, such as the Tec family kinase called Itk (see Box 8–3), and this occurs within minutes of ligand binding to the TCR. Phosphorylated PLCγ1 catalyzes the hydrolysis of a plasma membrane phospholipid called phosphatidylinositol 4,5-bisphosphate (PIP_2), generating two breakdown products, **inositol 1,4,5-trisphosphate** (IP_3) and **diacylglycerol** (DAG). IP_3 and DAG then activate two distinct downstream signaling pathways in T cells.

IP_3 produces a rapid increase in cytosolic free calcium within minutes after T cell activation. IP_3 diffuses through the cytosol to the endoplasmic reticulum, where it binds to its receptor and stimulates release of membrane-sequestered calcium stores. The released calcium causes a rapid rise (during a few minutes) in the cytosolic free calcium ion concentration, from a resting level of about 100 nM to a peak of 600 to 1000 nM. In addition, a plasma membrane calcium channel is opened in response to as yet incompletely understood TCR-generated signals, producing an influx of extracellular calcium. This influx of extracellular calcium allows the T cell to sustain an increase in cytosolic free calcium for more than an hour. Cytosolic free calcium acts as a signaling molecule by binding to a ubiquitous calcium-dependent regulatory protein called calmodulin. Calcium-calmodulin complexes activate several enzymes, including a protein serine/threonine phosphatase called **calcineurin** that is important for transcription factor activation, as discussed later.

DAG, the second breakdown product of PIP_2, activates the enzyme protein kinase C (PKC, which has several isoforms) that also participates in the generation of active transcription factors (see Fig. 8–11). DAG is hydrophobic, and it remains in the membrane where it is formed. The combination of elevated free cytosolic calcium and DAG activates membrane-associated PKC by inducing a conformational change that makes the catalytic site of the kinase accessible to substrate. The PKC-ϕ isoform is known to localize to the immunological synapse and is involved in the activation of several downstream signaling pathways. However, the substrates of PKC enzymes in T cells are not clearly defined.

The importance of PKC and calcium signals for the functional activation of T cells is supported by the observation that pharmacologic activators of PKC, such as phorbol myristate acetate, and calcium ionophores, such as ionomycin, which raise cytosolic free calcium ion concentrations, act together to stimulate T cell cytokine secretion and proliferation. These pharmacologic agents mimic the effects of antigen and induce T cell functional responses in the absence of antigen.

So far, we have described several signal transduction pathways initiated by ligand binding to the TCR that

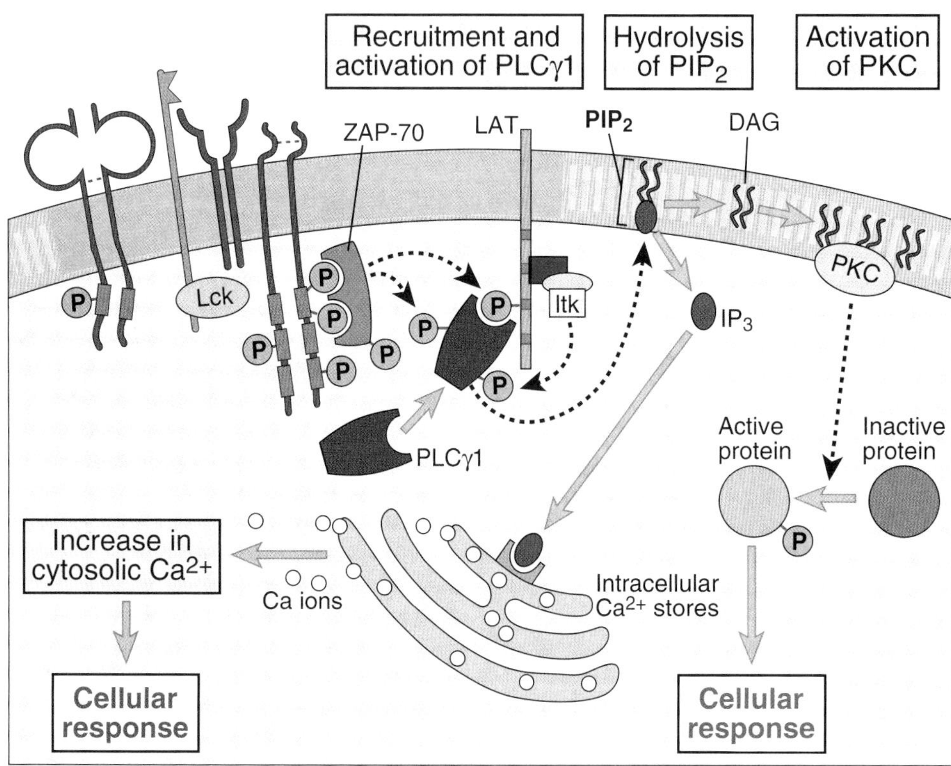

Figure 8–11 T cell signaling through membrane inositol phospholipid metabolism. The LAT adapter protein that is phosphorylated on T cell activation binds the cytosolic enzyme PLCγ1, which is phosphorylated by ZAP-70 and other kinases, such as Itk, and activated. Active PLCγ1 hydrolyzes membrane PIP_2 to generate IP_3, which stimulates an increase in cytosolic calcium, and DAG, which activates the enzyme PKC. Increased cytosolic calcium and PKC then activate various transcription factors, leading to cellular responses.

result in the activation of different types of enzymes: a Ras–MAP kinase pathway leading to activation of the kinases such as ERK and JNK, a PLCγ1-calcium–dependent pathway leading to activation of the phosphatase calcineurin, and a PLCγ1-DAG–dependent pathway leading to activation of PKC (see Fig. 8–7). Each of these pathways contributes to the expression of genes encoding proteins needed for T cell clonal expansion, differentiation, and effector functions. In the following section, we describe the mechanisms by which these different signaling pathways stimulate the transcription of various genes in T cells.

Activation of Transcription Factors That Regulate T Cell Gene Expression

The enzymes generated by TCR signaling activate transcription factors that bind to regulatory regions of numerous genes in T cells and thereby enhance transcription of these genes (Fig. 8–12). Much of our understanding of the transcriptional regulation of genes in T cells is based on analyses of cytokine genes. The transcriptional regulation of most cytokine genes in T cells is controlled by the binding of transcription factors to nucleotide sequences in the promoter and

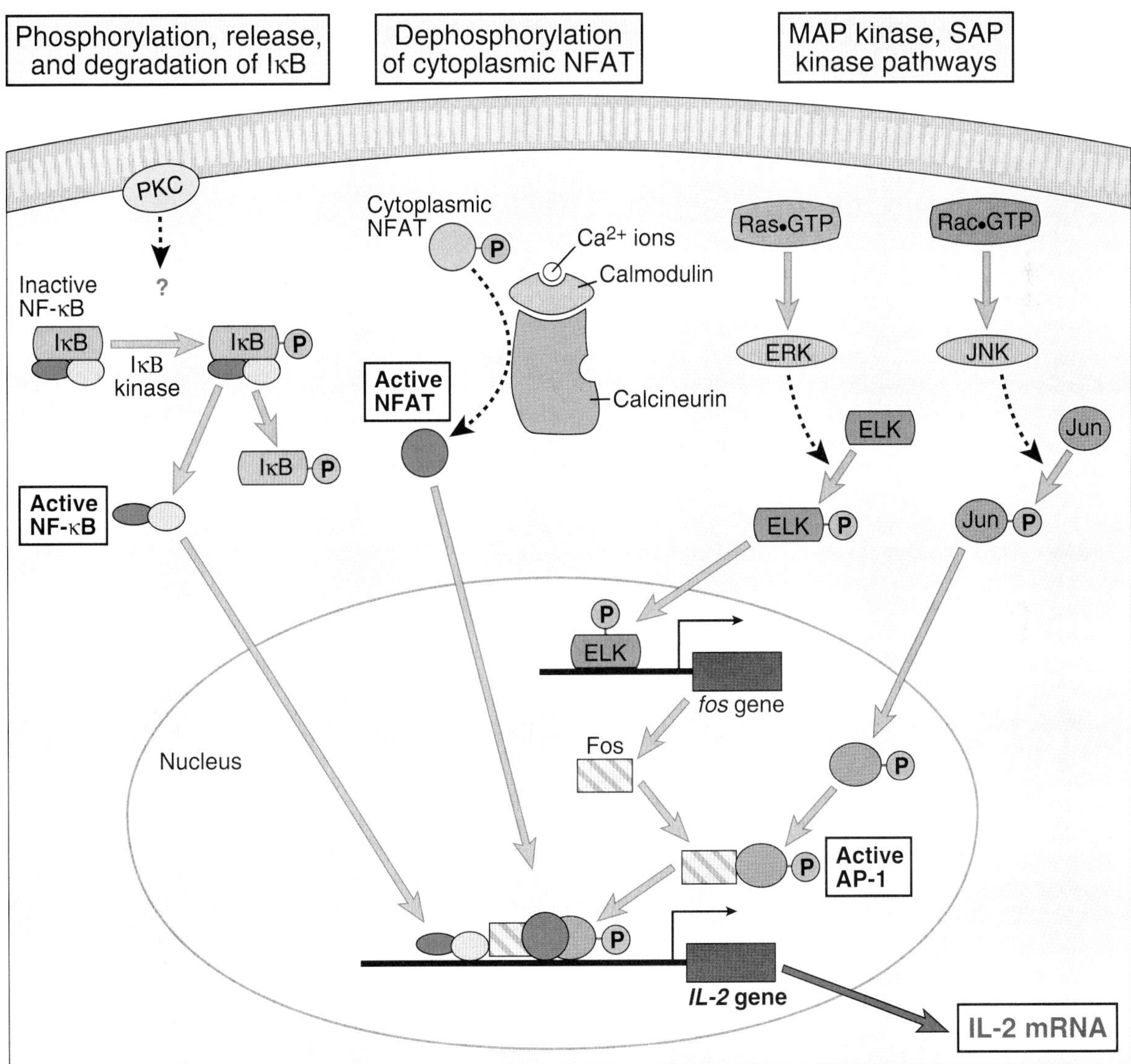

Figure 8–12 Activation of transcription factors in T cells.
Multiple signaling pathways converge in antigen-stimulated T cells to generate transcription factors that stimulate expression of various genes (in this case, the IL-2 gene). The calcium–calmodulin pathway activates NFAT, and the Ras and Rac pathways generate the two components of AP-1. Less is known about the link between TCR signals and NF-κB activation. (NF-κB is shown as a complex of two subunits, which in T cells are typically the p50 and p65 proteins, named for their molecular sizes in kilodaltons.) PKC is important in T cell activation, but it is not clear which transcription factors it induces, and its action is shown as a dashed arrow. These transcription factors function coordinately to regulate gene expression. Note also that the various signaling pathways are shown as activating unique transcription factors, but there may be considerable overlap, and each pathway may play a role in the activation of multiple transcription factors.

enhancer regions of these genes. For instance, the IL-2 promoter, located 5′ of the gene, contains a segment of approximately 300 base pairs in which are located binding sites for several different transcription factors. All these sites must be occupied by transcription factors for maximal transcription of the IL-2 gene. Different transcription factors are activated by different cytoplasmic signal transduction pathways, and the requirement for multiple transcription factors accounts for the need to activate multiple signal transduction pathways on antigen recognition. It is likely that the same principles are true for many genes in T cells, including genes encoding cytokine receptors and effector molecules, although different genes may be responsive to different combinations of transcription factors.

Three transcription factors that are activated in T cells by antigen recognition and appear to be critical for most T cell responses are nuclear factor of activated T cells (NFAT), AP-1, and nuclear factor κB (NF-κB).

NFAT is a transcription factor required for the expression of IL-2, IL-4, TNF, and other cytokine genes. There are four different NFATs, each encoded by separate genes; NFAT1 and NFAT2 are the types found in T cells. NFAT is present in an inactive, serine phosphorylated form in the cytoplasm of resting T lymphocytes. It is activated by the calcium-calmodulin–dependent phosphatase calcineurin. Calcineurin dephosphorylates cytoplasmic NFAT, thereby uncovering a nuclear localization signal that permits NFAT to translocate into the nucleus. Once in the nucleus, NFAT binds to the regulatory regions of IL-2, IL-4, and other cytokine genes, usually in association with other transcription factors, such as AP-1.

The mechanism of activation of NFAT was discovered indirectly by studies of the mechanism of action of the immunosuppressive drugs cyclosporine and FK-506 (see Chapter 16). These drugs, which are natural products of fungi, are the main therapeutic agents used to prevent allograft rejection, and they function largely by blocking T cell cytokine gene transcription. Cyclosporine binds to a cytosolic protein called cyclophilin, and FK-506 binds to a structurally homologous protein called FK-506–binding protein (FKBP). Cyclophilin and FKBP are also called immunophilins. Cyclosporine-cyclophilin complexes and FK-506–FKBP complexes bind to and inhibit calcineurin, and therefore they block translocation of NFAT into the nucleus.

AP-1 is a transcription factor found in many cell types; it is specifically activated in T lymphocytes by TCR-mediated signals. AP-1 is actually the name for a family of DNA-binding factors composed of dimers of two proteins that bind to one another through a shared structural motif called a leucine zipper. The best characterized AP-1 factor is composed of the proteins Fos and Jun. TCR-induced signals lead to the appearance of active AP-1 in the nucleus of T cells. Activation of AP-1 typically involves synthesis of the Fos protein and phosphorylation of preexisting Jun protein. Transcription and synthesis of Fos can be enhanced by the ERK pathway, as described before, and also by PKC. JNK phosphorylates c-Jun, and AP-1 complexes containing the phosphorylated form of Jun have increased transcriptional enhancing activity. AP-1 appears to physically associate with other transcription factors in the nucleus, including NFAT, and works best in combination with NFAT. Thus, AP-1 activation represents a convergence point of several TCR-initiated signaling pathways.

NF-κB is a transcription factor that is activated in response to TCR signals and is essential for cytokine synthesis. NF-κB proteins are homodimers or heterodimers of proteins that are homologous to the product of a cellular proto-oncogene called c-*rel* and are important in the transcription of many genes in diverse cell types, particularly in cells of innate immunity (Box 8–4). In resting T cells, NF-κB is present in the cytoplasm in a complex with other proteins called inhibitors of κB (IκBs), which block the entry of NF-κB into the nucleus. TCR signals lead to serine phosphorylation of IκB. The enzymes responsible for phosphorylation of IκB are called IκB kinases. In T cells, PKC, the MAP kinase pathway, and calcium may all lead to the phosphorylation of IκB, but how these signaling intermediates activate IκB kinases has not been defined. The phosphorylation of IκB is followed by attachment of multiple copies of a small protein called ubiquitin. This ubiquitination targets IκB for proteolysis in the cytosolic proteasome, the multienzyme protease complex that degrades many cytosolic proteins. Thus, NF-κB is released and translocates to the nucleus, where it contributes to the transcriptional activation of multiple cytokine genes and cytokine receptor genes.

Although we have described some of the major signaling pathways in T cells as generating distinct transcription factors, many experimental results suggest that these TCR signaling pathways may not be independent.

- Pharmacologic activators or inhibitors of one pathway appear to influence others. For instance, cyclosporine and FK-506, which inhibit calcineurin, not only inhibit the activation of NFAT but also inhibit the activation of NF-κB; and phorbol esters, which activate PKC, activate both NF-κB and AP-1.
- Components of one signaling pathway may also activate multiple transcription factors. For example, overexpression in T cell tumor lines of dominant negative forms of Ras (by gene transfection) not only blocks AP-1 activation, as expected, but also blocks NFAT activation.

The links between different signaling proteins, activation of transcription factors, and functional responses of T cells are often difficult to establish because there are complex and incompletely understood interactions between signaling pathways. Also, we have focused on selected pathways to illustrate how antigen recognition may lead to biochemical alterations, but it is likely that other signaling molecules are also involved in antigen-induced lymphocyte activation.

Biochemistry of Costimulation

Costimulatory signals delivered by T cell receptors, such as CD28, cooperate with TCR signals to augment

BOX 8–4

Transcriptional Regulation and NF-κB

A common theme in immunology is that activating stimuli, such as antigens and cytokines, result in the initiation of transcription of genes that were previously silent or transcribed at very low rates in the responding cells. The set of genes that can be transcribed in any given differentiated cell type is determined by numerous mechanisms, including the accessibility of the DNA encoding a gene to soluble protein factors (i.e., the "openness of the chromatin"), chemical modifications of the DNA in the regulatory regions of a gene (e.g., by methylation of particular nucleotides), and protein factors that bind to the DNA and promote or repress transcription. When a gene is available for active transcription, a complex of proteins, including the RNA polymerase enzyme, assemble near the site where transcription begins. The DNA sequence that binds this basal transcription complex of proteins is called the **promoter.** However, binding of the basal transcription complex to the promoter is not sufficient by itself to initiate transcription efficiently, and additional signals are provided by interactions with DNA-binding proteins called **transcription factors.** Transcription factors have dual functions: they must recognize and bind to specific DNA sequences, and they must interact with proteins of the basal transcription complex, either directly or through a coactivator protein. The specific DNA sequences that bind these transcription factors must be located on the same segment of DNA as the promoter and are therefore called cis-acting sequences. In some cases, these sequences must be near and in a particular orientation to the transcriptional start site and are often considered to be part of the promoter. In other cases, these cis-acting regulatory sequences can be as much as several thousand nucleotides away and will work in either orientation. Such movable regulatory DNA sequences are called **enhancers.** The transcription factors that bind to promoter or enhancer sequences are usually encoded by genes that are distant from the promoter or enhancer sequences (e.g., on a different chromosome), and therefore transcription factors are sometimes called trans-acting factors, meaning they need not be encoded by the same piece of DNA as the regulated gene. In fact, many transcription factors are multimeric proteins, and their subunits may be encoded by widely separated genes on separate chromosomes.

Transcription factors may be activated in different ways in response to various stimuli.

1. Transcription factors may not be present in a resting cell, and activation signals induce their *de novo* synthesis. An example of this kind of regulation is the synthesis of c-Fos, a component of transcription factor AP-1, in response to antigenic stimulation of lymphocytes.
2. Transcription factors may require assembly into multimeric complexes to bind to DNA, and this step may be regulated. An example of this kind of regulation is the assembly of cytokine-responsive STAT proteins into dimers, which is induced by the phosphorylation of these proteins by Janus kinases (see Chapter 11, Box 11–2).
3. Transcription factors may require covalent modification to interact with the proteins of the basal transcription complex, and this step may be regulated. For instance, in the case of c-Jun, regulation involves phosphorylation of an amino acid side chain in the amino terminal transactivating region of the protein by the enzyme c-Jun N-terminal kinase.
4. Transcription factors may preexist in a form that is capable of binding DNA and of mediating transactivation, but the factor may not have access to the cis-acting regulatory sequences of the target gene. In the case of nuclear factor of activated T cells (NFAT), regulation involves removal of a phosphate moiety from an amino acid side chain, thereby exposing an amino acid sequence required for the NFAT protein to enter the nucleus. The protein phosphatase that mediates this reaction, calcineurin, is activated in the T cell by antigen recognition (see text).

We discuss the transcription factor called **nuclear factor κB (NF-κB)** as a prototype because of its central role in many immunologic reactions. The functional NF-κB transcription factor is a dimer of either identical or structurally homologous protein subunits of about 50 to 75 kD. The common structural motif shared by these proteins is called a rel homology domain because this sequence was first identified in the retroviral transforming gene *v-rel.* The mammalian proteins that share this motif are p50 (also called NF-κB1), p52 (NF-κB2), p65 (RelA), c-Rel, and RelB. *Drosophila* express a member of this family called dorsal. Members of the NF-κB/Rel family are expressed in almost every cell type; RelB is expressed in lymphocytes and a few other cells. All of these proteins can participate in either homodimer or heterodimer formation, except for RelB, which only forms heterodimers with p50 or p52.

In resting cells, functional NF-κB dimers are present in an inactive state in the cytoplasm, bound to one or more inhibitory proteins called **inhibitors of κB (IκBs).** The activation of NF-κB is initiated by the signal-induced degradation of IκB proteins. The details of this process are not fully known, but it involves phosphorylation of specific serine residues in IκB by an enzymatic complex called IκB kinase (IKK). How IKK activation is linked to upstream signals generated by the TCR or cytokine receptors is not fully understood but probably involves additional kinases as well as TRAF family adapter molecules (see Box 11–1). IKK is composed of at least two kinases called IKK-α and IKK-β and a noncatalytic regulatory subunit called NF-κB essential modulator (NEMO) or IKK-γ. IKK-mediated phosphorylation targets IκB for ubiquitination and, finally, degradation of the polyubiquitinated IκB by the cytoplasmic proteasome. Once NF-κB is freed from IκB, it is able to enter the nucleus, where it binds to specific DNA sequences in target genes and stimulates their transcription. NF-κB may interact with other proteins to activate transcription optimally.

NF-κB was so named because the first identified binding site for this protein is located within an intronic enhancer in the Ig κ light chain gene. Although NF-κB is not required for Igκ chain expression, multiple roles for NF-κB in the immune system have been determined by molecular studies and the phenotype of several knockout mice (see Table). NF-κB is involved in T cell activation, contributing to IL-2 transcription (see text), and in the

Continued on following page

BOX 8–4

Transcriptional Regulation and NF-κB (*Continued*)

Molecule	Function	Phenotype of gene knockout in mice
p50	Component of NF-κB transcription factor	Defects in antibody and innate immune responses to infection
p52	Component of NF-κB transcription factor	Impaired antibody responses to T-dependent antigens; absence of B cell follicles, follicular dendritic cell networks, and germinal centers in secondary lymphoid organs
p65 (RelA)	Component of NF-κB transcription factor	Embryonic lethal due to hepatocyte apoptosis
RelB	Component of NF-κB transcription factor	Inflammation of multiple organs, myeloid hyperplasia and extramedullary hematopoiesis, impaired cellular immunity
c-Rel	Component of NF-κB transcription factor	Defects in lymphocyte proliferation, humoral immunity, and interleukin-2 expression
IκB-α	Inhibitor of NF-κB; blocks nuclear localization	Perinatal lethality with increased basal NF-κB activity in hematopoietic organs, excess granulopoiesis, and dermatitis
IκB-β	Inhibitor of NF-κB; blocks nuclear localization	
IκB-ε	Inhibitor of NF-κB; blocks nuclear localization	
Bcl-3	Inhibitor of NF-κB; blocks nuclear localization	Impaired antibody responses to T-dependent antigens; absence of B cell follicles, follicular dendritic cell networks, and germinal centers in secondary lymphoid organs
p100	Inhibitor of NF-κB; blocks nuclear localization	Gastric hyperplasia and an impaired proliferative response in lymphocytes
IKK-α	Catalytic component of IκB kinase, which phosphorylates IkB, leading to its degradation and activation of NF-κB	Perinatal lethality with defective differentiation of the epidermis and related keratinizing tissues
IKK-β	Catalytic component of IκB kinase, which phosphorylates IκB, leading to its degradation and activation of NF-κB	Embryonic lethal due to hepatocyte apoptosis
IKK-γ (NEMO)	Regulatory component of IκB kinase, which phosphorylates IκB, leading to its degradation and activation of NF-κB	Male embryonic lethality (X-linked) due to hepatocyte apoptosis; heterozygous female mice develop inflammatory and proliferative skin lesions similar to human genetic disorder incontinentia pigmenti

responses of many diverse cell types to microbial products and proinflammatory cytokines such as TNF and IL-1 (see Chapter 11). In fact, many of the cellular responses seen in innate immune reactions are dependent on the activity of this transcription factor. NF-κB also activates the transcription of genes whose products protect cells from apoptotic death and is thus a component of a basic survival mechanism of cells. Knockout of the genes encoding the p65 subunit (RelA) or IKK-β in mice results in embryonic lethality due to massive liver cell apoptosis. This supports the notion that NF-κB plays an important anti-apoptotic role *in vivo*.

the activation of transcription factors. CD28 engagement may enhance signaling by the TCR complex in part by stabilizing and prolonging the synapse between T cells and APCs. CD28 may also activate distinct signaling pathways that work with TCR-induced signals to stimulate the biologic responses of T cells. CD28 clustering induced by antibodies or by binding to B7 costimulators can activate PI-3 kinase and facilitate GTP/GDP exchange in Ras, resulting in activation of the MAP kinase pathway as well as activation of the Akt kinase. CD28 also provides an independent pathway for the activation of the adapter protein Vav and the associated Rac pathway. In some cultured T cell lines, CD28 signals have been shown to activate a form of NF-κB that binds to a site in the IL-2 gene promoter, called the CD28 response element, that is not activated by TCR-mediated signals. All these pathways promote T cell survival, cytokine production, and proliferation. CD28 may also block inhibitory signals in T cells. For instance, when the LAT or SLP-76 adapter is activated by TCR signaling, another adapter called Cbl-b may be recruited to the complex. Phosphorylation and activation of Cbl-b inhibit T cell activation, in part by blocking TCR-mediated signals that are dependent on PI-3 kinase. CD28 signals, through activation of Vav and the Rac pathway, block the inhibitory activity of Cbl-b and thus augment TCR signals. In knockout mice lacking Cbl-b, the T cells respond to antigen even without CD28-mediated costimulation and produce abnormally high amounts of IL-2, and the mice develop autoimmunity as a result of hyperactivation of the T cells. Which of these multiple CD28-triggered signaling pathways is essential for the function of this receptor is not known.

Even less is known about the biochemical mechanisms by which the second T cell receptor for B7 molecules, CTLA-4, inhibits T cell activation. There is some evidence that engagement of CTLA-4 blocks normal phosphorylation of TCR-associated ζ chains, perhaps by recruiting a phosphatase to the synapse. Whether a T cell uses CD28 or CTLA-4 to bind to B7 molecules on APCs is a key determinant of the outcome of antigen recognition, but how this choice is made is not known. One possibility is that because CTLA-4 binds to B7-1 and B7-2 with ~50-fold higher affinity than does CD28, APCs with low expression of B7 may preferentially engage CTLA-4. Normal resting APCs, which may be displaying self antigens but express little B7, engage CTLA-4 and induce tolerance in self-reactive T cells. Infections up-regulate B7 expression, leading to engagement of CD28 and T cell activation. It is also known that naive T cells express CD28, but CTLA-4 expression requires T cell activation. Therefore, naive T cells may use CD28 to initiate responses, but at later times, more CTLA-4 may be expressed, and its binding to B7 molecules may function to terminate the responses.

Altered Peptide Ligands

The signaling events and functional consequences of T cell antigen recognition may be altered by changing some of the TCR contact residues of a peptide antigen. As we discussed in Chapter 6, the TCRs on an individual T cell contact only a few amino acid residues of a particular MHC-bound peptide. Synthetic peptides in which one or two TCR contact residues have been changed induce only a subset of the functional responses, or entirely different responses, compared with the responses to the unaltered (native) peptide. For instance, some of these variant peptides may induce only some of the many cytokines that are induced by the native peptide or may induce quantitatively smaller responses than the native peptides do. These responses are called partial activation, and the peptides that induce them are called partial, or weak, agonists. Yet other variant peptides deliver negative signals to specific T cells that inhibit responses to native peptides; these are called antagonist peptides, and the phenomenon is referred to as T cell antagonism. Peptides with altered TCR contact residues that elicit responses different from the responses to the native antigen are called **altered peptide ligands** (APLs). The qualitatively and quantitatively different responses elicited by these APLs support the idea, mentioned earlier in the chapter, that the outcome of T cell antigen recognition is influenced by the quality of the TCR-antigen interaction. Many weak agonists and antagonist peptides have a more rapid dissociation from the TCR than do the native peptides. This result is consistent with the idea that the duration of TCR engagement by antigen may be a major determinant of the T cell response.

APLs are important for two main reasons. First, they represent a mechanism by which T cell activation can be regulated. It is possible, for example, that microbes produce altered versions of their own antigens that inhibit host immune responses to the microbe. APLs could theoretically be administered to patients to inhibit unwanted immune responses against defined antigens (e.g., in autoimmune diseases in which the pathogenic self antigen is known). Second, the analysis of intracellular biochemical events induced by APLs has provided further insights into how TCR signaling pathways work. There is already evidence that some APLs cause distinct patterns of tyrosine phosphorylation of the TCR-associated ζ chains and induce lower sustained levels of intracellular calcium than do the wild-type peptides from which they were derived.

Summary

- T cell responses are initiated by signals provided by clustering of TCR complexes through recognition of antigen on the surface of an APC and through signals provided by costimulators expressed on APCs. The response of the T cell varies with the nature of the antigen, the APC that presents the antigen, and the stage of maturation and differentiation of the T cells.

- The best defined costimulators for T cells are the B7 proteins, which are recognized by CD28 on T cells. B7 molecules are expressed on professional APCs, and their expression is enhanced by microbes and by cytokines produced during innate immune reactions to microbes. The requirement for costimulation, especially for activation of naive T cells, ensures that T cell responses are induced in lymphoid organs, where professional APCs are concentrated, and against microbes and microbial products.

- T cell responses to antigen and costimulators include synthesis of cytokines and effector molecules, cellular proliferation, differentiation into effector and memory cells, and performance of effector functions.

- Clustering of TCRs by antigen recognition triggers intracellular signaling pathways that result in the production of transcription factors, which activate a variety of genes in T cells. Intracellular signaling may be divided into membrane events, cytoplasmic signaling pathways, and nuclear transcription of genes. Membrane events include the recruitment and activation of protein tyrosine kinases into the TCR complex; the phosphorylation of TCR complex constituents (e.g., the ζ chains); and the recruitment of protein tyrosine kinases, especially ZAP-70, and adapter proteins. Cytoplasmic signaling pathways lead to the activation of effector enzymes, such as the kinases ERK, JNK, and PKC, and the phosphatase calcineurin. These enzymes contribute to the activation of transcription factors such as NFAT, AP-1, and NF-κB, which function to enhance gene expression in antigen-stimulated T cells.

- Some peptides in which the TCR contact residues are altered may induce partial T cell responses or inhibit T cell activation by poorly understood biochemical mechanisms.

Selected Readings

Acuto O, and D Cantrell. T cell activation and the cytoskeleton. Annual Review of Immunology 18:165–184, 2000.

Alegre ML, KA Frauwirth, and CB Thompson. T cell regulation by CD28 and CTLA-4. Nature Immunology Reviews 1:220–228, 2001.

Bromley SK, WR Burack, KG Johnson, K Somersalo, TN Sims, C Sumen, MM Davis, AS Shaw, PM Allen, and ML Dustin. The immunological synapse. Annual Review of Immunology 19:375–396, 2001.

Clements JL, NJ Boerth, JR Lee, and GA Koretzky. Integration of TCR-dependent signaling pathways by adapter proteins. Annual Review of Immunology 17:89–108, 1999.

Coyle AJ, and J-C Gutierrez-Ramos. The expanding B7 superfamily: increasing complexity in costimulatory signals regulating T cell function. Nature Immunology 2:203–209, 2001.

Dustin ML, and JA Cooper. The immunological synapse and the actin cytoskeleton: molecular hardware for T cell signaling. Nature Immunology 1:23–29, 2000.

Germain RN, and I Stefanova. The dynamics of T cell receptor signaling: complex orchestration and the key roles of tempo and cooperation. Annual Review of Immunology 19:467–522, 1999.

Ghosh S, JJ May, and EB Kopp. NF-κB and Rel proteins: evolutionarily conserved mediators of immune responses. Annual Review of Immunology 16:225–260, 1998.

Healy JI, and CC Goodnow. Positive vs negative signaling by lymphocyte antigen receptors. Annual Review of Immunology 16:645–670, 1998.

Jameson SC. Maintaining the norm: T Cell homeostasis. Nature Reviews Immunology 2:547–556, 2002.

Jenkins MK, A Khoruts, E Ingulli, DL Mueller, SJ McSorley, RL Reinhardt, A Itano, and KA Pape. In vivo activation of antigen-specific CD4 T cells. Annual Review of Immunology 19:23–45, 2001.

Kaech SM, EJ Wherry, and R Ahmed. Effector and memory T cell differentiation: implications for vaccine development. Nature Reviews Immunology 2:251–262, 2002.

Karin M, Z Liu, and E Zendi. AP-1 function and regulation. Current Opinion in Cell Biology 9:240–246, 1997.

Klenerman P, V Cerundolo, and PR Dunbar. Tracking T cells with tetramers: new tales from new tools. Nature Reviews Immunology 2:263–272, 2002.

Lanzavecchia A, and F Sallusto. Dynamics of T lymphocyte responses: intermediates, effectors, and memory cells. Science 290:92–97, 2000.

Lanzavecchia A, and F Sallusto. Antigen decoding by T lymphocytes: from synapses to fate determination. Nature Immunology 2:487–492, 2001.

Marrack P, J Bender, D Hildeman, M Jordan, T Mitchell, M Murakami, A Sakamoto, BC Schaefer, B Swanson, and J Kappler. Homeostasis of αβ TCR+ T cells. Nature Immunology 1:107–111, 2000.

Rao A, C Luo, and PG Hogan. Transcription factors of the NFAT family: regulation and function. Annual Review of Immunology 15:707–747, 1998.

Salomon B, and JA Bluestone. Complexities of CD28/B7: CTLA-4 costimulatory pathways in autoimmunity and transplantation. Annual Review of Immunology 19:225–252, 2001.

Samelson LE. Signal transduction mediated by the T cell antigen receptor: the role of adapter proteins. Annual Reviews of Immunology 20:371–394, 2002.

Sharpe AH, and GJ Freeman. The B7-CD28 superfamily. Nature Reviews Immunology 2:116–126, 2002.

Sloan-Lancaster J, and PM Allen. Altered peptide ligand-induced partial T cell activation: molecular mechanisms and role in T cell biology. Annual Review of Immunology 14:1–27, 1996.

Sprent J, and DF Tough. T cell death and memory. Science 293:245–248, 2001.

Yablonski D, and A Weiss. Mechanisms of signaling by the hematopoietic-specific adapter proteins SLP-76 and LAT and their B cell counterpart BLNK/SLP-65. Advances in Immunology 79:93–128, 2001.

Chapter 9

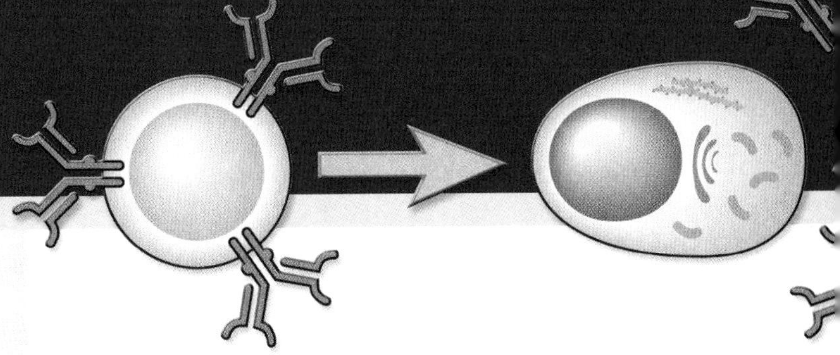

B Cell Activation and Antibody Production

Humoral immunity is mediated by secreted antibodies, which are produced by cells of the B lymphocyte lineage. Antibodies bind to the antigens of extracellular microbes and function to neutralize and eliminate these microbes. The elimination of different types of microbes requires several effector mechanisms, which are mediated by distinct classes, or isotypes, of antibodies. This chapter describes the molecular and cellular events of the humoral immune response, in particular the stimuli that induce B cell growth and differentiation and how these stimuli influence the type of antibody that is produced.

General Features of Humoral Immune Responses

The earliest studies of adaptive immunity were devoted to analyses of serum antibodies produced in response to microbes, toxins, and model antigens. Much of our current understanding of adaptive immune responses and the cellular interactions that take place during such responses has evolved from studies of antibody production. The type and amount of antibodies produced vary according to the type of antigen, involvement of T cells, prior history of antigen exposure, and anatomic site.

- ***The process of activation of B cells and the generation of antibody-producing cells consists of sequential phases*** (Fig. 9–1). As we discussed in Chapter 7, mature antigen-responsive B lymphocytes develop from bone marrow precursors before antigenic stimulation and populate peripheral lymphoid tissues, which are the sites of interaction with foreign antigens. Humoral immune responses are initiated by the recognition of antigens by B lymphocytes specific for each antigen. Antigen binds to the membrane IgM and IgD receptors on naive B cells and activates the cells. B cell activation consists of a series of responses that lead to **proliferation,** resulting in expansion of the clone of antigen-specific cells, and

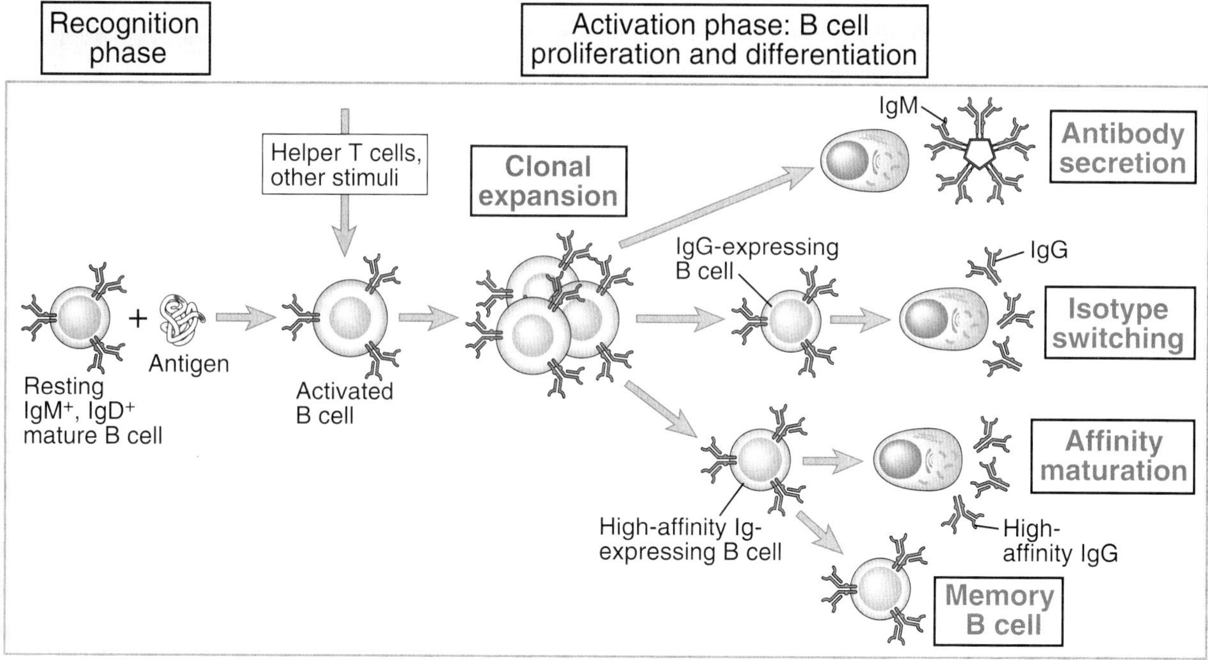

Figure 9–1 Phases of the humoral immune response.
The activation of B cells is initiated by specific recognition of antigens by the surface Ig receptors of the cells. Antigen and other stimuli, including helper T cells, stimulate the proliferation and differentiation of the specific B cell clone. Progeny of the clone may produce IgM or other Ig isotypes (e.g., IgG), may undergo affinity maturation, or may persist as memory cells.

differentiation, resulting in the generation of effector cells that actively secrete antibodies and memory B cells. Some activated B cells begin to produce antibodies other than IgM and IgD; this process is called heavy chain isotype (class) switching. Activated B cells may also produce antibodies that bind to antigens with higher and higher affinities; this process is called affinity maturation.

- ***Antibody responses to protein antigens require CD4⁺ helper T lymphocytes that recognize the antigen and play an essential role in activating B lymphocytes.*** For this reason, proteins are classified as thymus-dependent or T-dependent antigens. The term "helper" T lymphocyte arose from the realization that these cells stimulate, or help, B lymphocytes to produce antibodies. As we shall see later in this chapter, a great deal is known about the mechanisms of action of helper T cells.

- ***Antibody responses to nonprotein antigens, such as polysaccharides and lipids, do not require antigen-specific helper T lymphocytes.*** Therefore, polysaccharide and lipid antigens are called thymus-independent or T-independent (TI) antigens.

- ***Activated B cells differentiate into antibody-secreting cells, some of which continue to produce antibodies for long periods, and into long-lived memory cells*** (Fig. 9–2). Humoral immune responses are initiated in peripheral lymphoid organs, such as the spleen for blood-borne antigens, draining lymph nodes for antigens entering through the skin and other epithelia, and mucosal lymphoid tissues for some inhaled and ingested antigens. Antibodies enter the circulation or the lumens of mucosal organs and mediate their protective effects wherever antigens are present, even though antibody-producing cells remain resident mainly in the secondary lymphoid organs and the bone marrow. Some antibody-secreting cells migrate from the peripheral lymphoid organs to the bone marrow, where they live and produce low levels of antibodies that provide immediate protection on exposure to microbes. Some progeny of activated B cells may differentiate into memory cells, which mount rapid responses to subsequent encounters with the antigen.

- ***Heavy chain isotype switching and affinity maturation are typically seen in helper T cell–dependent humoral immune responses to protein antigens.*** As we shall discuss later, isotype switching is stimulated by helper T cell signals, including the membrane molecule CD40 ligand and cytokines, and affinity maturation is also dependent on T cells, but the signals involved are not as well defined. The humoral immune response is also different at various anatomic sites. For instance, mucosal lymphoid tissues are uniquely adapted to produce high levels of IgA in response to the same antigens that stimulate other antibody isotypes in nonmucosal lymphoid tissues.

- ***Primary and secondary antibody responses to protein antigens differ qualitatively and quantitatively*** (Table 9–1). Primary responses result from the activation of previously unstimulated naive B cells, whereas secondary responses are due to stimu-

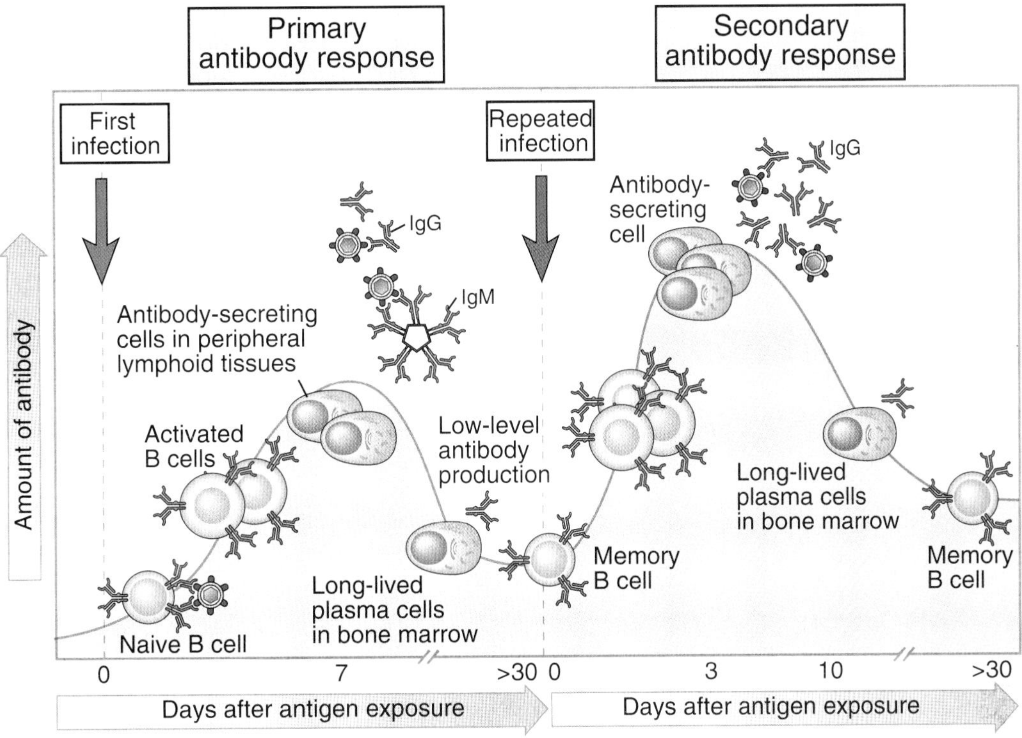

Figure 9–2 Kinetics of primary and secondary humoral immune responses. In a primary immune response, naive B cells are stimulated by antigen, become activated, and differentiate into antibody-secreting cells that produce antibodies specific for the eliciting antigen. Some of the antibody-secreting plasma cells survive in the bone marrow and continue to produce antibodies for long periods. Long-lived memory B cells are also generated during the primary response. A secondary immune response is elicited when the same antigen stimulates these memory B cells, leading to more rapid proliferation and differentiation and production of greater quantities of specific antibody than are produced in the primary response.

lation of expanded clones of memory B cells. Therefore, the secondary response develops more rapidly than does the primary response, and larger amounts of antibodies are produced in the secondary response (see Fig. 9–2). Heavy chain isotype switching and affinity maturation also increase with repeated exposures to protein antigens.

In the following sections, we first describe how antigens initiate the process of B cell activation. We then discuss the role of helper T cells in B cell responses to protein antigens and the changes in B lymphocyte physiology in response to these signals that occur during the activation phase. We will return to TI antigens at the end of the chapter.

Table 9–1. Features of Primary and Secondary Antibody Responses

Feature	Primary response	Secondary response
Time lag after immunization	Usually 5–10 days	Usually 1–3 days
Peak response	Smaller	Larger
Antibody isotype	Usually IgM > IgG	Relative increase in IgG and, under certain situations, in IgA or IgE
Antibody affinity	Lower average affinity, more variable	Higher average affinity (affinity maturation)
Induced by	All immunogens	Only protein antigens
Required immunization	Relatively high doses of antigens, optimally with adjuvants (for protein antigens)	Low doses of antigens; adjuvants may not be necessary

Antigen Recognition and Antigen-Induced B Cell Activation

The activation of antigen-specific B lymphocytes is initiated by the binding of antigen to membrane immunoglobulin (Ig) molecules, which are the antigen receptors of mature B cells. Naive B cells reside in and circulate through the follicles of peripheral lymphoid organs (the spleen, lymph nodes, and mucosal lymphoid tissues). These mature, naive B cells survive for limited periods until they encounter antigen (see Chapter 2). Antigens that enter these organs through the blood or lymph are located by specific B cells and bind to the antigen receptors of the B cells. The B lymphocyte antigen receptor serves two key roles in B cell activation. First, antigen-induced clustering of receptors delivers biochemical signals to the B cells that initiate the process of activation. Second, the receptor binds antigen and internalizes it into endosomal vesicles, and if the antigen is a protein, it is processed into peptides that are presented on the B cell surface for recognition by helper T cells. This antigen-presenting function of B cells will be discussed later. The biochemical and functional responses of B cells have been analyzed by a variety of methods (Box 9–1).

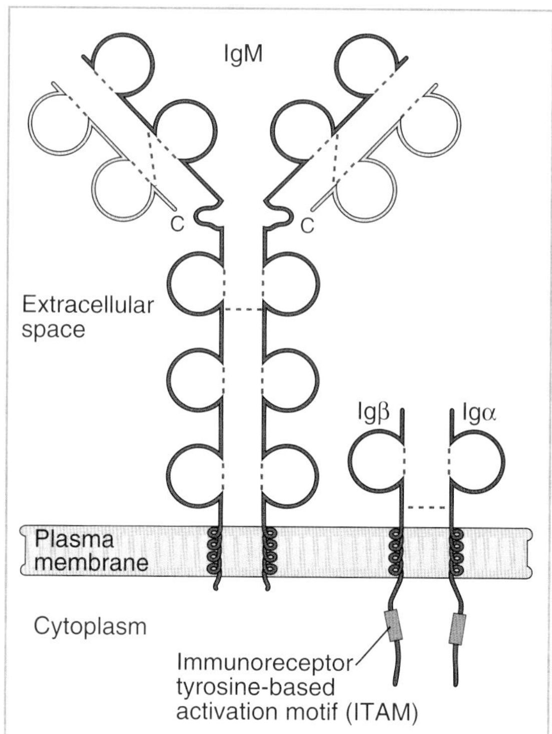

Figure 9–3 B cell antigen receptor complex. Membrane IgM (and IgD) on the surface of mature B cells is associated with the invariant Igα and Igβ molecules, which contain ITAMs in their cytoplasmic tails that mediate signaling functions. Note the similarity to the TCR complex (see Fig. 6–2, Chapter 6).

Signal Transduction by the B Lymphocyte Antigen Receptor Complex

The B cell antigen receptor delivers activating signals to a B cell when two or more receptor molecules are brought together, or cross-linked, by multivalent antigens. Membrane IgM and IgD, the antigen receptors of naive B cells, have short cytoplasmic tails consisting of only three amino acids (lysine, valine, and lysine). These tails are too small to transduce signals generated by the clustering of Ig. Ig-mediated signals are actually transduced by two other molecules, called Igα and Igβ, that are disulfide linked to one another and are expressed in B cells noncovalently associated with membrane Ig (Fig. 9–3). Igα and Igβ are also required for the surface expression of membrane Ig molecules and together with membrane Ig form the **B cell receptor (BCR) complex.** Thus, Igα and Igβ serve the same functions in B cells as the CD3 and ζ proteins do in T lymphocytes (see Chapter 6). The cytoplasmic domains of Igα and Igβ contain tyrosine-rich motifs (immunoreceptor tyrosine-based activation motifs, or ITAMs) that are also found in CD3 and ζ proteins and are required for signal transduction. Cross-linking of membrane Ig brings several ITAMs into proximity, and this triggers subsequent signaling events (Fig. 9–4).

The early signaling events initiated by the BCR complex are similar to the events described in TCR complex signaling (see Chapter 8).

- ***Antigen-mediated cross-linking of membrane Ig induces phosphorylation of the tyrosines in the ITAMs of Igα and Igβ.*** Cross-linked Ig receptors enter specialized membrane domains, or lipid rafts, where many adapter proteins and signaling molecules may be concentrated, as in T cells. The phosphorylation of Igα and Igβ is mediated by Src family protein tyrosine kinases such as Lyn, Blk, and Fyn, which are loosely associated with the BCR complex. The tyrosine kinase Syk then binds through its Src homology 2 (SH2) domains to the phosphotyrosine residues of Igα and Igβ. Syk is the B cell equivalent of ZAP-70 in T lymphocytes. Syk is activated when it associates with phosphorylated tyrosines of ITAMs and may itself be phosphorylated on specific tyrosine residues by BCR-associated Src family kinases, leading to further activation.
- ***Syk, and other tyrosine kinases, activate numerous downstream signaling pathways that are regulated by adapter proteins.*** In B cells, the adapter protein SLP-65 (for SH2-binding leukocyte phosphoprotein of 65 kD, also called BLNK for B cell linker protein) plays a central role in the formation of a scaffold of other adapter proteins, guanine nucleotide exchange proteins, and other enzymes, including phospholipase C and the Btk and Itk tyrosine kinases.
- ***The Ras–MAP kinase (mitogen-activated protein kinase) pathway is activated in antigen-stimulated B cells.*** The GTP/GDP exchange factor Sos is recruited to the SLP-65 complex, probably through the binding of the Grb-2 adapter protein; the subsequent activation of Ras proceeds in the same manner as in T cells (see Fig. 8–10, Chapter 8).
- ***The phosphatidylinositol-specific phospholipase C (PLC) is activated in response to BCR signaling***

BOX 9–1

Assays for B Lymphocyte Activation

It is technically difficult to study the effects of antigens on normal B cells because, as the clonal selection hypothesis predicted, very few lymphocytes in an individual are specific for any one antigen. To examine the effects of antigen binding to B cells, investigators have attempted to isolate antigen-specific B cells from complex populations of normal lymphocytes or to produce cloned B cell lines with defined antigenic specificities. These efforts have met with little success. However, transgenic mice have been developed in which virtually all B cells express a transgenic Ig of known specificity, so that most of the B cells in these mice respond to the same antigen. Another approach to circumventing this problem is to use anti-Ig antibodies as analogues of antigens, with the assumption that anti-Ig will bind to constant (C) regions of membrane Ig molecules on all B cells and will have the same biologic effects as an antigen that binds to the hypervariable regions of membrane Ig molecules on only the antigen-specific B cells. To the extent that precise comparisons are feasible, this assumption appears generally correct, indicating that anti-Ig antibody is a valid model for antigens. Thus, anti-Ig antibody is frequently used as a polyclonal activator of B lymphocytes. The same concept underlies the use of antibodies against framework determinants of TCRs or against receptor-associated CD3 molecules as polyclonal activators of T lymphocytes (see Chapter 8).

Much of our knowledge of B cell activation is based on *in vitro* experiments, in which different stimuli are used to activate B cells and their proliferation and differentiation can be measured accurately. The same assays may be done with B cells recovered from mice exposed to different antigens or with homogeneous B cells expressing transgene-encoded antigen receptors. The most frequently used assays for B cell responses are the following.

ASSAYS FOR B CELL PROLIFERATION The proliferation of B lymphocytes, like that of other cells, is measured *in vitro* by determining the amount of ^{3}H-labeled thymidine incorporated into the replicating DNA of cultured cells. Thymidine incorporation provides a quantitative measure of the rate of DNA synthesis, which is usually directly proportional to the rate of cell division. Cellular proliferation *in vivo* can be measured by injecting the thymidine analogue bromodeoxyuridine (BrdU) into animals and staining cells with anti-BrdU antibody to identify and enumerate nuclei that have incorporated BrdU into their DNA during DNA replication. The same assays may be used to measure the proliferation of T cells (see Box 8–1).

ASSAYS FOR ANTIBODY PRODUCTION Antibody production is measured in two different ways: with assays for cumulative Ig secretion, which measure the amount of Ig that accumulates in the supernatant of cultured lymphocytes or in the serum of an immunized individual; and with single-cell assays, which determine the number of cells in an immune population that secrete Ig of a particular specificity or isotype. The most accurate, quantitative, and widely used techniques for measuring the total amount of Ig in a culture supernatant or serum sample are radioimmunoassay (RIA) and enzyme-linked immunosorbent assay (ELISA), described in Appendix III. By use of antigens bound to solid supports, it is possible to use RIA or ELISA to quantitate the amount of a specific antibody in a sample. In addition, the availability of anti-Ig antibodies that detect Igs of different heavy or light chain classes allows measurement of the quantities of different isotypes in a sample. Other techniques for measuring antibody levels include hemagglutination for antierythrocyte antibodies and complement-dependent lysis for antibodies specific for known cell types. Both assays are based on the demonstration that if the amount of antigen (i.e., cells) is constant, the concentration of antibody determines the amount of antibody bound to cells, and this is reflected in the degree of cell agglutination or subsequent binding of complement and cell lysis. Results from these assays are usually expressed as antibody titers, which are the dilution of the sample giving half-maximal effects or the dilution at which the end point of the assay is reached.

A single-cell assay for antibody secretion that has been used in the past is the hemolytic plaque assay, in which the antigen is either an erythrocyte protein or a molecule covalently coupled to an erythrocyte surface. Such erythrocytes serve as "indicator cells." They are mixed with lymphocytes, among which are the specific antibody-producing cells, and are incubated in a semisolid supporting medium to allow secreted antibody to bind to the erythrocyte surface. If the antibody binds complement avidly, the subsequent addition of complement leads to lysis of the indicator cells that are coated with specific antibody. As a result, clear zones of lysis, called plaques, are formed around individual B lymphocytes or plasma cells that secrete the specific antibody. These antibody-secreting cells are also called plaque-forming cells. This assay can also be used to detect antibodies that do not fix complement by incorporating into the medium a complement-binding anti-Ig antibody that will coat indicator cells to which the specific Ig is bound first. Another technique for measuring the number of antibody-secreting cells is the ELISPOT assay. In this method, antigen is bound to the bottom of a well, antibody-secreting cells are added, and antibodies that have been secreted and are bound to the antigen are detected by an enzyme-linked anti-Ig antibody, as in an ELISA, in a semisolid medium. Each spot represents the location of an antibody-secreting cell. Single-cell assays provide a measure of the numbers of Ig-secreting cells, but they cannot accurately quantitate the amount of Ig secreted by each cell or by the total population.

and also activates downstream signaling pathways. (In B cells, the dominant isoform of PLC is the γ2 isoform, whereas T cells express the γ1 isoform of the enzyme. There are no known functional differences between these isoforms.) PLC becomes active when it binds to SLP-65 and is phosphorylated by Syk and Btk. Active PLC breaks down membrane phosphatidylinositol bisphosphate (PIP_2) to yield the signaling intermediates inositol trisphosphate (IP_3) and diacylglycerol (DAG). IP_3 mobilizes

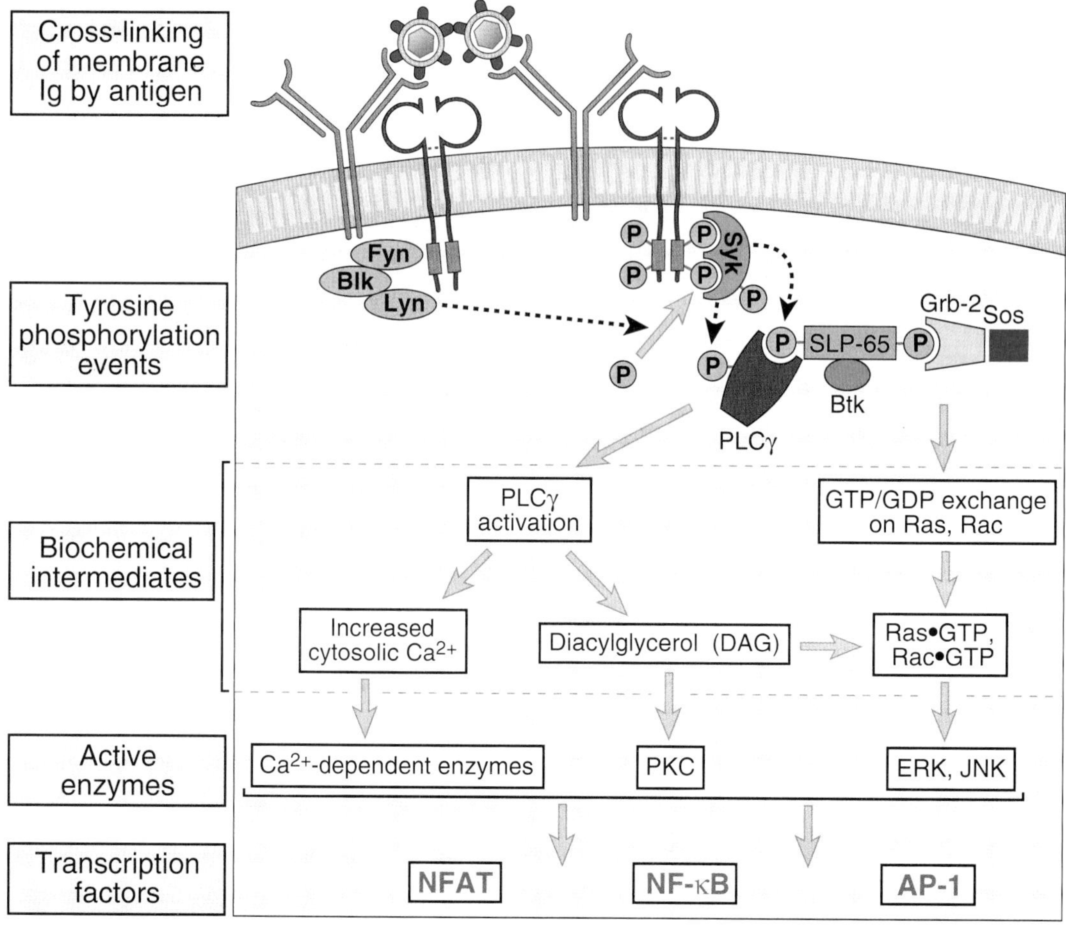

Figure 9–4 Signal transduction by the BCR complex. Antigen-induced cross-linking of membrane Ig on B cells leads to clustering of the Igα and Igβ molecules and tyrosine phosphorylation of the ITAMs in the cytoplasmic tails of these molecules. This leads to docking of Syk and subsequent tyrosine phosphorylation events as depicted. Several signaling cascades follow these events, as shown, leading to the activation of several transcription factors. These signal transduction pathways are similar to those described in T cells (Chapter 8).

calcium from intracellular stores, leading to a rapid elevation of cytoplasmic calcium, which may be augmented by an influx of calcium from the extracellular milieu. In the presence of calcium, DAG activates some isoforms of protein kinase C, which phosphorylate other proteins on serine/threonine residues.

These signaling cascades ultimately activate transcription factors that induce the expression of genes whose products are required for functional activation of B cells. Some of the transcription factors that are known to be activated by antigen receptor–mediated signal transduction in B cells are Fos, JunB, and nuclear factor κB (NF-κB). Various transcription factors are involved in stimulating proliferation of B cells and their differentiation into antibody-secreting cells.

As in T cells, our knowledge of the antigen-induced signaling pathways in B cells and their links with subsequent functional responses is incomplete. We have described some of these pathways to illustrate the main features, but others may play important roles in B cell activation. The same signaling pathways are used by membrane IgM and IgD on naive B cells and by IgG, IgA, and IgE on B cells that have undergone isotype switching because all these membrane isotypes appear to associate with Igα and Igβ. Also, other surface molecules, including complement protein receptors and Fc receptors, augment or inhibit signals transduced by the antigen receptors, as we will discuss shortly.

Second Signals for B Cells Provided by Complement Receptors

The activation of B cells requires, in addition to antigen, signals that are provided by complement proteins. The complement system consists of a collection of plasma proteins that are activated either by binding to antigen-complexed antibody molecules (the classical pathway) or by binding directly to some polysaccharides and microbial surfaces in the absence of antibodies (the alternative and lectin pathways) (see Chapter 14). Thus, microbes may activate the complement system directly, during innate immune responses, or after the binding of antibodies. Protein antigens may be bound by preexisting antibodies or by antibodies produced early in the response, and these antigen-antibody complexes activate complement by the classical pathway. Complement activation results in the proteolytic cleavage of complement proteins. The key component of the system is a protein called C3, and its cleavage results in the production of a molecule called C3b that binds covalently to the microbe or antigen-antibody complex. C3b is further degraded into a fragment called C3d, which remains bound to the microbial surface. B lymphocytes express a receptor for C3d that is called the type 2 complement receptor (CR2, or CD21). The complex of C3d and antigen or C3d and antigen-antibody complex binds to B cells, with the membrane Ig recognizing antigen and CR2 recognizing the bound C3d (Fig. 9–5). CR2 is expressed on mature B cells as a complex with two other membrane proteins, CD19 and CD81 (also called TAPA-1). The CR2-CD19-CD81 complex is often called the B cell coreceptor complex because CR2 binds to antigens through attached C3d at the same time that membrane Ig binds directly to the antigen. Binding of C3d to the B cell complement receptor brings CD19 into proximity of BCR-associated kinases, and the cytoplasmic tail of CD19 rapidly becomes phosphorylated. The phosphorylated CD19 activates several signaling pathways, notably one dependent on the enzyme PI-3 kinase, that augment the signaling pathways initiated by antigen binding to membrane Ig. In addition, Src family kinases linked to CD21 may phosphorylate ITAMs and augment BCR signaling. As a result, the response of the B cell is greatly enhanced.

The importance of the complement system in humoral immune responses has been established by several experiments.

- If C3d is covalently attached to a protein antigen, the modified antigen is about 1000-fold more immunogenic than the native antigen.
- Knockout of the C3, CR2, or CD19 gene in mice results in defects in antibody production.

The requirement for C3d as the second signal for B cell activation ensures that B cell responses will most likely occur when microbes and antigens that activate complement are encountered. It also provides an amplification mechanism for humoral immune responses because antibodies are able to activate complement and lead to more B cell stimulation. This role of complement is analogous to the idea, introduced in our discussion of T cell activation, that antigen is the first signal for activation and that costimulators, which are expressed in response to microbes, provide second signals (see Chapter 8). As we will see later, the complement system enhances antibody production not only by CR2-mediated B cell activation but also by promoting the display of antigens in germinal centers.

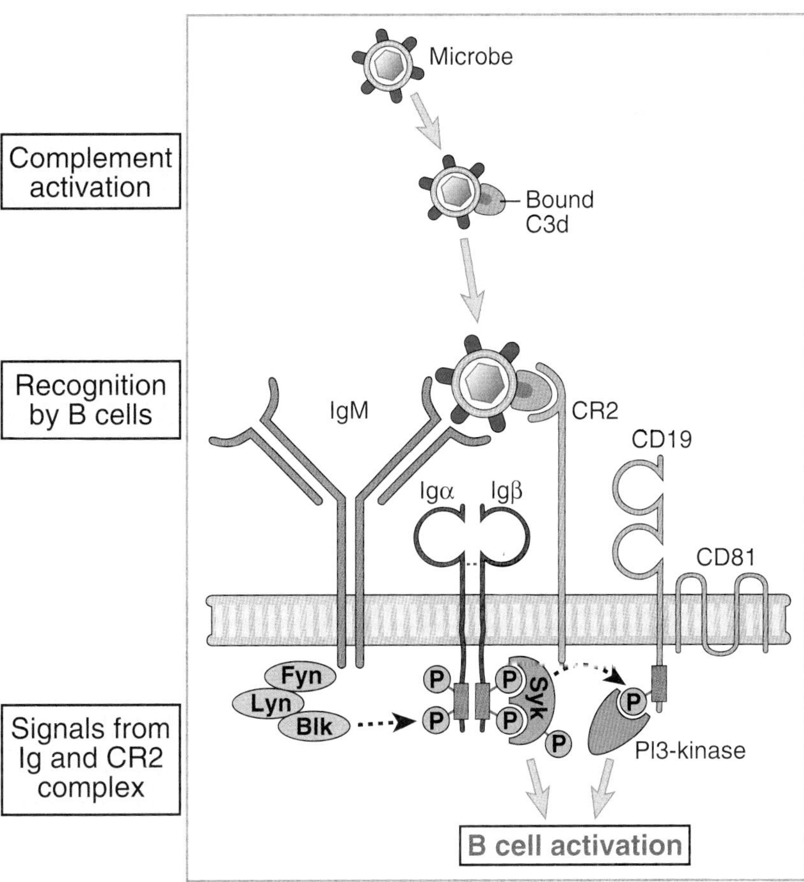

Figure 9–5 Role of complement in B cell activation.

B cells express a complex of the CR2 complement receptor, CD19, and CD81. Microbial antigens that have bound the complement fragment C3d can simultaneously engage both the CR2 molecule and the membrane Ig on the surface of a B cell. This leads to the initiation of signaling cascades from both the BCR complex and the CR2 complex, because of which the response to C3d-antigen complexes is greatly enhanced compared with the response to antigen alone.

Functional Responses of B Cells to Antigen Recognition

The early cellular events that are induced by antigen-mediated cross-linking of the BCR complex initiate B cell proliferation and differentiation and prepare the cells for subsequent interactions with helper T cells (Fig. 9–6). Antigen recognition stimulates the entry of previously resting cells into the G_1 stage of the cell cycle, accompanied by increases in cell size, cytoplasmic RNA, and biosynthetic organelles such as ribosomes. The survival of the B cells is enhanced as a result of the induction of various anti-apoptotic genes. The activated B cells also show low levels of proliferation and antibody secretion. As we will discuss later, although proliferation and Ig secretion can be induced in the absence of T cell help, they are greatly enhanced by signals from helper T cells. Activated B cells show increased expression of class II major histocompatibility complex (MHC) molecules and costimulators, first B7-2 (CD86) and later B7-1 (CD80), because of which antigen-stimulated B cells are more efficient activators of helper T lymphocytes than are naive B cells. The expression of receptors for several T cell–derived cytokines is also increased, which enables antigen-specific B lymphocytes to respond to T cell help. At the same time, the B cells change their expression of chemokine receptors, which enables them to migrate toward and interact with helper T cells (discussed in more detail later).

The importance of signaling by the BCR complex for the subsequent responses of the cells may vary with the nature of the antigen. Most TI antigens, such as polysaccharides and glycolipids, are polymers that display multiple identical epitopes in a polyvalent array on each molecule. Therefore, such antigens effectively cross-link B cell antigen receptors and initiate responses even though they are not recognized by helper T lymphocytes. In contrast, many naturally occurring globular protein antigens express only one copy of each epitope per molecule in their native conformation. Therefore, such protein antigens cannot simultaneously bind to and cross-link two Ig molecules and are unlikely to deliver activating signals to the B cells. However, such proteins may cross-link antigen receptors if they form aggregates, and this can happen if they become bound to previously produced antibodies. Importantly, protein antigens recruit T cell help, and helper T cells and their products are potent stimulators of B lymphocyte proliferation and differentiation. Therefore, protein antigens may need to trigger minimal or even no signals by the BCR complex to induce humoral immune responses. In such responses, a major function of membrane Ig may be to bind and internalize the antigen for subsequent presentation to helper T cells (discussed later).

Helper T Cell–Dependent Antibody Responses to Protein Antigens

Antibody responses to protein antigens require recognition of the antigen by helper T cells and cooperation between the antigen-specific B and T lymphocytes. The helper function of T lymphocytes was discovered by experiments done in the late 1960s, even before the

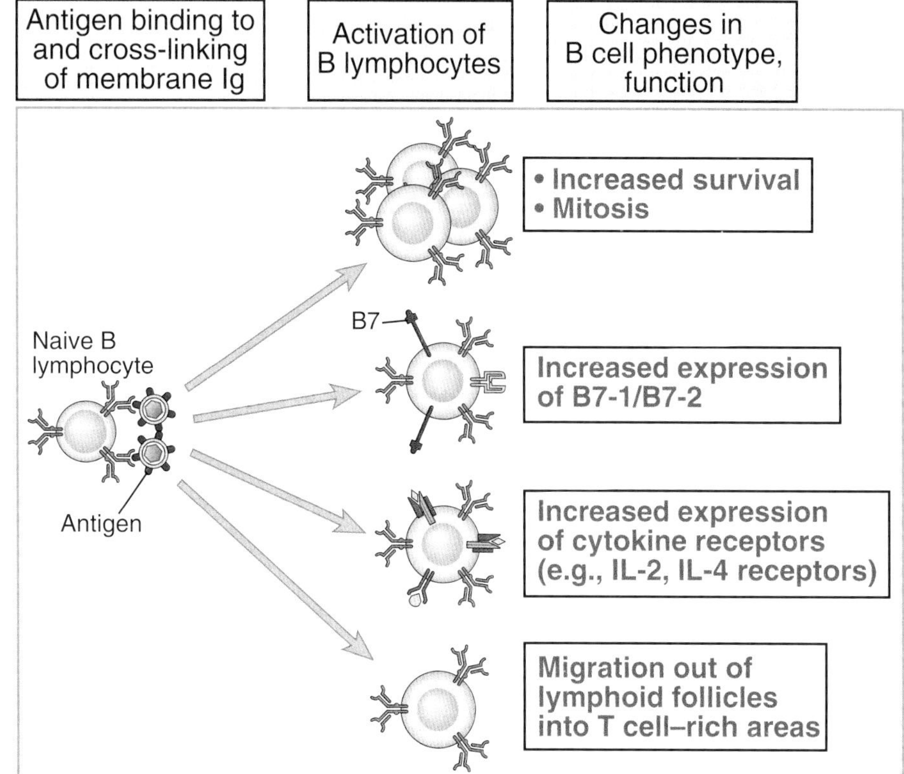

Figure 9–6 Functional responses induced by antigen-mediated cross-linking of the BCR complex. Antigen-mediated cross-linking of the B cell antigen receptor induces several cellular responses, including mitosis, expression of new surface molecules, including costimulators and cytokine receptors, and altered migration of the cells.

classification of lymphocytes into T and B cell subsets was established. Subsequent studies established that most helper T cells are $CD4^{+}CD8^{-}$ and recognize peptide antigens presented by class II MHC molecules.

- If mouse bone marrow lymphocytes, which include mature B cells but few or no mature T cells, are adoptively transferred into irradiated syngeneic recipients, they do not produce specific antibody on immunization with sheep red blood cells, a model protein antigen. If, however, mature thymocytes or thoracic duct lymphocytes (which include T lymphocytes but few B cells) are transferred at the same time, antibody responses develop after immunization (Table 9–2).
- Purified B cells proliferate and differentiate *in vitro* in response to protein antigens only if helper T lymphocytes are also present (see Table 9–2).
- Humans or knockout mice with reduced numbers of $CD4^{+}$ T cells show defective antibody responses to protein antigens.

Helper T lymphocytes stimulate B cell clonal expansion, isotype switching, affinity maturation, and differentiation into memory B cells (see Fig. 9–1). Different phases of T-dependent B cell activation occur in different anatomic regions within peripheral lymphoid organs (Fig. 9–7). The early phase occurs at the border of T cell–rich zones and primary follicles and results in B cell proliferation, initial antibody secretion, and some isotype (class) switching. The late phase of T-dependent humoral immune responses takes place in the specialized microenvironment of the germinal centers within lymphoid follicles and results in affinity maturation, memory B cell generation, and more isotype switching. The molecular and anatomic details of each of the early and late events in T-dependent B cell responses are described next.

Early Events in T Cell–Dependent Antibody Responses: T-B Cell Interaction, B Cell Proliferation, Antibody Secretion, and Isotype Switching

The interaction between helper T cells and B lymphocytes sequentially involves antigen-induced activation of the two cell types, physical contact between the cells, antigen presentation by B cells to differentiated helper T cells, activation of the helper T cells, and expression of membrane and secreted molecules by the helper T cells that bind to and activate the B cells. We have described the initial activation of T cells by antigen in Chapter 8 and of B cells earlier in this chapter. Here we describe the subsequent events in helper T cell–dependent B cell responses.

Table 9–2. Identification of a Role of Helper T Cells in Antibody Responses to Protein Antigens

Adoptive transfer (cells transferred into irradiated recipient)			
Source of B cells	Source of T cells	Antigen	Anti-SRBC antibody-producing cells in spleen
Bone marrow cells	None	SRBC	–
None	Thoracic duct cells	SRBC	–
Bone marrow cells	Thoracic duct cells	SRBC	+
Bone marrow cells	Thoracic duct cells	—	–

Cell culture		
Cells cultured	Antigen	Anti-SRBC antibody-producing cells in culture
Unfractionated spleen cells	SRBC	+
Splenic B cells	SRBC	–
Splenic T cells	SRBC	–
Splenic B cells and T cells	SRBC	+
Splenic B cells and T cells	—	–

Abbreviations: SRBC, sheep red blood cells.

Mouse B lymphocytes by themselves do not produce antibody against a T cell–dependent antigen, SRBC, *in vivo* (adoptive transfer) or *in vitro* (cell culture). The addition of T cells allows the B cells to respond to SRBC. A response does not occur in the absence of antigen.

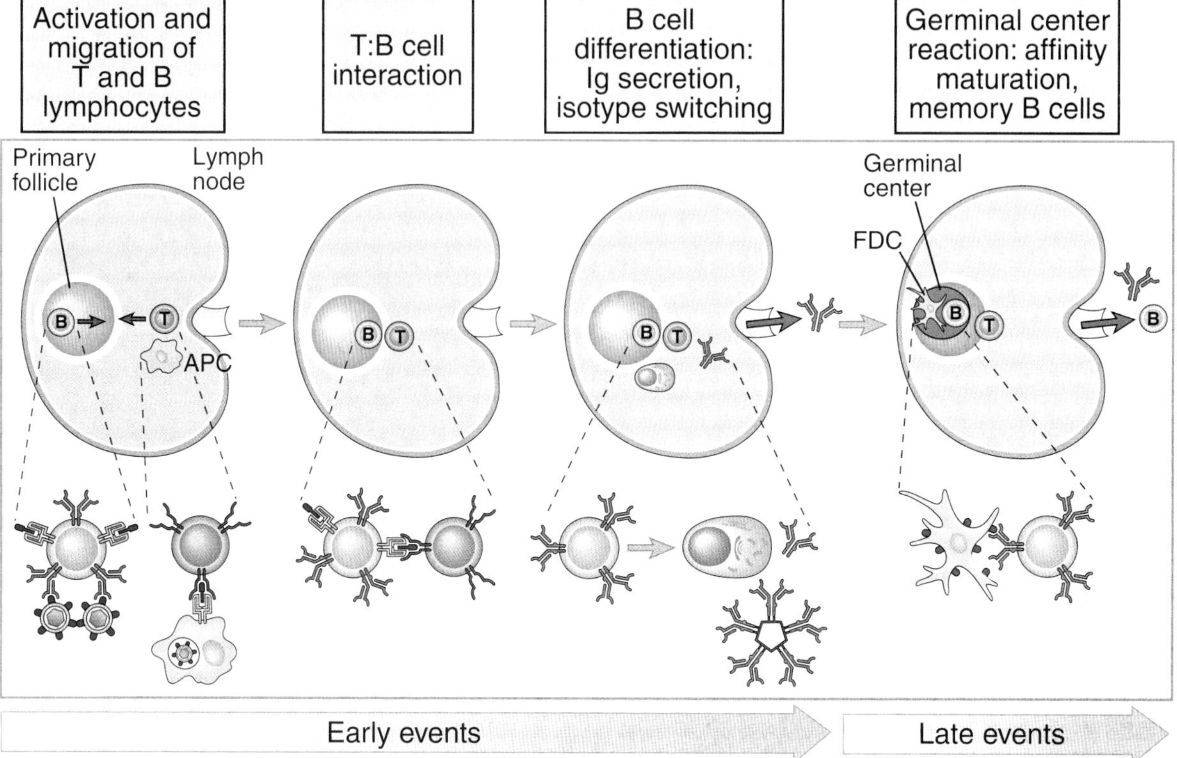

Figure 9–7 Early and late events in humoral immune responses to T cell–dependent protein antigens.

Immune responses are initiated by the recognition of antigens by B cells and helper T cells. The activated lymphocytes migrate toward one another and interact, resulting in B cell proliferation, differentiation into antibody-secreting cells, and early isotype switching. The late events occur in germinal centers and include affinity maturation of the response and additional isotype switching. APC, antigen-presenting cell; FDC, follicular dendritic cell.

Antigen-Induced Migration of B Cells and Helper T Cells

Protein antigens are recognized by specific B and T lymphocytes in peripheral lymphoid organs, and the activated cell populations come together in these organs to initiate humoral immune responses. The frequency of naive B cells or T cells with a particular antigen specificity is as low as 1 in 10^5 to 10^6, and even after the cells respond to antigen, they are rare in lymphoid organs. Therefore, it may seem highly unlikely that the necessary cells and antigen will all be in the right place at the same time. This problem is solved by the regulated movement of lymphocytes in lymphoid organs. Naive B and T cells are anatomically segregated in lymphoid organs (see Chapter 2) and are induced to migrate toward one another after activation by antigen, ensuring that the cells come together only when they need to. Within 1 or 2 days after antigen administration, naive $CD4^+$ T lymphocytes recognize antigens presented by professional antigen-presenting cells (APCs), such as dendritic cells, in the T cell zones of the lymphoid organs. The activated T cells reduce their expression of CCR7, the receptor that responds to chemokines produced in the T cell zones, and begin to leave these zones. At the same time, B lymphocytes recognize antigens in the follicles and are activated. The B cells increase expression of CCR7, the chemokine receptor that promotes migration of cells into the T cell zones of lymphoid organs (see Chapter 2). As a result, antigen-stimulated B cells begin to move out of the follicles toward the T cell zones. The initial encounters between antigen-stimulated B and T lymphocytes occur at the interface of the follicles and the T cell zones (Fig. 9–8). The activated helper T cells express surface molecules and secrete cytokines, discussed in detail later, that stimulate B cells to proliferate and differentiate into antibody-secreting cells. Thus, by 3 to 7 days after antigen exposure, antibody-producing B cells are found close to activated T lymphocytes.

A fundamental feature of T cell–B cell interactions is that the lymphocytes that interact with each other are the ones that have been stimulated by the antigen, because antigen recognition induces many of the reactions that promote these cellular interactions. This feature ensures that the ensuing response is specific for the eliciting antigen. The T cell–B cell interaction is called a cognate interaction because it is dependent on the specific recognition of antigen and several other surface molecules on the two cells. In the following section, we describe the sequential events in T cell–B cell interactions and the mechanisms by which helper T cells stimulate B lymphocytes.

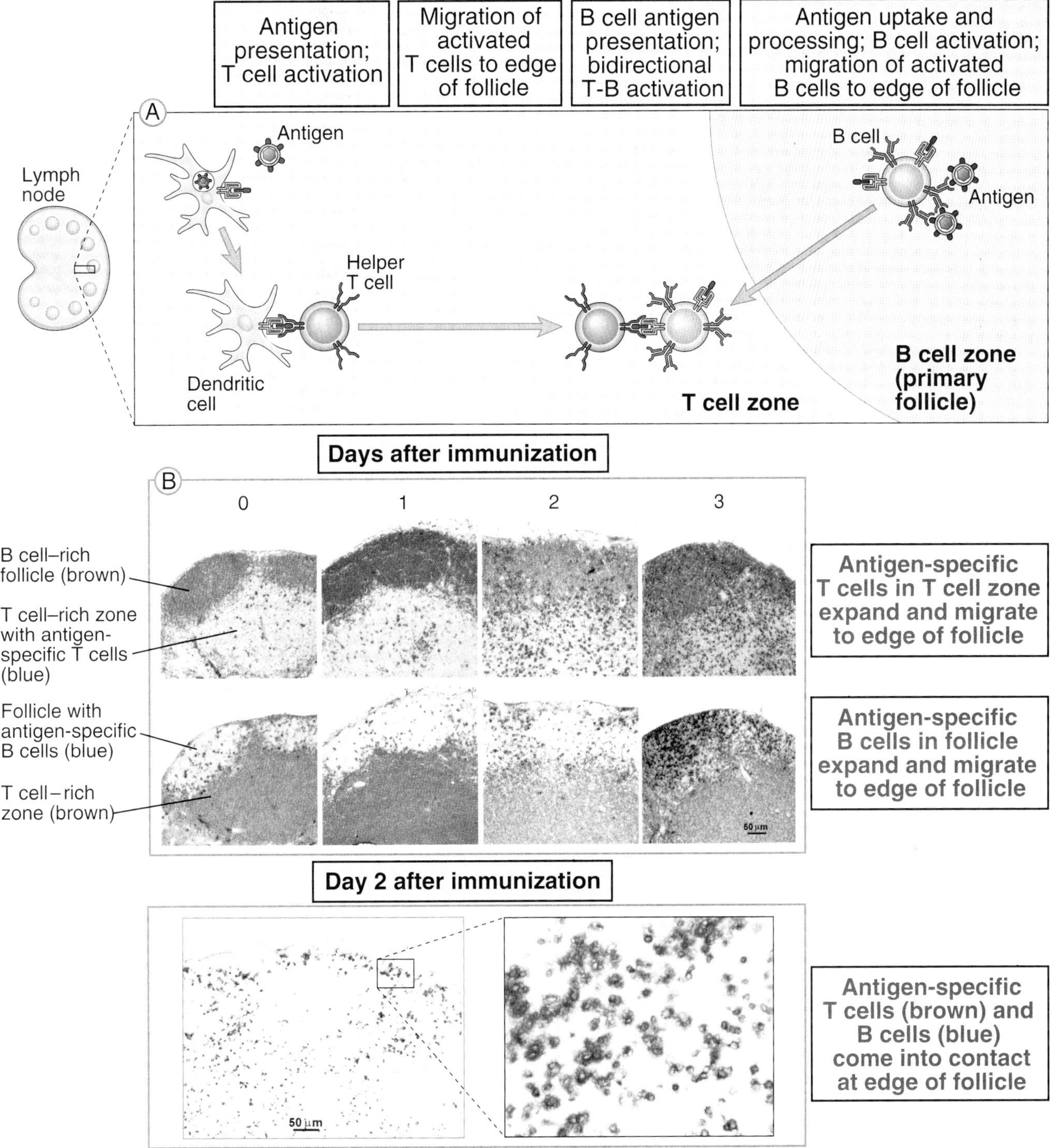

Figure 9–8 Migration and interactions of B cells and helper T cells.

A. The initiation of humoral immune responses to protein antigens in lymph nodes is shown schematically. Antigen-activated helper T cells and B cells move toward one another and make contact adjacent to the edge of primary follicles. In this location, the B cell presents antigen to the T cell, and the B cell receives activating signals from the T cell.

B. An immunohistochemical analysis of antigen-dependent T cell–B cell interactions in a lymph node is shown. In this experiment, T cells expressing a TCR specific for the protein antigen ovalbumin and B cells specific for the protein hen egg lysozyme were adoptively transferred into normal mice, and the mice were immunized with a conjugate of ovalbumin–hen egg lysozyme. (The T cells and B cells were obtained from TCR and Ig transgenic mice, respectively. See Appendix III for a description of antigen receptor transgenic mice.) The locations of the antigen-specific T cells and B cells in draining lymph nodes were followed after immunization with use of antibodies specific for the cell populations and two-color immunohistochemistry. (Adapted from Garside P, E Ingulli, RR Merica, JG Johnson, RJ Noelle, and MK Jenkins. Visualization of specific B and T lymphocyte interactions in the lymph node. Science 281:96–99, 1998. Copyright 1998. American Association for the Advancement of Science.)

Presentation of Protein Antigens by B Lymphocytes to Helper T Cells

Antigen-specific B lymphocytes bind the native antigen to membrane Ig molecules, internalize and process it in endosomal vesicles, and present on their surfaces peptide fragments of the antigen complexed with class II MHC molecules (Fig. 9–9). Thus, the B cells themselves function as APCs in humoral immune responses to protein antigens. The peptide-MHC complexes can then be recognized by specific CD4$^+$ helper T lymphocytes.

Analysis of antibody responses to **hapten-carrier conjugates** demonstrates how antigen presentation by B lymphocytes contributes to the development of humoral immune responses. Haptens, such as dinitrophenol, are small chemicals that can be bound by B cell membrane Ig and by secreted antibodies but are not immunogenic "by themselves. If, however, the haptens are coupled to proteins, which serve as carriers, the conjugates are able to induce antibody responses against the haptens. There are three important characteristics of antihapten antibody responses to hapten-protein conjugates. First, such responses require both hapten-specific B cells and protein (carrier)–specific helper T cells. Second, to stimulate a response, the hapten and carrier portions have to be physically linked and cannot be administered separately. Third, the interaction is class II MHC restricted (i.e., the helper T cells cooperate only with B lymphocytes that express class II MHC molecules recognized as self by the T cells). All these features of antibody responses to hapten-protein conjugates can be explained by the antigen-presenting functions of B lymphocytes. Hapten-specific B cells bind the antigen through the hapten determinant, endocytose the hapten-carrier conjugate, and present peptides derived from the carrier protein to carrier-specific helper T lymphocytes. Thus, the two cooperating lymphocytes recognize different epitopes of the same complex antigen. The hapten is responsible for efficient carrier uptake, which explains why hapten and carrier must be physically linked. The requirement for MHC-associated antigen presentation for T cell activation accounts for the MHC restriction of T cell–B cell interactions.

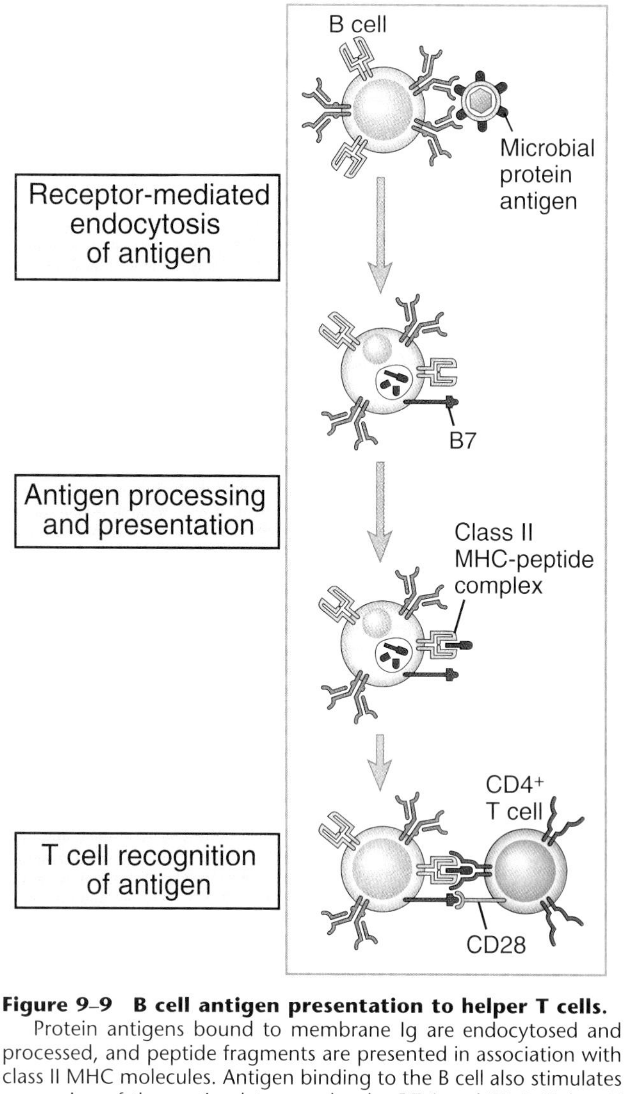

Figure 9–9 B cell antigen presentation to helper T cells. Protein antigens bound to membrane Ig are endocytosed and processed, and peptide fragments are presented in association with class II MHC molecules. Antigen binding to the B cell also stimulates expression of the costimulatory molecules B7-1 and B7-2. Helper T cells recognize the MHC-peptide complexes and costimulators and are activated to then stimulate B cell responses.

The membrane Ig of B cells is a high-affinity receptor for antigen that can efficiently internalize that antigen by receptor-mediated endocytosis and deliver the antigen to the endosomal compartment where proteins are processed and peptides bind to class II MHC molecules (see Fig. 9–9). The characteristics of humoral responses elucidated for hapten-carrier conjugates apply to all protein antigens in which one intrinsic determinant, usually a native conformational determinant, is recognized by B cells (and is, therefore, analogous to the hapten) and another determinant, in the form of a class II–associated peptide, is recognized by helper T cells (and is analogous to the carrier). In any humoral immune response, B cells specific for the antigen that initiates the response are preferentially activated compared with cells that are not specific for the antigen. There are several reasons for this. First, only B cells expressing specific membrane Ig molecules that bind the antigen receive the signals that initiate B cell activation. Second, B cells are able to present the antigen they recognize specifically at 10^4- to 10^6-fold lower concentrations than those of the antigens for which they do not express specific receptors. This efficiency of Ig-mediated antigen internalization and subsequent presentation is because membrane Ig molecules are able to bind the antigen even at low concentrations, and antigens endocytosed with Ig are delivered to the vesicular antigen-processing pathway that is efficient at generating peptide–class II MHC complexes (see Chapter 5). Third, specific antigen recognition induces surface molecules on the B cells and helper T lymphocytes that mediate bidirectional signaling and subsequent activation of the two cell types.

The B cells in T cell–B cell conjugates are exposed to signals delivered by T cell surface molecules and to the highest concentrations of T cell–derived cytokines. Therefore, antigen-specific B lymphocytes are the preferential recipients of T cell help and are stimulated to proliferate and differentiate. The antibodies that are subsequently secreted are specific for conformational determinants of the antigen because membrane Ig on B cells is capable of binding conformational epitopes of native antigens. This feature of B cell antigen recognition determines the fine specificity of the antibody response and is independent of the fact that helper T cells recognize only linear epitopes of processed peptides. In fact, a single B lymphocyte that binds and endocytoses a protein may present multiple different peptides complexed with class II MHC molecules to different helper T cells, but the resultant antibody response remains specific for the native protein.

Antigen binding to membrane Ig enhances the expression of costimulators that increase the ability of the B lymphocyte to activate helper T cells. This occurs at the same time that antigen is being processed and presented by the B lymphocytes (see Fig. 9–9). The principal costimulators that are expressed on activated B cells are B7-2 and B7-1, both of which bind to CD28 on the T cell (see Chapter 8). Helper T cells can then recognize peptide-MHC complexes (signal 1) and costimulators (signal 2) and are stimulated to perform their effector function, which is to promote B cell growth and differentiation.

Helper T Cell–Mediated Activation of B Lymphocytes: The Role of CD40:CD40 Ligand Interactions and Cytokines

Helper T cells activated by antigen and B7 costimulation express a surface molecule called CD40 ligand (CD40L) that engages its receptor, CD40, on the B cells that are presenting antigen, and this interaction stimulates B cell proliferation and differentiation (Fig. 9–10). The role of this ligand-receptor pair in humoral immune responses was defined by a series of experiments.

- The helper function of T lymphocytes cannot be replaced *in vitro* by their secreted products (cytokines), indicating a need for direct T cell–B cell contact.
- If helper T cells are first activated with antigen, chemically fixed to render them incapable of producing cytokines, and then cocultured with B cells, they are still able to induce proliferation of the B cells (Fig. 9–11). B cell proliferative responses are seen even if the B cells are cultured with purified plasma membranes of activated helper T lymphocytes. This result suggested that the helper function of CD4$^+$ T cells is mediated, at least in part, by T cell membrane proteins.
- Antibodies were generated against helper T cells and examined for their ability to block T cell–dependent B cell activation. One such antibody recognized a membrane protein on activated helper T cells that proved to be the ligand for CD40, a receptor expressed on B cells (see Fig. 9–11).
- Fibroblasts expressing CD40L (by gene transfection) stimulate B cells much as contact with helper T lymphocytes does (see Fig. 9–11).
- CD40 or CD40L gene knockout mice exhibit profound defects in antibody production, isotype switching, affinity maturation, and memory B cell generation in response to protein antigens. Similar abnormalities are found in humans with mutations in the CD40L gene, which results in a disease called the **X-linked hyper-IgM syndrome** (see Chapter 20).

CD40 is a member of a family of cell surface proteins whose prototypes are tumor necrosis factor (TNF) receptors. **CD40L** (CD154) is a T cell membrane protein that is structurally homologous to TNF and Fas

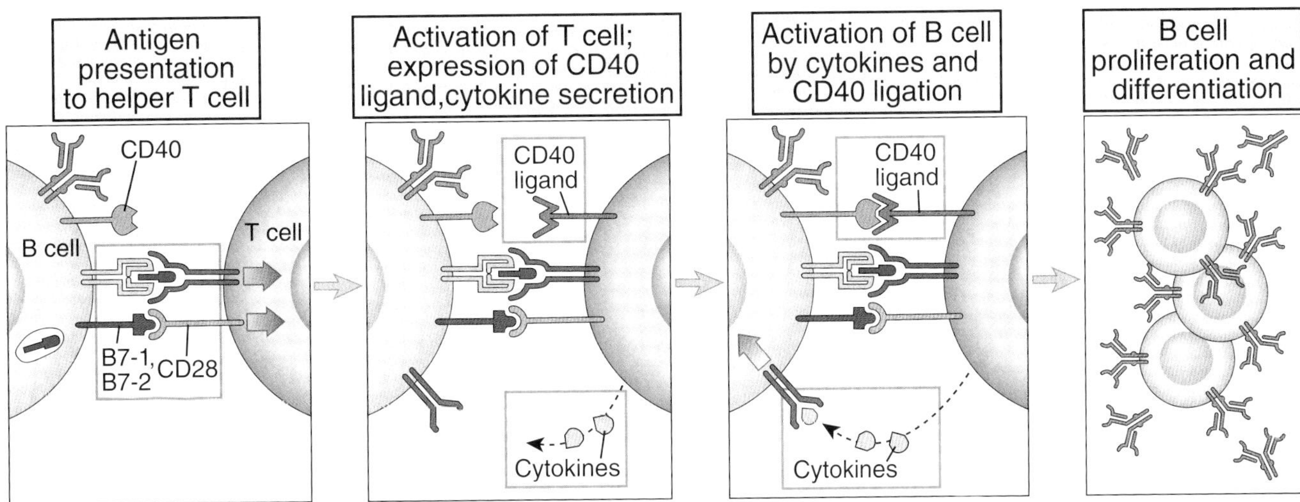

Figure 9–10 Mechanisms of helper T cell–mediated B cell activation.
B cells display processed peptides derived from endocytosed protein antigens and express the costimulators B7-1 and B7-2. Helper T cells recognize the antigen (in the form of peptide-MHC complexes) and the costimulators and are stimulated to express CD40 ligand and to secrete cytokines. CD40 ligand then binds to CD40 on the B cells and initiates B cell proliferation and differentiation. Cytokines bind to cytokine receptors on the B cells and also stimulate B cell responses.

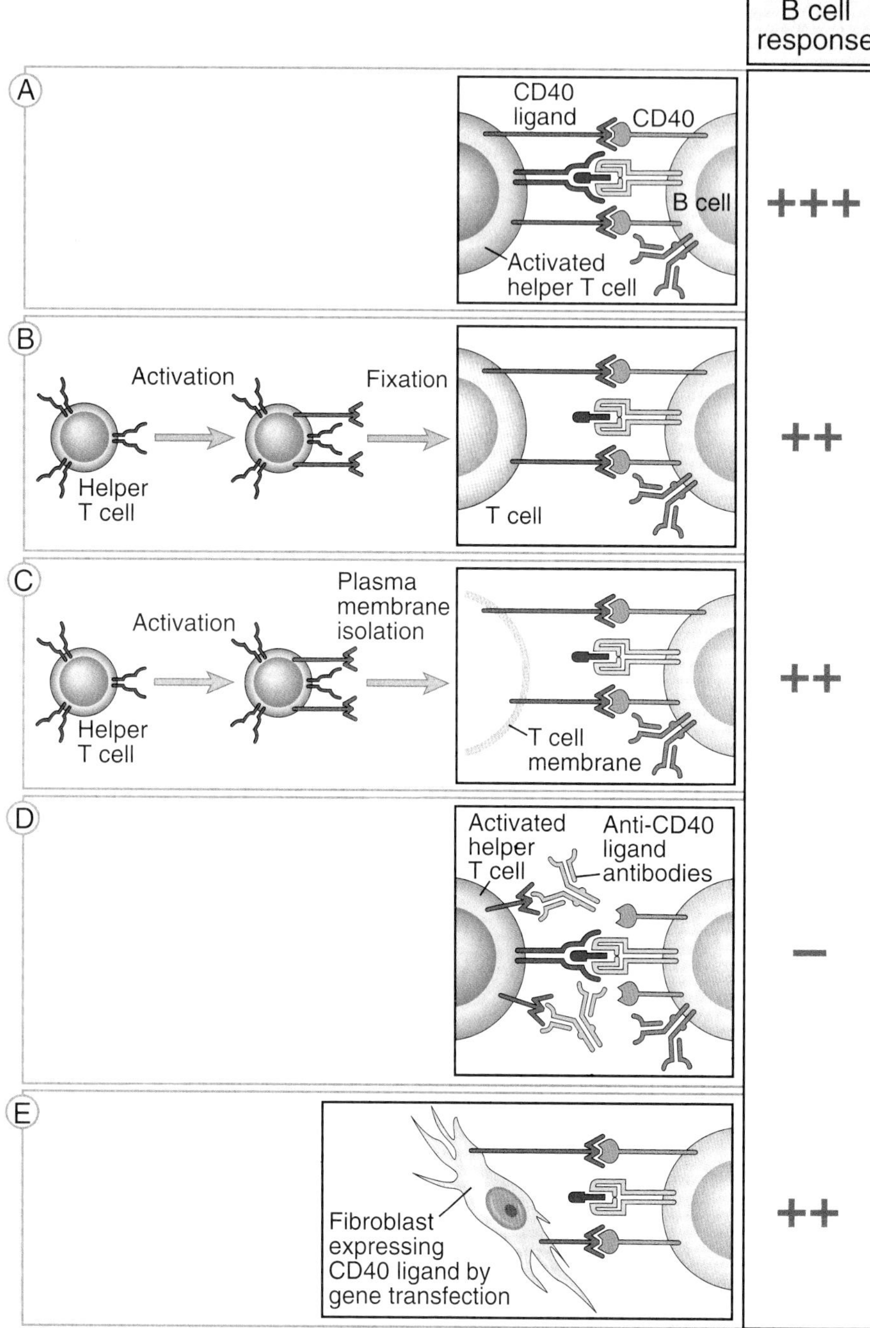

Figure 9–11 Role of CD40 in contact-dependent T cell help of B cells.

A. Activated helper T cells recognize antigen presented by B cells and express CD40 ligand (CD40L), which binds to CD40 on B cells and initiates B cell responses. (Note that sustained CD40 ligand expression on T cells requires recognition of costimulators in addition to antigen, as shown in Figure 9–10; costimulators are not shown in this diagram.)

B. Preactivated and fixed helper T cells also stimulate B cell responses by engaging CD40, even if they cannot recognize the antigen or secrete cytokines.

C. CD40 ligand–containing plasma membrane fractions of activated T cells can provide the necessary signals to activate B cells.

D. Blocking antibodies against CD40 ligand inhibit the T cell contact–mediated stimulation of B cells.

E. Fibroblasts expressing CD40 ligand as a transfected gene product can also stimulate B cells.

Note that the full growth and differentiation of B cells require T cell–derived cytokines as well as T cell contact.

ligand. CD40 is constitutively expressed on B cells, and CD40L is expressed on the surface of helper T cells after activation by antigen and costimulators. When these activated helper T cells bind to antigen-presenting B cells, CD40L interacts with CD40 on the B cells. CD40L binding to CD40 results in oligomerization of CD40 molecules, and this induces the association of cytoplasmic proteins (called TNF receptor–associated factors, or TRAFs) to the cytoplasmic domains of CD40. The TRAFs recruited to CD40 initiate enzyme cascades that lead to the activation and nuclear translocation of transcription factors, including NF-κB and AP-1. Similar signaling pathways are employed by TNF receptors (see Chapter 11, Box 11–1). The links between CD40-induced transcription factors and responses of B cells that are stimulated by T cell help, such as isotype switching, are not yet understood. T cell–mediated macrophage activation also involves the interaction of CD40L on T cells with CD40 on macrophages (see Chapter 13). Thus, this pathway of contact-mediated cellular responses is a general mechanism for the activation of target cells by helper T lymphocytes and is not unique to antibody production. Engagement of CD40 also leads to enhanced expression of B7 molecules on the B cells, causing more T cell activation. Because the expression of B7 on the B cell and of CD40L on the helper T cell is regulated (i.e., they are dependent on or enhanced by antigen-mediated stimulation), only lymphocytes specifically stimulated by antigen interact bidirectionally with one another, thus maintaining the specificity of the immune response.

Interestingly, a DNA virus called the Epstein-Barr virus (EBV) infects human B cells and induces their proliferation. This may lead to immortalization of the cells and the development of lymphomas (see Chapter 17, Box 17–2). The cytoplasmic domain of a transforming protein of EBV associates with the same TRAF molecules as does the cytoplasmic domain of CD40, and this apparently triggers B cell proliferation. Thus, the viral protein is functionally homologous to the physiologic B cell signaling molecule, and EBV has apparently co-opted a normal pathway of B lymphocyte activation for its own purpose, which is to promote survival and proliferation of cells that the virus has infected.

Activated helper T lymphocytes secrete cytokines that act in concert with CD40L to stimulate B cell proliferation and production of antibodies of different isotypes. We have mentioned cytokines previously as important secreted products of T lymphocytes and other cells of the immune system, and they will be discussed in much more detail in Chapter 11. The roles of these proteins in humoral immunity have been most clearly established by showing that various aspects of antibody responses can be inhibited by cytokine antagonists or are deficient in mice in which particular cytokine genes are knocked out by homologous recombination.

Cytokines serve two principal functions in antibody responses: they increase B cell proliferation and differentiation (which was initiated by CD40 signals), and they promote switching to different heavy chain isotypes. Different cytokines play distinct but often overlapping roles in antibody production, and their actions may be synergistic or antagonistic. Antigen recognition by B cells enhances the expression of receptors for cytokines, and as we have described earlier, B cells in direct contact with helper T lymphocytes are exposed to high concentrations of these secreted proteins. As a result, antigen-specific B cells respond to cytokines more than do bystander B cells that are not specific for the initiating antigen but that happen to be close to the antigen-stimulated lymphocytes. Three helper T cell–derived cytokines, IL-2, IL-4, and IL-5, enhance B cell proliferation. IL-6, which is produced by macrophages, T cells, and many other cell types, is a growth factor for already differentiated, antibody-secreting B cells. The effects of cytokines on isotype switching are described later.

B Cell Differentiation into Antibody-Secreting Cells

Some of the progeny of the B cells that have proliferated in response to antigen and T cell help differentiate into effector cells that actively secrete antibodies. Antibody synthesis and secretion in response to protein antigens, like B cell proliferation, are stimulated by CD40-mediated signals and cytokines. Both stimuli activate transcription factors that enhance the transcription of Ig genes and therefore Ig synthesis. Cytokines may also affect RNA processing to increase the amount of transcripts encoding the secretory form of Ig (discussed later). Multiple cytokines, including IL-2, IL-4, and IL-6, have been shown to stimulate antibody synthesis and secretion by activated B lymphocytes. Within lymphoid organs, antibody-secreting cells are found mainly in extrafollicular sites, such as the red pulp of the spleen and the medulla of the lymph nodes. Many of the antibody-secreting B cells change into plasma cells that are morphologically distinct B cells committed to abundant antibody production (see Chapter 2). These cells also migrate to the bone marrow, and at 2 to 3 weeks after immunization, the marrow may be a major site of antibody production. Plasma cells in the bone marrow may continue to secrete antibodies for months or even years after the antigen is no longer present. These antibodies can provide immediate protection if the antigen, such as a microbe, is encountered later. It is estimated that almost half the antibody in the blood of a healthy adult is produced by long-lived plasma cells and is specific for antigens that were encountered in the past. Secreted antibodies enter the circulation and mucosal secretions, but antibody-producing cells do not circulate actively.

The differentiation of B cells from antigen-recognizing cells that express membrane Ig receptors for antigens into effector cells that actively secrete antibodies involves a change in Ig expression from the membrane to the secreted form. Membrane and secreted Ig molecules differ in their carboxyl termini (see Chapter 3, Fig. 3–6). For instance, in secreted μ, the $C_\mu4$ domain is followed by a tail piece containing charged amino acids. In membrane μ, on the other hand, $C_\mu4$ is followed by a short spacer, 26 hydrophobic transmembrane residues, and a cytoplasmic tail of three amino acids (lysine, valine, and lysine). The transition from membrane to secreted Ig reflects a change in the processing of the heavy chain messenger RNA (mRNA). The primary RNA transcript in all IgM-producing B cells contains the rearranged VDJ (variable-diversity-joining) cassette, the four C_μ exons coding for the constant (C) region domains, and the two exons encoding the transmembrane and cytoplasmic domains. Alternative processing of this transcript, which is regulated by RNA cleavage and the choice of polyadenylation sites, determines whether the transmembrane and cytoplasmic exons are included in the mature mRNA (Fig. 9–12). If they are, the μ chain produced contains the amino acids that make up the transmembrane and cytoplasmic segments and is therefore anchored in the lipid bilayer of the plasma membrane. If, on the other hand, the transmembrane segment is excluded from the μ chain, the carboxyl terminus consists of about 20 amino acids constituting the tail piece. Because this protein does not have a stretch of hydrophobic amino acids or a positively charged cytoplasmic domain, it cannot remain anchored in the cell membrane and is secreted. Thus, each B cell can synthesize both membrane and secreted Ig. As differentiation proceeds, more and more of the Ig mRNA is of the form encoding secreted Ig. The biochemical signals initiated by antigen binding to membrane Ig and by helper T cells that regulate this process of alternative RNA splicing are not known. All C_H genes

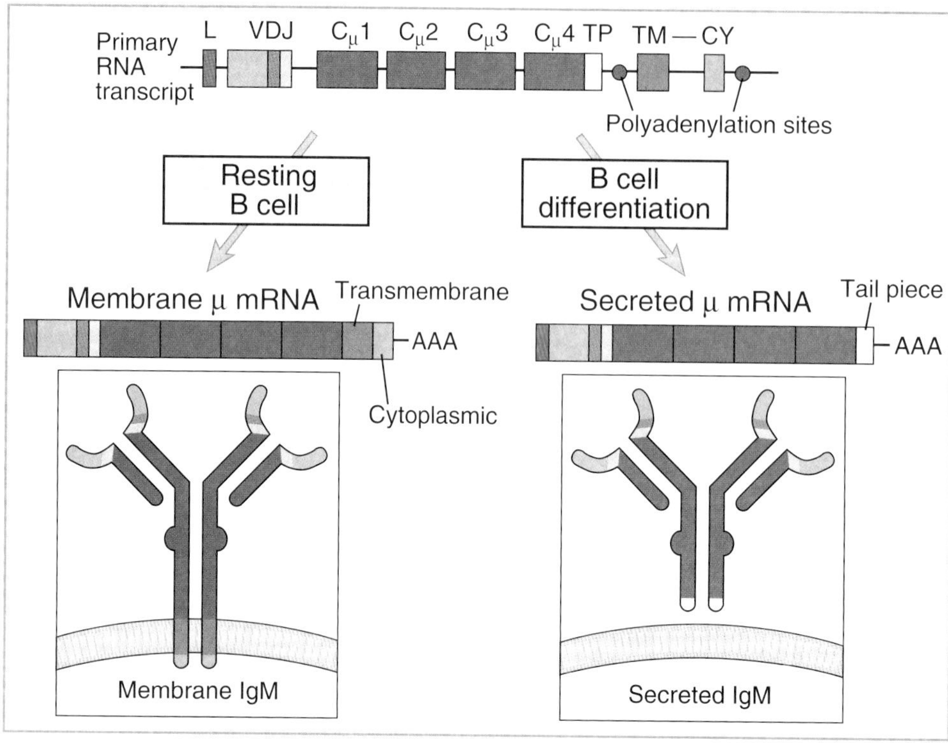

Figure 9–12 Production of membrane and secreted μ chains in B lymphocytes. Alternative processing of a primary RNA transcript results in the formation of mRNA for the membrane or secreted form of the μ heavy chain. B cell differentiation results in an increasing fraction of the μ protein produced as the secreted form. TP, TM, and CY refer to tail piece, transmembrane, and cytoplasmic segments, respectively. $C_\mu1$, $C_\mu2$, $C_\mu3$, and $C_\mu4$ are four exons of the C_μ gene.

contain similar membrane exons, and all heavy chains can apparently be expressed in membrane-bound and secreted forms. The secretory form of the δ heavy chain is rarely made, however, so that IgD is usually present only as a membrane-bound protein.

Heavy Chain Isotype (Class) Switching

In response to CD40 engagement and cytokines, some of the progeny of activated IgM- and IgD-expressing B cells undergo the process of heavy chain isotype (class) switching, leading to the production of antibodies with heavy chains of different classes, such as γ, α, and ε (Fig. 9–13). Isotype switching occurs in peripheral lymphoid tissues, in B cells that are activated at the edges of the follicles and in germinal centers. The requirement for CD40 signaling to promote isotype switching in B cells is well documented by analysis of mice and humans lacking CD40 or its ligand. In all these cases, the antibody response to protein antigens is dominated by IgM antibodies, and there is little switching to other isotypes. The mechanisms by which CD40 signals induce isotype switching are not defined.

Cytokines play essential roles in regulating switching to particular heavy chain isotypes. For instance, IL-4, which is produced mainly by $CD4^+$ T cells, is the principal switch factor for IgE in all species examined, and the production of IgG2a in mice is dependent on interferon-γ (IFN-γ), which is secreted by T cells and by NK (natural killer) cells.

- Addition of IL-4 or IFN-γ induces specific isotype switching in cultures of mature IgM- and IgD-expressing B cells stimulated with antigens or polyclonal activators (Table 9–3).
- IgE responses to antigen-specific or polyclonal stimulation are inhibited by antibodies that neutralize IL-4, and IgG2a responses are blocked by antibodies that neutralize IFN-γ.
- IL-4–deficient mice created by gene knockout have no serum IgE, and IFN-γ knockout mice have greatly reduced serum IgG2a.

The capacity of B cells to produce different antibody isotypes provides a remarkable plasticity in humoral immune responses by generating antibodies that perform distinct effector functions and are involved in defense against different types of infectious agents (see Fig. 9–13). Isotype switching in response to different types of microbes is regulated by the types of helper T cells that are activated by these microbes. For instance, the major protective humoral immune response to bacteria with polysaccharide-rich capsules consists of IgM antibodies, which bind to the bacteria, activate the complement system, and induce phagocytosis of the bacteria. Polysaccharide antigens, which do not elicit T cell help, stimulate mainly IgM antibodies, with little, if any, isotype switching to some IgG subclasses. The response to many viruses and bacteria consists of production of IgG antibodies, which block entry of the microbes into host cells and also promote phagocytosis by macrophages. Viruses and many bacteria activate helper T cells of the T_H1 subset, which produce the cytokine IFN-γ, the main inducer of B cell switching to opsonizing and complement-fixing IgG subclasses. The immune response to many helminthic parasites is mainly production of IgE, which participates in eosinophil-mediated killing of the helminths (see Chapter 15); IgE antibodies also mediate immediate

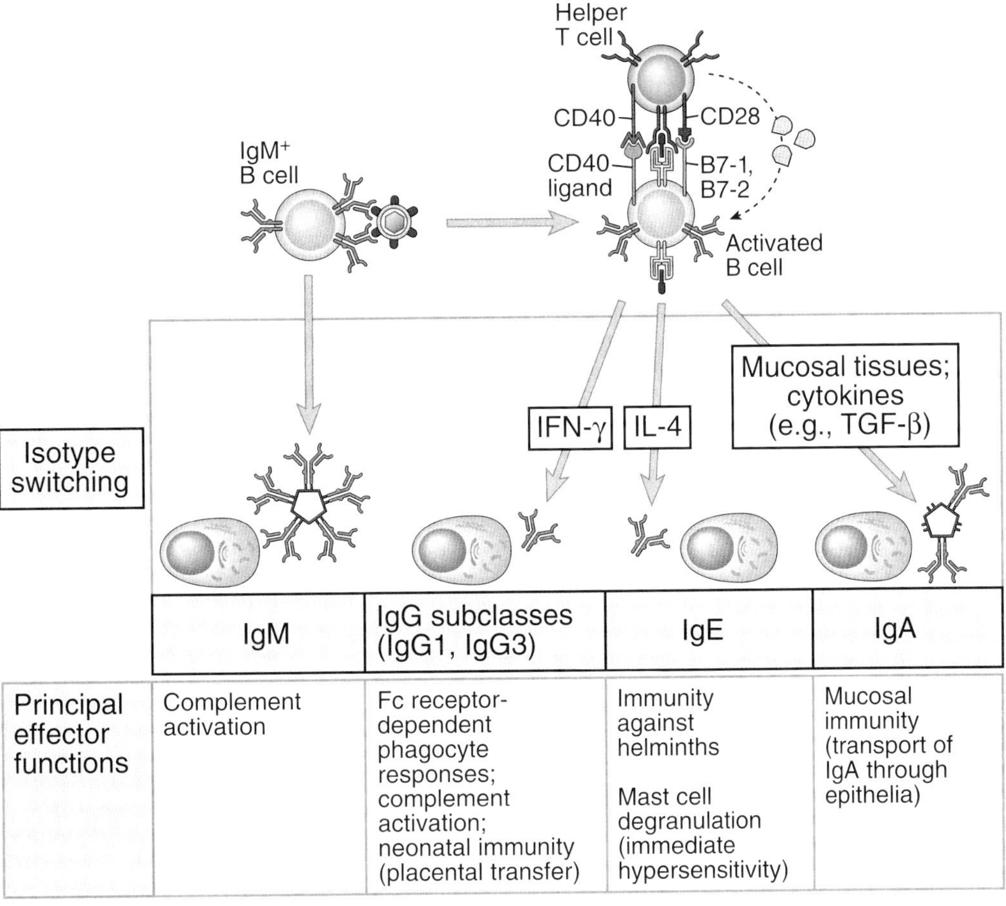

Figure 9–13 Ig heavy chain isotype switching.
B cells activated by helper T cell signals (CD40L, cytokines) undergo switching to different Ig isotypes, which mediate distinct effector functions. Selected examples of switched isotypes in humans are shown.

hypersensitivity (allergic) reactions (see Chapter 19). Helminths activate the T_H2 subset of helper T cells, which produces IL-4, the cytokine that induces switching to IgE. (We will discuss the development and functions of helper T cell subsets in more detail in Chapter 13.) In addition, B cells in different anatomic sites switch to different isotypes. Specifically, B cells in mucosal tissues switch to IgA, which is the antibody class that is most efficiently transported through epithelia into mucosal secretions, where it defends against microbes that try to enter through the epithelia. Switching to IgA is stimulated by transforming growth factor-

Table 9–3. Heavy Chain Isotype Switching Induced by Cytokines

B cells cultured with		**Ig isotype secreted (percent of total Ig produced)**				
Polyclonal activator	Cytokine	IgM	IgG1	IgG2a	IgE	IgA
LPS	None	85	2	<1	<1	<1
LPS	IL-4	70	**20**	<1	**5**	<1
LPS	IFN-γ	80	2	**10**	<1	<1
LPS	TGF-β + IL-5	75	2	<1	<1	**15**

Addition of various cytokines to purified IgM^+IgD^+ mouse B cells cultured with the polyclonal activator lipopolysaccharide (LPS) induces switching to different heavy chain isotypes. The values of the isotypes shown are approximations and do not add up to 100% because not all were measured. (Courtesy of Dr. Robert Coffman, DNAX Research Institute, Palo Alto, Calif.)

β, (TGF-β), which is produced by many cell types in mucosal and other tissues, acting in concert with T cell–derived IL-5. These examples of isotype switching illustrate how helper T cells function as controllers of immune responses—these T cells secrete different cytokines in response to different microbes, and the cytokines stimulate antibody responses that are best at combating those microbes.

The principal molecular mechanism of isotype switching is a process called **switch recombination,** in which the rearranged VDJ gene segment in a B cell recombines with a downstream C region gene and the intervening DNA is deleted. Switch recombination was first observed in myelomas, in which it was found that cells producing one Ig isotype have deleted all rearranged C_H genes 5′ of this isotype. Thus, if the C_μ and C_δ genes are deleted, the rearranged VDJ gene segment will be attached to the next C_H complex, giving rise to γ3 heavy chains (in the mouse); subsequent deletion of all γ subclass–encoding genes will result in the production of ε heavy chains, and so on (Fig. 9–14). These DNA recombination events involve nucleotide sequences called switch regions, which are located in the introns at the 5′ end of each C_H locus. Switch regions occupy distances of 1 to 10 kilobases and contain numerous tandem repeats of conserved DNA sequences. Upstream of each switch region is a small exon called the I exon (for initiator of transcription). CD40 and cytokines trigger isotype switching by increasing the accessibility of the DNA at a specific C region and then inducing transcription through the I exon, switch region, and C_H exons. This transcript is spliced to remove the switch region. The resulting RNA, composed of the I exon and the constant region exons, usually contains numerous stop codons and cannot be translated; it is therefore called a germline transcript. Germline transcription is accompanied by accessibility of a particular C gene to enzymes that mediate switch recombination. As a result, the rearranged VDJ complex in that B cell recombines with the transcriptionally active downstream C region. For instance, IL-4 induces germline transcription through the I_ε-S_ε-C_ε locus, and IFN-γ induces germline transcription in mice through the $I_\gamma2a$-$S_\gamma2a$-$C_\gamma2a$ locus (see Fig. 9–14). This leads first to the production of germline ε or γ2a transcripts in an IgM-expressing B cell (depending on which cytokine is present, IL-4 or IFN-γ) and then to switch recombination and the production of IgE or IgG2a, respectively, with the same VDJ exon and variable (V) region as that of the original IgM produced by that B cell. Knockout of the I exon or switch region for any heavy chain isotype leads to an inability to switch to that isotype. The enzymes that mediate switch recombination are not yet identified. One enzyme known to be required for isotype switching and affinity maturation is an RNA editing enzyme that functions as a cytosine deaminase and is called activation-induced deaminase. Humans with deficiency of this enzyme develop a disease similar to the hyper-IgM syndrome caused by mutations in CD40L, and knockout mice lacking this enzyme have profound defects in isotype switching and affinity maturation. What this enzyme does during either process is unknown.

Late Events in T Cell–Dependent Antibody Responses: Germinal Center Reactions

The late events in helper T cell–dependent antibody responses, including affinity maturation and the generation of memory B cells, occur in the germinal centers of lymphoid follicles. As we discussed before, the initial B cell response to protein antigens occurs at the boundaries between lymphoid follicles and T cell zones (see Fig. 9–7). Within 4 to 7 days after antigen exposure, some of the activated B cells migrate deep into the follicle and begin to proliferate rapidly, forming the lightly staining central region of the follicle, called the **germinal center** (Fig. 9–15). The doubling time of these proliferating germinal center B cells, also called centroblasts, is estimated to be 6 to 12 hours, so that within 5 days, a single lymphocyte may give rise to almost 5000 progeny. Each fully formed germinal center contains cells derived from only one or a few antigen-specific B cell clones. The progeny of the proliferating B cells in the germinal center are smaller cells, sometimes called centrocytes, that undergo differentiation and selection processes described next.

The architecture of lymphoid follicles and the germinal center reactions within follicles depend on the presence of **follicular dendritic cells** (Fig. 9–16). Follicular dendritic cells (FDCs) are found only in lymphoid follicles and express complement receptors (CR1, CR2, and CR3) and Fc receptors. All these molecules are involved in the selection of germinal center B cells (discussed later). FDCs do not express class II MHC molecules. The origin of FDCs is unclear. They are not derived from the bone marrow, and they are clearly different from the class II MHC–expressing dendritic cells that present peptide antigens to $CD4^+$ T lymphocytes. The long cytoplasmic processes of FDCs make up a meshwork around which germinal centers are formed. Proliferating B cells accumulate in a histologically identifiable light zone of the germinal center, which has few FDCs. The small nondividing progeny of the B cells migrate to an adjacent basal dark zone, where they come into close contact with the processes of the abundant FDCs and where the subsequent selection events occur (see Fig. 9–15).

The formation of germinal centers depends on the presence of helper T cells and the interactions between CD40 and CD40L and is therefore observed only in antibody responses to helper T cell–dependent protein antigens. Germinal center formation is impaired in humans and in mice with genetic defects in T cell development or activation (see Chapter 20) or with mutations of either CD40 or its ligand. This is partly because, as we discussed earlier, CD40:CD40L interactions are required during the early events of helper T cell–dependent B cell activation, and only activated B cells migrate into follicles to form germinal centers. In addition, germinal centers contain small numbers of helper T cells, which express CD40L and may stimulate the proliferation of germinal center B cells by CD40 engagement.

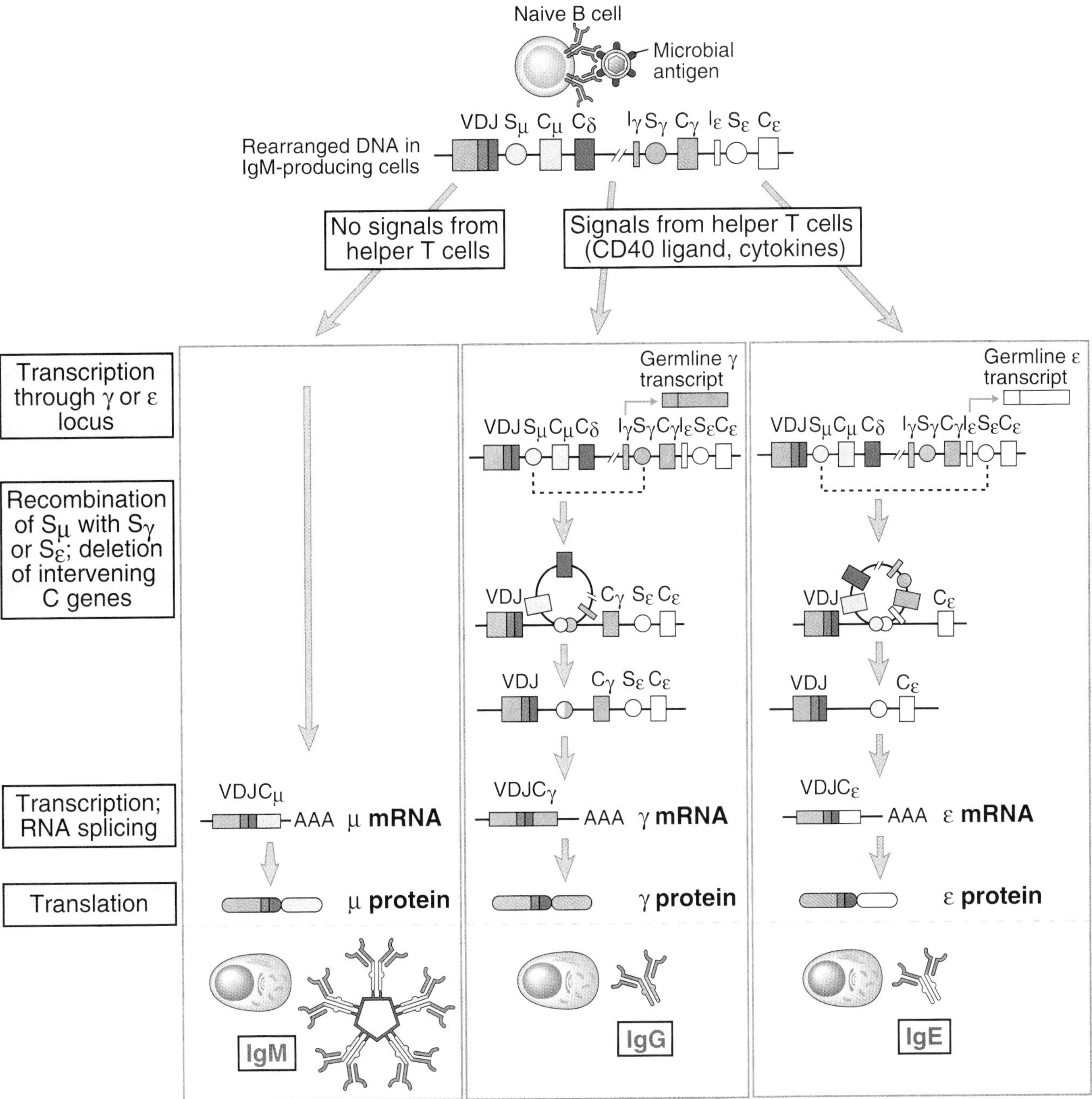

Figure 9–14 Molecular mechanisms of heavy chain isotype switching.
In the absence of helper T cell signals, B cells produce IgM. When antigen-activated B cells encounter helper T cell signals (CD40L and, in this example, IL-4), the B cells undergo switching to other Ig isotypes (in this example, IgE). These stimuli initiate germline transcription through the $I_ε$-$S_ε$-$C_ε$ locus. The proximal C_H genes are deleted in a circle of DNA, leading to recombination of the VDJ complex with the $C_ε$ gene. Switch regions are indicated by circles labeled $S_μ$ or $S_γ$. $I_γ$ represents an initiation site for germline transcription. (Note that there are multiple $C_γ$ genes located between $C_δ$ and $C_ε$, but these are not shown.)

Affinity Maturation: Somatic Mutations in Ig Genes and Selection of High-Affinity B Cells

Affinity maturation is the process that leads to increased affinity of antibodies for a particular antigen as a T-dependent humoral response progresses and is the result of somatic mutation of Ig genes followed by selective survival of the B cells producing the antibodies with the highest affinities. The process of affinity maturation generates antibodies with increasing capacity to bind antigens and thus to combat persistent or recurrent antigens. Helper T cells and CD40:CD40L interactions are required for affinity maturation to proceed, and therefore affinity maturation occurs only in antibody responses to helper T cell–dependent protein antigens.

In proliferating germinal center B cells, the Ig V genes undergo point mutations at an extremely high

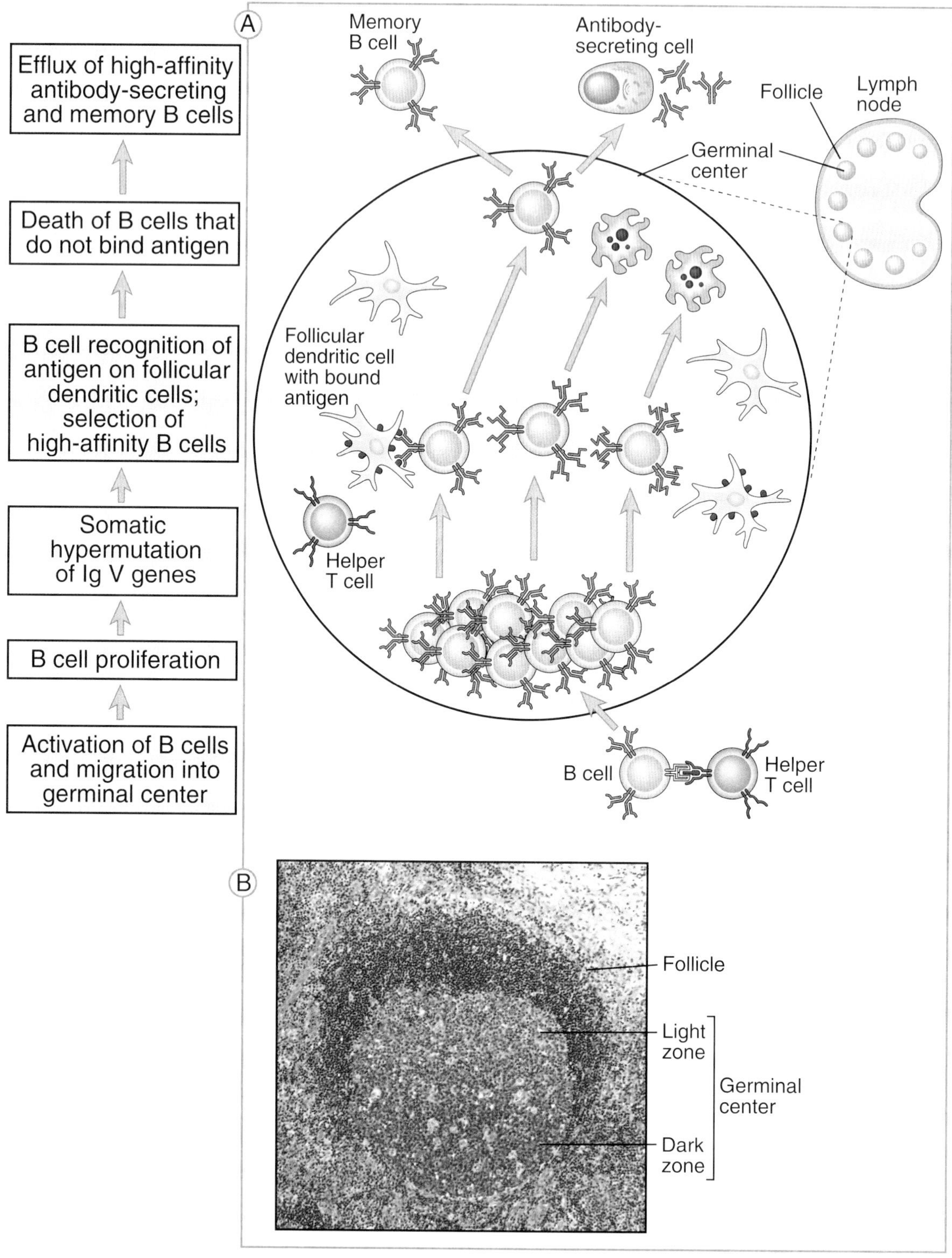

Figure 9–15 Germinal center reactions in T cell–dependent antibody responses.
A. Schematic diagram of germinal center reactions in a lymph node. B cells that have been activated by helper T cells at the edge of a primary follicle migrate into the follicle and proliferate, forming the dark zone. Somatic mutations of Ig V genes occur in these B cells, and they migrate into the light zone where they encounter follicular dendritic cells displaying antigen. B cells with the highest affinity Ig receptors are selected to survive, and they differentiate into antibody-secreting or memory B cells.
B. Histology of a secondary follicle with a germinal center in a lymph node. The germinal center is contained within the follicle and includes a basal dark zone and an adjacent light zone. (Courtesy of Dr. James Gulizia, Department of Pathology, Brigham and Women's Hospital, Boston.)

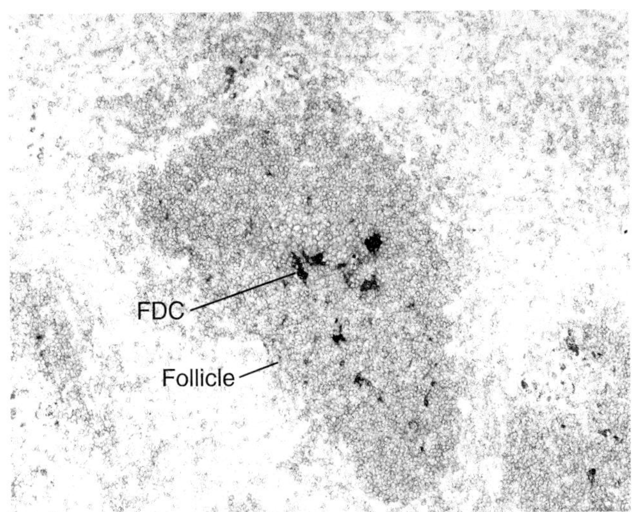

Figure 9–16 Follicular dendritic cells.
This immunohistochemical stain shows follicular dendritic cells (FDC, stained brown with a specific enzyme-labeled antibody) in the follicle of a spleen. B cells in the follicle are stained blue. (Courtesy of Dr. Garnett Kelsoe, Duke University, Durham, NC.)

rate. This rate is estimated to be 1 in 10^3 V gene base pairs per cell division, which is 10^3 to 10^4 times higher than the spontaneous rate of mutation in other mammalian genes. (For this reason, mutation in Ig V genes is also called hypermutation.) The V genes of expressed heavy and light chains in each B cell contain a total of about 700 nucleotides; this implies that mutations will accumulate in expressed V regions at an average rate of almost one per cell division. Ig V gene mutations continue to occur in the progeny of individual B cells. As a result, any B cell clone can accumulate more and more mutations during its life in the germinal centers. It is estimated that as a result of somatic mutations, the nucleotide sequences of IgG antibodies derived from one clone of B cells can diverge as much as 5% from the original germline sequence. This usually translates to up to 10 amino acid substitutions. The importance of somatic hypermutation in the process of affinity maturation is well established.

Analysis of the Ig genes of B cell clones isolated at different stages of antibody responses to proteins or hapten-protein conjugates first showed the accumulation of point mutations in the V regions of the antibodies (Fig. 9–17). Several features of these mutations are noteworthy. First, the mutations are clustered in the V regions, mostly in the antigen-binding comple-

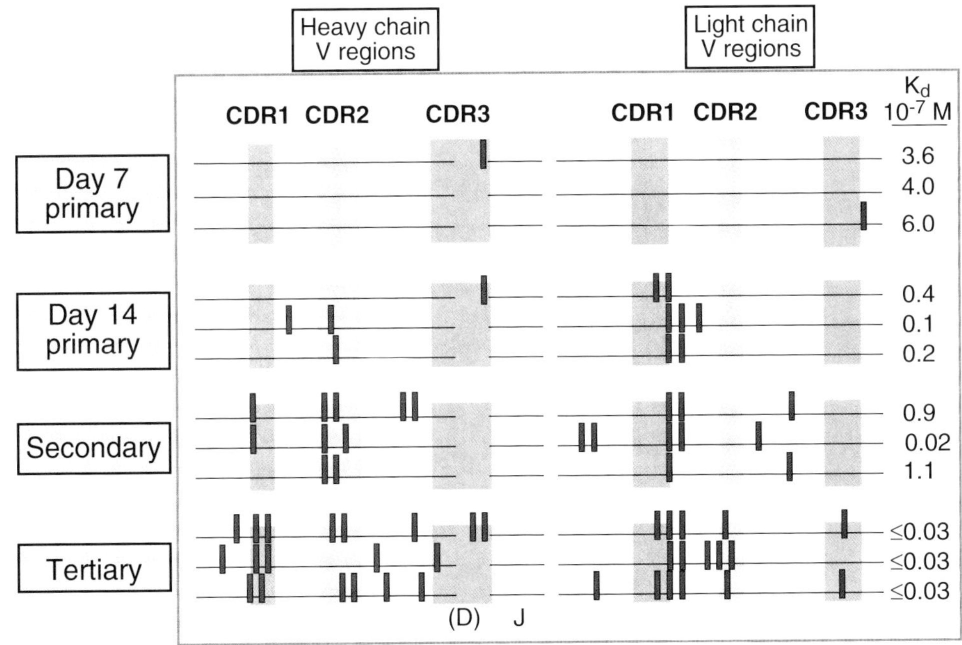

Figure 9–17 Somatic mutations in Ig V genes.
Hybridomas were produced from spleen cells of mice immunized 7 or 14 days previously with a hapten, oxazolone, coupled to a protein, and from spleen cells obtained after secondary and tertiary immunizations with the same antigen. Hybridomas producing oxazolone-specific monoclonal antibodies were isolated, and the nucleotide sequences of the V genes encoding the Ig heavy and light chains were determined. Mutations in V genes increase with time after immunization and with repeated immunizations and are clustered in the complementarity-determining regions (CDRs). The location of CDR3 in the heavy chains is approximate. The affinities of the antibodies produced also tend to increase with more mutations, as indicated by the lower dissociation constants (K_d) for hapten binding. (Adapted from Berek C, and C Milstein. Mutation drift and repertoire shift in the maturation of the immune response. Immunological Reviews 96:23–41, 1987. Munksgaard International Publishers Ltd, Copenhagen, Denmark.)

mentarity-determining regions. Second, there are more mutations in IgG than in IgM antibodies. Third, the presence of mutations correlates with the increasing affinities of the antibodies for the antigen that induced the response.

- Mutations in Ig genes were also found in clones of B cells isolated from germinal centers microdissected from the spleens of mice that had been immunized with hapten-protein conjugates. Analyses of these Ig genes showed that the progeny of a single B cell clone progressively accumulate mutations with time after immunization.

The mechanisms of somatic mutations in Ig genes are poorly understood. It is clear that the rearranged Ig VDJ DNA becomes highly susceptible to mutations, suggesting enhanced susceptibility of this region to DNA-binding factors that promote mutations. It is not known whether germinal center T cells provide specific contact-mediated signals or cytokines that stimulate somatic hypermutation in B cells. The enzyme activation-induced deaminase, which was mentioned earlier, plays an essential role in affinity maturation, but its mode of action is not known.

On the basis of the studies described, it is believed that repeated stimulation by T-dependent protein antigens leads to increasing numbers of mutations in the Ig genes of antigen-specific germinal center B cells. Some of these mutations are likely to be useful because they will generate high-affinity antibodies. However, many of the mutations may result in a decline or even in a loss of antigen binding. Therefore, the next and crucial step in the process of affinity maturation is the selection of the useful, high-affinity B cells.

FDCs in the germinal centers display antigens, and the B cells that bind these antigens with high affinity are selected to survive (Fig. 9–18). The early response to antigen results in the production of antibodies, some of which form complexes with residual antigen and may activate complement. FDCs express receptors for the Fc portions of antibodies and for products of complement activation, including C3b and C3d. These receptors bind and display antigens that are complexed with antibodies or complement products. Antigen may also be present in soluble form in the germinal center. Meanwhile, germinal center B cells that have undergone somatic hypermutation migrate into the FDC-rich light zone of the germinal center. These B cells die by apoptosis unless they are rescued by recognition of antigen. Therefore, the B cells that recognize antigen displayed by FDCs are selected to live. As more antibody is produced, more of the antigen is eliminated and less is available in the germinal centers. Therefore, the B cells that will be able to specifically bind this antigen and to be rescued from death need to express antigen receptors with higher and higher affinity for the antigen. As a result, as the antibody response to an antigen progresses, the B cells that are selected in germinal centers produce Ig of increasing affinity for the antigen. This selection process results in affinity maturation of the antibody response. Because somatic mutations leave many B cells that do not express high-affinity receptors for antigen and that cannot therefore be selected to survive, the germinal centers are sites of tremendous apoptosis.

The survivors of this antigen-driven selection process migrate from the basal light zone of the germinal center to the apical zone, where they may undergo additional isotype switching. The cells then exit the germinal center and develop into high-affinity antibody secretors outside the germinal centers, in the same lymphoid organ or in the bone marrow.

Generation of Memory B Cells and Secondary Humoral Immune Responses

Some of the antigen-activated B cells do not develop into antibody secretors. Instead, they acquire the ability to survive for long periods, apparently without antigenic stimulation. These are **memory cells,** capable of mounting rapid responses to subsequent introduction of antigen. We do not know why some of the progeny of an antigen-stimulated B cell clone differentiate into antibody-secreting cells whereas others become functionally quiescent, long-lived memory cells. Some memory B cells may remain in the lymph node. Others exit germinal centers, circulate in the blood, and may take up residence in other lymphoid tissues. Memory cells typically bear high-affinity (mutated) antigen receptors and Ig molecules of switched isotypes more commonly than do naive B lymphocytes. The production of large quantities of isotype-switched, high-affinity antibodies is greatly accelerated after secondary exposures to antigens, and this can be attributed to the activation of memory cells in germinal centers and the rapid formation of immune complexes that can be concentrated by FDCs.

Many of the features of secondary (i.e., memory) antibody responses to protein antigens, and their differences from primary responses (see Table 9–1), are due to the actions of $CD4^+$ helper T cells. Thus, heavy chain class switching, which is typical of secondary responses, is due to helper T cells and their cytokines. Affinity maturation, which increases with repeated antigenic stimulation, is also secondary to helper T cell–induced B cell activation. These features are usually seen in responses to protein antigens because only protein antigens stimulate specific helper T cells. High-affinity antibodies are required to neutralize the infectivity of many microbes and the pathogenicity of microbial toxins. Therefore, effective vaccines against these microorganisms must induce affinity maturation and memory B cell formation, and both reactions will occur only if the vaccines are able to activate helper T cells. This concept has been applied to the design of vaccines for some bacterial infections in which the target antigen is a capsular polysaccharide, which is incapable of stimulating T cells. In these cases, the polysaccharide is covalently linked to a foreign protein to form the equivalent of a hapten-carrier conjugate, which does activate helper T cells. Such vaccines, which are called **conjugate vaccines,** more readily induce high-affinity antibodies and memory than do polysaccharide vaccines without linked proteins.

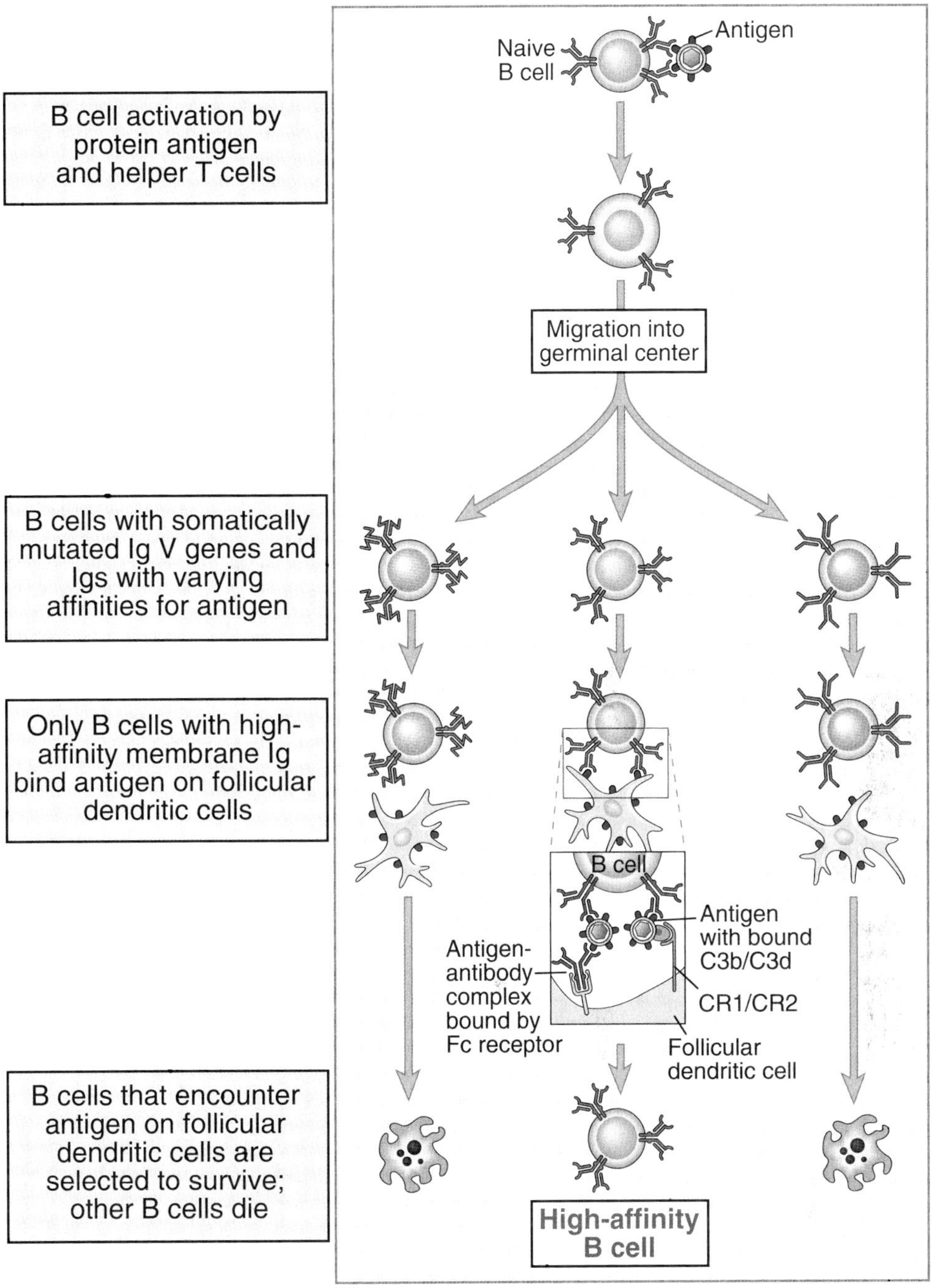

Figure 9–18 B cell selection in germinal centers.
Somatic mutation of variable (V) region genes in germinal center B cells generates antibodies with different affinities for antigen. Subsequently, binding of the B cells to antigen displayed on follicular dendritic cells is necessary to rescue the B cells from programmed cell death. The B cells with the highest affinity for antigen will have a selective advantage for survival as the amount of available antigen decreases during an immune response. This leads to an average increase in the affinity of antibodies for antigen as the humoral immune response progresses.

B cell activation by protein antigen and helper T cells

Naive B cell

Antigen

Migration into germinal center

B cells with somatically mutated Ig V genes and Igs with varying affinities for antigen

Only B cells with high-affinity membrane Ig bind antigen on follicular dendritic cells

B cell

Antigen-antibody complex bound by Fc receptor

Antigen with bound C3b/C3d

CR1/CR2

Follicular dendritic cell

B cells that encounter antigen on follicular dendritic cells are selected to survive; other B cells die

High-affinity B cell

Antibody Responses to T Cell–Independent Antigens

Many nonprotein antigens, such as polysaccharides and lipids, stimulate antibody production in the absence of helper T cells, and these antigens are termed thymus-independent or T-independent. These antibody responses differ in several respects from responses to T-dependent protein antigens (Table 9–4). As we have discussed in the previous sections, antibody responses to protein antigens require the participation of helper T cells, and helper T cells stimulate isotype switching, affinity maturation, and long-lived memory. In contrast, the antibodies that are produced in the absence of T cell help are generally of low affinity and consist mainly of IgM with limited isotype switching to some IgG subtypes. Some nonprotein antigens do induce Ig isotypes other than IgM, but the mechanism of isotype switching in the absence of T cell help is not known. In humans, the dominant antibody class induced by pneumococcal capsular polysaccharide is IgG2. In addition, despite their inability to specifically activate helper T cells, many polysaccharide vaccines, such as pneumococcal vaccine, induce long-lived protective immunity. A possible reason for this is that polysaccharides are not

Table 9–4. Properties of Thymus-Dependent and Thymus-Independent Antigens

	Thymus-dependent antigen	Thymus-independent antigen
Chemical nature	Proteins	Polymeric antigens, especially polysaccharides; also glycolipids, nucleic acids
Features of antibody response		
Isotype switching	Yes (IgM → IgG, IgE, IgA)	Little or no: may be some IgG (IgM, IgG)
Affinity maturation	Yes	Little or no
Secondary response (memory B cells)	Yes	Only seen with some antigens (e.g., polysaccharides)
Ability to induce delayed-type hypersensitivity	Yes	No

degraded efficiently, persist for long periods in lymphoid tissues, and continue to stimulate newly arising naive B cells. Although it is not known whether long-lived quiescent memory B cells are generated in response to these polysaccharide antigens, rapid and large secondary responses typical of memory (but without much isotype switching or affinity maturation) do occur on secondary exposure to these antigens.

The most important TI antigens are polysaccharides, glycolipids, and nucleic acids, all of which induce specific antibody production in T cell–deficient animals. These antigens cannot be processed and presented in association with MHC molecules, and therefore they cannot be recognized by helper T cells. Most TI antigens are polyvalent, being composed of multiple identical antigenic epitopes. Such polyvalent antigens may induce maximal cross-linking of membrane Ig on specific B cells, leading to activation without a requirement for cognate T cell help. B cell activation by TI antigens is one situation in which membrane Ig–mediated signal transduction may be critical for subsequent responses of the cells. In addition, many polysaccharides activate the complement system by the alternative pathway, generating C3d, which binds to the antigen and provides second signals for B cell activation (see Fig. 9–5). Experiments with mice suggest that antibody responses to polysaccharides do require the presence of small numbers of macrophages or helper T cells. These cells may secrete cytokines that augment B cell responses to TI antigens, but neither the nature of these cytokines nor the mechanisms leading to their production are understood.

Antibody responses to TI antigens may occur at particular anatomic sites in lymphoid tissues. Macrophages located in the marginal zones of lymphoid follicles in the spleen are particularly efficient at trapping polysaccharides when these antigens are injected intravenously. Marginal zone B cells are a distinct subset of B cells that respond mainly to polysaccharides and produce IgM. TI antigens may persist for prolonged periods on the surfaces of marginal zone macrophages, where they are recognized by specific B cells, or they may be transferred from the marginal zone to the adjacent follicle.

The practical significance of TI antigens is that many bacterial cell wall polysaccharides belong to this category, and humoral immunity is the major mechanism of host defense against infections by such encapsulated bacteria. For this reason, individuals with congenital or acquired deficiencies of humoral immunity are especially susceptible to life-threatening infections with encapsulated bacteria, such as pneumococcus, meningococcus, and *Haemophilus*. Other examples of responses to TI antigens are natural antibodies, which are present in the circulation of normal individuals and are apparently produced without overt antigen exposure. Most natural antibodies are low-affinity anticarbohydrate antibodies, postulated to be produced by B-1 peritoneal B cells stimulated by bacteria that colonize the gastrointestinal tract and by marginal zone B cells in lymphoid organs. Antibodies to the A and B glycolipid blood group antigens are examples of these natural antibodies.

Antibody Feedback: Regulation of Humoral Immune Responses by Fc Receptors

Secreted antibodies inhibit continuing B cell activation by forming antigen-antibody complexes that simultaneously bind to antigen receptors and Fcγ receptors on antigen-specific B cells (Fig. 9–19). This is the explanation for a phenomenon called **antibody feedback,** which refers to the down-regulation of antibody production by secreted IgG antibodies. IgG antibodies inhibit B cell activation by forming complexes with the antigen, and these complexes bind to a B cell receptor for the Fc portions of the IgG, called the Fcγ receptor II (FcγRIIB, or CD32). (The biology of Fc receptors is discussed in Chapter 14.) The cytoplasmic domain of FcγRIIB contains a six–amino acid (isoleucine-X-tyrosine-X-X-leucine) motif shared by other receptors in the immune system that mediate negative signals, including the killer inhibitory receptor on NK cells (see Chapter 12). By analogy to ITAMs, this inhibitory motif is called the **immunoreceptor tyrosine-based inhibition motif** (ITIM). When the Fcγ receptor of B cells is engaged, the ITIM of the receptor is phosphorylated on tyrosine residues, and it forms a docking site for the inositol 5-phosphatase SHIP (SH2

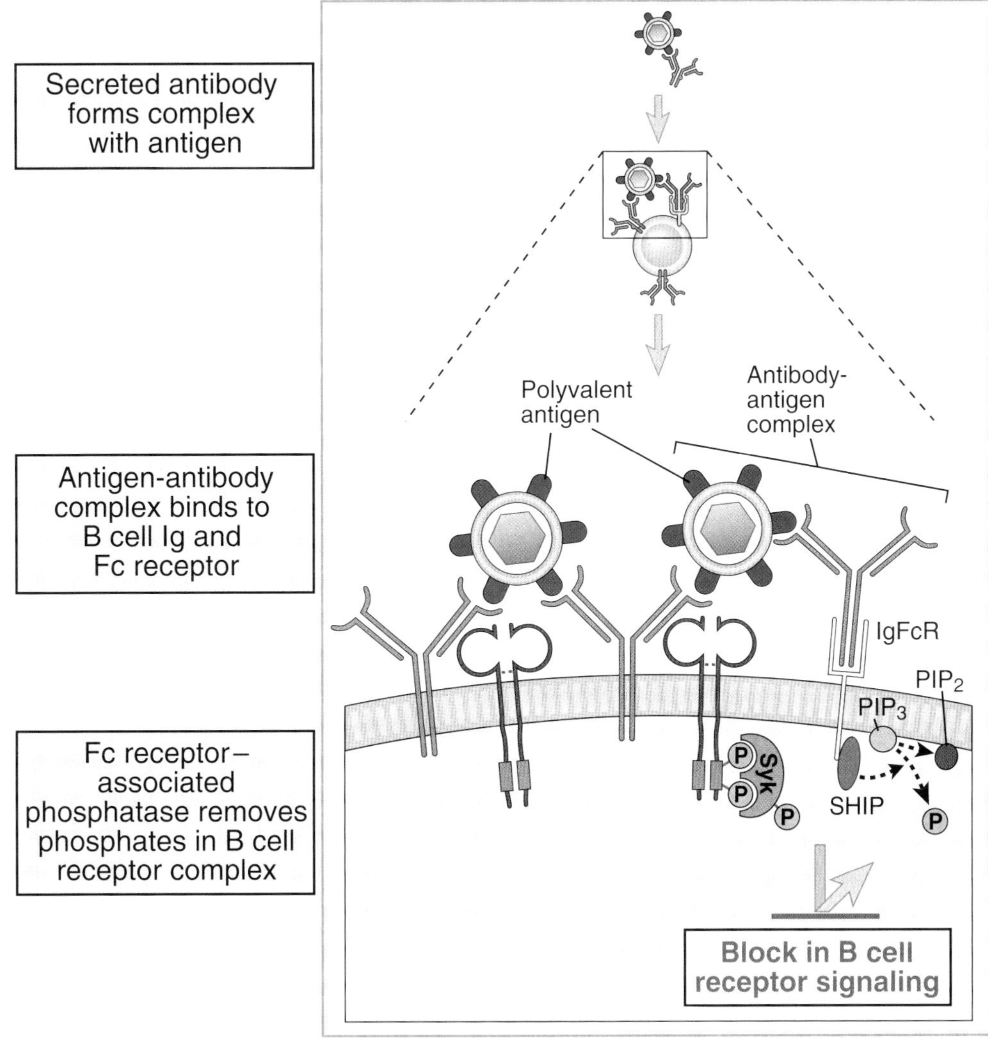

Figure 9–19 Regulation of B cell activation by Ig Fc receptors. Antigen-antibody complexes can simultaneously bind to membrane Ig (through antigen) and the FcγRIIB receptor through the Fc portion of the antibody. As a consequence of this simultaneous ligation of receptors, phosphatases associated with the cytoplasmic tail of the FcγRIIB inhibit signaling by the BCR complex and block B cell activation.

domain–containing inositol phosphatase). The recruited SHIP hydrolyses the 5′ phosphate of PIP_3, which is produced by clustering of the B cell antigen receptor and binds PLC and Btk, both of which are involved in BCR-mediated signaling. By this mechanism, engagement of FcγRII terminates the B cell response to antigen. The antigen-antibody complexes simultaneously interact with the antigen receptor (through the antigen) and the FcγRIIB (through the antibody), and this brings the inhibitory phosphatases close to the antigen receptors whose signaling is blocked.

Fc receptor–mediated antibody feedback is a physiologic control mechanism in humoral immune responses because it is triggered by secreted antibody and blocks further antibody production. We have stated earlier in the chapter that antibodies can also amplify antibody production by activating complement and generating C3d, a second signal for B cell activation. It is not clear under which circumstances secreted antibodies provide complement-mediated amplification or Fc receptor–mediated inhibition. A likely scenario is that early in humoral immune responses, IgM antibodies (which activate complement but do not bind to the Fcγ receptor) are involved in amplification, whereas increasing production of IgG leads to feedback inhibition.

B cells express another inhibitory receptor called CD22. CD22 is a sialic acid–binding lectin; its natural ligand is not known, and we do not know how it is engaged during physiologic B cell responses. However, knockout mice lacking CD22 show greatly enhanced B cell activation. The cytoplasmic domain of this molecule contains an ITIM, which binds the tyrosine phosphatase SHP-1. It is thought that SHP-1 removes phosphates from the tyrosine residues of critical BCR-associated signaling molecules. A mouse strain called moth-eaten, which develops severe autoimmunity with uncontrolled B cell activation and autoantibody production, has a mutation in SHP-1.

Summary

- In humoral immune responses, B lymphocytes are activated by antigen and secrete antibodies that act to eliminate the antigen. Both protein and nonprotein antigens can stimulate antibody responses. B cell responses to protein antigens require the contribution of $CD4^+$ helper T cells specific for the antigen.
- B cell activation is initiated by the clustering of antigen receptors (membrane IgM and IgD on naive B cells) by the binding of multivalent antigen. Membrane Ig–associated signaling molecules Igα and Igβ transduce signals on antigen binding to the Ig, and these signals lead to activation of transcription factors and expression of various genes.
- Helper T cell–dependent B cell responses to protein antigens require initial activation of naive T cells in the T cell zones and of B cells in lymphoid follicles in lymphoid organs. The activated lymphocytes migrate toward one another and interact at the edges of follicles, where the B cells present the antigen to helper T cells.
- Activated helper T cells express CD40L, which engages CD40 on the B cells, and the T cells secrete cytokines that bind to cytokine receptors on the B cells. The combination of CD40 and cytokine signals stimulates B cell proliferation and differentiation into antibody-secreting cells.
- Helper T cell–derived signals, including CD40L and cytokines, also induce isotype switching in B cells by a process of switch recombination, leading to the production of various Ig isotypes. Different isotypes mediate different effector functions.
- Germinal centers are formed inside the follicles of spleen and lymph node when activated B cells migrate into the follicles and proliferate. The late events in T cell–dependent antibody responses, including affinity maturation and generation of memory B cells, take place within germinal centers.
- Affinity maturation leads to increased affinity of antibodies during the course of a T cell–dependent humoral response. Affinity maturation is a result of somatic hypermutation of Ig heavy and light chain genes followed by selective survival of the B cells that produce the high-affinity antibodies and bind to antigen displayed by FDCs in the germinal centers.
- Some of the progeny of germinal center B cells differentiate into antibody-secreting cells that migrate to extrafollicular regions of secondary lymphoid organs and bone marrow. Other progeny become memory B cells that live for long periods, recirculate between lymph nodes and spleen, and respond rapidly to subsequent exposures of antigen by differentiating into high-affinity antibody secretors.
- Thymus-independent (TI) antigens are nonprotein antigens that induce humoral immune responses without the involvement of helper T cells. Many TI antigens, including polysaccharides, glycolipids, and nucleic acids, are polyvalent, can cross-link multiple membrane Ig molecules on a B cell, and activate complement, thereby activating the B cells without T cell help. TI antigens stimulate antibody responses in which there is limited or no heavy chain class switching, affinity maturation, or memory B cell generation because these features are dependent on helper T cells, which are not activated by nonprotein antigens.
- Antibody feedback is a mechanism by which humoral immune responses are down-regulated when enough antibody has been produced and soluble antibody-antigen complexes are present. B cell membrane Ig and the B cell receptor for the Fc portions of IgG, called FcγRIIB, are clustered together by antibody-antigen complexes. This activates an inhibitory signaling cascade through the cytoplasmic tail of FcγRII that terminates the activation of the B cell.

Selected Readings

Berland H, and HH Wortis. Origins and functions of B-1 cells with notes on the role of CD5. Annual Reviews of Immunology 20:253–300, 2002.

Carroll MC. The role of complement in B cell activation and tolerance. Advances in Immunology 74:61–88, 2000.

Clark EA, and JA Ledbetter. How B and T cells talk to each other. Nature 367:425–428, 1994.

DeFranco AL. B-cell activation 2000. Immunological Reviews 176:5–9, 2000.

Fagarasan S, and T Honjo. T-independent immune response: new aspects of B cell biology. Science 290:89–92, 2000.

Fearon DT, and MC Carroll. Regulation of B lymphocyte responses to foreign and self-antigens by the CD19/CD21 complex. Annual Review of Immunology 18:393–422, 2000.

Foy TM, A Aruffo, J Bajorath, JE Buhlman, and RJ Noelle. Immune regulation by CD40 and its ligand. Annual Review of Immunology 14:591–617, 1996.

Hayakawa K, and RR Hardy. Development and function of B-1 cells. Current Opinion in Immunology 12:346–353, 2000.

Heyman B. Regulation of antibody responses via antibodies, complement, and Fc receptors. Annual Review of Immunology 18:709–737, 2000.

Honjo T, K Kinoshita, and M Muramatsu. Molecular mechanism of class switch recombination: linkage with somatic hypermutation. Annual Review of Immunology 20: 165–196, 2002.

Hsueh RC, and RH Scheuermann. Tyrosine kinase activation in the decision between growth, differentiation, and death responses initiated from the B cell antigen receptor. Advances in Immunology 75:283–316, 2000.

Kurosaki T. Regulation of B cell signal transduction by adapter proteins. Nature Reviews Immunology 2:354–363, 2002.

Martin A, and MD Scharff. AID and mismatch repair in antibody diversification. Nature Reviews Immunology 2: 605–614, 2002.

Mond JJ, A Lees, and CM Snapper. T cell–independent antigens type 2. Annual Review of Immunology 13:665–692, 1995.

Pierce SK. Lipid rafts and B cell activation. Nature Reviews Immunology 2:96–15, 2002.

Przylepa J, C Himes, and G Kelsoe. Lymphocyte development and selection in germinal centers. Current Topics in Microbiology and Immunology 229:85–104, 1998.

Rajewsky K. Clonal selection and learning in the antibody system. Nature 381:751–758, 1996.

Ravetch JV, and LL Lanier. Immune inhibitory receptors. Science 290:84–89, 2000.

Stavnezer J. Antibody class switching. Advances in Immunology 61:79–146, 1996.

Chapter 10

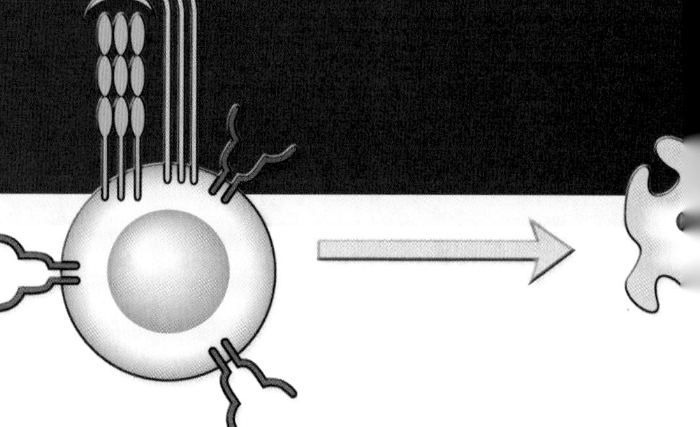

Immunologic Tolerance

Immunologic tolerance is defined as unresponsiveness to an antigen that is induced by previous exposure to that antigen. When specific lymphocytes encounter antigens, the lymphocytes may be activated, leading to immune responses, or the cells may be inactivated or eliminated, leading to tolerance (Fig. 10–1). Different forms of the same antigen may induce an immune response or tolerance. Antigens that induce tolerance are called **tolerogens,** or tolerogenic antigens, to distinguish them from immunogens, which generate immunity. Tolerance to self antigens, also called **self-tolerance,** is a fundamental property of the normal immune system. In this chapter, we discuss immunologic tolerance mainly in the context of self-tolerance and summarize how self-tolerance may fail. We also mention the relevance of this phenomenon to unresponsiveness to foreign antigens. We conclude with a discussion of the mechanisms by which normal immune responses are terminated.

Immunologic tolerance is important for several reasons.

- ***Normal individuals are tolerant of their own antigens (self antigens).*** All individuals inherit essentially the same antigen receptor genes, and these genes recombine and are expressed in lymphocytes as the lymphocytes arise from stem cells. The molecular mechanisms that generate functional antigen receptor genes from germline sequences are random and are not influenced by what is foreign or self for each individual. As a result, different clones of immature lymphocytes may express receptors capable of recognizing various foreign antigens as well as self antigens. Potentially immunogenic self antigens are present on the cells and in the circulation of every individual. An individual's lymphocytes may have free access to many of these self antigens, yet they normally do not mount immune responses against the antigens. This is because of self-tolerance, which is induced by the recognition of self antigens by specific lymphocytes under special conditions.

  The necessity of maintaining self-tolerance was appreciated from the early days of immunology. In Chapter 1, we introduced the concept of **self/**

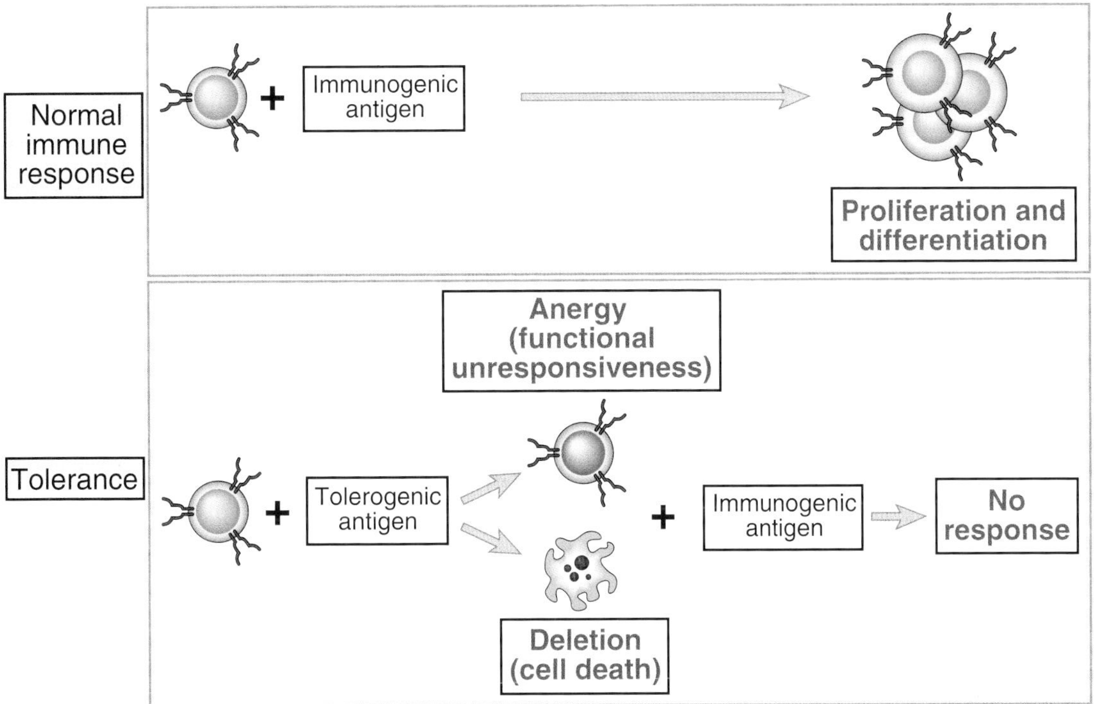

Figure 10–1 Fates of lymphocytes after encounter with antigens.
In a normal immune response, an immunogenic antigen stimulates the proliferation and differentiation of antigen-specific lymphocytes. (Immunogenic antigens are recognized by lymphocytes in the presence of second signals, or costimulators, which are not shown.) Tolerogenic antigens may induce functional unresponsiveness or death of antigen-specific lymphocytes, making these cells incapable of responding to the antigen (tolerance). Some antigens elicit no response (ignorance), but the lymphocytes are able to respond to subsequent antigen challenge (not shown). This illustration depicts T lymphocytes; the same principles apply to B lymphocytes. Note that T lymphocytes recognize antigens presented by antigen-presenting cells, which are not shown.

nonself discrimination, which is the ability of the normal immune system to recognize and respond to foreign antigens but not to self antigens. Burnet added to his clonal selection hypothesis the corollary that lymphocytes specific for self antigens are eliminated to prevent immune reactions against one's own antigens. As we shall see later in this chapter, self-tolerance is maintained by several different mechanisms that prevent the maturation and activation of potentially harmful self-reactive lymphocytes. Failure of self-tolerance results in immune reactions against self (autologous) antigens. Such reactions are called **autoimmunity,** and the diseases they cause are called autoimmune diseases. The pathogenesis and clinicopathologic features of autoimmune diseases will be discussed in Chapter 18. Defining the mechanisms of self-tolerance is the key to understanding the pathogenesis of autoimmune diseases.

- ***Foreign antigens may be administered in ways that inhibit immune responses by inducing tolerance in specific lymphocytes.*** Many of the mechanisms of tolerance to foreign antigens are similar to those of self-tolerance in mature lymphocytes. Effective immunization methods are designed to enhance the immunogenicity of antigens by administering them in ways that promote lymphocyte activation and prevent tolerance induction.

- ***The induction of immunologic tolerance may be exploited as a therapeutic approach for preventing harmful immune responses.*** A great deal of effort is being devoted to development of strategies for inducing tolerance to prevent the rejection of organ allografts and xenografts and to treat autoimmune and allergic diseases. Tolerance induction is also an approach for preventing immune reactions to the products of newly expressed genes in gene therapy protocols and preventing reactions to injected proteins in patients with deficiencies of these proteins (e.g., hemophiliacs treated with factor VIII).

General Features and Mechanisms of Immunologic Tolerance

There are several characteristics of self-tolerance in T and B lymphocyte populations, and many of these are also features of tolerance to foreign antigens.

- ***Tolerance is immunologically specific and results from the recognition of antigens by specific lymphocytes.*** The key advance that allowed immunologists to study the specificity and mechanisms of tolerance was the ability to induce this phenomenon in experimental animals.

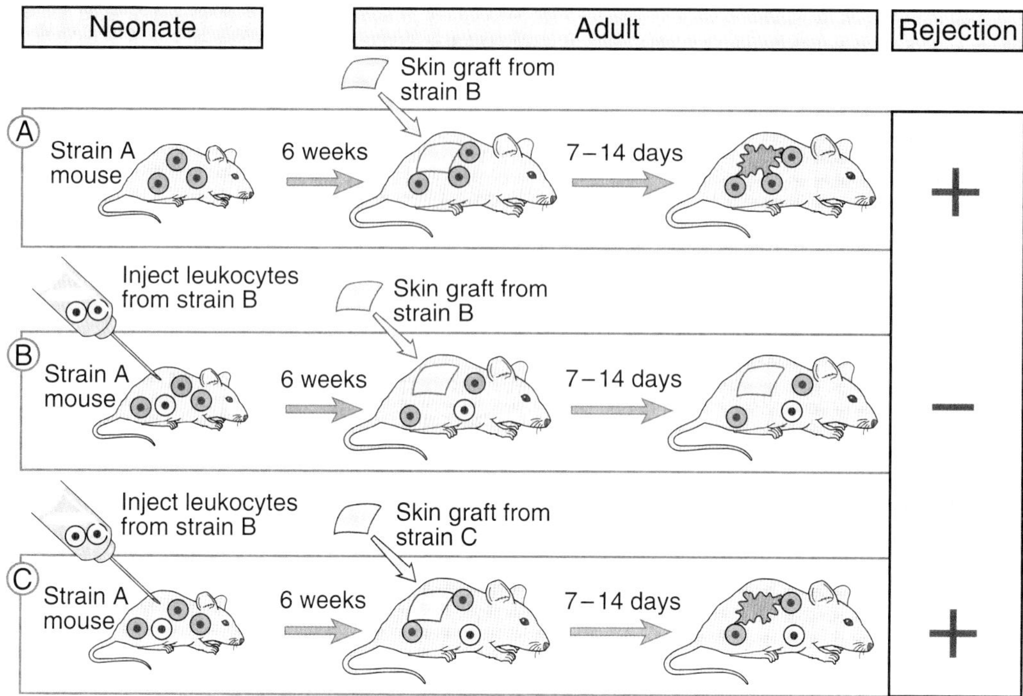

Figure 10–2 The induction of tolerance to tissue transplants. An adult strain A mouse rejects a graft from a strain B mouse (A). If a neonatal strain A mouse is injected with strain B leukocytes (shown in red), when the mouse becomes an adult, it fails to reject a strain B graft (B). This neonatally injected strain A mouse rejects grafts from other strains (e.g., strain C), indicating that tolerance is immunologically specific (C).

The results establishing tolerance as an immunologically specific phenomenon came from studies of graft rejection in inbred mice done by Peter Medawar and colleagues in the 1950s. An adult mouse of strain A will reject a skin graft from an allogeneic mouse of strain B that differs from strain A at the major histocompatibility complex (MHC). If the strain A mouse is injected with lymphocytes of strain B during neonatal life, the injected cells will not be rejected (because the neonate is immunodeficient), and small numbers will survive indefinitely in the recipient, which now becomes a chimera. This strain A recipient will accept a graft from strain B even after it becomes an immunocompetent adult (Fig. 10–2). However, the strain A recipient will reject skin grafts from all mouse strains whose MHC is different from that of strain B. Thus, tolerance to the graft is immunologically specific. Such experiments led to the concept that exposure of developing lymphocytes to foreign antigens induces tolerance to these antigens. The persistence of allogeneic lymphoid cells in a host is called hematopoietic microchimerism, and it is being studied as a possible approach for preventing graft rejection in humans. The mechanism of this form of tolerance remains poorly defined.

- ***Self-tolerance may be induced in generative lymphoid organs as a consequence of immature self-reactive lymphocytes recognizing self antigens, called central tolerance, or in peripheral sites as a result of mature self-reactive lymphocytes encountering self antigens under particular conditions, called peripheral tolerance*** (Fig. 10–3). Central tolerance ensures that the repertoire of mature lymphocytes cannot recognize ubiquitous, or widely disseminated, self antigens, which are the antigens most likely to be present in the generative lymphoid organs. This is the mechanism mainly responsible for the elimination of self-reactive lymphocytes from the mature repertoire and thus for self/nonself discrimination. However, central tolerance cannot explain why the immune system does not respond to antigens that are present only in peripheral tissues. Tolerance to such tissue-specific self antigens is maintained by the mechanisms of peripheral tolerance.

- ***Central tolerance occurs because during their maturation in the generative lymphoid organs, all lymphocytes pass through a stage in which encounter with antigen leads to tolerance rather than activation.*** The most tolerance-sensitive stages of lymphocyte maturation are anatomically confined to the generative (also called central) lymphoid organs, namely, the thymus for T cells and the bone marrow for B lymphocytes. The only antigens normally present at high concentrations in these organs are self antigens because foreign antigens that enter from the external environment are captured and transported to peripheral lymphoid organs, such as

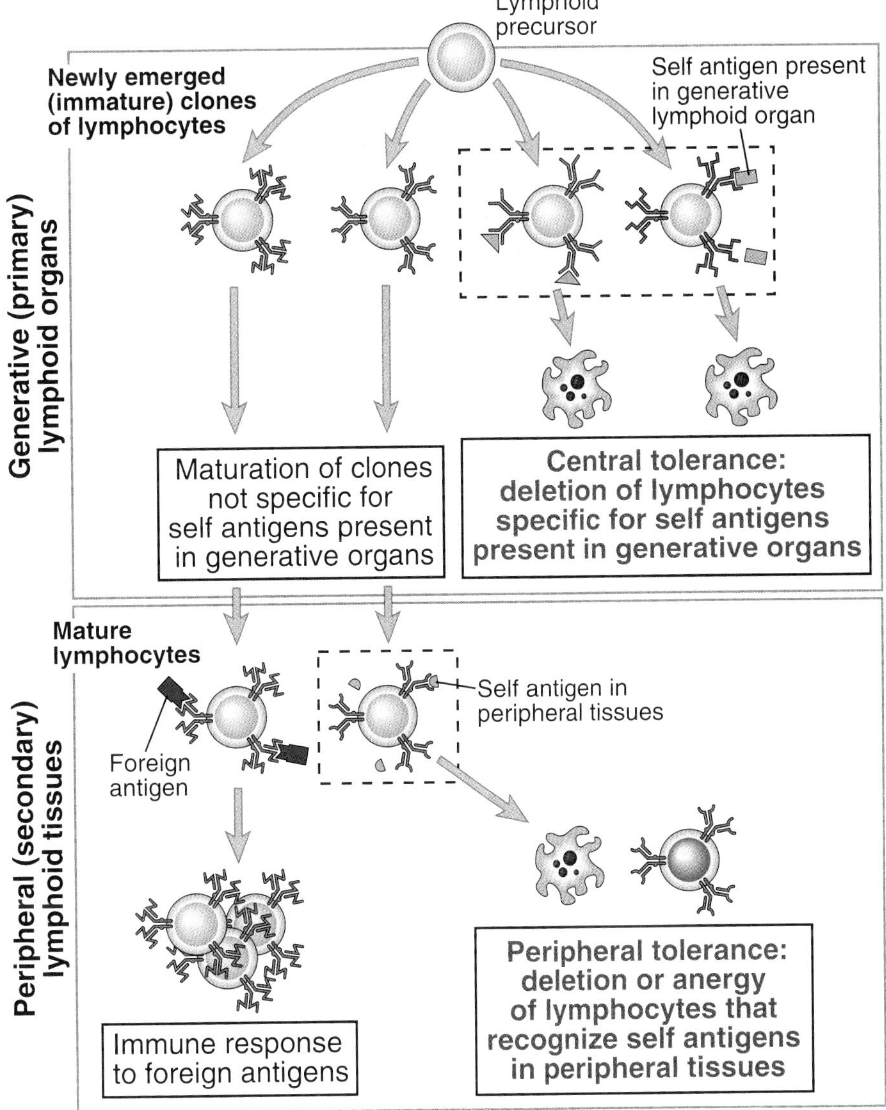

Figure 10–3 Central and peripheral tolerance to self antigens. Immature lymphocytes specific for self antigens may encounter these antigens in the generative lymphoid organs and are then deleted (central tolerance). Some self-reactive lymphocytes may mature and enter peripheral tissues and may be inactivated or deleted by encounter with self antigens in these tissues (peripheral tolerance). The illustration depicts B lymphocytes, but the same processes occur with T lymphocytes.

the lymph nodes, spleen, and mucosal lymphoid tissues. Therefore, in the generative lymphoid organs, immature lymphocytes normally encounter only self antigens at high concentrations, and clones of lymphocytes whose receptors recognize these self antigens with high affinity are killed (deleted). This process is also called **negative selection** (see Chapter 7). Central tolerance eliminates many of the potentially most dangerous lymphocytes (i.e., those with high-affinity receptors for ubiquitous self antigens). Some T cells that encounter self antigens in the thymus may develop into regulatory cells, whose function is to inhibit immune responses (discussed later in the chapter).

- ***Peripheral tolerance is induced when mature lymphocytes recognize antigens without adequate levels of the costimulators that are required for activation or as a result of persistent and repeated stimulation by self antigens in peripheral tissues.*** Peripheral tolerance is most important for maintaining unresponsiveness to self antigens that are expressed in peripheral tissues and not in the generative lymphoid organs. The mature lymphocyte repertoire contains cells capable of recognizing such tissue-specific self antigens, and the responses of the mature lymphocytes to these antigens either are not initiated or are tightly regulated to maintain self-tolerance.

- ***The principal mechanisms of lymphocyte tolerance are apoptotic cell death, called deletion; functional inactivation without cell death, called anergy; and suppression of lymphocyte activation and effector functions by regulatory lymphocytes.*** Central tolerance is mainly due to deletion, whereas all three mechanisms contribute to peripheral tolerance. The induction and relative importance of these mechanisms of tolerance are the main themes of this chapter.

- ***Some self antigens may be ignored by the immune system, so that lymphocytes encounter the self antigen but fail to respond in any detectable way and remain viable and functional.*** The importance of this postulated phenomenon for the maintenance of self-tolerance is not established, and we will not discuss it further.

We do not know how many or which self antigens induce central or peripheral tolerance (or are ignored). This is mainly because study of self-tolerance has been difficult; lymphocytes specific for self antigens either are not present in a normal individual or experimental animal or are functionally silent. In either case, these cells cannot be identified by examining their responses to a self antigen. New experimental approaches, especially the creation of transgenic mice and the identification of genes that influence the choice between tolerance and autoimmunity, have provided valuable experimental models for analyzing self-tolerance, and many of our current concepts are based on studies with such models (Box 10–1). A general principle that has emerged from these studies is that the choice between lymphocyte activation and tolerance is determined by the features of the antigens and by the regulation of lymphocyte responses. Therefore, autoimmunity may result from changes in the display of self antigens or from abnormalities in the selection and regulation of lymphocytes (see Chapter 18).

T Lymphocyte Tolerance

Tolerance in CD4$^+$ helper T lymphocytes is an effective mechanism for preventing immune responses to protein antigens because helper T cells are necessary inducers of both cell-mediated and humoral immune responses to proteins. This realization has been the impetus for a large amount of work on the mechanisms of tolerance in CD4$^+$ T cells. Immunologists have also developed many experimental models for studying tolerance in CD4$^+$ T cells. These systems have provided a great deal of information about CD4$^+$ T cell tolerance, and many of the therapeutic strategies that are being developed to induce tolerance to transplants and autoantigens are targeted to these T cells. Much less is known about tolerance in CD8$^+$ T cells.

Central Tolerance in T Cells

During their maturation in the thymus, immature T cells that recognize antigens with high avidity are deleted (Fig. 10–4). This process of negative selection of T lymphocytes was described in Chapter 7, when the maturation of T cells in the thymus was discussed. The two main factors that determine whether a particular self antigen will induce negative selection of self-reactive thymocytes are the concentration of that antigen in the thymus and the affinity of the thymocyte T cell receptors (TCRs) that recognize the antigen. Self proteins are processed and presented in association with MHC molecules on thymic antigen-presenting cells (APCs). The self antigens that are present in the thymus are diverse and include many circulating and cell-associated proteins. Among the immature T cells that arise from precursors in the thymus are some whose receptors specifically recognize self peptide–MHC complexes with high affinity. If double-positive thymocytes with such high-affinity receptors encounter self antigens in the thymus, the result is apoptotic death of the cells. A likely explanation for the tolerance sensitivity of immature lymphocytes is that antigen recognition triggers signals in these cells different from those in mature lymphocytes. However, we do not know what these signaling differences might be or how they determine the outcome of antigen recognition. This process affects both class I and class II MHC–restricted T cells and is therefore important for tolerance in both CD8$^+$

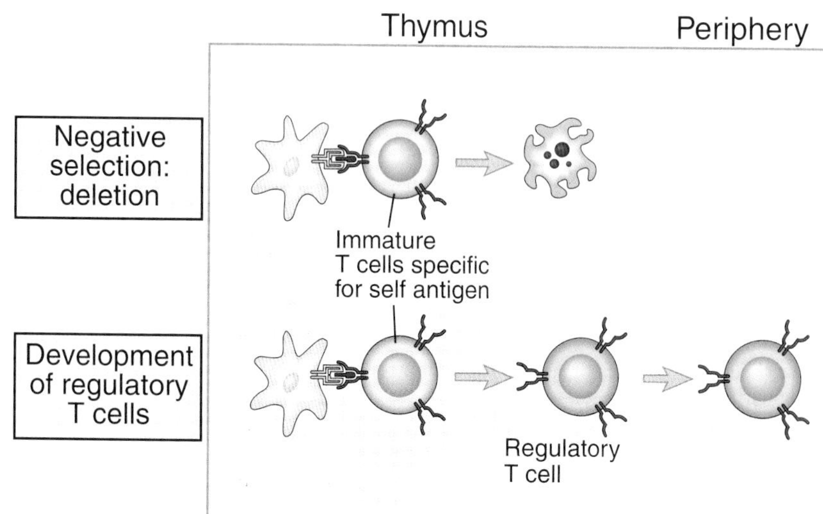

Figure 10–4 Central T cell tolerance. Recognition of self antigens by immature T cells in the thymus may lead to death of the cells (negative selection, or deletion) or the development of regulatory T cells that enter peripheral tissues.

BOX 10–1

Transgenic Mouse Models for the Analysis of Tolerance and Autoimmunity

The experimental analysis of self-tolerance is confounded by two important technical problems. First, it is not possible to identify self-reactive lymphocytes by functional assays because these cells are normally deleted or functionally inactive (anergic). Second, in normal animals or humans, it has been difficult or impossible to define the nature, tissue distribution, and levels of expression of self antigens, particularly MHC-associated peptide antigens for T cells. For these reasons, much of our early understanding of tolerance was based on administering tolerogenic forms of foreign antigens to animals and studying subsequent immune responses to immunogenic forms of the same antigens. Conclusions about self-tolerance were largely extrapolations from these studies with foreign antigens. Transgenic technology has provided a valuable tool for studying self-tolerance in mice. Rearranged antigen receptor genes can be expressed as transgenes in T or B lymphocytes (see Appendix III). Because these antigen receptor genes inhibit recombination at other, endogenous, antigen receptor gene loci (the phenomenon of allelic exclusion), a large fraction of the T or B lymphocytes in these mice express the introduced, transgene-encoded antigen receptor. Therefore, lymphocytes with a known specificity may be detected and followed quantitatively for the life of a mouse. The second application of transgenic technology is to express known proteins in different tissues. These transgene-encoded antigens are present throughout the development of the animal, and therefore they are effectively self antigens for the mouse.

Transgenic approaches may be used to study self-tolerance in many ways.

- The maturation and functional responsiveness of self antigen–specific lymphocytes may be followed in mice by expressing an antigen receptor specific for a normally expressed self antigen. This was first done by expressing a class I MHC–restricted TCR specific for the male antigen H-Y in $CD8^+$ T cells. The T cells fail to mature in male mice because they are negatively selected in the thymus when the immature cells encounter H-Y peptides (see Chapter 7, Fig. 7–21). The same principle has been exploited to study B cell tolerance to a self class I MHC molecule by expressing a membrane Ig specific for one class I allele in B cells. In mice containing that class I allele, the B cells are eliminated in the bone marrow or they change their specificity.
- A variation of this approach is to express transgenic antigen receptors specific for self antigens that are targets of autoimmune diseases. Examples include mice expressing a TCR specific for a protein in pancreatic islet β cells (a target for autoreactive T cells in type I diabetes), a TCR specific for myelin basic protein (which is a central nervous system autoantigen), and Ig specific for self DNA (involved in the autoimmune disease lupus). These transgenic mice are useful for defining not only the mechanisms of self-tolerance but also the pathogenesis of reactions that serve as models of human autoimmune diseases.
- Transgenic models may be made even more amenable to analysis by coexpressing both the antigen receptors of T or B lymphocytes and the antigen that is recognized by these receptors. Two examples we mention in the text are T cells specific for a viral glycoprotein expressed in islet β cells and B cells specific for hen egg lysozyme expressed in different tissues. By changing the promoters used to drive transgene expression, it is possible to vary the site of expression of the antigen. The use of inducible promoters allows investigators to turn the expression of the antigen on and off during the life of the mouse. It is also possible to express the same antigen in different forms (secreted, membrane bound, and cytoplasmic) and thus to analyze tolerance to different types of self antigens.
- Genes encoding particular immunoregulatory molecules, such as costimulators and cytokines, may be coexpressed with antigens, thus modeling the consequences of local alterations in the tissues where particular self antigens are present. In addition, by breeding antigen receptor transgenics with appropriate knockout mice, investigators have generated mice in which lymphocytes of known specificities lack genes encoding lymphocyte regulatory molecules, such as CTLA-4 and Fas ligand. This results in selective defects in lymphocyte regulation and provides models for studying the effects of such changes on defined lymphocyte populations as well as the pathogenesis of disorders associated with mutations in these regulatory genes.

Experimental systems using transgenic and knockout mice have allowed investigators to analyze the types of antigens that induce central and peripheral tolerance in T and B cells, the mechanisms of these pathways of tolerance, and the genetic control of self-tolerance. Experimental protocols have been developed to compare the consequences of self antigen recognition by immature or mature lymphocytes. For instance, as described in the text, by mating one mouse expressing a transgenic antigen receptor with another mouse expressing the antigen, in the offspring, the immature lymphocytes are exposed to the antigen throughout development. Alternatively, mature lymphocytes expressing the antigen receptor may be transferred into mice expressing the antigen as a self protein, and the consequences of this encounter may be analyzed.

Despite the value of transgenic technology, several important caveats should be mentioned. Expression of a single antigen receptor markedly limits the normal lymphocyte repertoire. Transgene-encoded protein antigens are often expressed at higher concentrations than are normal self proteins. Transgene-encoded immunoregulatory molecules not only are expressed at high levels but also are expressed constitutively and constantly, which is rarely the case with normal immunoregulatory molecules. Therefore, many of the normal controls on lymphocyte activation and regulation may be lost in these transgenic mice.

and CD4$^+$ lymphocyte populations. Negative selection of thymocytes is responsible for the fact that the repertoire of mature T cells that leave the thymus and populate peripheral lymphoid tissues is unresponsive to the self antigens that are present at high concentrations in the thymus. The mechanism of deletion during negative selection is apoptotic death, but the signals and receptors involved in this process are not known. Some self-reactive T cells that see self antigens in the thymus may not be deleted and instead may differentiate into regulatory T cells (see Fig. 10–4) that leave the thymus and inhibit responses against self tissues in the periphery (discussed later).

It is often hypothesized that autoimmunity results from a failure of negative selection in the thymus. However, little formal evidence supports this hypothesis in any human or experimental autoimmune disease. In fact, it is possible that even if central tolerance fails, peripheral mechanisms are adequate for maintaining unresponsiveness to many self antigens.

- In one animal model of diabetes, the nonobese diabetic (NOD) mouse, it is postulated that class II MHC molecules are structurally unstable and incapable of presenting self antigens in the thymus at concentrations high enough to induce negative selection. As a result, CD4$^+$ T cells specific for many self antigens may mature and enter peripheral tissues in NOD mice, and these T cells cause many autoimmune diseases (insulitis and diabetes, thyroiditis, sialadenitis, to name a few). However, this theory has not been formally proved, and it is not clear how the same MHC molecules that fail to induce negative selection in the thymus are able to present self peptides in peripheral tissues to activate mature T cells and produce autoimmune disease.

Peripheral T Cell Tolerance

Peripheral tolerance is the mechanism by which mature T cells that recognize self antigens in peripheral tissues become incapable of subsequently responding to these antigens. Peripheral tolerance mechanisms are responsible for T cell tolerance to tissue-specific self antigens that are not abundant in the thymus. The same mechanisms may induce unresponsiveness to tolerogenic forms of foreign antigens. Peripheral tolerance is due to anergy, deletion, or suppression of T cells, and each of these mechanisms has been defined for CD4$^+$ cells in several experimental models.

Anergy Induced by Antigen Recognition without Adequate Costimulation

If CD4$^+$ T cells recognize peptide antigens presented by APCs that are deficient in costimulators, the T cells survive but are rendered incapable of responding to the antigen even if it is later presented by competent APCs (Fig. 10–5). This type of functional unresponsiveness was first demonstrated by *in vitro* experiments with cloned lines of mouse T cells and was called **clonal anergy.** We previously introduced the concept that full activation of T cells requires the recognition of antigen by the TCR (signal 1) and recognition of costimulators, mainly B7-1 and B7-2, by CD28 (signal 2) (see Chapter 8). Signal 1 (i.e., antigen recognition) alone may lead to anergy. Antigen-induced anergy has been demonstrated in a variety of experimental systems.

- If cloned lines of mouse CD4$^+$ T cells are exposed to peptide-MHC complexes presented on synthetic lipid membranes, on APCs that lack costimulators like B7 molecules, or on APCs that are treated with chemicals that destroy costimulators, the T cells remain viable but are incapable of responding to the antigen even if it is subsequently presented by competent APCs (Fig. 10–6). The induction of anergy may be prevented during the first culture by adding APCs that do express costimulators or by stimulating CD28, the T lymphocyte receptor for B7 molecules, with specific antibodies. This type of anergy is also prevented and even reversed by adding interleukin (IL)-2 to the cultures, providing a growth stimulus to the antigen-responsive T cells. It has proved difficult to do such experiments with normal, naive T cells, because these cells die unless they encounter costimulators.

- T cell anergy can be induced by administering foreign antigens in ways that result in antigen recognition without costimulation. In one experimental model, small numbers of T cells from transgenic mice expressing a TCR specific for a known antigen are transferred into normal mice, and the recipients are exposed to the antigen in different forms. If the antigen is administered subcutaneously with adjuvants (the immunogenic form), antigen-specific T cells proliferate in the draining lymph nodes, differentiate into effector cells, and migrate toward lymphoid follicles, where T cell–B cell interactions occur. In contrast, if a large dose of the antigen is administered in aqueous form, without adjuvants (the tolerogenic form), the antigen-specific T cells remain viable but with a greatly reduced ability to proliferate, differentiate, or migrate toward follicles (Fig. 10–7). It is believed that in this model, the aqueous antigen induces anergy in the antigen-specific T cells, resulting in a block in the expansion and effector functions of the cells. These experiments also illustrate an important principle mentioned earlier in the chapter, that the same antigen may be immunogenic or tolerogenic, depending on how it is administered.

- An antigen, such as a viral glycoprotein, may be expressed in the tissues of a mouse as a transgene. This is often done by expressing the antigen under the control of the insulin promoter, in which case it is produced mainly by pancreatic islet β cells. In effect, this viral protein becomes a tissue-specific self antigen for the mouse. If the antigen-expressing transgenic mouse is bred with another mouse that expresses the antigen-specific TCR as a transgene, large numbers of the specific T cells encounter the self antigen. These T cells

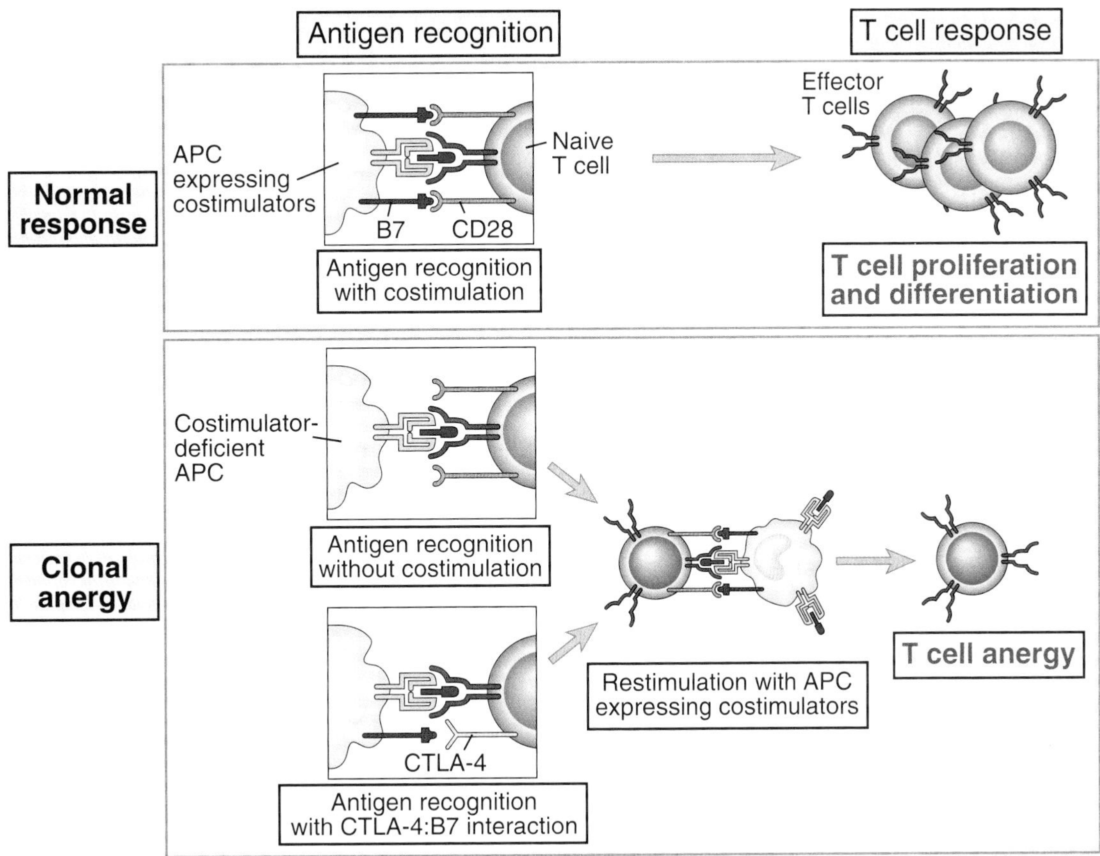

Figure 10–5 T cell anergy.
T cell responses are induced when the cells recognize an antigen presented by a costimulator-expressing antigen-presenting cell (APC) and recognize costimulators (such as B7) by activating receptors (CD28). If the T cell recognizes antigen without costimulation or in the presence of CTLA-4:B7 interaction, the T cell fails to respond and may be rendered incapable of responding even if the antigen is subsequently presented by costimulator-expressing APCs.

may become anergic and do not respond to the viral antigen even if they are removed from the mouse and exposed to the antigen *ex vivo* (Fig. 10–8). Presumably, the transgene-encoded viral glycoprotein is presented by APCs, in the pancreatic islets or draining lymph nodes, that do not express adequate levels of costimulators needed to elicit T cell responses, and recognition of antigen on these APCs leads to T cell anergy. In the same experimental model, coexpression of the viral antigen and B7 costimulators in islet cells results in the breakdown of anergy and immune responses against the islets. This result illustrates how aberrant expression of costimulators may trigger autoimmune reactions, a concept we will return to in Chapter 18.

Anergy may be induced if T cells use the inhibitory receptor for B7 molecules, CTLA-4, to recognize costimulators on APCs at the time that the cells are recognizing antigen (see Fig. 10–5). In this situation, anergy is not a consequence of antigen recognition without costimulation; rather, anergy is induced because the CTLA-4 receptor delivers active inhibitory signals to the T cells when this receptor encounters B7 costimulators on APCs.

- The importance of CTLA-4 in tolerance induction is illustrated by the finding that knockout mice lacking CTLA-4 develop uncontrolled lymphocyte activation with massively enlarged lymph nodes and spleen and fatal multiorgan lymphocytic infiltrates suggestive of systemic autoimmunity. In other words, eliminating this one control mechanism results in a severe T cell–mediated disease.
- Blocking CTLA-4 with antibodies also enhances autoimmune diseases in animal models, such as encephalomyelitis induced by immunization with myelin antigens and diabetes induced by injection of T cells reactive with antigens in the β cells of pancreatic islets.
- In the antigen-induced model of anergy described earlier (see Fig. 10–7), T cells lacking CTLA-4 are resistant to the induction of anergy.

These findings indicate that in normal animals, CTLA-4 functions continuously to keep T cells in check. We do not know the factors that determine why T cells recognize B7 molecules with the activating receptor CD28 to induce immune responses under some conditions and, at other times, recognize the same

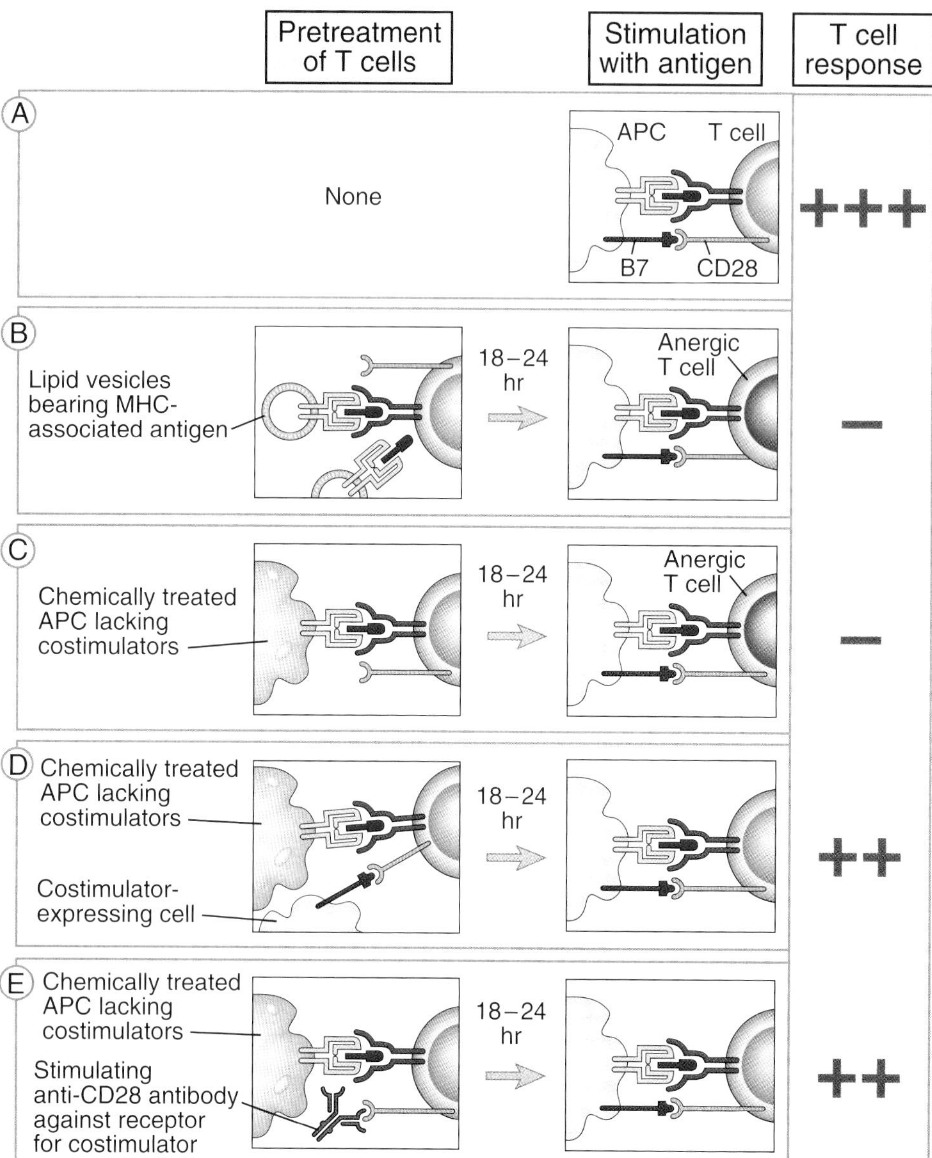

Figure 10–6 Role of B7 costimulators in T cell activation and anergy.
T cell activation requires antigen recognition and the interaction of CD28 on the T cell with B7 molecules on the antigen-presenting cell (APC) (A). Pretreatment of the T cells with lipid vesicles that display the antigen but lack B7 (B) or with APCs that are treated to destroy costimulators (C) results in T cell anergy and a failure to respond to antigen presented by normal APCs. Providing a costimulatory signal from another cell (D) or with an anti-CD28 antibody (E) prevents the induction of anergy. Such experiments are done with T cell clones specific for defined peptides.

B7 molecules with the inhibitory receptor CTLA-4 to induce tolerance. It is possible that APCs that express low levels of B7 normally engage CTLA-4 preferentially because CTLA-4 binds to B7 molecules with higher affinity than does CD28. Also, CD28 is expressed on naive T cells and may therefore be used to initiate immune responses, whereas CTLA-4 is expressed after T cells are activated and may function to terminate responses. It is not known whether self-reactive T cells start responding to self antigens, express CTLA-4, and are then prevented from responding further.

Such experimental results have led to the hypothesis that ***the nature of tissue APCs is an important determinant of whether self-tolerance or autoimmunity develops.*** APCs that are resident in peripheral lymphoid and nonlymphoid tissues are normally in a resting state and express few or no costimulators. Such APCs may be constantly presenting self antigens, and T cells that recognize these antigens become anergic. As we shall discuss in Chapter 18, local infections and inflammation may activate resident APCs, leading to increased expression of costimulators, breakdown of tolerance, and autoimmune reactions against the tissue antigens. However, which self antigens normally induce anergy in specific T cells, and the fates of anergic cells *in vivo*, are unknown.

The biochemical mechanisms of anergy also remain poorly defined. Anergic T cells fail to produce their growth factor, IL-2, and to proliferate in response to antigen. In T cell clones that are rendered anergic, cross-linking of the TCR fails to trigger signal transduction pathways that lead to the activation of the enzymes JNK and ERK, which are involved in the generation of the AP-1 transcription factor (see Chapter 8). It is interesting that not all TCR-mediated signals are lost in these functionally inactive T cells; the mechanism of this selective biochemical defect is not known.

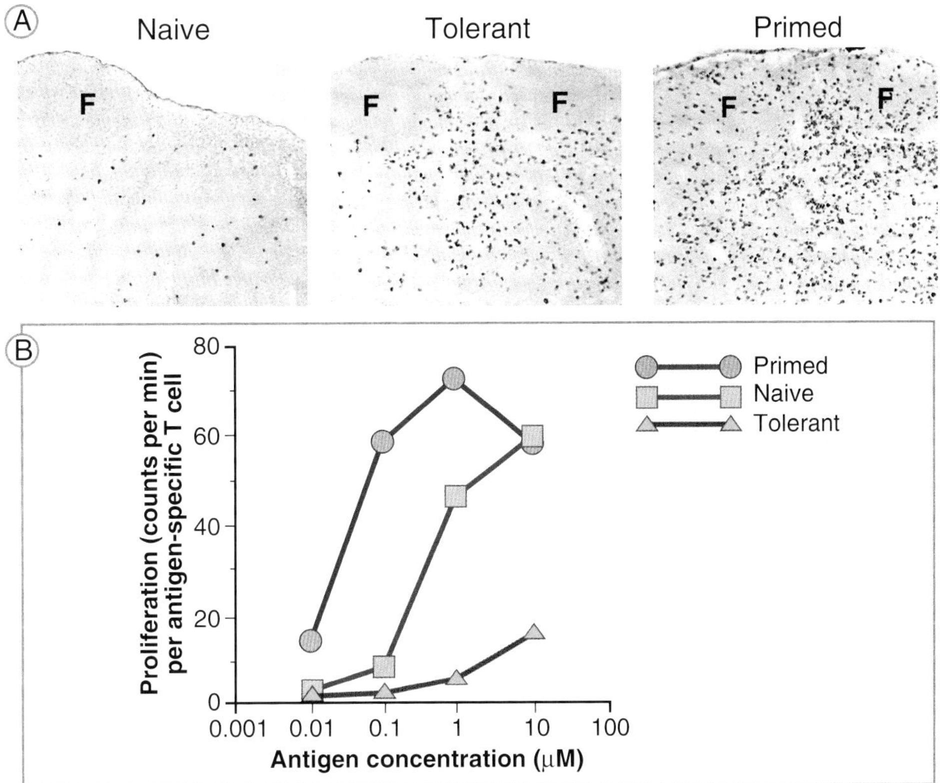

Figure 10–7 Induction of T cell tolerance by an aqueous antigen.

T cells from transgenic mice expressing an antigen receptor specific for a peptide of ovalbumin are transferred into normal recipient mice, and the recipients are left untreated or are exposed to the peptide in immunogenic form (with adjuvant) or in tolerogenic form (large dose of aqueous peptide without adjuvant).

A. Lymph nodes of the recipient mice are stained with an antibody that recognizes the ovalbumin-specific T cells. Untreated (naive) mice contain few of these T cells. In mice given tolerogenic antigen (tolerant), there is some expansion in the number of T cells, but the cells fail to enter the B cell–rich lymphoid follicles (F). In mice given immunogenic antigen (primed), there is greater expansion of T cells, and these cells do enter the follicles. (From Pape KA, ER Kearney, A Khoruts, A Mondino, R Mevica, ZM Chen, E Inguli, J White, JG Johnson, and MK Jenkins. Use of adoptive transfer of T cell-antigen-receptor-transgenic T cells for the study of T-cell activation *in vivo.* Immunological Reviews 156:67–78, 1997. Copyright 1997 by Munksgaard.)

B. The T cells are recovered from the transfer recipients and stimulated with ovalbumin peptide in culture, and their proliferative responses are measured by the incorporation of ^{3}H-thymidine into DNA (expressed as counts per minute per T cell). Naive T cells respond to antigen, cells from primed mice show an increased response, and cells from tolerant mice fail to respond, an indication of anergy. (From Kearney ER, KA Pape, DY Loh, and MK Jenkins. Visualization of peptide-specific T cell immunity and peripheral tolerance induction *in vivo.* Immunity 1:327–339, 1994. Copyright 1994, with permission from Elsevier Science.)

It has not been possible to carry out similar biochemical analyses in normal T cells that are rendered anergic by a transgene-encoded self antigen or by antigens administered in tolerogenic forms.

On the basis of experimental studies of anergy induced by antigen recognition without adequate costimulation, attempts are ongoing to promote the acceptance of organ allografts by blocking costimulators at the time of transplantation. In experimental animals, encouraging results have been seen in graft recipients treated with a combination of antagonists that block both B7 molecules and CD40 ligand (CD40L) (see Chapter 16) or with antagonists of CD40L used alone. The role of the CD40:CD40L pathway in tolerance is undefined. The important finding is that these antagonists induce prolonged graft acceptance, well beyond the half-lives of the administered antagonists. This suggests that the antagonists are inducing long-lived transplantation tolerance and not merely preventing acute graft rejection. Clinical trials with costimulator antagonists in transplant recipients are ongoing. The same strategy may be useful for treatment of autoimmune diseases, although here the challenge will be to inhibit established pathologic immune responses against self antigens.

Deletion of T Cells by Activation-Induced Cell Death

Repeated stimulation of T lymphocytes by persistent antigens results in death of the activated cells by a

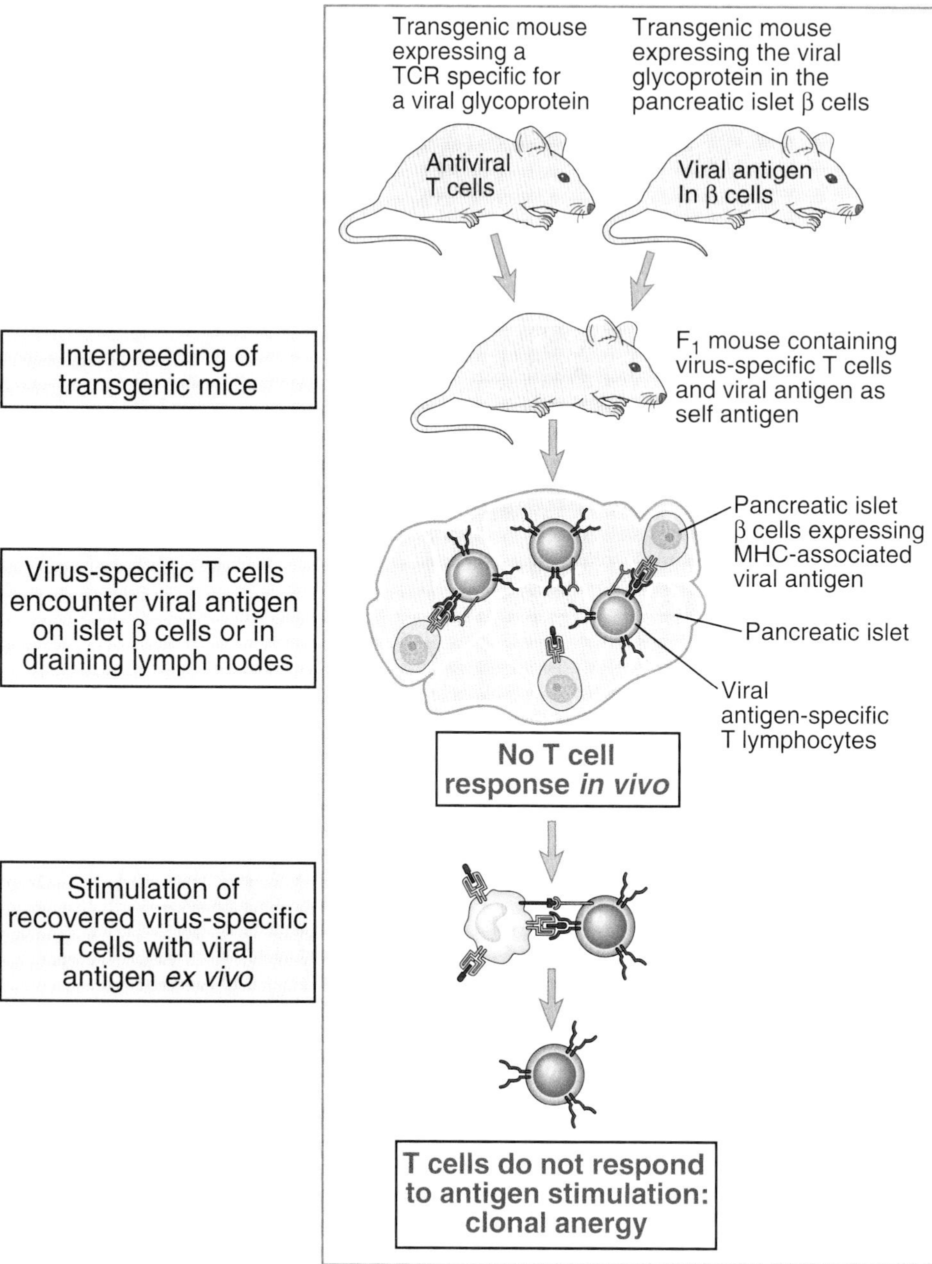

Figure 10–8 T cell anergy induced by a self antigen in transgenic mice.

Two sets of transgenic mice are created, one that expresses a TCR specific for a viral glycoprotein antigen and another that expresses the antigen in the β cells of pancreatic islets. When these two mice are interbred, in the F_1 offspring, the T cells encounter this islet self antigen, but there may not be a T cell response *in vivo*. If the T cells are recovered and challenged with the viral antigen, the cells fail to respond, indicating that the cells became anergic *in vivo*. In some similar experiments, the T cells fail to respond *in vivo* but remain functionally responsive, indicating that they have ignored the presence of the self antigen.

process of apoptosis (Fig. 10–9). This form of regulated cell death is called **activation-induced cell death.** It is induced when large numbers of recently activated T cells are reactivated by antigens or agents that mimic antigens.

- If $CD4^+$ T cells that have recently been activated *in vitro* with polyclonal activators, such as anti-CD3 antibodies, are restimulated with the same activators, the T cells undergo apoptosis. This also happens when recently activated antigen-specific T cell clones are cultured with high concentrations of the antigen.
- Some microbial proteins bind to and activate all T cells whose TCR β chain variable (V) regions belong to a particular family; such proteins are called superantigens (see Chapter 15, Box 15–1). In mice injected with a large dose of a superantigen, T cells expressing the V_β-containing TCRs first are activated and then die by apoptosis.
- If mice expressing a transgenic TCR on most of their T cells are injected with high doses of the antigen that is recognized by that TCR, again the T cells first are activated and then undergo apoptosis.

Activation-induced cell death is a form of apoptosis induced by signals from membrane death receptors (Box 10–2). In $CD4^+$ T cells, repeated activation leads to the coexpression of two molecules, a death-inducing receptor called Fas (CD95) and its ligand, Fas ligand (FasL). Fas is a member of the tumor necrosis factor

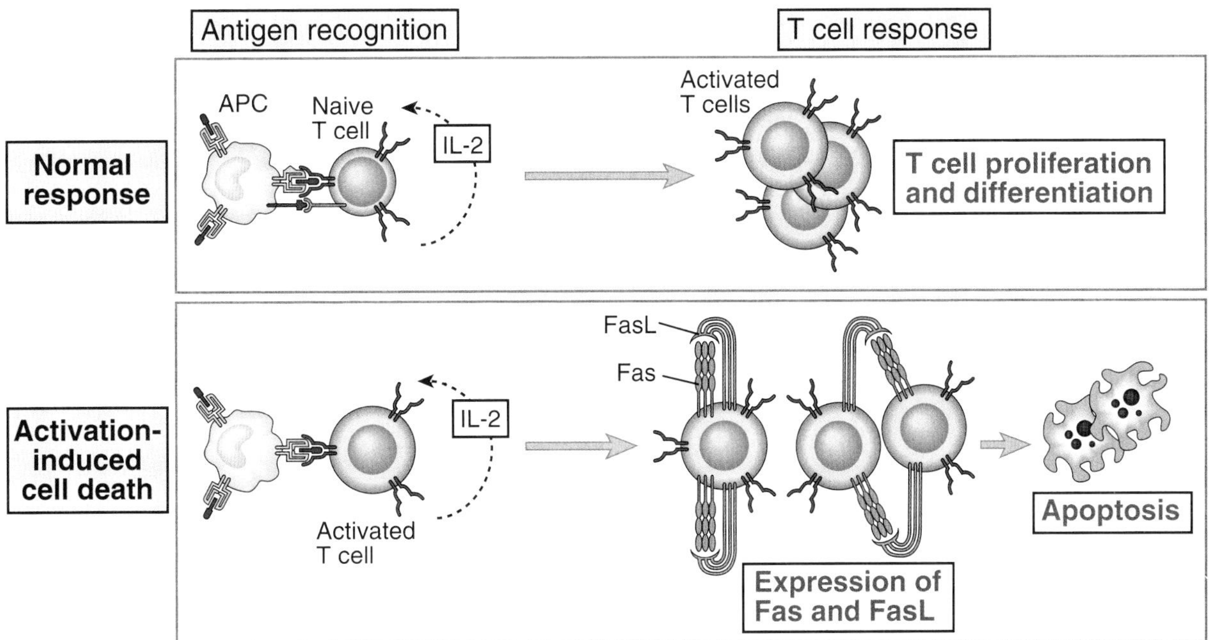

Figure 10–9 Fas-mediated activation-induced death of T lymphocytes. T cells respond to antigen presented by a normal antigen-presenting cell (APC) by secreting IL-2 and undergoing proliferation and differentiation. Restimulation of recently activated T cells by antigen leads to coexpression of the death receptor Fas and Fas ligand (FasL), engagement of Fas, and apoptotic death of the T cells. Note that FasL on one T cell may engage Fas either on the same cell or on another cell.

BOX 10–2

Apoptosis in Lymphocytes

There are many situations in biology when cells normally die and are eliminated by phagocytosis without eliciting harmful inflammatory reactions. For instance, the process of embryogenesis involves modeling of tissues and organs by balanced cell division and cell death, and physiologic reductions in circulating hormone levels lead to death of hormone-dependent cells. In these situations, cell death occurs by a process called **apoptosis,** which is characterized by DNA cleavage, nuclear condensation and fragmentation, plasma membrane blebbing, changes in membrane lipid distribution, and detachment of cells from the extracellular matrix. Apoptotic cells are rapidly phagocytosed because they express membrane molecules that are recognized by a variety of receptors on phagocytes. This type of physiologic cell death contrasts with necrosis, in which plasma membrane integrity breaks down and cellular contents are enzymatically degraded and released, resulting in pathologic inflammation. In the immune system, apoptosis is important for eliminating unwanted and potentially dangerous lymphocytes at many stages of maturation and after activation of mature cells. In the following sections, we describe the mechanisms and regulation of apoptosis, focusing on lymphocytes. The physiologic roles of apoptosis in the immune system are discussed in this and other chapters.

INDUCTION OF APOPTOSIS IN LYMPHOCYTES The induction of apoptosis involves the activation of cytosolic enzymes called **caspases.** Caspases are cysteine proteases (i.e., proteases with cysteines in their active sites), so named because they cleave substrates at aspartic acid residues. Caspases are present in the cytoplasm of most cells in an inactive form (also called a zymogen, referring to an inactive enzyme). In its inactive state, a caspase exists as a single polypeptide chain with a prodomain and a catalytic domain. Caspases are themselves activated by cleavage after aspartic residues, and the active caspase that is produced is a dimer with two catalytic subunits. Fourteen caspases have been identified, and the number is likely to increase. Some caspases function as initiators, to start the process of apoptosis often by cleaving and thereby activating more caspases. These activated caspases function as effectors or executioners, cleaving many substrates and leading to nuclear fragmentation and the other changes of apoptosis. In lymphocytes, caspase activation and subsequent apoptosis may be induced by two distinct pathways, one of which is associated with mitochondrial permeability changes and the other with signals from death receptors in the plasma membrane. The mechanisms of induction of these two pathways are illustrated in Figure A, and their biochemical mechanisms are in Figure B.

Passive cell death as a result of loss of survival stimuli: the intrinsic, or mitochondrial, pathway of apoptosis. If lymphocytes are deprived of necessary survival stimuli, such as growth factors or costimulators (for T cells), the result is rapid increase in the permeability of mitochondrial membranes and release of several proteins, including cytochrome *c*, into the cytoplasm. Cytochrome *c* functions

Continued on following page

BOX 10–2

Apoptosis in Lymphocytes (*Continued*)

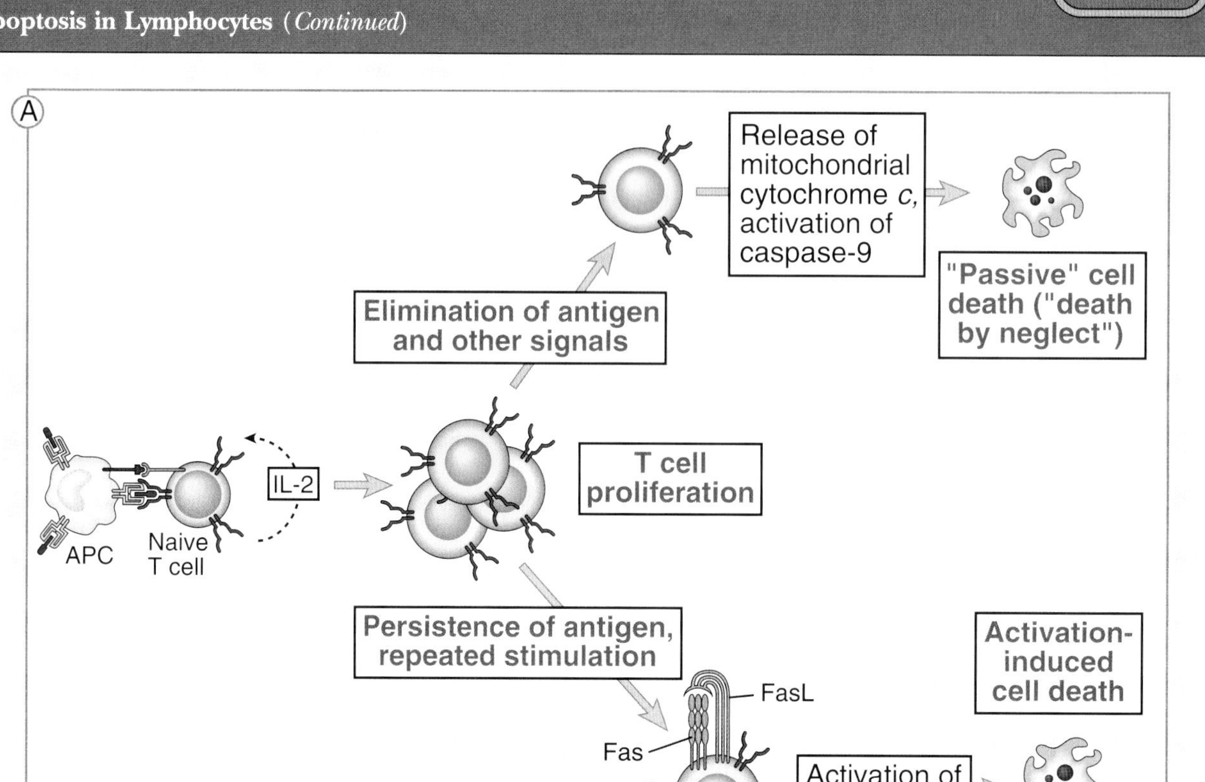

A. Pathways of T cell apoptosis.
Activated T cells die when antigens and other survival stimuli are lost (passive cell death), or they undergo activation-induced death as a result of repeated stimulation by antigen. Note that FasL on one T cell may engage Fas either on the same cell (as shown) or on another cell. These pathways are best described for $CD4^+$ T cells. APC, antigen-presenting cell.

as a cofactor with a protein called apoptosis activating factor-1 (Apaf-1) to activate an enzyme, called caspase-9, that initiates the apoptotic pathway. Other proteins released from mitochondria may directly block the normal anti-apoptotic activities of Bcl family members (described later), again resulting in cell death. This pathway of apoptosis is called passive cell death, implying that it does not require active signals resulting from the engagement of death receptors. (Note, however, that all pathways of apoptosis are actively induced by enzymes and protein degradation.) This form of apoptosis is also called **programmed cell death,** or death by neglect, implying that many cells are programmed to die unless protected by survival stimuli, and they will die if neglected (not provided survival stimuli). DNA damage caused by irradiation, certain chemotherapeutic drugs, and glucocorticoids may induce apoptosis of target cells by the mitochondrial pathway. In addition, antigen recognition alone may trigger mitochondrial translocation of pro-apoptotic members of the Bcl family (such as Bim, Bax, and Bak), which block the protective actions of the anti-apoptotic members, again resulting in cell death.

Activation-induced cell death mediated by death receptors: the extrinsic, or receptor-initiated, pathway of apoptosis. The second pathway of apoptosis in lymphocytes is triggered by the binding of ligands to death-inducing membrane receptors. The best defined death receptors belong to a family of proteins with homologous cysteine-rich extracellular domains. The first members of this family to be identified were receptors for the cytokine tumor necrosis factor (TNF), and the family includes a large number of proteins, such as Fas and CD40. The cytoplasmic regions of different members of this family contain either a conserved "death domain" or a domain that binds signaling molecules and activates transcription factors. (The pathway of transcriptional activation by TNF receptors is described in Chapter 11, Box 11–1.) The two best described death domain–containing receptors are Fas (CD95) and the type I TNF receptor; we focus on Fas as the prototype because its role in lymphocyte regulation is better established. Fas was identified as a 36-kD surface protein that, on cross-linking by specific antibodies, triggered apoptosis of cells that expressed it. Lymphoid cells and many other cell types express Fas. Fas ligand (FasL) is

Continued on following page

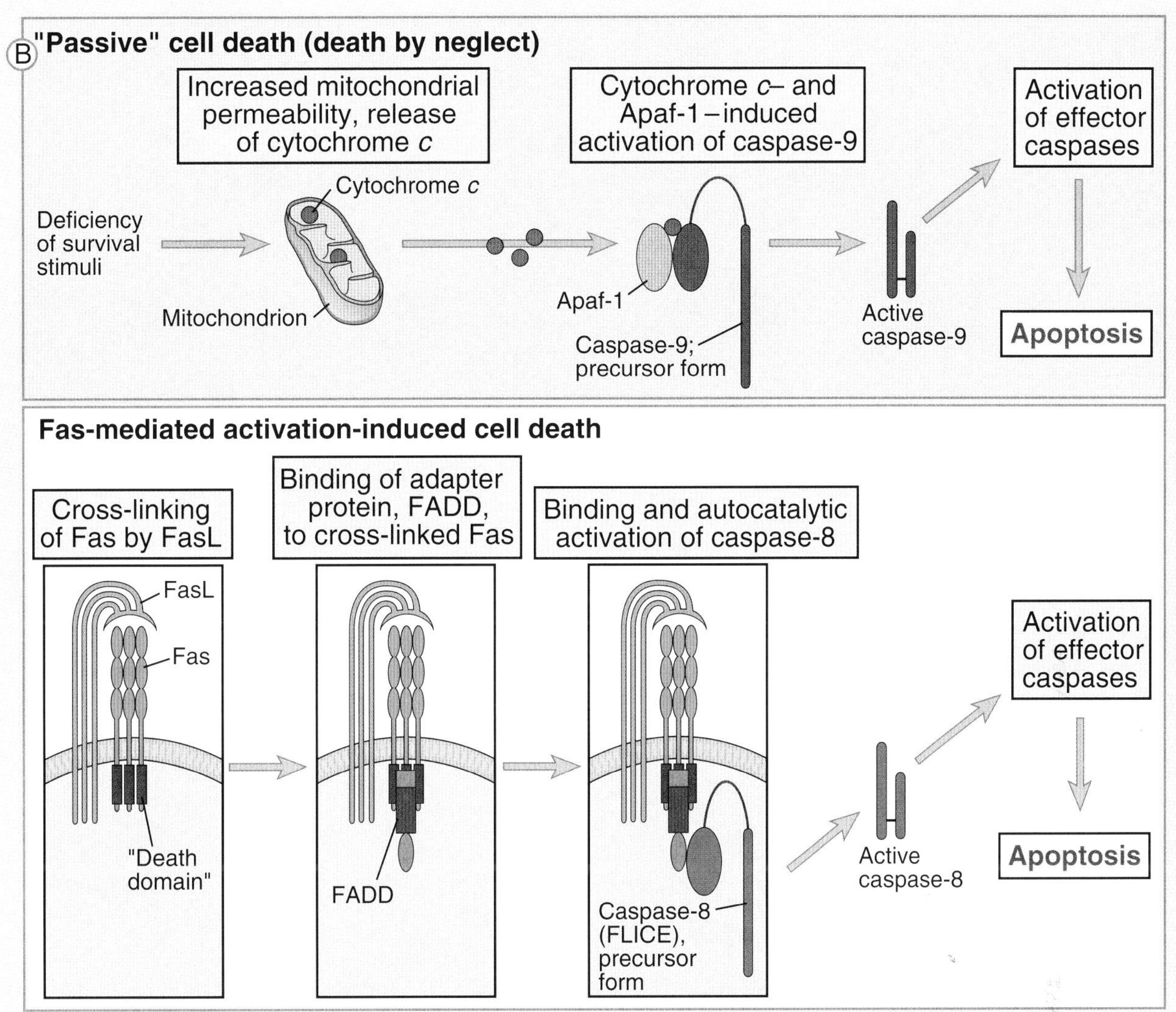

B. Biochemical mechanisms of apoptosis.
In passive cell death and activation-induced cell death, different mechanisms lead to activation of caspase-9 and caspase-8, respectively, and ultimately to apoptosis. Cytochrome *c* is one of several pro-apoptotic molecules released from mitochondria that become permeable because of deficiency of survival signals or damage. Note that FasL on one T cell may engage Fas either on the same cell (as shown) or on another cell.

a homotrimeric membrane protein that is expressed mainly on T lymphocytes after activation by antigen and IL-2. When mature T lymphocytes are repeatedly stimulated by antigens, they coexpress Fas and FasL. FasL binds to Fas on the same or adjacent cells, clustering three or more Fas molecules. The intracellular death domains of the clustered Fas receptors bind a cytosolic death domain–containing adapter protein called FADD (for Fas-associated death domain). FADD, in turn, binds the inactive form of a caspase, caspase-8 (see Figure B). Caspase-8 undergoes autocatalytic activation and is then able to activate effector caspases and trigger apoptosis. This pathway of apoptosis is called **activation-induced cell death** because it is induced by lymphocyte activation (and not by the absence of survival stimuli). The type I TNF receptor probably triggers a similar pathway of cell death. Although the type I TNF receptor does not bind FADD directly, its cytoplasmic domain does bind a homologous protein, called TRADD (for TNF receptor–associated death domain), that can recruit FADD to the complex. The physiologic role of TNF receptors in regulating lymphocyte survival and in self-tolerance is not established. Note that apoptosis induced by antigen recognition, and involving the mitochondrial pathway, has also been called activation-induced cell death, because it follows activation by the antigen.

Passive cell death by the mitochondrial pathway and activation-induced cell death by the death receptor pathway differ in how they are induced and, as we shall see, in their regulation and principal physiologic roles (see Table). In some nonlymphoid cells, such as hepatocytes, Fas-induced signals result in increased mitochondrial permeability, and the two death pathways may act cooperatively to trigger apoptosis. Many of the proteins known to

Continued on following page

BOX 10–2

Apoptosis in Lymphocytes (*Continued*)

induce and regulate apoptosis were identified as the products of genes that are homologous to genes first shown to regulate apoptosis in the worm *Caenorhabditis elegans.* During the development of this worm, particular cells die in a precise sequence, so that the consequences of genetic manipulations on death or survival of cells can be accurately defined. Several different *ced* genes (for "*ce*ll *d*eath abnormal" genes) are known, and their mammalian homologues have been identified. Caspase-9 is homologous to Ced-3, Apaf-1 to Ced-4, and the anti-apoptotic protein Bcl-2 (see below) to Ced-9.

Effector mechanisms of apoptosis. Once caspase-9 or caspase-8 becomes proteolytically active, it in turn cleaves and activates other downstream effector caspases, including caspase-3 and caspase-6. These enzymes act on a variety of substrates, including nucleases and proteins of the nuclear envelope, to initiate DNA fragmentation and nuclear breakdown, the hallmarks of apoptosis. (Note that not all mammalian caspases are involved in cell death. The first of these enzymes to be identified, now called caspase-1, functions to convert the precursor form of the cytokine IL-1β to its active form and was therefore originally called the IL-1–converting enzyme [ICE]. On the basis of this name, caspase-8 was originally called FADD-like ICE or FLICE.)

REGULATION OF APOPTOSIS Programmed death of lymphocytes (passive cell death) is prevented by various activating stimuli, including specific antigen recognition, growth factors (such as the cytokine IL-2), and costimulation (e.g., engagement of CD28 on T cells by B7 molecules on APCs). All these stimuli function by inducing the expression of anti-apoptotic proteins of the **Bcl** family. The first member of this family to be identified was called Bcl-2 because it was the second oncogene found in a human B cell lymphoma. Bcl-2, and its homologue Bcl-x, inhibit apoptosis by blocking the release of pro-apoptotic proteins like cytochrome *c* from mitochondria and by inhibiting the activation of caspase-9 (see Figure B). Several other Bcl family members have been identified that form homodimers and heterodimers and can be phosphorylated in response to growth factors, thereby regulating their activities. The details of these interactions are being investigated in many laboratories. Some proteins related to Bcl proteins are pro-apoptotic. For instance, a protein called Bid (which contains a domain that is homologous to domains found in Bcl proteins) binds to and blocks the activity of Bcl-2. Therefore, Bid promotes apoptosis. Another related protein called Bim, which may be induced by antigen recognition, antagonizes Bcl-2 and thus promotes apoptosis. Many other pro-apoptotic and anti-apoptotic members of this complex family are known. Bcl proteins do not appear to block Fas/TNF receptor–induced apoptosis in most cell types.

Activation-induced cell death by the Fas pathway is prevented by a protein called FLIP (for FLICE-inhibitory protein) that has a death domain but lacks a caspase domain. FLIP may bind to the adapter protein FADD or to inactive caspase-8 in the cytoplasm, but it cannot activate the caspase. Thus, it competitively inhibits the binding of caspase-8 to the Fas-associated protein complex and blocks the apoptotic signal. Naive T cells contain high levels of FLIP, and activation of the cells in the presence of IL-2 reduces the expression of FLIP. This is why the Fas pathway is inactive in naive T cells, allowing antigen-stimulated responses to develop, but becomes active after T cell stimulation, functioning to prevent responses to repeated antigen encounter.

PHYSIOLOGIC ROLES OF APOPTOSIS IN LYMPHOCYTES Programmed, or passive, cell death plays an essential role in controlling the size of the lymphocyte pool

Pathways of Apoptosis in Lymphocytes

Features	"Passive" cell death (death by neglect)	Activation-induced cell death
Induced by	Deficiency of survival stimuli (antigen, growth factors, costimulators)	Repeated lymphocyte activation
Membrane receptors involved	None	Death receptors (e.g., Fas)
Early caspases involved	Caspase-9	Caspase-8 (and caspase-10 in humans)
Effect of IL-2 on T cells	Prevents apoptosis	Enhances apoptosis
Role of Bcl proteins	Prevents apoptosis	No effect in most cell types
Principal physiologic roles	Death of immature lymphocytes that fail positive selection Death of mature cells that do not encounter antigen, and after antigen is eliminated	Elimination of some self-reactive mature lymphocytes that repeatedly encounter self antigens Negative selection of immature lymphocytes (largely not Fas or TNF-R mediated)

Abbreviation: TNF-R, tumor necrosis factor receptor.

Continued on following page

at many stages of lymphocyte maturation and activation. Immature lymphocytes that do not express functional antigen receptors or are not positively selected die by neglect (see Chapter 7). After their maturation, if naive lymphocytes do not encounter the antigen for which they are specific, the naive cells die by apoptosis. After activation by antigen, many of the progeny of the activated cells also die as the antigen is eliminated. In all these situations, the lymphocytes do not receive the survival stimuli that would protect them from programmed cell death. As expected, overexpression of Bcl-2 or Bcl-x as a transgene in T or B lymphocytes results in enhanced survival of immature lymphocytes and prolonged immune responses. Thus, this pathway of apoptosis is critical for maintaining homeostasis in the immune system.

Fas-mediated activation-induced cell death appears to be most important for preventing uncontrolled activation of lymphocytes (e.g., by abundant and persistent self antigens). Great interest in the function of Fas was spurred by the demonstration that in two inbred mouse strains that develop autoimmune disease as a result of recessive single-gene mutations, the defects lie in either Fas or FasL. These were the first systemic immune diseases shown to be a result of a failure of apoptosis. A small number of humans with similar disorders have been described. We will return to a discussion of these autoimmune disorders in Chapter 18. The negative selection of immature thymocytes that encounter high concentrations of self antigens is also due to activation-induced cell death, but it does not appear to rely on either Fas or TNF receptors. The Fas pathway may prevent uncontrolled lymphocyte activation in response to persistent infections (e.g., some viral infections), but the importance of this pathway in normal homeostasis is not established. In addition to its role in the maintenance of peripheral tolerance to self antigens, Fas:FasL-mediated cell death may serve other functions. Cytolysis by $CD8^+$ cytolytic T lymphocytes (CTLs) is in part mediated by FasL on the CTLs binding to Fas on target cells (see Chapter 13). Two tissues known to be sites of immune privilege, namely, the testes and the eyes, may constitutively express FasL. It is postulated that FasL kills leukocytes that enter the tissues, thus preventing local immune responses, which is the hallmark of immune privilege. However, these findings are controversial and may not apply to all species. The physiologic value of immune privilege in these tissues, and in the central nervous system, is not understood. The physiologic role of apoptosis induced by antigen recognition without second signals is not well understood; it is believed to be important in homeostasis and self-tolerance.

(TNF) receptor family, and FasL is homologous to the cytokine TNF. When T cells are repeatedly activated, FasL is expressed on the cell surface, and it binds to surface Fas on the same or adjacent T cells. This activates a cascade of intracellular cysteine proteases, called caspases, that ultimately cause the apoptotic death of the cells. Apoptotic cells are rapidly removed by phagocytes and do not induce inflammation. The net effect is that the population of mature lymphocytes is depleted of T cells specific for the antigen that induced repeated stimulation. High concentrations of the growth factor IL-2 enhance the sensitivity of antigen-stimulated T cells to Fas-mediated apoptosis. Therefore, this mechanism of deletion-induced tolerance is usually seen when large numbers of T cells are activated and produce IL-2. A different pathway of apoptosis is triggered by depletion of survival stimuli, including antigens and growth factors (see Box 10–2). This pathway appears to be more important for maintaining homeostasis than for self-tolerance, and it is discussed at the end of this chapter.

It is believed that Fas-mediated activation-induced cell death is responsible for the elimination of T cells specific for abundant peripheral self antigens, which are most likely to be the self antigens that trigger repeated T cell activation. The same pathway of apoptosis is involved in the elimination of self-reactive B lymphocytes (discussed later). Mice with defects in the expression of Fas or mutations in FasL, and children with Fas mutations, develop autoimmune diseases with some similarity to systemic lupus erythematosus (see Chapter 18). Surprisingly, knockout mice lacking IL-2 also develop autoimmunity (and not immunodeficiency, as would be expected from the absence of this growth-promoting cytokine). A possible mechanism of autoimmunity in IL-2 knockout mice is also failure of Fas-mediated apoptosis of self-reactive T cells.

The term *activation-induced cell death* is also used to describe apoptosis resulting from T cell stimulation by antigen in the absence of innate immunity or costimulation. It is believed that antigen recognition results in mitochondrial translocation of pro-apoptotic proteins, which are members of the Bcl family, without anti-apoptotic members of the family (see Box 10–2). In this situation, the death of the cells is by the mitochondrial pathway, and independent of the engagement of death receptors. Superantigens, and perhaps self antigens, may induce deletion of T cells by this pathway.

Tolerance Induced by Regulatory T Lymphocytes

Some immune responses are inhibited by cells that block the activation and functions of effector T lymphocytes (Fig. 10–10). These inhibitory cells are also T cells, and they are called **regulatory T cells.** Several experimental models support the importance of regulatory T cells in the maintenance of self-tolerance.

- If naive T cells from a normal mouse are transferred into a lymphocyte-deficient syngeneic mouse, the recipient develops multiorgan autoimmune disease involving the thyroid, colon, stomach, and other organs. If T cells expressing activation markers from the normal mouse are transferred together with the naive cells, the induction of the disease is prevented. The interpretation of this experiment is that in the normal mouse, there are naive T cells capable of reacting to self antigens, and they are kept in check by reg-

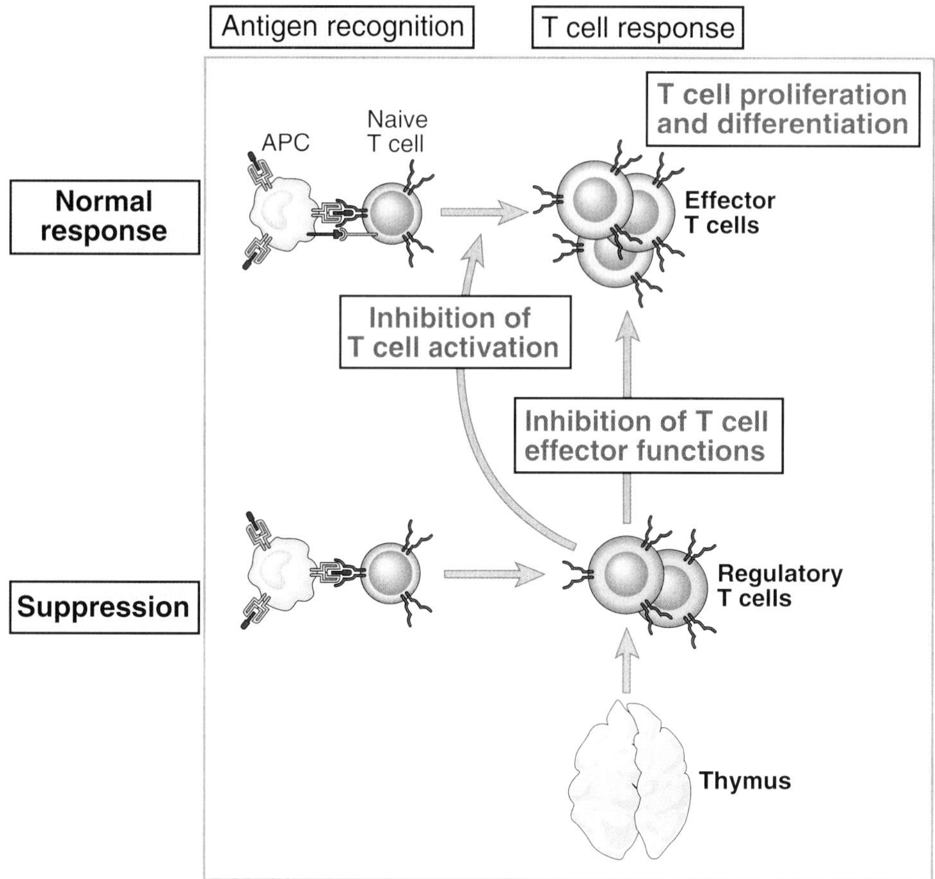

Figure 10–10 T cell–mediated suppression.
In a normal response, T cells recognize antigen and proliferate and differentiate into effector cells. Some T cells may differentiate into regulatory cells in the peripheral tissues or the thymus, and these regulatory cells inhibit the development or functions of effector cells. APC, antigen-presenting cell.

ulatory cells that have previously been activated by the same self antigens. When these naive T cells are transferred into a recipient that has no other lymphocytes, they cannot be controlled, and this leads to autoimmunity. Cotransfer of regulatory (previously activated) T cells prevents autoimmunity.

Studies indicate that in humans and mice, regulatory cells are CD4$^+$ T lymphocytes that express high levels of the IL-2 receptor α chain (CD25) but not other markers of activation. Regulatory T cells may be generated by self antigen recognition in the thymus or in peripheral lymphoid organs, but we do not know what special conditions of antigen exposure generate these cells. IL-2 may play a role in the development or function of regulatory T cells, and deficiency of IL-2 or IL-2 receptors may result in defects in regulatory cells. Such defects may contribute to autoimmunity in mice lacking IL-2 or IL-2 receptors. Presumably, regulatory T cells recognize self antigens, but their specificity is not defined. The mechanism of action of regulatory cells is also not well established. Some studies indicate that regulatory T cells inhibit immune responses by secreting immunosuppressive cytokines such as IL-10 and transforming growth factor-β (TGF-β) (Fig. 10–11). TGF-β is an inhibitor of T cell and B cell proliferation. IL-10, which is produced by some helper T lymphocytes (and other cells), inhibits macrophage activation and antagonizes the actions of the principal macrophage-activating cytokine interferon (IFN)-γ. Therefore, T cells that secrete these inhibitory cytokines may suppress the responses of other T cells. Other studies suggest that regulatory T cells function by directly interacting with APCs or with responding T cells, and not by secreting cytokines.

Peripheral Tolerance in CD8$^+$ T Lymphocytes

Most of our knowledge of peripheral T cell tolerance is limited to CD4$^+$ T cells, and much less is known about the mechanisms of tolerance in mature CD8$^+$ T cells. It is possible that if CD8$^+$ T cells recognize class I MHC–associated peptides without costimulation or T cell help, the CD8$^+$ cells become anergic. In this situation, the CD8$^+$ T cells would encounter signal 1 (antigen) without second signals, and the mechanism of anergy would be essentially the same as for helper T lymphocytes. The role of CTLA-4 in inducing anergy in CD8$^+$ T cells is not established. CD8$^+$ T cells that are exposed to high concentrations of self antigens may undergo activation-induced cell death, but this process does not appear to involve the Fas death receptor. It is not known whether regulatory T cells directly inhibit the activation of CD8$^+$ T cells.

Factors That Determine the Tolerogenicity of Self Antigens

Studies with a variety of experimental models have shown that many features of protein antigens deter-

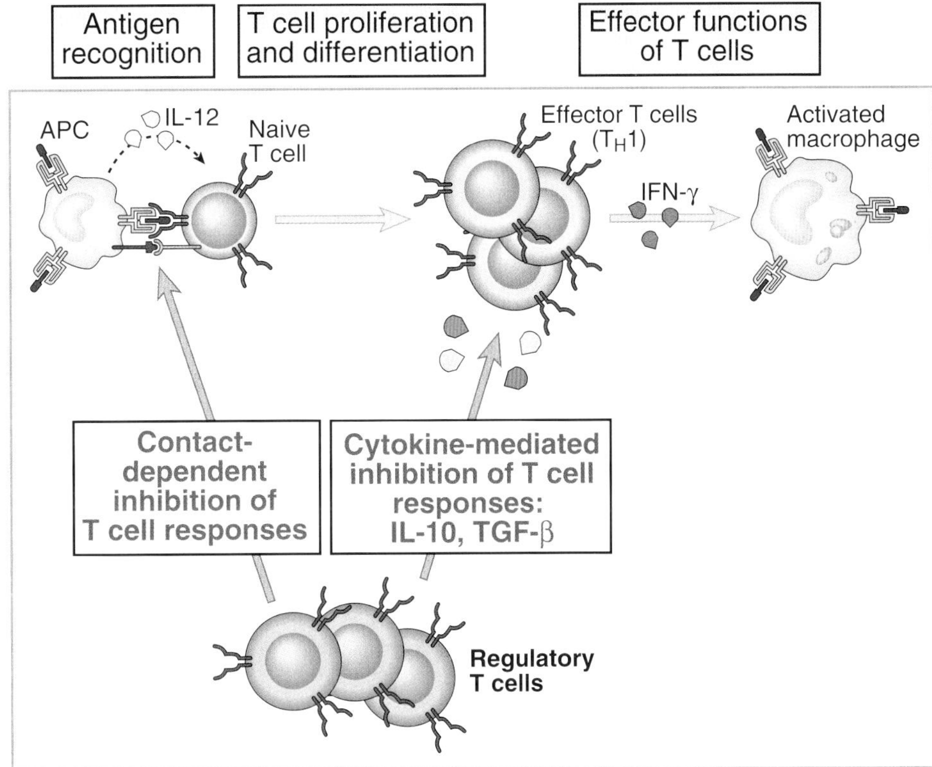

Figure 10–11 Mechanisms of action of regulatory T cells. The postulated mechanisms by which regulatory T cells may inhibit a typical T_H1 response are shown. In this type of T cell response, an antigen-presenting cell (APC) presents antigen to naive T cells and secretes the cytokine IL-12, which stimulates differentiation of the naive cells into T_H1 effectors. The T_H1 cells produce IFN-γ, which activates the macrophages in the effector phase of the response. Regulatory T cells may inhibit T cell activation by as yet undefined mechanisms that require contact between the regulatory cells and the responding T cells or APCs. Some regulatory T cells may secrete immunosuppressive cytokines, such as IL-10 (which inhibits APC function and macrophage activation) and TGF-β (which inhibits T cell proliferation and also macrophage activation).

mine whether these antigens will induce T cell activation or tolerance (Table 10–1). Self antigens have special properties that make them tolerogenic. Some self antigens are present at high concentrations in the generative lymphoid organs, and these antigens may induce central tolerance or the development of regulatory T cells. In the periphery, self antigens are normally displayed to the immune system without inflammation or innate immunity. Under these conditions, APCs express few or no costimulators, and antigen recognition may either elicit no response (ignorance) or induce anergy. Because self antigens cannot be eliminated, those that gain access to professional APCs are capable of repeatedly activating specific T lymphocytes, and repeated stimulation may trigger activation-induced cell death. These concepts are based largely on experimental models in which antigens are administered to mice or are expressed as transgenes in mice. One of the continuing challenges in this field is to define the characteristics of various normally expressed self antigens that make them tolerogenic, especially in humans.

Table 10–1. Factors That Determine the Immunogenicity and Tolerogenicity of Protein Antigens

Factor	Factors that favor stimulation of immune responses	Factors that favor tolerance
Amount	Optimal doses that vary for different antigens	High doses
Persistence	Short-lived (eliminated by immune response)	Prolonged (repeated T cell stimulation induces apoptosis)
Portal of entry; location	Subcutaneous, intradermal; absence from generative organs	Intravenous, oral; presence in generative organs
Presence of adjuvants	Antigens with adjuvants: stimulate helper T cells	Antigens without adjuvants: nonimmunogenic or tolerogenic
Properties of antigen-presenting cells	High levels of costimulators	Low levels of costimulators and cytokines

B Lymphocyte Tolerance

Tolerance in B lymphocytes is necessary for maintaining unresponsiveness to thymus-independent self antigens, such as polysaccharides and lipids. B cell tolerance may also play a role in preventing antibody responses to protein antigens. Experiments with transgenic mice have led to the concept that there are multiple "checkpoints" during B cell maturation and activation at which encounter with self antigens may abort these processes.

Central Tolerance in B Cells

Immature B lymphocytes that recognize self antigens in the bone marrow with high affinity either are deleted or change their specificity. As for T cells, the factors that determine whether immature B cells will be negatively selected are the nature and concentration of the self antigen in the bone marrow and the affinity of the B cell receptors for the antigen. Central tolerance is most likely to occur with multivalent self antigens, which bind to and cross-link many antigen receptors on each specific B cell and thus deliver strong immunoglobulin (Ig)–mediated signals to the B cells. Examples of such multivalent antigens are cell membrane molecules and polymeric molecules, such as double-stranded DNA.

- The mechanisms of self-tolerance in B lymphocytes have been examined mainly in experimental models using transgenic mice. In one such model (Fig. 10–12), one set of mice is created in which an Ig receptor specific for a model protein antigen, hen egg lysozyme (HEL), is expressed as a transgene. Most of the B cells in these transgenic mice are HEL specific and can be stimulated to produce anti-HEL antibody. The antigen HEL is expressed in another set of transgenic mice; because this protein is present throughout development, in effect it is a self antigen (like the viral protein expressed in pancreatic islets, referred to earlier). Moreover, in HEL antigen–expressing transgenic mice, HEL-specific helper T cells are tolerant (deleted or anergic). If the Ig transgenic mice and the HEL transgenic mice are mated, in the F_1 offspring, immature B cells specific for HEL are exposed to HEL in the absence of HEL-specific helper T cells. If the HEL is expressed as a membrane protein on all cells, including cells in the bone marrow, the immature B cells that encounter this self antigen are killed and do not attain maturity. If the HEL is present as a soluble protein, immature B cells recognize it with lower avidity than that with which they recognize the membrane form. These B cells do mature and exit the bone marrow, but they decrease their expression of antigen receptors and are unable to respond to the self antigen.
- In another transgenic system, if the genes encoding an Ig specific for a class I MHC allele are introduced into mice expressing that allele, B cells expressing the transgenic Ig fail to mature and exit the marrow. The class I MHC molecule is a good example of a membrane-bound self antigen that is displayed on cell surfaces in a multivalent form able to cross-link B cell Ig molecules.

The principal mechanism of central tolerance of immature B cells that encounter multivalent self antigens, such as membrane proteins, is apoptotic death. This is similar to the mechanism of negative selection of immature T cells in the thymus. B cells in the bone marrow that encounter self antigens may also respond to these antigens by reactivating their *RAG1* and *RAG2* genes and expressing a new Ig light chain, thus acquiring a new specificity. This process is called **receptor editing** (see Chapter 7) and is a potential mechanism for self-reactive B cells to lose this reactivity and survive.

Peripheral B Cell Tolerance

Mature B lymphocytes that recognize self antigens in peripheral tissues in the absence of specific helper T cells may be rendered functionally unresponsive or are excluded from lymphoid follicles. Many of these mechanisms of peripheral B cell tolerance have been analyzed in the HEL transgenic system mentioned before. In such experimental systems, specific B cells can be exposed to soluble self antigens in the periphery in the absence of T cell help (Fig. 10–13). The principal fate of these self-recognizing B cells is long-lived functional anergy, resulting in an inability to respond to antigen. If anergic B cells do encounter any antigen-specific helper T cells, the B cells may be killed by FasL on the T cells engaging Fas on the B cells. This mechanism of elimination of self-reactive B lymphocytes fails in mice and humans with mutations in Fas or FasL, and such a failure may contribute to autoantibody production. The biochemical mechanisms of B cell anergy are not well understood. Anergic B cells appear incapable of activating tyrosine kinases, such as Syk, or maintaining sustained increases in intracellular calcium on exposure to the antigen. B cells that encounter self antigens in the periphery also lose their capacity to migrate into lymphoid follicles and thus to be activated to produce antibodies against the self antigen. A likely mechanism of follicular exclusion is that the B cells receive a partial signal from the antigen that is not able to fully activate the cells but does lead to reduced expression of the chemokine receptor (CXCR5) that normally brings naive B lymphocytes into the follicles.

It is suspected that many diseases caused by autoantibodies are due to a failure of B cell tolerance, but little is known about which pathway of tolerance fails or why. Normal individuals do not produce autoantibodies against self protein antigens, and this may be due to deletion or tolerance of helper T lymphocytes even if functional B cells are present. In these cases, defects in the maintenance of T cell tolerance may result in autoantibody production.

The mechanisms of tolerance in T and B lymphocytes are similar in many respects, but there are also important differences (Table 10–2). Much has been learned from use of animal models, especially transgenic mice. Application of this knowledge to under-

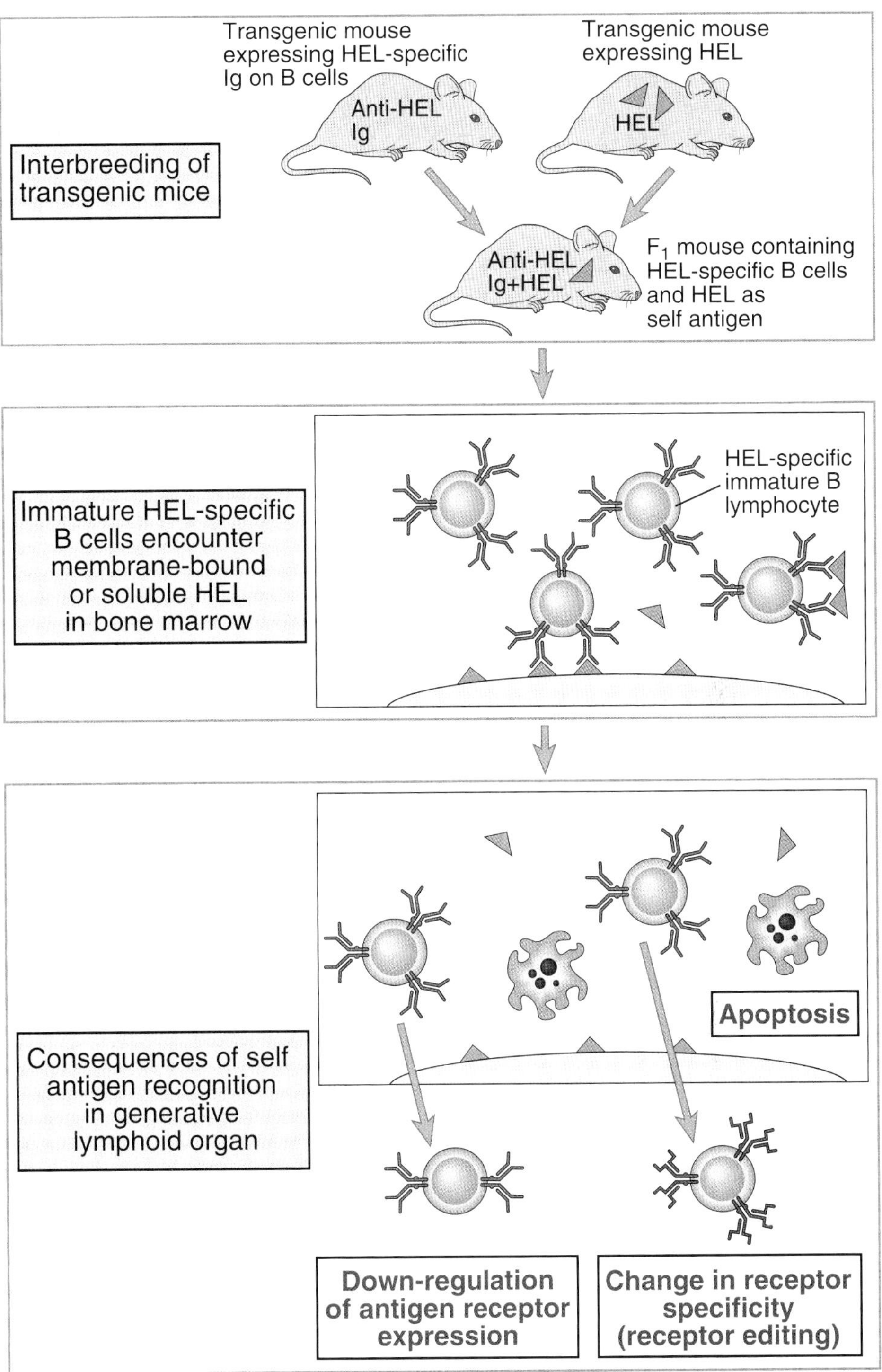

Figure 10–12 Central tolerance in B lymphocytes in a transgenic mouse model.
A transgenic mouse expressing an Ig specific for the antigen hen egg lysozyme (HEL) is bred with another transgenic mouse that produces HEL as a self antigen. In the "double transgenic" F_1 mouse, most B cells express HEL-specific receptors that recognize the self HEL. When immature B cells recognize the antigen in the bone marrow, the B cells may be deleted by apoptosis, the B cells may change the specificity of their antigen receptors (receptor editing), or the cells may leave the bone marrow with greatly reduced levels of receptor expression. Receptor editing has been demonstrated in several experimental models of central B cell tolerance but not in this particular model; it is included because it may be a frequent consequence of self antigen recognition during B cell maturation.

standing the mechanisms of tolerance to different self antigens in normal individuals, and to defining why tolerance fails, giving rise to autoimmune diseases, is an area of active investigation.

Tolerance Induced by Foreign Protein Antigens

Foreign antigens may be administered in ways that preferentially induce tolerance rather than immune responses. In general, protein antigens administered with adjuvants favor immunity, whereas high doses of antigens administered systemically without adjuvants tend to induce tolerance (see Fig. 10–7). The likely reason for this is that adjuvants stimulate the expression of costimulators on APCs, and in the absence of costimulation, T cells that recognize the antigen may become anergic. Tolerogenic antigens may also activate regulatory T cells or promote the differentiation of T cells into populations that produce cytokines such as IL-4, which does not induce cell-mediated immunity. Many

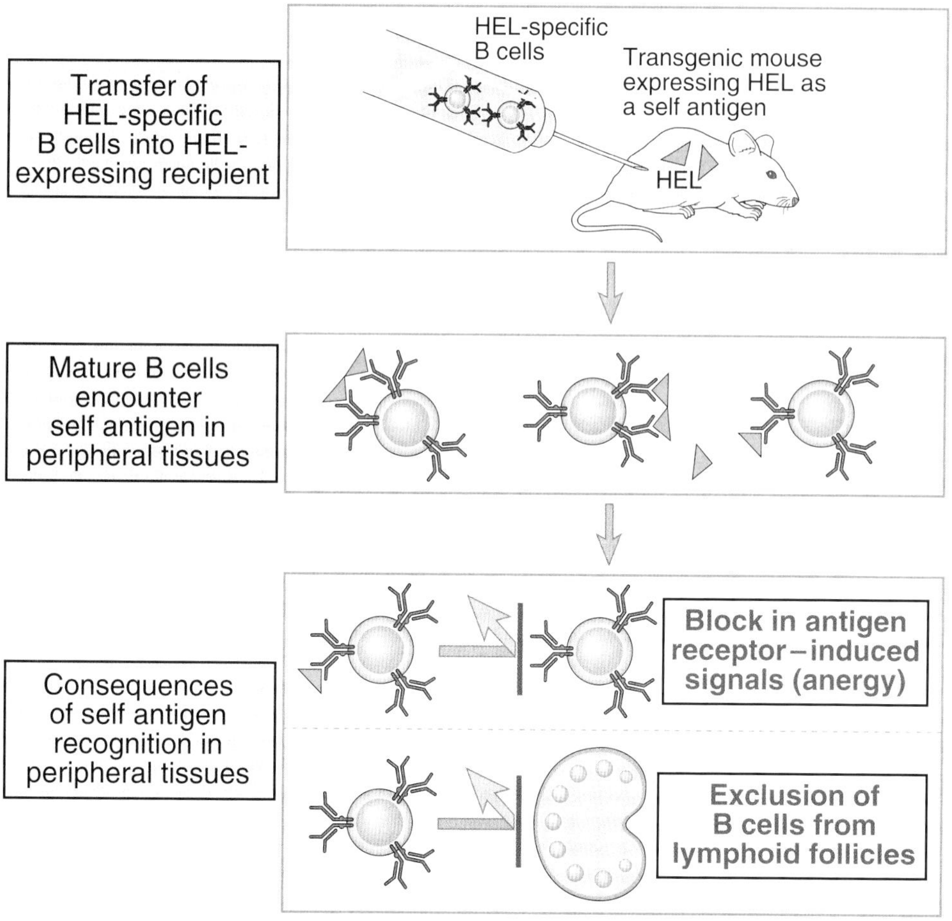

Figure 10–13 Peripheral B cell tolerance in a transgenic mouse model.
B cells specific for hen egg lysozyme (HEL) are transferred into mice that express HEL as a circulating self antigen. (HEL-specific T cells are deleted in these mice because HEL is present in the thymus.) When the B cells encounter the self antigen in the absence of T cell help, the B cells are excluded from lymphoid follicles, and they become incapable of responding to antigen recognition.

Table 10–2. Self-Tolerance in T and B Lymphocytes

Feature	T lymphocytes	B lymphocytes
Principal sites of tolerance induction	Thymus (cortex); periphery	Bone marrow; periphery
Tolerance-sensitive stage of maturation	$CD4^+CD8^+$ (double-positive) thymocyte	Immature (IgM^+IgD^-) B lymphocyte
Stimuli for tolerance induction	Central: high-avidity recognition of antigen in thymus	Central: high-avidity recognition of multivalent antigen in bone marrow
	Peripheral: antigen presentation by APCs lacking costimulators; repeated stimulation by self antigen	Peripheral: antigen recognition without T cell help
Principal mechanisms of tolerance	Central tolerance: clonal deletion (apoptosis)	Central tolerance: clonal deletion (apoptosis), receptor editing
	Peripheral tolerance: anergy, activation-induced cell death, suppression	Peripheral tolerance: block in signal transduction (anergy); failure to enter lymphoid follicles

Abbreviation: APCs, antigen-presenting cells.

other features of antigens, and how they are administered, may influence the balance between immunity and tolerance (see Table 10–1).

The oral administration of a protein antigen often leads to a marked suppression of systemic humoral and cell-mediated immune responses to immunization with the same antigen. This phenomenon is called **oral tolerance.** It has been postulated that the physiologic importance of oral tolerance may be as a mechanism for preventing immune responses to food antigens and to bacteria that normally reside as commensals in the intestinal lumen and are needed for digestion and absorption. Different doses of orally administered antigens may induce anergy in antigen-specific T cells or may stimulate the production of cytokines, such as TGF-β, that inhibit lymphocyte proliferation, resulting in the suppression of immune responses. In fact, TGF-β may participate in both distinctive responses to oral immunization, namely, production of IgA in mucosal tissues and systemic tolerance, because this cytokine induces B cell switching to IgA and inhibits lymphocyte proliferation. It is unclear why oral administration of some antigens, such as soluble proteins in large doses, induces systemic T cell tolerance, whereas oral immunization with other antigens, such as attenuated polio virus vaccines, induces protective T cell–dependent antibody responses and long-lived memory. Oral tolerance is a potential therapy for autoimmune diseases in which the autoantigen is known and for other clinical situations in which it may be desirable to inhibit specific immune responses to defined protein antigens, but clinical trials of orally administered antigens to treat autoimmune diseases have not been successful.

Homeostasis in the Immune System: Termination of Normal Immune Responses

So far in this chapter, we have discussed how the immune system becomes unresponsive to self antigens. Lymphocyte death and inactivation are also important for maintaining a fairly steady number of these cells throughout the life of an individual, despite the constant production of new lymphocytes in the generative lymphoid organs and the tremendous expansions that may occur during responses to potent immunogenic antigens. The maintenance of constant numbers of cells is called **homeostasis**. In the following section, we discuss the known mechanisms that function to maintain homeostasis after lymphocyte activation.

Immune responses to foreign antigens are self-limited and wane as the antigens are eliminated, returning the immune system to its basal resting state. In previous chapters, we discussed the expansion of T and B lymphocytes after stimulation with antigens and other signals and the differentiation of these lymphocytes into effector and memory cells. Lymphocytes that do not receive activating signals die "by neglect" (see Box 10–2). Antigens, costimulators, and cytokines (growth factors) produced during immune responses prevent lymphocytes from dying by this pathway of apoptosis. Survival stimuli for lymphocytes function mainly by inducing the expression of anti-apoptotic proteins, the most important of which are members of the Bcl family. Lymphocyte survival induced by antigen, costimulators, and cytokines is the prelude to clonal expansion and differentiation of the lymphocytes into effector cells. The effector cells that develop during adaptive immune responses function to eliminate the antigen, as a result of which the innate immune response also subsides. Therefore, the clones of lymphocytes that were activated by the antigen are deprived of the essential survival stimuli, and they die by apoptosis (Fig. 10–14). Much of the physiologic decline of immune responses, or homeostasis, is due to programmed death of lymphocytes resulting from the loss of survival signals. The effector cells that develop after antigen stimulation also have short half-lives and are usually not self-renewing. Therefore, after the antigen is eliminated, the only sign that it was present is the persistence of long-lived but functionally quiescent memory lymphocytes.

In addition to this decline of immune responses because of cell death, antigen-stimulated lymphocytes may trigger active regulatory mechanisms that also serve to terminate immune responses. Two of these mechanisms have been mentioned before as mechanisms of peripheral T cell tolerance. Activated T cells begin to express CTLA-4, which interacts with B7 molecules and inhibits continued lymphocyte proliferation. CTLA-4 appears after 3 or 4 days of T cell activation *in vitro,* and this may herald the decline of the T cell response. Thus, CTLA-4 may be a physiologic terminator of T cell activation. Activated T cells may also express death receptors such as Fas and ligands for these receptors, and the interaction of these molecules results in apoptosis (see Box 10–2). Because coexpression of Fas and FasL and Fas-mediated apoptosis are induced by repeated antigen stimulation, they are most likely to be triggered in situations of persistent antigen exposure (e.g., with self antigens, or during chronic infections). However, there is no good evidence that either CTLA-4 or death receptors function to terminate normal immune responses to foreign antigens, such as microbial proteins. Similarly, we do not know whether regulatory T cells play a role in limiting responses to foreign antigens.

The responses of B lymphocytes are also actively controlled because IgG antibodies produced by the B cells form complexes with the antigen, and the complexes bind to Fcγ receptors on the B cells and inhibit these cells. This process of **antibody feedback** was described in Chapter 9.

Another mechanism for regulating adaptive immune responses was proposed by Niels Jerne in the 1970s as the **network hypothesis.** This idea is based on the fact that lymphocyte antigen receptors are extremely diverse and that receptors of any one specificity have amino acid sequences different from the receptors of all other specificities. These unique sequences form determinants, called **idiotypes,** that may be recognized by other lymphocytes with complementary, or anti-idiotypic, specificities (see Chapter 3, Box 3–3). Thus,

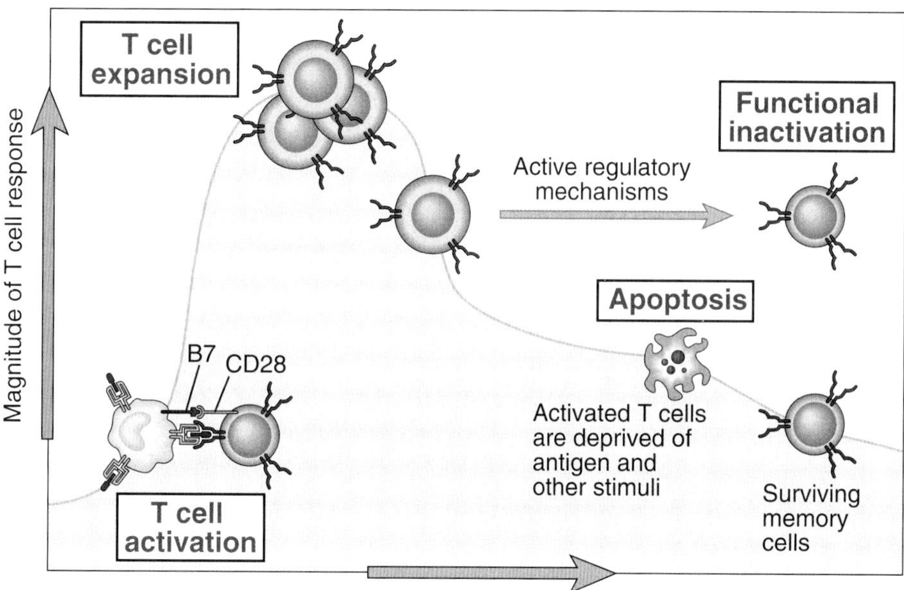

Figure 10–14 Mechanisms of the decline of normal immune responses (homeostasis). T lymphocytes proliferate and differentiate in response to antigen. As the antigen is eliminated, many of the activated T cells die by apoptosis. Some responses may be terminated by active regulatory mechanisms, such as CTLA-4–mediated inhibition or engagement of death receptors. At the end of the immune response, memory cells are the only surviving cells. Apoptosis is the principal mechanism for the decline of both T cell and B cell responses (only T cells are shown).

lymphocytes may respond to the unique antigen receptors of other lymphocytes; such responses are said to be anti-idiotypic. The basic tenet of the network hypothesis is that complementary interactions involving idiotypes and anti-idiotypes reach a steady state at which the immune system is at homeostasis. When a foreign antigen enters the system, one or a few clones of lymphocytes respond, their idiotypes are expanded, and anti-idiotype responses are triggered that function to shut off the antigen-specific (idiotype-expressing) lymphocytes. Although this concept remains an intriguing idea, it has not been proved experimentally that idiotypic networks are actually involved in regulating physiologic immune responses.

Summary

- Immunologic tolerance is unresponsiveness to an antigen induced by the exposure of specific lymphocytes to that antigen. Tolerance to self antigens is a fundamental property of the normal immune system, and the failure of self-tolerance leads to autoimmune diseases. Antigens may be administered in ways that induce tolerance rather than immunity, and this may be exploited for the prevention and treatment of transplant rejection and autoimmune and allergic diseases.

- Central tolerance is induced in the generative lymphoid organs (thymus and bone marrow) when immature lymphocytes encounter self antigens present in these organs. Peripheral tolerance occurs when mature lymphocytes recognize self antigens in peripheral tissues under particular conditions.

- The principal mechanisms of tolerance are deletion (apoptotic cell death), anergy (functional inactivation), and suppression by regulatory T cells. Some self antigens may be ignored by the immune system, and they elicit no detectable reaction.

- In T lymphocytes, central tolerance (negative selection) occurs when double-positive thymocytes with high-affinity receptors for self antigens recognize these antigens in the thymus.

- Several mechanisms account for peripheral tolerance in mature T cells. In $CD4^+$ T cells, anergy is induced by antigen recognition without adequate costimulation and by recognition of altered forms of the native antigen. Repeated stimulation of T cells by persistent antigens results in activation-induced cell death. Some self antigens activate regulatory T cells, which inhibit immune responses in part by producing immunosuppressive cytokines.

- In B lymphocytes, central tolerance is induced when immature B cells recognize multivalent self antigens in the bone marrow. The usual result is apoptotic death of the B cells or the acquisition of a new specificity, called receptor editing. Mature B cells that recognize self antigens in the periphery in the absence of T cell help may be rendered anergic or are excluded from lymphoid follicles and cannot be activated by antigen.

- Immune responses to foreign antigens decline with time after immunization. This is mainly because of apoptosis of activated lymphocytes that are deprived of survival stimuli as the antigen is eliminated and innate immunity wanes. Various active mechanisms of lymphocyte inhibition may also function to terminate immune responses.

Selected Readings

Anderton SM, and DC Wraith. Selection and fine-tuning of the autoimmune T cell repertoire. Nature Reviews Immunology 2:487–498, 2002.

Goodnow CC, JG Cyster, SB Hartley, SE Bell, MP Cooke, JI Healy, S Akkaraju, JC Rathmell, SL Pogue, and KP Shokat. Self-tolerance checkpoints in B lymphocyte development. Advances in Immunology 59:279–368, 1995.

Healy JI, and CC Goodnow. Positive versus negative signaling by lymphocyte antigen receptors. Annual Review of Immunology 16:645–670, 1998.

Klinman NR. The "clonal selection hypothesis" and current concepts of B cell tolerance. Immunity 5:189–195, 1996.

Matzinger P. Tolerance, danger, and the extended family. Annual Review of Immunology 12:991–1045, 1994.

Mondino A, A Khoruts, and MK Jenkins. The anatomy of T-cell activation and tolerance. Proceedings of the National Academy of Sciences USA 93:2245–2252, 1996.

Sakaguchi S. Regulatory T cells: key controllers of immunologic self-tolerance. Cell 101:455–458, 2000.

Salomon B, and JA Bluestone. Complexities of CD28/B7: CTLA-4 costimulatory pathways in autoimmunity and transplantation. Annual Review of Immunology 19:225–252, 2001.

Shevach EM. Regulatory T cells in autoimmunity. Annual Review of Immunology 18:423–449, 2000.

Shevach EM. $CD4^{+}CD25^{+}$ suppressor T cells: more questions than answess. Nature Reviews Immunology 2:389–400, 2002.

Siegel RM, FK-M Chan, and MJ Lenardo. The multifaceted role of Fas signaling in immune cell homeostasis and autoimmunity. Nature Immunology 1:469–474, 2000.

Thompson CB, and JP Allison. The emerging role of CTLA-4 as an immune attenuator. Immunity 7:445–450, 1997.

Van Parijs L, and AK Abbas. Homeostasis and self-tolerance in the immune system: shutting lymphocytes off. Science 280:243–248, 1998.

Walker LS, and AK Abbas. The enemy within: keeping self-reactive T cells at bay in the periphery. Nature Reviews Immunology 2:11–19, 2002.

Section IV

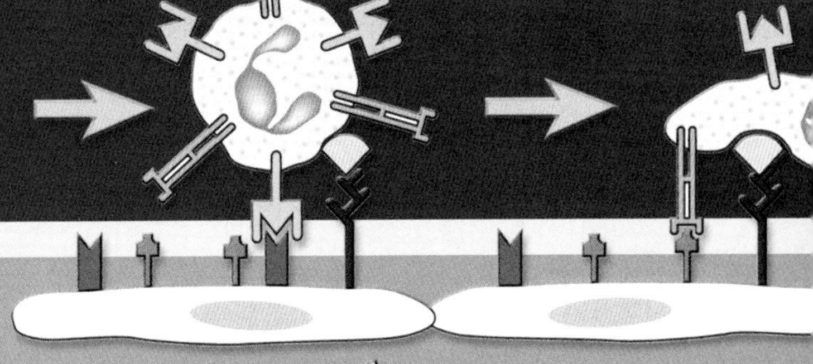

Effector Mechanisms of Immune Responses

The physiologic function of all immune responses is to eliminate microbes and other foreign antigens. The mechanisms by which specific lymphocytes recognize and respond to foreign antigens (i.e., the recognition and activation phases of adaptive immune responses) were discussed in Sections II and III. Section IV is devoted to the effector mechanisms that are activated during immune responses and how these mechanisms function in host defense.

In Chapter 11, we describe cytokines, the soluble mediators of innate and adaptive immunity, and the mechanisms by which leukocytes communicate with one another and with other cells. Chapter 12 deals with the effector mechanisms of innate immunity, the early defense against microbes. In Chapter 13, we describe the effector cells of cell-mediated immunity, namely, T lymphocytes and macrophages, which function as defense mechanisms against intracellular microbes. Chapter 14 is devoted to the effector mechanisms of antibody-mediated humoral immunity, including the complement system, that are involved in host defense against extracellular microbes. Chapter 15 is an overview of the mechanisms of innate and adaptive immunity against different types of microbes and the interplay between microbes and the immune system.

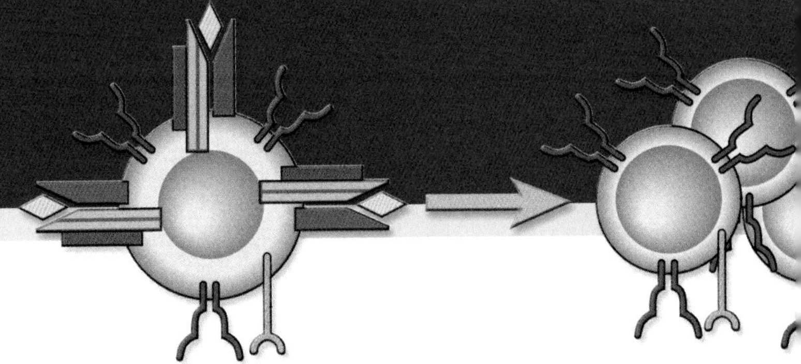

Chapter 11

Cytokines

Cytokines are proteins secreted by the cells of innate and adaptive immunity that mediate many of the functions of these cells. Cytokines are produced in response to microbes and other antigens, and different cytokines stimulate diverse responses of cells involved in immunity and inflammation. In the activation phase of adaptive immune responses, cytokines stimulate the growth and differentiation of lymphocytes, and in the effector phases of innate and adaptive immunity, they activate different effector cells to eliminate microbes and other antigens. Cytokines also stimulate the development of hematopoietic cells. In clinical medicine, cytokines are important as therapeutic agents and as targets for specific antagonists in numerous immune and inflammatory diseases.

The nomenclature of cytokines is often based on their cellular sources. Cytokines that are produced by mononuclear phagocytes were called **monokines,** and those produced by lymphocytes were called **lymphokines.** With the development of anticytokine antibodies and molecular probes, it became clear that the same protein may be synthesized by lymphocytes, monocytes, and a variety of tissue cells, including endothelial cells and some epithelial cells. Therefore, the generic term **cytokines** is the preferred name for this class of mediators. Because many cytokines are made by leukocytes (e.g., macrophages or T cells) and act on other leukocytes, they are also called **interleukins.** This term is imperfect because many cytokines that are synthesized only by leukocytes and that act only on leukocytes are not called interleukins, for historical reasons, whereas many cytokines called interleukins are made by or act on cells other than leukocytes. Nevertheless, the term has been useful because as new cytokines are molecularly characterized, they are assigned an interleukin (IL) number (e.g., IL-1, IL-2, and so on) to maintain a standard nomenclature. Cytokines are also increasingly used in clinical situations and in animal studies to stimulate or inhibit inflammation, immunity, and hematopoiesis. In this setting, cytokines are often referred to as biologic response modifiers. Throughout this book, we use the term *cytokine,* which does not imply restricted cellular sources or biologic activities.

In this chapter, we discuss the structure, production, and biologic actions of cytokines. Before describing the individual molecules, we begin with a summary of the general properties of cytokines.

General Properties of Cytokines

Cytokines are polypeptides produced in response to microbes and other antigens that mediate and regulate immune and inflammatory reactions (Fig. 11–1). Although cytokines are structurally diverse, they share several properties.

- ***Cytokine secretion is a brief, self-limited event.*** Cytokines are not usually stored as preformed molecules, and their synthesis is initiated by new gene transcription as a result of cellular activation. Such transcriptional activation is transient, and the messenger RNAs encoding most cytokines are unstable, so cytokine synthesis is also transient. The production of some cytokines may additionally be controlled by RNA processing and by post-transcriptional mechanisms, such as proteolytic release of an active product from an inactive precursor. Once synthesized, cytokines are rapidly secreted, resulting in a burst of release as needed.
- ***The actions of cytokines are often pleiotropic and redundant*** (Fig. 11–2). Pleiotropism refers to the ability of one cytokine to act on different cell types. This property allows a cytokine to mediate diverse biologic effects, but it greatly limits the therapeutic use of cytokines because administration of a cytokine for a desired clinical effect may result in numerous unwanted side effects. Redundancy refers to the property of multiple cytokines having the same functional effects. Because of this redundancy, antagonists against a single cytokine or mutation of one cytokine gene may not have functional consequences, as other cytokines may compensate.

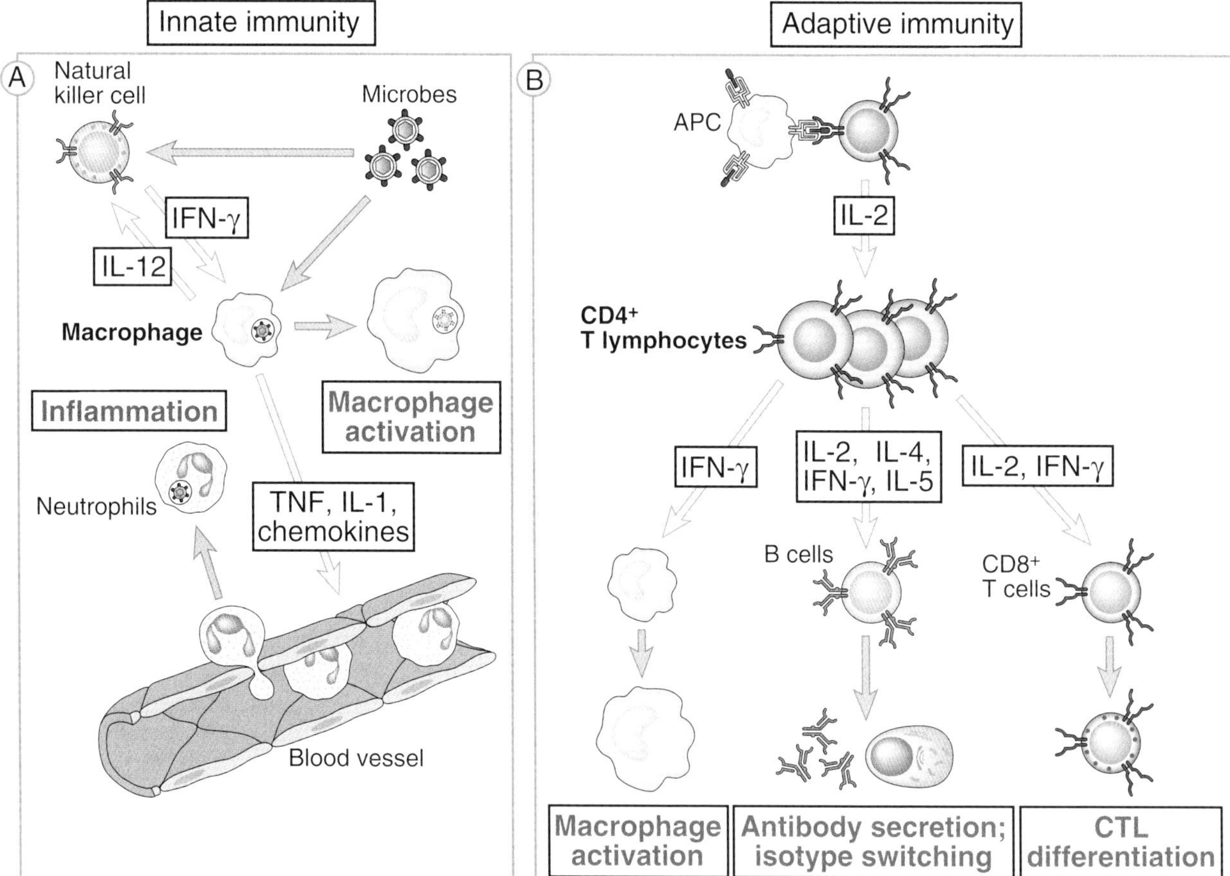

Figure 11–1 Functions of cytokines in host defense.
In innate immunity, cytokines produced by macrophages and NK cells mediate the early inflammatory reactions to microbes and promote the elimination of microbes. In adaptive immunity, cytokines stimulate proliferation and differentiation of antigen-stimulated lymphocytes and activate specialized effector cells, such as macrophages. The properties of the cytokines shown in this figure are discussed later in the chapter. APC, antigen-presenting cell; CTL, cytolytic T lymphocyte; IFN, interferon; IL, interleukin; NK, natural killer; TNF, tumor necrosis factor.

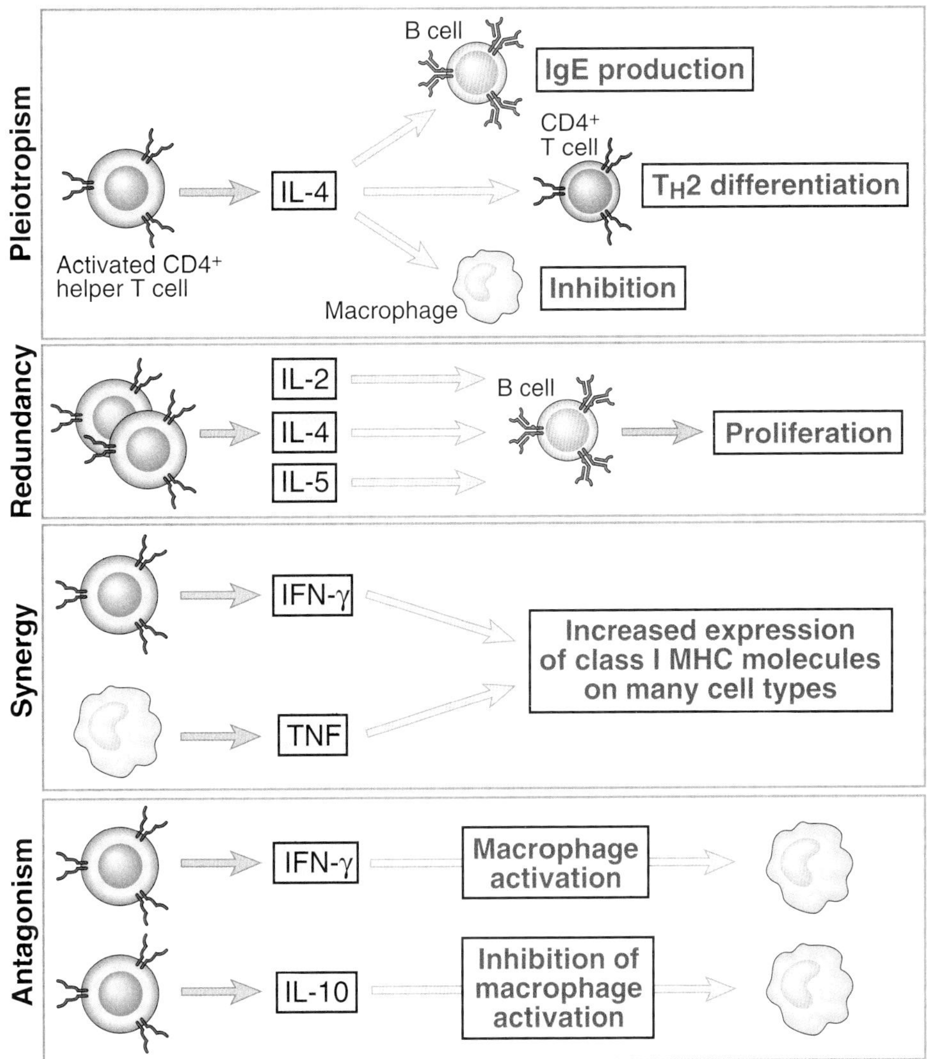

Figure 11–2 Properties of cytokines.

Selected examples are shown to illustrate the following properties of cytokines: pleiotropism, one cytokine having multiple effects on diverse cell types; redundancy, multiple cytokines having the same or overlapping actions; synergy, two or more cytokines having greater than additive effects; and antagonism, one cytokine inhibiting the action of another.

- ***Cytokines often influence the synthesis and actions of other cytokines.*** The ability of one cytokine to stimulate production of others leads to cascades in which a second or third cytokine may mediate the biologic effects of the first. Two cytokines may antagonize each other's action, produce additive effects, or, in some cases, produce greater than anticipated, or synergistic, effects.

- ***Cytokine actions may be local and systemic.*** Most cytokines act close to where they are produced, either on the same cell that secretes the cytokine **(autocrine action)** or on a nearby cell **(paracrine action).** T cells often secrete cytokines at the site of contact with antigen-presenting cells, the so-called immune synapse (see Chapter 8). This may be one reason that cytokines often act on cells in contact with the cytokine producers. When produced in large amounts, cytokines may enter the circulation and act at a distance from the site of production **(endocrine action).**

- ***Cytokines initiate their actions by binding to specific membrane receptors on target cells.*** Receptors for cytokines often bind their ligands with high affinities, with dissociation constants (K_d values) in the range of 10^{-10} to 10^{-12} M. (For comparison, recall that antibodies typically bind antigens with a K_d of 10^{-7} to 10^{-11} M and that major histocompatibility complex [MHC] molecules bind peptides with a K_d of only about 10^{-6} M.) As a consequence, only small quantities of a cytokine are needed to occupy receptors and elicit biologic effects. Most cells express low levels of cytokine receptors (on the order of 100 to 1000 receptors per cell), but this is adequate for inducing responses.

- ***External signals regulate the expression of cytokine receptors and thus the responsiveness of cells to cytokines.*** For instance, stimulation of T or B lymphocytes by antigens leads to increased expression of cytokine receptors. For this reason, during an immune response, the antigen-specific lymphocytes are the preferential responders to secreted cytokines. This is one mechanism for maintaining the specificity of immune responses, even though cytokines themselves are not antigen specific. Receptor expression is also regulated by cytokines themselves, including the same cytokine that binds to the receptor, permitting positive amplification or negative feedback.

- ***The cellular responses to most cytokines consist of changes in gene expression in target cells, resulting in the expression of new functions and sometimes in the proliferation of the target cells.*** Many of the changes in gene expression induced by cytokines result in differentiation of T and B lymphocytes and activation of effector cells such as macrophages. For instance, cytokines stimulate switching of antibody isotypes in B cells, differentiation of helper T cells into T_H1 and T_H2 subsets, and activation of microbicidal mechanisms in phagocytes. Exceptions to the rule that cytokines work by changing gene expression patterns are chemokines, which elicit rapid cell migration, and a cytokine called tumor necrosis factor (TNF), which induces apoptosis by activating cellular enzymes, without new gene transcription or protein synthesis.

Functional Categories of Cytokines

For our discussion, we classify cytokines into three main functional categories based on their principal biologic actions.

1. ***Mediators and regulators of innate immunity*** are produced mainly by mononuclear phagocytes in response to infectious agents. Bacterial products, such as lipopolysaccharide (LPS), and viral products, such as double-stranded RNA, directly stimulate macrophages to secrete these cytokines as part of innate immunity. The same cytokines may also be secreted by macrophages that are activated by antigen-stimulated T cells (i.e., as part of adaptive cell-mediated immunity). Most members of this group of cytokines act on endothelial cells and leukocytes to stimulate the early inflammatory reactions to microbes, and some function to control these responses. NK (natural killer) cells also produce cytokines during innate immune reactions.
2. ***Mediators and regulators of adaptive immunity*** are produced mainly by T lymphocytes in response to specific recognition of foreign antigens. Some T cell cytokines function primarily to regulate the growth and differentiation of various lymphocyte populations and thus play important roles in the activation phase of T cell–dependent immune responses. Other T cell–derived cytokines recruit, activate, and regulate specialized effector cells, such as mononuclear phagocytes, neutrophils, and eosinophils, to eliminate antigens in the effector phase of adaptive immune responses.
3. ***Stimulators of hematopoiesis*** are produced by bone marrow stromal cells, leukocytes, and other cells, and stimulate the growth and differentiation of immature leukocytes.

In general, the cytokines of innate and adaptive immunity are produced by different cell populations and act on different target cells (Table 11–1). However, these distinctions are not absolute because the same cytokine may be produced during innate and adaptive immune reactions, and different cytokines produced during such reactions may have overlapping actions.

Cytokine Receptors and Signaling

Before we describe the functions of individual cytokines, it is useful to summarize the characteristics of cytokine receptors and how they transduce signals as a consequence of the binding of the cytokines. All cytokine receptors consist of one or more transmembrane proteins whose extracellular portions are responsible for cytokine binding and whose cytoplasmic portions are responsible for initiating intracellular signaling pathways. These signaling pathways are typically activated by ligand-induced receptor clustering, bringing together the cytoplasmic portions of two or more receptor molecules in a process analogous to signaling by T and B cell receptors for antigens (see Chapters 8 and 9).

The most widely used classification of cytokine receptors is based on structural homologies among the extracellular cytokine-binding domains. According to this classification, cytokine receptors are divided into five families (Fig. 11–3A).

- ***Type I cytokine receptors,*** also called hemopoietin receptors, contain one or more copies of a domain with two conserved pairs of cysteine residues and a membrane proximal sequence of tryptophan-serine-X-tryptophan-serine (WSXWS), where X is any amino acid. These receptors typically bind cytokines that fold into four α-helical strands. The conserved features of the receptors presumably form structures that bind four α-helical cytokines, but the specificity for individual cytokines is determined by amino acid residues that vary from one receptor to another. These receptors consist of unique ligand-binding chains and one or more signal-transducing chains, which are often shared by receptors for different cytokines (Fig. 11–3B).
- ***Type II cytokine receptors*** are similar to type I receptors by virtue of two extracellular domains with conserved cysteines, but type II receptors do not contain the WSXWS motif. These receptors consist of one ligand-binding polypeptide chain and one signal-transducing chain.
- Some cytokine receptors contain extracellular immunoglobulin (Ig) domains and are therefore classified as members of the ***Ig superfamily.*** This group of receptors binds diverse cytokines that signal by different mechanisms.
- ***TNF receptors*** belong to a family of receptors (some of which are not cytokine receptors) with conserved cysteine-rich extracellular domains. On ligand

Table 11–1. Comparative Features of the Cytokines of Innate and Adaptive Immunity

Features	Innate immunity	Adaptive immunity
Examples	TNF-α, IL-1, IL-12, IFN-γ *	IL-2, IL-4, IL-5, IFN-γ *
Major cell source	Macrophages, NK cells	T lymphocytes
Principal physiologic functions	Mediators of innate immunity and inflammation (local and systemic)	Adaptive immunity: regulation of lymphocyte growth and differentiation; activation of effector cells (macrophages, eosinophils, mast cells)
Stimuli	LPS (endotoxin), bacterial peptidoglycans, viral RNA, T cell–derived cytokines (IFN-γ)	Protein antigens
Amounts produced	May be high; detectable in serum	Generally low; usually undetectable in serum
Local or systemic effects	Both	Usually local only
Roles in disease	Systemic diseases (e.g., septic shock)	Local tissue injury (e.g., granulomatous inflammation)
Inhibitors of synthesis	Corticosteroids	Cyclosporine, FK-506

*IFN-γ plays important roles in innate and adaptive immunity.

binding, these receptors activate associated intracellular proteins that induce apoptosis or stimulate gene expression, or both.

- ***Seven-transmembrane α-helical receptors*** are also called serpentine receptors, because their transmembrane domains appear to "snake" back and forth through the membrane, and G protein–coupled receptors, because their signaling pathways involve GTP-binding (G) proteins. The mammalian genome encodes many such receptors involved in sensing environmental stimuli. In the immune system, members of this receptor class mediate rapid and transient responses to a family of cytokines called chemokines.

Cytokine receptors can also be grouped according to the signal transduction pathways they activate (Table 11–2). Such a grouping will correspond to structural homologies in the cytoplasmic regions of the signaling chains of the receptors. In many cases, members of a family defined by extracellular domains engage similar signal transduction pathways. We describe the principal features of these different signaling pathways when we consider the individual cytokines.

With this introduction to the shared properties of cytokines, we proceed to discussions of individual cytokines. We conclude each section with an overview of the roles of the cytokines in the relevant host response.

Cytokines That Mediate and Regulate Innate Immunity

An important component of the early innate immune response to viruses and bacteria is the secretion of cytokines, which mediate many of the effector functions of innate immunity (see Chapter 12). In this section, we first describe the individual cytokines of innate immunity (Table 11–3), and then we summarize how these cytokines function in host defense and inflammation. One cytokine, IFN-γ, plays important roles in both innate and adaptive immunity; it is discussed later in the chapter.

Tumor Necrosis Factor (TNF)

TNF is the principal mediator of the acute inflammatory response to gram-negative bacteria and other infectious microbes and is responsible for many of the systemic complications of severe infections. (TNF is also called TNF-α for historical reasons and to distinguish it from the closely related TNF-β, or lymphotoxin.) TNF was originally identified (and was so named) as a substance present in the serum of animals treated with bacterial endotoxin (lipopolysaccharide, or LPS) that caused the necrosis of tumors *in vivo*. As we shall discuss later, this effect is due to a pathologic complication of high concentrations of TNF.

Production, Structure, Receptors

The major cellular source of TNF is activated mononuclear phagocytes, although antigen-stimulated T cells, NK cells, and mast cells can also secrete this protein. The most potent stimulus for eliciting TNF production by macrophages is LPS, and large amounts of this cytokine may be produced in infections by gram-negative bacteria, which release LPS. IFN-γ, produced by T cells and NK cells, augments TNF synthesis by LPS-stimulated macrophages.

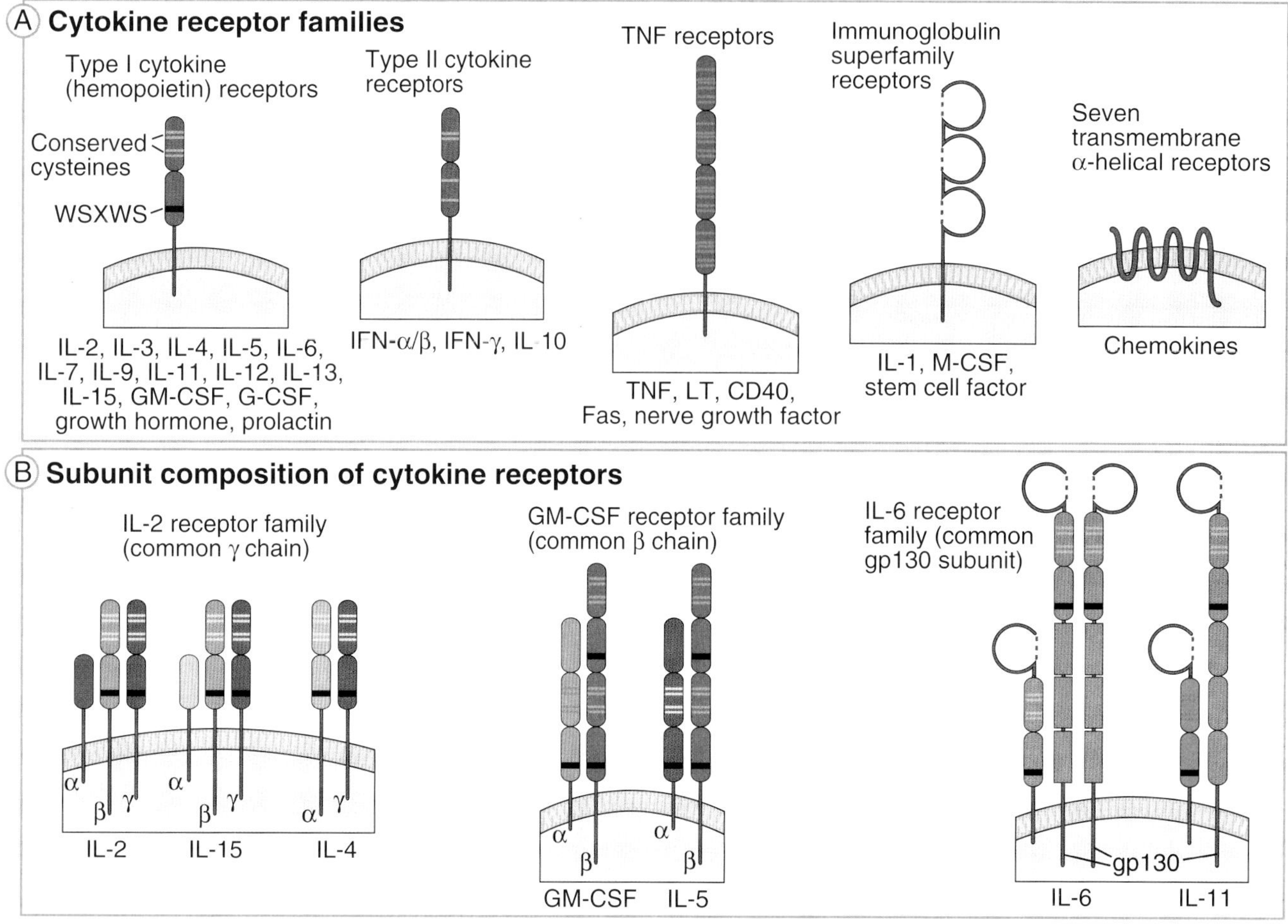

Figure 11–3 Structure of cytokine receptors.

A. Receptors for different cytokines are classified into families on the basis of conserved extracellular domain structures. The cytokines or other ligands that bind to each receptor family are listed below the schematic drawings. WSXWS, tryptophan-serine-X-tryptophan-serine.

B. Different cytokine receptors are composed of cytokine-specific ligand-binding chains (often the α chain) noncovalently associated with signaling subunits that are shared by receptors for different cytokines. Selected examples of cytokine receptors in each group are shown.

Table 11–2. Signal Transduction Mechanisms of Cytokine Receptors

Signal transduction pathway	Cytokine receptors using this pathway	Signaling mechanism
JAK/STAT pathway	Type I and type II cytokine receptors	JAK-mediated phosphorylation and activation of STAT transcription factors (see Box 11–2)
TNF receptor signaling by TRAFs	TNF receptor family: TNR-RII, CD40	Binding of adapter proteins, activation of transcription factors (see Box 11–1)
TNF receptor signaling by death domains	TNF receptor family: TNF-RI, Fas	Binding of adapter proteins, caspase activation (see Box 11–1)
Receptor-associated tyrosine kinases	M-CSF receptor, stem cell factor receptor	Intrinsic tyrosine kinase activity in receptor
G protein signaling	Chemokine receptors	GTP exchange and dissociation of Gα · GTP from Gβγ, Gα · GTP activates various cellular enzymes

Table 11–3. Cytokines of Innate Immunity

Cytokine	Size	Principal cell source	Principal cell targets and biologic effects
Tumor necrosis factor (TNF)	17 kD; 51-kD homotrimer	Macrophages, T cells	Endothelial cells: activation (inflammation, coagulation) Neutrophils: activation Hypothalamus: fever Liver: synthesis of acute-phase proteins Muscle, fat: catabolism (cachexia) Many cell types: apoptosis
Interleukin-1 (IL-1)	17 kD mature form; 33-kD precursors	Macrophages, endothelial cells, some epithelial cells	Endothelial cells: activation (inflammation, coagulation) Hypothalamus: fever Liver: synthesis of acute-phase proteins
Chemokines (see Table 11–4)	8–12 kD	Macrophages, endothelial cells, T cells, fibroblasts, platelets	Leukocytes: chemotaxis, activation; migration into tissues
Interleukin-12 (IL-12)	Heterodimer of 35-kD + 40-kD subunits	Macrophages, dendritic cells	T cells: T_H1 differentiation NK cells and T cells: IFN-γ synthesis, increased cytolytic activity
Type I IFNs (IFN-α, IFN-β)	IFN-α: 15–21 kD IFN-β: 20–25 kD	IFN-α: macrophages IFN-β: fibroblasts	All cells: antiviral state, increased class I MHC expression NK cells: activation
Interleukin-10 (IL-10)	Homodimer of 34–40 kD; 18-kD subunits	Macrophages, T cells (mainly T_H2)	Macrophages, dendritic cells: inhibition of IL-12 production and expression of costimulators and class II MHC molecules
Interleukin-6 (IL-6)	19–26 kD	Macrophages, endothelial cells, T cells	Liver: synthesis of acute-phase proteins B cells: proliferation of antibody-producing cells
Interleukin-15 (IL-15)	13 kD	Macrophages, others	NK cells: proliferation T cells: proliferation (memory $CD8^+$ cells)
Interleukin-18 (IL-18)	17 kD	Macrophages	NK cells and T cells: IFN-γ synthesis

In mononuclear phagocytes, TNF is synthesized as a nonglycosylated type II membrane protein, with an intracellular amino terminus and a large extracellular carboxyl terminus. Membrane TNF is expressed as a homotrimer and is able to bind to one type of TNF receptor (TNF-RII). The membrane form of TNF is cleaved by a membrane-associated metalloproteinase, releasing a 17-kD polypeptide. Three of these polypeptide chains polymerize to form the 51-kD circulating TNF protein. Secreted TNF assumes a triangular pyramid shape, each side of the pyramid being formed by one subunit (Fig. 11–4). The receptor-binding sites are at the base of the pyramid, allowing simultaneous binding of the cytokine to three receptor molecules.

There are two distinct TNF receptors of molecular sizes 55 kD (called type I TNF receptor [TNF-RI], or the p55 receptor) and 75 kD (called type II TNF receptor [TNF-RII], or the p75 receptor). The affinities of TNF for its receptors are unusually low for a cytokine, the K_d being only ~1×10^{-9} M for binding to TNF-RI and ~5×10^{-10} M for binding to TNF-RII. Both TNF receptors are present on almost all cell types examined. The TNF receptors are members of a large family of proteins, many of which are involved in immune and inflammatory responses (Box 11–1). Cytokine binding to some TNF receptor family members, such as TNF-RII, leads to the recruitment of proteins, called TNF receptor–associated factors (TRAFs), to the cytoplasmic domains of the receptors. The TRAFs ultimately activate transcription factors, notably nuclear factor κB (NF-κB) and activation protein-1 (AP-1). Cytokine binding to other family members, such as TNF-RI, leads to recruitment of an adapter protein that activates caspases and triggers apoptosis, although TNF-RI signaling also activates transcription factors. The mechanisms that determine whether cellular activation or apoptosis is the dominant effect of TNF are not well defined. TNF-RI knockout mice show more impaired host defense than do TNF-RII knockout mice, suggesting that TNF-RI is the more important for the functions of the cytokine.

BOX 11–1

Signaling by the TNF Receptor (TNF-R) Family

The TNF family of proteins includes secreted cytokines and membrane proteins that share sequence homologies and fold into homotrimeric triangular pyramidal complexes, which bind to structurally similar cell surface receptors. Members of this family include TNF, lymphotoxin (TNF-β), Fas ligand, CD40 ligand, OX-40, receptor activator of NF-κB ligand (RANK-L), TNF-related apoptosis-inducing ligand (TRAIL), and several other proteins. The cell surface receptors for the TNF family of proteins are type I membrane proteins that can also be grouped into a family, called the TNF-R family, on the basis of sequence homology in their cysteine-rich extracellular ligand-binding domains. Members of the TNF-R family include TNF-RI, TNF-RII, lymphotoxin-β receptor (LT-βR), Fas, CD40, OX-40 ligand, RANK, and others. The binding of TNF family members to their respective receptors initiates a wide variety of responses. Many of these responses are proinflammatory and depend on activation of the NF-κB and AP-1 transcription factors leading to new gene transcription. In contrast, some TNF-R family members (TNF-RI and Fas) deliver signals that cause apoptotic cell death. The specific responses to the cytokines depend on the particular receptor and cell type. Many of the molecular details of the signaling pathways engaged by TNF-R family molecules are now known. Although the members of this receptor family share structural features in their extracellular ligand-binding regions, they have widely divergent cytoplasmic domain structures. Nonetheless, there are shared features in the signaling pathways associated with these receptors. We discuss signaling by the TNF-R family, with an emphasis on how a protypical member of the family, TNF-RI, can induce anti-apoptotic and inflammatory responses in some circumstances or apoptosis in others.

As is the case with many membrane receptors in the immune system, the cytoplasmic tails of the TNF-R family members do not contain intrinsic enzymatic activities, but they do contain structural motifs that bind to cytoplasmic signaling molecules and promote the assembly of signaling complexes. One of these structural motifs is called the **death domain,** and it binds, by homotypic interactions, to death domains in a variety of cytoplasm signaling/adapter molecules. The cytoplasmic tails of both TNF-RI and Fas contain death domains, and mutation or deletion of this region prevents TNF-RI or Fas molecules from delivering apoptosis-inducing signals. However, death domain interactions are also essential for the anti-apoptotic, proinflammatory signaling pathways. The cytoplasmic signaling molecules that contain death domains and that are involved in TNF-R signaling include TRADD (TNF receptor–associated death domain), FADD (Fas-associated death domain), and RIP (receptor interacting protein).

The second type of motif that plays a key role in signaling by several TNF-R family members binds to one of a family of molecules called TNF receptor–associated factors (TRAFs) (see Figure). TNF-RII, LT-βR, and CD40 all bind TRAF proteins. To date, six TRAFs have been identified, and they are called TRAF-1 to TRAF-6. All TRAFs share a C-terminal region of homology called a TRAF domain, which mediates binding to the cytoplasmic domains of TNF-R family members, and TRAFs 2 to 6 have RING and zinc finger motifs that are involved in signaling.

Multiple different interactions of death domain proteins and TRAFs are known to occur in the signaling pathways associated with the different TNF-R family members. In the case of TNF-RI, a current model of these interactions illustrates how TNF may lead to either apoptosis or inflammatory responses (see Figure). In this model, the death domain protein TRADD binds directly to the TNF-RI death domain and acts as a pivotal adapter molecule leading to one of two different signaling cascades. In one of these pathways, the death domain protein FADD binds to TRADD, and the aspartyl-directed cysteine protease caspase-8 binds to FADD. Caspase-8 binding initiates the activation of a cascade of caspases that eventually causes apoptosis. In response to Fas ligand binding, Fas mediates apoptosis by a similar pathway, but in this case, FADD binds directly to the cytoplasmic tail of Fas (see Chapter 10, Box 10–2). The alternative proinflammatory and anti-apoptotic pathway involves the binding of TRAF-2 and RIP-1 to TRADD and results in NF-κB– and AP-1–dependent gene transcription. Both TRAF-2 and RIP-1 are involved in the activation of IκB kinases, which mediate the initial steps in NF-κB activation (see Chapter 8, Box 8–4). Gene knockout studies suggest that TRAF-5 may be able to substitute for TRAF-2 in NF-κB activation. TRAF-2 also activates the mitogen-activated protein kinase (MAP kinase) cascade that leads to JNK activation, phosphorylation of c-Jun, and formation of the AP-1 transcription factor composed of c-Fos and c-Jun. The combination of NF-κB and AP-1 activation promotes the transcription of a variety of genes involved in inflammation, including endothelial adhesion molecules, cytokines, and chemokines. Furthermore, NF-κB also enhances expression of a family of cellular inhibitors of apoptosis (cIAPs), which block the function of caspases. Therefore, when the proinflammatory pathway is engaged, there is active inhibition of the apoptotic pathway. It is still unclear what determines whether TNF binding to TNFR-1 will activate the inflammatory or apoptotic signaling pathways.

Other members of the TNF-R family use TRAF-dependent signaling pathways that lead to NF-κB and AP-1 activation similar to the TNF-RI pathway, but in contrast to TNF-RI, these other receptors directly bind TRAFs to their cytoplasmic tails. TRAF-1 and TRAF-2 interact with TNF-RII, TRAF-2 and TRAF-3 interact with CD40, and TRAF-4 interacts with LT-βR. CD40 delivers activating signals to B cells and macrophages through TRAF binding (see Chapters 9 and 13). TNF-RII, which lacks a death domain, can sometimes deliver apoptotic signals, but the mechanism is not understood. Interestingly, one of the transforming gene products of the Epstein-Barr virus encodes a self-aggregating TRAF domain–containing protein that binds TRAF molecules, and therefore infection by the virus mimics TNF- or CD40-induced signals.

Although the IL-1 receptor is not a member of the TNF-R family, many of the biologic effects of IL-1 are similar to the effects of TNF-α because the IL-1 signaling pathway shares biochemical intermediates with the TNF pathway. Binding of IL-1 to the type I IL-1 receptor (IL-1R) leads to the recruitment of an adapter protein, called MyD88, and

Continued on following page

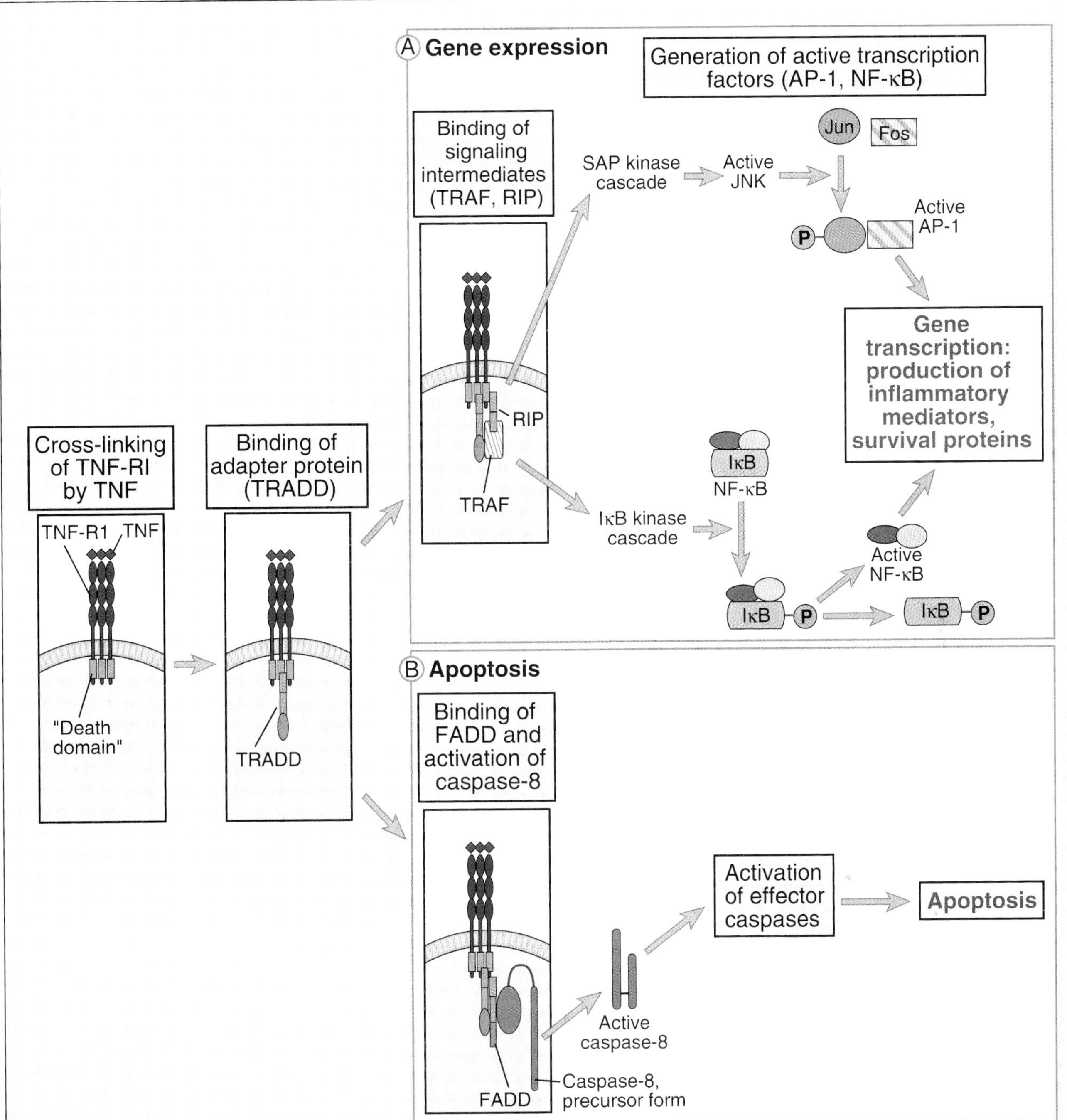

Signal transduction by TNF receptors.
The type I TNF receptor (TNF-RI) may stimulate gene expression (A) or induce apoptosis (B). These distinct effects are both initiated by the binding of the adapter protein TRADD followed by either TRAF and RIP, leading to new gene expression, or binding of the adapter protein FADD, leading to apoptosis. The cytoplasmic tails of other members of the TNF-R family may directly bind FADD (e.g., Fas), leading to apoptosis, or directly bind TRAFs (e.g., TNF-RII or CD40), leading to gene expression. The genes induced by TNF-R family members encode mainly mediators of inflammation and anti-apoptotic proteins.

a serine/threonine kinase called IL-1 receptor–associated kinase (IRAK). IRAK autophosphorylates and dissociates from the complex and subsequently binds TRAF-6. The IRAK–TRAF-6 complex activates both NF-κB and AP-1. This signaling pathway is also used by the Toll-like receptors that are involved in innate immunity (see Chapter 12, Box 12–1). IL-18 also signals by a similar mechanism, and the cytoplasmic regions of the receptors for IL-1 and IL-18 are homologous to each other.

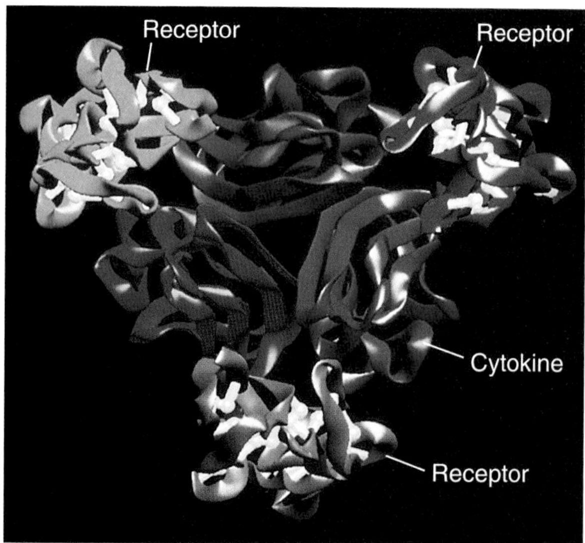

Figure 11–4 Structure of the TNF receptor with bound lymphotoxin.

The ribbon structure depicts a top view of a complex of three TNF receptors (TNF-RI) and one molecule of the bound cytokine, revealed by x-ray crystallography. Lymphotoxin (LT) is a homotrimer in which the three subunits are colored dark blue. The LT homotrimer forms an inverted three-sided pyramid with its base at the top and its apex at the bottom. Three TNF-RI molecules, colored magenta, cyan, and red, bind one homotrimer of LT, with each receptor molecule interacting with two different LT monomers in the homotrimer complex. Disulfide bonds in the receptor are colored yellow. TNF is homologous to LT and presumably binds to its receptors in the same way. (From Banner DW, A D'Arcy, W Jones, R Gentz, HJ Schoenfeld, C Broger, H Loetscher, and W Lesslauer. Crystal structure of the soluble human 55 kd TNF receptor-human TNFbeta complex; implications for TNF receptor activation. Cell 73:431–445, 1993. Copyright 1993, with permission from Elsevier Science.)

Biologic Actions

The principal physiologic function of TNF is to stimulate the recruitment of neutrophils and monocytes to sites of infection and to activate these cells to eradicate microbes (Fig. 11–5). TNF mediates these effects by several actions on vascular endothelial cells and leukocytes.

- TNF causes vascular endothelial cells to express adhesion molecules that make the endothelial surface adhesive for leukocytes, initially for neutrophils and subsequently for monocytes and lymphocytes. The most important of these adhesion molecules are selectins and ligands for leukocyte integrins (see Chapter 6, Boxes 6–2 and 6–3). The sequence of events in the recruitment of leukocytes to sites of infection will be described in more detail in Chapters 12 and 13.
- TNF stimulates endothelial cells and macrophages to secrete chemokines (discussed later) that enhance the affinity of leukocyte integrins for their ligands and induce leukocyte chemotaxis and recruitment. TNF also acts on mononuclear phagocytes to stimulate secretion of IL-1, which functions much like TNF itself (see later). This is an example of a cascade of cytokines that have similar or complementary biologic activities.
- In addition to its role in inflammation, TNF induces the apoptosis of some cell types. The physiologic significance of this response is not known.

The actions of TNF on endothelium and leukocytes are critical for local inflammatory responses to microbes. If inadequate quantities of TNF are present (e.g., in animals treated with neutralizing anti-TNF antibodies or in TNF gene knockout mice), a consequence may be failure to contain infections. TNF also contributes to local inflammatory reactions that are injurious to the host (e.g., in autoimmune diseases) (see Chapter 18). Neutralizing antibodies to TNF and soluble TNF receptors are in clinical use to reduce inflammation in patients with rheumatoid arthritis and inflammatory bowel disease.

In severe infections, TNF is produced in large amounts and causes systemic clinical and pathologic abnormalities. If the stimulus for TNF production is sufficiently strong, the quantity of the cytokine produced is so large that it enters the blood stream and acts at distant sites as an endocrine hormone (see Fig. 11–5). The principal systemic actions of TNF are the following.

- TNF acts on the hypothalamus to induce fever and is therefore called an endogenous (i.e., host-derived) pyrogen (to distinguish it from LPS, which functions as an exogenous, or microbe-derived, pyrogen). Fever production in response to TNF (and IL-1) is mediated by increased synthesis of prostaglandins by cytokine-stimulated hypothalamic cells. Prostaglandin synthesis inhibitors, such as aspirin, reduce fever by blocking this action of TNF and IL-1.
- TNF acts on hepatocytes to increase synthesis of certain serum proteins, such as serum amyloid A protein and fibrinogen. The combination of hepatocyte-derived plasma proteins induced by TNF and by IL-1 and IL-6, two other cytokines of innate immunity, constitutes the acute-phase response to inflammatory stimuli (see Chapter 12, Box 12–2).
- Prolonged production of TNF causes wasting of muscle and fat cells, called cachexia. This wasting results from TNF-induced appetite suppression and reduced synthesis of lipoprotein lipase, an enzyme needed to release fatty acids from circulating lipoproteins so that they can be used by the tissues.
- When large amounts of TNF are produced, with serum concentrations reaching 10^{-7} M or more, myocardial contractility and vascular smooth muscle tone are inhibited, resulting in a marked fall in blood pressure, or shock.
- TNF causes intravascular thrombosis, mainly as a result of loss of the normal anticoagulant properties of the endothelium. TNF stimulates endothelial cell expression of tissue factor, a potent activator of coagulation, and inhibits expression of thrombomodulin, an inhibitor of coagulation. These endothelial alterations are exacerbated by activation of neutrophils,

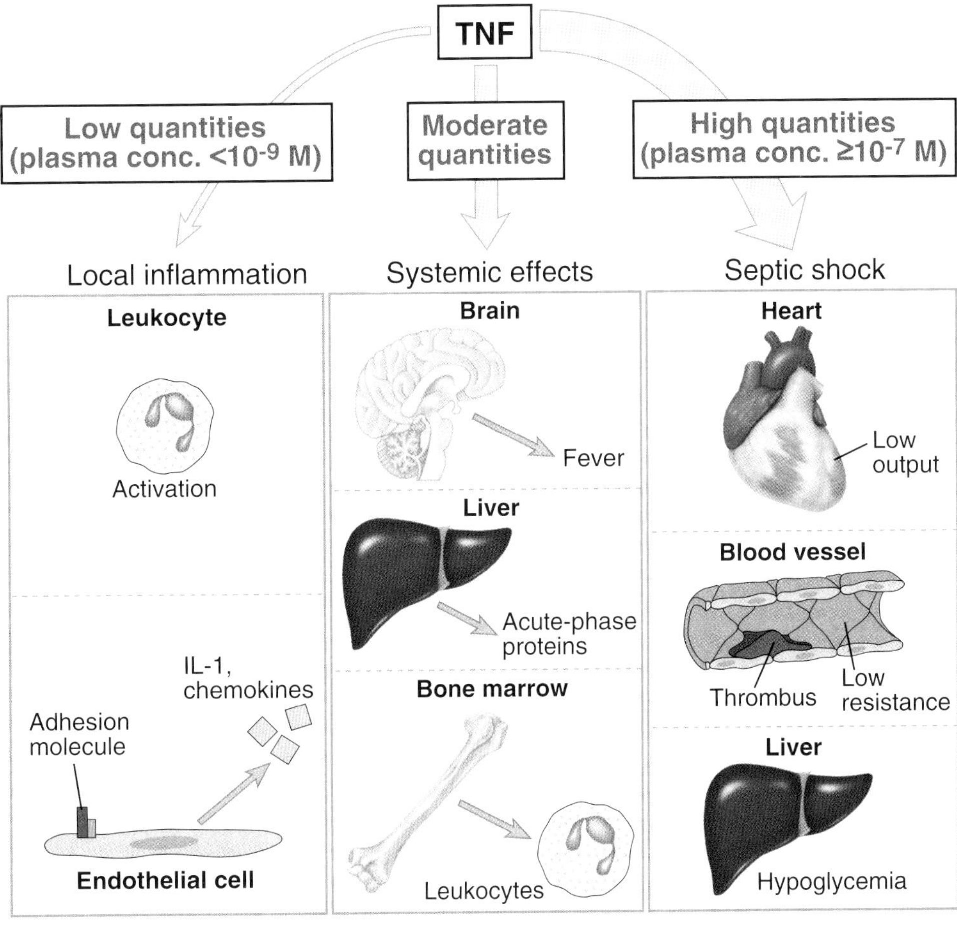

Figure 11–5 Biologic actions of TNF. At low concentrations, TNF acts on leukocytes and endothelium to induce acute inflammation. At moderate concentrations, TNF mediates the systemic effects of inflammation. At high concentrations, TNF causes the pathologic abnormalities of septic shock.

leading to vascular plugging by these cells. The ability of this cytokine to cause necrosis of tumors, which is the basis of its name, is mainly a result of thrombosis of tumor blood vessels.

- High circulating levels of TNF cause severe metabolic disturbances, such as a fall in blood glucose concentrations to levels incompatible with life. This is due to overuse of glucose by muscle and failure of the liver to replace the glucose.

A complication of severe gram-negative bacterial sepsis is a syndrome called **septic shock** (or endotoxin shock), which is characterized by vascular collapse, disseminated intravascular coagulation, and metabolic disturbances. This syndrome is due to LPS-induced production of TNF and other cytokines, including IL-12, IFN-γ, and IL-1 (the last also being produced in response to TNF itself, as part of a cytokine cascade). The concentration of serum TNF may be predictive of the outcome of severe gram-negative infections. This is one of the few examples of a disorder in which measuring levels of a circulating cytokine is informative. Septic shock can be reproduced in experimental animals by administration of LPS or TNF (see Chapter 12, Box 12–2). Antagonists of TNF can prevent mortality in the experimental models, but clinical trials with anti-TNF antibodies or with soluble TNF receptors have not shown benefit in patients with sepsis. The cause of this therapeutic failure is not known, but it may be because other cytokines elicit the same responses as TNF, an example of redundancy.

There are many cytokines and membrane proteins belonging to the TNF–TNF receptor families, and they serve important functions in innate and adaptive immune responses. Two membrane proteins that are members of the TNF-R family are CD40 and Fas; their functions are discussed in other chapters. A newly discovered member of the TNF-R family is a protein called osteoprotegerin (OPG) or receptor activator of NF-κB (RANK). The receptor is expressed on osteoclasts and some macrophages and dendritic cells. The cytokine that is the ligand for this receptor, called OPG ligand or RANK ligand, is made by activated T cells. Production of this cytokine plays an important role in bone resorption in many states, notably arthritis.

Interleukin-1 (IL-1)

The principal function of IL-1, similar to that of TNF, is as a mediator of the host inflammatory response to infections and other inflammatory stimuli. IL-1 functions together with TNF in innate immunity and inflammation.

Production, Structure, Receptors

The major cellular source of IL-1, like that of TNF, is activated mononuclear phagocytes. IL-1 production by mononuclear phagocytes is induced by bacterial products such as LPS and by other cytokines such as TNF. Unlike TNF, IL-1 is also produced by many cell types other than macrophages, such as neutrophils, epithelial cells (e.g., keratinocytes), and endothelial cells.

There are two forms of IL-1, called IL-1α and IL-1β, that are less than 30% homologous to each other, but they bind to the same cell surface receptors and mediate the same biologic activities. Both IL-1 polypeptides are synthesized as 33-kD precursors and are secreted as 17-kD mature proteins. The active form of IL-1β is the cleaved product, but IL-1α is active either as the 33-kD precursor or as the smaller cleaved product. IL-1β is proteolytically cleaved by a protease, called IL-1β–converting enzyme (ICE), to generate the biologically active secreted protein. ICE was the first described mammalian member of a family of cysteine proteases called caspases. Many members of this family are involved in apoptotic death in a variety of cells (see Chapter 10, Box 10–2). Unlike most secreted proteins, neither IL-1α nor IL-1β has a hydrophobic signal sequence to target the nascent polypeptide to the endoplasmic reticulum, and we do not know how these molecules are secreted. Most of the IL-1 found in the circulation is IL-1β.

Two different membrane receptors for IL-1 have been characterized, and both are members of the Ig superfamily. The type I receptor is expressed on almost all cell types and is the major receptor for IL-1–mediated responses. The type II receptor is expressed on B cells but may be induced on other cell types. It does not induce responses to IL-1, and its major function may be to act as a "decoy" that competitively inhibits IL-1 binding to the type I signaling receptor. The cytoplasmic portion of the type I IL-1 receptor is homologous to a domain of Toll-like receptors, which are involved in defense against infections (see Chapter 12, Box 12–1). Binding of IL-1 to the type I IL-1 receptor leads to the activation of a kinase called the IL-1 receptor–associated kinase (IRAK) and ultimately to activation of the NF-κB and AP-1 transcription factors (see Box 11–1).

Biologic Actions

The biologic effects of IL-1 are similar to those of TNF and depend on the quantity of cytokine produced.

- When secreted at low concentrations, IL-1 functions as a mediator of local inflammation. It acts on endothelial cells to increase expression of surface molecules that mediate leukocyte adhesion, such as ligands for integrins.
- When secreted in larger quantities, IL-1 enters the blood stream and exerts endocrine effects. Systemic IL-1 shares with TNF the ability to cause fever, to induce synthesis of acute-phase plasma proteins by the liver, and to initiate metabolic wasting (cachexia).

The similarities between IL-1 actions and those of TNF appear surprising at face value because the cytokines and their receptors are structurally different. The likely explanation for the similar biologic effects is that receptors for both cytokines signal by homologous proteins and activate the same transcription factors (see Box 11–1). However, there are several differences between IL-1 and TNF. For instance, IL-1 does not induce apoptotic death of cells, and even at high systemic concentrations, by itself it does not cause the pathophysiologic changes of septic shock.

Mononuclear phagocytes produce a natural inhibitor of IL-1 that is structurally homologous to the cytokine and binds to the same receptors but is biologically inactive, so that it functions as a competitive inhibitor of IL-1. It is therefore called IL-1 receptor antagonist (IL-1ra). IL-1ra may be an endogenous regulator of IL-1 action. Attempts to inhibit IL-1 action by IL-1ra or soluble receptors have not been of benefit in clinical trials of septic shock or arthritis to date, perhaps as a result of the redundancy of IL-1 actions with those of TNF.

Chemokines

Chemokines are a large family of structurally homologous cytokines that stimulate leukocyte movement and regulate the migration of leukocytes from the blood to tissues. The name "chemokine" is a contraction of "chemotactic cytokine." Some chemokines may be produced by various cells in response to inflammatory stimuli and recruit leukocytes to sites of inflammation; other chemokines are produced normally in various tissues and recruit leukocytes (mainly lymphocytes) to these tissues in the absence of inflammation.

Structure, Production, Receptors

All chemokines are 8- to 12-kD polypeptides that contain two internal disulfide loops. About 50 different chemokines have already been identified, and there may be many more. The chemokines are classified into families on the basis of the number and location of N-terminal cysteine residues. The two major families are the CC chemokines, in which the cysteine residues are adjacent, and the CXC family, in which these residues are separated by one amino acid. These differences correlate with organization of the subfamilies into separate gene clusters. In inflammation, the CXC chemokines act mainly on neutrophils, and the CC chemokines act mainly on monocytes, lymphocytes, and eosinophils. A small number of chemokines have a single cysteine (C family) or two cysteines separated by three amino acids (CX_3C). Chemokines were originally named on the basis of how they were identified and what responses they triggered. Attempts have recently been made to develop a standard nomenclature based in part on which receptors the chemokines bind to (see later).

Chemokines involved in inflammatory reactions are produced by leukocytes in response to external stimuli, and chemokines that regulate cell traffic through tissues are produced constitutively by various cells in these tissues. The chemokines of the CC and CXC subfamilies are produced by leukocytes and by several types of tissue cells, such as endothelial cells, epithelial cells, and fibroblasts. In many of these cells, secretion of chemokines is induced by microbes and by inflammatory cytokines, mainly TNF and IL-1. Several CC chemokines are also produced by antigen-stimulated T cells, providing a link between adaptive immunity and recruitment of inflammatory leukocytes. Some chemokines are produced constitutively (i.e., without any inflammatory stimulus) in lymphoid organs, and these are involved in the physiologic traffic of lymphocytes through the organs. Chemokines of both subfamilies bind to heparan sulfate proteoglycans on endothelial cells and are displayed in this way to circulating leukocytes. In fact, the cell-associated form may be the main functional form of chemokines. The cellular display apparently provides a high local concentration of chemokines, which function to stimulate motility of leukocytes that attach to the endothelium through adhesion molecules (see Chapter 13).

Eleven distinct receptors for CC chemokines (called CCR1 through CCR11) and six for CXC chemokines (called CXCR1 through CXCR6) have already been identified, and this list is almost certainly incomplete (Fig. 11–6). Chemokine receptors are expressed on leukocytes, with the greatest number of distinct chemokine receptors seen on T cells. The receptors exhibit overlapping specificity for chemokines within each subfamily, and the pattern of cellular expression of the receptors determines which cell types respond to which chemokines. All the chemokine receptors have a characteristic structure with seven-transmembrane α-helical domains. This feature is seen in other receptors that are coupled to trimeric guanosine triphosphate (GTP)–binding proteins (G proteins), and such receptors belong to the family of G protein–coupled receptors (GPCRs). When occupied by ligand, these receptors act as GTP exchange proteins, catalyzing the replacement of bound guanosine diphosphate (GDP) by GTP. The GTP-associated form of these G proteins can activate a variety of cellular enzymes, including some that stimulate cellular locomotion. Chemokine receptors may be rapidly down-regulated by exposure to the chemokine, and this is a likely mechanism for terminating responses.

Certain chemokine receptors, notably CCR5 and CXCR4, act as coreceptors for the human immunodeficiency virus (HIV) (see Chapter 20). Some activated T lymphocytes secrete chemokines that bind to CCR5 and block infection with HIV by competing with the virus.

Biologic Actions

Chemokines were discovered on the basis of their activities as leukocyte chemoattractants, but we now know that they serve many important functions in the immune system and in other systems.

- ***Chemokines recruit the cells of host defense to sites of infection.*** Leukocyte recruitment is a result of several sequential actions of chemokines on these cells. Chemokines that are expressed on endothelial cells bound to heparan act on leukocytes rolling on the endothelium and increase the affinity of leukocyte integrins for their ligands (see Chapter 6, Fig. 6–11). This step of integrin activation is critical for the firm adherence of the leukocytes to the endothelium, as a prelude to subsequent migration into extravascular tissue. Recall that TNF and IL-1 stimulate expression of integrin ligands on endothelium, and thus these two cytokines and chemokines act cooperatively in the process of leukocyte migration. Chemokines induce movement of leukocytes and their migration toward the chemical gradient of the cytokine by stimulating alternating polymerization and depolymerization of actin filaments. Different chemokines act on different cells and thus control the nature of the inflammatory infiltrate. For instance, the CXC chemokine IL-8 recruits neutrophils preferentially, and the CC chemokine eotaxin recruits eosinophils.
- ***Chemokines regulate the traffic of lymphocytes and other leukocytes through peripheral lymphoid tissues.*** Some of the most intriguing and surprising discoveries about chemokines have been their roles in the normal migration of immune cells into lymphoid organs. In Chapter 2, we mentioned the role of different chemokines in promoting the migration of T cells, B cells, and dendritic cells to different regions of peripheral lymphoid organs (see Fig. 2–11, Chapter 2). Various chemokines also promote migration of previously activated effector and memory T cells to nonlymphoid tissues, including mucosal organs and skin. The selectivity of different cell types for different tissues depends to a large extent on which chemokines are produced in the tissues and which chemokine receptors are expressed on the cell types.
- Chemokines are also involved in the development of diverse nonlymphoid organs. Knockout mice lacking the CXCR4 receptor have fatal defects in the development of the heart and the cerebellum. These roles of chemokines are unexpected and raise the possibility of many other as yet undiscovered functions in morphogenesis.

Interleukin-12 (IL-12)

IL-12 is a principal mediator of the early innate immune response to intracellular microbes and is a key inducer of cell-mediated immunity, the adaptive immune response to these microbes. IL-12 was originally identified as an activator of NK cell cytolytic function, but its most important action is to stimulate IFN-γ production by T cells as well as by NK cells.

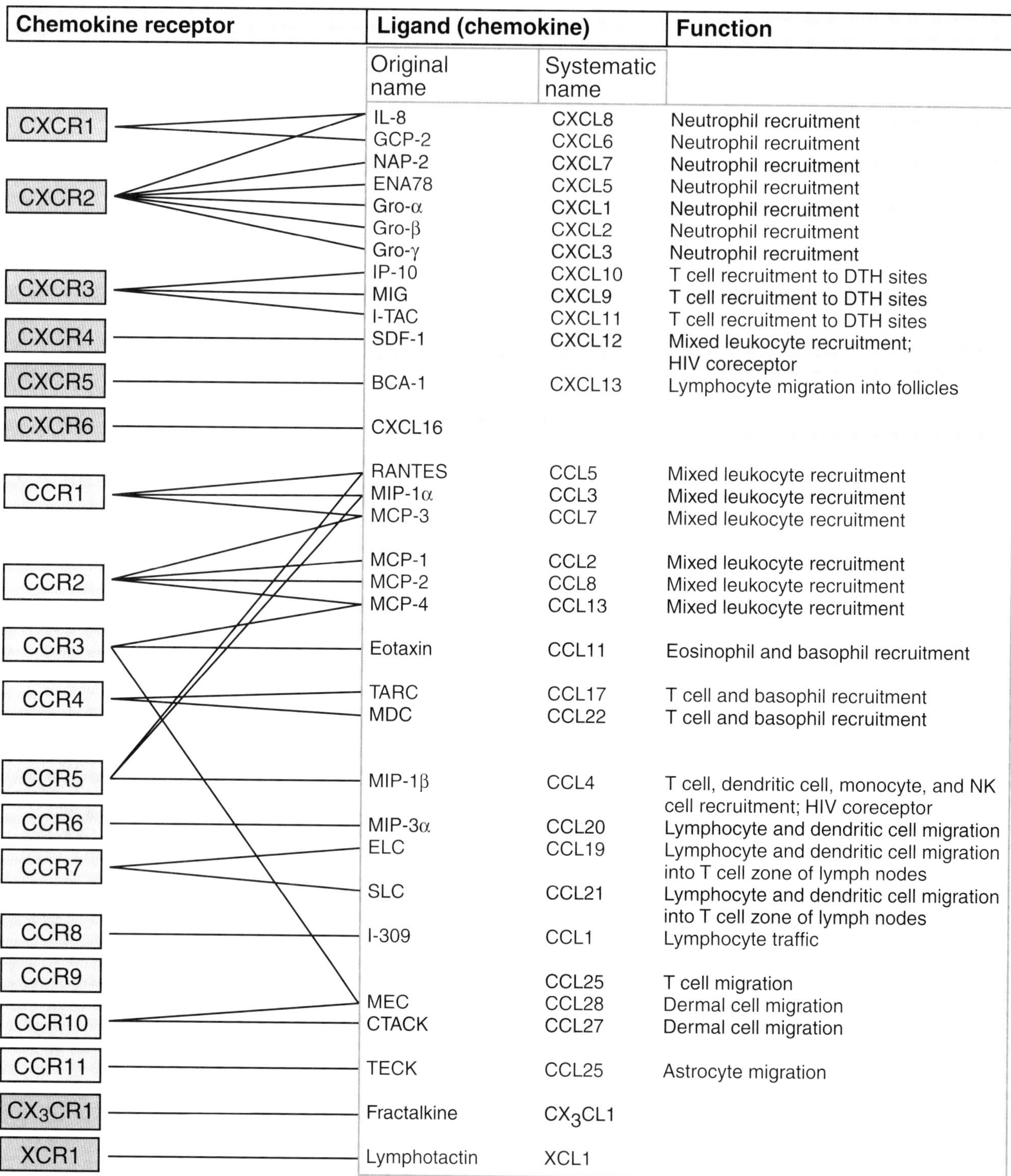

Figure 11–6 Chemokine receptors and their ligands.

The known chemokine receptors and the chemokines they bind are listed. (The new nomenclature of cytokines uses the names referred to as systematic names.) Only selected major functions of the chemokines are included.

Structure, Production, Receptors

IL-12 exists as a disulfide-linked heterodimer of 35-kD (p35) and 40-kD (p40) subunits. The p35 subunit has a four–α-helical globular domain structure. The p40 subunit is homologous not to other cytokines but to the receptor for IL-6, containing both an Ig-like domain and motifs characteristic of type I cytokine receptors.

The principal sources of IL-12 are activated mononuclear phagocytes and dendritic cells. Many cells appear to synthesize the p35 subunit, but only these antigen-presenting cells (APCs) produce the p40 component and therefore the biologically active cytokine. During innate immune reactions to microbes, IL-12 is produced in response to many microbial stimuli (including LPS), infection by intracellular bacteria (such as *Listeria* and mycobacteria), and virus infections. In addition, antigen-stimulated helper T cells induce the production of IL-12 from macrophages and dendritic cells, mainly by CD40 ligand on the T cells engaging CD40 on the macrophages and dendritic cells. IFN-γ produced by NK cells or T cells also stimulates IL-12 production. Thus, IL-12 is produced by APCs when they present antigens to T cells, during the induction and effector phases of cell-mediated immune responses (see Chapter 13).

The receptor for IL-12 is a heterodimer composed of β1 and β2 subunits. Both chains are required for high-affinity binding of the cytokine, and the β2 chain is involved in signaling. This receptor signals through a JAK/STAT pathway, in which cytokine binding to the receptor activates receptor-associated tyrosine kinases called Janus kinases (JAKs), and ultimately leads to the activation of transcription factors called signal transducers and activators of transcription (STATs). Many cytokines use this pathway to induce responses in target cells, and different cytokines activate different combinations of JAKs and STATs (Box 11–2); IL-12 is the main cytokine known to activate STAT4. Expression of the signaling chain of the IL-12 receptor is itself enhanced by cytokines, mainly IFN-γ (whose production is stimulated by IL-12), and this is an example of a positive amplification loop in immune responses.

BOX 11–2

Cytokine Signaling by Janus Kinases and Signal Transducers and Activators of Transcription

One of the best understood mechanisms by which cytokines transduce signals that elicit specific responses in target cells involves enzymes called Janus kinases (JAKs) and transcription factors called signal transducers and activators of transcription (STATs). The JAK/STAT signaling pathways are used by all type I and type II cytokine receptors. Studies of these pathways have revealed direct links between cytokine binding to receptors and transcriptional activation of target genes.

The discovery of the JAK/STAT pathways came from biochemical and genetic analyses of interferon (IFN) signaling. The promoter regions of genes responsive to IFNs contain sequences that bind cellular proteins that are phosphorylated upon IFN treatment of the cells. These proteins were shown to activate transcription of cytokine-responsive genes, and they were therefore called STAT proteins. Mutant cell lines were generated that were unresponsive to IFNs. Some of these mutant cell lines were found to lack particular STAT proteins, and introduction of the STATs by gene transfection restored cytokine responsiveness in the cells. This established the essential roles of the STATs in responses to the cytokines. Other mutant cell lines were found to be deficient in one or more related tyrosine kinases, which were called Janus kinases after the two-headed Roman god because of the presence of two kinase domains (only one of which is active). Subsequent studies, including analyses of knockout mice lacking the various STATs and JAKs, have shown that JAK/STAT pathways are involved in responses to many cytokines (see Table).

The sequence of events in the JAK/STAT signaling pathways is now well defined (see Figure). Inactive JAK enzymes are loosely attached to the cytoplasmic domains of type I and type II cytokine receptors. When two receptor molecules are brought together by binding of a cytokine molecule, the receptor-associated JAKs become active through transphosphorylation, and they phosphorylate tyrosine residues in the cytoplasmic portions of the clustered receptors. Some of these phosphotyrosine moieties of the receptors are recognized by Src homology 2 (SH2) domains of monomeric cytosolic STAT proteins, which become attached to the receptors. The STAT proteins are then phosphorylated by the receptor-associated JAK kinases. The SH2 domain of one STAT protein is able to bind to the phosphotyrosine residues of another STAT protein. As a result, two STAT proteins bind to each other and dissociate from the receptor. The STAT dimers migrate to the nucleus, where they bind to DNA sequences in the promoter regions of cytokine-responsive genes and activate gene transcription. After each round, new STAT proteins can bind to the cytokine receptor, become phosphorylated, dimerize, and again migrate to the nucleus.

One intriguing question that arises is, What determines the specificity of responses to many different cytokines, given the limited numbers of JAKs and STATs used by the various cytokine receptors? The likely answer is that unique amino acid sequences in the different cytokine receptors provide the scaffolding for specifically binding, and thereby activating, different combinations of JAKs and STATs. The SH2 domains of different STAT proteins selectively bind to the phosphotyrosine residues and flanking regions of different cytokine receptors. This is largely responsible for the activation of particular STATs by

Continued on following page

Cytokine Signaling by Janus Kinases and Signal Transducers (*Continued*)

BOX 11–2

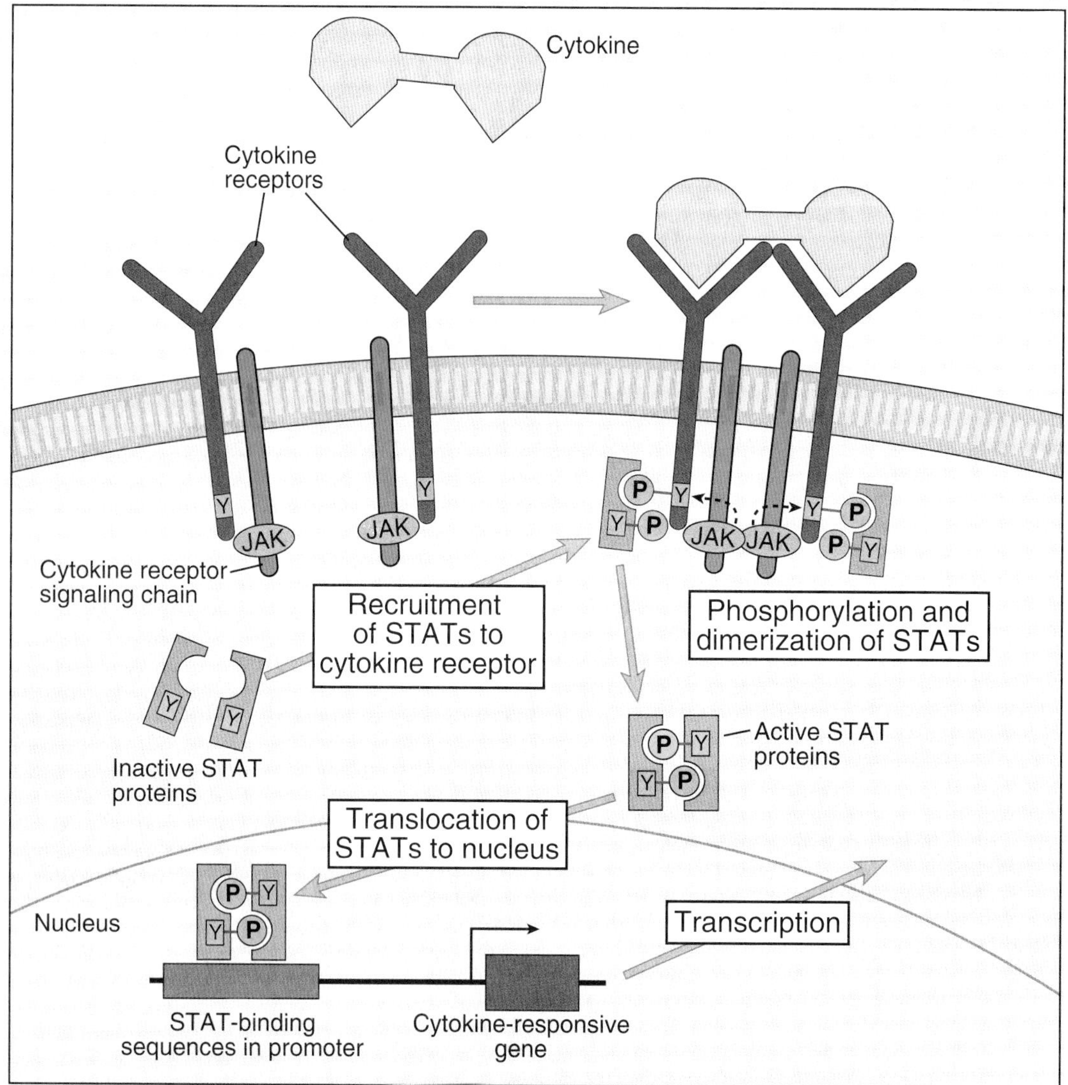

Cytokine signaling by the JAK/STAT pathway.
Cytokine-induced clustering of receptors leads to JAK-mediated phosphorylation of the receptor chains, attachment of inactive STATs, phosphorylation of the bound STATs (also by the JAKs), dimerization of STATs and migration to the nucleus, and stimulation of gene transcription.

various cytokine receptors and therefore for the specificity of cytokine signaling. In addition, cytokines activate signaling pathways and transcription factors other than STATs. For instance, the IL-2 receptor β chain activates Ras-dependent MAP kinase pathways that may be involved in gene transcription and growth stimulation. Other cytokine receptors may similarly activate other signaling pathways in concert with the JAK/STAT pathways to elicit biologic responses to the cytokines.

Several mechanisms of negative regulation of JAK/STAT pathways have been identified. Proteins called suppressors of cytokine signaling (SOCS) are a family of STAT pathway inhibitors. Members of this family are identified by the presence of an SH2 domain and a conserved 40–amino acid C-terminal region called a SOCS box. Eight different SOCS proteins have been identified; in addition, other SOCS box–containing proteins that do not have SH2 domains also exist. The mechanisms of SOCS protein inhibition of JAK/STAT signaling are not well understood, but they appear to target both cytokine receptors and JAK kinases. Interestingly, the more variable N-terminal ends of the SOCS, but not the conserved SOCS boxes, are required for their inhibitory activities. The SOCS box appears to be involved in targeting associated proteins for proteasomal degradation. SOCS gene knockout mice have begun to provide information on the physiologic role of this family. SOCS-1 knockout mice, for example, die at 3 weeks of age because of excessive actions of IFN-γ,

Continued on following page

JAK/STAT	Involved cytokines*	Phenotype of knockout mice
STAT1	IFN-α/β, IFN-γ	Defect in innate immunity; no reponse to IFNs
STAT2	IFN-α/β	Defective immunity to viruses
STAT3	IL-6, IL-10	Embryonic lethal
STAT4	IL-12	Defect in T_H1 development, IFN-γ production
STAT5a	Prolactin	Lactation defect
STAT5b	Growth hormone	Dwarfism
STAT5a and STAT5b	IL-2, IL-7, IL-9 (in addition to above)	Lactation defect, dwarfism, and defective T cell proliferation in response to IL-2
STAT6	IL-4	Defect in T_H2 development, IL-4–dependent Ig isotypes
JAK1	IFN-α/β, IFN-γ, cytokines using γ_c and gp130 (e.g., IL-2, IL-4, IL-6)	Perinatal lethal; defective innate immunity, possible defect in neuronal viability
JAK2	Epo, IL-3, IFN-γ	Embryonic lethal, hematopoietic failure
JAK3	Cytokines using γ_c chain (IL-7, IL-2, IL-4)	Defect in T cell maturation
Tyk2	IFN-α/β, IFN-γ, IL-12, IL-10, others	Defective IL-12 response of NK cells, defective immunity to viruses

*Selected examples of involved cytokines are shown.

and the phenotype can be corrected by crossing the mice with IFN-γ knockout mice. Other knockout mice studies suggest that SOCS-2 inhibits signaling by the receptors for growth hormone and insulin-like growth factor, whereas SOCS-3 regulates erythropoietin action. The expression of SOCS proteins is induced by the same cytokine stimuli that activate JAK/STAT pathways, and thus they are negative feedback inhibitors. Other inhibitors of cytokine signaling include tyrosine phosphatases, such as SHP-1, which can dephosphorylate and therefore deactivate JAK molecules, and members of the protein inhibitors of activated STAT (PIAS) family, which bind phosphorylated STAT proteins and prevent their interaction with DNA.

Biologic Actions

IL-12 is critical for initiating a sequence of responses involving macrophages, NK cells, and T lymphocytes that results in the eradication of intracellular microbes (Fig. 11–7).

- ***IL-12 stimulates the production of IFN-γ by NK cells and T lymphocytes.*** Macrophages produce IL-12 in response to many microbes. Secreted IL-12 stimulates NK cells and T cells to produce IFN-γ, which then activates the macrophages to kill the phagocytosed microbes. Thus, innate immunity against many microbes is mediated by cytokines acting in the following sequence: microbes → macrophage response → IL-12 → IFN-γ → macrophage activation → killing of microbes. Large amounts of IL-12 are produced in severe gram-negative sepsis, resulting in the production of IFN-γ, which synergizes with bacterial LPS to stimulate macrophage production of TNF, the principal mediator of septic shock. IL-12 antagonists prevent lethality in experimental models of LPS-induced septic shock. We will return to IFN-γ when we discuss the cytokines of adaptive immunity.
- ***IL-12 stimulates the differentiation of CD4⁺ helper T lymphocytes into IFN-γ–producing T_H1 cells.*** The T_H1 subset of helper T cells activates phagocytes in cell-mediated immunity. This effect of IL-12 will be discussed more fully in Chapter 13.
- ***IL-12 enhances the cytolytic functions of activated NK cells and CD8⁺ cytolytic T lymphocytes (CTLs).*** This action of IL-12 is also important in cell-mediated immunity (see Chapter 13).

Knockout mice lacking the p40 component of IL-12, and hence the functional cytokine, are defective in IFN-γ production and T_H1 cell development and therefore in cell-mediated immunity to intracellular microbes. However, IFN-γ synthesis is not completely abrogated in these mice, probably because of the actions of other compensatory cytokines (notably IL-18, described later). IL-12 knockout mice also have defects in NK cell function. A few patients with mutations in

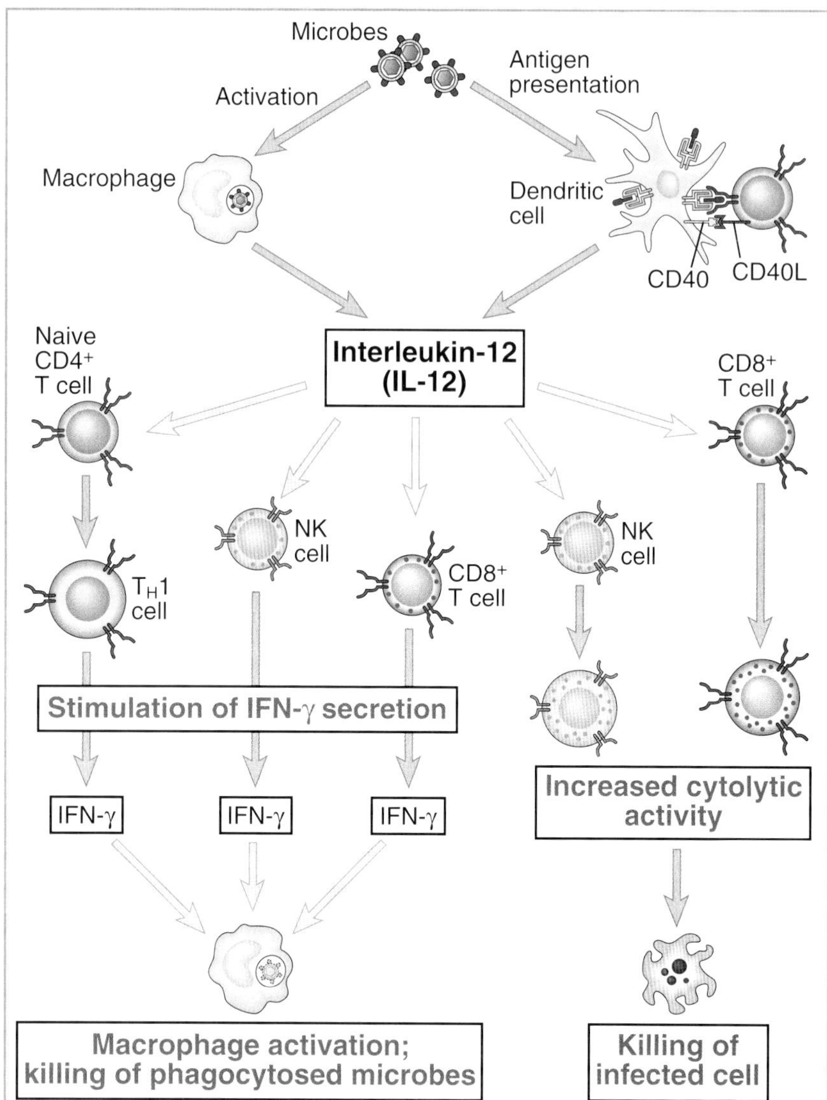

Figure 11–7 Biologic actions of IL-12. IL-12 is produced by macrophages and dendritic cells that respond to microbes or to T cell signals such as CD40 ligand engaging CD40. IL-12 acts on T lymphocytes and NK cells to stimulate IFN-γ production and cytolytic activity, both of which function to eradicate intracellular microbes.

the IL-12 receptor have been described; they are highly susceptible to infections with intracellular bacteria, notably *Salmonella* and atypical mycobacteria.

IL-12 is an important link between innate and adaptive immunity, being produced during early innate immune reactions against intracellular microbes and stimulating adaptive immune responses that protect the host against these microbes. This illustrates a concept, introduced in Chapter 1, that innate immune reactions stimulate subsequent adaptive immune responses (see also Chapter 12). Recombinant IL-12 is in clinical trials to boost protective cell-mediated immune responses in patients with defects in cell-mediated immunity and cancer, both as systemic therapy and as a component of vaccines.

Type I Interferons (IFNs)

Type I IFNs mediate the early innate immune response to viral infections. The term *interferon* derives from the ability of these cytokines to interfere with viral infection.

Structure, Production, Receptors

Type I IFNs consist of two distinct groups of proteins called IFN-α and IFN-β. IFN-α is actually a family of about 20 structurally related polypeptides, each encoded by a separate gene. Mononuclear phagocytes are the major source of IFN-α, and IFN-α is sometimes called leukocyte interferon. IFN-β is a single protein produced by many cells, such as fibroblasts, and it is sometimes called fibroblast interferon. The most potent stimulus for type I IFN synthesis is viral infection, specifically double-stranded RNA that is produced by viruses during their replication in infected cells. Experimentally, production of type I IFN is commonly elicited by synthetic double-stranded RNA, which mimics the signal produced during viral infection. Antigen-activated T cells also stimulate mononuclear phagocytes to synthesize type I IFNs.

Although IFN-α and IFN-β are structurally different, they bind to the same cell surface receptor and induce similar biologic responses. The type I IFN receptor is a heterodimer of two structurally related polypeptides;

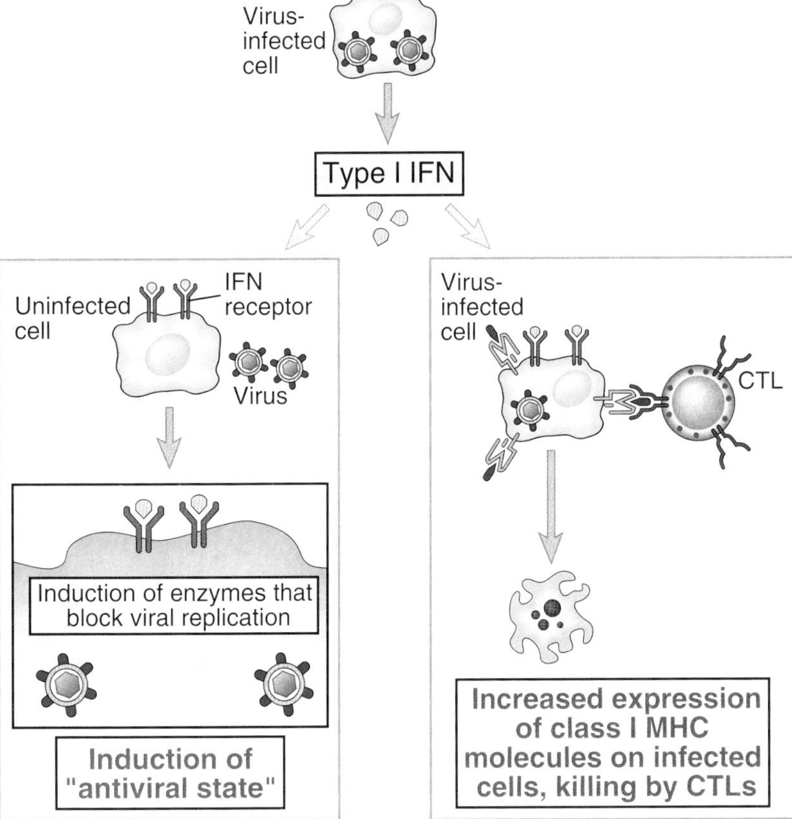

Figure 11–8 Biologic actions of type I interferons.
Type I IFNs (IFN-α, IFN-β) are produced by virus-infected cells and macrophages (not shown). Type I IFNs inhibit virus infection and enhance CTL activity against virus-infected cells.

one binds the cytokine, and the other transduces signals through a JAK/STAT pathway. Both chains are members of the type II cytokine receptor family.

Biologic Actions

The actions of type I IFNs protect against viral infections and promote cell-mediated immunity against intracellular microbes (Fig. 11–8).

- ***Type I IFN inhibits viral replication.*** IFN causes cells to synthesize a number of enzymes, such as 2′,5′ oligoadenylate synthetase, that interfere with transcription of viral RNA or DNA and viral replication. The antiviral action of type I IFN is primarily a paracrine action, in that a virally infected cell secretes IFN to protect neighboring cells that are not yet infected. A cell that has responded to IFN and is resistant to viral infection is said to be in an "antiviral state." IFN secreted by an infected cell may also act in an autocrine fashion to inhibit viral replication in that cell.
- ***Type I IFN increases expression of class I MHC molecules.*** Because $CD8^+$ CTLs recognize foreign antigens bound to class I MHC molecules, type I IFN enhances the recognition of class I–associated viral antigens on infected cells and therefore the efficiency of CTL-mediated killing of these cells.
- Type I IFN stimulates the development of T_H1 cells in humans. This effect is mainly due to the ability of type I IFN to promote in T cells the expression of functional receptors for the major T_H1-inducing cytokine IL-12. Type I IFN may also increase the cytolytic activity of NK cells.
- Type I IFN inhibits the proliferation of many cell types, including lymphocytes, *in vitro*. This is likely due to induction of the same enzymes that block viral replication, but it may also involve other enzymes that alter the metabolism of amino acids, such as tryptophan. The physiologic importance of this antiproliferative action is not known.

Thus, the principal activities of type I IFN function in concert to eradicate viral infections. Knockout mice lacking the receptor for type I IFN are susceptible to viral infections. IFN-α is in clinical use as an antiviral agent in certain forms of viral hepatitis. IFN-β is used as a therapy for multiple sclerosis, but the mechanism of its beneficial effect in this disease is not known.

Interleukin-10 (IL-10)

IL-10 is an inhibitor of activated macrophages and dendritic cells and is thus involved in the control of innate immune reactions and cell-mediated immunity. So far, we have described cytokines that stimulate innate immunity. IL-10, in contrast, is an inhibitor of host immune responses, particularly responses involving macrophages.

Production, Structure, Receptors

IL-10 has a four–α-helical globular domain structure and binds to a type II cytokine receptor. IL-10 is produced mainly by activated macrophages, and because it inhibits macrophage functions, it is an excellent example of a negative feedback regulator. It is not clear whether different stimuli may act on macrophages to induce the production of a regulatory cytokine like IL-10 and effector cytokines like TNF and IL-12, or whether the same stimuli elicit production of all these cytokines but with different kinetics. T lymphocytes also secrete IL-10, and it is produced by some nonlymphoid cell types (e.g., keratinocytes) as well.

Biologic Actions

The biologic effects of IL-10 result from its ability to inhibit many of the functions of activated macrophages. As we have discussed previously, macrophages respond to microbes by secreting cytokines and by expressing costimulators that enhance T cell activation and cell-mediated immunity. IL-10 acts on the activated macrophages to terminate these responses and return the system to its resting state as the microbial infection is eradicated.

- ***IL-10 inhibits the production of IL-12 by activated macrophages and dendritic cells.*** Because IL-12 is a critical stimulus for IFN-γ secretion and is an inducer of innate and cell-mediated immune reactions against intracellular microbes, IL-10 functions to down-regulate all such reactions. In fact, IL-10 was discovered as an inhibitor of IFN-γ production.
- ***IL-10 inhibits the expression of costimulators and class II MHC molecules on macrophages and dendritic cells.*** Because of these actions, IL-10 serves to inhibit T cell activation and terminate cell-mediated immune reactions.

Knockout mice lacking IL-10 develop inflammatory bowel disease, probably as a result of uncontrolled activation of macrophages reacting to enteric microbes. These mice also show excessive inflammation and tissue injury in response to chemical irritants.

The Epstein-Barr virus contains a gene homologous to human IL-10, and viral IL-10 has the same activities as the natural cytokine. This raises the intriguing possibility that acquisition of the IL-10 gene during the evolution of the virus has given the virus the ability to inhibit host immunity and thus a survival advantage in the infected host.

Other Cytokines of Innate Immunity

IL-6 is a cytokine that functions in both innate and adaptive immunity. It is synthesized by mononuclear phagocytes, vascular endothelial cells, fibroblasts, and other cells in response to microbes and to other cytokines, notably IL-1 and TNF. It is also made by some activated T cells. The functional form of IL-6 is a homodimer, with each subunit forming a four–α-helical globular domain. The receptor for IL-6 consists of a cytokine-binding protein and a signal-transducing subunit, both of which belong to the type I cytokine receptor family. The 130-kD signal-transducing subunit is called gp130; it activates a JAK/STAT signaling pathway and is also the signaling component of other cytokine receptors (see Fig. 11–3B).

IL-6 has several diverse actions. In innate immunity, it stimulates the synthesis of acute-phase proteins by hepatocytes and thus contributes to the systemic effects of inflammation, the so-called acute-phase response (see Chapter 12, Box 12–2). IL-6 stimulates production of neutrophils from bone marrow progenitors, usually acting in concert with colony-stimulating factors (discussed later in the chapter). In adaptive immunity, IL-6 stimulates the growth of B lymphocytes that have differentiated into antibody producers. IL-6 similarly acts as a growth factor for neoplastic plasma cells (myelomas), and many myeloma cells that grow autonomously secrete IL-6 as an autocrine growth factor. Moreover, IL-6 can promote the growth of monoclonal antibody–producing hybridomas, which are derived from myelomas.

IL-15 is a cytokine produced by mononuclear phagocytes and probably many other cell types in response to viral infection, LPS, and other signals that trigger innate immunity. IL-15 is structurally homologous to IL-2 (discussed later). The receptor for IL-15 has a unique cytokine-binding α chain, which is homologous to the α chain of the IL-2 receptor, and the same signal-transducing β and γ chains as in the IL-2 receptor.

The best documented function of IL-15 is to stimulate the proliferation of NK cells. Because IL-15 is synthesized early in response to viral infections, it stimulates expansion of NK cells within the first few days after infection. Once the adaptive immune response develops, this function may be taken over by T cell–derived IL-2. Thus, IL-15 may be thought of as the equivalent of IL-2 in the early innate immune response (i.e., it serves the functions in innate immunity that are served by IL-2 in adaptive immunity). IL-15 also acts as a T cell growth and survival factor, especially for long-lived memory $CD8^+$ T cells. Knockout mice lacking IL-15 or the IL-15 receptor α chain have greatly reduced numbers of NK cells and a partial reduction of $CD8^+$ T cells.

IL-18 is structurally homologous to IL-1 and signals by a similar receptor-associated kinase (IRAK), but it has a different function than IL-1. IL-18 is produced by macrophages in response to LPS and other microbial products. It stimulates the production of IFN-γ by NK cells and T cells and synergizes with IL-12 in this response. Thus, IL-18 is an inducer of cell-mediated immunity, especially in combination with IL-12. Knockout mice lacking IL-18 are deficient in IFN-γ production, and mice lacking both IL-12 and IL-18 are almost completely lacking in IFN-γ and in T_H1 responses to intracellular microbes. Like IL-1β, IL-18 is synthesized as a precursor that has to be cleaved by the enzyme ICE to generate the biologically active protein. Knockout mice lacking ICE show defects in LPS-induced IFN-γ production, which is attributable to the absence of active IL-18.

Several other cytokines have been identified from DNA sequence information (e.g., from the Human Genome Project), but the biology of these cytokines remains to be fully explored. IL-19, IL-20, IL-22, and IL-24 are homologous to IL-10. The limited studies done to date indicate that many of these may be involved in inflammatory reactions in the skin; no function for IL-19 has been described so far. IL-21 is homologous to IL-15 and stimulates the proliferation of NK cells. IL-23 is similar to IL-12 and consists of a 19-kD subunit associated with the IL-12 p40 chain. Like IL-12, IL-23 may be a stimulus for cell-mediated immune responses.

Roles of Cytokines in Innate Immunity and Inflammation

Now that we have discussed the individual cytokines of innate immunity, it is useful to integrate this information and consider how these cytokines contribute to innate immune reactions against microbes. Different cytokines play key roles in innate immunity to different classes of microbes. In infections by pyogenic (pus-forming) extracellular bacteria, macrophages respond to bacterial endotoxins and perhaps to other bacterial products by producing TNF, IL-1, and chemokines (Fig. 11–9). TNF and IL-1 act on vascular endothelium at the site of the infection to induce the expression of adhesion molecules that promote stable attachment of blood neutrophils and monocytes to the endothelium at this site. Chemokines produced by the macrophages and by endothelial cells stimulate the extravasation of the leukocytes to the infection, where the innate immune reaction is mounted to eliminate the infectious microbes.

Macrophages also respond to many microbes, including intracellular bacteria and LPS-producing bacteria, by secreting IL-12, which induces the local production of IFN-γ from NK cells and T lymphocytes. IFN-γ then activates the macrophages to destroy phagocytosed microbes. IL-12 also stimulates the subsequent adaptive immune response and directs it toward T_H1 cells, which are the mediators of cellular immunity and the most effective response for destroying intracellular bacteria. These actions of IL-12 are complemented by IL-18. Cytokine-mediated leukocyte recruitment and activation are responsible for the injury to normal tissues that often accompanies innate immune reactions to infections. These macrophage-derived cytokines, especially TNF, IL-1, and IL-12, are also responsible for the systemic manifestations of infection.

In viral infections, type I IFNs are secreted by infected cells and macrophages and function to inhibit viral replication and infection. IL-15 stimulates the

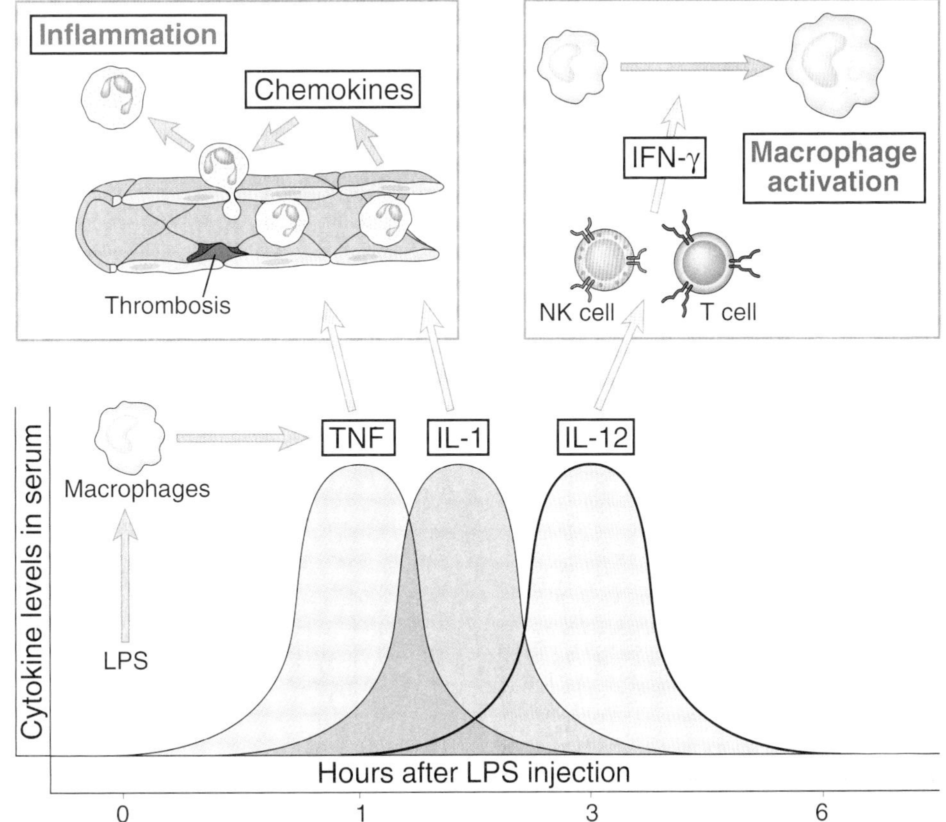

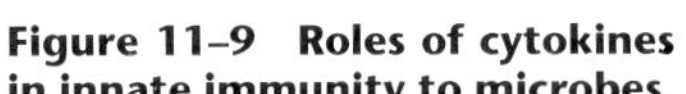

Figure 11–9 Roles of cytokines in innate immunity to microbes. This figure illustrates the role of cytokines in host responses to bacteria that produce LPS (endotoxin). LPS acts on macrophages to induce the secretion of multiple cytokines, including TNF, IL-1, and IL-12, which can be measured in the serum of individuals treated with LPS or infected with LPS-producing bacteria. TNF and IL-1 stimulate acute inflammation by their actions on endothelial cells and leukocytes. IL-12 stimulates the production of IFN-γ, which can also be measured in the serum. Note that chemokines may be produced by many cell populations; only endothelial cells are shown as the source in this illustration. Antagonists against TNF, IL-12, and IFN-γ reduce the pathologic complications of sepsis and decrease the mortality associated with septic shock.

expansion of NK cells, and IL-12 enhances the cytolytic activity of NK cells. NK cell–mediated killing of virus-infected cells eliminates the reservoir of infection.

The dominant cytokines produced in response to different microbes account for the nature of the innate immune reactions to these microbes. For instance, the early response to pyogenic bacteria consists mainly of neutrophils, the response to intracellular bacteria is dominated by activated macrophages, and the response to viruses consists of NK cells in addition to other inflammatory cells. There may be considerable overlap, however, and these varied cellular reactions may be seen to different degrees in many infections.

Cytokines That Mediate and Regulate Adaptive Immunity

Cytokines mediate the proliferation and differentiation of lymphocytes after antigen recognition in the activation phase of adaptive immune responses and mediate the activation of specialized effector cells in the effector phase of adaptive immunity. Cytokine production is one of the principal responses of T lymphocytes to antigen recognition. Different types of microbes and antigen exposures may induce CD4$^+$ helper T cells to differentiate into distinct effector populations, such as T_H1 and T_H2 subsets, that produce different sets of cytokines and serve different functions. In the following section, we first describe the major cytokines of adaptive immunity (Table 11–4) and conclude by describing how cytokines contribute to specialized effector cell responses against different microbes.

Interleukin-2 (IL-2)

IL-2 is a growth factor for antigen-stimulated T lymphocytes and is responsible for T cell clonal expansion after antigen recognition. For this reason, IL-2 was originally called T cell growth factor. IL-2 acts mainly on the same cells that produce it (i.e., it functions as an autocrine growth factor).

Table 11–4. Cytokines of Adaptive Immunity

Cytokine	Size	Principal cell source	Principal cell targets and biologic effects
Interleukin-2 (IL-2)	14–17 kD	T cells	T cells: proliferation, increased cytokine synthesis; potentiates Fas-mediated apoptosis NK cells: proliferation, activation B cells: proliferation, antibody synthesis (*in vitro*)
Interleukin-4 (IL-4)	18 kD	CD4$^+$ T cells (T_H2), mast cells	B cells: isotype switching to IgE T cells: T_H2 differentiation, proliferation Macrophages: inhibition of IFN-γ–mediated activation Mast cells: proliferation (*in vitro*)
Interleukin-5 (IL-5)	45–50 kD; homodimer of 20-kD subunits	CD4$^+$ T cells (T_H2)	Eosinophils: activation, increased production B cells: proliferation, IgA production
Interferon-γ (IFN-γ)	50 kD (glycosylated); homodimer of 21- to 24-kD subunits	T cells (T_H1, CD8$^+$ T cells), NK cells	Macrophages: activation (increased microbicidal functions) B cells: isotype switching to opsonizing and complement-fixing IgG subclasses T cells: T_H1 differentiation Various cells: increased expression of class I and class II MHC molecules, increased antigen processing and presentation to T cells
Transforming growth factor-β (TGF-β)	25 kD; homodimer of 12.5-kD subunits	T cells, macrophages, other cell types	T cells: inhibition of proliferation and effector functions B cells: inhibition of proliferation; IgA production Macrophages: inhibition
Lymphotoxin (LT)	21–24 kD; secreted as homotrimer or associated with $LT\beta_2$ on the cell membrane	T cells	Recruitment and activation of neutrophils Lymphoid organogenesis
Interleukin-13 (IL-13)	15 kD	CD4$^+$ T cells (T_H2)	B cells: isotype switching to IgE Epithelial cells: increased mucus production Macrophages: inhibition

Production, Structure, Receptors

IL-2 is produced by $CD4^+$ T lymphocytes and, in lesser amounts, by $CD8^+$ T cells. Activation of T cells by antigens and costimulators stimulates transcription of the IL-2 gene and synthesis and secretion of the protein (see Chapter 8). IL-2 production is transient, with peak secretion occurring about 8 to 12 hours after activation.

Secreted IL-2 is a 14- to 17-kD glycoprotein that folds into a globular protein containing four α-helices. It is the prototype of the four–α-helical cytokines that interact with type I cytokine receptors (Fig. 11–10).

The expression of functional IL-2 receptors is enhanced by antigen stimulation; therefore, T cells that recognize antigens are the cells that proliferate preferentially in response to IL-2 produced during adaptive immune responses. The IL-2 receptor (IL-2R) consists of three noncovalently associated proteins called α, β, and γ, the last two being members of the type I cytokine receptor family. The α and β chains are involved in cytokine binding, and the β and γ chains are involved in signal transduction (see Fig. 11–10). IL-2Rα is a 55-kD polypeptide that appears on T cell activation (Fig. 11–11) and was originally called Tac (for T activation) antigen. IL-2 binds to the α chain alone with low affinity, and this does not lead to any detectable biologic response. The IL-2Rβ protein is expressed at low levels on resting T cells (and on NK cells) associated with a polypeptide called the common γ (γ_c) chain because it is also a component of receptors for other cytokines, including IL-4, IL-7, and IL-15. IL-2 induces growth of cells expressing this IL-2Rβγ_c complex, with half-maximal growth stimulation occurring at the same concentration of cytokine that produces half-maximal binding (~10^{-9}M). Cells that express IL-2Rα and form IL-2Rαβγ_c complexes can bind IL-2 much more tightly, with a K_d of ~10^{-11}M, and growth stimulation of such cells occurs at a similarly low IL-2 concentration. Upon antigen receptor–mediated T cell activation, IL-2Rα is rapidly expressed, thereby reducing the concentration of IL-2 needed for growth stimulation (see Fig. 11–11). Therefore, antigen-stimulated T cells are more responsive to IL-2 than are naive T cells. Binding of IL-2 to its receptor results in the activation of multiple signal transduction pathways, including the JAK/STAT pathway (mainly JAK1 and JAK3 activating STAT5), which is unique to cytokines, and phosphatidylinositol-3 kinase and Ras–MAP kinase signaling pathways, which are activated by many types of receptors (see Chapter 8). Chronic T cell stimulation leads to shedding of IL-2Rα. Clinically, an increased level of shed IL-2Rα in the serum is a marker of strong antigenic stimulation (e.g., acute rejection of a transplanted organ).

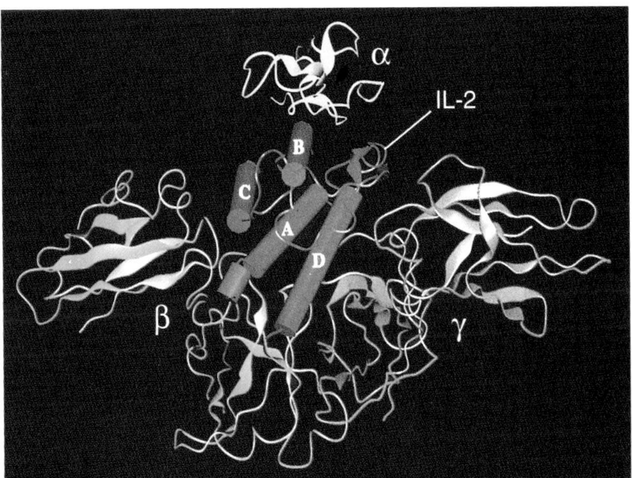

Figure 11–10 Model for the binding of IL-2 to its receptor.

This ribbon diagram is modeled after the known x-ray crystal structure of growth hormone with its receptor and the structural similarity of growth hormone and IL-2. IL-2 is colored red, and the α, β, and γ chains of the receptor are colored yellow, green, and blue, respectively. The four α-helices of the IL-2 molecule are labeled A, B, C, and D. IL-2 interacts with all three chains of the heterotrimeric receptor, and the β and γ chains of the receptor interact with each other. (From Theze J, PM Alzari, and J Bertoglio. Interleukin 2 and its receptors: recent advances and new immunological functions. Immunology Today 17:481–486, 1996. Copyright 1996, with permission from Elsevier Science.)

Biologic Actions

IL-2 was discovered as a T cell growth factor, but it plays several other important roles in adaptive immune responses (Fig. 11–12).

- ***IL-2, produced by T cells on antigen recognition, is responsible for the proliferation of the antigen-specific cells.*** On exposure to IL-2, T cells show a rapid rise in the concentrations of cyclins that associate with and activate different cyclin-dependent kinases. The kinases phosphorylate and activate a variety of cellular proteins, such as Rb, that stimulate transition from the G_1 to the S phase of the cell cycle. In addition, IL-2 induces a fall in the level of a protein called p27 that inhibits the actions of cyclin-kinase complexes. Thus, IL-2 promotes cell cycle progression through cyclin synthesis and relieves a block in cell cycle progression through p27 degradation. IL-2 also promotes survival of cells by inducing the anti-apoptotic protein Bcl-2. The major action of IL-2 is autocrine, but it may stimulate proliferation of some adjacent T cells, functioning as a paracrine growth factor. In addition to stimulating T cell growth, IL-2 increases production of other cytokines, such as IFN-γ and IL-4, by the T cells.
- ***IL-2 promotes the proliferation and differentiation of other immune cells.*** It stimulates the growth of NK cells and enhances their cytolytic function, producing so-called lymphokine-activated killer cells (see Chapter 12). Because NK cells, like resting T cells, express IL-2Rβγ_c (but not IL-2Rα), they can be stimulated only by high levels of IL-2. (As mentioned earlier, in NK cells, the βγ_c complex is associated with the α chain of the IL-15 receptor; for this reason, IL-15 is a potent growth factor for NK cells.) IL-2 acts on B cells both as a growth factor and as a stimulus for antibody synthesis.

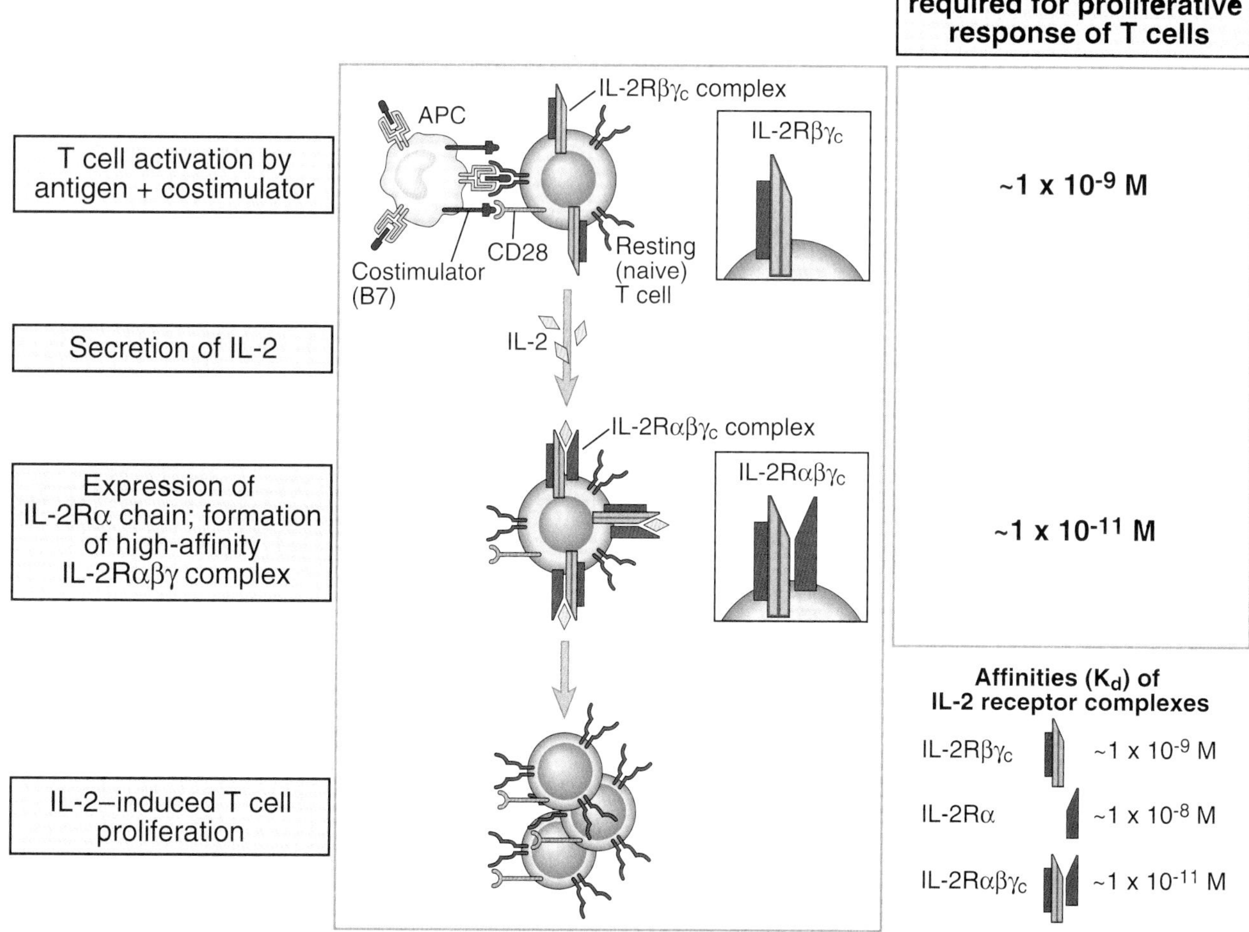

Figure 11–11 Regulation of IL-2 receptor expression.
Resting (naive) T lymphocytes express the IL-2Rβγ complex, which has a moderate affinity for IL-2. Activation of the T cells by antigen, costimulators, and IL-2 itself leads to expression of the IL-2Rα chain and high levels of the high-affinity IL-2Rαβγ complex. APC, antigen-presenting cell.

- ***IL-2 potentiates apoptotic death of antigen-activated T cells.*** Repeated activation of CD4⁺ T cells in the presence of IL-2 makes these cells sensitive to apoptosis by the Fas pathway (see Chapter 10, Box 10–2). It is intriguing that the same cytokine can stimulate T cell survival and proliferation on the one hand and promote cell death on the other. It appears that if an immune response is persistent and T cells are exposed to increasing quantities of IL-2, the pro-apoptotic actions become dominant, contributing to termination of the response. IL-2 may also stimulate the development of regulatory T cells, providing another mechanism for shutting off immune responses (see Chapter 10). Knockout mice lacking IL-2, IL-2Rα, or IL-2Rβ develop autoimmunity, and this may reflect an obligatory role of IL-2 in the elimination or regulation of T cells that are specific for self antigens. Knockout mice lacking γ_c, and humans with γ_c mutations, instead show defects in lymphocyte maturation; the human disease is called **X-linked severe combined immunodeficiency** (see Chapter 20). This maturation block is presumably due to an inability of immature T cells lacking γ_c to respond to the lymphopoietic cytokine IL-7, whose receptor also uses the γ_c chain for signaling.

Interleukin-4 (IL-4)

IL-4 is the major stimulus for the production of IgE antibodies and for the development of T_H2 cells from naive CD4⁺ helper T cells. IL-4 is the signature cytokine of the T_H2 subset and functions as both the inducer and an effector cytokine of these cells.

Structure, Production, Receptors

IL-4 is a member of the four–α-helical cytokine family. The principal cellular sources of IL-4 are CD4⁺ T lymphocytes of the T_H2 subset as well as activated mast cells and basophils.

The IL-4 receptor of lymphoid cells consists of a cytokine-binding α chain that is a member of the type

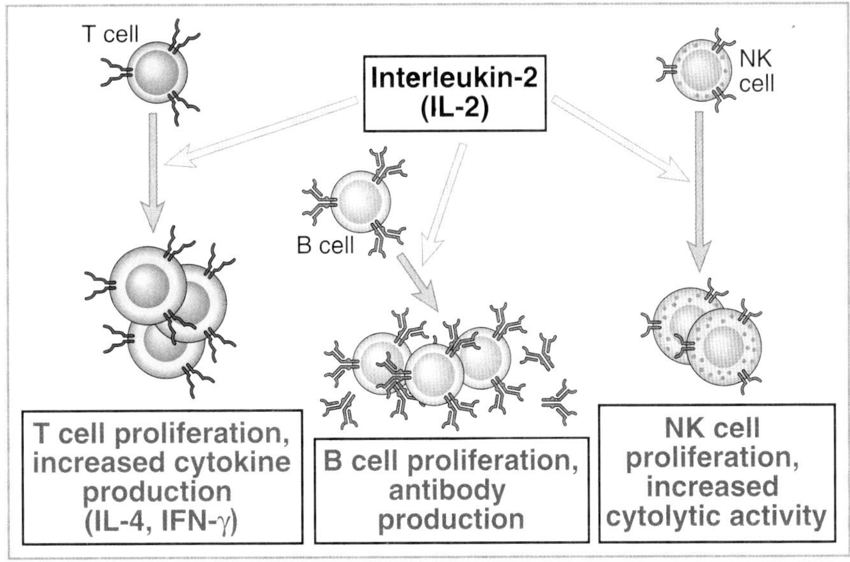

Figure 11–12 Biologic actions of IL-2. IL-2 stimulates the proliferation and differentiation of T and B lymphocytes and NK cells. As discussed in the text, IL-2 also functions to inhibit immune responses (e.g., against self antigens) by promoting Fas-mediated apoptosis of T cells and stimulating the activity of regulatory T cells (not shown here).

I cytokine receptor family, associated with the γ_c chain shared by other cytokine receptors. This IL-4 receptor signals by the JAK/STAT pathway (JAK3 or 4/STAT6) and by a pathway that involves the insulin response substrate (IRS) called IRS-2. IL-4 is the only cytokine that activates the STAT6 protein, which induces transcription of genes that account for many of the actions of IL-4, such as T_H2 differentiation and B cell switching to IgE. Activation of the IRS-2 pathway is responsible for IL-4–induced cellular proliferation. In nonlymphoid cells, the IL-4 receptor α chain is associated not with the γ_c chain but with a signaling chain that is also a component of the receptor for IL-13 (discussed later).

Biologic Actions

The biologic actions of IL-4 include stimulation of IgE and mast cell/eosinophil-mediated reactions and suppression of macrophage-dependent reactions (Fig. 11–13).

- ***IL-4 is the principal cytokine that stimulates B cell Ig heavy chain class switching to the IgE isotype.*** The mechanisms of class switching were described in Chapter 9. Knockout mice lacking IL-4 have less than 10% of normal IgE levels. IgE antibodies play a role in eosinophil-mediated defense against helminthic or arthropod infections, this being the major function of T_H2 cells in host defense. IgE is also the principal mediator of immediate hypersensitivity (allergic) reactions, and production of IL-4 is important for the development of allergies (see Chapter 19). IL-4 also enhances switching to IgG4 (in humans, or the homologous IgG1 in mice) and inhibits switching to the IgG2a and IgG3 isotypes in mice, both of which are stimulated by IFN-γ. This is one of several reciprocal antagonistic actions of IL-4 and IFN-γ.
- ***IL-4 stimulates the development of T_H2 cells from naive $CD4^+$ T cells and functions as an autocrine growth factor for differentiated T_H2 cells.*** Thus,

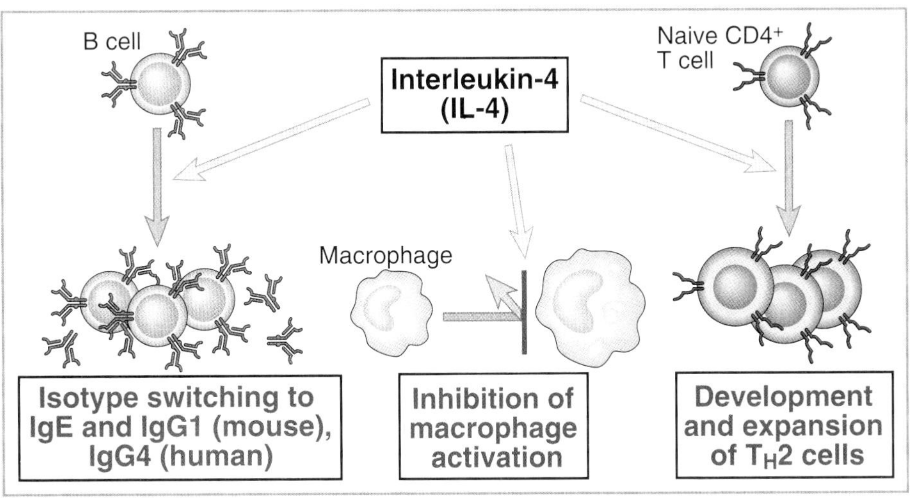

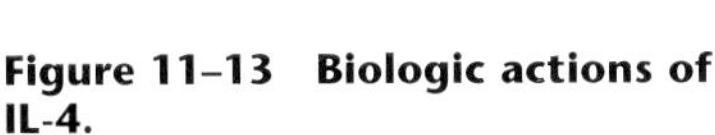
Figure 11–13 Biologic actions of IL-4. IL-4 stimulates B cell isotype switching to some immunoglobulin classes, notably IgE, and differentiation of naive T cells to the T_H2 subset. IL-4 is also an inhibitor of IFN-γ–induced macrophage activation and a growth factor for mast cells, particularly in combination with IL-3.

IL-4 is responsible for the induction and expansion of this subset. Knockout mice lacking IL-4 or STAT6 show a deficiency in the development and maintenance of T_H2 cells, even after stimuli (such as helminthic infections) that are normally potent inducers of this subset. This role of IL-4 is discussed in Chapter 13.

- IL-4 antagonizes the macrophage-activating effects of IFN-γ and thus inhibits cell-mediated immune reactions.

Interleukin-5 (IL-5)

IL-5 is an activator of eosinophils and serves as the link between T cell activation and eosinophilic inflammation.

Structure, Production, Receptors

IL-5 is a homodimer, with each subunit containing a four–α-helical domain. It is produced by the T_H2 subset of $CD4^+$ T cells and by activated mast cells. The IL-5 receptor is a type I cytokine receptor. It is associated with a 150-kD signal-transducing subunit that is shared with receptors for IL-3 and GM-CSF and is sometimes called the common β chain. IL-5 signaling is mediated through a JAK/STAT pathway.

Biologic Actions

The major actions of IL-5 are to activate mature eosinophils and stimulate the growth and differentiation of eosinophils. Activated eosinophils are able to kill helminths. Eosinophils express Fc receptors specific for IgE antibodies and are thereby able to bind to IgE-coated microbes, such as helminths. Thus, the two main T_H2 cytokines, IL-4 and IL-5, function in concert: IL-4 stimulates production of IgE, which opsonizes helminths and binds eosinophils, and IL-5 activates the eosinophils to destroy the parasites. Knockout mice lacking IL-5 are defective in eosinophil responses and are susceptible to some helminthic infections.

IL-5 stimulates the proliferation of B cells and the production of IgA antibodies (see Chapter 9). IL-5 was first identified as a cytokine that stimulated proliferation of mouse B cells, but this action is shared by other cytokines, as shown by the normal B cell expansion in IL-5 knockout mice.

Interferon-γ (IFN-γ)

IFN-γ is the principal macrophage-activating cytokine and serves critical functions in innate immunity and in adaptive cell-mediated immunity. IFN-γ is also called immune, or type II, IFN. It has some antiviral activity, but it is not a potent antiviral interferon, and it functions mainly as an effector cytokine of immune responses.

Structure, Production, Receptors

IFN-γ is a homodimeric protein produced by NK cells, $CD4^+$ T_H1 cells, and $CD8^+$ T cells; it is the signature cytokine of the T_H1 subset of helper T cells. NK cells secrete IFN-γ in response to recognition of unknown components of microbes or in response to IL-12; in this setting, IFN-γ functions as a mediator of innate immunity. In adaptive immunity, T cells produce IFN-γ in response to antigen recognition, and production is enhanced by IL-12 and IL-18. As we have mentioned previously and will discuss in more detail in Chapter 13, the sequence of reactions involving IL-12 and IFN-γ is central to cell-mediated immunity against intracellular microbes.

The receptor for IFN-γ is composed of two structurally homologous polypeptides belonging to the type II cytokine receptor family; one binds the cytokine, and the other participates in signaling. Binding of the cytokine activates STAT1, which then stimulates transcription of IFN-γ–responsive genes (including genes encoding MHC molecules and B7 costimulators), enzymes that synthesize microbicidal substances such as nitric oxide, and cytokines such as the p40 subunit of IL-12. Different IFN-γ–responsive genes are activated by STAT1 alone or by STAT1 acting with two other transcription factors, IFN response factor-1 and class II transactivator, that are themselves induced by STAT1. STAT1 knockout mice are completely insensitive to the actions of IFN-γ.

Biologic Actions

The functions of IFN-γ are important in cell-mediated immunity against intracellular microbes (Fig. 11–14).

- ***IFN-γ is the macrophage-activating cytokine that provides the means by which T lymphocytes and NK cells activate macrophages to kill phagocytosed microbes.*** IFN-γ enhances the microbicidal function of macrophages by stimulating the synthesis of reactive oxygen intermediates and nitric oxide. IFN-γ mediates these effects mainly by activating transcription of the genes that encode the enzymes required for generating reactive oxygen intermediates and reactive nitrogen intermediates. These enzymes are phagocyte oxidase and inducible nitric oxide synthase, respectively. The reactive molecules are produced within lysosomes, and they destroy microbes that are contained within phagolysosomes. We will return to a more detailed discussion of macrophage activation in Chapter 12.
- ***IFN-γ stimulates expression of class I and class II MHC molecules and costimulators on APCs.*** IFN-γ also stimulates the production of many proteins involved in antigen processing, including the transporter associated with antigen processing (TAP), the LMP-2 and LMP-7 components of the proteasome, and HLA-DM. Thus, IFN-γ enhances MHC-associated antigen presentation and amplifies the recognition phase of immune responses by increasing expression of the ligands that T cells recognize (see Chapter 4, Fig. 4–11). IFN-γ is also an activator of vascular endothelial cells, and it potentiates many of the actions of TNF on endothelial cells, promoting T

Figure 11–14 Biologic actions of IFN-γ.

IFN-γ activates phagocytes and APCs and induces B cell switching to some immunoglobulin isotypes (that often bind complement and Fc receptors on phagocytes and are distinct from the isotypes induced by IL-4). The T_H1-inducing effect of IFN-γ may be indirect, mediated by increased IL-12 production and receptor expression.

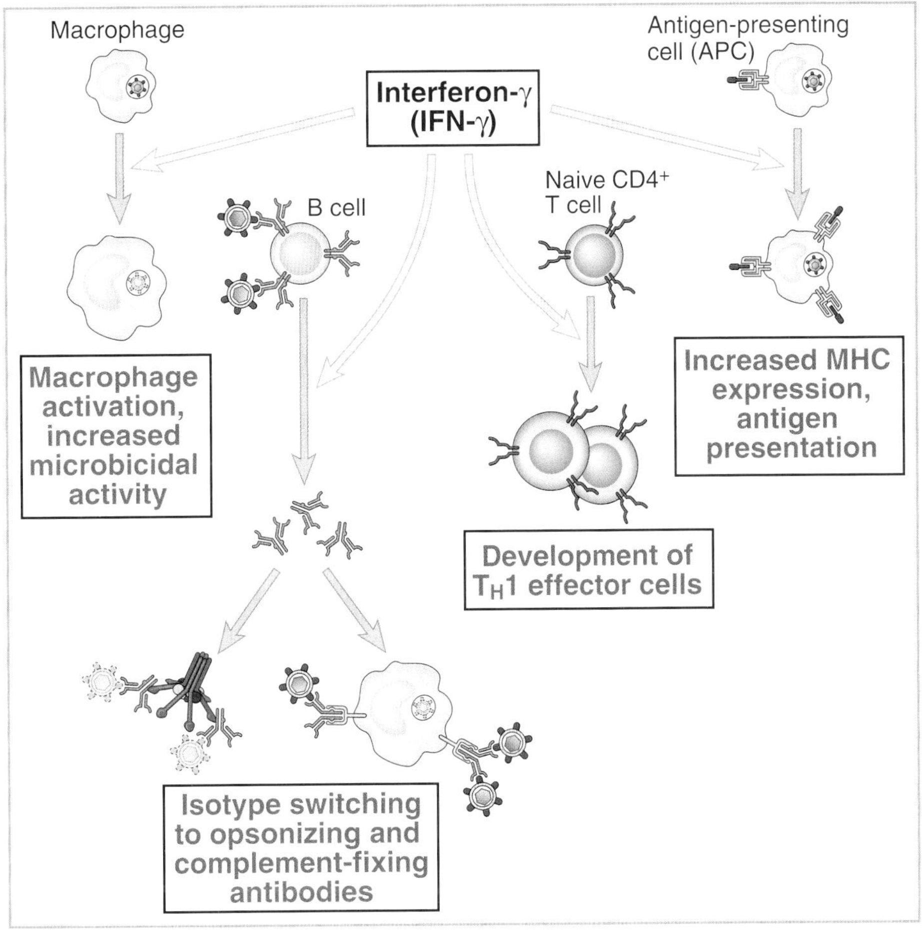

lymphocyte adhesion and extravasation to sites of infection.

- ***IFN-γ promotes the differentiation of naive CD4⁺ T cells to the T_H1 subset and inhibits the proliferation of T_H2 cells.*** Part of the T_H1-inducing effect of INF-γ is mediated indirectly by activating mononuclear phagocytes to produce IL-12, which is the major T_H1-inducing cytokine. In addition, IFN-γ stimulates production of a transcription factor that directly promotes T_H1 differentiation (see Chapter 13). In mice, IFN-γ also enhances expression of the signaling chain of the IL-12 receptor.
- ***IFN-γ acts on B cells to promote switching to certain IgG subclasses, notably IgG2a in mice, and to inhibit switching to IL-4–dependent isotypes, such as IgE and IgG1 in mice.*** The IgG subclasses induced by IFN-γ bind to Fcγ receptors on phagocytes and activate complement, and both these mechanisms promote the phagocytosis of opsonized microbes. Thus, IFN-γ induces antibody responses that also participate in phagocyte-mediated elimination of microbes, in concert with the direct macrophage-activating effects of this cytokine.
- IFN-γ activates neutrophils and stimulates the cytolytic activity of NK cells.

The net effect of these activities of IFN-γ is to promote macrophage-rich inflammatory reactions while inhibiting IgE-dependent eosinophil-rich reactions. Knockout mice lacking IFN-γ or the IFN-γ receptor are susceptible to infections with intracellular microbes, such as mycobacteria, because of defective macrophage activation.

Transforming Growth Factor-β (TGF-β)

The principal action of TGF-β in the immune system is to inhibit the proliferation and activation of lymphocytes and other leukocytes. TGF-β was discovered as a tumor product that promoted the survival of cells in semisolid culture media. It is actually a family of closely related molecules encoded by distinct genes, commonly designated TGF-β1, TGF-β2, and TGF-β3. Cells of the immune system synthesize mainly TGF-β1.

Production, Structure, Receptors

TGF-β1 is a homodimeric protein that is synthesized as a precursor and activated by proteolytic cleavage. It is secreted by antigen-stimulated T cells, LPS-activated mononuclear phagocytes, and many other cell types. Some regulatory T cells produce TGF-β, and the same cells may also produce IL-10, which, like TGF-β, has immunosuppressive activities (see Chapter 10, Fig. 10–11). TGF-β receptors include two high-affinity polypeptide receptors (type I and type II) that signal through a serine/threonine kinase domain that phosphorylates transcription factors called SMADs.

Biologic Actions

TGF-β inhibits the proliferation and differentiation of T cells and the activation of macrophages. TGF-β also acts on other cells, such as neutrophils and endothelial cells, largely to counteract the effects of proinflammatory cytokines. By these actions, TGF-β functions to inhibit immune and inflammatory responses. Mice in which the TGF-β1 gene has been knocked out develop uncontrolled inflammatory lesions and lymphoproliferation.

TGF-β stimulates production of IgA antibodies by inducing B cells to switch to this isotype. IgA is the antibody isotype required for mucosal immunity (see Chapter 14).

TGF-β has many diverse actions outside the immune system. It may inhibit proliferation of some cell types and stimulate others. Often, TGF-β can either inhibit or stimulate growth of the same cell type *in vitro,* depending on culture conditions. TGF-β causes synthesis of extracellular matrix proteins such as collagens, of matrix-modifying enzymes such as matrix metalloproteinases, and of cellular receptors for matrix proteins such as integrins. These actions may promote tissue repair after local immune and inflammatory reactions have been controlled.

Other Cytokines of Adaptive Immunity

Lymphotoxin (LT) is a cytokine produced by T lymphocytes and other cells. It is approximately 30% homologous to macrophage-derived TNF and serves many of the same functions. (For this reason, LT is also called TNF-β.) The secreted form of LT (sometimes called LTα) is a homotrimer, similar to TNF, and it binds to TNF receptors. LT is also expressed as a membrane protein, in which one chain of the secreted form associates with two subunits of a structurally related membrane protein called LTβ. The LTβ membrane form binds to a different receptor also belonging to the TNF receptor family.

LT activates endothelial cells and neutrophils and is thus a mediator of the acute inflammatory response, providing a link between T cell activation and inflammation. These biologic effects of LT are the same as those of TNF, consistent with their binding to the same receptors. However, because the quantity of LT synthesized by antigen-stimulated T cells is much less than the amounts of TNF made by LPS-stimulated mononuclear phagocytes, LT is not readily detected in the circulation. Therefore, LT is usually a locally acting cytokine and not a mediator of systemic injury.

Studies in transgenic and knockout mice have shown that LT is required for the normal development of lymphoid organs (see Chapter 2). Knockout mice lacking membrane LTβ or the receptor for LTβ show various defects in the formation of lymph nodes, Peyer's patches, and splenic white pulp. In these animals, the B cell areas in the lymphoid organs do not develop normally, and no germinal centers are seen in the spleen. LT may function in lymphoid organogenesis by inducing the production of chemokines that promote lymphocyte migration into particular areas of lymphoid organs.

IL-13 is a cytokine structurally similar to IL-4 that is produced by T_H2 $CD4^+$ T cells and by some epithelial cells. The IL-13 receptor is found mainly on nonlymphoid cells, such as macrophages, and can be activated by either IL-13 or IL-4. IL-13 mimics the effects of IL-4 on nonlymphoid cells, such as macrophages, but appears to have less of an effect on T or B lymphocytes than does IL-4. The major action of IL-13 on macrophages is to inhibit their activation and to antagonize IFN-γ. IL-13 stimulates mucus production by lung epithelial cells and may play a role in asthma. Knockout mice lacking IL-13 show decreased IgE production and allergic reactions.

Several other T cell–derived cytokines have been described, but their physiologic functions are unclear. IL-16 is a T cell–derived cytokine that acts as a specific chemoattractant of eosinophils. However, it appears to be derived from a fragment of an intracellular protein, and it is not known whether it is secreted under physiologic conditions. IL-17 consists of a family of cytokines that are produced by activated and memory T cells and induce the production of other proinflammatory cytokines, such as TNF, IL-1, and chemokines. IL-25 is structurally homologous to IL-17 but is secreted by T_H2 cells and stimulates the production of other T_H2 cytokines, including IL-4, IL-5, and IL-13. Thus, IL-17 and IL-25 are believed to play a role in amplifying different T cell–dependent inflammatory reactions, but their essential *in vivo* functions are unknown. Migration inhibition factor (MIF) is a T cell–derived activity that immobilizes mononuclear phagocytes, an effect that might cause the cells to be retained at sites of inflammation. This was the first cytokine activity to be described, but it has proved difficult to biochemically characterize a cytokine with this function.

Roles of T Cell Cytokines in Specialized Adaptive Immune Responses

The cytokines of adaptive immunity are critical for the development of immune responses and for the activation of effector cells that serve to eliminate microbes and other antigens. In Chapter 1, we mentioned a cardinal feature of adaptive immunity, that responses are specialized to eliminate different types of microbes. Much of this specialization is due to the actions of cytokines, which may be produced by subpopulations of helper T cells. Different types of microbes stimulate naive $CD4^+$ T cells to differentiate into effector cells that produce distinct sets of cytokines and perform distinct functions. The best defined of these subsets are the T_H1 and T_H2 cells, which have been mentioned previously. We will describe the properties and functions of these subsets in Chapter 13, when we discuss the effector mechanisms of cell-mediated immunity. Here we summarize some salient features to illustrate the diverse roles of different cytokines. Many intracellular microbes (bacteria and viruses) induce the development of T_H1 cells, which produce IFN-γ, the cytokine that activates phagocytes to destroy intracellular microbes and stimulates the production of opsonizing antibodies that promote more phagocytosis. Helminthic parasites, in contrast, stimulate the development of T_H2 cells, which produce IL-4 and IL-5. IL-4 enhances production of helminth-specific IgE antibodies, which coat the parasites, and IL-5 activates eosinophils, which bind to the IgE-coated parasites and destroy them. Thus, cytokines are essential for the development and effectiveness of adaptive immune responses.

Cytokines That Stimulate Hematopoiesis

Cytokines are necessary for normal hematopoiesis in the bone marrow and provide a means of fine-tuning bone marrow function in response to stimulation. Several of the cytokines generated during both innate and adaptive immune responses stimulate the growth and differentiation of bone marrow progenitor cells. Thus, immune and inflammatory reactions, which consume leukocytes, also elicit production of new leukocytes.

Mature leukocytes arise from pluripotent stem cells by commitment to a particular lineage (differentiation) and progressive expansion of the progeny (Fig. 11–15). The differentiation and expansion of bone marrow progenitor cells are stimulated by cytokines, which are called **colony-stimulating factors** (CSFs) because they

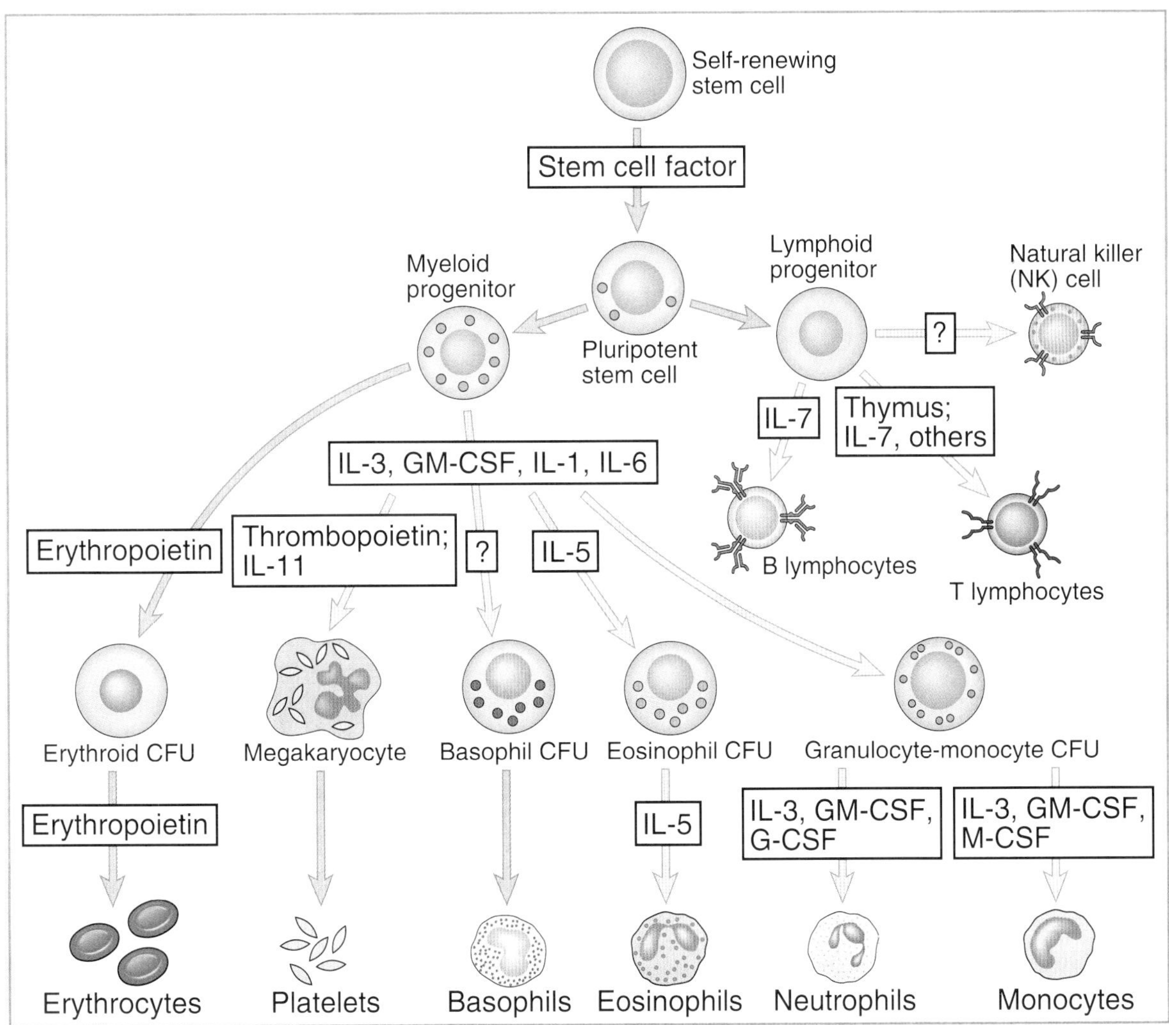

Figure 11–15 Roles of cytokines in hematopoiesis.
Different cytokines stimulate the growth and maturation of different lineages of blood cells. CFU, colony-forming unit; CSF, colony-stimulating factor.

Table 11–5. Hematopoietic Cytokines

Cytokine	Size	Principal cell sources	Principal cell targets	Principal cell populations induced
Stem cell factor (c-Kit ligand)	24 kD	Bone marrow stromal cells	Pluripotent stem cells	All
Interleukin-7 (IL-7)	25 kD	Fibroblasts, bone marrow stromal cells	Immature lymphoid progenitors	B and T lymphocytes
Interleukin-3 (IL-3)	20–26 kD	T cells	Immature progenitors	All
Granulocyte-monocyte CSF (GM-CSF)	18–22 kD	T cells, macrophages, endothelial cells, fibroblasts	Immature and committed progenitors, mature macrophages	Granulocytes and monocytes, macrophage activity
Monocyte CSF (M-CSF)	Dimer of 70–90 kD; 40-kD subunits	Macrophages, endothelial cells, bone marrow cells, fibroblasts	Committed progenitors	Monocytes
Granulocyte CSF (G-CSF)	19 kD	Macrophages, fibroblasts, endothelial cells	Committed progenitors	Granulocytes

Abbreviation: CSF, colony-stimulating factor.

are often assayed by their ability to stimulate the formation of cell colonies in bone marrow cultures. Under the influence of different CSFs, these colonies acquire characteristics of specific cell lineages (e.g., granulocytes, mononuclear phagocytes, or lymphocytes). The names assigned to CSFs reflect the types of colonies that arise in these assays. In this section, we focus on cytokines that are important for the development of lymphocytes (Table 11–5); those that stimulate maturation of other hematopoietic lineages are topics for hematology texts.

Stem Cell Factor (c-Kit Ligand)

Pluripotent stem cells express a tyrosine kinase membrane receptor that is the protein product of the cellular proto-oncogene *c-kit.* The cytokine that interacts with this receptor is called c-Kit ligand, or stem cell factor because it acts on immature stem cells. Therefore, c-Kit is also called the stem cell factor receptor. Stem cell factor is synthesized by stromal cells of the bone marrow as a transmembrane protein or a secreted protein, both produced from the same gene by alternative splicing of the RNA. It is believed that stem cell factor is needed to make bone marrow stem cells responsive to other CSFs but that it does not cause colony formation by itself. It may also play a role in sustaining the viability and proliferative capacity of immature T cells in the thymus and of mast cells in mucosal tissues. The soluble form of stem cell factor is absent in a mutant mouse strain called steel. The steel mouse has defects in mast cell production but not in most other lineages, suggesting that the membrane form of the factor is more important than the soluble form for stimulating stem cells to mature into various hematopoietic lineages. Elimination of both forms of stem cell factor by gene knockout is lethal.

Interleukin-7 (IL-7)

IL-7 is a four–α-helical cytokine secreted by bone marrow stromal cells that stimulates survival and expansion of immature precursors committed to the B and T lymphocyte lineages (see Chapter 7). The IL-7 receptor consists of a unique IL-7–binding α chain associated with the γ_c chain first identified as a component of the IL-2 receptor. Knockout mice lacking IL-7 or the IL-7 receptor α chain or its associated JAK3 kinase are lymphopenic, with decreased number of T and B cells. It is likely that the immunodeficiencies seen in knockout mice lacking γ_c or its associated JAK3 kinase and in humans with mutations in these genes also result mainly from IL-7 signaling defects (see Chapter 20). *In vitro,* IL-7 is also a growth factor for mature T cells, mimicking this action of IL-2.

Interleukin-3 (IL-3)

IL-3, also known as multilineage colony-stimulating factor (multi-CSF), is a product of CD4$^+$ T cells that acts on immature marrow progenitors and promotes the expansion of cells that differentiate into all known mature cell types. IL-3 is a member of the four–α-helical family of cytokines. In humans, the IL-3 receptor consists of a cytokine-binding component that is a member of the type I cytokine receptor family and a signal-transducing subunit that is shared with IL-5 and GM-CSF receptors. In the mouse, the signal-transducing subunit of the IL-3 receptor is unique. Signal transduction in both species involves a JAK/STAT pathway. Most functional analyses of IL-3 have been performed in mice. In addition to its effect on multiple cell lineages, IL-3 promotes the growth and development of mast cells from bone marrow–derived progenitors, an action enhanced by IL-4. However, knockout of either the IL-3 receptor or its signal-transducing subunit in mice does not cause noticeable impairment of hematopoiesis. Human IL-3 has been identified by the complementary DNA cloning of a molecule homologous to mouse IL-3, but it has been difficult to establish a role for this cytokine in hematopoiesis in humans. In fact, many actions attributed to mouse IL-3 appear to be performed by human GM-CSF.

Other Hematopoietic Cytokines

Granulocyte-monocyte colony-stimulating factor (GM-CSF), monocyte colony-stimulating factor (M-CSF), and granulocyte colony-stimulating factor (G-CSF) are cytokines made by activated T cells, macrophages, endothelial cells, and bone marrow stromal cells that act on bone marrow progenitors to increase production of inflammatory leukocytes. GM-CSF promotes the maturation of bone marrow cells into dendritic cells and monocytes. G-CSF is generated at sites of infection and acts as an endocrine hormone to mobilize neutrophils from the marrow to replace those consumed in inflammatory reactions. Recombinant GM-CSF and G-CSF are used to stimulate bone marrow recovery after cancer chemotherapy and bone marrow transplantation. These are some of the most successful clinical applications of cytokines.

IL-9 is a cytokine that supports the growth of some T cell lines and of bone marrow–derived mast cell progenitors. IL-9 uses the γ_c chain signaling subunit and a JAK/STAT pathway. Its physiologic role is unknown.

IL-11 is produced by bone marrow stromal cells. It uses the same gp130 signaling subunit used by IL-6 and signals by a JAK/STAT pathway. It stimulates megakaryocytopoiesis and is in clinical use to treat patients with platelet deficiencies resulting from cancer chemotherapy.

Summary

- Cytokines are a family of proteins that mediate many of the responses of innate and adaptive immunity. The same cytokines may be produced by many cell types, and individual cytokines often act on diverse cell types. Cytokines are synthesized in response to inflammatory or antigenic stimuli and usually act locally, in an autocrine or paracrine fashion, by binding to high-affinity receptors on target cells. Certain cytokines may be produced in sufficient quantity to circulate and exert endocrine actions. For many cell types, cytokines serve as growth factors.
- Cytokines mediate their actions by binding with high affinity to receptors belonging to a limited number of structural families. Different cytokines use specialized signaling pathways, such as the JAK/STAT pathway.
- The cytokines that mediate innate immunity are produced mainly by activated macrophages and include the following: TNF and IL-1 are mediators of acute inflammatory reactions to microbes; chemokines recruit leukocytes to sites of inflammation; IL-12 stimulates production of the macrophage-activating cytokine IFN-γ; type I IFNs are antiviral cytokines; and IL-10 is an inhibitor of macrophages. These cytokines function in innate immune responses to different classes of microbes.
- The cytokines that mediate and regulate adaptive immune responses are produced mainly by antigen-stimulated T lymphocytes, and they include the following: IL-2 is the principal T cell growth factor; IL-4 stimulates IgE production and the development of T_H2 cells from naive helper T cells; IL-5 activates eosinophils; IFN-γ is an activator of macrophages; and TGF-β inhibits the proliferation of T lymphocytes and the activation of leukocytes.
- The colony-stimulating factors (CSFs) consist of cytokines produced by bone marrow stromal cells, T lymphocytes, and other cells that stimulate the growth of bone marrow progenitors, thereby providing a source of additional inflammatory leukocytes. Several of these (e.g., stem cell factor and IL-7) play important roles in lymphopoiesis.
- Cytokines serve many functions that are critical to host defense against pathogens and provide links between innate and adaptive immunity. Cytokines contribute to the specialization of immune responses by activating different types of effector cells. Cytokines also regulate the magnitude and nature of immune responses by influencing the growth and differentiation of lymphocytes. Finally, cytokines provide important amplification mechanisms that enable small numbers of lymphocytes specific for any one antigen to activate a variety of effector mechanisms to eliminate the antigen.
- Excessive production or actions of cytokines can lead to pathologic consequences. The administration of cytokines or their inhibitors is a potential approach for modifying biologic responses associated with immune and inflammatory diseases.

Selected Readings

Alexander WS. Suppressors of cytokine signalling (SOCS) in the immune system. Nature Reviews Immunology 2:410–416, 2002.

Gately MK, LM Renzetti, J Magram, AS Stern, L Adorini, U Gubler, and DH Presky. The interleukin-12/interleukin-12 receptor system: role in normal and pathologic immune responses. Annual Review of Immunology 16:495–521, 1998.

Ihle JN. The Stat family in cytokine signaling. Current Opinion in Cell Biology 13:211–217, 2001.

Imada K, and WJ Leonard. The Jak-Stat pathway. Molecular Immunology 37:1–11, 2000.

Letterio JJ, and AB Roberts. Regulation of immune responses by TGF-beta. Annual Review of Immunology 16:137–161, 1998.

Locksley RM, N Killeen, and MJ Lenardo. The TNF and TNF receptor superfamilies: integrating mammalian biology. Cell 104:487–501, 2001.

Moore KW, R de W Malefyt, RL Coffman, and A O'Garra. Interleukin-10 and the interleukin-10 receptor. Annual Review of Immunology 19:683–765, 2001.

Nelson BH, and DM Willerford. Biology of the interleukin-2 receptor. Advances in Immunology 70:1–81, 1998.

O'Shea JJ, M Gadina, and RD Schreiber. Cytokine signaling in 2002: new surprises in the Jak/Stat pathway. Cell 109:S121–S131, 2002.

Rossi D, and A Zlotnik. The biology of chemokines and their receptors. Annual Review of Immunology 18:217–243, 2000.

Stark GR, IM Kerr, BR Williams, RH Silverman, and RD Schreiber. How cells respond to interferons. Annual Review of Biochemistry 67:227–264, 1998.

Sugamura KH, H Asao, M Kondo, N Tanaka, N Ishii, K Ohno, M Nakamura, and T Takeshita. The interleukin-2 receptor γ chain: its role in the multiple cytokine receptor complexes and T cell development in XSCID. Annual Review of Immunology 14:179–205, 1996.

Trinchieri G, and P Scott. Interleukin-12: basic principles and clinical applications. Current Topics in Microbiology and Immunology 238:57–78, 1999.

Waldmann TA, and Y Tagaya. Multifaceted regulation of interleukin-15 expression and its role in NK cell differentiation and host response to intracellular pathogens. Annual Review of Immunology 17:19–49, 1999.

Yasukawa H, A Sasaki, and A Yoshimura. Negative regulation of cytokine signaling pathways. Annual Review of Immunology 18:143–164, 2000.

Yoshie O, T Imai, and H Nomiyama. Chemokines in immunity. Advances in Immunology 78:57–110, 2001.

Zlotnik A, and O Yoshie. Chemokines: a new classification system and their role in immunity. Immunity 12:121–127, 2001.

Chapter 12

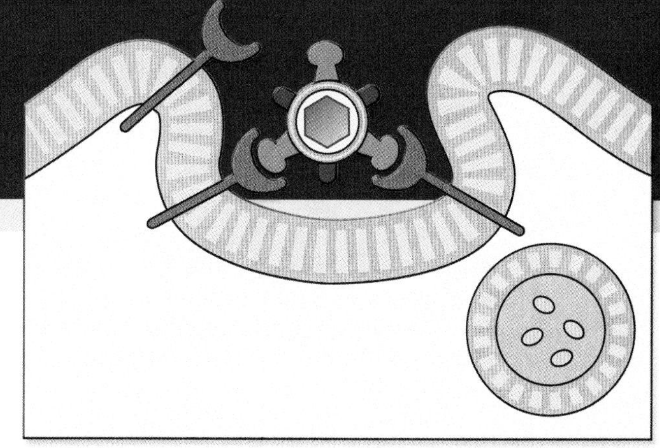

Innate Immunity

Innate immunity is the first line of defense against infections. The mechanisms of innate immunity exist before encounter with microbes and are rapidly activated by microbes before the development of adaptive immune responses (see Chapter 1, Fig. 1–1). Innate immunity is also the phylogenetically oldest mechanism of defense against microbes and is present in all multicellular organisms, including plants and insects. Adaptive immunity mediated by T and B lymphocytes appeared in jawed vertebrates and is superimposed on innate immunity to improve host defense against microbes. In Chapter 1, we introduced the concept that the adaptive immune response enhances the antimicrobial functions of innate immunity and provides both memory of antigen encounter and specialization of effector mechanisms. In this chapter, we describe the components, specificity, and functions of the innate immune system.

Innate immunity serves three important functions.

- ***Innate immunity is the initial response to microbes that prevents infection of the host and, in many instances, can eliminate the microbes.*** The importance of innate immunity in host defense is illustrated by studies showing that inhibiting or eliminating any of several mechanisms of innate immunity markedly increases susceptibility to infections, even when the adaptive immune system is intact and functional. We will review examples of such studies later in this chapter and in Chapter 15 when we discuss immunity to different types of microbes. Many pathogenic microbes have evolved strategies to resist innate immunity, and these strategies are crucial for the virulence of the microbes. Adaptive immune responses, being more potent and specialized, are critical for eliminating microbes that are able to resist the defense mechanisms of innate immunity.
- ***The effector mechanisms of innate immunity are often used to eliminate microbes even in adaptive immune responses.*** For instance, in cell-mediated immunity, antigen-specific T lymphocytes produce cytokines that activate an important effector mechanism of innate immunity, namely, phagocytes (see Chapter 13). In humoral immunity, B lymphocytes

produce antibodies that use two effector mechanisms of innate immunity, phagocytes and the complement system, to eliminate microbes (see Chapter 14).

- ***Innate immunity to microbes stimulates adaptive immune responses and can influence the nature of the adaptive responses to make them optimally effective against different types of microbes.*** Thus, innate immunity not only serves defensive functions early after infection but also provides the "warning" that an infection is present against which a subsequent adaptive immune response has to be mounted. Moreover, different components of the innate immune response often react in distinct ways to different microbes (e.g., intracellular versus extracellular microbes) and thereby influence the type of adaptive immune response that develops (e.g., cell mediated versus humoral, respectively). We will return to this concept at the end of the chapter.

Some components of innate immunity are functioning at all times, even before infection; these components include barriers to microbial entry provided by epithelial surfaces, such as the skin and lining of the gastrointestinal and respiratory tracts. Other components of innate immunity are normally inactive but poised to respond rapidly to the presence of microbes; these components include phagocytes and the complement system. The innate immune response, like the adaptive immune response, can be divided into recognition, activation, and effector phases. We begin our discussion of innate immunity by describing, in general terms, how the innate immune system recognizes microbes and then proceed to the individual components of innate immunity and their functions in host defense.

Features of Innate Immune Recognition

The innate immune response has a unique specificity for the products of microbes that differs from the specificity of the adaptive immune system in several respects (Table 12–1).

The components of innate immunity recognize structures that are characteristic of microbial pathogens and are not present on mammalian cells. The innate immune system is unable to recognize nonmicrobial substances, whereas the adaptive immune system is capable of recognizing a much wider array of foreign substances whether or not they are products of microbes. Different innate immune responses may be specific for structures that are shared by particular classes of microbes (Table 12–2). These structures include nucleic acids that are unique to microbes, such as double-stranded RNA found in replicating viruses or unmethylated CpG DNA sequences found in bacteria; features of proteins that are found in microbes, such as initiation by *N*-formylmethionine, which is typical of bacterial proteins; and complex lipids and carbohydrates that are synthesized by microbes but not by mammalian cells, such as lipopolysaccharides (LPS) in gram-negative bacteria, teichoic acids in gram-positive bacteria, and mannose-rich oligosaccharides found in microbial but not mammalian glycoproteins. The microbial targets of innate immunity have been described as molecular patterns, and the receptors that bind these conserved structures are called pattern recognition receptors. Different classes of microbes (e.g., viruses, gram-negative bacteria, gram-positive bacteria, fungi) express different molecular patterns that are recognized by different pattern recognition receptors on host cells and in the circulation.

Because of this specificity for microbial structures, the innate immune system, like the adaptive immune system, is able to distinguish self from nonself. The mechanisms of innate immunity have evolved to recognize microbes (nonself) and not mammalian (self) molecules. In contrast, in the adaptive immune system, self/nonself discrimination is based not on inherited specificity for microbes but on the selection of lymphocytes for recognition of foreign antigens. In fact, the innate immune response is not known to react against self structures and is thus even better at discriminating between self and nonself than the adaptive immune system is. As we shall see in Chapter 18, adaptive immune responses can occur against autologous antigens and result in autoimmune diseases, but this problem does not appear to happen with innate immunity.

The innate immune system has evolved to recognize microbial products that are often essential for survival of the microbes. This host adaptation is important because it ensures that the targets of innate immunity cannot be discarded by microbes in an effort to evade recognition by the host. In contrast, as we shall see in Chapter 15, microbes may mutate or lose many of the antigens that are recognized by the adaptive immune system, thereby enabling the microbes to evade host defense without compromising their own survival. An example of a target of innate immunity that is essential for microbes is double-stranded viral RNA, which plays a critical role in the replication of certain viruses. Because double-stranded RNA is necessary for the replication of some viruses, these viruses are unable to evade recognition by the innate immune system by failing to express this molecule. Similarly, LPS and teichoic acid are structural components of bacterial cell walls that are required for bacterial survival and cannot be discarded.

The receptors of the innate immune system are encoded in the germline. In contrast, T and B lymphocytes, the principal components of adaptive immunity, use somatic gene recombination to generate their antigen receptors (see Chapter 7). Because many fewer receptors can be encoded in the germline than can be generated through gene rearrangements, the innate immune system has a limited repertoire of specificities. It is estimated that the innate immune system can recognize about 10^3 molecular patterns of microbes. In contrast, the adaptive immune system is capable of recognizing 10^7 or more distinct antigens. Furthermore, whereas the adaptive immune system can distinguish

Table 12–1. Specificity of Innate and Adaptive Immunity

	Innate immunity	Adaptive immunity
Specificity	For structures shared by classes of microbes ("molecular patterns") Different microbes; Identical mannose receptors	For structural detail of microbial molecules (antigens); may recognize nonmicrobial antigens Different microbes; Distinct antibody molecules
Receptors	Encoded in germline; limited diversity LPS receptor; *N*-formyl-methionyl receptor; Mannose receptor; Scavenger receptor	Encoded by genes produced by somatic recombination of gene segments; greater diversity TCR; Ig
Distribution of receptors	Nonclonal: identical receptors on all cells of the same lineage	Clonal: clones of lymphocytes with distinct specificities express different receptors
Discrimination of self and nonself	Yes; host cells are not recognized or they may express molecules that prevent innate immune reactions	Yes; based on selection against self-reactive lymphocytes; may be imperfect (giving rise to autoimmunity)

between antigens of different microbes of the same class and even different antigens of one microbe, innate immunity can distinguish only classes of microbes.

With this general introduction to innate immunity, we proceed to a discussion of the individual components of innate immunity and their functions in host defense.

Components of the Innate Immune System

The innate immune system consists of epithelial barriers and circulating cells and proteins that recognize microbes or substances produced in infections and initiate responses that eliminate the microbes (Table 12–3). The principal effector cells of innate immunity are neutrophils, mononuclear phagocytes, and NK (natural killer) cells. These cells attack microbes that have breached epithelial barriers and entered into tissues or the circulation. Each of these cell types plays a distinct role in the response to microbes. Some of the cells of innate immunity, notably macrophages and NK cells, secrete cytokines that activate phagocytes and stimulate the cellular reaction of innate immunity, called **inflammation.** Inflammation consists of recruitment of leukocytes and extravasation of several plasma proteins into a site of infection and activation of the leukocytes and proteins to eliminate the infectious agent. As we shall see later, inflammation can also injure normal tissues. If microbes enter the circulation, they are combated by various plasma proteins. The major circulating proteins of innate immunity are the proteins of the complement system and other plasma proteins that recognize microbial structures, such as mannose-binding lectin. In the following sections, we describe the properties and functions of each of these components of innate immunity.

Table 12–2. Examples of Molecular Patterns of Microbes and Pattern Recognition Receptors of Innate Immunity

Molecular pattern of microbe	Source	Pattern recognition receptor of innate immunity	Principal innate immune response
dsRNA	Replicating viruses	Toll-like receptor?	Type I interferon production by infected cells
LPS	Gram-negative bacterial cell wall	Toll-like receptor/CD14	Macrophage activation
Unmethylated CpG nucleotides	Bacterial DNA	Toll-like receptor	Macrophage activation
N-formylmethionyl peptides	Bacterial proteins	*N*-formylmethionyl peptide receptors	Neutrophil and macrophage activation
Mannose-rich glycans	Microbial glycoproteins or glycolipids	1. Macrophage mannose receptor 2. Plasma mannose-binding lectin	1. Phagocytosis 2. Opsonization, complement activation
Phosphorylcholine and related molecules	Microbial membranes	Plasma C-reactive protein	Opsonization, complement activation

Abbreviations: dsRNA, double-stranded RNA; LPS, lipopolysaccharide.

Epithelial Barriers

Intact epithelial surfaces form physical barriers between microbes in the external environment and host tissue (Fig. 12–1). The three main interfaces between the environment and the host are the skin and the mucosal surfaces of the gastrointestinal and respiratory tracts. All three are protected by continuous epithelia that prevent the entry of microbes, and loss of integrity of these epithelia commonly predisposes to infection.

Epithelia produce peptides that have a natural antibiotic function. The best known of these peptides are **defensins,** cysteine-rich peptides made up of 29 to 34 amino acids that are present in the skin of many species, including mammals. Defensins are also abundant in neutrophil granules and constitute about 5% of all the cellular proteins of human neutrophils. Defensins are broad-spectrum antibiotics that kill a wide variety of bacteria and fungi. Synthesis of defensins is increased in response to inflammatory cytokines such as interleukin (IL)-1 and tumor necrosis factor (TNF), which are produced by macrophages and other cells in response to microbes. The epithelium of the intestine secretes potent antimicrobial peptides, called cryptocidins, that are capable of locally sterilizing the lumen, for example, within the crypts of the intestine. The mechanisms of action of these natural antibiotics are not fully known. Epithelia also secrete several cytokines that function in innate immunity, and this property may assist in host defense against microbes. For example, keratinocytes in the epidermis produce IL-1 and many other cytokines. How epithelial cells recognize the presence of microbes is not understood.

Barrier epithelia and serosal cavities contain intraepithelial T lymphocytes and the B-1 subset of B cells, respectively, and these cells may recognize and respond to commonly encountered microbes. The unique locations and specificities of these classes of lymphocytes suggest that they serve as sentinels at common sites of microbial invasion. **Intraepithelial T lympho-**

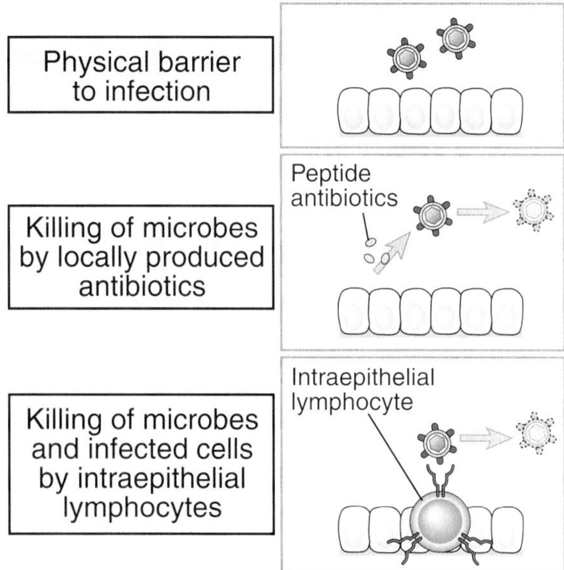

Figure 12–1 Epithelial barriers.
Epithelia at the portals of entry of microbes provide physical barriers, produce antimicrobial substances, and harbor intraepithelial lymphocytes that are believed to kill microbes and infected cells.

Table 12–3. Components of Innate Immunity

Components	Principal functions
Barriers	
Epithelial layers	Prevent microbial entry
Defensins	Microbial killing
Intraepithelial lymphocytes	Microbial killing
Circulating effector cells	
Neutrophils	Early phagocytosis and killing of microbes
Macrophages	Efficient phagocytosis and killing of microbes, secretion of cytokines that stimulate inflammation
NK cells	Lysis of infected cells, activation of macrophages
Circulating effector proteins	
Complement	Killing of microbes, opsonization of microbes, activation of leukocytes
Mannose-binding lectin (collectin)	Opsonization of microbes, activation of complement (lectin pathway)
C-reactive protein (pentraxin)	Opsonization of microbes, activation of complement
Coagulation factors	Walling off infected tissues
Cytokines	
TNF, IL-1, chemokines	Inflammation
IFN-α, -β	Resistance to viral infection
IFN-γ	Macrophage activation
IL-12	IFN-γ production by NK cells and T cells
IL-15	Proliferation of NK cells
IL-10, TGF-β	Control of inflammation

cytes are present in the epidermis of the skin and in mucosal epithelia (see Chapter 2). These cells are T lymphocytes with antigen receptors like other T cells and, by this criterion, they belong to the adaptive immune system. However, intraepithelial T cells typically express a limited diversity of antigen receptors that are formed from germline sequences without great variation in complementarity-determining regions (see Chapter 7). In some species, such as mice and chickens, the majority of intraepithelial lymphocytes express γδ T cell receptors. Some intraepithelial T lymphocytes recognize glycolipid antigens of microbes, which are displayed bound to CD1 molecules expressed on certain epithelia, such as in the intestine. CD1 molecules are β_2-microglobulin–associated, class I major histocompatibility complex (MHC)–like proteins, but they are encoded by genes located outside the MHC and are nonpolymorphic. Some CD1-restricted T cells belong to the NK-T cell subset. Thus, the unusual nature of the receptors and the antigens that they recognize place intraepithelial T lymphocytes into a special category of T cells that is akin more to effector cells of innate immunity than to cells of adaptive immunity. Intraepithelial lymphocytes may function in host defense by secreting cytokines, activating phagocytes, and killing infected cells.

The peritoneal cavity contains a population of B lymphocytes, called **B-1 cells** (see Chapter 7), whose antigen receptors are immunoglobulin molecules that are produced by somatic gene recombination, as in other B lymphocytes, but have limited diversity, much like the antigen receptors of intraepithelial T lymphocytes. Many B-1 cells produce IgM antibodies specific for polysaccharide and lipid antigens, such as phosphorylcholine and LPS that are shared by many types of bacteria. In fact, normal individuals contain circulating antibodies against such bacteria, most of which are present in the intestines, without any evidence of infection. These antibodies are called **natural antibodies** and are largely the product of B-1 cells. Natural antibodies serve as a preformed defense mechanism for microbes that succeed in penetrating epithelial barriers.

A third population of cells present under many epithelia and in serosal cavities are **mast cells.** Mast cells respond to microbes and various mediators by secreting substances that stimulate inflammation. We will return to a discussion of mast cells in Chapter 19.

Phagocytes: Neutrophils and Macrophages

Phagocytes, including neutrophils and macrophages, are cells whose primary function is to identify, ingest, and destroy microbes. Neutrophils, also called polymorphonuclear leukocytes, are the most abundant population of circulating white blood cells and mediate the earliest phases of inflammatory responses. Neutrophils circulate as spherical cells about 12 to 15 μm in diameter with numerous membranous projections. The nucleus of a neutrophil is segmented into three to five connected lobules, hence the term polymorphonuclear leukocytes. The cytoplasm contains granules of two types. The majority, called specific granules, are filled with enzymes such as lysozyme, collagenase, and elastase. These granules do not stain strongly with either basic or acidic dyes (hematoxylin and eosin, respectively), which distinguishes neutrophil granules from those of basophils and eosinophils, respectively. The remainder of the granules of neutrophils, called azurophilic granules, are lysosomes containing enzymes and other microbicidal substances. Neutrophils are produced in the bone marrow and arise from a common lineage with mononuclear phagocytes. Production of neutrophils is stimulated by granulocyte colony-stimulating factor. An adult human produces more than 1×10^{11} neutrophils per day, each of which circulates in the blood for only about 6 hours. Neutrophils may migrate to sites of infection within a few hours after the entry of microbes. If a circulating neutrophil is not recruited into a site of inflammation within this period, it undergoes programmed cell death and is usually phagocytosed by resident macrophages in the liver or spleen.

Macrophages and their circulating precursors, called monocytes, play central roles in innate and adaptive immunity and are important effector cells for the elimination of microbes. Macrophage-like cells are phylogenetically the oldest mediators of innate immunity. *Drosophila* responds to infection by surrounding microbes with "hemocytes," which are similar to macrophages, and these cells phagocytose the microbes and wall off the infection by inducing coagulation of the surrounding hemolymph. Similar phagocyte-like cells have been identified even in plants. The morphologic features of mononuclear phagocytes were described in Chapter 2. Blood monocytes develop in the bone marrow and may remain in the circulation for extended periods. After entering into tissue, monocytes differentiate into tissue macrophages. Macrophages are resident in subepithelial connective tissue, in the interstitia of parenchymal organs, in the lining of the vascular sinusoids in the liver and spleen, and in the lymphatic sinuses of lymph nodes. Thus, these phagocytic cells are strategically placed at all the sites where microbes may gain entry into the host. Macrophages typically respond to microbes nearly as rapidly as neutrophils do but persist much longer at sites of inflammation. Therefore, macrophages are the dominant effector cells of the later stages of the innate immune response, 1 or 2 days after infection. Macrophages are longer lived than neutrophils, and unlike neutrophils, macrophages are not terminally differentiated and can undergo cell division at an inflammatory site.

The functional responses of phagocytes in host defense consist of sequential steps—active recruitment of the cells to the sites of infection, recognition of microbes, phagocytosis, and destruction of ingested microbes. In addition, macrophages produce cytokines that serve many important roles in innate and adaptive immune responses. Next we describe each of the steps in phagocyte-mediated eradication of microbes.

Recruitment of Leukocytes to Sites of Infection

Neutrophils and monocytes are recruited from the blood to sites of infection by binding to adhesion molecules on endothelial cells and by chemoattractants produced in response to the infection. These leukocytes normally circulate in the blood and do not migrate into tissues. Their recruitment to sites of infection is a multistep process involving attachment to endothelial cells and migration through the endothelium (Fig. 12–2). Resident tissue macrophages that recognize microbes secrete the cytokines TNF, IL-1, and chemokines. TNF and IL-1 act on the endothelial cells of postcapillary venules adjacent to the infection and induce the expression of several adhesion molecules. Within 1 to 2 hours, the endothelial cells begin to express E-selectin (see Chapter 6, Box 6–3). Leukocytes express at the tips of their microvilli carbohydrate ligands for the selectins, which bind to the endothelial selectins. These are low-affinity interactions (K_d ~100 μm) with a fast off-rate, and they are easily disrupted by the force of the flowing blood. As a result, the leukocytes detach and bind again and thus begin to roll along the endothelial surface. TNF and IL-1 also induce endothelial expression of ligands for integrins, mainly vascular cell adhesion molecule-1 (VCAM-1, the ligand for the VLA-4 integrin) and intercellular adhesion molecule-1 (ICAM-1, the ligand for the LFA-1 and Mac-1 integrins) (see Chapter 6, Box 6–2). Leukocytes express these integrins in a low-affinity state. Meanwhile, chemokines that were produced at the infection site enter the blood vessel, bind to endothelial cell heparan sulfate glycosaminoglycans, and are displayed at high concentrations. These chemokines act on the rolling leukocytes and activate the leukocytes. One of the consequences of activation is the conversion of VLA-4 and LFA-1 integrins on the leukocytes to a high-affinity state (see Chapter 6, Fig. 6–11). The combination of induced expression of integrin ligands on the endothelium and activation of integrins on the leukocytes results in firm integrin-mediated binding of the leukocytes to the endothelium at the site of infection. The leukocytes stop rolling, their cytoskeleton is reorganized, and they spread out on the endothelial surface. Chemokines then act on the adherent leukocytes and stimulate the cells to migrate through interendothelial spaces toward the chemical concentration gradient (i.e., toward the infection site). The net result of this process is that leukocytes, first neutrophils

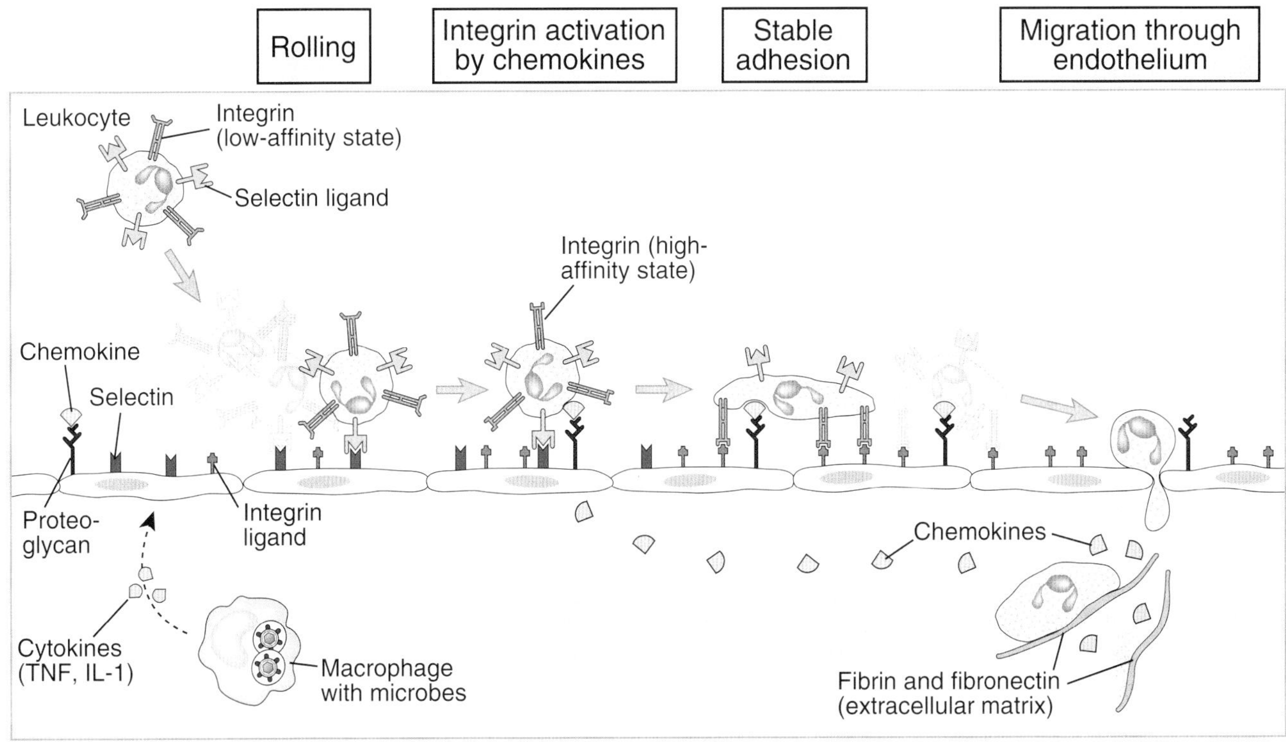

Figure 12–2 Recruitment of leukocytes.
At sites of infection, macrophages that have encountered microbes produce cytokines (such as TNF and IL-1) that activate the endothelial cells of nearby venules to produce selectins, ligands for integrins, and chemokines. Selectins mediate weak tethering and rolling of blood leukocytes, such as neutrophils, on the endothelium; integrins mediate firm adhesion of neutrophils; and chemokines increase the affinity of neutrophil integrins and stimulate the migration of the cells through the endothelium to the site of infection. Blood neutrophils, monocytes, and activated T lymphocytes use essentially the same mechanisms to migrate to sites of infection.

and then monocytes, rapidly accumulate around the infectious microbes. This reaction is the central component of inflammation. It is typically elicited by microbes, but it may be seen in response to a variety of noninfectious stimuli as well.

In the tissues, the neutrophils and monocytes (now called macrophages) recognize microbes and function to eradicate the infection.

Recognition of Microbes by Neutrophils and Macrophages

Neutrophils and macrophages express surface receptors that recognize microbes in the blood and tissues and stimulate the phagocytosis and killing of the microbes. The microbicidal mechanisms of phagocytes are largely confined to intracellular vesicles (lysosomes and phagolysosomes) to protect the cells themselves from injury. Therefore, ingestion of microbes into these vesicles is a necessary prelude to microbial killing, and the first step in ingestion is recognition of the microbes by various cell surface receptors. Neutrophils and macrophages also express some receptors that activate the cells to produce cytokines and microbicidal substances and receptors that stimulate the migration of the cells to sites of infection.

There are several classes of phagocyte receptors that bind microbes and mediate their internalization (Fig. 12–3).

- **Mannose receptors and scavenger receptors** function to bind and ingest microbes. The mannose receptor is a macrophage lectin that binds terminal mannose and fucose residues of glycoproteins and glycolipids. These sugars are typically part of molecules found on microbial cell walls, whereas mammalian glycoproteins and glycolipids contain terminal sialic acid or *N*-acetylgalactosamine. Therefore, the macrophage mannose receptor recognizes microbes and not host cells. Scavenger receptors were originally defined as molecules that bind and mediate endocytosis of oxidized or acetylated low-density lipoprotein (LDL) particles that can no longer interact with the conventional LDL receptor. Macrophage scavenger receptors bind a variety of microbes as well as modified LDL particles. Macrophage integrins, notably Mac-1 (CD11bCD18), may also bind microbes for phagocytosis.
- **Receptors for opsonins** promote phagocytosis of microbes coated with various proteins. The process of coating a microbe to target it for phagocytosis is called **opsonization,** and substances that

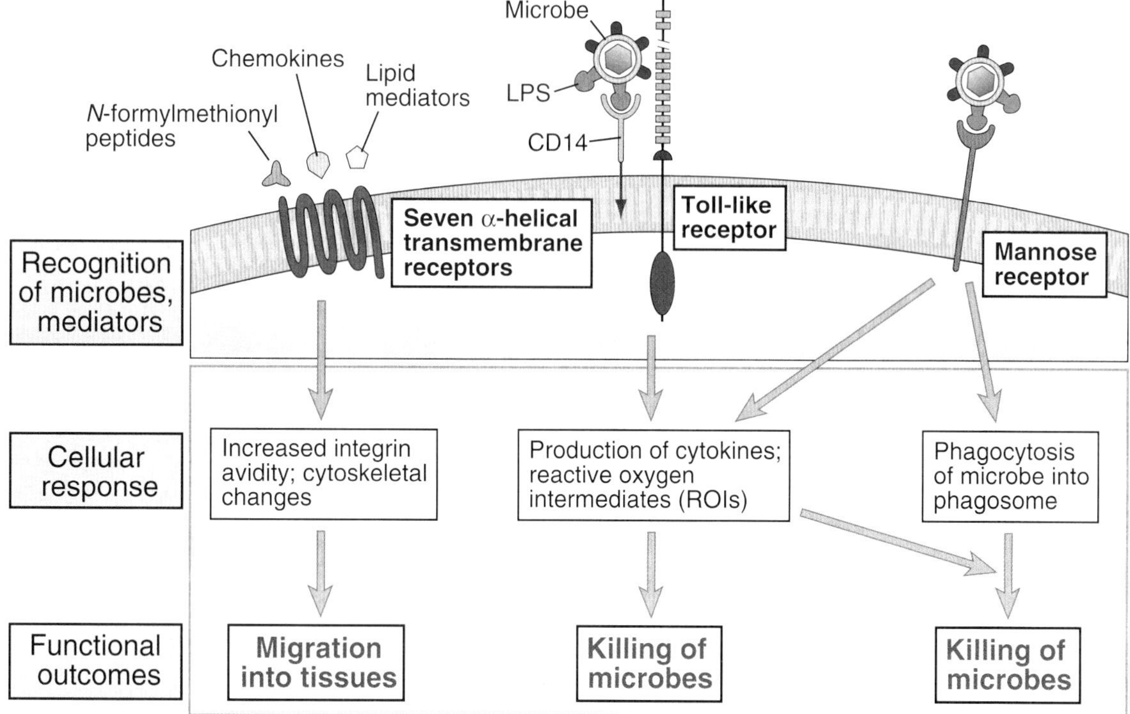

Figure 12–3 Receptors and responses of phagocytes. Neutrophils and macrophages use diverse membrane receptors to recognize microbes, microbial products, and substances produced by the host in infections. These receptors activate cellular responses that function to stimulate inflammation and eradicate microbes. Note that only selected examples of receptors of different classes are shown. LPS, lipopolysaccharide.

coat the microbes are **opsonins.** These substances include antibodies, complement proteins, and lectins. One of the most efficient systems for opsonizing particles is coating the particles with IgG antibodies, which are termed specific opsonins and are recognized by the high-affinity Fcγ receptor of phagocytes, called FcγRI (see Chapter 14). Components of the complement system, especially fragments of the complement protein C3, are also potent opsonins because phagocytes express a receptor, called the type 1 complement receptor (CR1), that recognizes a breakdown product of C3 (see Chapter 14). These complement fragments are produced when complement is activated by either the classical (antibody-dependent) or the alternative (antibody-independent) pathway. Many bacteria can activate the alternative pathway and produce complement proteins that efficiently opsonize the bacteria in the absence of antibody molecules. A number of plasma proteins, including mannose-binding lectin, fibronectin, fibrinogen, and C-reactive protein, can coat microbes and are recognized by receptors on phagocytes. For example, a macrophage cell surface receptor called the C1q receptor binds microbes opsonized with plasma mannose-binding lectin, and integrins bind fibrinogen-coated particles. Both Fc receptors and C3b receptors also deliver signals that activate the phagocytes.

Other phagocyte receptors function to activate the phagocytes but do not participate directly in ingestion of microbes (see Fig. 12–3).

- **Toll-like receptors (TLRs)** are homologous to a *Drosophila* protein called Toll and function to activate phagocytes in response to different types and components of microbes. To date, 10 mammalian TLRs have been identified, and each appears to be required for responses to a different class of infectious pathogen (Box 12–1). Different TLRs play essential roles in cellular responses to LPS, other bacterial proteoglycans, and unmethylated CpG nucleotides, all of which are found only in bacteria. These receptors function by receptor-associated kinases to stimulate the production of microbicidal substances and cytokines in the phagocytes (see Box 12–1). TLRs may associate with other molecules that participate in the direct recognition of microbial products. The host response to LPS illustrates many of the functional consequences of recognition of a microbial product by a TLR and associated proteins (Box 12–2).
- **Different seven-transmembrane α-helical receptors, also called G protein–coupled receptors,** are expressed on leukocytes, recognize microbes and some mediators that are produced in response to infections, and function mainly to stimulate migra-

tion of the leukocytes to sites of infection. These receptors are found on neutrophils, macrophages, and most other types of leukocytes, and they are specific for diverse ligands. Receptors of this class recognize short peptides containing *N*-formylmethionyl residues. Because all bacterial proteins and few mammalian proteins (only those synthesized within mitochondria) are initiated by *N*-formylmethionine, this receptor allows neutrophils to detect and respond to bacterial proteins. Neutrophils and, at lower levels, macrophages also express seven-transmembrane α-helical receptors for certain CXC chemokines, especially IL-8 (see Chapter 11); for proteolytic products of complement proteins, such as C5a (see Chapter 14); and for a variety of lipid mediators of inflammation, including platelet-activating factor, prostaglandin E, and leukotriene B_4. Binding of ligands, such as microbial products and chemokines, to the

BOX 12–1

Toll-like Receptors

The Toll-like receptors (TLRs) are a family of membrane proteins that serve as pattern recognition receptors for a variety of microbe-derived molecules and stimulate innate immune responses to the microbes expressing these molecules. The first protein to be identified in this family was the *Drosophila* Toll protein, which is involved in establishing the dorsal-ventral axis during embryogenesis of the fly as well as mediating antimicrobial responses. Ten different mammalian TLRs have so far been identified on the basis of sequence homology to *Drosophila* Toll, and they are named TLR 1 to 10, but more members of the family may exist. All these receptors contain leucine-rich repeats flanked by characteristic cysteine-rich motifs in their extracellular regions and a Toll/IL-1 receptor (TIR) homology domain in their cytoplasmic region, which is essential for signaling. TIR domains are also found in the cytoplasmic tails of the IL-1 and IL-18 receptors, and similar signaling pathways are engaged by TLRs, IL-1, and IL-18. The TLRs are expressed on many different cell types that are important components of the innate immune system, including macrophages, dendritic cells, neutrophils, mucosal epithelial cells, and endothelial cells.

Mammalian TLRs are involved in responses to widely divergent types of molecules that are commonly expressed by microbial but not mammalian cells (see Figure). The innate immune response to one species of microbe may reflect an integration of the responses of several TLRs to different molecules produced by the microbe. Some of the microbial products that stimulate TLRs include gram-negative bacterial lipopolysaccharide (LPS), gram-positive bacterial peptidoglycan, bacterial lipoproteins, lipoteichoic acid, lipoarabinomannan, zymosan, the bacterial flagellar protein flagellin, heat shock protein 60, respiratory syncytial virus fusion protein, unmethylated CpG motifs, and double-stranded RNA. In many cases, a single TLR is responsible for stimulating inflammatory responses to a particular microbial ligand, such as TLR9-mediated responses to CpG. However, the repertoire of specificities of the TLR system is apparently extended by the ability of TLRs to heterodimerize with one another. For example, dimers of TLR2 and TLR6 are required for responses to peptidoglycan. In some cases, one of the TLRs of a heterodimer may confer ligand-binding specificity, and the other TLR may be required for signaling. Specificities of the TLRs are also influenced by various non-TLR adapter molecules. This is most thoroughly understood for TLR4 and its ligand LPS. LPS first binds to soluble LPS-binding protein (LBP) in the blood or extracellular fluid, and this complex serves to facilitate LPS binding to CD14, which exists as both a soluble plasma protein and a glycophosphatidylinositol-linked membrane protein on most cells except endothelium. Once LPS binds to CD14, LBP dissociates, and the LPS-CD14 complex physically associates with TLR4. An additional extracellular accessory protein called MD2 also binds to the complex with CD14. LPS, CD14, and MD2 are all required for efficient LPS-induced signaling, but it is not yet clear if direct physical interaction of LPS with TLR4 is necessary. Different combinations of accessory molecules in TLR complexes may serve to broaden the range of microbial products that can induce innate immune responses. For example, both CD14 and MD2 are associated with complexes of other TLRs (e.g., TLR2), and TLR4 may form complexes with other accessory molecules, such as MD1 and RP105, in certain cell types, such as B lymphocytes.

The predominant signaling pathway used by TLRs results in the activation of NF-κB (see Figure). In this pathway, ligand binding to the TLR at the cell surface leads to recruitment of several cytoplasmic signaling molecules through specific domain-domain interactions. The first protein to be recruited is the cytoplasmic adapter protein MyD88, which contains a TIR domain that probably binds to the TIR domain of the TLR. MyD88 also contains a death domain, homologous to those found in TNF receptor family signaling molecules (see Chapter 11, Box 11–1). A second protein to be recruited into the signaling complex is called IL-1 receptor–associated kinase (IRAK). IRAK contains a death domain that mediates interactions with the death domain of MyD88 and a serine/threonine protein kinase domain. On recruitment, IRAK undergoes autophosphorylation, dissociates from MyD88, and activates TNF-R–associated factor-6 (TRAF-6). TRAF-6 then activates the IκB kinase cascade, leading to NF-κB activation. This same pathway is involved in IL-1– and IL-18–induced activation of NF-κB. In some cell types, certain TLRs also engage other signaling pathways, such as the MAP kinase cascade, leading to activation of the AP-1 transcription factor. The relative importance of these additional pathways of TLR signaling and the way the "choice" of pathways is made are not well understood.

The genes that are expressed in response to TLR signaling encode proteins important in many different components of innate immune responses. These include inflammatory cytokines (TNF-α, IL-1, and IL-12), endothelial adhesion molecules (E-selectin), and proteins involved in microbial killing mechanisms (inducible nitric oxide synthase). The particular genes expressed will depend on the responding cell type.

Continued on following page

BOX 12–1

Toll-like Receptors (*Continued*)

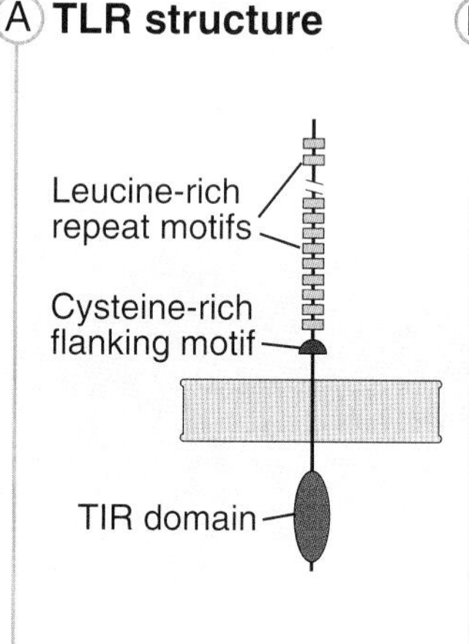

B Specificities of TLRs

TLR	Ligand	Microbial source
TLR2	Lipoproteins Peptidoglycan Zymosan LPS GPI anchor Lipoarabinomannan Phosphatidylinositol dimannoside	Bacteria Gram-positive bacteria Fungi Leptospira Trypanosomes Mycobacteria Mycobacteria
TLR3	? Double-stranded RNA	Viruses
TLR4	LPS HSP60	Gram-negative bacteria Chlamydia
TLR5	Flagellin	Various bacteria
TLR9	CpG DNA	Bacteria, protozoans

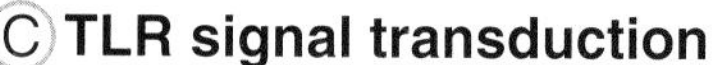

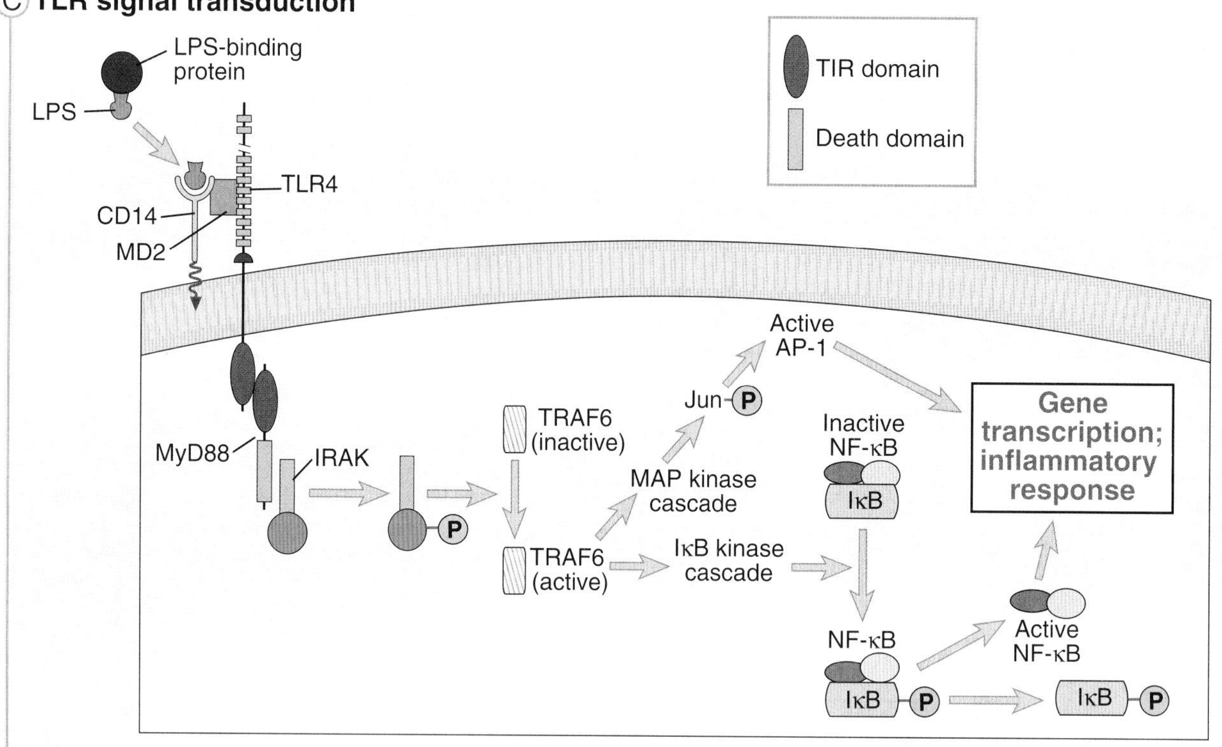

Mammalian Toll-like receptors (TLRs).

A. A typical TLR contains conserved extracellular and cytoplasmic domains. Different TLRs contain different numbers and arrangements of the extracellular leucine-rich and cysteine-rich motifs. TIR, Toll/IL-1 receptor.

B. Different TLRs are involved in responses to different microbial products. Some of the specificities listed may require heterodimerization with other TLRs (e.g., TLR2 with TLR6).

C. The signaling pathway triggered by TLRs that results in the generation of the NF-κB transcription factor is shown. Intracellular adapter proteins other than MyD88 may also be involved in some TLR signaling pathways. In addition to NF-κB activation, TLRs are also linked to AP-1 activation.

seven-transmembrane α-helical receptors induces migration of the cells from the blood through the endothelium and production of microbicidal substances by activation of the respiratory burst. The receptors initiate intracellular responses through associated trimeric guanosine triphosphate (GTP)–binding (G) proteins. In a resting cell, the receptor-associated G proteins form a stable inactive complex containing guanosine diphosphate (GDP) bound to Gα subunits. Occupancy of the receptor by ligand results in an exchange of GTP for GDP. The GTP-bound form of the G protein activates numerous cellular enzymes, including an isoform of phosphatidylinositol-specific phospholipase C that functions to increase intracellular calcium and activate protein kinase C. The G proteins also stimulate cytoskeletal changes, resulting in increased cell motility.

- Phagocytes express receptors for cytokines that are produced in reactions to microbes. One of the most important of these cytokines is interferon-γ (IFN-γ), which is secreted by NK cells during innate immune responses and by antigen-activated T lymphocytes during adaptive immune responses. IFN-γ is the major macrophage-activating cytokine.

Phagocytosis of Microbes

Neutrophils and macrophages ingest bound microbes into vesicles, where the microbes are destroyed (Fig. 12–4). Phagocytosis is a cytoskeleton-dependent process of engulfment of large particles (>0.5 μm in diameter). A phagocyte uses various surface receptors to bind a microbe and extends a cup-shaped membrane projection around the microbe. When the protruding membrane cup extends beyond the diameter of the particle, the top of the cup closes over, or "zips up," and pinches off the interior of the cup to form an "inside-out" intracellular vesicle. This vesicle, called a phagosome, contains the ingested foreign particle and breaks away from the plasma membrane. Cell surface receptors of phagocytes (discussed earlier) attach the particle to the phagocyte membrane and deliver activating signals that are involved in ingesting the particle and turning on the microbicidal activities of phagocytes. Phagocytosed microbes are destroyed, as described next; at the same time, peptides are generated from microbial proteins and presented to T lymphocytes to initiate adaptive immune responses (see Chapter 5).

Killing of Phagocytosed Microbes

Activated neutrophils and macrophages kill phagocytosed microbes by producing microbicidal molecules in phagolysosomes (see Fig. 12–4). Several receptors that recognize microbes, including TLRs, G protein–coupled receptors, Fc and C3 receptors, and receptors for cytokines, mainly IFN-γ, function cooperatively to activate phagocytes to kill ingested microbes. Fusion of phagocytic vacuoles (phagosomes) with lysosomes results in the formation of phagolysosomes, where the microbicidal mechanisms are concentrated. Activated macrophages and neutrophils convert molecular oxygen into **reactive oxygen intermediates** (ROIs), which are highly reactive oxidizing agents that destroy microbes (and other cells). The primary free radical–generating system is the phagocyte oxidase system. Phagocyte oxidase is a multisubunit enzyme that is assembled in activated phagocytes mainly in the phagolysosomal membrane. Phagocyte oxidase is

BOX 12–2

Physiologic and Pathologic Responses to Bacterial Lipopolysaccharide

Bacterial lipopolysaccharide (LPS or endotoxin) is a product of gram-negative bacteria, and a potent stimulator of innate immune responses that enhance killing of the bacteria, but it may also cause significant pathologic changes in the host. LPS is a mixture of fragments of the outer cell walls of gram-negative bacteria and contains both lipid components and polysaccharide moieties. The polysaccharide groups can be highly variable and are the major antigens of gram-negative bacteria recognized by the adaptive immune system. The lipid moiety, by contrast, is highly conserved and is an example of a molecular pattern recognized by the innate immune system.

LPS induces local and systemic inflammation, and many of the features of tissue injury observed in infection by gram-negative bacteria can be mimicked by administration of LPS. LPS is a potent activator of macrophages, and the cellular response involves the LBP/CD14/mammalian Toll-like receptor 4 system, as described in Box 12–1. Macrophages, which synthesize and express CD14, can respond to minute quantities of LPS, as little as 10 pg/mL, and cells that lack CD14 are generally unresponsive to LPS. However, some CD14 is shed and circulates as a plasma protein. Addition of soluble CD14 to cells that are normally unresponsive to LPS, such as vascular endothelial cells, allows such cells to respond to LPS, but usually at 100- to 1000-fold higher concentrations than $CD14^+$ macrophages. The genes in macrophages that are induced by LPS encode cytokines and enzymes of the respiratory burst. The functions of these proteins in innate immunity are described in the text.

The systemic changes observed in patients who have disseminated bacterial infections, sometimes called the systemic inflammatory response syndrome (SIRS), are reactions to cytokines whose production is stimulated by LPS. In mildly affected patients, the response consists of neutrophilia, fever, and a rise in acute-phase reactants in the plasma. Neutrophilia is a response of the bone marrow to circulating cytokines, especially G-CSF, resulting in

Continued on following page

BOX 12–2

Physiologic and Pathologic Responses to Bacterial Lipopolysaccharide (*Continued*)

increased production and release of neutrophils to replace those consumed during inflammation. An elevated circulating neutrophil count, especially one accompanied by the presence of immature neutrophils prematurely released from the bone marrow, is a clinical sign of infection. Fever is produced in response to substances called pyrogens that act to elevate prostaglandin synthesis in the vascular and perivascular cells of the hypothalamus. Bacterial products such as LPS (called exogenous pyrogens) stimulate leukocytes to release cytokines such as IL-1 and TNF (called endogenous pyrogens) that increase the enzymes, especially cyclooxygenase-2, that convert arachidonic acid into prostaglandins. Nonsteroidal anti-inflammatory drugs, including aspirin, reduce fever by inhibiting cyclooxygenase-2 and thus blocking prostaglandin synthesis. An elevated body temperature has been shown to help amphibians ward off microbial infections, and it is assumed that fever does the same for mammals, although the mechanism is unknown. One hypothesis is that fever may induce heat shock proteins that are recognized by some intraepithelial lymphocytes, promoting inflammation. Acute-phase reactants are plasma proteins, mostly synthesized in the liver, whose plasma concentrations increase as part of the response to LPS. Three of the best known examples of these proteins are C-reactive protein, fibrinogen, and serum amyloid A protein. Synthesis of these molecules by liver hepatocytes is up-regulated by cytokines, especially IL-6 (for C-reactive protein and fibrinogen) and IL-1 or TNF (for serum amyloid A protein). During the SIRS, serum amyloid A protein replaces apolipoprotein A, a component of high-density lipoprotein particles. This may alter the targeting of high-density lipoproteins from liver cells to macrophages, which can use these particles as a source of energy-producing lipids. The rise in fibrinogen causes erythrocytes to form stacks (rouleaux) that sediment more rapidly at unit gravity than do individual erythrocytes. This is the basis for measuring erythrocyte sedimentation rate as a simple test for the systemic inflammatory response due to any number of stimuli including LPS.

When a severe bacterial infection leads to the presence of organisms and LPS in the blood, a condition called sepsis, circulating cytokine levels increase and the form of the host response changes. High levels of cytokines produced in response to LPS can result in disseminated intravascular coagulation (DIC), caused by mechanisms described below. Multiple organs show inflammation and intravascular thrombosis, which can produce organ failure. Tissue injury in response to LPS can also result from the activation of neutrophils before they exit the vasculature, thus causing damage to endothelial cells and reduced blood flow. The lungs and liver are particularly susceptible to injury by neutrophils. Lung damage in the SIRS is commonly called the adult respiratory distress syndrome (ARDS) and results when neutrophil-mediated endothelial injury allows fluid to escape from the blood into the airspace. Liver injury and impaired liver function result in a failure to maintain normal blood glucose levels due to a lack of gluconeogenesis from stored glycogen. The kidney and the bowel are also injured, largely as a result of reduced perfusion. Overproduction of nitric oxide by cytokine-activated cardiac myocytes and vascular smooth muscle cells leads to heart failure and loss of perfusion pressure, respectively, resulting in hemodynamic shock. The clinical triad of DIC, hypoglycemia, and cardiovascular failure is described as **septic shock.** This condition is often fatal.

TNF produced by LPS-activated macrophages is a major mediator of LPS-induced injury. This is known because many of the effects of LPS can be mimicked by TNF and because anti-TNF antibodies or soluble TNF receptors can attenuate or completely block responses to LPS. IL-12 and IFN-γ also contribute to LPS-induced injury because IL-12 stimulates IFN-γ production by NK cells and T cells, and IFN-γ increases TNF secretion by LPS-activated macrophages and synergizes with TNF in effects on endothelium. Because septic shock is the result of cytokine overproduction, many clinical trials have been introduced to neutralize cytokines, such as TNF and IL-1, with antibodies, soluble receptors, or natural antagonists. The results of these trials have been disappointing, probably because of cytokine redundancy (i.e., the fact that many cytokines contribute to the systemic response in fulminant sepsis). It remains to be seen whether "cocktails" of multiple cytokine antagonists will be more effective.

The mechanisms by which LPS induces tissue injury were extensively studied in the rabbit initially by Robert Shwartzman, who had observed that when a rabbit is given a low-dose (subinjurious) intravenous injection of LPS, it will succumb to a second low-dose injection of LPS administered intravenously 24 hours later. The dead animal shows evidence of multiorgan injury and widespread intravascular thrombus formation, a condition that mimics clinical DIC. Thrombosis results from a simultaneous initiation of coagulation by LPS-induced tissue factor (TF) expression and from a down-regulation of natural anticoagulation mechanisms, including a decrease in expression of tissue factor pathway inhibitor (TFPI) and endothelial cell thrombomodulin. A localized form of LPS-mediated tissue injury may be induced by injecting a small dose of LPS into a skin site on a rabbit, followed 24 hours later by a second low dose of LPS administered intravenously. This causes hemorrhagic necrosis of the skin at the site of the first injection. On histologic examination, the tissue shows intravascular thrombosis as well as neutrophil influx, endothelial damage, and hemorrhage. In the local Shwartzman model of skin injury in the mouse, TNF can replace the second dose of LPS, and TNF antagonists prevent tissue injury, further supporting the central role of this cytokine in responses to LPS. Interestingly, the first description of TNF (and the origin of its name) was as an LPS-induced serum factor that mediated hemorrhagic necrosis of experimental tumor implants. TNF-mediated necrosis of tumors histopathologically resembles the local Shwartzman reaction. The current interpretation of these data is that tumors release a factor or factors that act on local endothelium to produce the same changes as the first injection of LPS does in the localized Shwartzman reaction. Intravenous administration of TNF then replaces the second intravenous injection of LPS, invoking a Shwartzman reaction with vascular thrombosis in the tumor and subsequent tumor necrosis.

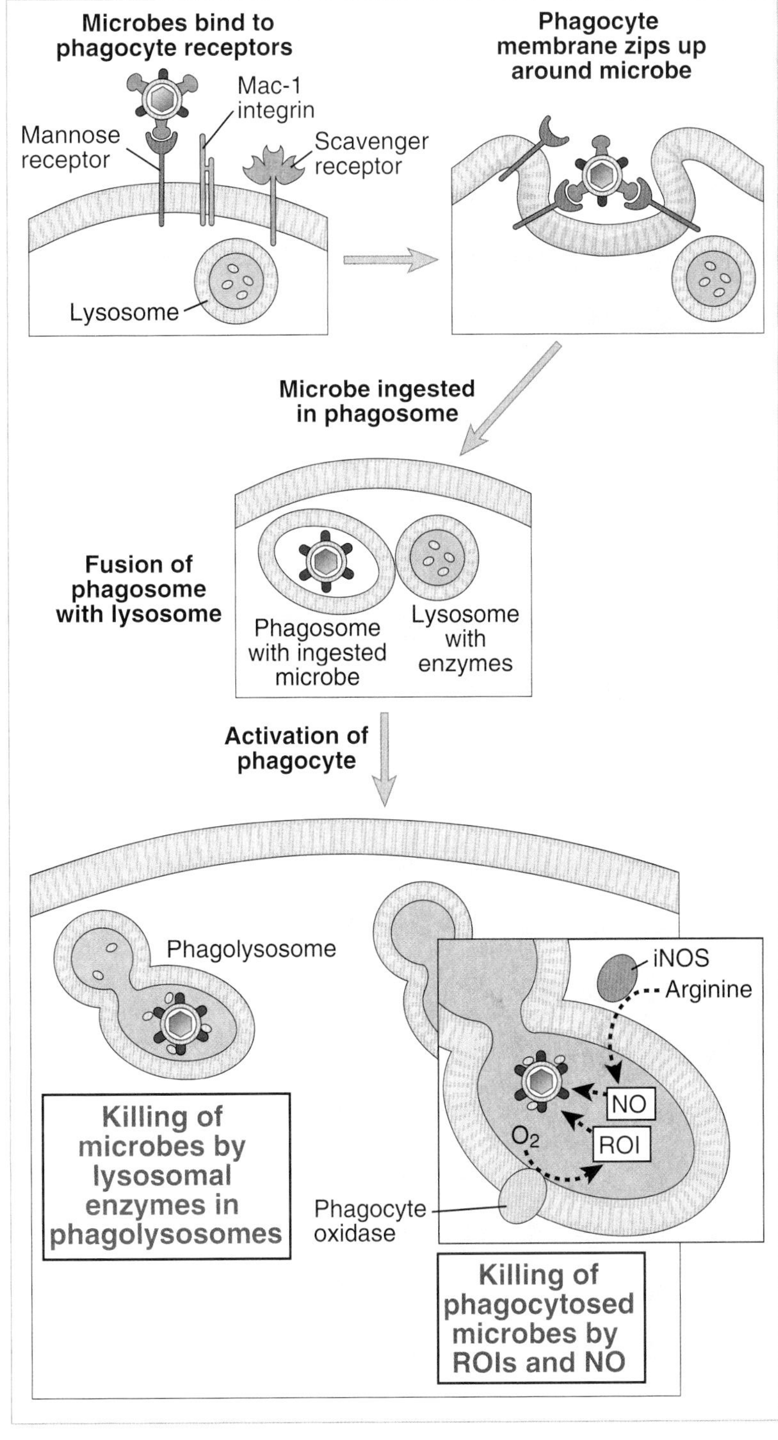

Figure 12–4 Phagocytosis and intracellular destruction of microbes.

Microbes may be ingested by different membrane receptors of phagocytes; some directly bind microbes, and others bind opsonized microbes. (Note that the Mac-1 integrin binds microbes opsonized with complement proteins, not shown.) The microbes are internalized into phagosomes, which fuse with lysosomes to form phagolysosomes, where the microbes are killed by reactive oxygen and nitrogen intermediates. iNOS, inducible nitric oxide synthase; NO, nitric oxide; ROIs, reactive oxygen intermediates.

induced and activated by many stimuli, including IFN-γ and signals from TLRs. The function of this enzyme is to reduce molecular oxygen into ROIs such as superoxide radicals, with the reduced form of nicotinamide adenine dinucleotide phosphate (NADPH) acting as a cofactor. Superoxide is enzymatically dismutated into hydrogen peroxide, which is used by the enzyme myeloperoxidase to convert normally unreactive halide ions into reactive hypohalous acids that are toxic for bacteria. The process by which ROIs are produced is called the respiratory burst. A disease called **chronic granulomatous disease** is caused by an inherited deficiency of one of the components of phagocyte oxidase; this deficiency compromises the capacity of neutrophils to kill gram-positive bacteria (see Chapter 20).

In addition to ROIs, macrophages produce reactive nitrogen intermediates, mainly **nitric oxide,** by the action of an enzyme called inducible nitric oxide synthase (iNOS). iNOS is a cytosolic enzyme that is absent in resting macrophages but can be induced in response to LPS and other microbial products that activate TLRs, especially in combination with IFN-γ. iNOS catalyzes the conversion of arginine to citrulline, and freely diffusible nitric oxide gas is released. Within phagolysosomes, nitric oxide may combine with hydrogen peroxide or superoxide, generated by phagocyte oxidase, to produce highly reactive peroxynitrite radicals that can kill microbes. The cooperative and redundant function of ROIs and nitric oxide is demonstrated by the finding that knockout mice lacking both iNOS and phagocyte oxidase are more susceptible to bacterial infections than single phagocyte oxidase or iNOS knockout animals are.

Activated neutrophils and macrophages also produce several proteolytic enzymes in the phagolysosomes, which function to destroy microbes. One of the important enzymes in neutrophils is elastase, a broad-spectrum serine protease known to be required for killing many types of bacteria.

When neutrophils and macrophages are strongly activated, they can injure normal host tissues by release of ROIs, nitric oxide, and lysosomal enzymes. The microbicidal products of these cells do not distinguish between self tissues and microbes. As a result, if these products enter the extracellular environment, they are capable of causing tissue injury.

Other Effector Functions of Activated Macrophages

In addition to killing phagocytosed microbes, macrophages serve many other functions in defense against infections (Fig. 12–5). Many of these functions are mediated by cytokines that were described in Chapter 11 as the cytokines of innate immunity. We have already referred to the role of TNF, IL-1, and chemokines in inducing inflammatory reactions to microbes. In addition to these cytokines, macrophages produce IL-12, which stimulates NK cells and T cells to produce IFN-γ. High concentrations of LPS induce a systemic disease characterized by disseminated coagulation, vascular collapse, and metabolic abnormalities, all of which are pathologic effects of high levels of cytokines secreted by activated macrophages (see Box 12–2). Activated macrophages also produce growth factors for fibroblasts and endothelial cells that participate in the remodeling of tissues after infections and injury. The effector functions of macrophages, and their role

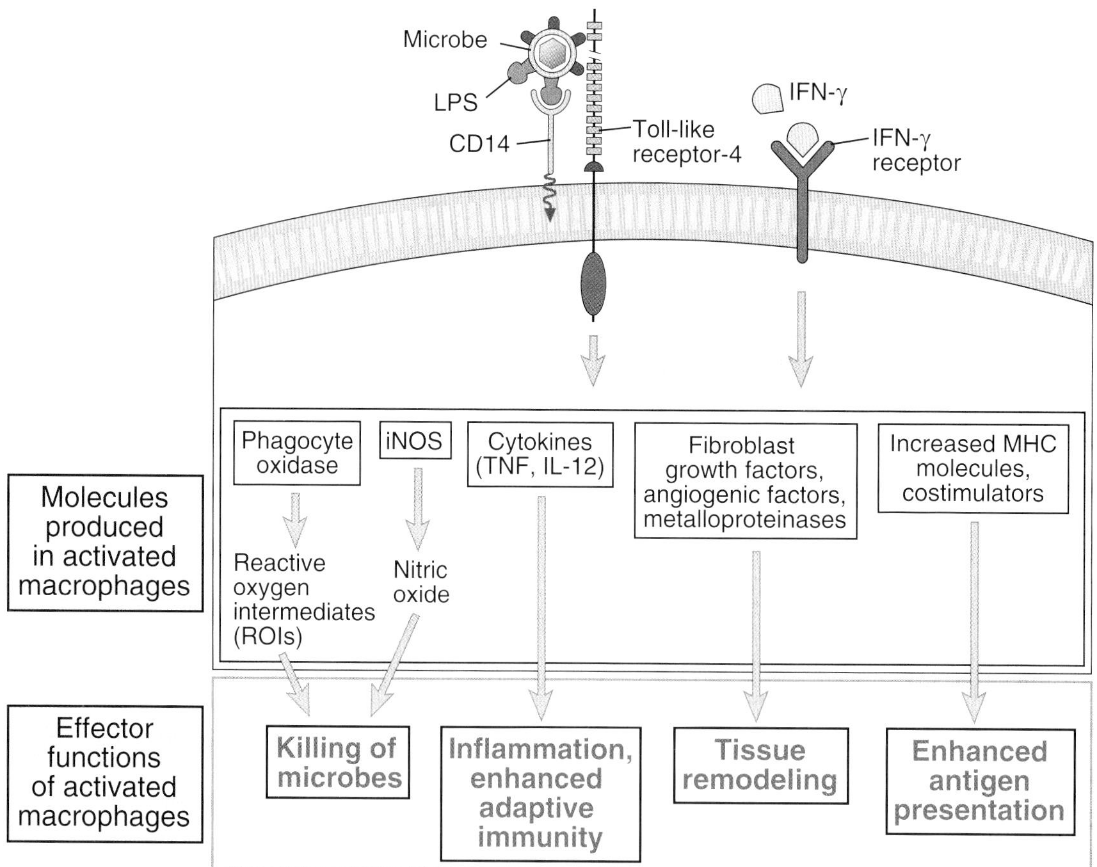

Figure 12–5 Effector functions of macrophages.
Macrophages are activated by microbial products such as lipopolysaccharide (LPS) and by NK cell–derived IFN-γ. The process of macrophage activation leads to the activation of transcription factors, the transcription of various genes, and the synthesis of proteins that mediate the functions of these cells. In adaptive cell-mediated immunity, macrophages are activated by stimuli from T lymphocytes (CD40 ligand and IFN-γ) and respond in essentially the same way (Chapter 13, Fig. 13–14).

in host defense, are described in more detail in Chapter 13.

NK Cells

NK (natural killer) cells are a subset of lymphocytes that kill infected cells and cells that have lost expression of class I MHC molecules, and they secrete cytokines, mainly IFN-γ (Fig. 12–6). The principal physiologic role of NK cells is in defense against infections by viruses and some other intracellular microbes. The term *natural killer* derives from the fact that if these cells are isolated from the blood or spleen, they kill various target cells without a need for additional activation. (In contrast, CD8⁺ T lymphocytes need to be activated before they differentiate into cytolytic T lymphocytes [CTLs] with the ability to kill targets.) NK cells are derived from bone marrow precursors and appear as large lymphocytes with numerous cytoplasmic granules, because of which they are sometimes called large granular lymphocytes. By surface phenotype and lineage, NK cells are neither T nor B lymphocytes, and they do not express somatically rearranged, clonally distributed antigen receptors like immunoglobulin or T cell receptors. NK cells constitute 5% to 20% of the mononuclear cells in the blood and spleen and are rare in other lymphoid organs.

Recognition of Infected Cells by NK Cells

NK cell activation is regulated by a balance between signals that are generated from activating receptors and inhibitory receptors (Fig. 12–7). There are several families of these receptors, which are described in detail in Box 12–3. The receptors are composed of ligand-binding chains and signaling chains. The ligands for the activating receptors are not well defined but may include molecules that are commonly expressed on the surfaces of most cells and some microbial products. The inhibitory receptors of NK cells bind to self class I MHC molecules, which are expressed on most normal cells. When both activating and inhibitory receptors are engaged, the influence of the inhibitory receptors is dominant, and the NK cell is not activated. This mechanism prevents killing of normal host cells. Infection of the host cells, especially by some viruses, often leads to an inhibition of class I MHC expression, and therefore the ligands for the inhibitory NK cell receptors are lost. As a result, the NK cells are released from their normal state of inhibition, and the infected cells are killed.

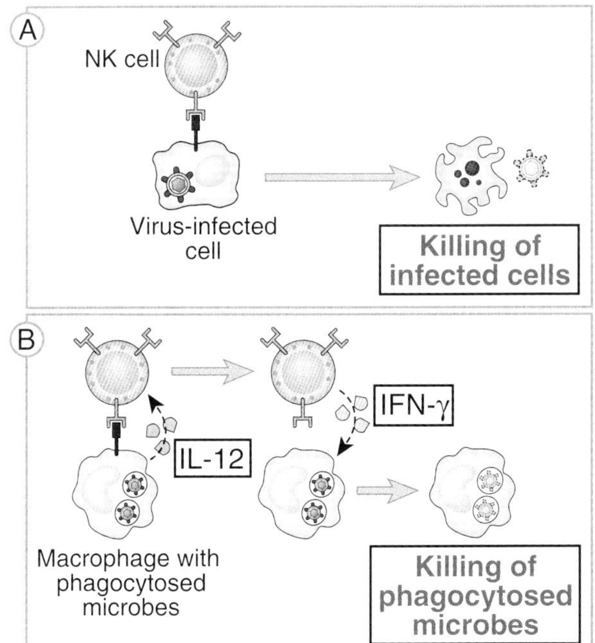

Figure 12–6 Functions of NK cells.
A. NK cells kill host cells infected by intracellular microbes, thus eliminating reservoirs of infection.
B. NK cells respond to IL-12 produced by macrophages and secrete IFN-γ, which activates the macrophages to kill phagocytosed microbes.

A common feature of NK cell–activating receptors is the presence of signaling molecules with immunoreceptor tyrosine-based activation motifs (ITAMs) in their cytoplasmic tails, as is the case for the signaling components of antigen receptors of T and B lymphocytes (see Chapters 8 and 9). Not surprisingly, the signaling pathways engaged by the NK cell–activating receptors involve recruitment and activation of tyrosine kinases and adapter proteins and activation of gene transcription and cytoskeletal reorganization, similar to the events that occur in T and B lymphocytes on antigen recognition. A common feature of the inhibitory receptors of NK cells are signaling chains with immunoreceptor tyrosine-based inhibitory motifs (ITIMs) in their cytoplasmic tails. On ligand binding to the receptors, these ITIMs become phosphorylated on tyrosine residues and bind tyrosine phosphatases, such as SHP-1, which in turn dephosphorylate signaling intermediates of the activation pathways.

NK cells also recognize antibody-coated targets by FcγRIIIa (CD16), a low-affinity receptor for the Fc portions of IgG1 and IgG3 antibodies. As a result of this recognition, NK cells kill target cells that have been coated with antibody molecules. This process, called antibody-dependent cell-mediated cytotoxicity, will be described in more detail in Chapter 14 when we consider the effector mechanisms of humoral immunity.

The expansion and activities of NK cells are also stimulated by cytokines, mainly IL-15 and IL-12. IL-15, which is produced by macrophages and many other cell types, is a growth factor for NK cells, and knockout mice lacking IL-15 or its receptors show a profound deficiency in the number of NK cells. The macrophage-derived cytokine IL-12 is a powerful inducer of NK cell IFN-γ production and cytolytic activity. IL-18 may augment these actions of IL-12. Recall that IL-12 and IL-18 also stimulate IFN-γ production by T cells and are thus central participants in IFN-γ production and the subsequent IFN-γ–mediated activation of macrophages in both innate and adaptive immunity. The type I IFNs, IFN-α and IFN-β, also activate the cytolytic potential of NK cells, perhaps by increasing

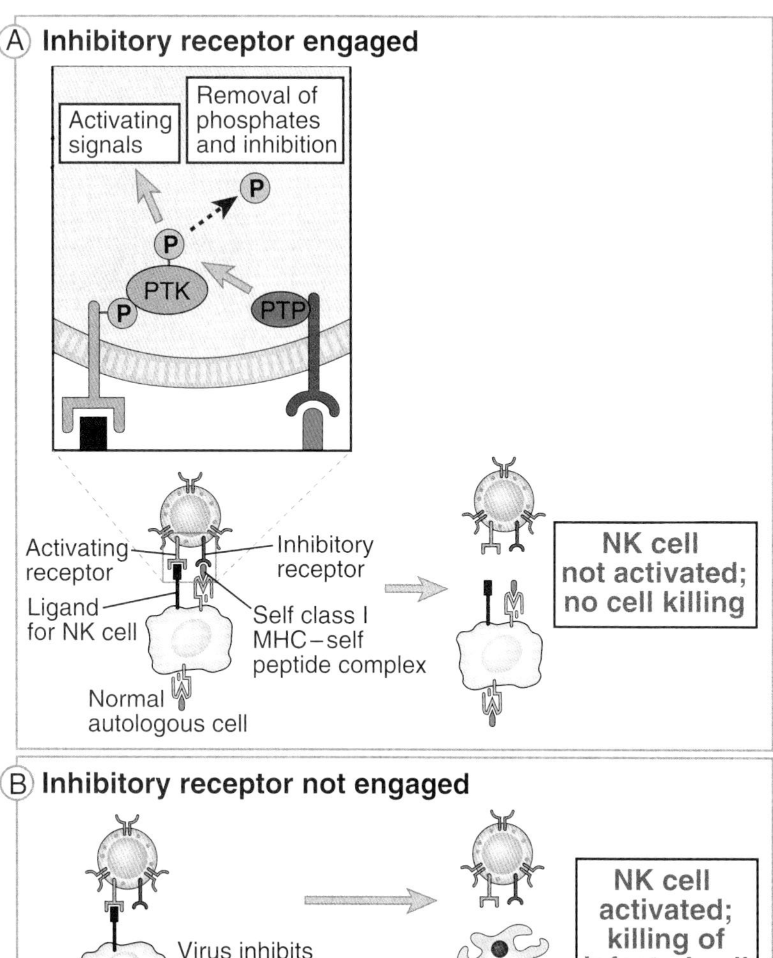

Figure 12–7 Activating and inhibitory receptors of NK cells.

A. Activating receptors of NK cells recognize ligands on target cells and activate protein tyrosine kinase (PTK), whose activity is inhibited by inhibitory receptors that recognize class I MHC molecules and activate protein tyrosine phosphatase (PTP). As a result, NK cells do not efficiently kill class I MHC–expressing targets.

B. If a virus infection inhibits class I MHC expression on infected cells, the NK cell inhibitory receptor is not engaged and the activating receptor functions unopposed to trigger responses of NK cells, such as cytolysis and cytokine secretion.

the expression of IL-12 receptors and therefore responsiveness to IL-12. IL-15, IL-12, and type I IFNs are produced by macrophages in response to infection, and thus all three cytokines activate NK cells in innate immunity. High concentrations of IL-2 also stimulate the activities of NK cells, and by this means NK cells may function in adaptive T cell–mediated immunity.

Effector Functions of NK Cells

The effector functions of NK cells are to kill infected cells and to activate macrophages to destroy phagocytosed microbes (see Fig. 12–6). The mechanism of NK cell–mediated cytolysis is essentially the same as that of cytolysis by CTLs (see Chapter 13). NK cells, like CTLs, have granules that contain a protein called perforin, which creates pores in target cell membranes, and enzymes called granzymes, which enter through perforin pores and induce apoptosis of target cells. By killing cells infected by viruses and intracellular bacteria, NK cells eliminate reservoirs of infection. Some tumors, especially those of hematopoietic origin, are targets of NK cells, perhaps because the tumor cells do not express normal levels or types of class I MHC molecules. NK cell–derived IFN-γ serves to activate macrophages, like IFN-γ produced by T cells, and increases the capacity of macrophages to kill phagocytosed bacteria (see Chapter 13).

NK cells play several important roles in defense against intracellular microbes. They kill virally infected cells before antigen-specific CTLs can become fully active, that is, during the first few days after viral infection. Early in the course of a viral infection, NK cells are expanded and activated by cytokines of innate immunity, such as IL-12 and IL-15, and they kill infected cells, especially those that display reduced levels of class I molecules. In addition, the IFN-γ secreted by NK cells activates macrophages to destroy phagocytosed microbes. This IFN-γ–dependent NK cell–macrophage reaction can control an infection with intracellular bacteria such as *Listeria monocytogenes* for several days or weeks and thus allow time for T cell–mediated immunity to develop and eradicate the infection. Depletion of NK cells leads to increased susceptibility to infection by some viruses and intracellular bacteria. In mice lacking T cells, the NK cell response may be adequate to keep infection with such microbes in check for some time, but the animals eventually succumb in the absence of T cell–mediated immunity. NK cells may also kill infected cells that attempt to escape CTL-mediated

BOX 12–3

Inhibitory and Activating Receptors of NK Cells

NK cells recognize and kill infected or malignantly transformed cells, but they do not usually harm normal cells. This ability to distinguish potentially dangerous targets from healthy self is dependent on the expression of both inhibitory and activating receptors. Inhibitory receptors on NK cells recognize class I MHC molecules, which are normally and constitutively expressed on most healthy cells in the body but are often not expressed by cells infected with virus or cancer cells. For the most part, activating receptors on NK cells recognize structures that are present on both dangerous target cells and normal cells, but the influence of the inhibitory pathways dominates when class I MHC is recognized. Some activating receptors recognize class I MHC–like molecules that are expressed only on stressed or transformed cells. Different families of NK cell receptors exist, and many of these receptors have evolved recently, as indicated by their absence in rodents and their structural divergence between chimpanzees and humans. The following discussion focuses on the properties of human NK cell inhibitory and activating receptors, with only brief consideration of murine NK receptors.

Numerous human NK inhibitory receptors have been identified, all of which have immunoreceptor tyrosine inhibitory motifs (ITIMs) in their cytoplasmic tails (see Figure). ITIMs recruit cytoplasmic protein tyrosine phosphatases SHP-1 and SHP-2, which dephosphorylate and thereby inactivate signaling intermediates generated by activating receptors on the same cell. Inhibitory NK receptors fall into three main families. The first family to be discovered is called the killer Ig-like receptor (KIR) family because its members contain two or three extracellular Ig-like domains. The KIRs recognize different alleles of HLA-A, -B, and -C molecules. Structural and binding studies indicate that the sequence of the peptides bound to the MHC molecules is important for KIR recognition of MHC molecules. HLA molecule binding to KIRs is characterized by very fast on-rates and off-rates, which would be consistent with the ability of NK cells to rapidly "test" for the presence of MHC expression on many cells in a short time. Furthermore, the inhibitory signals generated in an NK cell by KIR recognition of an MHC molecule are not long-lived, and the same NK cell can quickly go on to kill an MHC-negative target cell. Some members of the KIR family have short cytoplasmic tails without ITIMs, and these function as activating receptors, as discussed in more detail below. Mice do not express KIRs but instead use the Ly49 family of proteins, which have similar class I MHC specificities and ITIMs in their cytoplasmic tails.

A second family of inhibitory receptors consists of the Ig-like transcripts (ILTs), which also contain Ig-like domains. One member of this family, ILT-2, has a broad specificity for many class I MHC alleles and contains four ITIMs in its cytoplasmic tail. Interestingly, cytomegalovirus encodes a molecule called UL18 that is homologous to human class I MHC and that can bind to ILT-2. This may represent a decoy mechanism by which the virus engages an inhibitory receptor and protects its cellular host from NK cell–mediated killing.

The third NK inhibitory receptor family consists of heterodimers composed of either of the C-type lectins NKG2A or NKG2B covalently bound to CD94. NKG2A and NKG2B have two ITIMs in their cytoplasmic tails. The CD94/NKG2 receptors bind HLA-E, a nonclassical MHC molecule. Stable expression of HLA-E on the surface of cells depends on the binding of signal peptides derived from HLA-A, -B, -C, or -G. Therefore, the CD94/NKG2 inhibitory receptors perform a surveillance function for the absence of HLA-E, classical class I MHC, and HLA-G molecules. As is the case for the KIR receptors, some CD49/NKG2 receptors do not have cytoplasmic ITIM motifs, and these function as NK-activating receptors, as discussed below.

The activating receptors on NK cells include several structurally distinct groups of molecules, and only some of the ligands they bind are known. A shared feature of these receptors is their association with signaling molecules that contain immunoreceptor tyrosine-based activation motifs (ITAMs), including FcεRIγ, ζ, and DAP12 proteins. The activating NK receptors engage signaling pathways involving protein tyrosine kinases Syk and ZAP-70 and adapter molecules that are also part of the signaling pathways associated with lymphocyte antigen receptors and Ig Fc receptors (see Chapter 8). CD16, one of the first activating receptors identified on NK cells, is a low-affinity IgG Fc receptor that associates with FcεRIγ and ζ proteins and is responsible for NK cell–mediated antibody-dependent cellular cytotoxicity. A more recently discovered group of human NK-activating receptors, called natural cytotoxicity receptors, includes NKp46, NKp30, and NKp44. These are members of the Ig superfamily; they associate with FcRγ and ζ proteins and are expressed exclusively on NK cells. Although their ligands are not yet known, antibody-blocking studies suggest that they play a dominant role in NK-mediated killing of various tumor target cells. Ligand binding to activating NK cell receptors leads to cytokine production, enhanced migration to sites of infection, and killing activity against the ligand-bearing target cells.

As mentioned, some members of the KIR and CD94/NKG2 families of MHC-specific receptors do not contain ITIMs but rather associate with ITAM-bearing accessory molecules (such as DAP12) and deliver activating signals to NK cells. These include KIR2DS, CD49/NKG2C, CD49/NKG2E, and CD49/NKG2H. All these receptors are known to recognize normal class I MHC molecules, and it is not clear why these potentially dangerous receptors exist on NK cells. These activating receptors bind class I MHC molecules with lower affinities than the structurally related

Continued on following page

BOX 12–3

Inhibitory and Activating Receptors of NK Cells (*Continued*)

inhibitory receptors, and it is possible that the activating receptors actually bind MHC-related molecules specifically associated with pathological conditions. This is the case for NKG2D, which is expressed on NK cells, as well as on T cells, and is distantly related to the other NKG2 proteins. NKG2D associates with DAP10, a molecule homologous to DAP12, which contains a PI-3 kinase–binding motif in its cytoplasmic tail rather than an ITAM motif. This receptor recognizes the MICA, MICB, and ULBP molecules in humans and the RAE-1 and H-60 molecules in mice, all of which are encoded in the MHC, have domains homologous to class I MHC α and β domains, but do not display peptides or associate with β_2-microglobulin. These NKG2 ligands are not abundantly expressed on normal cells but are up-regulated by stress and are often found on tumor cells. Thus, NK cells may use these receptors to eliminate stressed (injured) host cells and tumor cells.

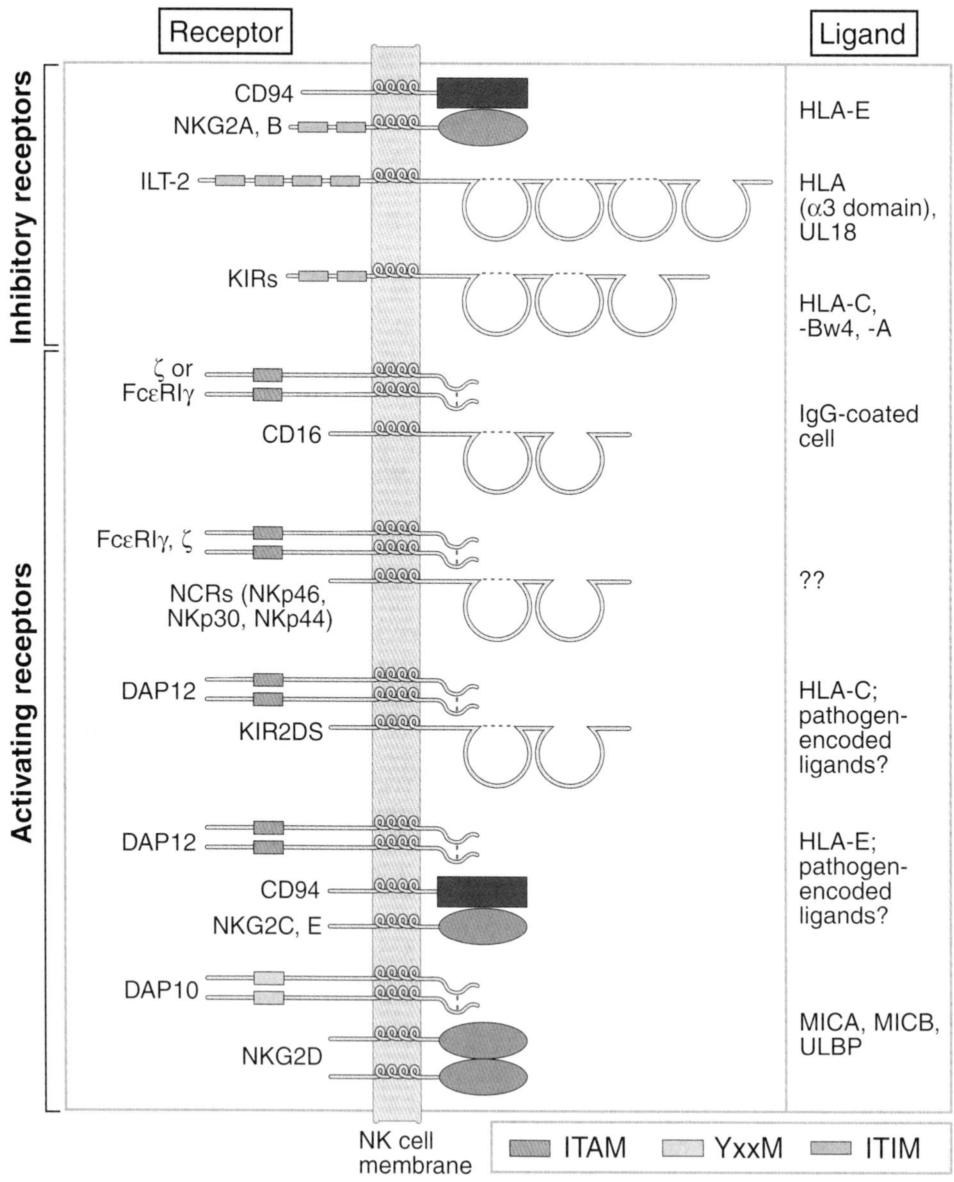

Examples of inhibitory and activating NK cell receptors and their ligands are shown. CD16 and the natural cytotoxic receptors (NCRs) associate with ζ chain homodimers, FcRγ homodimers, or ζ-FcRγ heterodimers. There are at least seven different KIRs, with varying ligand specificities.

immune attack by reducing expression of class I MHC molecules.

Because NK cells can kill certain tumor cells, it has also been proposed that NK cells serve to kill malignant clones *in vivo*. However, tumor-associated inflammatory infiltrates typically do not contain large numbers of NK cells.

The Complement System

The complement system consists of several plasma proteins that are activated by microbes and promote destruction of the microbes and inflammation. Recognition of microbes by complement occurs in three ways (Fig. 12–8). The **classical pathway,** so called because it was discovered first, uses a plasma protein called C1 to detect IgM, IgG1, or IgG3 antibodies bound to the surface of a microbe or other structure. The **alternative pathway,** which was discovered later but is phylogenetically older than the classical pathway, is triggered by direct recognition of certain microbial surface structures and is thus a component of innate immunity. The **lectin pathway** is triggered by a plasma protein called mannose-binding lectin (MBL), which recognizes terminal mannose residues on microbial glycoproteins and glycolipids. MBL bound to microbes activates one of the proteins of the classical pathway, in the absence of antibody, by the action of an associated serine protease. Recognition of microbes by any of these pathways results in sequential recruitment and assembly of additional complement proteins into protease complexes. The central protein of the complement system, C3, is cleaved, and its larger C3b fragment is deposited on the microbial surface where complement is activated. C3b becomes covalently attached to the microbes and serves as an opsonin to promote phagocytosis of the microbes. A smaller fragment, C3a, is released and stimulates inflammation by acting as a chemoattractant for neutrophils. C3b binds other complement proteins to form a protease that cleaves a protein called C5, generating a secreted peptide (C5a) and a larger fragment (C5b) that remains attached to the microbial cell membranes. C5a stimulates the influx of neutrophils to the site of infection as well as the vascular component of acute

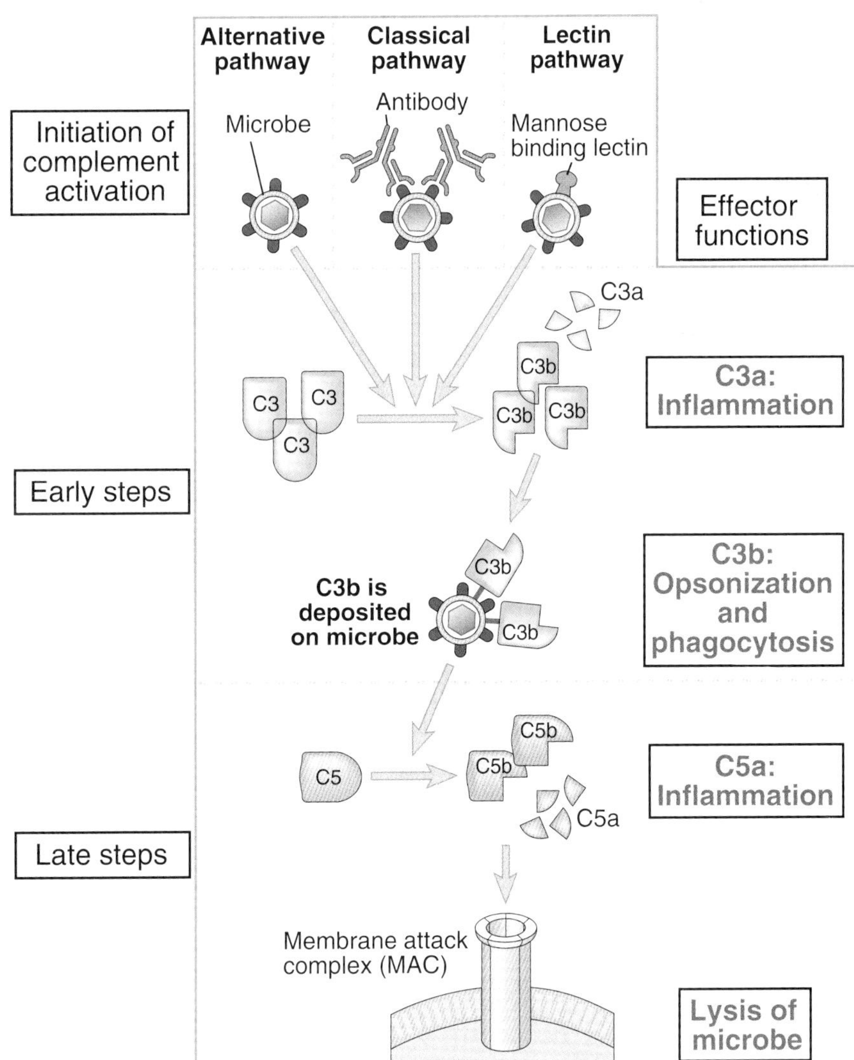

Figure 12–8 Pathways of complement activation.

The activation of the complement system may be initiated by three distinct pathways, all of which lead to the production of C3b (the early steps). C3b initiates the late steps of complement activation, culminating in the production of peptides that stimulate inflammation (C5a) and polymerized C9, which forms the membrane attack complex, so called because it creates holes in plasma membranes. The principal functions of major proteins produced at different steps are shown. The activation, functions, and regulation of the complement system are discussed in much more detail in Chapter 14.

inflammation. C5b initiates the formation of a complex of the complement proteins C6, C7, C8, and C9, which are assembled into a membrane pore that causes lysis of the cells where complement is activated. Mammalian cells express several regulatory proteins that block complement activation and thus prevent injury to host cells. The complement system will be discussed in more detail in Chapter 14.

Other Circulating Effector Proteins of Innate Immunity

Many plasma proteins, in addition to members of the complement system, are involved in innate immune responses to microbes (see Table 12–3). **Mannose-binding lectin,** which was mentioned before, is a plasma protein that functions as an opsonin. It belongs to the collectin family, so named because these proteins contain a collagen-like domain separated by a neck region from a calcium-dependent (C-type) lectin (i.e., carbohydrate-binding) domain. Plasma MBL, like the macrophage mannose receptor, binds carbohydrates with terminal mannose and fucose, which are typically found in microbial cell surface glycoproteins and glycolipids. Thus, MBL is a soluble pattern recognition receptor that binds to microbial but not mammalian cells. MBL is a hexamer that is structurally similar to the C1q component of the complement system (see Chapter 14). MBL binds to a macrophage surface receptor that is called the C1q receptor because it also binds C1q. This receptor mediates the phagocytosis of microbes that are opsonized by MBL. Moreover, MBL can activate the complement system, as discussed earlier and in Chapter 14.

C-reactive protein is a plasma protein that was identified and named because of its ability to bind to the capsules of pneumococcal bacteria. It belongs to the pentraxin family of plasma proteins, so named because they contain five identical globular subunits. C-reactive protein typically binds to bacterial phospholipids such as phosphorylcholine. It functions as an opsonin by binding C1q and interacting with phagocyte C1q receptors or by binding directly to Fcγ receptors. C-reactive protein may also contribute to complement activation through its attachment to C1q and activation of the classical pathway. C-reactive protein is called an acute-phase reactant because its plasma levels increase during the acute stages of many infections.

Coagulation factors are plasma proteins that mainly function to prevent hemorrhage by forming a thrombus at sites where blood vessel integrity is broken. Coagulation may also serve to wall off microbial infections and prevent spread of the microbes. In addition to circulating proteins, surfactant proteins in the lung, which also belong to the collectin family, protect the airways from infection.

Cytokines

The cytokines of innate immunity recruit and activate leukocytes and produce systemic alterations, including increases in the synthesis of effector cells and proteins that potentiate antimicrobial responses. In innate immunity, the principal sources of cytokines are macrophages, neutrophils, and NK cells, but endothelial cells and some epithelial cells such as keratinocytes produce many of the same proteins. As in adaptive immunity, cytokines serve to communicate information among inflammatory cells and between inflammatory cells and responsive tissue cells, such as vascular endothelial cells.

The cytokines of innate immunity were described in Chapter 11 and include cytokines that control viral infections, namely, IFN-α and IFN-β; cytokines that mediate inflammation, namely, TNF, IL-1, and chemokines; cytokines that stimulate the proliferation and activity of NK cells, namely, IL-15 and IL-12; cytokines that activate macrophages, especially NK cell–derived IFN-γ; and cytokines that serve to limit macrophage activation, especially IL-10. In addition, some cytokines of innate immunity, such as IL-6, increase bone marrow production of neutrophils and the synthesis of various proteins involved in host defense, such as C-reactive protein.

Role of Innate Immunity in Local and Systemic Defense Against Microbes

The early local reaction of innate immunity is the inflammatory response, in which leukocytes are recruited to the site of infection and activated to eradicate the infection. The function of inflammation is to destroy invading microbes by bringing activated effector cells into contact with invading microbes in an infected tissue. As discussed earlier in the chapter, inflammation in response to microbes is initiated by cytokines, especially TNF, IL-1, and chemokines, that act on endothelial cells and leukocytes to recruit and activate the leukocytes. Microbial products, such as LPS, and activated coagulation factors, such as thrombin, may also act directly on endothelial cells to promote the same kinds of changes that are induced by cytokines. Cytokines stimulate the expression of adhesion molecules on endothelial cells; these adhesion molecules bind blood leukocytes and initiate the recruitment of these cells to the sites of infection. Microbial products (e.g., *N*-formylmethionyl peptides), chemokines, complement-derived peptides (e.g., C5a), and lipid mediators such as leukotriene B_4 act on leukocytes to stimulate migration and activate microbicidal functions. The composition of inflammatory leukocytes within tissues changes with time from neutrophil rich to mononuclear cell rich, which is a reflection of both a change in the recruitment of different leukocytes and the short life span of neutrophils. Macrophages that are recruited to sites of infection are activated by microbial products and by NK cell–derived IFN-γ to phagocytose and kill microbes.

The importance of innate immunity in controlling infections is well illustrated by the course of *L. monocytogenes* infection in mice with severe combined immunodeficiency. These mice lack T and B lymphocytes. *L. monocytogenes* infection elicits a rapid neutrophil response, followed by a macrophage response, which can control the infection for several days or weeks. However, in the absence of adaptive immunity, the infection is never completely eradicated, and the animals eventually succumb.

Inflammation usually causes little tissue damage beyond that produced by the microbe itself. In some instances, the host inflammatory response itself exacerbates the amount of damage produced by the microbe. A typical example is the injury produced by LPS, which may damage endothelial cells and cause vascular thrombosis and ischemic injury to infected tissues (see Box 12–2).

Inflammation produces a variety of systemic changes in the host that enhance the ability of the innate immune system to eradicate infection and, in severe infections, can contribute to systemic tissue injury or death. These changes are thought to be mediated by the endocrine actions of cytokines and are collectively described as the acute-phase response or the systemic inflammatory response syndrome (see Box 12–2). This response consists of increased production of leukocytes; fever, which increases resistance to infection by unknown mechanisms; and changes in the levels of several plasma proteins. Plasma concentrations of complement proteins, fibrinogen, C-reactive protein, and serum amyloid A protein are typically increased. As discussed earlier, complement, fibrinogen, and C-reactive protein all play direct roles in host defense. In extreme cases of severe infection, the systemic response leads to shock, disseminated coagulation with multiorgan failure, and even death.

Role of Innate Immunity in Stimulating Adaptive Immune Responses

The innate immune response provides signals that function in concert with antigen to stimulate the proliferation and differentiation of antigen-specific T and B lymphocytes (Fig. 12–9). The two-signal hypothesis

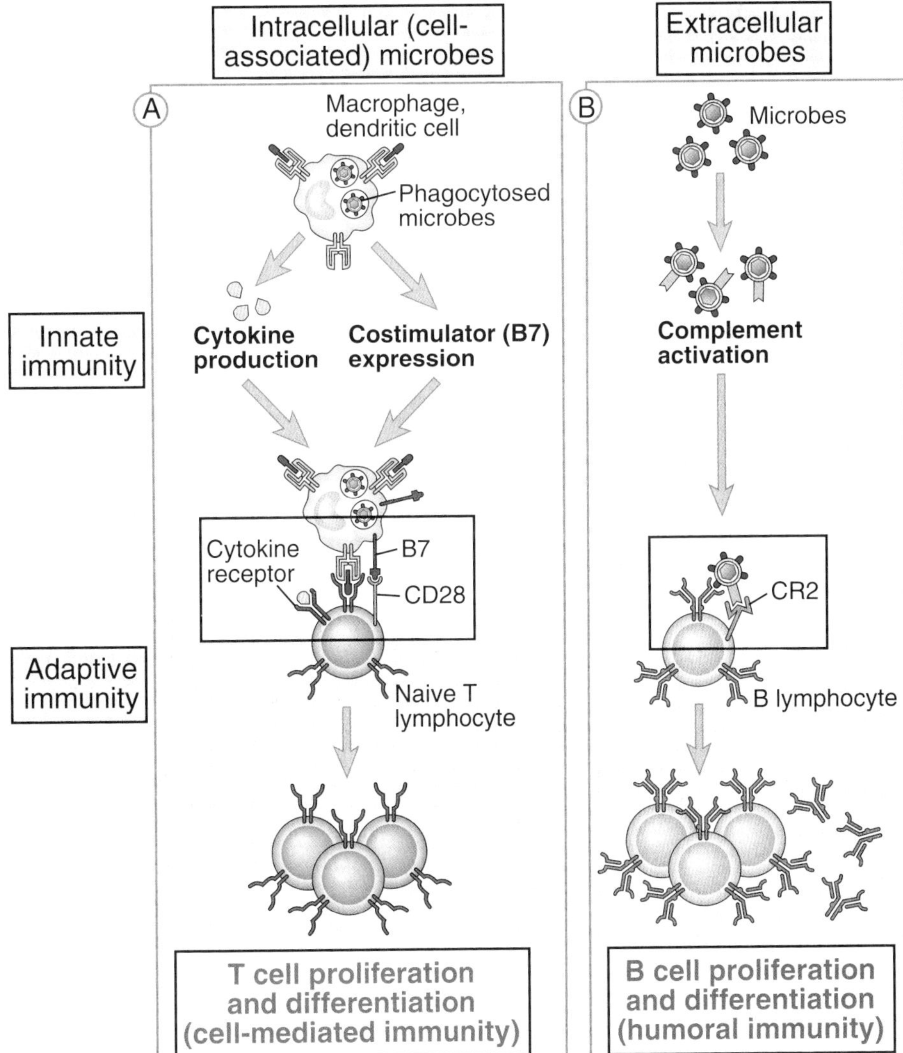

Figure 12–9 Stimulation of adaptive immunity by innate immune responses.

A. Macrophages and dendritic cells respond to phagocytosed (cell-associated) microbes by expressing costimulators (such as B7 proteins, which are recognized by the CD28 receptor of T cells) and by secreting cytokines (such as IL-12). Costimulators and IL-12 function, together with antigen recognition, to activate T lymphocytes.

B. The complement system is activated by extracellular microbes and generates proteins, such as C3d, which become attached to the microbes. B lymphocytes recognize microbial antigens by their antigen receptors and recognize C3d by a receptor called the type 2 complement receptor (CR2). Signals from the antigen receptor and CR2 function cooperatively to activate the B cells.

Note that in both examples, the second signals act on lymphocytes that also specifically recognize antigens of microbes; this recognition provides signal 1.

of lymphocyte activation was introduced in Chapter 1, as was the concept that signal 1 is always the antigen and signal 2 is either a product of a microbe or a component of the innate immune response that identifies the antigen as a microbial product (see Chapter 1, Fig. 1–8). Thus, innate immunity serves as the initial warning signal for the adaptive immune system to mount a protective host response. Microbes that colonize their hosts without eliciting an innate immune reaction with local inflammation may also fail to stimulate subsequent adaptive immunity. The molecules produced during innate immune reactions that function as second signals for lymphocyte activation are costimulators, cytokines, and complement breakdown products.

Costimulators are membrane proteins expressed on antigen-presenting cells (APCs) that function together with displayed antigens to stimulate specific T lymphocytes. In Chapters 6 and 8, we described the costimulators for T cells, the best defined of which are two structurally similar proteins called B7-1 (CD80) and B7-2 (CD86). When APCs encounter microbial products, such as LPS, and IFN-γ produced by NK cells, the APCs respond by expressing high levels of B7-1 and B7-2 and thus acquire the ability to stimulate T cell responses. In response to microbes, macrophages and dendritic cells also produce cytokines that promote the growth and differentiation of T lymphocytes. The prototype of such cytokines is IL-12, which stimulates naive T lymphocytes to develop into T_H1 effector cells that produce IFN-γ. Thus, phagocyte-derived IL-12 is a key inducer of cell-mediated immunity, the reaction that functions primarily to eradicate phagocytosed microbes (see Chapter 13, Fig. 13–8).

The best defined second signal for B cell activation is a complement protein called C3d, a breakdown product of C3. Microbes activate the complement system, either directly or after binding antibodies or plasma MBL, and the microbes become coated with C3 breakdown products, including C3d. Receptors for C3d, called type 2 complement receptors (CR2 or CD21), are expressed on mature B lymphocytes. When B lymphocytes recognize a microbial antigen by their antigen receptors and simultaneously recognize bound C3d by the complement receptor, the B cells are activated. Such activation results in an antibody response against the antigen (see Chapter 9, Fig. 9–5). The critical role of the complement system in humoral immune responses is demonstrated by the absence of such responses in gene knockout mice lacking either the C3 complement protein or CR2.

The second signals generated during innate immune responses to different microbes not only enhance the magnitude of the subsequent adaptive immune response but also influence the nature of the adaptive response (see Fig. 12–9). In infections by intracellular microbes, macrophages phagocytose or recognize the microbes and respond by expressing costimulators and producing cytokines that stimulate T cell–mediated immunity. The main function of cell-mediated immunity is to activate macrophages to kill intracellular microbes. In contrast, many extracellular microbes that enter the blood activate circulating complement proteins, which in turn enhances the production of antibodies by B lymphocytes. This humoral immune response serves to eliminate extracellular microbes. Thus, the cooperation between innate immunity and adaptive immunity is bidirectional, with each relying on components of the other to optimize host defense against infections.

The role of innate immunity in stimulating adaptive immune responses is the basis of the action of **adjuvants** (see Chapter 5), which are substances that need to be administered together with protein antigens to elicit maximal T cell–dependent immune responses. Many powerful adjuvants in experimental use are microbial products, such as killed mycobacteria and LPS, that elicit strong innate immune reactions and inflammation at the site of antigen entry. Thus, adjuvants stimulate the expression of costimulators on macrophages and other APCs and the secretion of cytokines such as IL-12. Consequently, the administration of protein antigens with adjuvants promotes cell-mediated immunity and T cell–dependent antibody production. In this way, adjuvants effectively convert an inert, nonmicrobial antigen to a mimic of a microbe. Vaccines are most effective for generating specific immune responses when they are administered subcutaneously or intradermally together with adjuvants. Adjuvants for use in humans are designed to stimulate innate immunity with the minimal amount of pathologic inflammation.

Summary

- The innate immune system provides the first line of host defense against microbes. The mechanisms of innate immunity exist before exposure to microbes. The components of the innate immune system include epithelial barriers, leukocytes (neutrophils, macrophages, and NK cells), circulating effector proteins (complement, collectins, pentraxins), and cytokines (e.g., TNF, IL-1, chemokines, IL-12, type I IFNs, and IFN-γ).

- The innate immune system uses pattern recognition receptors to recognize structures that are shared by microbes, are not present on mammalian cells, and are often essential for survival of the microbes, thus limiting the capacity of microbes to evade detection.

- Neutrophils and macrophages are phagocytes that kill ingested microbes by producing ROIs, nitric oxide, and enzymes in phagolysosomes. Macrophages also produce cytokines that stimulate inflammation and promote tissue remodeling at sites of infection. Phagocytes recognize and respond to microbial products by several different types of receptors, including Toll-like receptors, mannose receptors, and G protein–coupled receptors.

- NK cells are lymphocytes that defend against intracellular microbes by killing infected cells and providing a source of the macrophage-activating cytokine IFN-γ. NK cell recognition of infected cells is regulated by a combination of activating and inhibitory receptors. Inhibitory receptors recognize class I MHC molecules, because of which NK cells do not kill normal host cells but do kill cells in which class I MHC expression is reduced, such as virus-infected cells.

- The complement system is activated by microbes, and products of complement activation promote phagocytosis and killing of microbes and simulate inflammation. Other plasma proteins of innate immunity include mannose-binding lectin and C-reactive protein.
- Different cytokines of innate immunity recruit and activate leukocytes (e.g., TNF, IL-1, chemokines), enhance the microbicidal activities of phagocytes (IFN-γ), and stimulate NK cell and T cell responses (IL-12). In severe infections, excess systemic cytokine production is harmful and may even cause death of the host.
- Molecules produced during innate immune responses stimulate adaptive immunity and influence the nature of adaptive immune responses. Macrophages activated by microbes and by IFN-γ produce costimulators that enhance T cell activation and IL-12, which stimulates IFN-γ production by T cells and the development of IFN-γ–producing effector T cells. Complement fragments generated by the alternative pathway provide second signals for B cell activation and antibody production.

Selected Readings

Aderem A, and RJ Ulevitch. Toll-like receptors in the induction of the innate immune response. Nature 406:782–787, 2000.

Akira S, K Takeda, and T Kaisho. Toll-like receptors: critical proteins linking innate and acquired immunity. Nature Immunology 2:675–680, 2001.

Biron CA, LP Cosuens, KB Nguyen, GC Pien, and TP Salazar-Mather. Natural killer cells in antiviral defense: function and regulation by innate cytokines. Annual Review of Immunology 17:189–220, 1999.

Hack CE, LA Aarden, and LG Thijs. Role of cytokines in sepsis. Advances in Immunology 66:101–195, 1997.

Hoffman JA, FC Kafatos, CA Janeway, and RAB Ezekowitz. Phylogenetic perspectives in innate immunity. Science 284:1313–1318, 1999.

Janeway CA, and R Medzhitov. Innate immune recognition. Annual Review of Immunology 20:197–216, 2002.

Krieg A. CpG motifs in bacterial DNA and their immune effects. Annual Review of Immunology 20:709–760, 2002.

Lanier LL. On guard–activating NK cell receptors. Nature Immunology 2:23–27, 2001.

Lehrer RI, and T Ganz. Defensins of vertebrate animals. Current Opinion in Immunology 14:96–102, 2002.

Long EO. Regulation of immune responses through inhibitory receptors. Annual Review of Immunology 17: 875–904, 1999.

MacMicking J, Q-W Xie, and CF Nathan. Nitric oxide and macrophage function. Annual Review of Immunology 15:323–350, 1997.

Medzhitov R. Toll-like receptors and innate immunity. Nature Reviews Immunology 1:135–145, 2001.

Medzhitov R, and CA Janeway Jr. Innate immunity. New England Journal of Medicine 343:338–344, 2000.

Natarajan K, N Dimasi, J Wang, RA Mariuzza, and D Margulies. Structure and function of natural killer cell receptors: multiple molecular solutions to self, non-self. Annual Review of Immunology 20:853–885, 2002.

Underhill DM, and A Ozinsky. Phagocytosis of microbes: complexity in action. Annual Review of Immunology 20: 825–852, 2002.

Vilches C, and Parhan P. KIR: diverse, rapidly evolving receptors of innate and adaptive immunity. Annual Review of Immunology 20:217–251, 2002.

Chapter 13

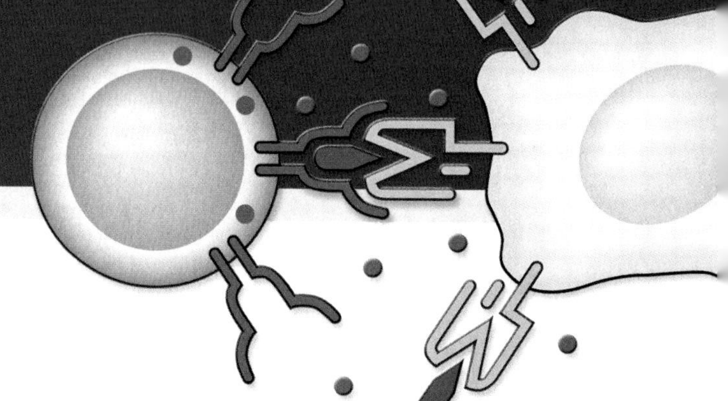

Effector Mechanisms of Cell-Mediated Immunity

Cell-mediated immunity (CMI) is the effector function of T lymphocytes, and it serves as the defense mechanism against microbes that survive within phagocytes or infect nonphagocytic cells. Historically, immunologists have divided adaptive immunity into humoral immunity, which can be adoptively transferred from an immunized donor to a naive host by antibodies in the absence of cells, and CMI, which can be adoptively transferred only by viable T lymphocytes. The effector phase of humoral immunity is triggered by the recognition of antigen by secreted antibodies; therefore, humoral immunity neutralizes and eliminates extracellular microbes and toxins that are accessible to antibodies, but it is not effective against microbes that survive and replicate inside infected cells. In contrast, in CMI, the effector phase is initiated by the recognition of antigens by T cells. T lymphocytes recognize protein antigens of intracellular microbes that are displayed on the surfaces of infected cells as peptides bound to self major histocompatibility complex (MHC) molecules. Defects in CMI result in increased susceptibility to infection by viruses and intracellular bacteria. Cell-mediated immune reactions are also important in allograft rejection (see Chapter 16) and in antitumor immunity (see Chapter 17). In this chapter, we discuss the development of effector T cells and the effector mechanisms of cell-mediated immune reactions. Antigen presentation to T lymphocytes and the process of T cell activation are described in Chapters 5, 6, and 8.

Types of Cell-Mediated Immune Reactions

Different types of microbes elicit distinct protective T cell responses (Fig. 13–1).

- ***The adaptive immune response to microbes residing within the phagosomes of phagocytes is mediated by T lymphocytes that recognize microbial antigens and activate the phagocytes to destroy the ingested***

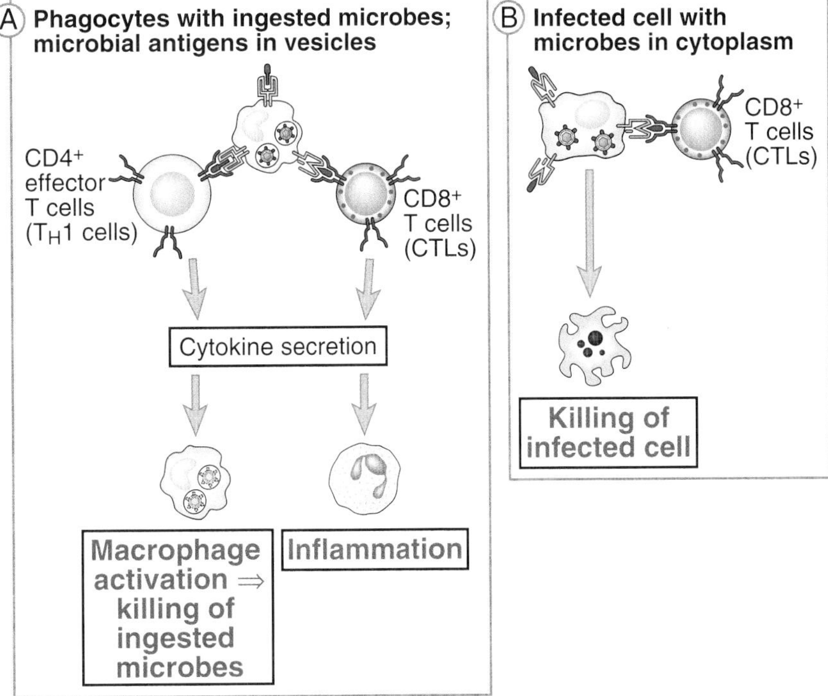

Figure 13–1 Types of T cell–mediated immune reactions.

A. $CD4^+$ T_H1 cells and $CD8^+$ T cells recognize class II MHC–associated or class I MHC–associated peptide antigens of phagocytosed microbes, respectively, and produce cytokines that activate the phagocytes to kill the microbes and stimulate inflammation.

B. $CD8^+$ cytolytic T lymphocytes (CTLs) recognize class I MHC–associated peptide antigens of microbes residing in the cytoplasm of infected cells and kill the cells.

microbes. Phagocytes are the major cells of host defense early after infection, during innate immunity (see Chapter 12). The function of phagocytes is to ingest and kill microbes. Many microbes have developed mechanisms that enable them to survive and even replicate within phagocytes, so innate immunity is unable to eradicate infections by such microbes. In these situations, CMI functions to enhance the microbicidal actions of phagocytes and thus to eliminate the microbes. T cell–mediated activation of phagocytes is dependent on the cytokine interferon-γ (IFN-γ). The major sources of IFN-γ are differentiated $CD4^+$ helper T cells of the T_H1 subset as well as $CD8^+$ T lymphocytes. T cells also produce tumor necrosis factor (TNF) and lymphotoxin, which promote leukocyte recruitment and inflammation. In CMI against phagocytosed microbes, the specificity of the response is due to T cells, but the actual effector function, that is, killing of microbes, is mediated by phagocytes. This cooperation of T lymphocytes and phagocytes illustrates an important link between adaptive and innate immunity: by means of cytokine secretion, T cells stimulate the function and focus the activity of nonspecific effector cells of innate immunity (phagocytes), thereby converting these cells into agents of adaptive immunity.

The fundamental concept that T cells are responsible for specific recognition of microbes but that phagocytes actually destroy the microbes in many cell-mediated immune responses was established with the original description of CMI to the intracellular bacterium *Listeria monocytogenes*. In the 1950s, George Mackaness showed that mice infected with a low dose of *Listeria* were protected from challenge with higher, lethal doses. Protection could be transferred to naive animals with lymphocytes (later shown to be T lymphocytes) from the infected mice, but not with serum (Fig. 13–2). *In vitro*, the bacteria were killed not by T cells from immune animals but by activated macrophages, emphasizing the central role of T cells in recognition and the roles of macrophages in the execution of effector function.

T cell–dependent macrophage activation and inflammation may cause tissue injury. This reaction is called **delayed-type hypersensitivity** (DTH), the term *hypersensitivity* referring to tissue injury caused by an immune response. DTH is a commonly used assay for cell-mediated immune reactions and a frequent accompaniment of protective CMI against microbes.

The adaptive immune response to microbes that infect and replicate in the cytoplasm of various cell types, including nonphagocytic cells, is mediated by $CD8^+$ cytolytic T lymphocytes (CTLs), which kill infected cells and eliminate the reservoirs of infection (see Fig. 13–1). CTLs are the principal defense mechanism against viruses that infect various cell types and replicate in the cytoplasm. If the infected cells lack the capacity to kill microbes, the infection can be eradicated only by destroying these cells. CTL-mediated killing is also a mechanism for eliminating microbes that are taken up by phagocytes but escape from phagosomes into the cytosol, where they are not susceptible to the microbicidal activities of phagocytes.

The adaptive immune response to helminthic parasites is mediated by T_H2 cells, which stimulate the production of IgE antibodies and activate

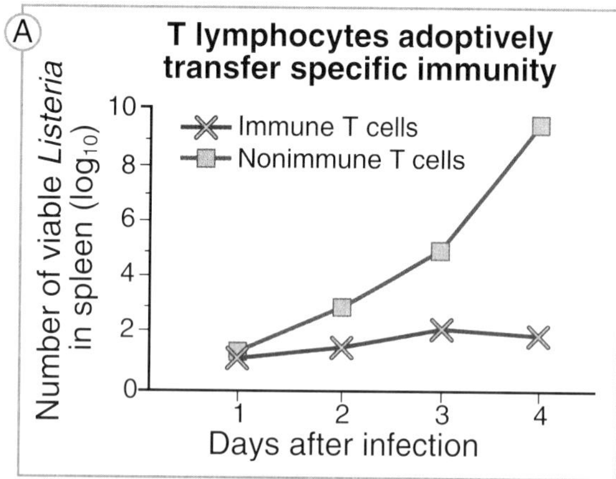

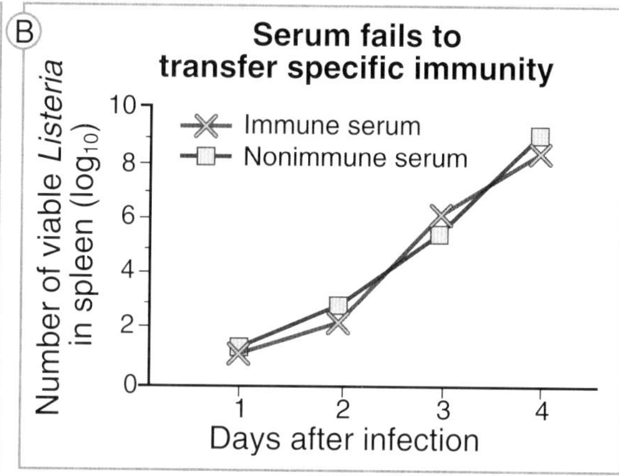

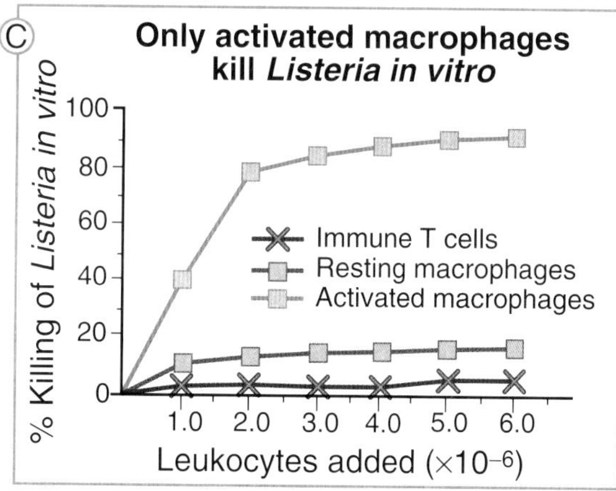

Figure 13–2 Cell-mediated immunity to *Listeria monocytogenes*.
Immunity to *L. monocytogenes* is measured by inhibition of bacterial growth in the spleens of animals inoculated with a known dose of viable bacteria. Such immunity can be transferred to normal mice by T lymphocytes (A) but not by serum (B) from syngeneic mice previously immunized with killed or low doses of *L. monocytogenes*. In an *in vitro* assay of cell-mediated immunity, the bacteria are actually killed by activated macrophages and not by T cells (C).

eosinophils that bind to and destroy IgE-coated helminths. The T_H2 subset of helper T cells also inhibits macrophage activation and is therefore important for limiting DTH reactions.

- The protective immune response to viruses and other intracellular microbes also consists of NK (natural killer) cells, which destroy infected cells early in the infection, as a component of innate immunity (see Chapter 12).

Development of Effector T Cells

Cell-mediated immune responses consist of the development of effector T cells from naive cells in peripheral lymphoid organs, migration of these effector T cells and other leukocytes to sites of infection, and either cytokine-mediated activation of leukocytes to destroy microbes or direct killing of infected cells (Fig. 13–3). We first describe the differentiation of naive T cells into effector cells and then the mechanisms by which these effector cells eradicate microbes.

Naive T cells do not produce effector cytokines or the molecules required to kill other cells; to eradicate microbes, the naive T cells must differentiate into effector cells with these functional capabilities. The development of the effector T cells of CMI involves the sequence of antigen recognition, clonal expansion, and differentiation that was discussed in Chapter 8 and is summarized here. Cell-mediated immune reactions are elicited by protein antigens of intracellular microbes and by soluble protein antigens that are administered with adjuvants. $CD4^+$ cells respond to antigens that are internalized into vesicles by antigen-presenting cells (APCs) because protein antigens in vesicles are degraded and presented in association with class II MHC molecules and recognized by $CD4^+$ (class II–restricted) T cells (see Chapter 5). $CD8^+$ T cell responses are elicited by microbes that reside in the cytosol of infected cells because cytoplasmic proteins are degraded in the cytosol, presented in association with class I MHC molecules, and recognized by $CD8^+$ (class I–restricted) T cells. The microbes that produce cytosolic antigens are typically viruses, which express proteins in the cytoplasm of infected cells. $CD8^+$ T cells may also respond to some phagocytosed bacteria and viruses because these microbes or their protein antigens may be transported or escape from phagosomes into the cytosol. Some chemicals introduced through the skin also elicit DTH reactions, called contact sensitivity reactions. It is believed that contact-sensitizing chemicals bind to and modify self proteins, creating new antigenic determinants that are presented to $CD4^+$ or $CD8^+$ T cells.

T Cell Antigen Recognition and Costimulation

The differentiation of naive T lymphocytes into effector cells of CMI requires antigen recognition and costimulation. When a microbe infects an individual or

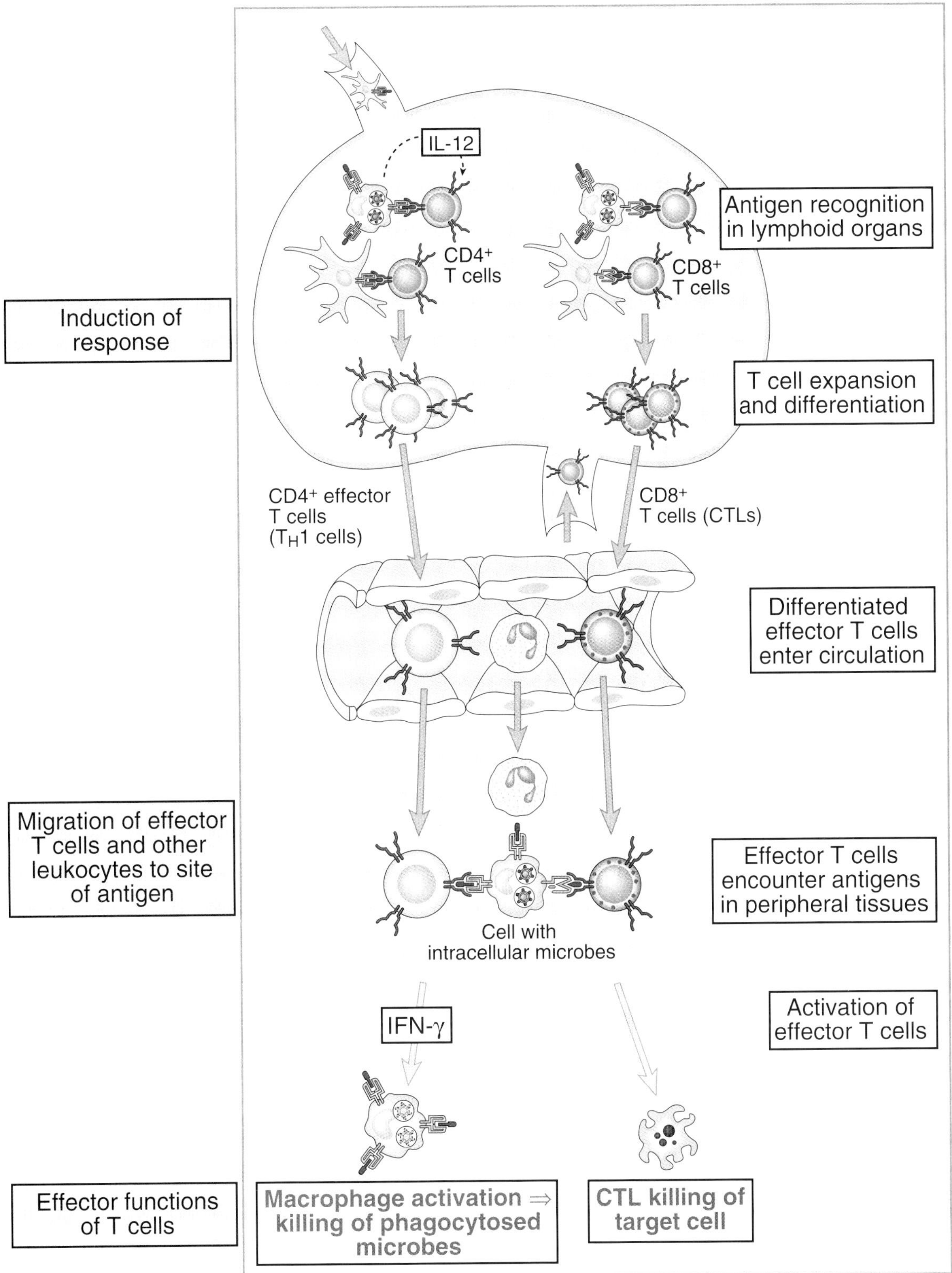

Figure 13–3 The induction and effector phases of cell-mediated immunity.

Induction of response: $CD4^+$ T cells and $CD8^+$ T cells recognize peptides that are derived from protein antigens and presented by professional antigen-presenting cells in peripheral lymphoid organs. The T lymphocytes are stimulated to proliferate and differentiate, and effector cells enter the circulation.

Migration of effector T cells and other leukocytes to the site of antigen: Effector T cells and other leukocytes migrate through blood vessels in peripheral tissues by binding to endothelial cells that have been activated by cytokines produced in response to infection in these tissues.

Effector functions of T cells: Effector T cells recognize the antigen in the tissues and respond by secreting cytokines that activate phagocytes to eradicate the infection. T cell–derived cytokines also stimulate inflammation.

a protein antigen is injected into the skin, specialized APCs, mainly dendritic cells in the skin and other epithelia, bind microbial antigens and transport these antigens from the portals of entry to the draining lymph nodes. During their migration to the lymph nodes, dendritic cells mature and become efficient APCs (see Chapter 5, Fig. 5–4). In the lymph nodes, these APCs present class II–associated peptides derived from the protein antigens for recognition by CD4$^+$ T lymphocytes. At the same time as the antigens are being presented by the APCs, the microbe or the adjuvant administered with the antigen elicits an innate immune response. This reaction stimulates the APCs to express high levels of costimulators, such as B7-1 and B7-2 proteins, which provide second signals for T cell activation, and to secrete cytokines such as interleukin (IL)-12, which stimulate differentiation of the T cells (see Chapter 8, Fig. 8–3).

The activation of CD8$^+$ T cells is also initiated by recognition of antigens on specialized APCs in peripheral lymphoid organs. However, CD8$^+$ T cells respond to microbes that may infect any nucleated cell (and to the antigens of tumors that may develop from any cell type; see Chapter 16). It is likely that dendritic cells ingest infected cells or tumor cells and process and present the antigens of the microbes or tumors for recognition by CD8$^+$ T lymphocytes. This process, called cross-presentation, was described in Chapter 5 (see Fig. 5–7). The differentiation of naive CD8$^+$ T cells into functional CTLs requires costimulation and the participation of CD4$^+$ helper cells (Fig. 13–4). CD4$^+$ helper T cells may stimulate the differentiation of CD8$^+$ T lymphocytes by several mechanisms. Helper T cells may secrete cytokines, such as IL-2, that stimulate the clonal expansion and differentiation of CD8$^+$ T cells. Antigen-stimulated helper T cells express CD40L, which binds to CD40 on APCs and activates these APCs to make them more efficient at stimulating the differentiation of CD8$^+$ T cells. The importance of CD4$^+$ T cells in the development of CTL responses is illustrated by studies with CD4 knockout mice, which lack helper T cells. In these mice, some viral infections fail to generate effective CTLs and are not eradicated. This role of CD4$^+$ T cells is also the accepted explanation for

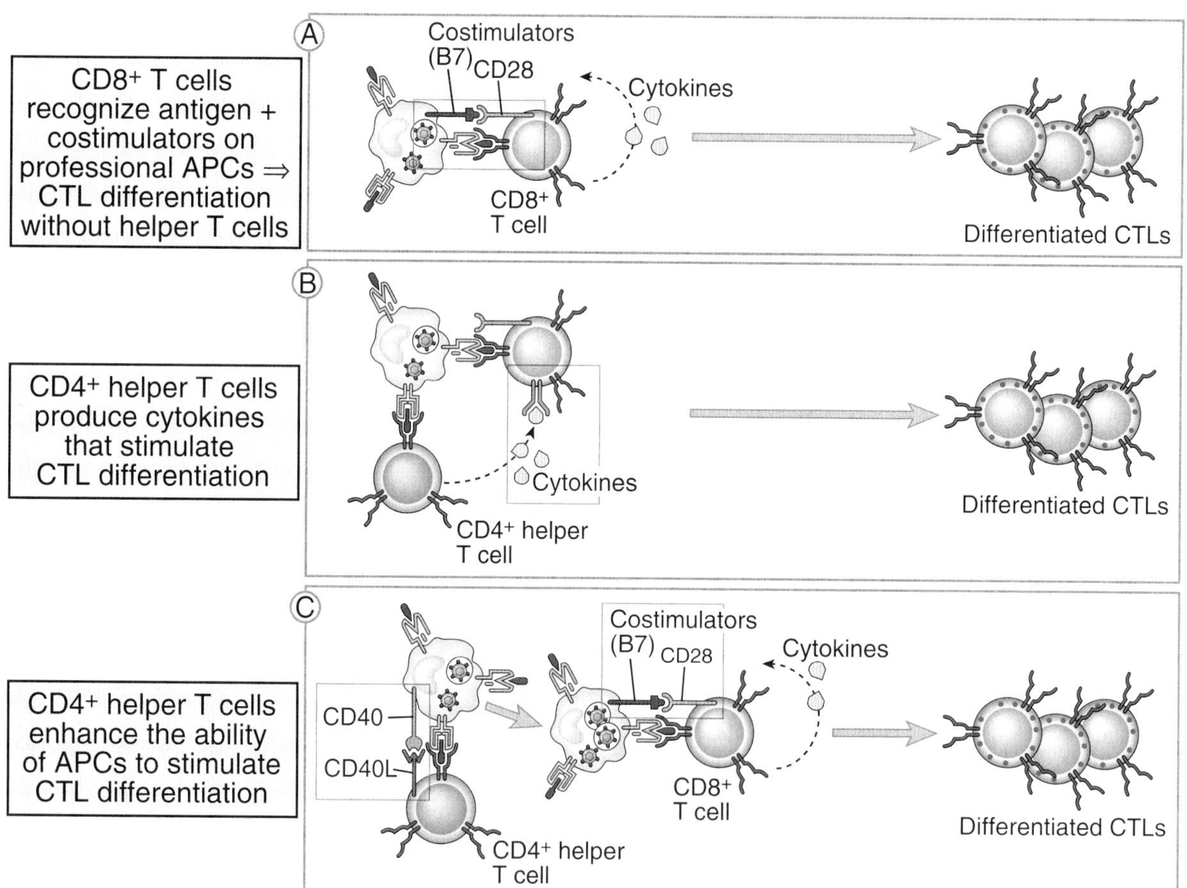

Figure 13–4 Role of costimulation and helper T cells in the differentiation of CD8$^+$ T lymphocytes.

Differentiation of naive CD8$^+$ T cells into effector cytolytic T lymphocytes (CTLs) requires antigen recognition (signal 1) and additional stimuli (signal 2). The second signal may be provided by costimulators, such as B7 molecules, expressed on professional antigen-presenting cells (APCs) (A) or by cytokines produced by CD4$^+$ helper T cells (B). CD4$^+$ helper T cells may also activate APCs and make them able to stimulate CTL development, for example, by stimulating expression of B7 molecules (C).

the defects in CTL generation seen in individuals infected with human immunodeficiency virus (HIV), in which the virus infects and eliminates only $CD4^+$ T cells. However, many viruses and tissue allografts are capable of inducing nearly normal levels of CTLs in mice lacking $CD4^+$ helper cells. It may be that if infected cells are ingested and presented by professional APCs (i.e., by the process of cross-presentation), the APCs will provide the signals that stimulate the development of CTLs without T cell help, but with less effective cross-presentation, the role of helper cells becomes critical.

Clonal Expansion of T Cells

After naive T cells encounter antigen and costimulators in peripheral lymphoid organs, they proliferate mainly in response to the autocrine growth factor IL-2. Antigen-stimulated T cells may undergo great proliferation, providing a large population of antigen-specific lymphocytes with the capacity to differentiate into effector cells (Fig. 13–5). Methods for estimating the frequency of antigen-specific T lymphocytes in a normal individual reveal an astonishing expansion of virus-specific $CD8^+$ T cells after viral infections (see Chapter 8, Box 8–1). At the peak of a viral infection in mice, a 50,000- to 100,000-fold increase in the number of antigen-specific $CD8^+$ T cells may be detected, and up to a third of the $CD8^+$ T cells in the spleen of the infected mouse may be specific for the antigens of that virus. Similarly, in humans infected with Epstein-Barr virus or HIV, up to 10% of the circulating $CD8^+$ T cells are specific for the virus during the acute phase of the infection. The magnitude of clonal expansion of $CD4^+$ T cells is considerably less, estimated to be 100- to 1000-fold. Some of the T cells that have proliferated differentiate into effector cells. As the antigens are eliminated, many of the activated T cells die by apoptosis, thereby providing a homeostatic mechanism that returns the immune system to its basal state of rest after the infection is cleared (see Chapter 10). Other progeny of the antigen-stimulated lymphocytes differentiate into memory cells, which are long-lived and poised to respond rapidly to antigen challenge.

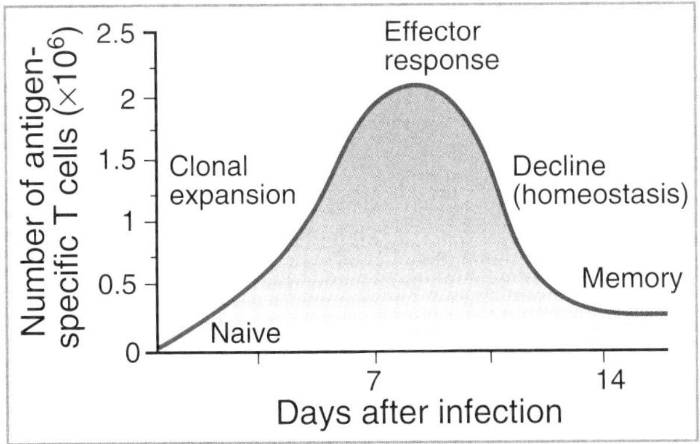

Figure 13–5 Clonal expansion of T cells.
T cells expand in response to infection, some of the progeny differentiate into effector cells, the majority die, and memory cells persist. The kinetics and numbers of cells are typical of the response of $CD8^+$ T cells in the spleen of a mouse infected with a virus, such as lymphocytic choriomeningitis virus; other intracellular microbes elicit qualitatively similar responses.

Differentiation of Naive $CD4^+$ T Cells into Subsets of Effector Cells

$CD4^+$ T cells may differentiate into subsets of effector cells that produce distinct sets of cytokines and therefore perform distinct effector functions (Fig. 13–6). One of the best examples of specialization of adaptive immunity is the ability of $CD4^+$ T lymphocytes to activate diverse effector mechanisms in response to different types of microbes. The basis of this specialization is the heterogeneity of $CD4^+$ T cells, illustrated by the existence of subsets that differ in how they are induced, what cytokines they produce, and what effector mechanisms they activate. We have referred to these subpopulations in previous chapters and now describe them in more detail.

Properties of T_H1 and T_H2 Subsets of Effector T Lymphocytes

The best defined subsets of effector T cells of the $CD4^+$ helper lineage are T_H1 and T_H2 cells; IFN-γ is the signature cytokine of T_H1 cells, and IL-4 and IL-5 are the defining cytokines of T_H2 cells (see Fig. 13–6). Populations of helper T cells that could be distinguished on the basis of their secreted cytokines were discovered in the 1980s by studying large panels of cloned cell lines derived from antigen-stimulated mouse $CD4^+$ T cells. It is now clear that individual T cells may express various mixtures of cytokines, and there may be many subpopulations with more heterogeneous patterns of cytokine production, especially in humans. However, chronic immune reactions are often dominated by either T_H1 or T_H2 populations. The relative proportions of these subsets induced during an immune response are major determinants of the protective functions and pathologic consequences of the response.

T_H1 and T_H2 populations are distinguished most clearly by the cytokines they produce (see Fig. 13–6). To date, no other phenotypic markers provide definitive classification. These subsets do show differences in the expression of various cytokine receptors, but such differences may reflect the activation status of the cells and may not be stable. The cytokines produced by these T cell subsets not only determine their effector functions but also participate in the development and expansion of the respective subsets. For instance, IFN-γ secreted by T_H1 cells promotes further T_H1 differentiation and inhibits the proliferation of T_H2 cells. Conversely, IL-4 produced by T_H2 cells promotes T_H2 differentiation, and IL-10, also produced by T_H2 cells (as well as by other cells), inhibits activation of T_H1 cells. Thus, each subset amplifies itself and cross-regulates the reciprocal subset. For this reason, once an immune response develops along one pathway, it becomes increasingly polarized in that direction, and

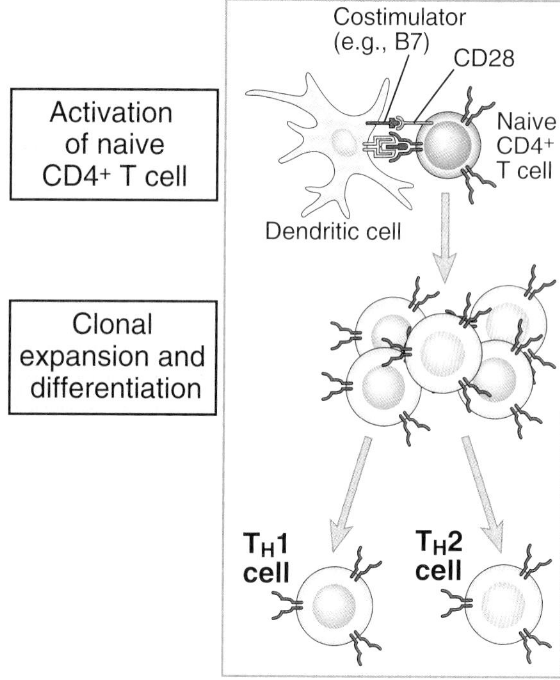

Property	T_H1 subset	T_H2 subset
Cytokines produced		
IFN-γ	+++	–
IL-4, IL-5, IL-13	–	+++
IL-10	+/–	++
IL-3, GM-CSF	++	++
Cytokine receptor expression		
IL-12R β chain	++	–
IL-18R	++	–
Chemokine receptor expression		
CCR4	+/–	++
CXCR3, CCR5	++	+/–
Ligands for E- and P-selectin	++	+/–
Antibody isotypes stimulated	IgG2a (mouse)	IgE, IgG1 (mouse)/IgG4 (humans)
Macrophage activation	+++	–

Figure 13–6 Properties of T_H1 and T_H2 subsets of $CD4^+$ helper T cells.

Naive $CD4^+$ T cells may differentiate into distinct subsets, such as T_H1 and T_H2 cells, in response to antigen, costimulators, and cytokines. The table lists the major differences between these two subsets.

the most extreme polarization is seen in chronic infections or in chronic exposure to environmental antigens, when the immune stimulation is persistent. These T cell populations show distinct patterns of migration to sites of infection as a result of differences in their binding to endothelial selectins and in their responsiveness to various chemokines (see Fig. 13–6).

Development of T_H1 and T_H2 Subsets

T_H1 and T_H2 subsets develop from the same precursors, which are naive $CD4^+$ T lymphocytes, and the pattern of differentiation is determined by stimuli present early during immune responses. The most important differentiation-inducing stimuli are cytokines, with IL-12 being the major inducer of T_H1 cells and IL-4 of T_H2 cells (Fig. 13–7). The same cytokines may function as growth factors to expand the respective subsets.

The T_H1 differentiation pathway is the response to microbes that infect or activate macrophages and to those that activate NK cells. The differentiation of antigen-activated $CD4^+$ T cells to T_H1 effectors is stimulated by many intracellular bacteria, such as *Listeria* and mycobacteria, and by some parasites, such as *Leishmania,* all of which infect macrophages. It is also stimulated by viruses and by protein antigens administered with strong adjuvants. A common feature of all these infections and immunization conditions is that they elicit innate immune reactions, with the production of IL-12. Some microbes engage Toll-like receptors on macrophages and dendritic cells and directly activate these cells to secrete IL-12 (Fig. 13–8). Other microbes may trigger IL-12 secretion indirectly, for instance, by stimulating NK cells to produce IFN-γ, which in turn acts on macrophages to induce IL-12 secretion. T cells may further enhance IL-12 production, by virtue of CD40L on the T cells engaging CD40 on APCs and stimulating IL-12 gene transcription. IL-12 is the major cytokine responsible for the induction of CMI, and knockout mice lacking IL-12 are extremely susceptible to infections with intracellular microbes. IL-12 binds to receptors on antigen-stimulated $CD4^+$ T cells and activates the transcription factor STAT4, and STAT4 promotes the differentiation of the T cells into T_H1 cells (see Fig. 13–7). A transcription factor called T-bet also plays a critical role in T_H1 development. T-bet is induced by IFN-γ, thus providing an amplification mechanism for T_H1 responses. T lymphocyte differentiation into T_H1 cells is impaired in knockout mice lacking STAT4 or T-bet, and these mice are susceptible to infections by intracellular microbes. IFNs, such as IFN-γ, also promote T_H1 development by stimulating the production of IL-12 by macrophages and the expression of functional IL-12 receptors on T lymphocytes. (In humans, IFN-α may stimulate IL-12 receptor expression.)

T_H2 differentiation occurs in response to helminths and allergens, which cause chronic T cell stimulation, often without a significant innate immune response or macrophage activation. The differentiation of antigen-stimulated T cells to the T_H2 subset is dependent on IL-4, which functions by activating STAT6, a transcription

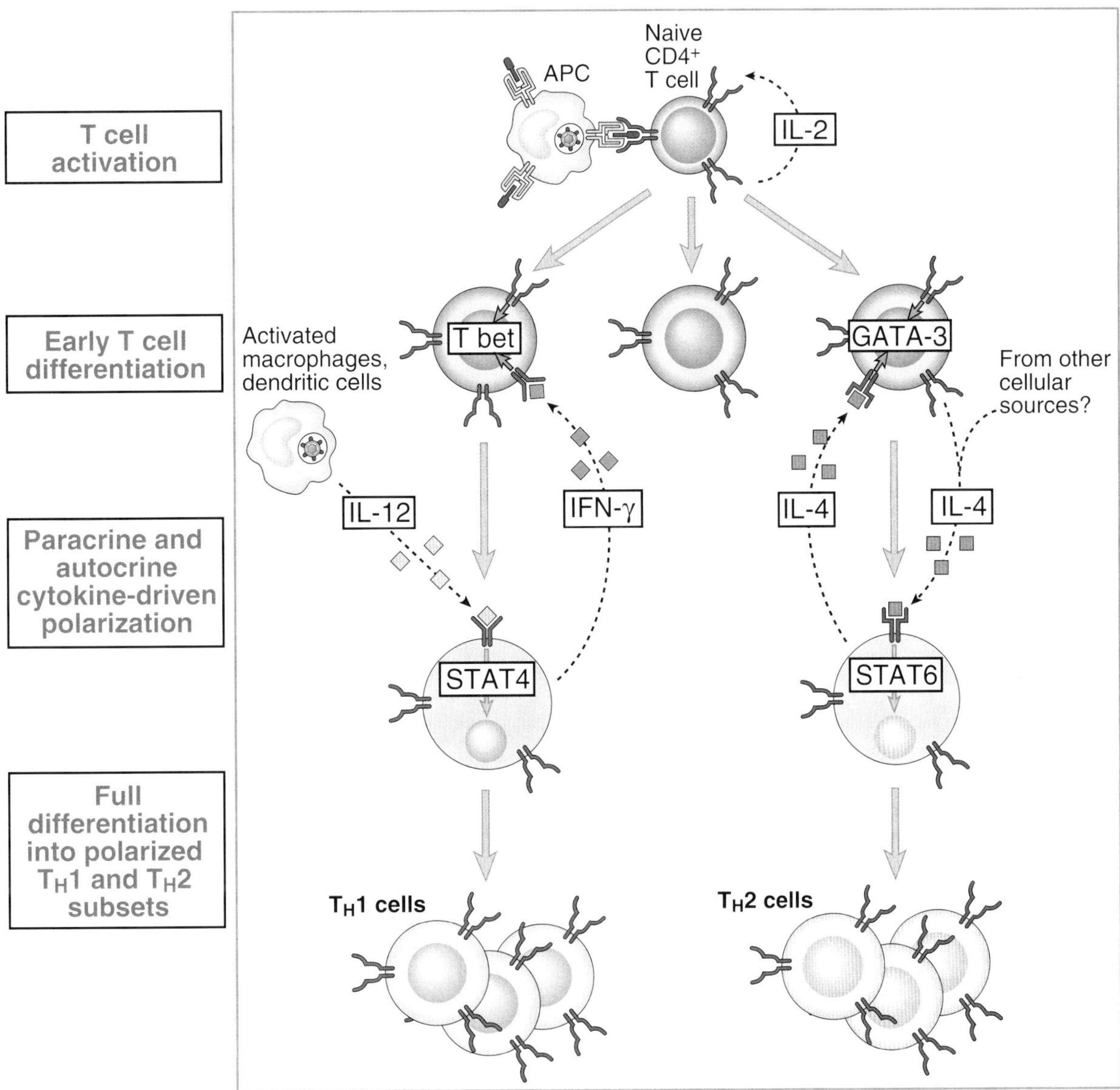

Figure 13–7 Development of T_H1 and T_H2 subsets.
Cytokines produced in the innate immune response to microbes or early in adaptive immune responses influence the differentiation of naive CD4+ T cells into T_H1 or T_H2 cells. IL-12, made by activated macrophages and dendritic cells, induces T_H1 cell development through a STAT4-dependent pathway. IL-4, which may be produced mainly by T cells themselves, favors induction of T_H2 cells through a STAT6-dependent pathway. The transcription factor T-bet, produced in response to IFN-γ, amplifies T_H1 responses, and GATA-3 is critical for T_H2 differentiation. Other cytokines that may influence helper T cell differentiation are not shown.

factor that stimulates T_H2 development (see Fig. 13–7). Another transcription factor called GATA-3 also plays an important role in T_H2 development by activating transcription of T_H2 cytokine genes. GATA-3 may be produced in response to antigen recognition, and its production may be enhanced by IL-4, providing an amplification mechanism for T_H2 responses. Knockout mice lacking IL-4, STAT6, or GATA-3 are profoundly deficient in T_H2 responses. The obligatory role of IL-4 in T_H2 differentiation raises an interesting question: Because differentiated T_H2 cells are the major source of IL-4 during immune responses to protein antigens, where does the IL-4 come from before T_H2 cells develop? A likely explanation is that antigen-stimulated $CD4^+$ T cells secrete small amounts of IL-4 from their initial activation. If the antigen is persistent and present at high concentrations, the local concentration of IL-4 gradually increases. If the antigen also does not trigger inflammation with attendant IL-12 production, the result is increasing differentiation of T cells to the T_H2 subset. Thus, T_H2 cells may develop in response to helminthic parasites and environmental allergens because these microbes and antigens cause persistent or repeated T cell stimulation with little inflammation or macrophage activation. In some situations, IL-4 produced by mast cells and a rare population of $CD4^+$

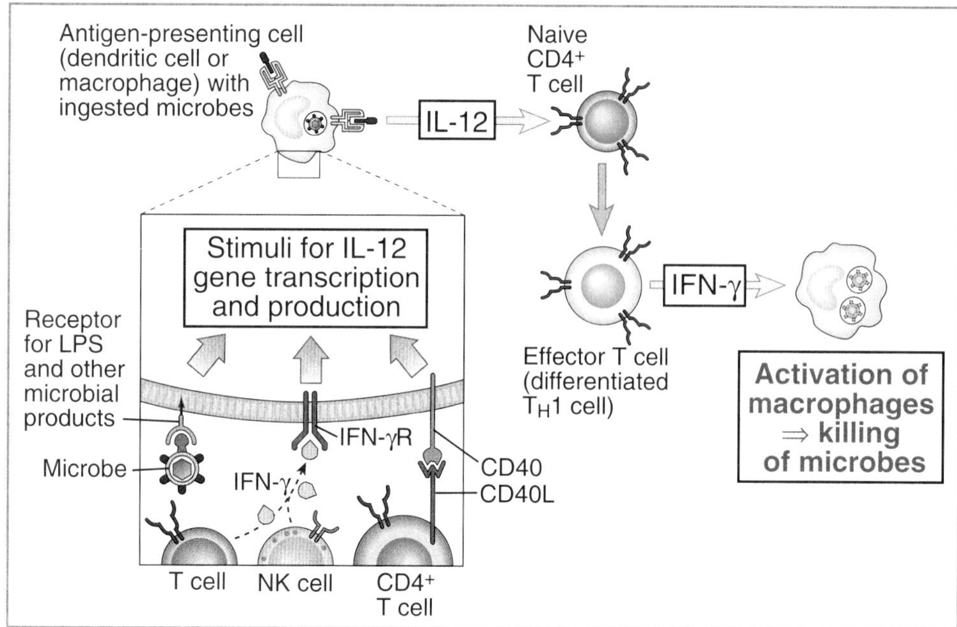

Figure 13–8 Role of IL-12 and IFN-γ in cell-mediated immunity.

Antigen-presenting cells secrete IL-12 in response to microbial products such as lipopolysaccharide (LPS), IFN-γ produced by NK cells and T cells, and CD40 engagement by T cell CD40L. IL-12 stimulates the differentiation of CD4⁺ helper T cells to T_H1 effectors, which produce IFN-γ. IFN-γ then activates macrophages to kill phagocytosed microbes (and to secrete more IL-12).

T cells that express markers of NK cells may contribute to T_H2 development.

Stimuli other than cytokines also influence the pattern of helper T cell differentiation. These stimuli include the amount of the antigen and the costimulators expressed on APCs. In addition, the genetic makeup of the host is an important determinant of the pattern of T cell differentiation. Inbred mice of some strains develop T_H2 responses to the same microbes that stimulate T_H1 differentiation in most other strains. Mice that develop T_H2 dominant responses are susceptible to infections by intracellular microbes (see Chapter 15).

Effector Functions of T_H1 and T_H2 Subsets

The principal function of T_H1 cells is in phagocyte-mediated defense against infections, especially with intracellular microbes (Fig. 13–9). As we shall discuss in more detail later, IFN-γ produced by T_H1 cells stimulates the microbicidal activities of phagocytes, thereby promoting the intracellular destruction of phagocytosed microbes. IFN-γ also stimulates the production of opsonizing and complement-fixing IgG antibodies, which promote the phagocytosis of microbes. Many organ-specific autoimmune diseases (see Chapter 18) and inflammatory reactions such as granulomas are due to excessive activation of T_H1 cells.

The principal effector function of T_H2 cells is in IgE- and eosinophil/mast cell–mediated immune reactions (Fig. 13–10). These reactions are induced by IL-4, IL-5, and IL-13 and are described later. T_H2 cells are responsible for defense against helminthic and arthropod infections and for allergic reactions (see Chapter 19). The antibodies stimulated by T_H2 cytokines do not promote phagocytosis or activate complement efficiently. In addition, several of the cytokines produced by T_H2 cells (notably IL-4, IL-13, and IL-10) antagonize the actions of IFN-γ and inhibit macrophage activation. This is the reason that T_H2 development is associated with deficient CMI to infections with intracellular microbes, such as *Leishmania* and mycobacteria (see Chapter 15).

Differentiation of Naive CD8⁺ T Cells into CTLs

Naive CD8⁺ T cells differentiate into CTLs, which are effector T cells that recognize and kill target cells expressing foreign peptide antigens in association with class I MHC molecules. Differentiation of pre-CTLs to active CTLs involves acquisition of the machinery to perform target cell killing. The most specific feature of CTL differentiation is the development of membrane-bound cytoplasmic granules that contain proteins, including perforin and granzymes, whose function is to kill other cells (described later). In addition, differentiated CTLs, like T_H1 cells, are capable of secreting cytokines, mostly IFN-γ, lymphotoxin, and TNF, which function to activate phagocytes and induce inflammation. The signals that stimulate differentiation of naive CD8⁺ T cells into CTLs are antigen, costimulators, and helper T cells, and these are described earlier in the chapter.

Migration of Effector T Cells and Other Leukocytes to Sites of Antigen

Effector T cells migrate to sites of infection and are retained at these sites (Fig. 13–11). To trigger the

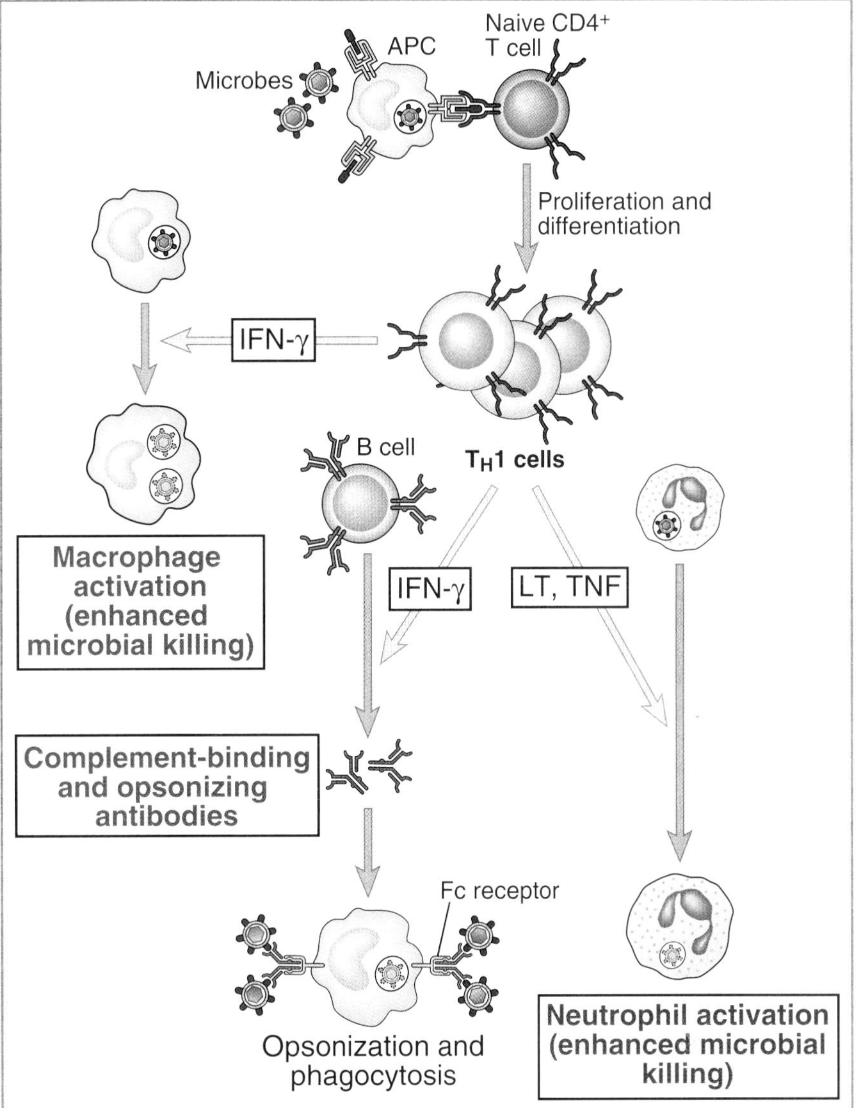

Figure 13–9 Effector functions of T_H1 cells.

$CD4^+$ T cells that differentiate into T_H1 cells secrete IFN-γ, lymphotoxin (LT) and tumor necrosis factor (TNF), and IL-2. IFN-γ acts on macrophages to increase phagocytosis and killing of microbes in phagolysosomes and on B lymphocytes to stimulate production of IgG antibodies that opsonize microbes for phagocytosis. LT and TNF activate neutrophils and stimulate inflammation. IL-2 is the autocrine growth factor made by this subset of T cells (not shown). APC, antigen-presenting cell.

effector phase of CMI, effector T cells have to come into contact with phagocytes or infected cells presenting the antigens that initiated the response. To locate microbes at any site, effector T cells that developed in lymphoid organs, such as lymph nodes, and entered the circulation have to leave the vasculature and enter the site of infection. (Noninfectious protein antigens elicit essentially the same reactions as do microbes, particularly if the proteins are introduced with adjuvants.) The directed migration of effector T lymphocytes to sites of infection is part of a more general process of leukocyte recruitment to these sites, the net result of which is the development of local inflammation. An initial phase of leukocyte influx may occur before T cells enter the site and are activated; this early inflammation is part of the innate immune response to microbes (see Chapter 12). After T cells enter the site of infection and are activated by antigen, they stimulate much greater leukocyte migration. This later, enhanced inflammation is sometimes called immune inflammation to indicate the role of T lymphocytes (immune cells) in the process.

The sequence of leukocyte migration and subsequent macrophage activation in CMI has been defined largely by analyses of DTH reactions in experimental animals. In the classical animal model, a guinea pig is first immunized by the administration of a protein antigen in adjuvant; this step is called the sensitization phase. About 2 weeks later, the animal is challenged subcutaneously with the same antigen and the subsequent reaction is analyzed; this step is called the elicitation phase. Humans may be sensitized for DTH reactions by microbial infection, by contact sensitization with chemicals and environmental antigens, or by intradermal or subcutaneous injection of protein antigens (Fig. 13–12). Subsequent exposure to the same antigen (also called challenge) elicits the reaction. For example, purified protein derivative (PPD), a protein antigen of *Mycobacterium tuberculosis,* elicits a DTH reaction, called the tuberculin reaction, when it is injected into individuals who have been exposed to *M. tuberculosis.* The characteristic response of DTH evolves during 24 to 48 hours. About 4 hours after the injection of antigen, neutrophils

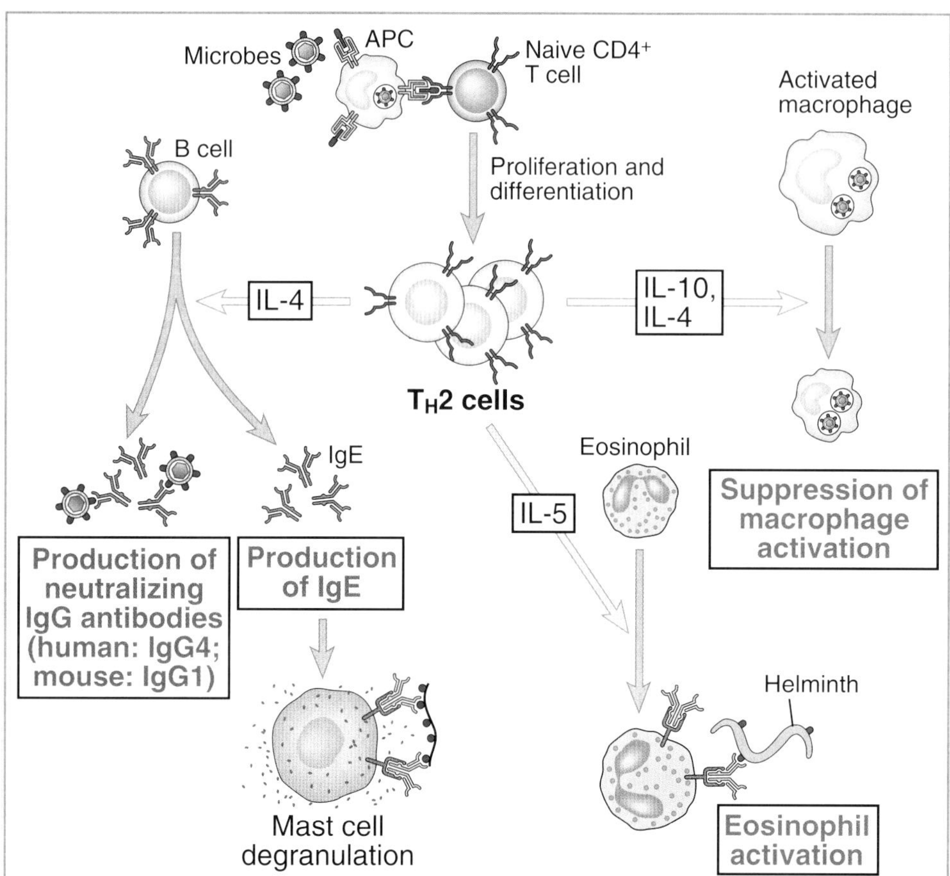

Figure 13–10 Effector functions of T_H2 cells. $CD4^+$ T cells that differentiate into T_H2 cells secrete IL-4 and IL-5. IL-4 acts on B cells to stimulate production of antibodies that bind to mast cells, such as IgE. IL-4 is also an autocrine growth and differentiation cytokine for T_H2 cells. IL-5 activates eosinophils, a response that is important for defense against helminthic infections. Cytokines from T_H2 cells also inhibit macrophage activation and T_H1-mediated reactions. APC, antigen-presenting cell.

accumulate around the postcapillary venules at the injection site. By about 12 hours, the injection site becomes infiltrated by T cells and blood monocytes, also organized in a perivenular distribution (Fig. 13–13). The endothelial cells lining these venules become plump, show increased biosynthetic organelles, and become leaky to plasma macromolecules. Fibrinogen escapes from the blood vessels into the surrounding tissues, where it is converted into fibrin. The deposition of fibrin and, to a lesser extent, the accumulation of T cells and monocytes within the extravascular tissue space around the injection site cause the tissue to swell and become hard (indurated). Induration, the hallmark of DTH, is detectable by about 18 hours after the injection of antigen and is maximal by 24 to 48 hours. This lag in the onset of palpable induration is the reason for calling the response "delayed type." A positive tuberculin skin test response is a widely used clinical indicator for evidence of previous or active tuberculosis infection. In clinical practice, loss of DTH responses to universally encountered antigens (e.g., *Candida* antigens) is an indication of deficient T cell function, a condition known as **anergy.** (This general loss of immune responsiveness is different from clonal anergy, a mechanism for maintaining tolerance to specific antigens, discussed in Chapter 10.)

Migration of leukocytes to sites of infection is stimulated by cytokines, which induce the expression of adhesion molecules on endothelial cells and the chemotaxis of leukocytes (see Fig. 13–11). Cytokines are produced by macrophages and endothelial cells stimulated by microbial products and, later in the reaction, by T lymphocytes responding to antigen. The most important cytokines in this reaction are TNF, IL-1, and chemokines. TNF and IL-1 activate endothelial cells to express ligands for leukocyte adhesion molecules, thereby resulting in the attachment of leukocytes to the endothelium at the site of infection. Chemokines increase the affinity of leukocyte integrins for their endothelial ligands and promote the transendothelial migration of the attached leukocytes into the extravascular tissue. This process of leukocyte migration was described in Chapter 12 (see Fig. 12–2). Cytokines have several other actions that contribute to DTH reactions. TNF activates endothelial cells to produce vasodilator substances, such as prostacyclin, that cause increased local blood flow and increased delivery of leukocytes to the site of inflammation. TNF and IFN-γ cause endothelial cells to undergo shape changes and basement membrane remodeling, which favors extravasation of cells and leakage of macromolecules. Leakage of plasma macromolecules, especially fibrinogen, is the basis of the induration seen in DTH reactions. The deposition of fibrinogen (and its insoluble cleavage product fibrin), as well as plasma fibronectin, in the tissues also forms a scaffold that facilitates the migration and subsequent retention of leukocytes in extravascular tissues.

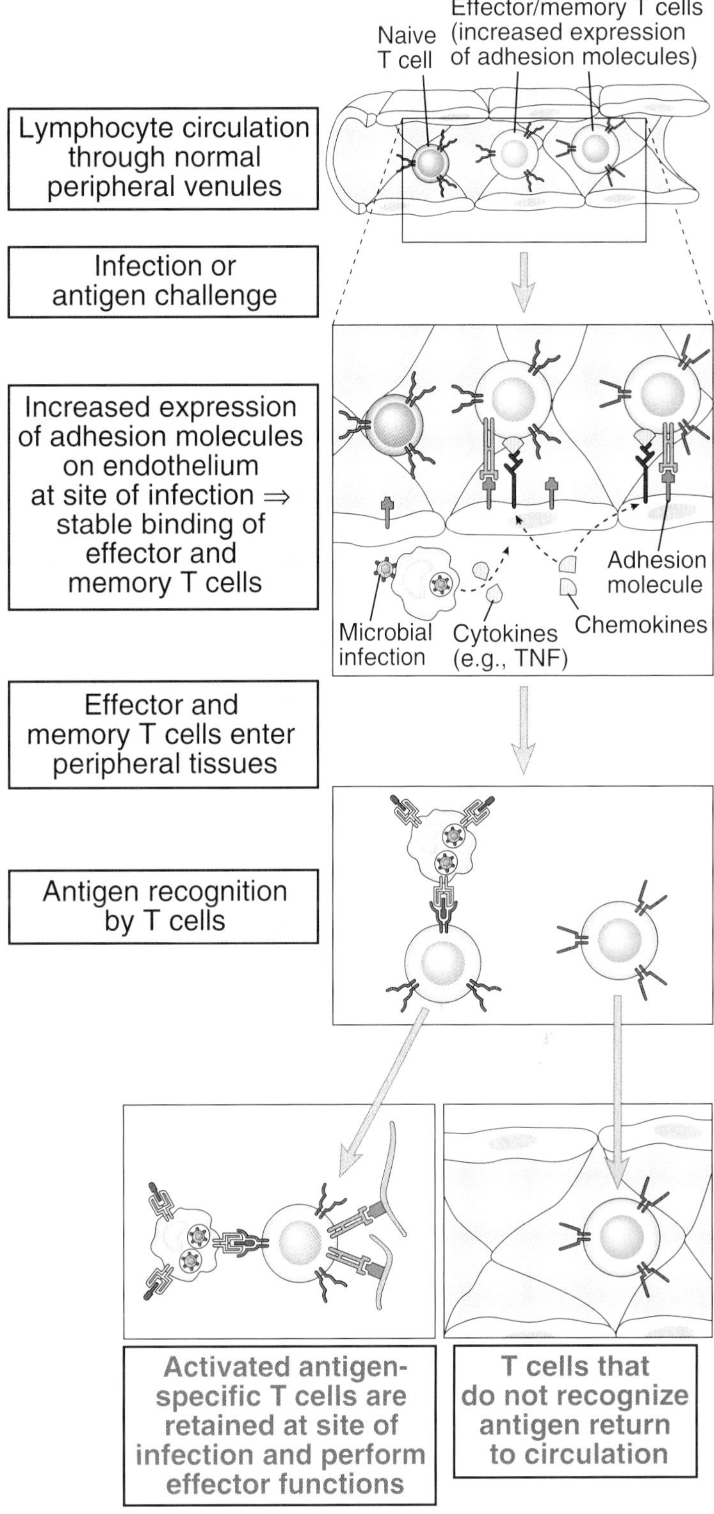

Figure 13–11 Migration and retention of effector and memory T cells at sites of infection.

Previously activated effector and memory T cells, but not naive cells, migrate through endothelium that is activated by cytokines (e.g., TNF) produced at a site of infection. In extravascular tissue, the T cells that specifically recognize antigen are activated and retained, whereas T cells that do not encounter the antigen for which they are specific return to the circulation, largely through lymphatic vessels (not shown).

Effector T lymphocytes express adhesion molecules and chemokine receptors that promote the migration of the cells to sites of infection and inflammation (see Fig. 13–11). Migration of activated T cells to peripheral tissues is mediated by the same adhesion molecules, the selectins and integrins, that are responsible for the migration of other leukocytes through cytokine-activated endothelium. Previously activated effector T cells migrate preferentially to peripheral tissues at sites of infection, in contrast to naive T lymphocytes, which migrate preferentially to peripheral lymph nodes, where immune responses are initiated. The reason for this difference is that compared with naive cells, activated T cells express higher levels of functional ligands

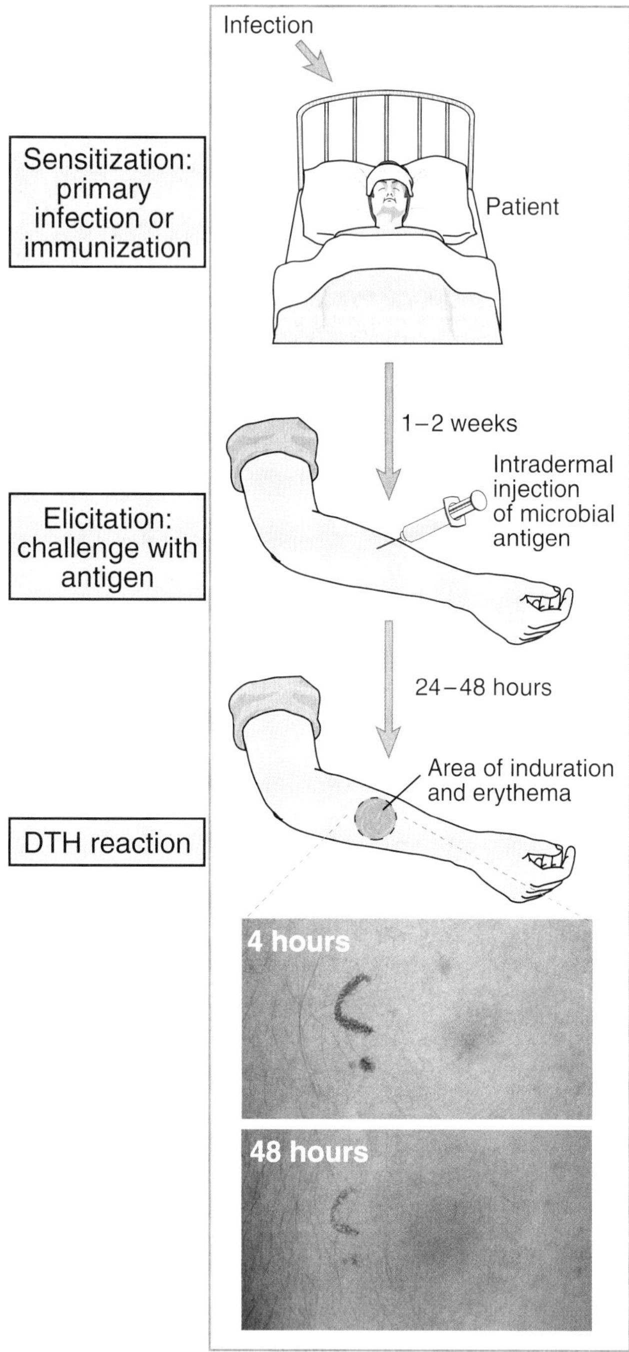

Figure 13–12 Delayed-type hypersensitivity reaction. Infection or immunization (vaccination) sensitizes an individual, and subsequent challenge with an antigen from the infectious agent elicits a delayed-type hypersensitivity (DTH) reaction. The reaction is manifested by induration with redness and swelling at the site of the challenge, which is undetectable at ~4 hours and peaks at ~48 hours. (Courtesy of Dr. J. Faix, Department of Pathology, Stanford University School of Medicine, Palo Alto, Calif.)

for E-selectin and P-selectin and higher levels of integrins (mainly LFA-1 and VLA-4). The endothelium at sites of infection expresses higher levels of selectins and the ligands for these integrins. Moreover, distinct populations of effector T cells may migrate to different tissues (skin, gut) because of the expression of distinct adhesion molecules. T cells that migrate preferentially to the skin express a carbohydrate ligand called cutaneous lymphocyte antigen (CLA) that binds E-selectin, and T cells that migrate to the intestines express an integrin called $\alpha_4\beta_7$, the ligand for which is present on the endothelium in the intestine. Effector T cell recruitment to peripheral sites of inflammation is also dependent on chemokines. Chemokines produced by endothelial cells or tissue macrophages at these sites bind to glycosaminoglycans on the endothelial cell surface and are displayed to effector (and memory) T cells that have engaged in low-affinity selectin-dependent rolling interactions with the endothelial cells. If the chemokines bind to receptors on the rolling T cells, the T cell integrin affinity for endothelial adhesion molecules is increased, and the T cell stops rolling, spreads out, and crawls to the interendothelial junctions. The T cells can then react to a chemical gradient of the chemokines in the extravascular tissue and migrate to the inflammatory site. Several different chemokine receptors and their chemokine ligands may be involved in T cell recruitment. Helper T cell subsets differ in some of the chemokine receptors they express, and therefore different chemokines can promote selective T_H1 or T_H2 recruitment to inflammatory sites. For example, T_H1 cells express CCR5 and CXCR3 and respond to the chemokines IP-10, iTAC, Mip1-α, Mip1-β, and RANTES, all of which are produced in response to microbes and stimuli generated during innate immune responses to microbes (such as the cytokine IFN-γ). T_H2 cells express the chemokine receptors CCR4 and CCR8 and respond to other chemokines that are often produced by epithelial cells (see Chapter 19). In contrast to effector T cells, naive T lymphocytes express high levels of L-selectin, whose ligand is expressed on the high endothelial venules of lymph nodes, and the chemokine receptor CCR7, which recognizes chemokines produced in the T cell zones of lymph nodes (see Chapter 2).

The migration of effector T cells from the circulation to peripheral sites of infection is largely independent of antigen, but cells that recognize antigen in extravascular tissues are preferentially retained there (see Fig. 13–11). T cell migration through blood and lymphatic vessels is controlled mainly by adhesion molecules and not by engagement of antigen receptors. Therefore, this process of migration results in the recruitment of circulating effector T cells to inflammatory sites, regardless of antigen specificity. This adhesion-dependent migration ensures that the maximum possible number of previously activated T cells have the opportunity to locate infectious microbes and eradicate the infection. Some memory T cells also migrate to peripheral tissues, even in the absence of infection, and survey the tissues for microbes. Once in the tissues, T cells encounter microbial antigens presented by macrophages and other APCs. T cells that specifically recognize antigens receive signals through their antigen receptors that increase the affinity of integrins for their ligands (see Chapter 6, Fig. 6–11). Two of these integrins, VLA-4 and VLA-5, bind to fibronectin in extracellular matrices, and a third adhesion mole-

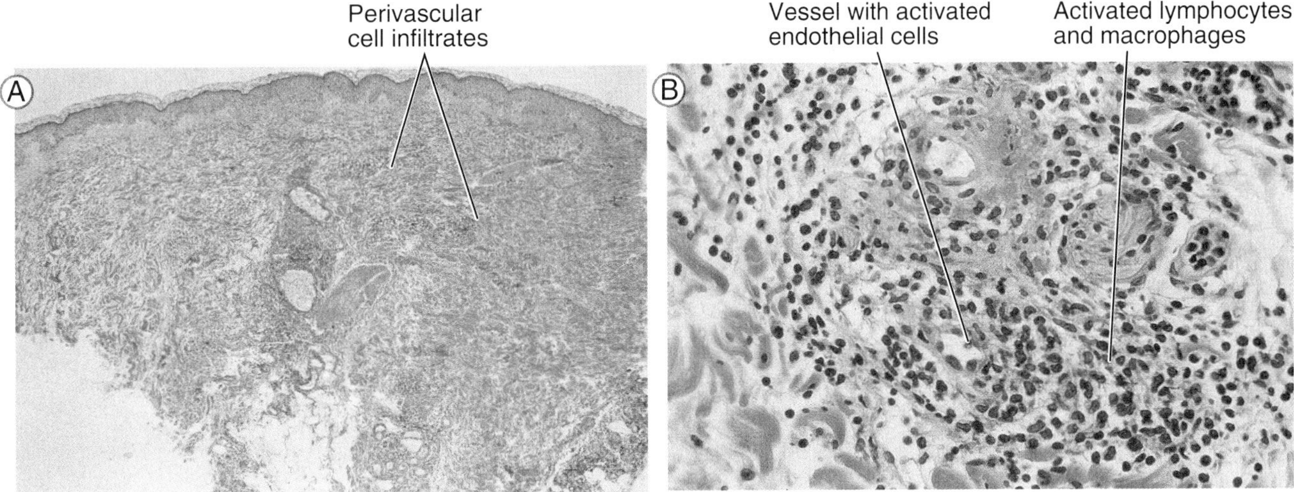

Figure 13–13 Morphology of a delayed-type hypersensitivity reaction. Histopathologic examination of the reaction illustrated in Figure 13–12 shows perivascular mononuclear cell infiltrates in the dermis (A). At higher magnification, the infiltrate is seen to consist of activated lymphocytes and macrophages surrounding small blood vessels in which the endothelial cells are also activated (B). (Courtesy of Dr. J. Faix, Department of Pathology, Stanford University School of Medicine, Palo Alto, Calif.)

cule, CD44, which is also expressed at high levels on effector and memory T cells, binds to hyaluronate. As a result, antigen-specific effector and memory T cells that encounter the antigen are preferentially retained at the extravascular site where the antigen is present. T cells not specific for the antigen may return through lymphatic vessels to the circulation.

Effector Mechanisms of Cell-Mediated Immunity

After effector T cells migrate to peripheral sites of infection or antigen challenge and recognize the antigen for which they are specific, the cells are activated to perform their effector functions. In CMI, the principal effector function of CD4$^+$ T cells is to stimulate the microbicidal activities of macrophages and other leukocytes, and the effector functions of CD8$^+$ CTLs are to kill infected cells and activate phagocytes.

T Cell–Mediated Activation of Macrophages and Other Leukocytes

Activated macrophages are the effector cells of CMI that function to eliminate phagocytosed microbes. Monocytes are recruited from blood into tissues and are exposed to signals from T_H1 effector cells and CD8$^+$ effector cells responding to antigen in the tissues. This interaction results in conversion of the monocytes to activated macrophages that are able to kill microbes. Activation consists of quantitative changes in the expression of various proteins that endow activated macrophages with the capacity to perform some functions that cannot be performed by resting monocytes. A macrophage is considered to be activated if it performs a function measured in a specific assay, for example, microbial killing. In the following sections, we describe the T cell signals that activate macrophages in cell-mediated immune reactions and the effector functions of these macrophages.

Stimuli for Macrophage Activation

CD4$^+$ T_H1 and CD8$^+$ T cells activate macrophages by contact-mediated signals delivered by CD40L-CD40 interactions and by the cytokine IFN-γ (Fig. 13–14). (Recall that helper T cells stimulate B lymphocyte proliferation and differentiation also by CD40-mediated signals and cytokines; see Chapter 9, Fig. 9–10.) When effector T_H1 cells and CD8$^+$ T cells are stimulated by antigen, the cells secrete cytokines, notably IFN-γ, and they express CD40L. IFN-γ is the major macrophage-activating cytokine. It activates some macrophage responses by itself and functions together with bacterial LPS or CD40 signals to elicit other responses. Knockout mice lacking IFN-γ or the IFN-γ receptor are extremely susceptible to infection by intracellular microbes. CD40L engages CD40 on macrophages that are presenting antigen to the T cells and activates an intracellular signal transduction pathway that is similar to the pathway activated by TNF receptors (see Chapter 11, Box 11–1). The importance of CD40 in macrophage activation is demonstrated by the immunologic defects in humans with inherited mutations in CD40L **(X-linked hyper-IgM syndrome)** and mice in which the gene for CD40 or CD40L is knocked out (see Chapter 20). All these disorders are characterized by severe deficiencies in CMI to intracellular microbes, and children with the X-linked hyper-IgM syndrome often succumb to infection by the intracellular pathogen *Pneumocystis carinii*. As expected, these patients and knockout mice also have defects in helper T cell–dependent antibody

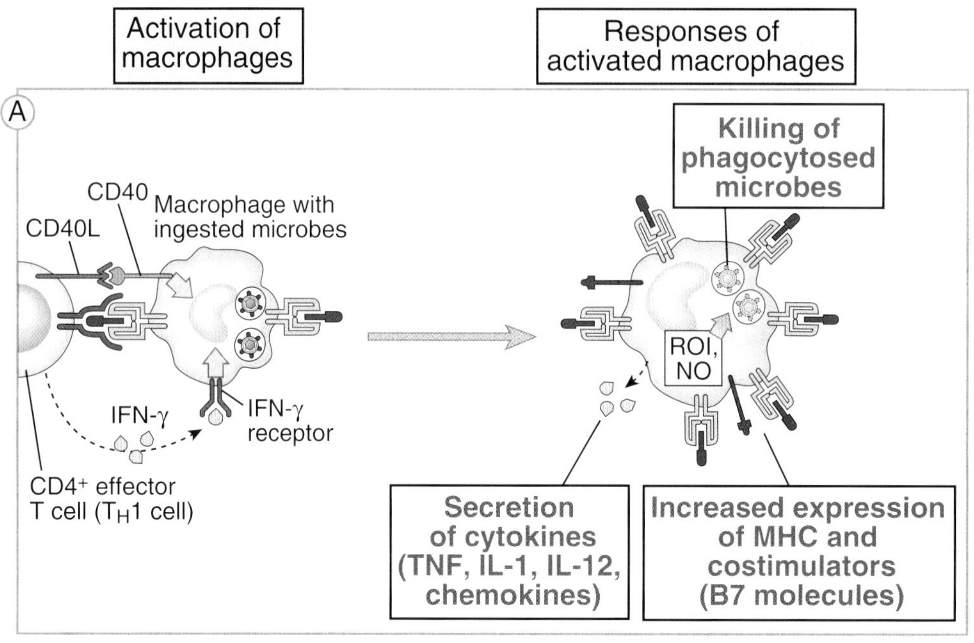

(B) Macrophage response	Role in cell-mediated immunity
Production of reactive oxygen intermediates, nitric oxide, increased lysosomal enzymes	Killing of microbes in phagolysosomes (effector function of macrophages)
Secretion of cytokines (TNF, IL-1, IL-12)	TNF, IL-1: leukocyte recruitment (inflammation) IL-12: T_H1 differentiation, IFN-γ production
Increased expression of B7 costimulators, MHC molecules	Increased T cell activation (amplification)

Figure 13–14 Activation and functions of macrophages in cell-mediated immunity. In cell-mediated immunity, macrophages are activated by CD40L-CD40 interactions and by IFN-γ and perform several functions that kill microbes, stimulate inflammation, and enhance the antigen-presenting capacity of the cells. Macrophages are also activated during innate immune reactions and perform the same functions (see Chapter 12, Fig. 12–5).

production. The requirement for CD40L-CD40 interactions for macrophage activation ensures that macrophages that are presenting antigens to the T cells (i.e., the macrophages that are harboring intracellular microbes) are also the macrophages that are most efficiently activated by the T cells. $CD8^+$ T cells can activate macrophages by the same mechanisms and with the same functional outcomes. In this case, the T cells recognize microbial antigens that are present in the cytosol of the antigen-presenting macrophages. In innate immune reactions, the same process of macrophage activation is triggered by microbial products such as LPS, which turn on some of the same biochemical pathways as CD40, and by IFN-γ secreted by NK cells (see Chapter 12).

Functions of Activated Macrophages

In response to CD40 signals and IFN-γ, production of several proteins in macrophages is increased. CD40 ligation activates the transcription factors NF-κB and AP-1, and IFN-γ activates the transcription factors STAT1 and IRF-1. As a result of these signals, activated macrophages produce increased amounts of the proteins that are responsible for the effector functions of these cells in CMI (see Fig. 13–14). The effector functions of activated macrophages include the following.

- ***Activated macrophages kill phagocytosed microbes, mainly by producing microbicidal reactive oxygen intermediates, nitric oxide, and lysosomal enzymes.*** The microbicidal mechanisms of macrophages were described in Chapter 12. To reiterate the key points, macrophage activation leads to increased synthesis of reactive oxygen intermediates and nitric oxide, which are potent microbicidal agents that are produced within the lysosomes of macrophages and kill ingested microbes. Activated macrophages contain increased amounts of lysosomal enzymes, which destroy phagocytosed microbes after phagosomes fuse with lysosomes. Reactive oxygen intermediates, nitric oxide, and lysosomal enzymes may also be released into adjacent tissue, where they kill extracellular microbes and may cause damage to normal tissue.

- Activated macrophages stimulate acute inflammation through the secretion of cytokines, mainly TNF, IL-1, and chemokines, and short-lived lipid mediators such as platelet-activating factor, prostaglandins, and leukotrienes. The collective action of these macrophage-derived cytokines and lipid mediators is to produce a local inflammation that is rich in neutrophils, which phagocytose and destroy infectious organisms.
- Activated macrophages (and neutrophils) remove dead tissues to facilitate repair after the infection is controlled. Activated macrophages also induce the formation of repair tissue by secreting growth factors that stimulate fibroblast proliferation (platelet-derived growth factor), collagen synthesis (transforming growth factor-β), and new blood vessel formation or angiogenesis (fibroblast growth factor). Thus, the activated macrophage acts as an endogenous surgeon to cauterize the wound and thereby eliminate antigen and resolve the inflammatory reaction.

Even though macrophages can respond directly to microbes in innate immune reactions, the ability of macrophages to kill ingested microorganisms is greatly enhanced by T cells. This is why CMI is able to eradicate microbes that have evolved to survive within macrophages in the absence of adaptive immunity. In addition to these effector functions, activated macrophages become more efficient APCs because of increased levels of molecules involved in antigen processing (such as components of the proteasome and cathepsins), increased surface expression of class II MHC molecules and costimulators, and production of cytokines (such as IL-12) that stimulate T lymphocyte proliferation and differentiation. These macrophage responses function to enhance T cell activation, thus serving as amplification mechanisms for CMI.

Some tissue injury may normally accompany cell-mediated immune reactions to microbes because the microbicidal products released by activated macrophages and neutrophils are capable of injuring normal tissue and do not discriminate between microbes and host tissue. However, this tissue injury is usually limited in extent and duration, and it resolves as the infection is cleared. If the activated macrophages fail to eradicate the infection, they continue to produce cytokines and growth factors, which progressively modify the local tissue environment. As a result, tissue injury is followed by replacement with connective tissue (fibrosis), and fibrosis is a hallmark of chronic DTH reactions. In chronic DTH reactions, activated macrophages also undergo changes in response to persistent cytokine signals. These macrophages develop increased cytoplasm and cytoplasmic organelles and histologically may resemble skin epithelial cells, because of which they are sometimes called epithelioid

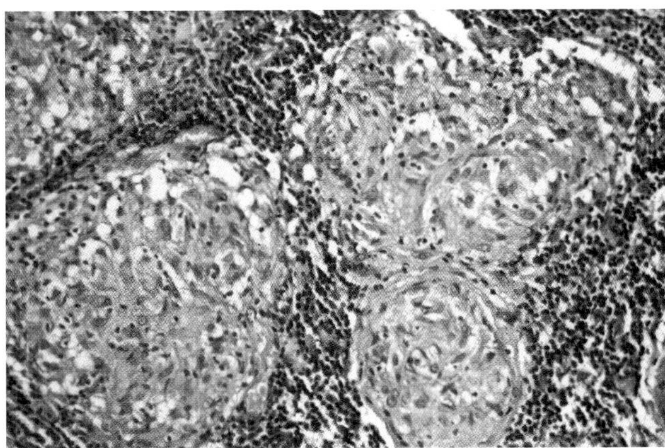

Figure 13–15 Granulomatous inflammation. Histopathologic examination of a lymph node shows a granuloma with activated macrophages and lymphocytes. In some granulomas, there may be a central area of necrosis. Immunohistochemical studies would identify the lymphocytes as T cells. This type of inflammation is a chronic delayed-type hypersensitivity reaction against persistent microbial and other antigens. (Courtesy of Dr. Henry Sanchez, Department of Pathology, UCSF School of Medicine, San Francisco.)

cells. Activated macrophages may fuse to form multinucleate giant cells. Clusters of activated macrophages, often surrounding particulate sources of antigen, produce nodules of inflammatory tissue called granulomas (Fig. 13–15). Granulomatous inflammation is a characteristic response to some persistent microbes, such as *M. tuberculosis* and some fungi, and represents a form of chronic DTH. Granulomatous inflammation is frequently associated with tissue fibrosis. Although fibrosis is normally a "healing reaction" to injury, it can also interfere with normal tissue function. In fact, much of the respiratory difficulty associated with tuberculosis or chronic fungal infection of the lung is caused by replacement of normal lung with fibrotic tissue and not directly attributable to the microbes.

Role of T_H2 Cells and Eosinophils in Defense Against Helminths

T_H2 cells induce inflammatory reactions that are dominated by eosinophils and mast cells (see Fig. 13–10). This type of immune response functions to eliminate helminthic infections and may play a role in defense against some ectoparasites. Helminths are too large to be phagocytosed and may be more resistant to the microbicidal activities of macrophages than are most bacteria and viruses. The immune response to helminths consists largely of T_H2 cells, which secrete IL-4, IL-5, and IL-13. IL-4 (and IL-13) stimulates the production of helminth-specific IgE antibodies, which opsonize the helminths. IL-5 activates eosinophils, which bind to the IgE-coated helminths by virtue of Fc receptors specific for the ε heavy chain. Activated eosinophils release their granule contents, including major basic protein and major cationic protein, which are capable of destroying even the tough integuments of helminths. Mast cells also express Fcε receptors and react to IgE-associated antigens by degranulating. The granule contents of mast cells include vasoactive amines, cytokines such as TNF, and lipid mediators that induce local inflammation. We will return to the pathologic consequences of T_H2-mediated inflammatory reactions in Chapter 19, when we discuss immediate hypersensitivity diseases.

T_H2 cells also inhibit CMI by the actions of cytokines that suppress macrophage activation. This role of T_H2 cells is mediated by the secretion of IL-4 and IL-13, which are antagonists of IFN-γ and therefore block T cell–mediated macrophage activation, and by the secretion of IL-10, which is a direct inhibitor of macrophage activation.

Mechanisms of CTL-Mediated Killing of Infected Cells

Intracellular microbes that find a haven outside phagosomes, and in nonphagocytic cells, cannot be eliminated by T cell–mediated activation of phagocytes. The only way to eradicate established infections by such microbes is to kill the infected cells, and this is the function of CTLs. Cell killing by CTLs is antigen specific and contact dependent. CTLs kill targets that express the same class I–associated antigen that triggered the proliferation and differentiation of pre-CTLs and do not kill adjacent uninfected cells that do not express this antigen. In fact, even the CTLs themselves are not injured during the killing of antigen-expressing targets. This specificity of CTL effector function ensures that normal cells are not killed by CTLs reacting against infected cells. This highly specific killing occurs because CTL activity is triggered by physical contact with their targets and is directed toward the targets.

The process of CTL-mediated killing of targets consists of antigen recognition, activation of the CTLs, delivery of the "lethal hit" that kills the target cells, and release of the CTLs (Fig. 13–16). Each of these steps is controlled by specific proteins and molecular interactions.

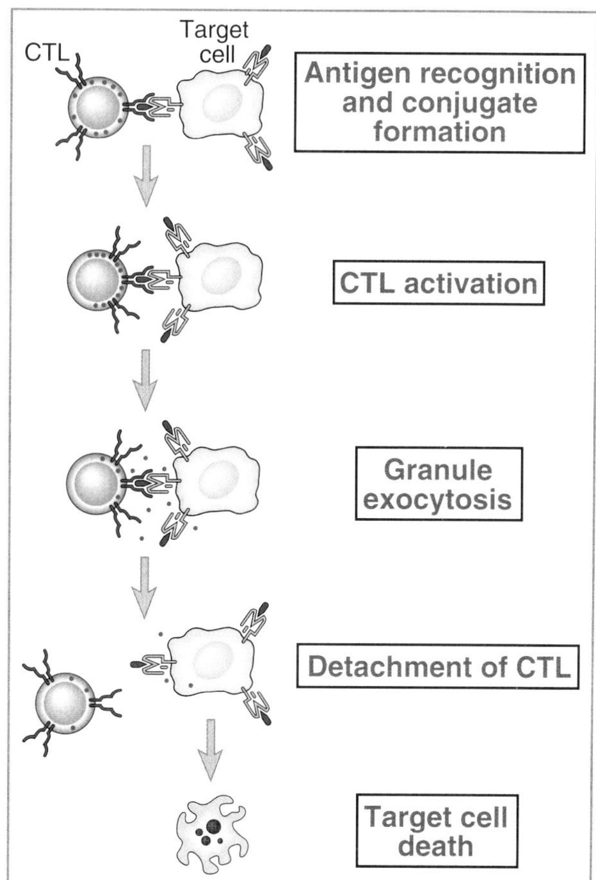

Figure 13–16 Steps in CTL-mediated lysis of target cells. A CTL recognizes the antigen-expressing target cell and is activated. Activation results in the release of granule contents from the CTL, which delivers a lethal hit to the target. The CTL may detach and kill another target cell while the first target goes on to die. Note that formation of conjugates between a CTL and its target and activation of the CTL also require interactions between accessory molecules (LFA-1, CD8) on the CTL and their specific ligands on the target cell; these are not shown.

Recognition of Antigen and Activation of CTLs

The CTL binds to the target cell by using its antigen receptor and accessory molecules, such as CD8 and the LFA-1 integrin. To be efficiently recognized by CTLs, target cells must express class I MHC molecules complexed to a peptide (the complex serving as the ligand for the T cell receptor and the CD8 coreceptor) and intercellular adhesion molecule-1 (the principal ligand for LFA-1).

- Conjugates of CTLs attached to target cells can be visualized by microscopy, and conjugate formation is the prelude to target cell lysis (Fig. 13–17).
- Antibodies that block any of these interactions inhibit CTL-mediated lysis *in vitro,* thus indicating that all these interactions function cooperatively in the process of CTL recognition of targets.

In the CTL–target cell conjugate, the antigen receptors of the CTL recognize MHC-associated peptides on the target cell. This recognition induces clustering of T cell receptors into a synapse and generates biochemical signals that activate the CTL. The biochemical signals are similar to the signals involved in the activation of helper T cells (see Chapter 8). Costimulators and cytokines, which are required for the differentiation of naive $CD8^+$ T cells into active CTLs, are not necessary for triggering the effector function of CTLs (i.e., target cell killing). Therefore, once $CD8^+$ T cells specific for an antigen have differentiated into fully functional CTLs, they can kill any nucleated cell that displays that antigen.

Killing of Target Cells by CTLs

Within a few minutes of a CTL's recognizing its target, the target cell undergoes changes that induce it to die

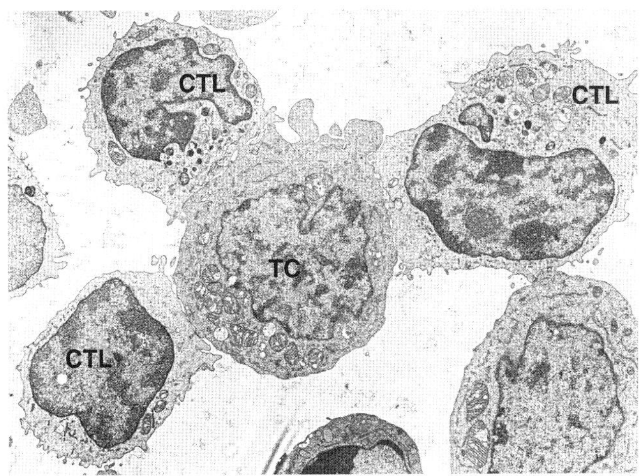

Figure 13–17 Conjugate formation between CTLs and a target cell.
Three CTLs from a cloned cell line specific for the human MHC molecule HLA-A2 bind to an HLA-A2–expressing target cell (TC) within 1 minute after the CTLs and targets are mixed. Note that in the CTL on the upper left, the granules have been redistributed toward the target cell. (Courtesy of Dr. P. Peters, Netherlands Cancer Institute, Amsterdam.)

by apoptosis. Target cell death occurs during the next 2 to 6 hours and proceeds even if the CTL detaches. Thus, the CTL is said to deliver a lethal hit to the target that results in cytolysis.

The principal mechanism of CTL-mediated cytolysis is the delivery of cytotoxic granule proteins to the target cell that is recognized by the CTL (Fig. 13–18). When the antigen receptors of the CTL recognize MHC-associated peptides on the target cell, the cytoskeleton of the CTL is reorganized such that the microtubule organizing center of the CTL moves to the area of the cytoplasm near the contact with the target cell. The cytoplasmic granules of the CTL become concentrated in this same region, and the granule membrane fuses with the plasma membrane. Membrane fusion results in exocytosis of the CTL's granule contents onto the surface of the target cell.

The two granule proteins that are the most important for CTL killing function are **perforin** and **granzymes.** Perforin is a pore-forming protein that is present as a monomer in the granules of CTLs (and NK cells). When it is exocytosed from the granules, the per-

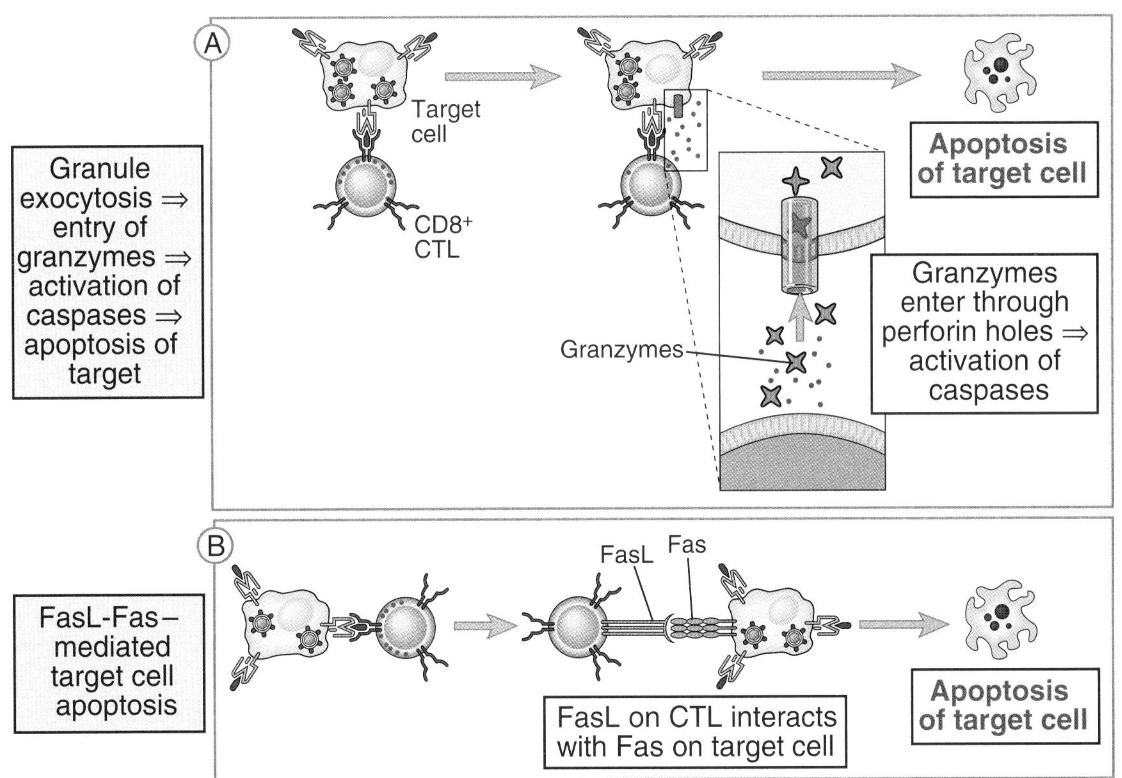

Figure 13–18 Mechanisms of CTL-mediated lysis of target cells.
CTLs kill target cells by two main mechanisms.
A. Perforin is exocytosed in CTL granules and polymerizes in the target cell plasma membrane to form pores. Granzymes are also exocytosed in CTL granules, enter target cells through the perforin pores, and induce target cell apoptosis.
B. Fas ligand (FasL) is expressed on activated CTLs, engages Fas on the surface of target cells, and induces apoptosis.

forin monomer comes into contact with high extracellular concentrations of calcium (typically 1 to 2 mM) and undergoes polymerization. Polymerization of perforin preferentially occurs in the lipid bilayer of the target cell plasma membrane, and here the polymerized perforin forms an aqueous channel. Granzymes (granule enzymes) are serine proteases that enter the target cell through these channels. Granzyme B, the most important of these enzymes, proteolytically cleaves and thereby activates cellular enzymes called caspases (see Chapter 10, Box 10–2), which in turn cleave several substrates and induce target cell apoptosis. In addition, if a sufficient number of perforin pores is created in the target cell membrane, the cell will be unable to exclude ions and water. The target cell dies partly because the influx of water induces osmotic swelling and partly because the high concentration of calcium ion that enters the cell may trigger apoptosis. This mechanism of cell killing is analogous to that used by the membrane attack complex of complement, and perforin is structurally homologous to the ninth component of complement, the principal constituent of the membrane attack complex (see Chapter 14).

CTLs use another mechanism of killing that is mediated by interactions of membrane molecules on the CTLs and target cells. On activation, CTLs express a membrane protein, called **Fas ligand (FasL),** that binds to its target protein Fas, which is expressed on many cell types. This interaction also results in activation of caspases and apoptosis of targets (Chapter 10, Box 10–2). Studies with knockout mice lacking perforin, granzyme B, or FasL indicate that granule proteins are the principal mediators of killing by $CD8^+$ CTLs. Some $CD4^+$ T cells are also capable of killing target cells (which, of course, must express class II MHC–associated peptides to be recognized by the $CD4^+$ cells). $CD4^+$ T cells are deficient in perforin and granzymes, and FasL may be more important for their killing activity.

In infections by intracellular microbes, the killing activity of CTLs is important for eradicating the reservoir of infection. In addition, the caspases that are activated in target cells by granzymes and FasL cleave many substrates, including nucleoproteins, and activate enzymes that degrade DNA, but they do not distinguish between host and microbial proteins. Therefore, by activating an apoptotic death pathway in target cells, CTLs can initiate the destruction of microbial DNA as well as the target cell genome, thereby eliminating potentially infectious DNA. Another protein found in human CTL (and NK cell) granules, called granulysin, can alter the permeability of target cell and microbial membranes.

After delivering the lethal hit, the CTL is released from its target cell, a process that may be facilitated by decreases in the affinity of accessory molecules for their ligands. This release usually occurs even before the target cell goes on to die. CTLs themselves are not injured during target cell killing. The probable reason for CTLs not being injured is that the directed granule exocytosis process during CTL-mediated killing preferentially delivers granule contents into the target cell and away from the CTL.

Summary

- CMI is the adaptive immune response against intracellular microbes. It is mediated by T lymphocytes and can be transferred from immunized to naive individuals by T cells and not by antibodies.
- There are two main forms of cell-mediated immune reactions. In one, which is exemplified by DTH reactions, $CD4^+$ T_H1 cells, as well as $CD8^+$ T cells, recognize antigens of microbes that have been ingested by phagocytes and activate the phagocytes to kill the microbes. In the second type of CMI, $CD8^+$ CTLs kill any nucleated cell that contains foreign antigens (microbial or tumor antigens) in the cytosol.
- Cell-mediated immune reactions consist of several steps: naive T cell recognition of cell-associated antigens in peripheral lymphoid organs, clonal expansion of the T cells and their differentiation into effector cells, migration of the effector T cells to the site of infection or antigen challenge, and elimination of the microbe or antigen.
- $CD4^+$ helper T lymphocytes may differentiate into specialized effector T_H1 cells that secrete IFN-γ, which favors phagocyte-mediated immunity, or into T_H2 cells that secrete IL-4 and IL-5, which favor IgE- and eosinophil/mast cell–mediated immune reactions. The differentiation of naive $CD4^+$ T cells into T_H1 and T_H2 populations is controlled by cytokines produced by APCs and by the T cells themselves.
- $CD8^+$ T lymphocytes differentiate into effector CTLs, acquiring the capacity to kill targets, under the influence of costimulators and help from $CD4^+$ T cells.
- The migration of T cells to sites of infection is mediated by chemokines and by the binding of adhesion molecules to their ligands on activated endothelium.
- The activation of macrophages by T_H1 cells is mediated by IFN-γ and CD40L-CD40 interactions. Activated macrophages kill phagocytosed microbes, stimulate inflammation, and repair damaged tissues. If the infection is not fully resolved, activated macrophages cause tissue injury and fibrosis.
- $CD8^+$ CTLs kill cells that express peptides derived from cytosolic antigens (e.g., viral antigens) that are presented in association with class I MHC molecules. CTL-mediated killing is mediated mainly by granule exocytosis, which releases perforin, a membrane pore-forming protein that forms pores in the target cell membrane, and granzymes, which enter the target cell through the perforin channel and induce apoptotic death of the target cell. CTLs also express FasL, which engages Fas on the target cell membrane and triggers apoptosis of the target cell.

Selected Readings

Boehm U, T Klamp, M Groot, and JC Howard. Cellular responses to interferon-gamma. Annual Review of Immunology 15:749–795, 1997.

Butcher EC, M Williams, K Youngman, I Roitt, and M Briskin. Lymphocyte trafficking and regional immunity. Advances in Immunology 72:209–253, 1999.

Grewal IS, and RA Flavell. CD40 and CD154 in cell-mediated immunity. Annual Review of Immunology 16:111–135, 1998.

Heath WR, and FR Carbone. Cross-presentation, dendritic cells, tolerance, and immunity. Annual Review of Immunology 19:47–64, 2001.

Kunkel EJ, and EC Butcher. Chemokines and the tissue-specific migration of lymphocytes. Immunity 16:1–4, 2002.

Murphy KM, W Ouyang, JD Farrar, J Yang, S Ranganath, H Asnagli, M Afkarian, and TL Murphy. Signaling and transcription in T helper development. Annual Review of Immunology 18:451–494, 2000.

O'Garra A. Cytokines induce the development of functionally heterogeneous T helper cell subsets. Immunity 8:275–283, 1998.

Oxenius A, RM Zinkernagel, and H Hengartner. $CD4^+$ T cell induction and effector functions: a comparison of immunity against soluble antigens and viral infections. Advances in Immunology 70:313–367, 1998.

Romagnani S. The Th1/Th2 paradigm. Immunology Today 18:263–267, 1997.

Russell JH, and TJ Ley. Lymphocyte-mediated cytotoxicity. Annual Review of Immunology 20:323–370, 2002.

Von Andrian UH, and CR Mackay. T-cell function and migration. New England Journal of Medicine 343:1020–1034, 2000.

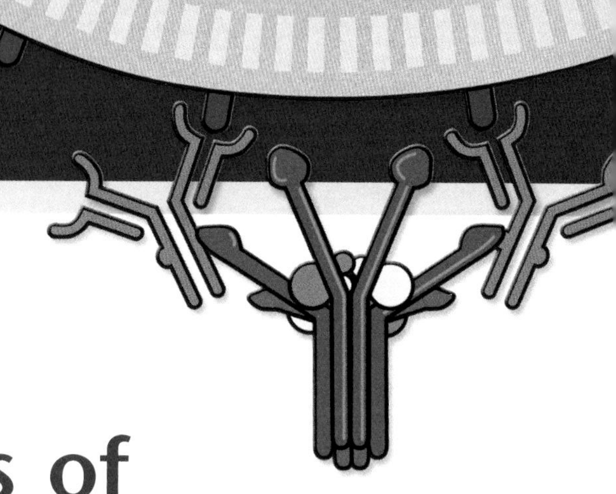

Chapter 14

Effector Mechanisms of Humoral Immunity

Humoral immunity is mediated by secreted antibodies, and its physiologic function is defense against extracellular microbes and microbial toxins. This type of immunity contrasts with cell-mediated immunity, the other effector arm of the adaptive immune system, which is mediated by T lymphocytes and functions to eradicate microbes that infect and live within host cells (see Chapter 13). Humoral immunity against microbial toxins was discovered in the early 1900s as a form of immunity that could be transferred from immunized to naive individuals by serum. The types of microbes that are combated by humoral immunity are extracellular bacteria, fungi, and even obligate intracellular microbes such as viruses, which are targets of antibodies before they infect cells or when they are released from infected cells. Defects in antibody production result in increased susceptibility to infection with extracellular microbes, notably bacteria and fungi. In this chapter, we discuss the effector mechanisms that are used by antibodies to eliminate antigens. The structure of antibodies is described in Chapter 3 and the process of antibody production in Chapter 9.

Overview of Humoral Immunity

The effector functions of antibodies are the neutralization and elimination of infectious microbes and microbial toxins (Fig. 14–1). As we shall see later, antibody-mediated elimination of antigens requires the participation of other effector systems, including phagocytes and complement proteins. Before these individual effector mechanisms are described, it is useful to summarize the important general features of the effector functions of antibodies.

- ***Antibodies are produced by B lymphocytes and plasma cells in the lymphoid organs and bone marrow, but antibodies perform their effector functions at sites distant from their production.*** Antibodies enter mucosal secretions, where they provide defense against ingested and inhaled microbes, and

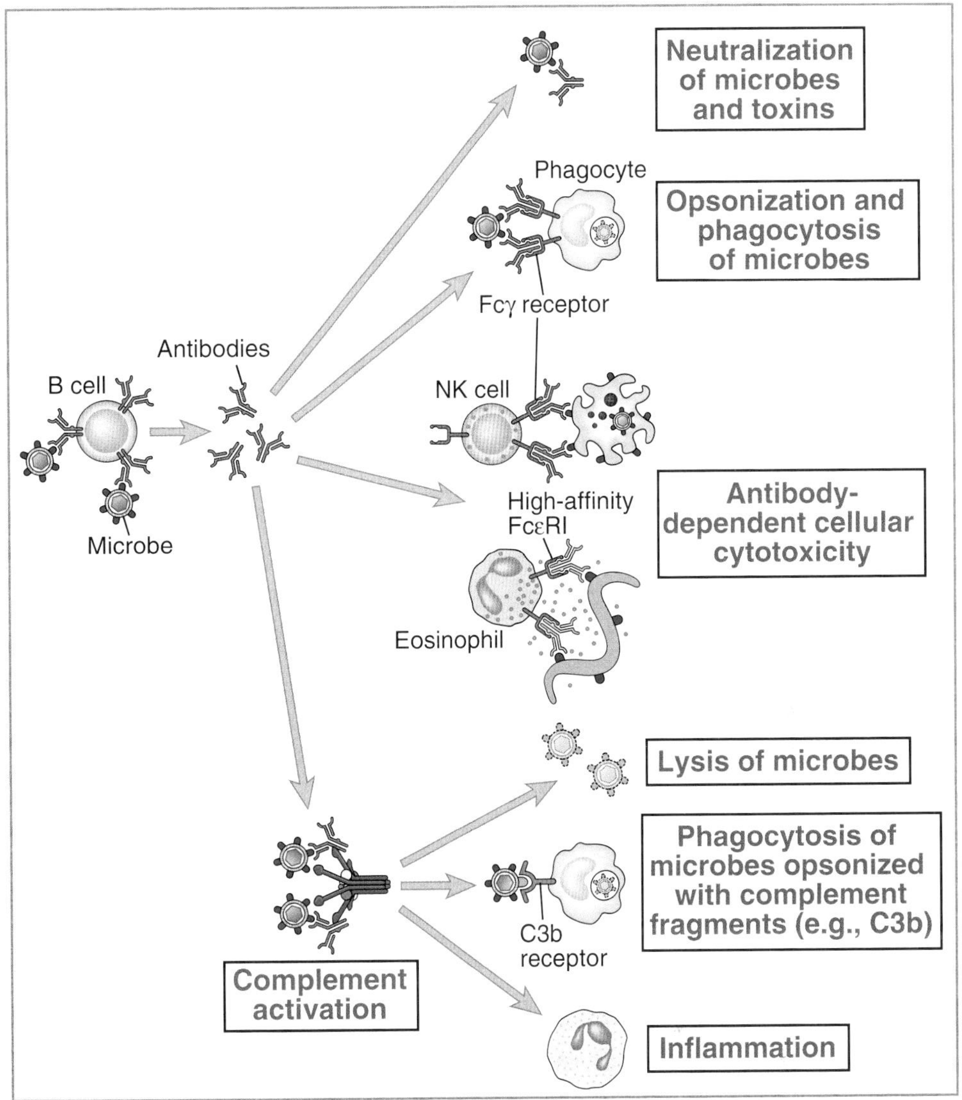

Figure 14–1 Effector functions of antibodies.
Antibodies against microbes (and their toxins, not shown here) neutralize these agents, opsonize them for phagocytosis and antibody-dependent cellular cytotoxicity, and activate the complement system. These various effector functions may be mediated by different antibody isotypes.

the blood, from which they are able to circulate to any site where antigen is located. Therefore, the effector phase of humoral immunity is systemic, even though the initial recognition and activation phases occur in the spleen, lymph nodes, and mucosal lymphoid tissue. Antibodies are also actively transported across the placenta into the circulation of the developing fetus. In cell-mediated immunity, activated T lymphocytes are able to migrate to peripheral sites of infection and inflammation, but they are not transported into mucosal secretions or across the placenta.

- ***The antibodies that mediate protective immunity may be derived from long-lived antibody-producing plasma cells generated by previous antigen exposure and, in secondary immune responses, by the activation of memory B cells*** (see Chapter 9, Fig. 9–2). The first exposure to a microbe or antigen, either by infection or by vaccination, leads to the activation of naive B lymphocytes and their differentiation into antibody-producing cells and memory cells. Some of the antibody-producing cells migrate to the bone marrow and live in this site, where they continue to produce antibodies for years after the antigen is eliminated. It is estimated that more than half the IgG found in the serum of normal individuals is derived from these long-lived antibody-producing cells, which were induced by exposure to various antigens throughout the life of the individual. If a previously immunized individual encounters the antigen, such as a microbe, the level of circulating antibody produced by the persisting antibody-producing cells provides immediate protection against the infection. At the same time, the antigen activates long-lived memory B cells, which generates a larger burst of antibody that provides the second and more effective wave of protection.

- ***Many of the effector functions of antibodies are mediated by the heavy chain constant regions of immunoglobulin (Ig) molecules, and different Ig heavy chain isotypes serve distinct effector functions*** (Table 14–1). For instance, some IgG subclasses bind to phagocyte Fc receptors and promote the phagocytosis of antibody-coated particles, IgM

Table 14–1. Functions of Antibody Isotypes

Antibody isotope	Isotype-specific effector functions
IgG	Opsonization of antigens for phagocytosis by macrophages and neutrophils Activation of the classical pathway of complement Antibody-dependent cell-mediated cytotoxicity mediated by natural killer cells and macrophages Neonatal immunity: transfer of maternal antibody across the placenta and gut Feedback inhibition of B cell activation
IgM	Activation of the classical pathway of complement Antigen receptor of naive B lymphocytes*
IgA	Mucosal immunity: secretion of IgA into the lumens of the gastrointestinal and respiratory tracts
IgE	Antibody-dependent cell-mediated cytotoxicity involving eosinophils Mast cell degranulation (immediate hypersensitivity reactions)
IgD	Antigen receptor of naive B lymphocytes*

*These functions are mediated by membrane-bound and not secreted antibodies.

and some IgG antibodies activate the complement system, and IgE binds to the Fc receptors of mast cells and eosinophils and triggers their activation. Each of these effector mechanisms will be discussed later in the chapter. The humoral immune system is specialized in such a way that different microbes or antigen exposures stimulate B cell switching to the Ig isotypes that are best for combating these microbes. The major stimuli for isotype switching during the process of B cell activation are helper T cell–derived cytokines together with CD40 ligand expressed by helper T cells (see Chapter 9). Different types of microbes stimulate the development of helper T cells, such as T_H1 and T_H2 subsets, that produce distinct sets of cytokines and therefore induce switching of B cells to different heavy chain isotypes. For instance, viruses and many bacteria stimulate the production of T_H1-dependent IgG isotypes that bind to phagocytes and NK (natural killer) cells and activate complement, whereas helminthic parasites stimulate the production of T_H2-dependent IgE antibody, which binds to and activates eosinophils. Phagocytes, NK cells, and complement are effective at eliminating many viruses and bacteria, and eosinophils are especially potent in destroying helminths. Neutralization is the only function of antibodies that is mediated entirely by binding of antigen and does not require participation of the Ig constant regions.

- ***Although many effector functions of antibodies are mediated by the Ig heavy chain constant regions, all these functions are triggered by the binding of antigens to the variable regions.*** The binding of antibodies to multiple copies of an antigen brings the Fc regions of antibodies close together, and this leads to complement activation and enhanced interactions of the antibodies with Fc receptors on phagocytes. The requirement for antigen binding ensures that antibodies activate various effector mechanisms only when they are needed, that is, when the antibodies encounter and specifically bind antigens, not when the antibodies are circulating in an antigen-free form.

With this introduction to humoral immunity, we proceed to a discussion of the various functions of antibodies in host defense.

Neutralization of Microbes and Microbial Toxins

Antibodies against microbes and microbial toxins block the binding of these microbes and toxins to cellular receptors (Fig. 14–2). In this way, antibodies inhibit, or "neutralize," the infectivity of microbes as well as the potential injurious effects of infection. Many microbes enter host cells by the binding of particular surface molecules to proteins of host cells. For example, influenza viruses use their envelope hemagglutinin to infect respiratory epithelial cells, and gram-negative bacteria use pili to attach to and infect a variety of host cells. Antibodies that bind to these microbial structures interfere with the ability of the microbes to interact with cellular receptors; these are examples of steric hindrance. In some cases, very few antibody molecules may bind to a microbe and induce conformational changes in surface molecules that prevent the microbe from interacting with cellular receptors; such interactions are examples of the allosteric effects of antibodies. Many microbial toxins mediate their pathologic effects also by binding to specific cellular receptors. For instance, tetanus toxin binds to receptors in the motor end plate of neuromuscular junctions and inhibits neuromuscular transmission, which leads to paralysis, and diphtheria toxin binds to cellular receptors and enters various cells, where it inhibits protein synthesis. Antitoxin antibodies sterically hinder the interactions of toxins with host cells and prevent the toxins from causing tissue injury and disease.

Antibody-mediated neutralization of microbes and toxins requires only the antigen-binding regions of the antibodies. Therefore, such neutralization may be mediated by antibodies of any isotype in the circulation and in mucosal secretions and can experimentally also

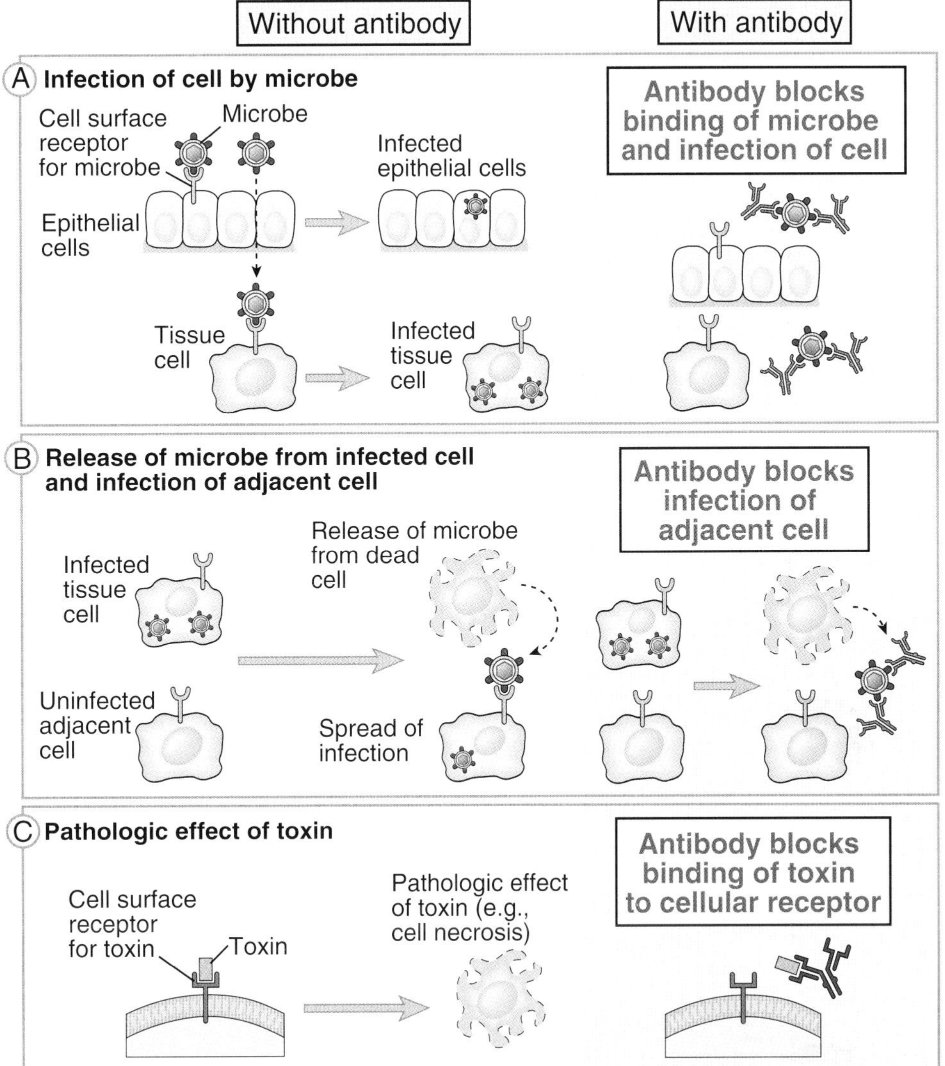

Figure 14–2 Neutralization of microbes and toxins by antibodies.

A. Antibodies prevent the binding of microbes to cells and thus block the ability of the microbes to infect host cells.

B. Antibodies inhibit the spread of microbes from an infected cell to an adjacent uninfected cell.

C. Antibodies block the binding of toxins to cells and thus inhibit the pathologic effects of the toxins.

be mediated by Fab or $F(ab')_2$ fragments of specific antibodies. Most neutralizing antibodies in the blood are of the IgG isotype; in mucosal organs, they are of the IgA isotype. The most effective neutralizing antibodies are those with high affinities for their antigens. High-affinity antibodies are produced by the process of affinity maturation (see Chapter 9). Many prophylactic vaccines work by stimulating the production of high-affinity neutralizing antibodies (Table 14–2). A mechanism that microbes have developed to evade host immunity is to mutate the surface antigens that are the targets of neutralizing antibodies (see Chapter 15).

Antibody-Mediated Opsonization and Phagocytosis

Antibodies of the IgG isotype coat (opsonize) microbes and promote their phagocytosis by binding to Fc receptors on phagocytes. Mononuclear phagocytes and neutrophils ingest microbes as a prelude to intracellular killing and degradation. These phagocytes express a variety of surface receptors that directly bind microbes and ingest them, even without antibodies, providing one mechanism of innate immunity (see Chapter 12). The efficiency of this process is markedly enhanced if the phagocyte can bind the particle with high affinity (Fig. 14–3). Mononuclear phagocytes and neutrophils express receptors for the Fc portions of IgG antibodies that specifically bind antibody-coated (opsonized) particles. Microbes may also be opsonized by a product of complement activation called C3b and are phagocytosed by binding to a leukocyte receptor for C3b. This process is described later in the chapter. The process of coating particles for phagocytosis is called **opsonization**, and substances that perform this function, including antibodies and complement proteins, are called specific opsonins.

Phagocyte Fc Receptors

Leukocyte Fc receptors promote the phagocytosis of opsonized particles and deliver signals that stimulate the microbicidal activities of the leukocytes. Fc recep-

Table 14–2. Vaccine-Induced Humoral Immunity

Infectious disease	Vaccine	Mechanism of protective immunity
Polio	Oral attenuated polio virus	Neutralization of virus by mucosal IgA antibody
Tetanus, diphtheria	Toxoids	Neutralization of toxin by systemic IgG antibody
Hepatitis, A or B	Recombinant viral envelope proteins	Neutralization of virus by systemic IgG antibody
Pneumococcal pneumonia, *Haemophilus*	Conjugate vaccines composed of bacterial capsular polysaccharide and protein	Opsonization and phagocytosis mediated by IgM and IgG antibodies, directly or secondary to complement activation

Selected examples of vaccines that work by stimulating protective humoral immunity are listed.

tors for different Ig heavy chain isotypes are expressed on many leukocyte populations and serve diverse functions in immunity (Box 14–1). Of these Fc receptors, the ones that are most important for phagocytosis of opsonized particles are receptors for the heavy chains of IgG antibodies, called Fcγ receptors. There are three types of Fcγ receptors, which have different affinities for the heavy chains of different IgG subclasses and are expressed on different cell types. The major high-affinity phagocyte Fcγ receptor is called FcγRI (CD64). It binds human IgG1 and IgG3 strongly, with a K_d of 10^{-8} to 10^{-9} M. (In mice, the high-affinity FcγRI receptor preferentially binds IgG2a and IgG2b antibodies.) FcγRI is composed of an Fc-binding α chain expressed in association with a disulfide-linked homodimer of a signaling protein called the FcR γ chain, which is homologous to the signal-transducing ζ chain of the T cell receptor (TCR) complex. The FcR γ chain, like the TCR ζ chain, contains immunoreceptor tyrosine-based activation motifs (ITAMs) in its cytoplasmic portion and is required for signal transduction and surface expression of the complete Fc receptor.

Phagocytosis of IgG-coated particles is mediated by binding of the Fc portions of opsonizing antibodies to Fcγ receptors on phagocytes. Therefore, the IgG subtypes that bind best to these receptors (IgG1 and IgG3) are the most efficient opsonins for promoting phagocytosis. Antibody molecules attached to the surface of a microbe or macromolecular antigen form multivalent arrays and are bound by phagocyte Fc receptors with much higher avidity than are free circulating antibodies. For this reason, FcγRI binds antibodies attached to antigens better than it binds free antibodies. Sequential binding of Fc receptors to antibody-coated particles leads to engulfment of the particles and their

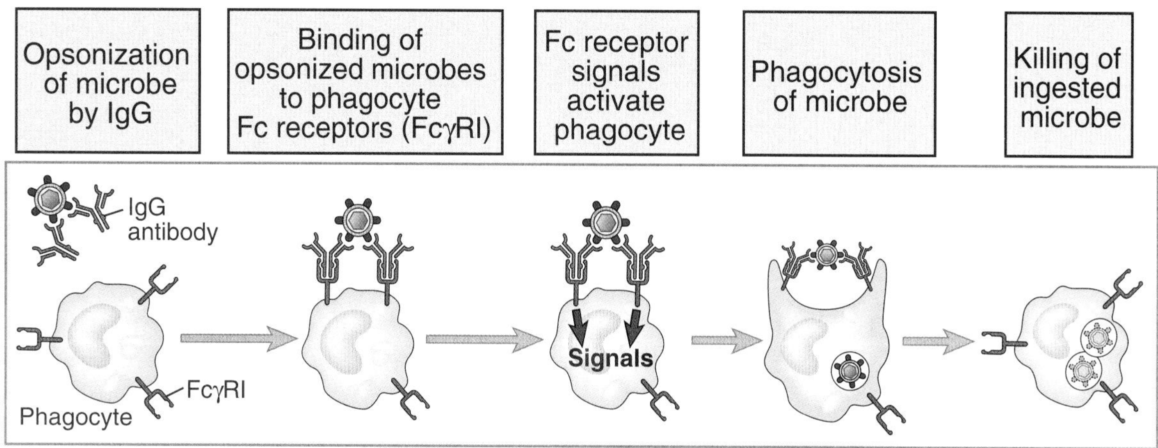

Figure 14–3 Antibody-mediated opsonization and phagocytosis of microbes. Antibodies of certain IgG subclasses bind to microbes and are then recognized by Fc receptors on phagocytes. Signals from the Fc receptors promote the phagocytosis of the opsonized microbes and activate the phagocytes to destroy these microbes.

BOX 14–1

Leukocyte Fc Receptors

Leukocytes express cell surface receptors that specifically bind the Fc portions of various Ig isotypes and subtypes. The Fc receptors on neutrophils and macrophages mediate the phagocytosis of opsonized particles and the activation of leukocytes to destroy phagocytosed particles. Fc receptors on NK cells are involved in activation of these cells to kill antibody-coated target cells. Fc receptors on B cells negatively regulate antibody responses. Two non-leukocyte Fc receptors are expressed on epithelial cells and mediate transepithelial transport of antibodies. Here we discuss the specific Fc receptors of leukocytes that mediate functional responses, namely, FcγRI, FcγRII, FcγRIII, FcεRI, FcεRII, and FcαR (see Table).

Each of the leukocyte FcRs contains one Fc-binding polypeptide chain, called the α chain, which is a member of the Ig superfamily. Differences in specificities or affinities of each FcR for the various IgG isotypes are based on differences in the structure of these α chains. In all the FcRs except FcγRII, the α chain is associated with one or more additional polypeptide chains involved in signal transduction, called β and γ chains (see Figure). Signaling functions of FcγRII are mediated by the cytoplasmic tail of the α chain.

There are three distinct types of Fcγ receptors, which have different affinities for heavy chains of different IgG subclasses. The major phagocyte Fcγ receptor, FcγRI (CD64), is expressed on macrophages and neutrophils and is a high-affinity receptor for IgG1 and IgG3 (in humans). The large extracellular amino terminal region of the receptor polypeptide folds into three tandem Ig-like domains. The Fc-binding α chain of FcγRI is associated with a disulfide-linked homodimer of a signaling protein called the FcR γ chain. This γ chain is also found in the signaling complexes associated with FcγRIII, FcαR, and FcεRI. The γ chain has only a short extracellular amino terminus but a large cytoplasmic carboxyl terminus, with structural homology to the ζ chain of the TCR complex. Like the TCR ζ chain, the FcR γ chain contains an immunoreceptor tyrosine-based activation motif (ITAM) that couples receptor clustering to activation of protein tyrosine kinases. Transcription of the FcγRI gene is stimulated by the macrophage-activating cytokine IFN-γ, and for this reason activated macrophages express higher levels of the receptor than do resting monocytes.

Both humans and mice express two different classes of low-affinity receptors for IgG, called FcγRII (CD32) and FcγRIII (CD16). FcγRII is expressed on phagocytes and other cell types and binds human IgG subtypes (IgG1 and IgG3) with sufficiently low affinity (K_d 10^{-6}M) that monomeric IgG molecules are unable to occupy this receptor at physiologic antibody concentrations. Therefore, FcγRII binds IgG mainly when the antibody is in immune complexes or on opsonized microbes or cells, which display arrays of Fc regions. In humans, there are three different isoforms of FcγRII (called A, B and C) that arise from alternative RNA splicing. These isoforms have similar intracellular domains and ligand specificities but differ in cytoplasmic tail structure, cell distribution, and functions.

FcR	Affinity for immunoglobulin	Cell distribution	Function
FcγRI (CD64)	High (K_d ~ 10^{-9} M); binds IgG1 and IgG3, can bind monomeric IgG	Macrophages, neutrophils; also eosinophils	Phagocytosis; activation of phagocytes
FcγRIIA (CD32)	Low (K_d > 10^{-7} M)	Macrophages, neutrophils; eosinophils, platelets	Phagocytosis; cell activation (inefficient)
FcγRIIB (CD32)	Low (K_d > 10^{-7} M)	B lymphocytes	Feedback inhibition of B cells
FcγRIIIA (CD16)	Low (K_d > 10^{-6} M)	NK cells	Antibody-dependent cell-mediated cytotoxicity
FcγRIIIB (CD16)	Low (K_d > 10^{-6} M); GPI-linked protein	Neutrophils, other cells	Phagocytosis (inefficient)
FcεRI	High (K_d > 10^{-10} M); binds monomeric IgE	Mast cells, basophils, eosinophils	Cell activation (degranulation)
FcεRII (CD23)	Low (K_d > 10^{-7} M)	B lymphocytes, eosinophils, Langerhans cells	Unknown
FcαR (CD89)	Low (K_d > 10^{-6} M)	Neutrophils, eosinophils, monocytes	Cell activation?

Continued on following page

BOX 14–1

Leukocyte Fc Receptors (*Continued*)

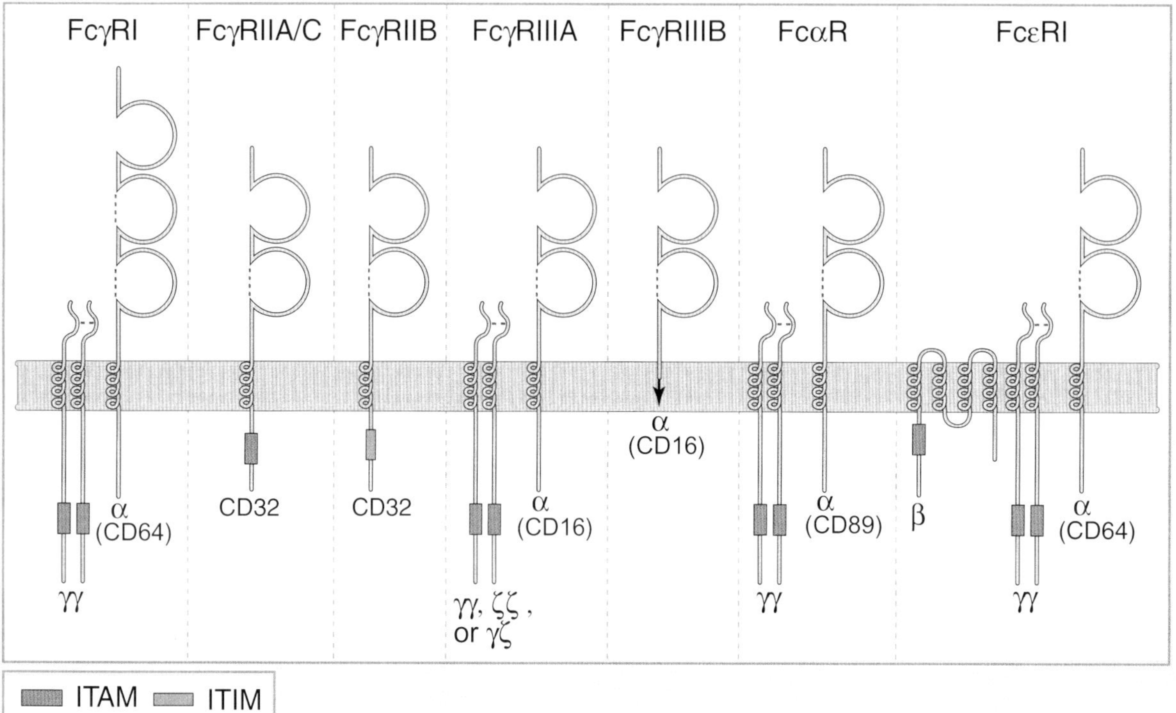

Subunit composition of Fc receptors.
Schematic models of the different human Fc receptors illustrate the Fc-binding α chains and the signaling subunits.

FcγRIIA is expressed by neutrophils and mononuclear phagocytes and probably participates in the phagocytosis of opsonized particles. FcγRIIA is also expressed by certain vascular endothelia and other cell types in which its function is unknown; it may play a role in the binding of molecules other than Ig, such as lipoproteins. The carboxyl termini of FcγRIIA and FcγRIIC contain ITAMs and, on clustering by IgG1- or IgG3-coated particles or cells, can deliver an activation signal to phagocytes. FcγRIIB is expressed exclusively by lymphocytes, especially B cells. The intracellular carboxyl terminus of this isoform contains an immunoreceptor tyrosine-based inhibition motif (ITIM) that can deliver inhibitory signals, counteracting the positive signals delivered to B cells by the antigen-induced cross-linking of membrane Ig. Thus, FcγRIIB clustering, induced by occupancy with polyvalent IgG1 or IgG3, may shut off B cell activation (see Chapter 9, Fig. 9–19).

The extracellular ligand-binding portion of FcγRIII (CD16) is similar to FcγRII in structure and affinity and specificity for IgG. Two separate genes code for this molecule in humans. The FcγRIIIA isoform, the product of the A gene, is a transmembrane protein expressed mainly on NK cells. FcγRIIIA associates with homodimers of the FcR γ chain, homodimers of the TCR ζ chain, or heterodimers composed of the FcR γ chain and the ζ chain. This association is necessary for cell surface expression and, through the ITAMs in these signaling chains, can deliver intracellular activating signals. Receptor clustering induced by occupancy with IgG1 or IgG3 bound to a target cell surface activates NK cells to kill the targets, thereby mediating antibody-dependent cell-mediated cytotoxicity (ADCC). The FcγRIIIB isoform, a product of the B gene, is a glycosylphosphatidylinositol (GPI)–linked protein expressed on neutrophils; it does not mediate phagocytosis or trigger neutrophil activation.

FcεRI is an IgE receptor expressed mainly on mast cells and basophils (see Chapter 19). The affinity of this receptor for IgE is extremely high (K_d 10^{-10} M), and therefore it readily binds monomeric IgE molecules even at the low normal plasma concentrations of this antibody isotype. The IgE-binding α chain is associated with a β chain and an FcR γ chain homodimer. The β chain spans the plasma membrane four times; both its amino terminus and carboxyl terminus are intracellular, and its carboxyl terminus contains an ITAM. Antigen-mediated cross-linking of IgE that is prebound to FcεRI results in activation and degranulation of the mast cells or basophils, leading to immediate hypersensitivity reactions (Chapter 19). FcεRI is also expressed on eosinophils, where it can mediate IgE-directed ADCC, a mechanism of defense against helminths. FcεRI is variably expressed on antigen-presenting cells such as monocytes, Langerhans cells, and tissue dendritic cells. The function of FcεRI on these antigen-presenting cells is not known.

Human FcεRII (CD23) is a C-type lectin that binds IgE with low affinity. It exists in two forms: CD23a is constitutively expressed on B cells, and CD23b is induced by IL-4

Continued on following page

on T cells, Langerhans cells, monocytes, macrophages, and eosinophils. Both forms mediate endocytosis of IgE-coated particles. The physiologic function of this receptor is not known.

FcαR (CD89) is an IgA receptor expressed on neutrophils, monocytes, and eosinophils. Its ligand-binding α chain is associated with an FcR γ homodimer.

As noted before, on binding of Ig molecules, most of the FcRs serve to activate the cells on which they are expressed. Activation requires cross-linking of the FcRs by several linked Ig molecules (e.g., on Ig-coated microbes or in immune complexes). Cross-linking of the ligand-binding α chains of an FcR results in signal transduction events that are similar to those that occur after antigen-receptor cross-linking in lymphocytes (see Chapter 8). These include Src kinase–mediated tyrosine phosphorylation of the ITAMs in the signaling chains of the FcRs; SH2 domain–mediated recruitment of Syk family kinases to the ITAMs; activation of PI-3 kinase; recruitment of adapter molecules, including SLP-76 and BLNK; and recruitment of enzymes such as phospholipase cγ and Tec family kinases. These events lead to generation of inositol trisphosphate and diacylglycerol and sustained calcium mobilization. Responses to these mediators in leukocytes include transcription of genes encoding cytokines, inflammatory mediators, and microbicidal enzymes and mobilization of the cytoskeleton leading to phagocytosis, granule exocytosis, and cell migration.

Immune complex–mediated cross-linking of the inhibitory FcγRIIB on B cells leads to tyrosine phosphorylation of the ITIM in the cytoplasmic tail, recruitment and activation of the SHIP phosphatase, and subsequent inhibition of B cell receptor–mediated, ITAM-dependent activation pathways. FcγRIIB may also generate ITIM-independent pro-apoptotic signals, which may be one mechanism of maintaining peripheral B cell tolerance. In addition, FcγRIIB is expressed on neutrophils, macrophages, and mast cells and may play a role in regulating the responses of these cells generated by activating FcRs.

The physiologic roles of FcRs have been addressed by generating knockout mice that fail to express these molecules. Knockout of the FcR γ chain in mice results in loss of expression of FCγRI, FcγRII, and FcεRI. These animals are impaired in their ability to clear opsonized microbes and to mount inflammatory reactions to immune complexes.

internalization in phagocytic vesicles. These phagosomes fuse with lysosomes, and the phagocytosed particles are destroyed in the phagolysosomes (see Chapter 12, Fig. 12–4).

Binding of opsonized particles to phagocyte Fc receptors, particularly FcγRI, also activates phagocytes by virtue of signals transduced by the FcR γ chain. These signals result in the activation of several tyrosine kinases in the phagocytes, which stimulate production of various microbicidal molecules. One consequence of phagocyte activation is production of the enzyme phagocyte oxidase, which catalyzes the intracellular generation of reactive oxygen intermediates that are cytotoxic for phagocytosed microbes. In addition, leukocytes that are activated by their Fc receptors secrete hydrolytic enzymes and reactive oxygen intermediates into the external milieu that are capable of killing extracellular microbes too large to be phagocytosed. The same toxic products may damage tissues; this mechanism of antibody-mediated tissue injury is important in hypersensitivity diseases (Chapter 18). Knockout mice lacking the Fc-binding chain of FcγRI or the signal-transducing FcR γ chain are defective in antibody-mediated defense against microbes and do not develop some forms of IgG antibody–mediated tissue injury, thus demonstrating the essential role of Fc receptors in these processes.

Expression of FcγRI on macrophages is stimulated by the macrophage-activating cytokine interferon-γ (IFN-γ). The antibody isotypes that bind best to Fcγ receptors (such as IgG2a in mice) are also produced as a result of IFN-γ–mediated isotype switching of B cells. In addition, IFN-γ directly stimulates the microbicidal activities of phagocytes (see Chapter 13). Thus, IFN-γ is an excellent example of a cytokine that has multiple actions that function cooperatively in one mechanism of host defense, namely, elimination of microbes by phagocytes.

Antibody-Dependent Cell-Mediated Cytotoxicity

NK cells and other leukocytes bind to antibody-coated cells by Fc receptors and destroy these cells. This process is called **antibody-dependent cell-mediated cytotoxicity** (ADCC) (Fig. 14–4). It was first described as a function of NK cells, which use their Fc receptor, FcγRIII, to bind to antibody-coated cells. FcγRIII is a low-affinity receptor that binds clustered IgG molecules displayed on cell surfaces and does not bind circulating monomeric IgG. Therefore, ADCC occurs only when the target cell is coated with antibody molecules, and free IgG in plasma neither activates NK cells nor competes effectively with cell-bound IgG for binding to FcγRIII. Engagement of FcγRIII by antibody-coated target cells activates the NK cells to synthesize and secrete cytokines such as IFN-γ as well as to discharge the contents of their granules, which mediate the killing functions of this cell type (see Chapter 12). ADCC can readily be demonstrated *in vitro*, but its role in host defense against microbes is not definitively established.

Eosinophils mediate a special type of ADCC directed against some helminthic parasites (see Fig. 14–4). Helminths are too large to be engulfed by phagocytes, and their integument is relatively resistant to the microbicidal products of neutrophils and macrophages, but they can be killed by a basic protein present in the

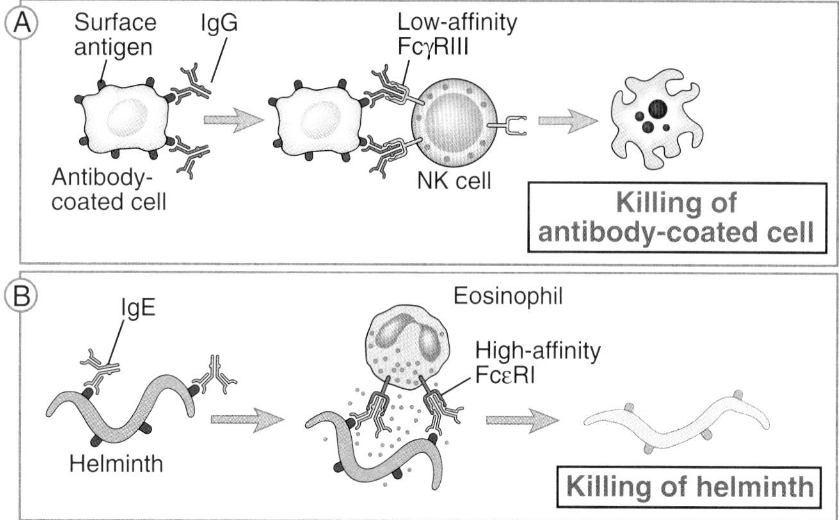

Figure 14–4 Antibody-dependent cell-mediated cytotoxicity.

A. Antibodies of certain IgG subclasses bind to cells (e.g., infected cells), and the Fc regions of the bound antibodies are recognized by an Fcγ receptor on NK cells. The NK cells are activated and kill the antibody-coated cells. Presumably, NK cells can lyse even class I MHC–expressing targets when these target cells are opsonized because the Fc receptor–mediated stimulation may overcome the inhibitory actions of class I MHC–recognizing NK cell inhibitory receptors (see Chapter 12).

B. IgE antibodies bind to helminthic parasites, and the Fc regions of the bound antibodies are recognized by Fcε receptors on eosinophils. The eosinophils are activated to release their granule contents, which kill the parasites.

granules of eosinophils. IgE coats the helminths, and eosinophils can then bind to the IgE through their FcεRI. The eosinophils are activated by FcεRI-induced signals and release their granule contents, which results in killing of the helminths.

The Complement System

The complement system is one of the major effector mechanisms of humoral immunity and is also an important effector mechanism of innate immunity. We briefly discussed the role of complement in innate immunity in Chapter 12. Here we describe the activation and regulation of complement in more detail.

The name of the complement system is derived from experiments performed by Jules Bordet shortly after the discovery of antibodies. He demonstrated that if fresh serum containing an antibacterial antibody was added to the bacteria at physiologic temperature (37°C), the bacteria were lysed. If, however, the serum was heated to 56°C or more, it lost its lytic capacity. This loss of lytic capacity was not due to decay of antibody activity because antibodies are heat stable, and even heated serum was capable of agglutinating the bacteria. Bordet concluded that the serum must contain another heat-labile component that assists, or complements, the lytic function of antibodies, and this component was later given the name complement.

The complement system consists of serum and cell surface proteins that interact with one another and with other molecules of the immune system in a highly regulated manner. Complement proteins are plasma proteins that are normally inactive; they are activated only under particular conditions to generate products that mediate various effector functions of complement. Several features of complement activation are essential for its normal function.

- ***Activation of complement involves the sequential proteolysis of proteins to generate enzymes with proteolytic activity.*** Proteins that acquire proteolytic enzymatic activity by the action of other proteases are called zymogens. The process of sequential zymogen activation, that is, an enzymatic cascade, is also characteristic of the coagulation and kinin systems. Proteolytic cascades allow tremendous amplification because each enzyme molecule activated at one step can generate multiple activated enzyme molecules at the next step.
- ***The products of complement activation become covalently attached to microbial cell surfaces or to antibodies bound to microbes and to other antigens.*** In the fluid phase, complement proteins are inactive or only transiently active (for seconds), and they become stably activated after they are attached to microbes or to antibodies. Many of the biologically active cleavage products of complement proteins also bind covalently to microbes, antibodies, and tissues in which the complement is activated. This characteristic ensures that the full activation and therefore the biologic functions of the complement system are limited to microbial cell surfaces or to sites of antibodies bound to antigens and do not occur in the blood.
- ***Complement activation is inhibited by regulatory proteins that are present on normal host cells and absent from microbes.*** The regulatory proteins are an adaptation of normal cells that minimize complement-mediated damage to host cells. Microbes lack these regulatory proteins, which allows complement activation to occur on microbial surfaces.

Pathways of Complement Activation

There are three major pathways of complement activation: the classical pathway, which is activated by certain isotypes of antibodies bound to antigens; the alternative pathway, which is activated on microbial cell surfaces in the absence of antibody; and the lectin pathway, which is activated by a plasma lectin that binds to mannose residues on microbes (see Fig. 12–8, Chapter 12). The names classical and alternative arose

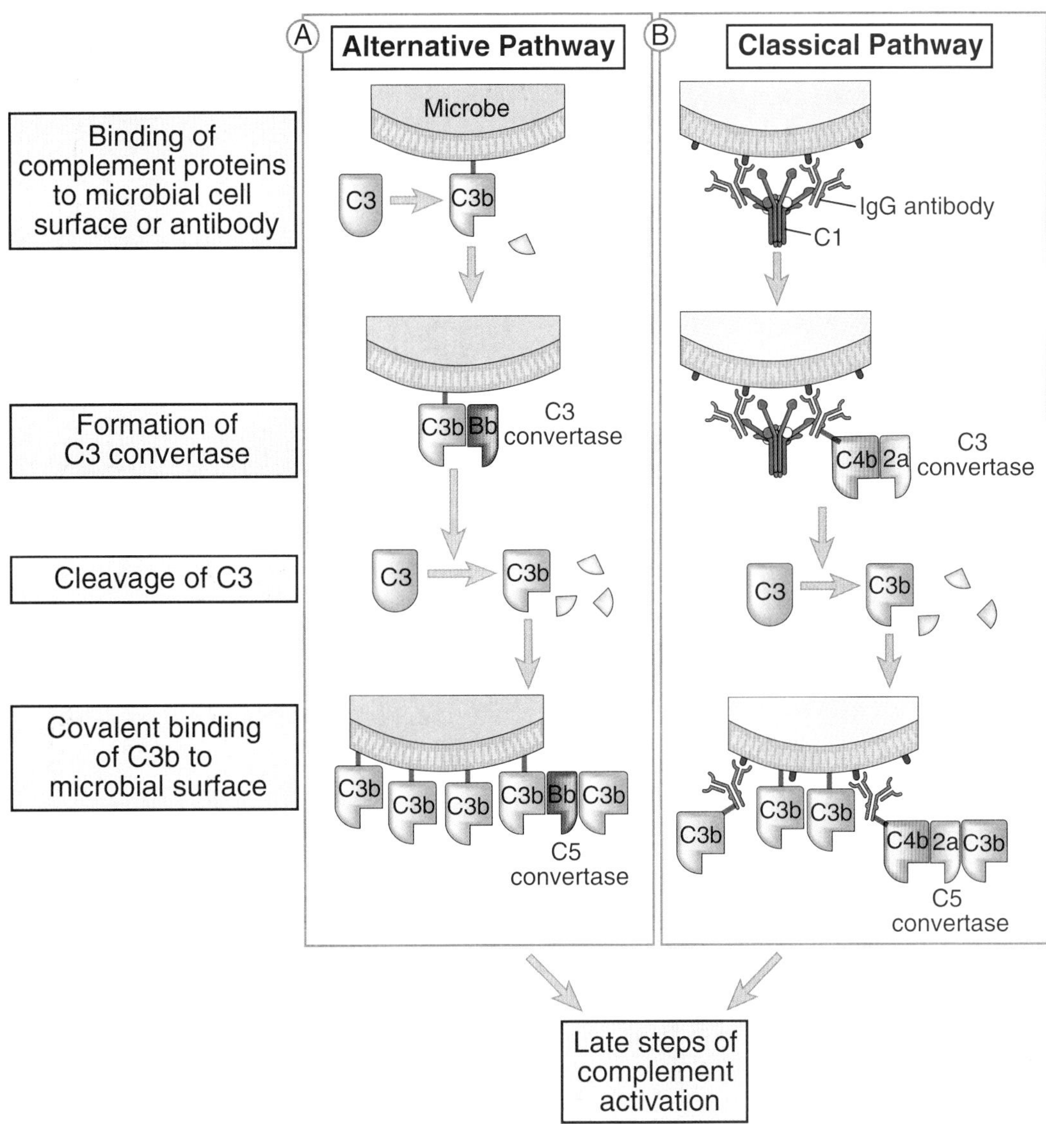

Figure 14–5 The early steps of complement activation by the alternative and classical pathways.

The alternative pathway (A) is activated by C3b binding to various activating surfaces, such as microbial cell walls, and the classical pathway (B) is initiated by C1 binding to antigen-antibody complexes. The C3b that is generated by the action of the C3 convertase binds to the microbial cell surface or the antibody and becomes a component of the enzyme that cleaves C5 (C5 convertase) and initiates the late steps of complement activation. The late steps of both pathways are the same (not shown here), and complement activated by both pathways serves the same functions. The lectin pathway (not shown) activates C1 in the absence of antibody, and the remaining steps are the same as in the classical pathway.

because the classical pathway was discovered and characterized first, but the alternative pathway is phylogenetically older. Although the pathways of complement activation differ in how they are initiated, all of them result in the generation of enzyme complexes that are able to cleave the most abundant complement protein, C3. The alternative and lectin pathways are effector mechanisms of innate immunity, whereas the classical pathway is a mechanism of humoral immunity.

The central event in complement activation is proteolysis of the complement protein C3 to generate biologically active products and the subsequent covalent attachment of a product of C3, called C3b, to microbial cell surfaces or to antibody bound to antigen (Fig. 14–5). Complement activation consists of early steps, which result in the proteolysis of C3, and late steps, which lead to the formation of a protein complex that lyses cells. The early steps of complement activation generate two proteolytic products of C3 called C3a and C3b. (By convention, the proteolytic products of each complement protein are identified by lowercase letter suffixes, *a* referring to the smaller product and *b* to the larger one.) C3b becomes covalently attached to the microbial cell surface or to the antibody molecules where complement is activated, and here it binds to other complement proteins and initiates the late steps

Spontaneous cleavage of C3

Hydrolysis and inactivation of C3b in fluid phase

C3b binds covalently to microbial surfaces, binds factor B

Cleavage of factor B by factor D; stabilization by properdin

Cleavage of additional C3 molecules by cell-associated C3 convertase

C3b covalently binds to cell surface, binds to C3bBb to form C5 convertase

Cleavage of C5; initiation of late steps of complement activation

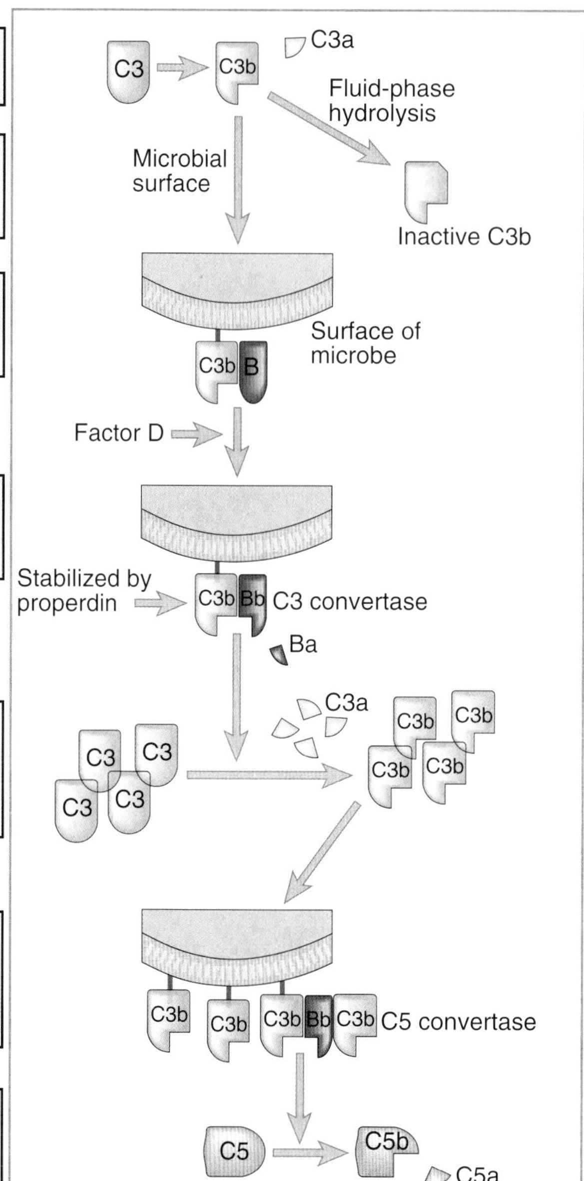

Figure 14–6 The alternative pathway of complement activation. Soluble C3 in plasma undergoes slow spontaneous hydrolysis of its internal thioester bond, which leads to the formation of a fluid-phase C3 convertase (not shown) and the generation of C3b. If the C3b is deposited on the surfaces of microbes, it binds factor B and forms the alternative pathway C3 convertase. This convertase cleaves C3 to produce more C3b, which binds to the microbial surface and participates in the formation of a C5 convertase. The C5 convertase cleaves C5 to generate C5b, the initiating event in the late steps of complement activation.

Table 14–3. Proteins of the Alternative Pathway of Complement

Protein	Structure	Serum concentration (μg/mL)	Function
C3	185 kD (α-subunit, 110 kD; β-subunit, 75 kD)	1000-1200	C3b binds to the surface of the microbe, where it functions as an opsonin and as a component of C3 and C5 convertases C3a stimulates inflammation (anaphylatoxin)
Factor B	93-kD monomer	200	Bb is a serine protease and the active enzyme of the C3 and C5 convertases
Factor D	25-kD monomer	1-2	Plasma serine protease, cleaves factor B when it is bound to C3b
Properdin	Composed of up to four 56-kD subunits	25	Stabilizes C3 convertases (C3bBb) on microbial surfaces

of complement activation. The pathways of complement activation differ in how C3b is produced, that is, in the early steps, but they share the same late steps. All the biologic functions of complement are dependent on proteolytic cleavage of C3. For example, complement activation promotes phagocytosis because leukocytes express receptors for C3b. Peptides produced by proteolysis of C3 (and other complement proteins) stimulate inflammation. With this background, we proceed to more detailed descriptions of the alternative and classical pathways.

The Alternative Pathway

The alternative pathway of complement activation results in the proteolysis of C3 and the stable attachment of its breakdown product C3b to microbial surfaces, without a role for antibody (Fig. 14–6 and Table 14–3). Normally, C3 in plasma is being continuously cleaved at a low rate to generate C3b in a process that is called C3 tickover. A small amount of the C3b may become covalently attached to the surfaces of cells, including microbes. An internal thioester bond in C3 becomes unstable when the molecule is cleaved, and it reacts with the amino or hydroxyl groups of cell surface proteins or polysaccharides to form amide or ester bonds (Fig. 14–7). If these bonds are not formed, the C3b remains in the fluid phase, its thioester is quickly hydrolyzed, and it becomes inactive, and complement activation stops. The bound C3b next binds a plasma protein called Factor B, and after it is bound, Factor B is cleaved by a plasma serine protease called Factor D to generate a fragment called Bb that remains attached

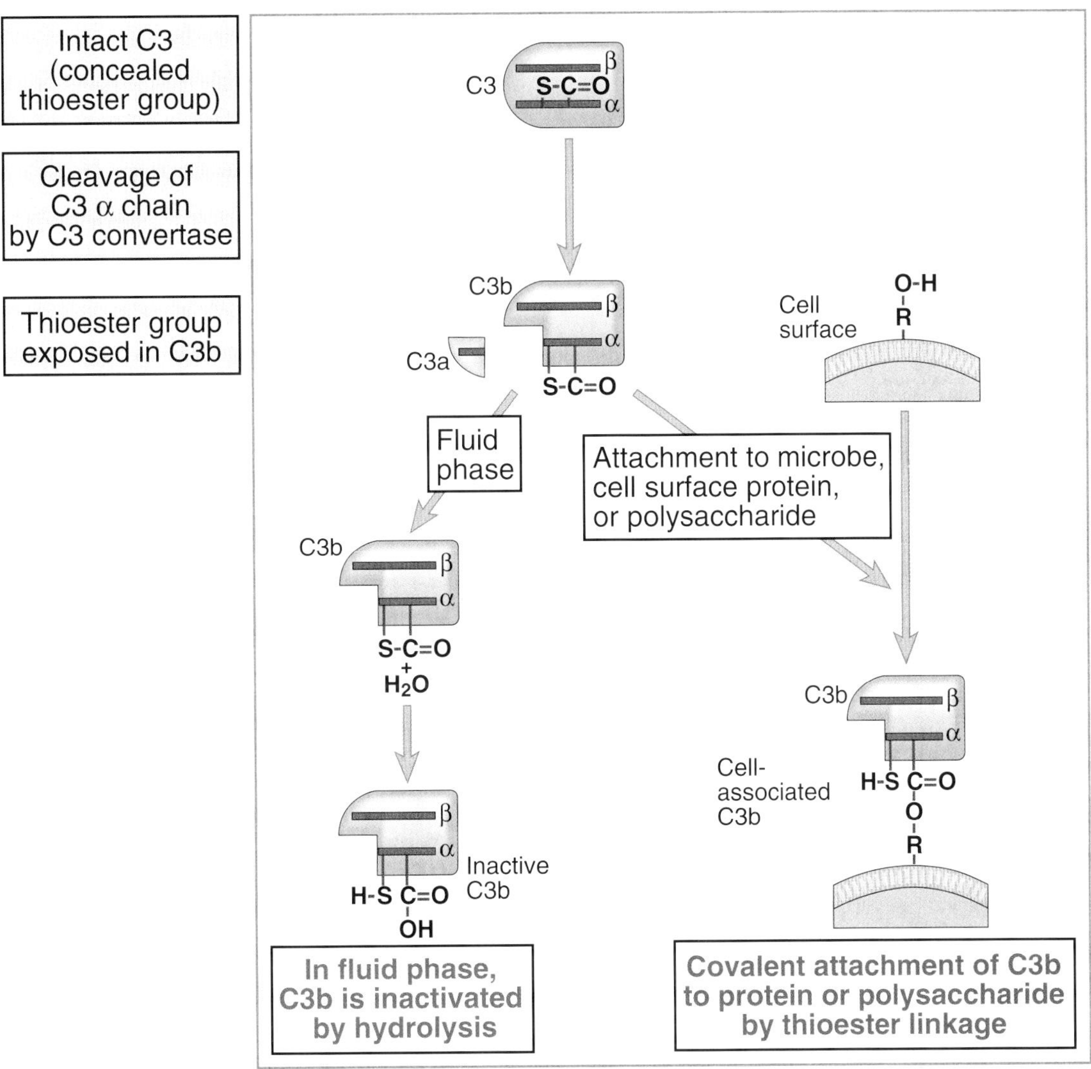

Figure 14–7 Internal thioester bonds of C3 molecules.
A schematic view of the internal thioester groups in C3 and their role in forming covalent bonds with other molecules is shown. Proteolytic cleavage of the α chain of C3 converts it into a metastable form in which the internal thioester bonds are exposed and susceptible to nucleophilic attack by oxygen (as shown) or nitrogen atoms. The result is the formation of covalent bonds with proteins or carbohydrates on the cell surfaces. C4 is structurally homologous to C3 and has an identical thioester group.

to C3b (and releases a smaller fragment called Ba). The C3bBb complex is the **alternative pathway C3 convertase,** and it functions to cleave more C3 molecules, thus setting up an amplification sequence. Even when C3b is generated by the classical pathway, it can form a complex with Bb, and this complex is able to cleave more C3. Thus, the alternative pathway C3 convertase functions to amplify complement activation when it is initiated by either the alternative or the classical pathway. When C3 is broken down and C3b remains attached to cells, C3a is released, and it has several biologic activities that are discussed later in the chapter.

Stable alternative pathway activation occurs on microbial cell surfaces and not on mammalian cells. If the C3bBb complex is formed on mammalian cells, it is rapidly degraded and the reaction is terminated by the action of several regulatory proteins present on

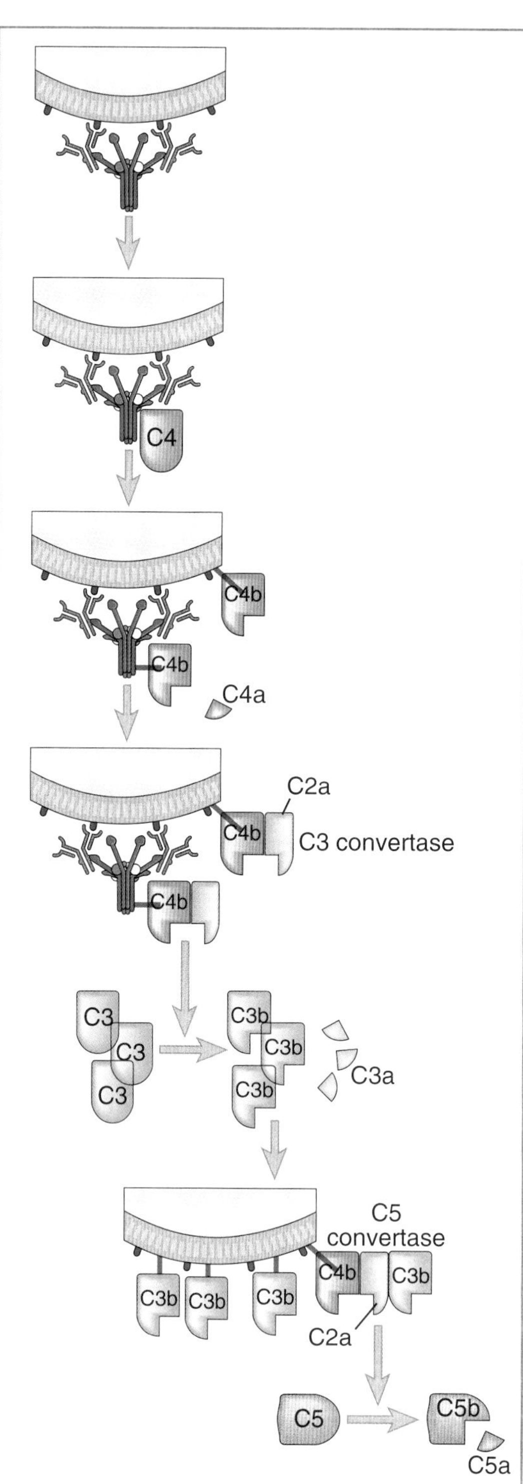

Figure 14–8 The classical pathway of complement activation. Antigen-antibody complexes that activate the classical pathway may be soluble, fixed on the surface of cells (as shown), or deposited on extracellular matrices. The classical pathway is initiated by the binding of C1 to antigen-complexed antibody molecules, which leads to the production of C3 and C5 convertases attached to the surfaces where the antibody was deposited. The C5 convertase cleaves C5 to begin the late steps of complement activation.

these cells (discussed later in the chapter). Lack of the regulatory proteins on microbial cells allows binding and activation of the alternative pathway C3 convertase. In addition, another protein of the alternative pathway, called properdin, can bind to and stabilize the C3bBb complex, and the attachment of properdin is favored on microbial as opposed to normal host cells.

Some of the C3b molecules generated by the alternative pathway C3 convertase bind to the convertase itself. This results in the formation of a C3bBb3b complex, which functions as the **alternative pathway C5 convertase** to cleave C5 and initiate the late steps of complement activation.

The Classical Pathway

The classical pathway is initiated by binding of the complement protein C1 to the C_H2 domains of IgG or the C_H3 domains of IgM molecules that have bound antigen (Fig. 14–8 and Table 14–4). Among IgG antibodies, IgG3 and IgG1 (in humans) are more efficient activators of complement than other subclasses are. C1 is a large, multimeric protein complex composed of C1q, C1r, and C1s subunits; C1q binds to the antibody, and C1r and C1s are proteases. The C1q subunit is made up of an umbrella-like radial array of six chains, each of which has a globular head connected by a collagen-like arm to a central stalk (Fig. 14–9). This hexamer performs the recognition function of the molecule and binds specifically to the Fc regions of μ and some γ heavy chains. Each Ig Fc region has a single C1q-binding site, and each C1q molecule must bind to two Ig heavy chains to be activated. This requirement explains why antibodies bound to antigens and not free circulating antibodies can initiate classical pathway activation (Fig. 14–10). Because each IgG molecule has only one Fc region, multiple IgG molecules must be brought close together before C1q can bind, and multiple IgG antibodies are brought together only when they bind to a multivalent antigen. Even though free (circulating) IgM is pentameric, it does not bind C1q, apparently because the Fc regions of free IgM are inaccessible to C1q. Binding of the IgM to an antigen induces a conformational change that exposes the C1q binding sites in the Fc regions and allows C1q to bind. Because of its pentameric structure, a single molecule of IgM can bind two C1q molecules, and this is one reason that IgM is a more efficient complement-binding (also called complement-fixing) antibody than IgG is.

C1r and C1s are serine esterases that form a tetramer containing two molecules of each. Binding of two or

Table 14–4. Proteins of the Classical Pathway of Complement

Protein	Structure	Serum concentration (μg/mL)	Function
C1 ($C1qr_2s_2$)	750 kD		Initiates the classical pathway
C1q	460 kD; hexamer of three pairs of chains (22, 23, 24 kD)	75-150	Binds to the Fc portion of antibody that has bound antigen
C1r	85-kD dimer	50	Serine protease, cleaves C1s to make it an active protease
C1s	85-kD dimer	50	Serine protease, cleaves C4 and C2
C4	210 kD, trimer of 97-, 75-, and 33-kD chains	300-600	C4b covalently binds to the surface of a microbe or cell, where antibody is bound and complement is activated C4b binds C2 for cleavage by C1s C4a stimulates inflammation (anaphylatoxin)
C2	102-kD monomer	20	C2a is a serine protease and functions as the active enzyme of C3 and C5 convertases to cleave C3 and C5
C3	See Table 14-3		

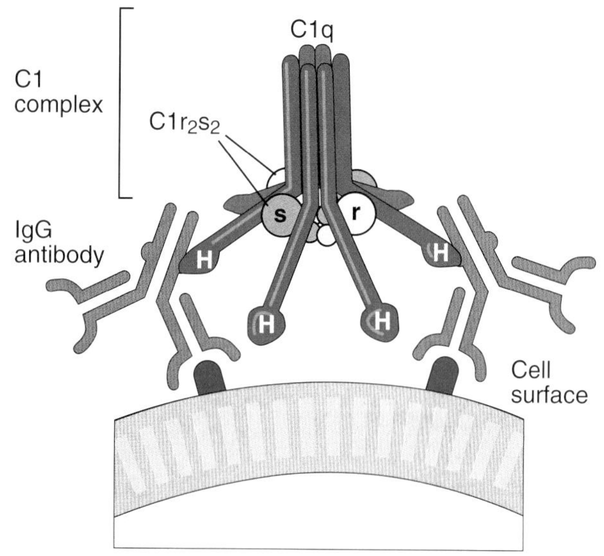

Figure 14–9 Structure of C1.

C1q consists of six identical subunits arranged to form a central core and symmetrically projecting radial arms. The globular heads at the end of each arm, designated H, are the contact regions for immunoglobulin. C1r and C1s form a tetramer composed of two C1r and two C1s molecules. The ends of C1r and C1s contain the catalytic domains of these proteins. One $C1r_2s_2$ tetramer wraps around the radial arms of the C1q complex in a manner that juxtaposes the catalytic domains of C1r and C1s.

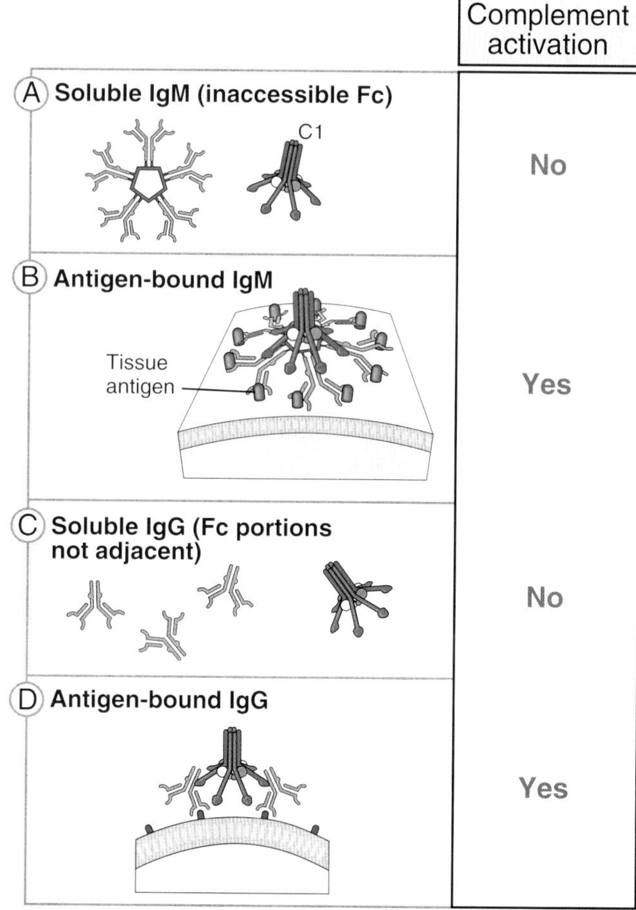

Figure 14–10 C1 binding to the Fc portions of IgM and IgG.

C1 must bind to two or more Fc portions to initiate the complement cascade. The Fc portions of soluble pentameric IgM are not accessible to C1 (A). After IgM binds to surface-bound antigens, it undergoes a shape change that permits C1 binding and activation (B). Soluble IgG molecules will also not activate C1 because each IgG has only one Fc region (C), but after binding to cell surface antigens, adjacent IgG Fc portions can bind and activate C1 (D).

more of the globular heads of C1q to the Fc regions of IgG or IgM leads to enzymatic activation of the associated C1r, which cleaves and activates C1s (see Fig. 14–8). Activated C1s cleaves the next protein in the cascade, C4, to generate C4b. (The smaller C4a fragment is released and has biologic activities that are described later.) C4 is homologous to C3, and C4b has an internal thioester bond, as in C3b, that forms covalent amide or ester linkages with the antigen-antibody complex or with the adjacent surface of a cell to which the antibody is bound. This attachment of C4b ensures that classical pathway activation proceeds on a cell surface or immune complex. The next complement protein, C2, then complexes with the cell surface–bound C4b and is cleaved by a nearby C1s molecule to generate a soluble C2b fragment of unknown importance and a larger C2a fragment that remains physically associated with C4b on the cell surface. (Note that in C2, the smaller fragment is called C2b and the larger one is called C2a for historical reason, an exception to the rule.) The resulting C4b2a complex is the **classical pathway C3 convertase** and has the ability to bind to and proteolytically cleave C3. Binding of this enzyme complex to C3 is mediated by the C4b component, and proteolysis is catalyzed by the C2a component. Cleavage of C3 results in the removal of the small C3a fragment, and C3b can form covalent bonds with cell surfaces or with the antibody where complement activation was initiated. Once C3b is deposited, it can bind factor B and generate more C3 convertase by the alternative pathway, as discussed before. The net effect of the multiple enzymatic steps and amplification is that a single molecule of C3 convertase can lead to the deposition of hundreds or thousands of molecules of C3b on the cell surface where complement is activated. The key early steps of the alternative and classical pathways are analogous: C3 in the alternative pathway is homologous to C4 in the classical pathway, and factor B is homologous to C2.

Some of the C3b molecules generated by the classical pathway C3 convertase bind to the convertase (as in the alternative pathway) and form a C4b2a3b complex. This complex functions as the **classical pathway C5 convertase**; it cleaves C5 and initiates the late steps of complement activation.

The Lectin Pathway

The **lectin pathway** of complement activation is triggered in the absence of antibody by the binding of microbial polysaccharides to circulating lectins, such as plasma mannose (or mannan)–binding lectin (MBL). MBL binds to mannose residues on polysaccharides, and because it is structurally similar to C1q, it triggers the complement system either by activating the C1r–C1s enzyme complex (like C1q) or by associating with another serine esterase, called mannose-binding protein–associated serine esterase, which cleaves C4. Apart from being activated in the absence of antibody, the rest of this pathway is the same as the classical pathway.

Late Steps of Complement Activation

C5 convertases generated by the alternative, classical, or lectin pathway initiate activation of the late components of the complement system, which culminates in formation of the cytocidal membrane attack complex (MAC) (Table 14–5 and Fig. 14–11). C5 convertases cleave C5 into a small C5a fragment that is released and a two-chain C5b fragment that remains bound to the complement proteins deposited on the cell surface. (C5a has potent biologic effects on several cells that are discussed later in the chapter.) The remaining components of the complement cascade, C6, C7, C8, and C9, are structurally related proteins without enzymatic activity. C5b transiently maintains a conformation capable of binding the next proteins in the cascade, C6 and C7. The C7 component of the resulting C5b,6,7 complex is hydrophobic, and it inserts into the lipid bilayer of cell membranes, where it becomes a high-affinity receptor for one C8 molecule. The C8 protein is a trimer composed of three chains, one of which binds to the C5b,6,7 complex; another inserts into the lipid bilayer of the membrane. This stably inserted C5b,6,7,8 complex (C5b–8) has a limited ability to lyse cells. The formation of a fully active MAC is accomplished by the binding of C9, the final component of the complement cascades, to the C5b–8 complex. C9 is a serum protein that polymerizes at the site of the bound C5b–8 to form pores in plasma membranes. These pores are about 100 Å in diameter, and they form channels that allow free movement of water and ions (Fig. 14–12). The entry of water results in osmotic swelling and rupture of the cells on whose surface the MAC is deposited. Calcium, which is present at much higher concentrations outside cells than inside, also enters, and high calcium concentrations can induce apoptosis in nucleated cells. The pores formed by polymerized C9 are similar to the membrane pores formed by perforin, the cytolytic granule protein found in cytolytic T lymphocytes (CTLs) and NK cells (see Chapter 13), and C9 is structurally homologous to perforin.

Receptors for Complement Proteins

Many of the biologic activities of the complement system are mediated by the binding of complement

Table 14–5. Proteins of the Late Steps of Complement Activation

Protein	Structure	Serum concentration (μg/mL)	Function
C5	190-kD dimer of 115- and 75- kD chains	80	C5b initiates assembly of the MAC C5a stimulates inflammation (anaphylatoxin)
C6	110-kD monomer	45	Component of the MAC: binds to C5b and accepts C7
C7	100-kD monomer	90	Component of the MAC: binds to C5b,6 and inserts into lipid membranes
C8	155-kD trimer of 64-, 64-, and 22-kD chains	60	Component of the MAC: binds to C5b,6,7 and initiates the binding and polymerization of C9
C9	79-kD monmer	60	Component of the MAC: binds to C5b,6,7,8 and polymerizes to form membrane pores

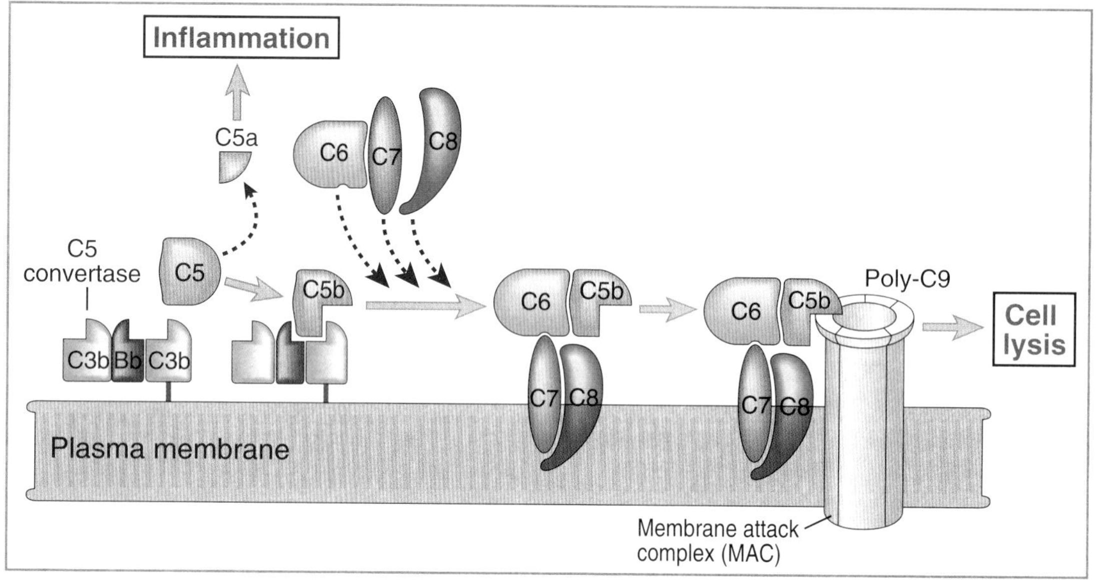

Figure 14–11 Late steps of complement activation and formation of the MAC. A schematic view of the cell surface events leading to formation of the MAC is shown. Cell-associated C5 convertase cleaves C5 and generates C5b, which becomes bound to the convertase. C6 and C7 bind sequentially, and the C5b,6,7 complex becomes directly inserted into the lipid bilayer of the plasma membrane, followed by stable insertion of C8. Up to 15 C9 molecules may then polymerize around the complex to form the MAC, which creates pores in the membrane and induces cell lysis. C5a released on proteolysis of C5 stimulates inflammation.

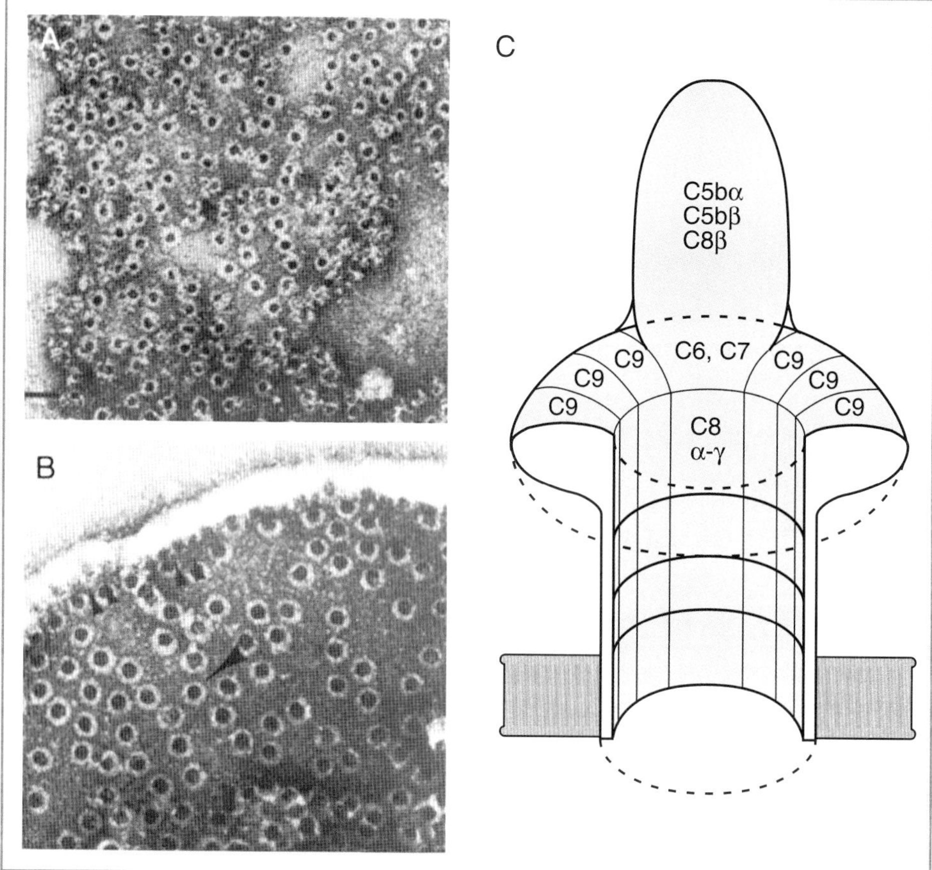

Figure 14–12 Structure of the MAC in cell membranes. A. Complement lesions in erythrocyte membranes are shown in this electron micrograph. The lesions consist of holes approximately 100 Å in diameter that are formed by poly-C9 tubular complexes.

B. For comparison, membrane lesions induced on a target cell by a cloned CTL line are shown in this electron micrograph. The lesions appear morphologically similar to complement-mediated lesions, except for a larger internal diameter (160 Å). CTL- and NK cell–induced membrane lesions are formed by tubular complexes of a polymerized protein (perforin), which is homologous to C9 (see Chapter 13).

C. A model of the subunit arrangement of the MAC is shown. The transmembrane region consists of 12 to 15 C9 molecules arranged as a tubule, in addition to single molecules of C6, C7, and C8 α and γ chains. The C5bα, C5bβ, and C8β chains form an appendage that projects above the transmembrane pore. (From Podack ER. Molecular mechanisms of cytolysis by complement and cytolytic lymphocytes. Journal of Cellular Biochemistry 30:133–170, 1986. Copyright 1986. Reprinted by permission of Wiley-Liss, Inc., a subsidiary of John Wiley & Sons, Inc.)

fragments to membrane receptors expressed on various cell types. The best characterized of these receptors are specific for fragments of C3 and are described here (Table 14–6). Other receptors include those for C3a, C4a, and C5a, which stimulate inflammation, and some that regulate complement activation.

The type 1 complement receptor (CR1, or CD35) functions mainly to promote phagocytosis of C3b- and C4b-coated particles and clearance of immune complexes from the circulation. CR1 is a high-affinity receptor for C3b and C4b. It is expressed mainly on blood cells, including erythrocytes, neutrophils, monocytes, eosinophils, and T and B lymphocytes; it is also found on follicular dendritic cells in the follicles of peripheral lymphoid organs. Phagocytes use this receptor to bind and internalize particles opsonized with C3b or C4b. The binding of C3b- or C4b-coated particles to CR1 also transduces signals that activate the microbicidal mechanisms of the phagocytes, especially when the Fcγ receptor is simultaneously engaged by antibody-coated particles. CR1 on erythrocytes binds circulating immune complexes with attached C3b and C4b and transports the complexes to the liver and spleen. Here, the immune complexes are removed from the erythrocyte surface by phagocytes, and the erythrocytes continue to circulate. CR1 is also a regulator of complement activation (see later).

The type 2 complement receptor (CR2, or CD21) functions to stimulate humoral immune responses by enhancing B cell activation by antigen and by promoting the trapping of antigen-antibody complexes in germinal centers. CR2 is present on B lymphocytes, follicular dendritic cells, and some epithelial cells. It specifically binds the cleavage products of C3b, called C3d, C3dg, and iC3b (*i* referring to inactive), which are generated by factor I–mediated proteolysis (discussed later). On B cells, CR2 is expressed as part of a trimolecular complex that includes two other noncovalently attached proteins called CD19 and target of antiproliferative antibody-1 (TAPA-1, or CD81). This complex delivers signals to B cells that enhance the responses of B cells to antigen (see Chapter 9, Fig. 9–5). On follicular dendritic cells, CR2 serves to trap iC3b- and C3dg-coated antigen-antibody complexes in germinal centers. The functions of CR2 in B cell activation are described later.

In humans, CR2 is the cell surface receptor for Epstein-Barr virus, a herpesvirus that causes infectious mononucleosis and is also linked to several human malignant tumors (see Chapter 17, Box 17–2). Epstein-Barr virus infects B cells and can remain latent for life.

The type 3 complement receptor, also called Mac-1 (CR3, CD11bCD18), is an integrin that functions as a receptor for the iC3b fragment generated by proteolysis of C3b. Mac-1 is expressed on neutrophils, mononuclear phagocytes, mast cells, and NK cells. It is a member of the integrin family of cell surface receptors

Table 14–6. Receptors for Fragments of C3

Receptor	Structure	Ligands	Cell distribution	Function
Type 1 complement receptor (CR1, CD35)	160-250 kD; multiple CCPRs	C3b > C4b > iC3b	Mononuclear phagocytes, neutrophils, B and T cells, erythrocytes, eosinophils, FDCs	Phagocytosis Clearance of immune complexes Promotes dissociation of C3 convertases by acting as cofactor for cleavage of C3b,C4b
Type 2 complement receptor (CR2, CD21)	145 kD; multiple CCPRs	C3d, C3dg > iC3b	B lymphocytes, FDCs, nasopharyngeal epithelium	Coreceptor for B cell activation Trapping of antigens in germinal centers Receptor for EBV
Type 3 complement receptor (CR3, Mac-1, CD11b/ CD18)	Integrin, with 165-kD α chain and 95-kD β_2 chain	iC3b, ICAM-1; also binds microbes	Mononuclear phagocytes, neutrophils, NK cells	Phagocytosis Leukocyte adhesion to endothelium (via ICAM-1)
Type 4 complement receptor (CR4, p150/95, CD11c/CD18)	Integrin, with 150-kD α chain and 95-kD β_2 chain	iC3b	Mononuclear phagocytes, neutrophils, NK cells	Phagocytosis, cell adhesion?

Abbreviations: CCPR, complement control protein repeat; FDC, follicular dendritic cell; ICAM-1, intercellular adhesion molecule-1.

(see Chapter 6, Box 6–2) and consists of an α chain (CD11b) noncovalently linked to a β chain (CD18) that is identical to the β chains of two closely related integrin molecules, leukocyte function–associated antigen-1 (LFA-1) and p150,95 (see next). Mac-1 on neutrophils and monocytes promotes phagocytosis of microbes opsonized with iC3b. In addition, Mac-1 may directly recognize bacteria for phagocytosis by binding to some unknown microbial molecules (see Chapter 12). It also binds to intercellular adhesion molecule-1 (ICAM-1) on endothelial cells and promotes stable attachment of the leukocytes to endothelium, even without complement activation. This binding leads to the recruitment of leukocytes to sites of infection and tissue injury.

The type 4 complement receptor (CR4, p150,95, CD11cCD18) is another integrin with a different α chain (CD11c) and the same β chain as Mac-1. It also binds iC3b, and the function of this receptor is probably similar to that of Mac-1. CD11c is also abundantly expressed on dendritic cells and is used as a marker for this cell type.

Regulation of Complement Activation

Activation of the complement cascade and the stability of active complement proteins are tightly regulated to prevent complement activation on normal host cells and to limit the duration of complement activation even on microbial cells and antigen-antibody complexes. Regulation of complement is mediated by several circulating and cell membrane proteins (Table 14–7). Many of these proteins, as well as several proteins of the classical and alternative pathways, belong to a family called regulators of complement activity (RCA) and are encoded by homologous adjacent genes.

Complement activation needs to be regulated for two reasons. First, low-level complement activation goes on spontaneously, and if such activation is allowed to proceed on normal cells, the result can be damage to normal cells and tissues. Second, even when complement is activated where needed, such as on microbial cells or antigen-antibody complexes, it needs to be controlled because degradation products of complement

Table 14–7. Regulators of Complement Activation

Receptor	Structure	Distribution	Interacts with	Function
C1 inhibitor (C1 INH)	104 kD	Plasma protein; conc. 200 μg/mL	C1r, C1s	Serine protease inhibitor; binds to C1r and C1s and dissociates them from C1q
Factor I	88-kD dimer of 50- and 38-kD subunits	Plasma protein; conc. 35 μg/mL	C4b, C3b	Serine protease; cleaves C3b and C4b by using factor H, MCP, C4BP, or CR1 as cofactors
Factor H	150 kD; multiple CCPRs	Plasma protein; conc. 480 μg/mL	C3b	Binds C3b and displaces Bb Cofactor for factor I–mediated cleavage of C3b
C4-binding protein (C4BP)	570 kD; multiple CCPRs	Plasma protein; conc. 300 μg/mL	C4b	Binds C4b and displaces C2 Cofactor for factor I–mediated cleavage of C4b
Membrane cofactor for protein (MCP, CD46)	45-70 kD; four CCPRs	Leukocytes, epithelial cells, endothelial cells	C3b,C4b	Cofactor for factor I–mediated cleavage of C3b and C4b
Decay-accelerating factor (DAF)	70 kD; GPI linked, four CCPRs	Blood cells, endothelial cells, epithelial cells	C4b2b, C3bBb	Displaces C2b from C4b and Bb from C3b (dissociation of C3 convertases)
CD59	18 kD; GPI linked	Blood cells, endothelial cells, epithelial cells	C7, C8	Blocks C9 binding and prevents formation of the MAC

Abbreviations: CCPR, complement control protein repeat; conc., concentration; GPI, glycophosphatidylinositol; MAC, membrane attack complex.

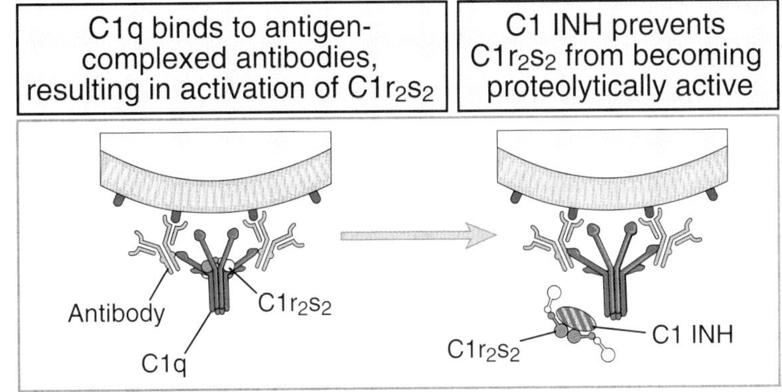

Figure 14–13 Regulation of C1 activity by C1 inhibitor (C1 INH).

C1 INH displaces $C1r_2s_2$ from C1q and terminates classical pathway activation.

proteins can diffuse to adjacent cells and injure them. Different regulatory mechanisms inhibit the formation of C3 convertases in the early steps of complement activation, break down and inactivate C3 and C5 convertases, and inhibit formation of the MAC in the late steps of the complement pathway.

The proteolytic activity of C1r and C1s is inhibited by a plasma protein called C1 inhibitor (C1 INH). C1 INH is a serine protease inhibitor (serpin) that mimics the normal substrates of C1r and C1s. If C1q binds to an antibody and begins the process of complement activation, C1 INH becomes a target of the enzymatic activity of the bound $C1r_2$–$C1s_2$. C1 INH is cleaved by and becomes covalently attached to these complement proteins, and as a result, the $C1r_2$–$C1s_2$ tetramer dissociates from C1q, thus stopping activation by the classical pathway (Fig. 14–13). In this way, C1 INH prevents the accumulation of enzymatically active $C1r_2$–$C1s_2$ in the plasma and limits the time for which active $C1r_2$–$C1s_2$ is available to activate subsequent steps in the complement cascade. An autosomal dominant inherited disease called **hereditary angioneurotic edema** is due to a deficiency of C1 INH. Clinical manifestations of the disease include intermittent acute accumulation of edema fluid in the skin and mucosa, which causes abdominal pain, vomiting, diarrhea, and potentially life-threatening airway obstruction. In these patients, the plasma levels of C1 INH protein are sufficiently reduced (<20% to 30% of normal) that activation of C1 by immune complexes is not properly controlled and increased breakdown of C4 and C2 occurs. The mediators of edema formation in patients with hereditary angioneurotic edema include a proteolytic fragment of C2, called C2 kinin, and bradykinin. C1 INH is an inhibitor of other plasma serine proteases besides C1, including kallikrein and coagulation factor XII, and both activated kallikrein and factor XII can promote increased formation of bradykinin.

Assembly of the components of C3 and C5 convertases is inhibited by the binding of regulatory proteins to C3b and C4b deposited on cell surfaces (Fig. 14–14). If C3b is deposited on the surfaces of normal mammalian cells, it may be bound by several membrane proteins, including membrane cofactor protein (MCP, or CD46), type 1 complement receptor (CR1), and decay-accelerating factor (DAF), and a plasma protein called Factor H. C4b deposited on cell surfaces is similarly bound by DAF, CR1, and another plasma protein called C4-binding protein (C4BP). By binding to C3b or C4b, these proteins competitively inhibit the binding of other components of the C3 convertase, such as Bb of the alternative pathway and C2a of the classical pathway, thus blocking further progression of the complement cascade. (Factor H inhibits binding of only Bb to C3b and is thus a regulator of the alternative but not the classical pathway.) MCP, CR1, and DAF are produced by mammalian cells but not by microbes. Therefore, these regulators of complement selectively inhibit complement activation on host cells and allow complement activation to proceed on microbes. In addition, cell surfaces rich in sialic acid favor binding of the reg-

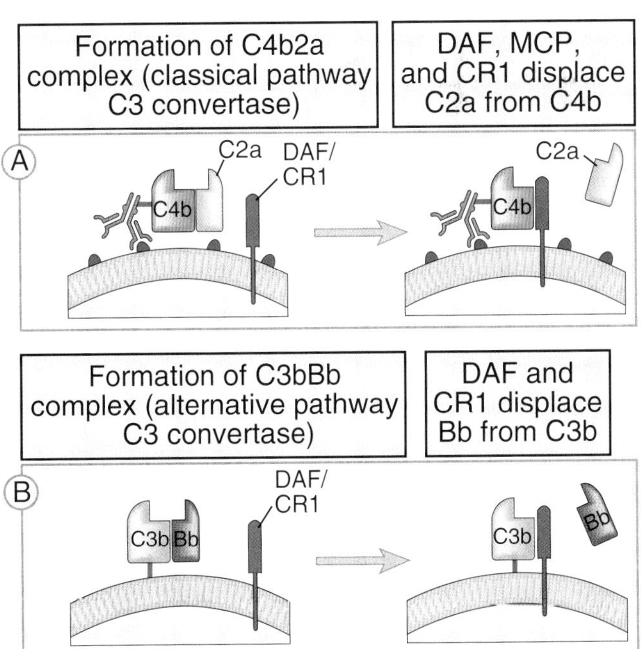

Figure 14–14 Inhibition of the formation of C3 convertases.

Several membrane proteins present on normal cells displace either C2a from the classical pathway C3 convertase (A) or Bb from the alternative pathway C3 convertase (B) and stop complement activation. CR1, type 1 complement receptor; DAF, decay-accelerating factor; MCP, membrane cofactor protein.

ulatory protein Factor H over the alternative pathway protein Factor B. Mammalian cells express higher levels of sialic acid than microbes do, which is another reason that complement activation is prevented on normal host cells and permitted on microbes.

DAF is a glycophosphatidylinositol-linked membrane protein expressed on endothelial cells and erythrocytes. Deficiency of an enzyme required to form such protein-lipid linkages results in failure to express many glycophosphatidylinositol-linked membrane proteins, including DAF and CD59 (see following), and causes a disease called **paroxysmal nocturnal hemoglobinuria**. This disease is characterized by recurrent bouts of intravascular hemolysis, at least partly attributable to unregulated complement activation on the surface of erythrocytes. Recurrent intravascular hemolysis in turn leads to chronic hemolytic anemia and venous thrombosis.

Cell-associated C3b is proteolytically degraded by a plasma serine protease called factor I, which is active only in the presence of regulatory proteins (Fig. 14–15). MCP, factor H, C4BP, and CR1 all serve as cofactors for Factor I–mediated cleavage of C3b (and C4b). Thus, these regulatory host cell proteins promote proteolytic degradation of complement proteins; as discussed before, the same regulatory proteins cause dissociation of C3b (and C4b)–containing complexes. Factor I–mediated cleavage of C3b generates fragments called iC3b, C3d, and C3dg, which do not participate in complement activation but may be recognized by receptors on phagocytes.

Formation of the MAC is inhibited by a membrane protein called CD59. CD59 is a glycophosphatidylinositol-linked protein expressed on many cell types. It works by incorporating itself into growing MACs after the membrane insertion of C5b–8, thereby inhibiting the subsequent addition of C9 molecules (Fig. 14–16). CD59 is present on normal host cells, where it limits MAC formation, but it is not present on microbes. Formation of the MAC is also inhibited by plasma proteins such as S protein, which functions by binding to soluble C5b,6,7 complexes and thereby preventing their insertion into cell membranes near the site where the complement cascade was initiated. Growing MACs can insert into any neighboring cell membrane besides the membrane on which they were generated. Inhibitors of MAC in the plasma and in host cell membranes ensure that lysis of innocent bystander cells does not occur near the site of complement activation.

Much of the analysis of the function of complement regulatory proteins has relied on *in vitro* experiments, and most of these experiments have focused on assays that measure MAC-mediated cell lysis as an end point. On the basis of these studies, a hierarchy of importance for inhibiting complement activation is believed to be CD59 > DAF > MCP, and this hierarchy may reflect the relative abundance of these proteins on cell surfaces.

The function of regulatory proteins may be overcome by increasing amounts of complement activation. We have emphasized the importance of these regulatory proteins in preventing complement activation on normal cells. However, complement-mediated phagocytosis and damage to normal cells are important pathogenetic mechanisms in many immunologic diseases (Chapter 18). In these diseases, large amounts of antibodies may be deposited on host cells, generating enough active complement proteins that the regulatory molecules are unable to control complement activation.

Functions of Complement

The principal effector functions of the complement system in innate immunity and specific humoral immunity are to promote phagocytosis of microbes on which complement is activated, to stimulate inflammation, and to induce the lysis of these microbes. In addition, products of complement activation provide second signals for the activation of B lymphocytes and the production of antibodies. Phagocytosis, inflammation, and stimulation of humoral immunity are all mediated by the binding of proteolytic fragments of complement proteins to various cell surface receptors, whereas cell lysis is mediated by the MAC. In the following section, we describe each of these functions of the complement system and their role in host defense.

Opsonization and Phagocytosis

Microbes on which complement is activated by the alternative or classical pathway become coated with

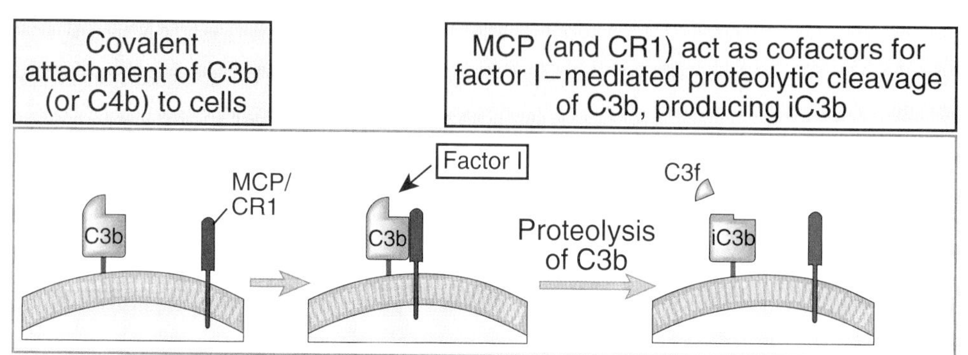

Figure 14–15 Factor I–mediated cleavage of C3b. In the presence of cell membrane-bound cofactors (membrane cofactor protein [MCP] or type 1 complement receptor [CR1]), plasma Factor I proteolytically cleaves C3b attached to cell surfaces, leaving an inactive form of C3b (iC3b). Factor H and C4-binding protein can also serve as cofactors for Factor I–mediated cleavage of C3b. The same process is involved in the proteolysis of C4.

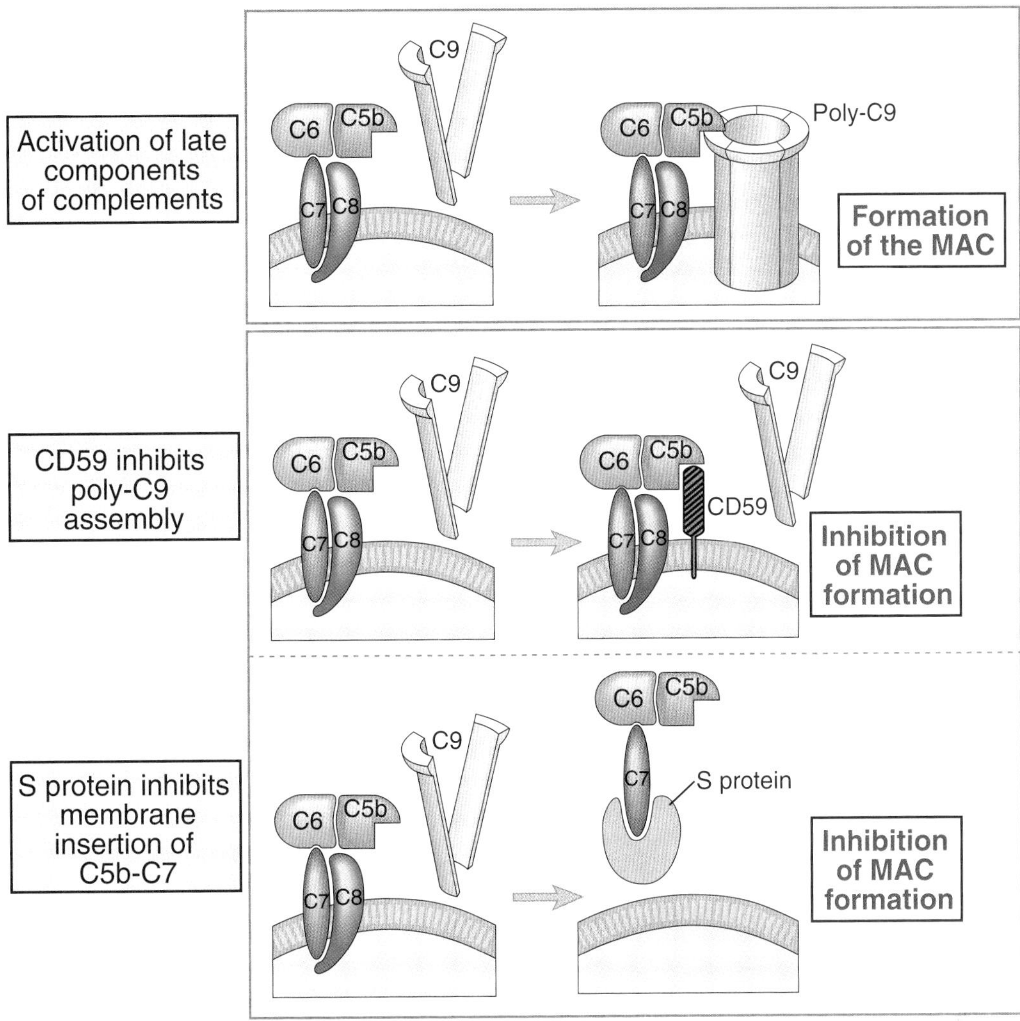

Figure 14–16 Regulation of formation of the MAC.
The MAC is formed on cell surfaces as an end result of complement activation. The membrane protein CD59 and plasma S protein inhibit formation of the MAC.

C3b, iC3b, or C4b and are phagocytosed by the binding of these proteins to specific receptors on macrophages and neutrophils (Fig. 14–17A). As discussed previously, activation of both the alternative and classical pathways leads to the generation of C3b and iC3b covalently bound to cell surfaces. Both C3b and iC3b act as opsonins by virtue of the fact that they specifically bind to receptors on neutrophils and macrophages. C3b and C4b (the latter generated by the classical pathway only) bind to CR1, and iC3b binds to CR3 (Mac-1) and CR4. By itself, CR1 is inefficient at inducing the phagocytosis of C3b-coated microbes, but its ability to do so is enhanced if the microbes are coated with IgG antibodies that simultaneously bind to Fcγ receptors. Macrophage activation by the cytokine IFN-γ also enhances CR1-mediated phagocytosis. C3b- and iC3b-dependent phagocytosis of microorganisms is a major defense mechanism against infections in innate and adaptive immunity. One example of the importance of complement is host defense against bacteria with polysaccharide-rich capsules, such as pneumococci and meningococci, which is mediated entirely by humoral immunity. IgM antibodies against capsular polysaccharides bind to the bacteria, activate the classical pathway of complement, and cause phagocytic clearance of the bacteria in the spleen. This is why individuals lacking the spleen (e.g., as a result of surgical removal after traumatic rupture) are susceptible to disseminated pneumococcal and meningococcal septicemia. C3-deficient humans and mice are extremely susceptible to lethal bacterial infections.

Stimulation of Inflammatory Responses

The proteolytic complement fragments C5a, C4a, and C3a induce acute inflammation by activating mast cells and neutrophils (Fig. 14–17B). All three peptides bind to mast cells and induce degranulation, with the release of vasoactive mediators such as histamine. These peptides are also called **anaphylatoxins** because the mast cell reactions they trigger are characteristic of anaphylaxis (see Chapter 19). In neutrophils, C5a stimu-

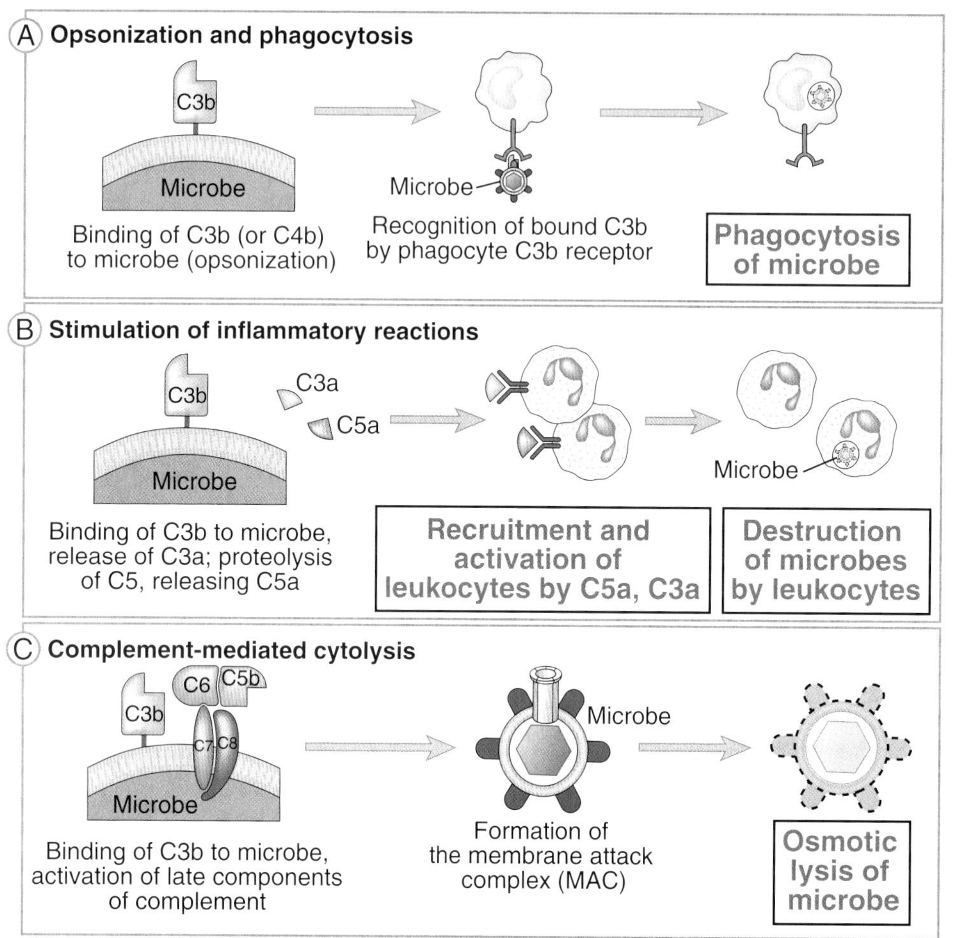

Figure 14–17 Functions of complement.

The major functions of the complement system in host defense are shown. Cell-bound C3b is an opsonin that promotes phagocytosis of coated cells (A); the proteolytic products C5a, C3a, and (to a lesser extent) C4a stimulate leukocyte recruitment and inflammation (B); and the MAC lyses cells (C).

lates motility, firm adhesion to endothelial cells, and, at high doses, stimulation of the respiratory burst and production of reactive oxygen intermediates. In addition, C5a may act directly on vascular endothelial cells and lead to increased vascular permeability and the expression of P-selectin, which promotes neutrophil binding. This combination of C5a actions on mast cells, neutrophils, and endothelial cells contributes to inflammation at sites of complement activation. C5a is the most potent mediator of mast cell degranulation, C3a is about 20-fold less potent, and C4a is about 2500-fold less. The proinflammatory effects of C5a, C4a, and C3a are mediated by binding of the peptides to specific receptors on various cell types. The C5a receptor is the most thoroughly characterized. It is a member of the seven–α-helical transmembrane receptor family and uses trimeric guanosine triphosphate (GTP)–binding proteins (G proteins) for coupling to signal transduction pathways. The C5a receptor is expressed on many cell types, including neutrophils, eosinophils, basophils, monocytes, macrophages, mast cells, endothelial cells, smooth muscle cells, epithelial cells, and astrocytes. The C3a receptor is also a member of the G protein–coupled receptor family.

Complement-Mediated Cytolysis

Complement-mediated lysis of foreign organisms is mediated by the MAC (Fig. 14–17C). This mechanism appears to be important for defense against only a few types of microbes because genetic defects in MAC components result in increased susceptibility only to infections by bacteria of the genus *Neisseria.*

Other Functions of the Complement System

By binding to antigen-antibody complexes, complement proteins promote the solubilization of these complexes and their clearance by phagocytes. Small numbers of immune complexes are frequently formed in the circulation when an individual mounts a vigorous antibody response to a circulating antigen. If the immune complexes accumulate in the blood, they may be deposited in vessel walls and lead to inflammatory reactions that damage surrounding tissue. The formation of immune complexes may require not only the multivalent binding of Ig Fab regions to antigens but also noncovalent interactions of Fc regions of juxtaposed Ig molecules. Complement activation on Ig molecules can sterically block these Fc-Fc interactions, thereby promoting dissolution of the immune complexes. In addition, as discussed before, immune complexes with attached C3b are bound to CR1 on erythrocytes, and the complexes are cleared by phagocytes in the liver.

The C3d protein generated from C3 binds to CR2 on B cells, activates the B cells, and provides a signal for

initiating humoral immune responses. C3d is generated when complement is activated by an antigen, either directly (for instance, when the antigen is a microbial polysaccharide) or after the binding of antibody. Complement activation results in the covalent attachment of C3b and its cleavage product C3d to the antigen. B lymphocytes can bind the antigen through their Ig receptors and simultaneously bind the attached C3d through CR2. The combined signals result in B cell activation (see Chapter 9, Fig. 9–5). Opsonized antigens are also bound by follicular dendritic cells in the germinal centers of lymphoid organs. Follicular dendritic cells display antigens to B cells in the germinal centers, and this process is important for the selection of high-affinity B cells (see Chapter 9, Fig. 9–15). The importance of complement in humoral immune responses is illustrated by the severe impairment in antibody production and germinal center formation seen in knockout mice lacking C3 or C4 or the CR2 receptor.

Although our discussion has emphasized the physiologic functions of complement as an effector mechanism of host defense, the complement system is also involved in several pathologic conditions (Box 14–2). Some autoimmune diseases are associated with the production of autoantibodies specific for self proteins expressed on cell surfaces (see Chapter 18). Binding of

BOX 14–2

The Complement System in Disease

The complement system may be involved in human disease in two general ways. First, deficiencies in any of the protein components may lead to abnormal patterns of complement activation. The absence of a component of the classical or alternative pathway or absence of the late steps may result in deficient complement activation. If regulatory components are absent, too much complement activation may occur at the wrong time or wrong site, leading to excess inflammation and cell lysis, and may also cause a deficiency in plasma complement proteins because of excessive consumption. Second, an intact, normally functioning complement system may be activated in response to abnormal stimuli such as persistent microbes, antibodies against self antigens, or immune complexes deposited in tissues. In these infectious and autoimmune diseases, the inflammatory and lytic effects of complement may significantly contribute to the pathologic changes of the disease.

COMPLEMENT DEFICIENCIES Inherited and spontaneous deficiencies in many of the complement proteins have been described in humans.

Genetic deficiencies in classical pathway components, including C1q, C1r, C4, C2, and C3, have been described; C2 deficiency is the most commonly identified human complement deficiency. A disease that resembles the autoimmune disease systemic lupus erythematosus develops in more than 50% of patients with C2 and C4 deficiencies. The reason for this association is unknown, but defects in complement activation may lead to failure to clear circulating immune complexes. If normally generated immune complexes are not cleared from the circulation, they may be deposited in blood vessel walls and tissues, where they activate leukocytes by Fc receptor–dependent pathways and produce local inflammation. In addition, complement proteins regulate antigen-mediated signals received by B cells; in their absence, self antigens may not induce B cell tolerance, and autoimmunity results. Somewhat surprisingly, C2 and C4 deficiencies are not usually associated with increased susceptibility to infections, which suggests that the alternative pathway and Fc receptor–mediated effector mechanisms are adequate for host defense against most microbes. Deficiency of C3 is associated with frequent serious pyogenic bacterial infections that may be fatal, illustrating the central role of C3 and its importance in opsonization, enhanced phagocytosis, and destruction of these organisms.

Deficiencies in components of the alternative pathway, including properdin and factor D, result in increased susceptibility to infection with pyogenic bacteria. C3 deficiency is mentioned above.

Deficiencies in the terminal complement components, including C5, C6, C7, C8, and C9, have also been described. Interestingly, the only consistent clinical problem in these patients is a propensity for disseminated infections by *Neisseria* bacteria, including *Neisseria meningitidis* and *Neisseria gonorrhoeae*, indicating that complement-mediated bacterial lysis is particularly important for defense against these organisms.

Deficiencies in complement regulatory proteins are associated with abnormal complement activation and a variety of related clinical abnormalities. Deficiencies in C1 inhibitor and decay-accelerating factor are mentioned in the text. In patients with Factor I deficiency, plasma C3 is depleted as a result of the unregulated formation of fluid-phase C3 convertase (by the normal "tickover" mechanism). The clinical consequence is increased infections with pyogenic bacteria. Factor H deficiency is rare and is characterized by excess alternative pathway activation, consumption of C3, and glomerulonephritis caused by inadequate clearance of immune complexes and renal deposition of complement by-products. The effects of a lack of Factor I or Factor H are similar to the effects of an autoantibody called C3 nephritic factor (C3NeF), which is specific for alternative pathway C3 convertase (C3bBb). CeNeF stabilizes C3bBb and protects the complex from Factor H–mediated dissociation, which results in unregulated consumption of C3. Patients with this antibody often have glomerulonephritis, possibly caused by inadequate clearing of circulating immune complexes.

Deficiencies in complement receptors include the absence of type 3 complement receptor (CR3) and CR4, both resulting from rare mutations in the β chain (CD18) gene common to the CD11CD18 family of integrin molecules. The congenital disease caused by this gene defect is called leukocyte adhesion deficiency (see Chapter 20). This disorder is characterized by recurrent pyogenic infections and is caused by inadequate adherence of neutrophils to endothelium at tissue sites of infection

Continued on following page

BOX 14–2

The Complement System in Disease (*Continued*)

and perhaps by impaired iC3b-dependent phagocytosis of bacteria.

PATHOLOGIC EFFECTS OF A NORMAL COMPLEMENT SYSTEM Even when it is properly regulated and appropriately activated, the complement system can cause significant tissue damage. Some of the pathologic effects associated with bacterial infections may be due to complement-mediated acute inflammatory responses to infectious organisms. In some situations, complement activation is associated with intravascular thrombosis and can lead to ischemic injury to tissues. For instance, antiendothelial antibodies against vascularized organ transplants and the immune complexes produced in autoimmune diseases may bind to vascular endothelium and activate complement, thereby leading to inflammation and generation of the membrane attack complex (MAC) with damage to the endothelial surface, which favors coagulation. There is also evidence that some of the late complement proteins may activate prothrombinases in the circulation that initiate thrombosis independent of MAC-mediated damage to endothelium.

It has long been believed that the clearest example of complement-mediated pathology is immune complex disease. Systemic vasculitis and immune complex glomerulonephritis result from the deposition of antigen-antibody complexes in the walls of vessels and kidney glomeruli (see Chapter 18). Complement activated by the immunoglobulin in these deposited immune complexes initiates the acute inflammatory responses that destroy the vessel walls or glomeruli and lead to thrombosis, ischemic damage to tissues, and scarring. However, as mentioned in the text, studies with knockout mice lacking the complement proteins C3 or C4 or lacking Fcγ receptors suggest that Fc receptor–mediated leukocyte activation may cause inflammation and tissue injury as a result of IgG deposition even in the absence of complement activation.

these antibodies results in complement-dependent lysis and phagocytosis of the cells. In other diseases, immune complexes deposit in tissues and induce inflammation by complement-mediated recruitment and activation of leukocytes. Primary abnormalities of complement proteins and regulatory proteins are the causes of various human diseases.

The similarities in the roles of complement and Fc receptors in phagocytosis and inflammation raise the question of which is the more important effector mechanism of humoral immunity. Surprisingly, knockout mice lacking C3 or C4 show virtually no defects in IgG antibody–mediated phagocytosis of opsonized erythrocytes or in immune complex–mediated vasculitis. Both these reactions are abolished in knockout mice lacking the high-affinity Fcγ receptor. These results suggest that in IgG antibody–mediated phagocytosis and inflammation, Fc receptor–dependent reactions may be more important than complement-mediated reactions. Whether this phenomenon is true in humans remains to be established. Also, IgM antibody–mediated protective immunity and pathologic reactions are dependent only on the complement system because IgM is an efficient activator of complement but does not bind to leukocyte Fc receptors.

Functions of Antibodies at Special Anatomic Sites

So far, we have described the effector functions of antibodies that are systemic and do not show any particular features related to location. Antibodies serve special defense functions as a result of active transport into two anatomic compartments, the lumens of mucosal organs and the developing fetus. In these sites, the principal mechanism of protective immunity against microbes is antibody-mediated neutralization because lymphocytes and other effector cells do not pass through mucosal epithelia or the placenta.

Mucosal Immunity

IgA is the major class of antibody that is produced in the mucosal immune system. The gastrointestinal and respiratory tracts are two of the most common portals of entry of microbes. Defense against microbes that enter by these routes is provided by antibody, largely IgA, that is produced in mucosal lymphoid tissues and secreted through the mucosal epithelium into the lumens of the organs. In mucosal secretions, IgA binds to microbes and toxins present in the lumen and neutralizes them by blocking their entry into the host (see Fig. 14–2). Secretory immunity is the mechanism of protective immunity induced by oral vaccines such as the polio vaccine.

The mucosal immune system is a collection of lymphocytes and accessory cells, often organized into discrete anatomic structures resembling lymphoid follicles that are located underneath the epithelia of the gastrointestinal and respiratory tracts (see Chapter 2). IgA is produced in larger amounts than any other antibody isotype, mainly because of the size of the intestinal surface. It is estimated that a normal 70-kg adult secretes about 2 g of IgA per day, which accounts for 60% to 70% of the total output of antibodies. Because IgA synthesis occurs mainly in mucosal lymphoid tissue and transport into the mucosal lumen is efficient, this isotype constitutes less than one quarter of the antibody in plasma and is a minor component of systemic humoral immunity compared with IgG and IgM. Antibody responses to antigens encountered by ingestion or inhalation are typically dominated by IgA. In antigen-stimulated B cells, switching to the IgA isotype is stimulated by transforming growth factor-β (which may be produced by T cells as well as by nonlymphoid stromal cells) and the T_H2 cytokine interleukin (IL)-5. The probable reason that larger amounts of IgA are produced in the mucosal immune system than in other tissues is that isotype switching to IgA occurs most efficiently in mucosal lymphoid tissue, in part because IL-5–producing helper T cells are more numerous in mucosal than in other lymphoid tissue. IgA-producing B cells may also have a special propensity to home to mucosal tissues.

Secreted IgA is transported through epithelial cells into the intestinal lumen by an IgA-specific Fc receptor called the poly-Ig receptor. IgA is produced by B cells in the lamina propria and secreted in the form of a dimer that is held together by the coordinately produced J chain. (In contrast, serum IgA is usually a monomer lacking the J chain.) From the lamina propria, the IgA must be transported across the epithelium into the lumen, and this function is mediated by the poly-Ig receptor. This receptor is synthesized by mucosal epithelial cells and expressed on their basal and lateral surfaces. The membrane-associated form is a glycoprotein with five extracellular domains homologous to Ig domains and is thus a member of the Ig superfamily. The secreted, dimeric IgA containing the J chain binds to the membrane-associated poly-Ig receptor on mucosal epithelial cells (Fig. 14–18). This complex is endocytosed into the epithelial cell and actively transported in vesicles to the luminal surface. Here the poly-Ig receptor is proteolytically cleaved, its transmembrane and cytoplasmic domains are left attached to the epithelial cell, and the extracellular domain of the receptor, which carries the IgA molecule, is released into the intestinal lumen. The IgA-associated component of the receptor is called the **secretory component.** The poly-Ig receptor is also responsible for the secretion of IgA into bile, milk, sputum, saliva, and sweat. Although its ability to transport IgA has been studied most extensively, the receptor is capable of transporting IgM into intestinal secretions as well. (Note that secreted IgM is also a polymer associated with the J chain.) This is the reason that this receptor is called the poly-Ig receptor.

Neonatal Immunity

Neonatal mammals are protected from infection by maternally produced antibodies transported across the placenta into the fetal circulation and by antibodies in ingested milk transported across the gut epithelium of newborns. Neonates lack the ability to mount effective immune responses against microbes, and for several months after birth, their major defense against infection is passive immunity provided by maternal antibodies. Maternal IgG is transported across the placenta, and maternal IgA and IgG in breast milk are ingested by the nursing infant. Ingested IgA and IgG can neutralize pathogenic organisms that attempt to colonize the infant's gut, and ingested IgG antibodies are also transported across the gut epithelium into the circulation of the newborn. Thus, a newborn contains essentially the same IgG antibodies as the mother.

Transport of maternal IgG across the placenta and across the neonatal intestinal epithelium is mediated by an IgG-specific Fc receptor called the **neonatal Fc receptor** (FcRn). The FcRn is unique among Fc receptors in that it resembles a class I major histocompatibility complex (MHC) molecule containing a transmembrane heavy chain that is noncovalently associated with β_2-microglobulin. However, the interaction of IgG with FcRn does not involve the peptide-binding cleft used by class I MHC molecules to display peptides for T cell recognition.

Adults express an Fc receptor homologous to FcRn that functions to protect plasma IgG antibodies from catabolism. This Fc receptor is expressed on many epithelial cell types. It binds circulating IgG, promotes endocytosis of the IgG complexed with the receptor in a form that protects the antibody from intracellular degradation, and returns the antibody to the circulation. Knockout mice lacking β_2-microglobulin have 10-fold lower levels of serum IgG than normal mice do because of increased catabolism of the antibody resulting from failure to express the protective β_2-microglobulin–associated Fc receptor.

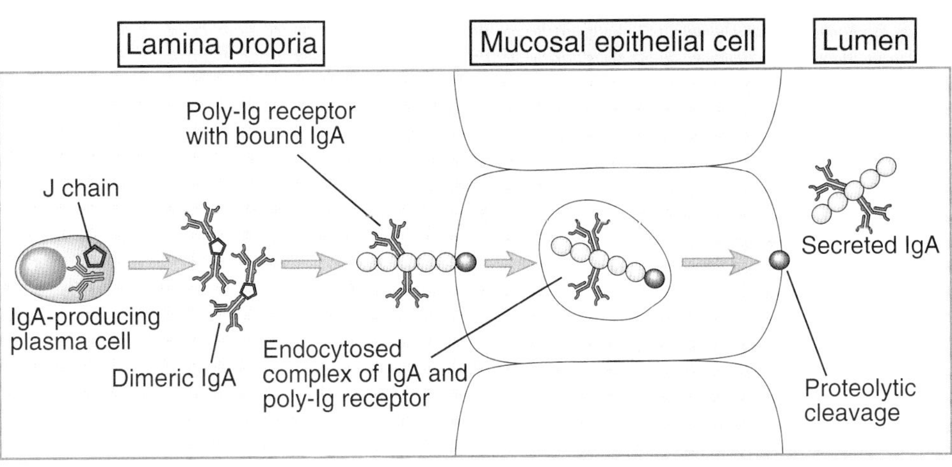

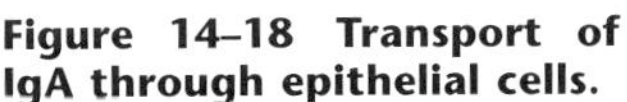

Figure 14–18 Transport of IgA through epithelial cells. IgA is produced by plasma cells in the lamina propria of mucosal tissue and binds to the poly-Ig receptor at the base of an epithelial cell. The complex is actively transported through the epithelial cell, and the bound IgA is released into the lumen by proteolytic cleavage. The process of active transport through the cell is called transcytosis.

Summary

- Humoral immunity is mediated by antibodies and is the effector arm of the adaptive immune system responsible for defense against extracellular microbes and microbial toxins. The antibodies that provide protection against infection may be produced by long-lived antibody-secreting cells generated by the first exposure to microbial antigen or by reactivation of memory B cells by the antigen.
- The effector functions of antibodies include neutralization of antigens, Fc receptor–dependent phagocytosis of opsonized particles, and activation of the complement system.
- Antibodies block, or neutralize, the infectivity of microbes by binding to the microbes and sterically hindering interactions of the microbes with cellular receptors. Antibodies similarly block the pathologic actions of toxins by preventing binding of the toxins to host cells.
- Antibody-coated (opsonized) particles are phagocytosed by binding of the Fc portions of the antibodies to phagocyte Fc receptors. There are several types of Fc receptors specific for different subclasses of IgG and for IgA and IgE antibodies, and different Fc receptors bind the antibodies with varying affinities. Attachment of antigen-complexed Ig to phagocyte Fc receptors also delivers signals that stimulate the microbicidal activities of phagocytes.
- The complement system consists of serum and membrane proteins that interact in a highly regulated manner to produce biologically active protein products. The two major pathways of complement activation are the alternative pathway, which is activated on microbial surfaces in the absence of antibody, and the classical pathway, which is activated by antigen-antibody complexes. The two pathways generate enzymes that cleave the C3 protein, and products of C3 become covalently attached to microbial surfaces or antibodies, so subsequent steps of complement activation are limited to these sites. Both pathways converge after C3 proteolysis, and the late steps consist of the proteolysis and association of several complement proteins, culminating in MAC formation.
- Complement activation is regulated by various plasma and cell membrane proteins that inhibit different steps in the cascades.
- The biologic functions of the complement system include opsonization of organisms and immune complexes by proteolytic fragments of C3, followed by binding to phagocyte receptors for complement fragments and phagocytic clearance, activation of inflammatory cells by proteolytic fragments of complement proteins called anaphylatoxins (C3a, C4a, C5a), cytolysis mediated by MAC formation on cell surfaces, solubilization and clearance of immune complexes, and enhancement of humoral immune responses.
- Defense against microbes and toxins in the lumens of mucosal organs is provided by IgA antibody produced in mucosal lymphoid tissue and actively transported through epithelial cells into the lumen.
- Protective immunity in neonates is a form of passive immunity provided by maternal antibodies transported across the placenta or ingested and transported across gut epithelium by a specialized neonatal Fc receptor.

Selected Readings

Barrington R, M Zhang, M Fischer, and MC Carroll. The role of complement in inflammation and adaptive immunity. Immunological Reviews 180:5–15, 2001.

Boes M. Role of natural and immune IgM antibodies in immune responses. Molecular Immunology 37:1141–1149, 2000.

Carroll MC. The role of complement and complement receptors in induction and regulation of immunity. Annual Review of Immunology 16:545–568, 1998.

Crawford K, and CA Alper. Genetics of the complement system. Reviews in Immunogenetics 2:323–338, 2000.

Kohl J. Anaphylatoxins and infectious and noninfectious inflammatory disorders. Molecular Immunology 38:175–187, 2001.

Krych-Goldberg M, and JP Atkinson. Structure-function relationships of complement receptor type 1. Immunological Reviews 180:112–122, 2001.

Liszewski MK, TC Farries, DM Lublin, IA Rooney, and JP Atkinson. Control of the complement system. Advances in Immunology 61:201–283, 1996.

Parren PW, and DR Burton. The antiviral activity of antibodies in vitro and in vivo. Advances in Immunology 77:195–262, 2001.

Petersen SV, S Thiel, and JC Jensenius. The mannan-binding lectin pathway of complement activation: biology and disease association. Molecular Immunology 38:133–149, 2001.

Radaev S, and P Sun. Recognition of immunoglobulins by Fcγ receptors. Molecular Immunology 38:1073–1083, 2002.

Ravetch JV, and S Bolland. IgG Fc receptors. Annual Review of Immunology 19:275–290, 2001.

Smith GP, and RA Smith. Membrane-targeted complement inhibitors. Molecular Immunology 38:249–255, 2001.

Walport MJ. Complement. New England Journal of Medicine 344:1058–1066 and 1141–1144, 2001.

Chapter 15

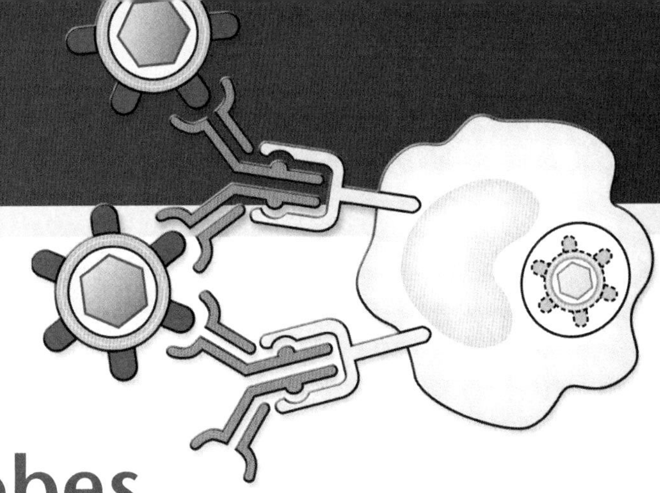

Immunity to Microbes

In the preceding chapters, we have described the components of the immune system and the generation and functions of immune responses. In this chapter, we integrate the information and discuss how the immune system performs its major physiologic function, which is to protect the host against microbial infections. We illustrate the physiologic relevance of various aspects of immune system function by describing the main features of immunity to different types of pathogenic microorganisms and how microbes try to resist the mechanisms of host defense.

The development of an infectious disease in an individual involves complex interactions between the microbe and the host. The key events during infection include entry of the microbe, invasion and colonization of host tissues, evasion from host immunity, and tissue injury or functional impairment. Some microbes produce disease by liberating toxins, even without extensive colonization of host tissues. Many features of microorganisms determine their virulence, and many diverse mechanisms contribute to the pathogenesis of infectious diseases. The topic of microbial pathogenesis is beyond the scope of this book and will not be discussed in detail. Rather, our discussion focuses on host immune responses to pathogenic microorganisms.

General Features of Immune Responses to Microbes

Although antimicrobial host defense reactions are numerous and varied, there are several important general features of immunity to microbes.

- ***Defense against microbes is mediated by the effector mechanisms of innate and adaptive immunity.*** The innate immune system provides early defense, and the adaptive immune system provides a more sustained and stronger response. Many pathogenic microbes have evolved to resist innate defense mechanisms, and protection against such microbes is critically dependent on adaptive immune responses. Adaptive immunity enhances the protective mechanisms of innate immunity and directs these mechanisms to sites of infection. Adaptive immune responses to microbes induce effector cells that eliminate the microbes and memory cells that protect the individual from subsequent infections.

- ***The immune system responds in distinct and specialized ways to different types of microbes to most effectively combat these infectious agents.*** Because microbes differ greatly in patterns of host invasion and colonization, their elimination requires diverse effector systems. The specialization of adaptive immunity allows the host to respond optimally to each type of microbe.
- ***The survival and pathogenicity of microbes in a host are critically influenced by the ability of the microbes to evade or resist the effector mechanisms of immunity.*** Infectious microbes and their hosts are engaged in a constant struggle for survival, and the balance between host immune responses and microbial strategies for resisting immunity often determines the outcome of infections. As we shall see later in the chapter, microorganisms have developed a variety of mechanisms for surviving in the face of powerful immunologic defenses. A common strategy used by many microbes is antigenic variation, by which the microbial structures recognized by the adaptive immune system are changed over successive generations of the microbe so that the microbes are not recognized.
- ***In many infections, tissue injury and disease may be caused by the host response to the microbe and its products rather than by the microbe itself.*** Immunity, like many other defense mechanisms, is necessary for host survival but also has the potential of causing injury to the host.

This chapter considers five types of pathogenic microorganisms that illustrate the main features of immunity to microbes: extracellular bacteria, intracellular bacteria, fungi, viruses, and protozoan and multicellular parasites. Our discussion of the immune responses to these microbes illustrates the diversity of antimicrobial immunity and the physiologic significance of the effector functions of lymphocytes discussed in earlier chapters.

Immunity to Extracellular Bacteria

Extracellular bacteria are capable of replicating outside host cells, for example, in the circulation, in connective tissues, and in tissue spaces such as the airways and intestinal lumens. Many different species of extracellular bacteria are pathogenic, and disease is caused by two principal mechanisms (Table 15–1). First, these bacteria induce inflammation, which results in tissue destruction at the site of infection. This is how pyogenic (pus-forming) cocci cause a large number of suppurative infections in humans. Second, many of these bacteria produce **toxins**, which have diverse pathologic effects. Such toxins may be endotoxins, which are components of bacterial cell walls, or exotoxins, which are actively secreted by the bacteria. The endotoxin of gram-negative bacteria, also called lipopolysaccharide (LPS), has been mentioned in earlier chapters as a potent activator of macrophages. Many exotoxins are cytotoxic, and they kill cells by various biochemical mechanisms. Other exotoxins interfere with normal cellular functions without killing cells, and yet other exotoxins stimulate the production of cytokines that cause disease.

Innate Immunity to Extracellular Bacteria

The principal mechanisms of innate immunity to extracellular bacteria are complement activation,

Table 15–1. Examples of Pathogenic Microbes

Microbe	Examples of human diseases	Mechanisms of pathogenicity
Extracellular bacteria		
Staphylococcus aureus	Skin and soft tissue infections, lung abscess Systemic: toxic shock syndrome, food poisoning	Skin infections; acute inflammation induced by toxins; cell death caused by pore-forming toxins Systemic: enterotoxin ("superantigen")-induced cytokine production by T cells causing skin necrosis, shock, diarrhea
Streptococcus pyogenes (group A)	Pharyngitis Skin infections: impetigo, erysipelas; cellulitis Systemic: scarlet fever	Acute inflammation induced by various toxins, e.g., streptolysin O damages cell membranes (antiphagocytic action of capsular polysaccharides)
Streptococcus pyogenes (pneumococcus)	Pneumonia, meningitis	Acute inflammation induced by cell wall constituents; pneumolysin is similar to streptolysin O
Escherichia coli	Urinary tract infections, gastroenteritis, septic shock	Toxins act on intestinal epithelium and cause increased chloride and water secretion; endotoxin (LPS) stimulates cytokine secretion by macrophages

Table 15–1. (*Continued*)

Microbe	Examples of human diseases	Mechanisms of pathogenicity
Vibrio cholerae	Diarrhea	Cholera toxin ADP ribosylates G protein subunit, which leads to increased cyclic AMP in intestinal epithelial cells and results in chloride secretion and water loss
Clostridium tetani	Tetanus	Tetanus toxin binds to the motor end plate at neuromuscular junctions and causes irreversible muscle contraction
Neisseria meningitidis (meningococcus)	Meningitis	Acute inflammation and systemic disease caused by potent endotoxin
Corynebacterium diphtheriae	Diphtheria	Diphtheria toxin ADP ribosylates elongation factor-2 and inhibits protein synthesis
Intracellular bacteria		
Mycobacteria	Tuberculosis, leprosy	Macrophage activation resulting in granulomatous inflammation and tissue destruction
Listeria monocytogenes	Listeriosis	Listeriolysin damages cell membranes
Legionella pneumophila	Legionnaires' disease	Cytotoxin lyses cells and causes lung injury and inflammation
Fungi		
Candida albicans	Candidiasis	Unknown; binds complement proteins
Aspergillus fumigatus	Aspergillosis	Invasion and thrombosis of blood vessels causing ischemic necrosis and cell injury
Histoplasma capsulatum	Histoplasmosis	Lung infection causes granulomatous inflammation
Viruses		
Polio	Poliomyelitis	Inhibits host cell protein synthesis (tropism for motor neurons in the anterior horn of the spinal cord)
Influenza	Influenza pneumonia	Inhibits host cell protein synthesis (tropism for ciliated epithelial cells)
Rabies	Rabies encephalitis	Inhibits host cell protein synthesis (tropism for peripheral nerves)
Herpes simplex	Various herpes infections (skin, systemic)	Inhibits host cell protein synthesis; functional impairment of immune cells
Hepatitis B	Viral hepatitis	Host CTL response to infected hepatocytes
Epstein-Barr virus	Infectious mononucleosis; B cell proliferation, lymphomas	Acute infection: cell lysis (tropism for B lymphocytes) Latent infection: stimulates B cell proliferation
Human immunodeficiency virus	Acquired immunodeficiency syndrome	Multiple: killing of $CD4^+$ T cells; functional impairment of immune cells (see Chapter 20)

Abbreviations: ADP, adenosine diphosphate; AMP, adenosine monophosphate; CTL, cytolytic T lymphocyte; LPS, lipopolysaccharide.

Examples of pathogenic microbes of different classes are listed, with brief summaries of known or postulated mechanisms of tissue injury and disease.

This table was compiled with the assistance of Dr. Arlene Sharpe, Department of Pathology, Harvard Medical School and Brigham and Women's Hospital, Boston.

phagocytosis, and the inflammatory response. Gram-positive bacteria contain a peptidoglycan in their cell walls that activates the alternative pathway of complement by promoting formation of the alternative pathway C3 convertase (see Chapter 14). LPS in the cell walls of gram-negative bacteria also activates the alternative complement pathway in the absence of antibody. Bacteria that express mannose on their surface may bind mannose-binding lectin, which is homologous to C1q, thereby leading to complement activation by the lectin pathway. One result of complement activation is opsonization and enhanced phagocytosis of the bacteria. In addition, the membrane attack complex lyses bacteria, especially *Neisseria* species, and complement by-products participate in inflammatory responses by recruiting and activating leukocytes. Phagocytes bind extracellular bacteria by various surface receptors, including mannose receptors and scavenger receptors, and bind opsonized bacteria by complement receptors. Toll-like receptors of phagocytes participate in the activation of the phagocytes as a result of encounter with microbes. These various receptors promote the phagocytosis of the microbes and stimulate the microbicidal activities of the phagocytes (see Chapter 12). In addition, activated phagocytes secrete cytokines, which induce leukocyte infiltration into sites of infection (inflammation). Injury to normal tissue is a pathologic side effect of inflammation. Cytokines also induce the systemic manifestations of infection, including fever and the synthesis of acute-phase proteins.

Adaptive Immune Responses to Extracellular Bacteria

Humoral immunity is the principal protective immune response against extracellular bacteria, and it functions to eliminate the microbes and neutralize their toxins (Fig. 15–1). Antibody responses against extracellular bacteria are directed against cell wall antigens and secreted and cell-associated toxins, which may be polysaccharides or proteins. The polysaccharides are prototypic thymus-independent antigens, and a major function of humoral immunity is defense against polysaccharide-rich encapsulated bacteria. The effector mechanisms used by antibodies to combat these infections include neutralization, opsonization and phago-

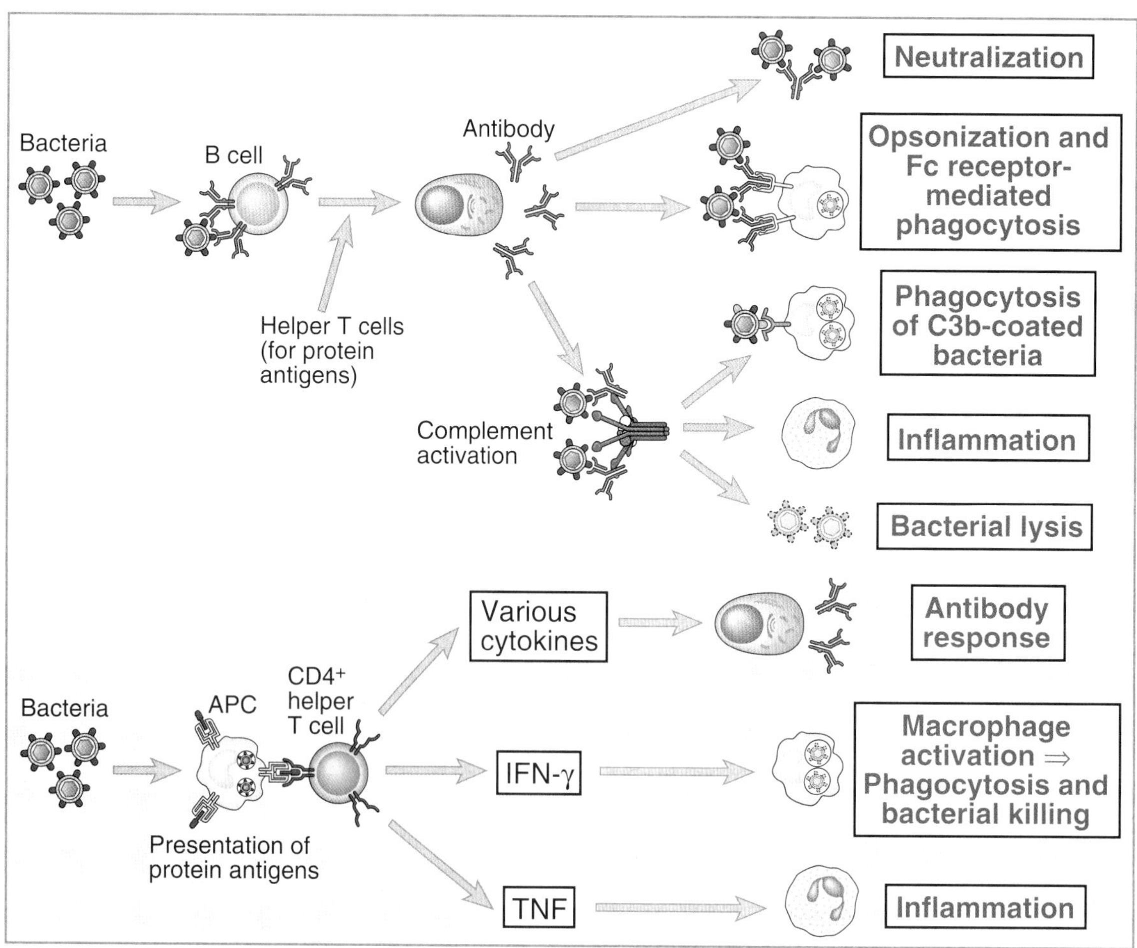

Figure 15–1 Adaptive immune responses to extracellular microbes. Adaptive immune responses to extracellular microbes, such as bacteria, and their toxins consist of antibody production and the activation of $CD4^+$ helper T cells. Antibodies neutralize and eliminate microbes and toxins by several mechanisms. Helper T cells produce cytokines that stimulate B cell responses, macrophage activation, and inflammation. APC, antigen-presenting cell; IFN-γ, interferon-γ; TNF, tumor necrosis factor.

cytosis, and activation of complement by the classical pathway (see Chapter 14). Neutralization is mediated by high-affinity IgG and IgA isotypes, opsonization by some subclasses of IgG, and complement activation by IgM and subclasses of IgG. The protein antigens of extracellular bacteria also activate CD4$^+$ helper T cells, which produce cytokines that stimulate antibody production, induce local inflammation, and enhance the phagocytic and microbicidal activities of macrophages (see Fig. 15–1). Interferon-γ (IFN-γ) is the T cell cytokine responsible for macrophage activation, and tumor necrosis factor (TNF) and lymphotoxin trigger inflammation.

The principal injurious consequences of host responses to extracellular bacteria are inflammation and septic shock, which are caused by cytokines produced mainly by activated macrophages. Septic shock is the most severe cytokine-induced pathologic consequence of infection by gram-negative and some gram-positive bacteria. It is a syndrome characterized by circulatory collapse and disseminated intravascular coagulation (see Chapter 12, Box 12–2). TNF is the principal mediator of septic shock. In fact, serum levels of TNF are predictive of the outcome of severe gram-negative bacterial infections. Some bacterial toxins stimulate all the T cells in an individual that express a particular family of V_β T cell receptor genes. Such toxins are called **superantigens** (Box 15–1). Their importance lies in their ability to activate many T cells, with the subsequent production of large amounts of cytokines and clinicopathologic abnormalities that are similar to septic shock.

A late complication of the humoral immune response to bacterial infection may be the generation of disease-producing antibodies. The best defined examples are two rare sequelae of streptococcal infections of the throat or skin that are manifested weeks or even months after the infections are controlled. Rheumatic fever is a sequel to pharyngeal infection with some serologic types of β-hemolytic streptococci. Infection leads to the production of antibodies against a bacterial cell wall protein (M protein). Some of these antibodies cross-react with myocardial sarcolemmal proteins and myosin and are deposited in the heart and subsequently cause inflammation (carditis). Poststreptococcal glomerulonephritis is a sequel to infection of the skin or throat with other serotypes of β-hemolytic streptococci. Antibodies produced against these bacteria form complexes with bacterial antigen, which may be deposited in kidney glomeruli and cause nephritis.

Evasion of Immune Mechanisms by Extracellular Bacteria

The virulence of extracellular bacteria has been linked to a number of mechanisms that resist host immunity (Table 15–2), including antiphagocytic mechanisms and inhibition of complement or inactivation of complement products. Bacteria with polysaccharide-rich capsules resist phagocytosis and are therefore much more virulent than homologous strains lacking a capsule. The capsules of many gram-positive and gram-negative bacteria contain sialic acid residues that inhibit complement activation by the alternative pathway.

Table 15–2. Mechanisms of Immune Evasion by Bacteria

Mechanism of immune evasion	Examples
Extracellular bacteria	
Antigenic variation	*Neisseria gonorrhoeae, Escherichia coli, Salmonella typhimurium*
Inhibition of complement activation	Many bacteria
Resistance to phagocytosis	Pneumococcus
Scavenging of reactive oxygen intermediates	Catalase-positive staphylococci
Intracellular bacteria	
Inhibition of phagolysosome formation	*Mycobacterium tuberculosis, Legionella pneumophila*
Scavenging of reactive oxygen intermediates	*Mycobacterium leprae* (phenolic glycolipid)
Disruption of phagosome membrane, escape into cytoplasm	*Listeria monocytogenes* (hemolysin protein)

The major mechanism used by bacteria to evade humoral immunity is genetic variation of surface antigens. Some surface antigens of bacteria such as gonococci and *Escherichia coli* are contained in their pili, which are the structures responsible for bacterial adhesion to host cells. The major antigen of the pili is a protein called pilin. The pilin genes of gonococci undergo extensive gene conversion, because of which the progeny of one organism can produce up to 10^6 antigenically distinct pilin molecules. This ability to alter antigens helps the bacteria evade attack by pilin-specific antibodies, although its principal significance for the bacteria may be to select for pili that are more adherent to host cells so that the bacteria are more virulent. In other bacteria, such as *Haemophilus influenzae*, changes in the production of glycosidases lead to chemical alterations in surface LPS and other polysaccharides, which enable the bacteria to evade humoral immune responses against these antigens.

Immunity to Intracellular Bacteria

A characteristic of facultative intracellular bacteria is their ability to survive and even replicate within phagocytes. Because these microbes are able to find a niche where they are inaccessible to circulating antibodies, their elimination requires the mechanisms of cell-mediated immunity (Fig. 15–2). As we shall discuss later in this section, the pathologic consequences of infection by many intracellular bacteria are due to the host response to these microbes (see Table 15–1).

BOX 15–1

Bacterial Superantigens

Some microbial toxins are called superantigens because they stimulate large numbers of T cells (more than conventional antigens) but not all T cells (which distinguishes them from polyclonal activators). Staphylococcal enterotoxins are exotoxins produced by the gram-positive bacterium *Staphylococcus aureus* and consist of five serologically distinct groups of proteins: SEA, SEB, SEC, SED, and SEE. These toxins are the most common cause of food poisoning in humans. A related toxin, TSST, causes a disease called toxic shock syndrome (TSS), which has been associated with tampon use and surgical wounds. Pyrogenic exotoxins of streptococci and exotoxins produced by mycoplasmas may be structurally and functionally related to these enterotoxins.

The immune response to staphylococcal enterotoxins and related proteins has a number of features that make these bacterial products unique in terms of biologic and pathologic effects:

- Staphylococcal enterotoxins are among the most potent naturally occurring T cell mitogens known. They are capable of stimulating the proliferation of normal T lymphocytes at concentrations of 10^{-9} M or less. As many as one in five normal T cells in mouse lymphoid tissue or human peripheral blood may respond to a particular enterotoxin.
- Enterotoxins bind to the V_β region of T cell receptors (TCRs), and each toxin stimulates T cells that express antigen receptors whose V_β regions are encoded by a single V_β gene or gene family. In other words, the specificity of T cells for different enterotoxins is encoded in the V_β region and is not related to other components of the TCR, such as the V_α, J, or D segments, because enterotoxins bind directly to the β chains of TCR molecules close to but outside the antigen-binding (complementarity-determining) regions. Different enterotoxins stimulate T cells expressing V_β genes from different families (see Table). The specificity of enterotoxins for V_β regions explains why they stimulate many but not all T cells.

Superantigens bind to class II MHC molecules on antigen-presenting cells (APCs) at a site that is away from the peptide-binding cleft. Superantigens do not need to undergo intracellular processing, as do conventional protein antigens, to bind to these MHC molecules. The same enterotoxin binds to class II molecules of different alleles, indicating that the polymorphism of the MHC does not influence the presentation of these antigens. Each staphylococcal enterotoxin molecule possesses two binding sites for class II MHC molecules. This characteristic allows each enterotoxin molecule to cross-link MHC molecules on APCs, and the enterotoxin-MHC molecule dimer may cross-link two antigen receptors on each T cell and thus initiate T cell responses.

The high frequency of staphylococcal enterotoxin–responding T cells, particularly CD4⁺ cells, has several functional implications. Acutely, exposure to high concentrations of enterotoxin leads to systemic reactions such as fever, disseminated intravascular coagulation, and cardiovascular shock. These abnormalities are probably mediated by cytokines, such as TNF, produced directly by the T cells or by macrophages that are activated by the T cells. In many respects, these reactions resemble systemic reactions to endotoxin (lipopolysaccharide), as in septic shock, which are also mediated by cytokines (see Chapter 12, Box 12–2). The secretion of large amounts of inflammatory cytokines is the likely pathogenesis of TSS, which is characterized by shock, skin exfoliation, conjunctivitis, and diarrhea and can progress to renal and pulmonary failure and death. Prolonged administration of enterotoxins to mice results in wasting, thymic atrophy, and profound immunodeficiency, also probably secondary to chronic high levels of TNF.

Staphylococcal enterotoxins are useful tools for analyzing T lymphocyte maturation, activation, and tolerance. Administration of SEB to neonatal mice leads to intrathymic deletion of all immature T cells that express the $V_\beta 3$ and $V_\beta 8$ TCR genes. This deletion mimics self antigen–induced negative selection of self-reactive T cells during thymic maturation. Superantigens also induce death of mature $CD4^+$ and $CD8^+$ T cells, either by engaging Fas or TNF receptors or by delivering pro-apoptotic signals to T cells without survival signals (see Chapter 10, Box 10–2). This type of cell death is postulated to be a model of deletion of mature T cells that are exposed to self antigens.

Viral gene products may also function as superantigens. In certain inbred strains of mice, different mouse mammary tumor virus genes have become incorporated into the genome. Viral antigens produced by the cells of one strain are capable of activating T lymphocytes from other strains that express particular V_β segments in their antigen receptors. The result is a form of "mixed lymphocyte reaction" that is not caused by MHC disparity. This was discovered long before viral superantigens were identified, and the interstrain reactions were attributed to Mls (minor lymphocyte stimulating) loci. We now know that Mls "loci" are actually different retroviral superantigen genes that are stably incorporated into the genome and inherited in different inbred strains.

Enterotoxin	Mice	Humans
SEB	V_β7, 8.1-8.3,17	V_β3,12,14,15,17, 20
SEC 2	V_β8.2,10	V_β12,13,14,15,17, 20
SEE	V_β11,15,17	V_β5.1, 6.1-6.3, 8, 18
TSST-1	V_β15,16	V_β2

Abbreviations: SE, staphylococcal enterotoxin; TSST, toxic shock syndrome toxin

Innate Immunity to Intracellular Bacteria

The innate immune response to intracellular bacteria consists mainly of phagocytes and NK (natural killer) cells. Phagocytes, initially neutrophils and later macrophages, ingest and attempt to destroy these microbes, but pathogenic intracellular bacteria are resistant to degradation within phagocytes. Intracellular bacteria activate NK cells either directly or by stimulating macrophage production of IL-12, a powerful NK cell–activating cytokine. The NK cells produce IFN-γ, which in turn activates macrophages and promotes killing of the phagocytosed bacteria. Thus, NK cells provide an early defense against these microbes, before the development of adaptive immunity. In fact, mice with severe combined immunodeficiency, which lack T and B cells, are able to control infection with the intracellular bacterium *Listeria monocytogenes* by NK cell–derived IFN-γ production. Innate immunity may limit bacterial growth for some time but usually fails to eradicate these infections, and eradication requires adaptive cell-mediated immunity.

Adaptive Immune Responses to Intracellular Bacteria

The major protective immune response against intracellular bacteria is cell-mediated immunity. Individuals with deficient cell-mediated immunity, such as patients with acquired immunodeficiency syndrome (AIDS), are extremely susceptible to infections with intracellular bacteria (and viruses). Cell-mediated immunity was first identified by George Mackaness in the 1950s as protection against the intracellular bacterium *L. monocytogenes.* This form of immunity could be adoptively transferred to naive animals with lymphoid cells but not with serum from infected or immunized animals (see Chapter 13, Fig. 13–2).

As we discussed in Chapter 13, cell-mediated immunity consists of two types of reactions—macrophage activation by the T cell–derived signals CD40 ligand and IFN-γ, which results in killing of phagocytosed microbes, and lysis of infected cells by cytolytic T lymphocytes (CTLs). Both CD4^{+} T cells and CD8^{+} T cells respond to protein antigens of phagocytosed microbes,

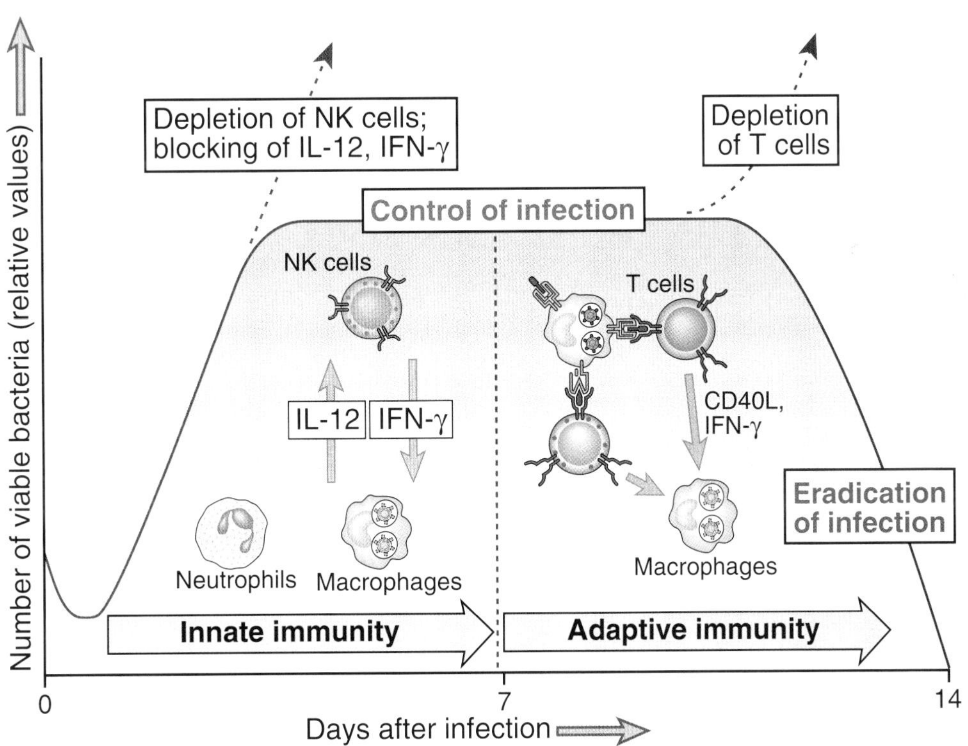

Figure 15–2 Innate and adaptive immunity to intracellular bacteria.
The innate immune response to intracellular bacteria consists of phagocytes and NK cells, interactions among which are mediated by cytokines (IL-12 and IFN-γ). The typical adaptive immune response to these microbes is cell-mediated immunity, in which T cells activate phagocytes to eliminate the microbes. Innate immunity may control bacterial growth, but elimination of the bacteria requires adaptive immunity. Depletion or blocking of various immune effector mechanisms at different stages of infection leads to unchecked bacterial growth, shown as dashed lines. These principles are based largely on analysis of *Listeria monocytogenes* infection in mice; the numbers of viable bacteria shown on the y-axis are relative values of bacterial colonies that can be grown from the tissues of infected mice. (From Unanue ER. Studies in listeriosis show the strong symbiosis between the innate cellular system and the T-cell response. Immunological Reviews 158: 11–25, 1997.)

which are displayed as peptides associated with class II and class I major histocompatibility complex (MHC) molecules, respectively. $CD4^+$ T cells differentiate into T_H1 effectors under the influence of IL-12, which is produced by macrophages and dendritic cells. The T cells express CD40 ligand and secrete IFN-γ, and these two stimuli activate macrophages to produce several microbicidal substances, including reactive oxygen intermediates, nitric oxide, and lysosomal enzymes. IFN-γ also stimulates the production of antibody isotypes (e.g., IgG2a in mice) that activate complement and opsonize bacteria for phagocytosis, thus aiding the effector functions of macrophages.

The importance of IL-12 and IFN-γ in immunity to intracellular bacteria has been demonstrated in several experimental models. For instance, knockout mice lacking either of these cytokines are extremely susceptible to infection with intracellular bacteria such as *Mycobacterium tuberculosis* and *L. monocytogenes* (Fig. 15–3).

Phagocytosed bacteria stimulate $CD8^+$ T cell responses if bacterial antigens are transported from phagosomes into the cytosol or if the bacteria escape from phagosomes and enter the cytoplasm of infected cells. In the latter case, the microbes are no longer susceptible to the microbicidal mechanisms of phagocytes,

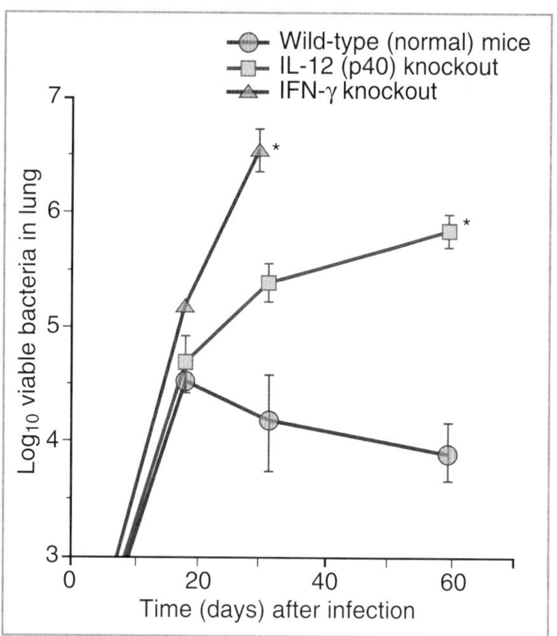

Figure 15–3 Role of IL-12 and IFN-γ in defense against an intracellular bacterial infection.

In this experiment, wild-type (normal control) mice and knockout mice lacking the p40 subunit of IL-12 or IFN-γ were infected with the intracellular bacterium *Mycobacterium tuberculosis* by aerosol. Lungs were examined at different times after infection for the number of bacteria capable of forming colonies in culture. Normal mice control bacterial growth, mice lacking IL-12 have a reduced ability to control the infection (and die by day 60), and IFN-γ knockout mice are incapable of limiting bacterial growth (and die by day 30 to 35). Asterisks indicate the time of death. (Data courtesy of Dr. Andrea Cooper, Department of Microbiology, Colorado State University, Fort Collins.)

and the infection is eradicated by the killing of infected cells by CTLs. Thus, the effectors of cell-mediated immunity, namely, $CD4^+$ T cells that activate macrophages and $CD8^+$ CTLs, function cooperatively in defense against intracellular bacteria (Fig. 15–4).

The role of different T cell subsets in defense against intracellular bacteria has been analyzed by adoptively transferring T cells from *L. monocytogenes*–infected mice to normal mice and challenging the recipients with the bacteria. By depleting particular cell types, it is possible to determine which effector population is responsible for protection. Such experiments have shown that both $CD4^+$ T cells and $CD8^+$ T cells function cooperatively to eliminate infection by wild-type *L. monocytogenes*. The $CD4^+$ cells produce large amounts of IFN-γ, which activates macrophages to kill phagocytosed microbes. However, *L. monocytogenes* produces a protein called hemolysin that allows bacteria to escape from the phagolysosomes of macrophages into the cytoplasm. In their cytoplasmic haven, the bacteria are protected from the microbicidal mechanisms of macrophages, such as reactive oxygen intermediates, which are produced mainly within phagolysosomes. $CD8^+$ T cells are then activated and function by killing any macrophages that may be harboring bacteria in their cytoplasm. A mutant of *L. monocytogenes* that lacks hemolysin remains confined to phagolysosomes. Such mutant bacteria can be completely eradicated by $CD4^+$ T cell–derived IFN-γ production and macrophage activation.

The macrophage activation that occurs in response to intracellular microbes is also capable of causing tissue injury. This injury may be manifested as delayed-type hypersensitivity (DTH) reactions to microbial protein antigens, such as purified protein derivative (PPD) of *M. tuberculosis* (see Chapter 13). Because intracellular bacteria have evolved to resist killing within phagocytes, they often persist for long periods and cause chronic antigenic stimulation and T cell and macrophage activation, which may result in the formation of **granulomas** surrounding the microbes (see Chapter 13, Fig. 13–15). The histologic hallmark of infection with some intracellular bacteria is granulomatous inflammation. This type of inflammatory reaction may serve to localize and prevent spread of the microbes, but it is also associated with severe functional impairment caused by tissue necrosis and fibrosis. The concept that protective immunity and pathologic hypersensitivity may coexist because they are manifestations of the same type of adaptive immune response is clearly exemplified in mycobacterial infections (Box 15–2).

Differences among individuals in the patterns of T cell responses to intracellular microbes are important determinants of disease progression and clinical outcome (Fig. 15–5). An example of this relationship between the type of T cell response and disease outcome is leprosy, which is caused by *Mycobacterium leprae*. There are two polar forms of leprosy, the lepromatous and tuberculoid forms, although many patients fall into less clear intermediate groups. In lepromatous

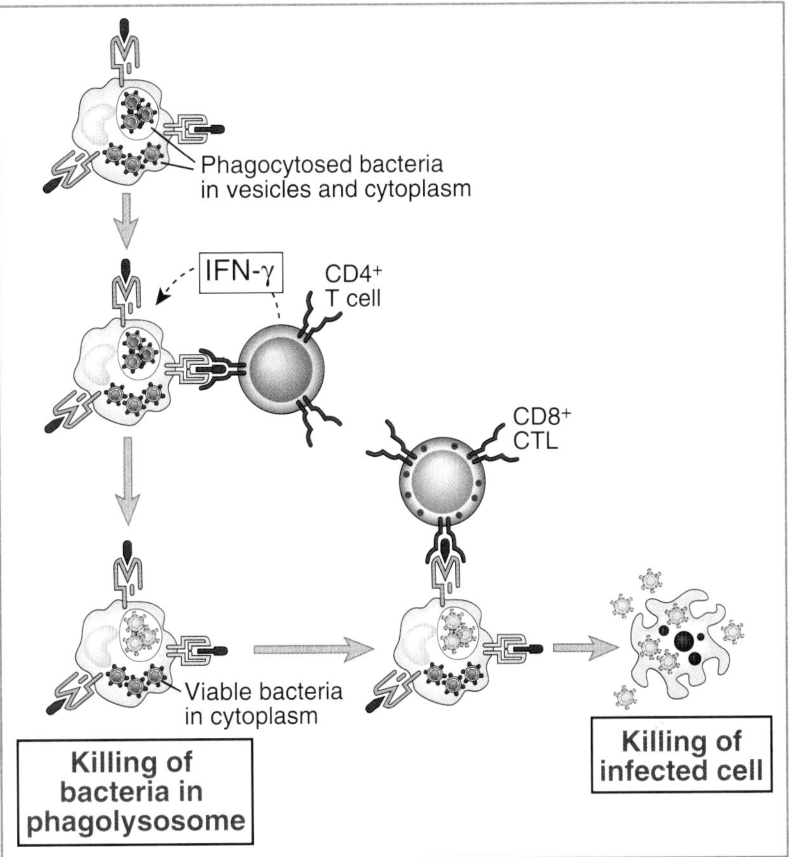

Figure 15–4 Cooperation of $CD4^+$ and $CD8^+$ T cells in defense against intracellular microbes.

Intracellular bacteria such as *Listeria monocytogenes* are phagocytosed by macrophages and may survive in phagosomes and escape into the cytoplasm. $CD4^+$ T cells respond to class II MHC–associated peptide antigens derived from the intravesicular bacteria. These T cells produce IFN-γ, which activates macrophages to destroy the microbes in phagosomes. $CD8^+$ T cells respond to class I–associated peptides derived from cytosolic antigens and kill the infected cells.

leprosy, patients have high specific antibody titers but weak cell-mediated responses to *M. leprae* antigens. Mycobacteria proliferate within macrophages and are detectable in large numbers. The bacterial growth and persistent, but inadequate, macrophage activation result in destructive lesions in the skin and underlying tissue. In contrast, patients with tuberculoid leprosy have strong cell-mediated immunity but low antibody levels. This pattern of immunity is reflected in granulomas that form around nerves and produce peripheral

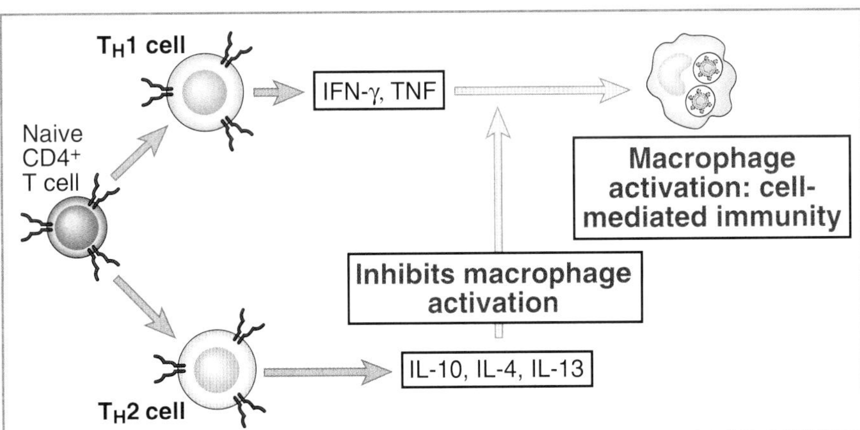

Infection	Response	Outcome
Leishmania major	Most mouse strains: T_H1	⇒ Recovery
	BALB/c mice: T_H2	⇒ Disseminated infection
Mycobacterium leprae	Some patients: T_H1	⇒ Tuberculoid leprosy
	Some patients: Defective T_H1 or dominant T_H2	⇒ Lepromatous leprosy (high bacterial count)

Figure 15–5 Role of T cells and cytokines in determining outcome of infections.

Naive $CD4^+$ T lymphocytes may differentiate into T_H1 cells, which activate phagocytes to kill ingested microbes, and T_H2 cells, which inhibit macrophage activation. The balance between these two subsets may influence the outcome of infections, as illustrated by *Leishmania* infection in mice and leprosy in humans.

BOX 15–2

Immunity to *Mycobacterium tuberculosis*

Mycobacteria are slow-growing, aerobic, facultative intracellular bacilli whose cell walls contain high concentrations of lipids. These lipids are responsible for the acid-resistant staining of the bacteria with the red dye carbol fuchsin, because of which these organisms are also called acid-fast bacilli. The two common human pathogens in this class of bacteria are *Mycobacterium tuberculosis* and *Mycobacterium leprae*; in addition, atypical mycobacteria such as *Mycobacterium avium-intracellulare* cause opportunistic infections in immunodeficient hosts (e.g., AIDS patients). *Mycobacterium bovis* infects cattle and may infect humans, and bacillus Calmette-Guérin (BCG) is an attenuated, nonvirulent strain of *M. bovis* that is used as a vaccine against tuberculosis.

Tuberculosis is an example of an infection with an intracellular bacterium in which protective immunity and pathologic hypersensitivity coexist, and the lesions are caused mainly by the host response. *M. tuberculosis* does not produce any known exotoxin or endotoxin. Infection usually occurs by the respiratory route and is transmitted from person to person. In a primary infection, bacilli multiply slowly in the lungs and cause only mild inflammation. The infection is contained by alveolar macrophages. More than 90% of infected patients remain asymptomatic, but bacteria survive in lungs and can be reactivated. By 6 to 8 weeks after infection, regional lymph nodes are involved, and $CD4^+$ T cells are activated. These T cells produce IFN-γ, which activates macrophages and enhances their ability to kill phagocytosed bacilli. TNF produced by T cells and macrophages also plays a role in local inflammation and macrophage activation, and TNF receptor knockout mice are highly susceptible to mycobacterial infections. However, *M. tuberculosis* is capable of surviving within macrophages because components of its cell wall inhibit the fusion of lysosomes with phagocytic vacuoles.

Continuing T cell activation leads to the formation of granulomas, with central necrosis, called caseous necrosis, that is caused by macrophage products such as lysosomal enzymes and reactive oxygen intermediates. This is a form of DTH reaction to the bacilli. It is postulated that necrosis serves to eliminate infected macrophages and provides an anoxic environment in which the bacilli cannot divide. Thus, even the tissue injury may serve a protective function. Caseating granulomas and the fibrosis (scarring) that accompanies granulomatous inflammation are the principal causes of tissue injury and clinical disease in tuberculosis. Only a minority of infected individuals (probably less than 10%) develop clinical symptoms. Previously infected persons show cutaneous DTH reactions to skin challenge with a bacterial antigen preparation (PPD, or tuberculin). Bacilli may survive for many years even without overt clinical manifestations and may be reactivated at any time. This is the reason for treating individuals who convert from PPD negative to PPD positive with antibiotics such as isoniazid and rifampin, even though they may have no symptoms of the disease. Although the prevalence of tuberculosis was markedly reduced with the use of such antibiotics, the incidence of the disease has recently been increasing. This is mainly because of the emergence of antibiotic-resistant strains and the increased incidence of immunodeficiency caused by HIV infection and immunosuppressive therapies. The efficacy of BCG as a prophylactic vaccine remains controversial. In rare cases, *M. tuberculosis* may cause lesions in extrapulmonary sites. In chronic tuberculosis, sustained production of TNF leads to cachexia.

Different inbred strains of mice vary in their susceptibility to infection with *M. tuberculosis* (and with other intracellular microbes, such as the protozoan *Leishmania major*). Susceptibility or resistance to *M. tuberculosis* maps to a single gene, originally called *bcg* or *lsh* before molecular characterization and now identified as a polymorphic *NRAMP1* (NRAMP, natural resistance–associated macrophage protein) gene. NRAMP1 is expressed on phagolysosomal membranes in macrophages and is involved in divalent cation transport. It is hypothesized that NRAMP1 contributes to microbial killing by depleting the phagosome of divalent cations and that allelic variants of *NRAMP1* are defective in this function. Studies in humans suggest that some allelic variants of NRAMP1 are also associated with susceptibility to mycobacterial infection.

Some studies have shown that both *in vivo* and *in vitro*, *M. tuberculosis* stimulates T cells expressing the γδ form of the antigen receptor. These T cells may be reacting to mycobacterial antigens that are homologous to heat shock proteins. Heat shock proteins are evolutionarily conserved, with little structural variations between prokaryotes and eukaryotes. They are induced on exposure to many kinds of stress, including heat; depletion of oxygen, nutrients, and essential ions; and exposure to free radicals. Their function may be as chaperones to promote refolding of proteins after cell injury. In infected cells, heat shock proteins may be produced by the stressed cells or by the bacteria. It is postulated that the response of γδ T cells to these proteins is a primitive defense mechanism against some microbes. Some γδ cells, as well as $CD4^-CD8^-TCR\alpha\beta$-expressing cells, recognize mycobacterial lipid antigens presented in association with nonpolymorphic CD1 molecules. However, the effector functions of these cells, their frequencies *in vivo*, and their roles in protective immunity against mycobacteria are not yet known.

Atypical mycobacteria constitute a heterogeneous group of mycobacteria that are widely distributed in the animal kingdom and in nature. They frequently colonize humans but rarely cause disease in immunocompetent individuals. However, they cause severe disease in immunodeficient individuals, such as AIDS patients. Unlike *M. tuberculosis* infection in patients with intact immune systems, *M. avium-intracellulare* infection in AIDS patients does not lead to well-formed granulomas, but rather disease is due to unchecked bacterial proliferation.

M. leprae is the cause of leprosy. The nature of the T cell response and specifically the types of cytokines produced by activated T cells are important determinants of the lesions and clinical course of *M. leprae* infection (see text).

sensory nerve defects and secondary traumatic skin lesions but less tissue destruction and a paucity of bacteria in the lesions. One possible reason for the differences in these two forms of disease caused by the same organism may be that there are different patterns of T cell differentiation and cytokine production in individuals. Some studies indicate that patients with the tuberculoid form of the disease produce IFN-γ and IL-2 in lesions (indicative of T_H1 cell activation), whereas patients with lepromatous leprosy produce more IL-4 and IL-10 (typical of T_H2 cells). In lepromatous leprosy, both the deficiency of IFN-γ and the macrophage suppressive effects of IL-10 and IL-4 may result in weak cell-mediated immunity and failure to control bacterial spread. The role of T_H1- and T_H2-derived cytokines in determining the outcome of infection has been most clearly demonstrated in infection by the protozoan parasite *Leishmania major* in different strains of inbred mice (discussed later in the chapter).

Evasion of Immune Mechanisms by Intracellular Bacteria

Different intracellular bacteria have developed various strategies to resist elimination by phagocytes (see Table 15–2). The outcome of infection by these organisms often depends on whether the T cell–stimulated microbicidal mechanisms of macrophages or microbial resistance to killing gains the upper hand. Resistance to phagocytosis is also the reason that such bacteria tend to cause chronic infections that may last for years, often recur or recrudesce after apparent cure, and are difficult to eradicate.

Immunity to Fungi

Fungal infections, also called mycoses, are important causes of morbidity and mortality in humans. Some fungal infections are endemic, and these infections are usually caused by fungi that are present in the environment and whose spores are inhaled by humans. Other fungal infections are said to be opportunistic because the causative agents cause mild or no disease in healthy individuals but may infect and cause severe disease in immunodeficient persons. A recent increase has been noted in opportunistic fungal infections secondary to an increase in immunodeficiencies caused mainly by AIDS and by therapy for disseminated cancer and transplant rejection, which inhibits bone marrow function and suppresses immune responses.

Different fungi infect humans and may live in extracellular tissue and within phagocytes. Therefore, the immune responses to these microbes are often combinations of the responses to extracellular and intracellular bacteria. However, much less is known about antifungal immunity than about immunity against bacteria and viruses. This lack of knowledge is partly due to the paucity of animal models for mycoses and partly due to the fact that these infections frequently occur in individuals who are incapable of mounting effective immune responses.

Innate and Adaptive Immunity to Fungi

The principal mediators of innate immunity against fungi are neutrophils and macrophages. Patients with neutropenia are extremely susceptible to opportunistic fungal infections. Neutrophils presumably liberate fungicidal substances, such as reactive oxygen intermediates and lysosomal enzymes, and phagocytose fungi for intracellular killing. Virulent strains of *Cryptococcus neoformans* inhibit the production of cytokines such as TNF and IL-12 by macrophages and stimulate production of IL-10, thus inhibiting macrophage activation.

Cell-mediated immunity is the major mechanism of adaptive immunity against fungal infections. *Histoplasma capsulatum,* a facultative intracellular parasite that lives in macrophages, is eliminated by the same cellular mechanisms that are effective against intracellular bacteria. $CD4^+$ and $CD8^+$ T cells cooperate to eliminate the yeast forms of *C. neoformans,* which tend to colonize the lungs and brain in immunodeficient hosts. *Candida* infections often start at mucosal surfaces, and cell-mediated immunity is believed to prevent spread of the fungi into tissues. In all these situations, T_H1 responses are protective and T_H2 responses are detrimental to the host. Not surprisingly, granulomatous inflammation is an important cause of host tissue injury in some intracellular fungal infections, such as histoplasmosis. Fungi often elicit specific antibody responses that are useful for serologic diagnosis. However, the protective efficacy of humoral immunity is not established.

Immunity to Viruses

Viruses are obligatory intracellular microorganisms that replicate within cells, often using the nucleic acid and protein synthetic machinery of the host. Viruses typically infect a wide variety of cell populations by using normal cell surface molecules as receptors to enter the cells. After entering cells, viruses can cause tissue injury and disease by any of several mechanisms. Viral replication interferes with normal cellular protein synthesis and function and leads to injury and ultimately death of the infected cell. This result is one type of cytopathic effect of viruses, and the infection is said to be "lytic" because the infected cell is lysed. Noncytopathic viruses may cause latent infections, during which viral DNA persists in host cells and produces proteins that may or may not alter cellular functions. Innate and adaptive immune responses to viruses are aimed at blocking infection and eliminating infected cells (Fig. 15–6).

Innate Immunity to Viruses

The principal mechanisms of innate immunity against viruses are inhibition of infection by type I IFNs and NK cell–mediated killing of infected cells. Infection by many viruses is associated with production of double-stranded RNA, which stimulates the production of type I IFN by infected cells probably by engaging a Toll-like receptor. Type I IFNs function to inhibit viral replication in both infected and uninfected cells by inducing

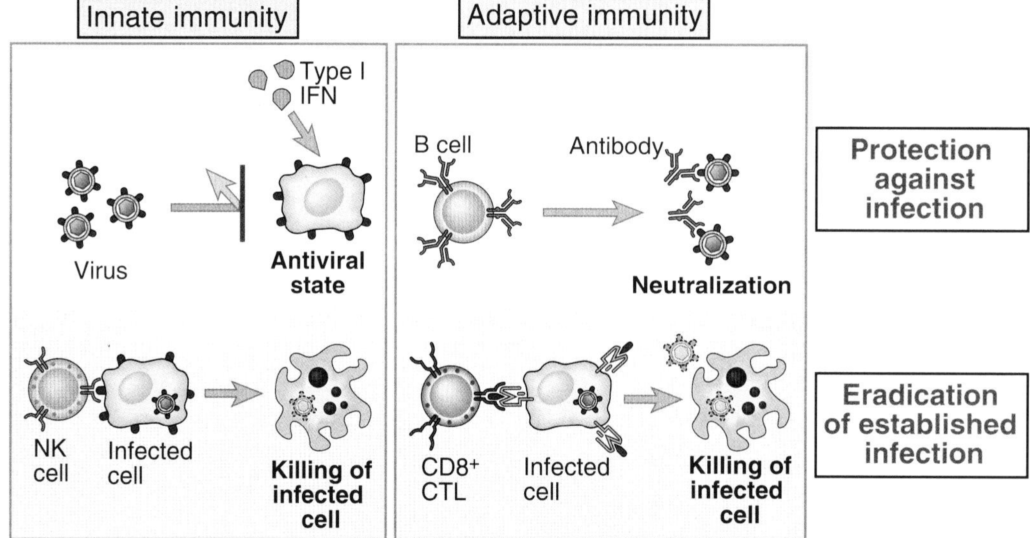

Figure 15–6 Innate and adaptive immune responses against viruses. Immunity against viruses functions to prevent infection and to eradicate established infection. Innate immunity is mediated by type I IFNs, which prevent infection, and NK cells, which eliminate infected cells. Adaptive immunity is mediated by antibodies and CTLs, which also block infection and kill infected cells, respectively.

an "antiviral state" (see Chapter 11). NK cells kill cells infected with a variety of viruses and are an important mechanism of immunity against viruses early in the course of infection, before adaptive immune responses have developed. NK cells also recognize infected cells in which the virus has shut off class I MHC expression (discussed later) because the absence of class I releases NK cells from a normal state of inhibition (see Chapter 12, Fig. 12–7).

Adaptive Immune Responses to Viruses

Adaptive immunity against viral infections is mediated by antibodies, which block virus binding and entry into host cells, and by CTLs, which eliminate the infection by killing infected cells (see Fig. 15–6). Antibodies are produced and are effective against viruses only during the extracellular stage of the lives of these microbes. Viruses may be extracellular early in the course of infection, before they enter host cells, or, in the case of cytopathic viruses, when they are released from lysed infected cells. Antiviral antibodies function mainly as neutralizing antibodies to prevent virus attachment and entry into host cells. These neutralizing antibodies bind to viral envelope or capsid antigens. Secreted antibodies of the IgA isotype are important for neutralizing viruses that enter through the respiratory and intestinal mucosa. Oral immunization against poliomyelitis works by inducing mucosal immunity. In addition to neutralization, antibodies may opsonize viral particles and promote their clearance by phagocytes. Complement activation may also participate in antibody-mediated viral immunity, mainly by promoting phagocytosis and possibly by direct lysis of viruses with lipid envelopes.

The importance of humoral immunity in defense against viral infections is supported by the observation that resistance to a particular virus, induced by either infection or vaccination, is often specific for the serologic (antibody-defined) type of the virus. An example is influenza virus, in which exposure to one serologic type does not confer resistance to other serotypes of the virus. Neutralizing antibodies block viral infection of cells and spread of viruses from cell to cell, but once the viruses enter cells and begin to replicate intracellularly, they are inaccessible to antibodies. Therefore, humoral immunity induced by previous infection or vaccination is able to protect individuals from viral infection but cannot by itself eradicate established infection.

Elimination of viruses that reside within cells is mediated by CTLs, which kill the infected cells. As we have mentioned in previous chapters, the principal physiologic function of CTLs is surveillance against viral infection. Most virus-specific CTLs are $CD8^+$ T cells that recognize cytosolic, usually endogenously synthesized, viral antigens in association with class I MHC molecules on any nucleated cell. Full differentiation of $CD8^+$ CTLs requires cytokines produced by $CD4^+$ helper cells or costimulators expressed on infected cells. If the infected cell is a tissue cell and not a professional antigen-presenting cell (APC), the infected cell may be phagocytosed by a professional APC, such as a dendritic cell, which processes the viral antigens and presents them to naive $CD8^+$ T cells. This process of cross-presentation, or cross-priming, was described in Chapter 5 (see Fig. 5–7). As discussed in Chapters 8 and 13, $CD8^+$ T cells undergo massive proliferation during viral infection, and most of the proliferating cells are specific for a few viral peptides. Some of the activated T cells differentiate into effector CTLs, which can kill any infected nucleated cell. The antiviral effects of CTLs are mainly due to killing of infected cells, but other mechanisms include activation of nucleases within infected cells that degrade viral genomes and secretion of cytokines, such as IFN-γ, which has some antiviral activity.

The importance of CTLs in defense against viral infection is demonstrated by the increased susceptibility to such infections seen in patients and animals that are deficient in T lymphocytes. Mice can be protected against influenza virus by adoptive transfer of virus-specific, class I–restricted CTLs and by cloned lines of such T cells.

In some viral infections, especially with noncytopathic viruses, CTLs may be responsible for tissue injury. An experimental model of a disease caused by the host immune response is lymphocytic choriomeningitis virus (LCMV) infection in mice, which induces inflammation of the spinal cord meninges. LCMV infects meningeal cells, but it is noncytopathic and does not injure the infected cells directly. The virus stimulates the development of virus-specific CTLs that kill infected meningeal cells during a physiologic attempt to eradicate the infection. Therefore, T cell–deficient mice infected with LCMV become chronic carriers of the virus, but pathologic lesions do not develop, whereas in normal mice, meningitis develops. This observation appears to contradict the usual situation, in which immunodeficient individuals are more susceptible to infectious diseases than normal individuals are. Hepatitis B virus infection in humans shows some similarities to murine LCMV in that immunodeficient persons who become infected do not develop the disease but become carriers who can transmit the infection to otherwise healthy persons. The livers of patients with acute and chronic active hepatitis contain large numbers of $CD8^+$ T cells, and hepatitis virus–specific, class I MHC–restricted CTLs can be isolated from liver biopsy specimens and propagated *in vitro*.

Immune responses to viral infections may be involved in producing disease in other ways (see Chapter 18). A consequence of persistent infection with some viruses, such as hepatitis B, is the formation of circulating immune complexes composed of viral antigens and specific antibodies. These complexes are deposited in blood vessels and lead to systemic vasculitis. Some viral proteins contain amino acid sequences that are also present in some self antigens. It has been postulated that because of this "molecular mimicry," antiviral immunity can lead to immune responses against self antigens.

Table 15–3. Mechanisms of Immune Evasion by Viruses

Mechanism of immune evasion	Examples
Antigenic variation	Influenza, rhinovirus, HIV
Inhibition of antigen processing	
Blockade of TAP transporter	Herpes simplex
Removal of class I MHC molecules from the ER	Cytomegalovirus
Production of cytokine receptor homologues	Vaccinia, poxviruses (IL-1, IFN-γ) Cytomegalovirus (chemokine)
Production of immunosuppressive cytokine	Epstein-Barr virus (IL-10)
Infection of immunocompetent cells	HIV

Abbreviations: ER, endoplasmic reticulum; HIV, human immunodeficiency virus; TAP, transporter associated with antigen processing.

Representative examples of different mechanisms used by viruses to resist host immunity are listed.

Evasion of Immune Mechanisms by Viruses

Viruses have evolved numerous mechanisms for evading host immunity (Table 15–3).

- ***Viruses can alter their antigens by point mutations or by reassortment of RNA genomes in RNA viruses.*** The antigens affected may be targets of antibodies or T cells, and large numbers of antigenically different strains of many viruses are known to exist. Because of antigenic variation, a virus may become resistant to immunity generated in the population by previous infections. The influenza pandemics that occurred in 1918, 1957, and 1968 were due to different strains of the virus, and subtler variants arise more frequently. There are so many serotypes of rhinovirus that specific immunization against the common cold may not be a feasible preventive strategy. Human immunodeficiency virus 1 (HIV-1), the virus that causes AIDS, is also capable of tremendous antigenic variation (see Chapter 20). In these situations, prophylactic vaccination may have to be directed against invariant viral proteins.
- ***Some viruses inhibit class I MHC–associated presentation of cytosolic protein antigens.*** Several mechanisms that inhibit antigen presentation have been described with different viruses (Box 15–3). Inhibition of antigen processing and presentation blocks the assembly and expression of stable class I MHC molecules and the display of viral peptides. As a result, cells infected by such viruses cannot be recognized or killed by $CD8^+$ CTLs. NK cells may be a host adaptation to kill these infected cells because NK cells are activated by the absence of class I MHC molecules.
- ***Some viruses produce molecules that inhibit innate and adaptive immunity.*** Poxviruses encode molecules that bind to several cytokines, including IFN-γ, TNF, IL-1, IL-18, and chemokines, and these molecules are secreted by infected cells. The secreted cytokine-binding proteins may function as competitive antagonists of the cytokines. Some

BOX 15–3

Inhibition of Antigen Processing by Viruses

As viruses have co-evolved with their hosts, they have developed many strategies to evade immune responses. A large variety of viral genes have been identified that encode proteins that modulate host immune responses. Some of these viral proteins inhibit the presentation of viral antigens to T cells. CD8$^+$ class I MHC–restricted CTLs are the major mechanisms of defense against viral infections of cells. If a virus could inhibit the class I–restricted antigen presentation pathway, that virus would become invisible to CTLs and would be able to replicate in infected cells. In Chapter 5, we described the steps in the processing of cytosolic antigens and the presentation of antigenic peptides bound to class I molecules (see Fig. 5–14). Each of these steps may be targeted for inhibition by a viral product. Some examples are shown in the Figure and listed here.

- The transcription of class I MHC genes is inhibited by the E1A protein of pathogenic strains of adenovirus.
- Herpes simplex viruses 1 and 2 produce a protein, called ICP-47, that binds to the peptide-binding site of the TAP transporter and prevents the transporter from capturing cytosolic peptides and transporting them into the endoplasmic reticulum for binding to class I molecules.
- The adenovirus E3 19-kD protein binds to and retains class I molecules in the endoplasmic reticulum, preventing these molecules from exiting with their peptide cargo.
- The human cytomegalovirus (CMV) US3 protein sequesters class I molecules in the endoplasmic reticulum, and murine CMV gp40 (40-kD glycoprotein) retains class I molecules in the cis-Golgi compartment.
- Human CMV produces two proteins, US2 and US11, which bind to class I molecules in the endoplasmic reticulum and actively carry, or "dislocate," these molecules into the cytosol, where they cannot be loaded with antigenic peptides and are degraded in the proteasome.
- Kaposi's sarcoma herpes virus (KSHV) K3 and K5 proteins induce rapid internalization of class I MHC molecules from the cell surface.
- Two proteins of HIV, Vpu and Nef, also inhibit class I expression in infected cells; Nef appears to do this by forcing internalization of class I molecules from the surface of infected cells, and Vpu destabilizes newly synthesized class I molecules.

The consequence of blocking class I–peptide association in all these cases is that infected cells show reduced expression of stable class I molecules on the surface and do not display viral peptides for T cell recognition. However, it is difficult to prove that the viral genes encoding proteins that inhibit antigen presentation are actually virulence genes, required for the infectivity or pathogenicity of the viruses.

An excellent example of the constant struggle between microbes and their hosts is the adaptation of the mammalian immune system to recognize class I–deficient cells. Thus, viruses try to evade recognition by CTLs by inhibiting class I MHC expression, but NK cells have evolved to respond specifically to the absence of class I MHC on virus-infected cells (see Chapter 12). Not surprisingly, there is emerging evidence that some viruses may produce proteins that act as ligands for NK cell inhibitory receptors and thus inhibit NK cell activation.

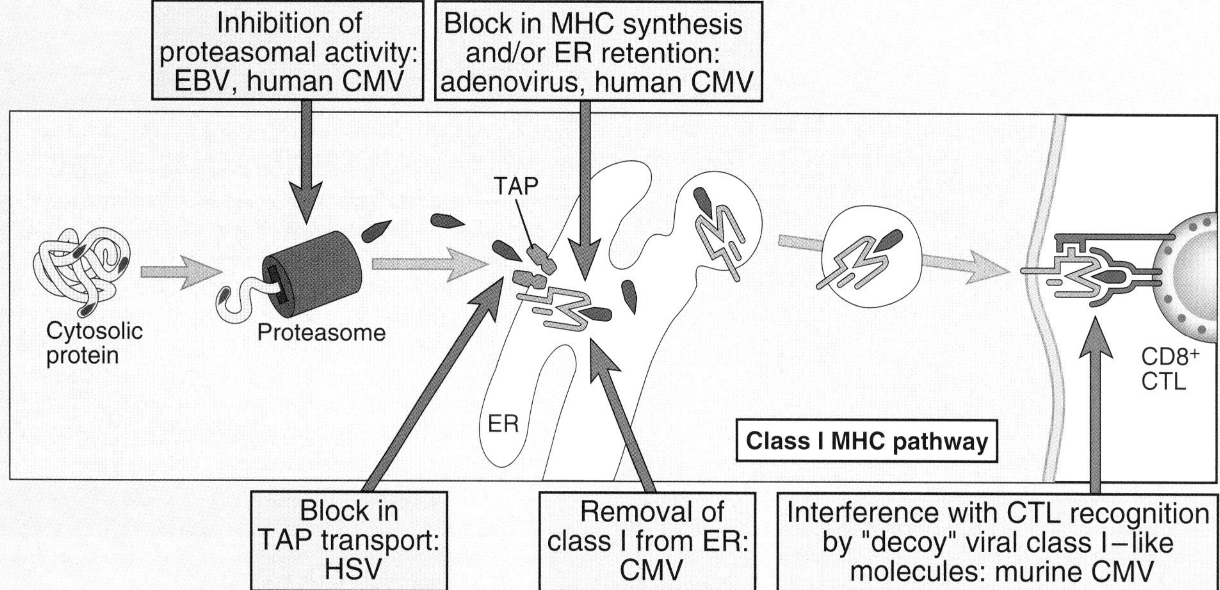

The pathway of class I MHC–associated antigen presentation is shown, with examples of viruses that block different steps in this pathway. CMV, cytomegalovirus; CTL, cytolytic T lymphocyte; EBV, Epstein-Barr virus; ER, endoplasmic reticulum; HSV, herpes simplex virus; TAP, transporter associated with antigen processing.

cytomegaloviruses produce a molecule that is homologous to class I MHC proteins and may compete for binding and presentation of peptide antigens. Epstein-Barr virus produces a protein that is homologous to the macrophage-suppressive cytokine IL-10 and may function to inhibit macrophage function and cell-mediated immunity. These examples probably represent a small fraction of immunosuppressive viral molecules. Identification of these molecules raises the intriguing possibility that viruses have acquired genes encoding inhibitors of immune responses during their passage through human hosts and have thus evolved to infect and colonize humans.

- ***Viruses may infect and either kill or inactivate immunocompetent cells.*** The obvious example is HIV, which survives by infecting and eliminating $CD4^+$ T cells, the key regulators of immune responses to protein antigens.

Immunity to Parasites

In infectious disease terminology, parasitic infection refers to infection with animal parasites such as protozoa, helminths, and ectoparasites (e.g., ticks and mites). Such parasites currently account for greater morbidity and mortality than any other class of infectious organisms, particularly in developing countries. It is estimated that about 30% of the world's population suffers from parasitic infestations. Malaria alone affects more than 100 million people worldwide and is responsible for about 1 million deaths annually. The magnitude of this public health problem is the principal reason for the great interest in immunity to parasites and for the development of immunoparasitology as a distinct branch of immunology.

Most parasites go through complex life cycles, part of which occurs in humans (or other vertebrates) and part of which occurs in intermediate hosts, such as flies, ticks, and snails. Humans are usually infected by bites from infected intermediate hosts or by sharing a particular habitat with an intermediate host. For instance, malaria and trypanosomiasis are transmitted by insect bites, and schistosomiasis is transmitted by exposure to water in which infected snails reside. Most parasitic infections are chronic because of weak innate immunity and the ability of parasites to evade or resist elimination by adaptive immune responses. Furthermore, many antiparasite antibiotics are not effective at killing the organisms. Individuals living in endemic areas require repeated chemotherapy because of continued exposure, and such treatment is often not possible because of expense and logistic problems. Therefore, the development of prophylactic vaccines for parasites has long been considered an important goal for developing countries.

Innate Immunity to Parasites

Although different protozoan and helminthic parasites have been shown to activate different mechanisms of innate immunity, these organisms are often able to survive and replicate in their hosts because they are well adapted to resisting host defenses. The principal innate immune response to protozoa is phagocytosis, but many of these parasites are resistant to phagocytic killing and may even replicate within macrophages. Phagocytes also attack helminthic parasites and secrete microbicidal substances to kill organisms that are too large to be phagocytosed. Many helminths have thick teguments that make them resistant to the cytocidal mechanisms of neutrophils and macrophages. Some helminths may also activate the alternative pathway of complement, although as we shall discuss later, parasites recovered from infected hosts appear to have developed resistance to complement-mediated lysis.

Adaptive Immune Responses to Parasites

Different protozoa and helminths vary greatly in their structural and biochemical properties, life cycles, and pathogenic mechanisms. It is therefore not surprising that different parasites elicit distinct adaptive immune responses (Table 15–4). In general, pathogenic protozoa have evolved to survive within host cells, so protective immunity against these organisms is mediated by mechanisms similar to those that eliminate intracellular bacteria and viruses. In contrast, metazoa such as helminths survive in extracellular tissues, and their elimination is often dependent on special types of antibody responses.

The principal defense mechanism against protozoa that survive within macrophages is cell-mediated immunity, particularly macrophage activation by T_H1 cell–derived cytokines. Infection of mice with *Leishmania major*, a protozoan that survives within the endosomes of macrophages, is the best documented example of how dominance of T_H1 or T_H2 responses determines disease resistance or susceptibility (see Fig. 15–5). Resistance to the infection is associated with activation of *Leishmania*-specific T_H1 $CD4^+$ T cells, which produce IFN-γ and thereby activate macrophages to destroy intracellular parasites. Conversely, activation of T_H2 cells by the protozoa results in increased parasite survival and exacerbation of lesions because of the macrophage-suppressive actions of T_H2 cytokines, notably IL-4.

Most inbred strains of mice are resistant to infection with *L. major*, but inbred BALB/c mice are highly susceptible and die if they are infected with large numbers of parasites. After infection, the resistant strains produce large amounts of IFN-γ in response to leishmanial antigens, whereas the strains that are susceptible to fatal leishmaniasis produce more IL-4 in response to the parasite. IFN-γ activates macrophages and enhances intracellular killing of *Leishmania*, and high levels of IL-4 inhibit the activation of macrophages by IFN-γ. Treatment of resistant mice with anti–IFN-γ antibody makes them susceptible, and conversely, treatment of susceptible mice with anti–IL-4 antibody induces resistance. The same results are seen in knockout mice lacking IFN-γ or IL-4. Treatment of susceptible mice with IL-12 at the time of infection also induces resist-

Table 15–4. Immune Responses to Disease-Causing Parasites

Parasite	Diseases	Principal mechanisms of protective immunity
Protozoa		
Plasmodium	Malaria	Antibodies and $CD8^+$ CTLs
Leishmania	Leishmaniasis (mucocutaneous, disseminated)	$CD4^+$ T_H1 cells activate macrophages to kill phagocytosed parasites
Trypanosoma	African trypanosomiasis	Antibodies
Entamoeba histolytica	Amebiasis	Antibodies, phagocytosis
Metazoa		
Schistosoma	Schistosomiasis	ADCC mediated by eosinophils, macrophages
Filaria	Filariasis	Cell-mediated immunity; role of antibodies?

Abbreviations: ADCC, antibody-dependent cell-mediated cytotoxicity; CTLs, cytolytic T lymphocytes.

Selected examples of parasites and immune responses to them are listed.

ance to the infection. IL-12 enhances the production of IFN-γ and the development of T_H1 cells. This result is the basis for the suggested use of IL-12 as a vaccine adjuvant, not only for leishmaniasis but also for other infections that are combated by cell-mediated immunity.

Multiple genes appear to control protective versus harmful immune responses to intracellular parasites in inbred mice and presumably in humans as well. Attempts to identify these genes are ongoing in many laboratories.

Protozoa that replicate inside various host cells and lyse these cells stimulate specific antibody and CTL responses, similar to cytopathic viruses. An example of such an organism is the malaria parasite. It was thought for many years that antibodies were the major protective mechanism against malaria, and early attempts at vaccinating against this infection focused on generating antibodies. It is now apparent that the CTL response is an important defense against the spread of this intracellular protozoan (Box 15–4).

Defense against many helminthic infections is mediated by the activation of T_H2 cells, which results in production of IgE antibodies and activation of eosinophils. IgE antibodies bind to the surface of the helminth, eosinophils then attach through Fcε receptors, and the eosinophils are activated to secrete granule enzymes that destroy the parasites (see Chapter 14, Fig. 14–4). Production of specific IgE antibody and eosinophilia are frequently observed in infections by helminths. These responses are attributed to the propensity of helminths to stimulate the T_H2 subset of $CD4^+$ helper T cells, which secrete IL-4 and IL-5. IL-4 stimulates the production of IgE, and IL-5 stimulates the development and activation of eosinophils. Eosinophils may be more effective at killing helminths than other leukocytes are because the major basic protein of eosinophil granules may be more toxic for helminths than the proteolytic enzymes and reactive oxygen intermediates produced by neutrophils and macrophages. The expulsion of some intestinal nematodes may be due to IL-4–dependent mechanisms that are not well defined but apparently do not require IgE.

Adaptive immune responses to parasites can also contribute to tissue injury. Some parasites and their products induce granulomatous responses with concomitant fibrosis. *Schistosoma mansoni* eggs deposited in the liver stimulate $CD4^+$ T cells, which in turn activate macrophages and induce DTH reactions. DTH reactions result in the formation of granulomas around the eggs. The granulomas serve to contain the schistosome eggs, but severe fibrosis associated with this chronic cell-mediated immune response leads to disruption of venous blood flow in the liver, portal hypertension, and cirrhosis. In lymphatic filariasis, lodging of the parasites in lymphatic vessels leads to chronic cell-mediated immune reactions and ultimately to fibrosis. Fibrosis results in lymphatic obstruction and severe lymphedema. Chronic and persistent parasitic infestations are often associated with the formation of complexes of parasite antigens and specific antibodies. The complexes can be deposited in blood vessels and kidney glomeruli and produce vasculitis and nephritis, respectively (see Chapter 20). Immune complex disease has been described in schistosomiasis and malaria.

BOX 15–4

Immunity to Malaria

Malaria is a disease caused by a protozoan parasite (*Plasmodium*) that infects more than 100 million people and causes 1 to 2 million deaths annually. Malaria, especially that caused by infection with *Plasmodium falciparum*, continues to be one of the most widespread and prevalent diseases today. Infection is initiated when sporozoites are inoculated into the blood stream by the bite of an infected mosquito (*Anopheles*). The sporozoites rapidly disappear from the blood and invade the parenchymal cells of the liver. In the hepatocytes, sporozoites develop into merozoites by a multiple-fission process termed *schizogony*. One to 2 weeks after infection, the infected hepatocytes burst and release thousands of merozoites, thereby initiating the erythrocytic stage of the life cycle. The merozoites invade red blood cells by a process that involves multiple ligand-receptor interactions, such as binding of the *P. falciparum* protein EBA-175 to glycophorin A on erythrocytes. Merozoites develop sequentially into ring forms, trophozoites, and schizonts, each of which expresses both shared and unique antigens. The erythrocytic cycle continues when schizont-infected red blood cells burst and release merozoites that invade other erythrocytes. Sexual stage gametocytes develop in some cells and are taken up by mosquitoes during a blood meal, after which they fertilize and develop into oocysts. Immature sporozoites develop in the mosquitoes within 2 weeks and travel to the salivary glands, where they mature and become infective.

The clinical features of malaria caused by the four species of *Plasmodium* that infect humans include fever spikes, anemia, and splenomegaly. Many pathologic manifestations of malaria may be due to the activation of T cells and macrophages and production of TNF. The development of cerebral malaria in a murine model is prevented by depletion of $CD4^+$ T lymphocytes or by injection of neutralizing anti-TNF antibody.

The immune response to malaria is complex and stage specific; that is, immunization with antigens derived from sporozoites, merozoites, or gametocytes protects only against the particular stage. On the basis of this observation, it is postulated that a vaccine consisting of combined immunogenic epitopes from each of these stages should stimulate more effective immunity than a vaccine that incorporates antigens from only one stage. The best characterized malaria vaccines are directed against sporozoites. Because of the stage-specific nature of sporozoite antigens, such vaccines must provide sterilizing immunity to be effective. Protective immunity may be induced in humans by injection of radiation-inactivated sporozoites. This type of protection is partially mediated by antibodies that inhibit sporozoite invasion of liver cells *in vitro*. Such antibodies recognize the circumsporozoite (CS) protein, which mediates the binding of parasites to liver cells. The CS protein contains a central region of about 40 tandem repeats of the sequence Asn-Ala-Asn-Pro (NANP), which makes up the immunodominant B cell epitope of the protein. Anti-(NANP)n antibodies neutralize sporozoite infectivity, but such antibodies provide only partial protection against infection. The antibody response to CS protein is dependent on helper T cells. Most CS-specific helper T cells recognize epitopes outside the NANP region, and some of these T cell epitopes correspond to the most variable residues of the CS protein, which suggests that variation of the antigens of the surface coat may have arisen in response to selective pressures imposed by specific T cell responses.

$CD8^+$ T cells play an important role in immunity to the hepatic stages of infection. If sporozoite-immunized mice are depleted of $CD8^+$ T cells by injection of anti-CD8 antibodies, they are unable to resist a challenge infection. The protective effects of $CD8^+$ T cells may be mediated by direct killing of sporozoite-infected hepatocytes or indirectly by the secretion of IFN-γ and activation of hepatocytes to produce nitric oxide and other agents that kill parasites. IL-12 induces resistance to sporozoite challenge in rodents and nonhuman primates, presumably by stimulating IFN-γ production. Conversely, resistance of *Plasmodium berghei* sporozoite–immunized mice to a challenge infection is abrogated by treatment with anti–IFN-γ antibodies.

The sexual blood stage of malaria is an important target for vaccine development. The major goal of this form of immunization is to kill infected erythrocytes or to block merozoite invasion of new red cells. Although infected individuals mount strong immune responses against blood stage antigens during natural malaria infections, most of these responses do not appear to affect parasite survival or to result in the selection of new antigenic variants. Nevertheless, some merozoite proteins may be good vaccine candidates. Of particular interest is the major merozoite surface antigen MSP-1, which contains a highly conserved carboxyl terminal region. Immunization with recombinant DNA–derived carboxyl terminal peptides has been shown to confer significant protection against malaria in rodents and has shown promising results in primate trials with human malaria parasite strains. The resistance induced by MSP-1 vaccination appears to involve antibody-dependent mechanisms.

Transmission-blocking vaccines are being developed to act on stages of the parasite life cycle that are found in mosquitoes. Such vaccines provide no protection for an immunized individual but act to reduce the number of parasites available for development in the mosquito vector. One such vaccine is an antigen, Pfs25, that is located on the surface of zygotes and ookinetes and is involved in parasite invasion of mosquito gut epithelium. In individuals immunized against this parasite antigen, the antibodies that develop are ingested by the mosquito during a blood meal and block the ability of the parasite to infect and mature in the mosquito. These parasite stages are found only in the mosquito vector and are not exposed to host immune responses. Therefore, the antigens expressed in the mosquito do not undergo the high rates of variation that are typical of immunodominant parasite antigens in the vertebrate host.

For a review on malaria vaccines, see Miller LH, and SL Hoffman. Research towards vaccines against malaria. Nature Medicine 4:520–524, 1998.

This box was written with the assistance of Drs. Alan Sher and Louis Miller, National Institutes of Health, Bethesda, Md.

Table 15–5. Mechanisms of Immune Evasion by Parasites

Mechanism of immune evasion	Examples
Antigenic variation	Trypanosomes, *Plasmodium*
Acquired resistance to complement, CTLs	Schistosomes
Inhibition of host immune responses	Filaria (secondary to lymphatic obstruction), trypanosomes
Antigen shedding	Entamoeba

Abbreviation: CTL, cytolytic T lymphocyte.

Evasion of Immune Mechanisms by Parasites

Parasites evade protective immunity by reducing their immunogenicity and by inhibiting host immune responses. Different parasites have developed remarkably effective ways of resisting immunity (Table 15–5).

- Parasites change their surface antigens during their life cycle in vertebrate hosts. Two forms of antigenic variation are well defined. The first is a stage-specific change in antigen expression, such that the mature tissue stages of parasites produce different antigens than the infective stages do. For example, the infective sporozoite stage of malaria parasites is antigenically distinct from the merozoites that reside in the host and are responsible for chronic infection. By the time that the immune system has responded to infection by sporozoites, the parasite has differentiated, expresses new antigens, and is no longer a target for immune elimination. The second and most remarkable example of antigenic variation in parasites is the continuous variation of major surface antigens seen in African trypanosomes such as *Trypanosoma brucei* and *Trypanosoma rhodesiense.* Continuous antigenic variation in trypanosomes is probably due to programmed variation in expression of the genes encoding the major surface antigen. Infected individuals show waves of blood parasitemia, and each wave consists of parasites expressing a surface antigen that is different from the previous wave (Fig. 15–7). Thus, by the time the host produces antibodies against the parasite, an antigenically different organism has grown out. More than a hundred such waves of parasitemia can occur in an infection. One consequence of antigenic variation in parasites is that it is difficult to effectively vaccinate individuals against these infections.
- Parasites become resistant to immune effector mechanisms during their residence in vertebrate hosts. Perhaps the best examples are schistosome larvae, which travel to the lungs of infected animals and during this migration develop a tegument that is resistant to damage by complement and by CTLs. The biochemical basis of this change is not known.
- Protozoan parasites may conceal themselves from the immune system either by living inside host cells or by developing cysts that are resistant to immune effectors. Some helminthic parasites reside in intestinal lumens and are sheltered from cell-mediated immune effector mechanisms. Parasites may also shed their antigenic coats, either spontaneously or after binding specific antibodies. Shedding of antigens renders the parasites resistant to immune effector mechanisms.
- Parasites inhibit host immune responses by multiple mechanisms. T cell anergy to parasite antigens has been observed in severe schistosomiasis involving the liver and spleen and in filarial infections. The mechanisms of immunologic unresponsiveness in these infections are not well understood. In lymphatic filariasis, infection of lymph nodes with subsequent architectural disruption may contribute to deficient immunity. More nonspecific and generalized immunosuppression is observed in malaria and African trypanosomiasis. This immune deficiency has been

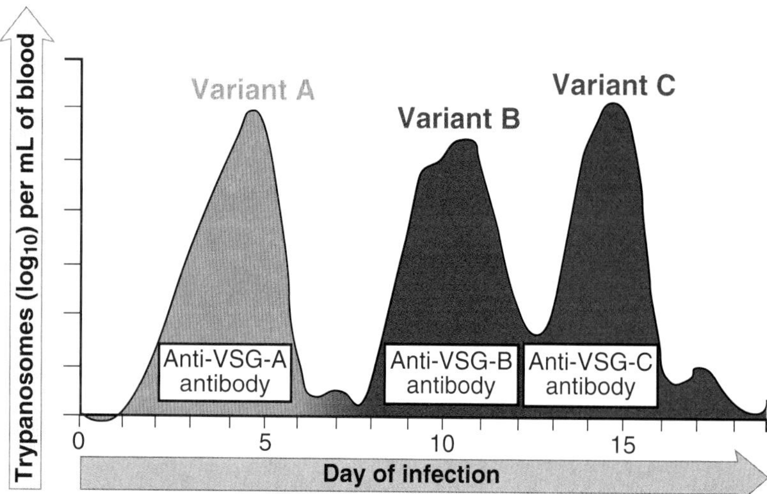

Figure 15–7 Antigenic variation in trypanosomes.
In a mouse infected experimentally with a single clone of *Trypanosoma rhodesiense,* the blood parasite counts show cyclic waves. Each wave is due to a new antigenic variant of the parasite (labeled variants A, B, and C) that expresses a new variable surface glycoprotein (VSG, the immunodominant antigen of the parasite), and each decline is a result of a specific antibody response to that variant. (Courtesy of Dr. John Mansfield, University of Wisconsin, Madison.)

attributed to the production of immunosuppressive cytokines by activated macrophages and T cells and defects in T cell activation.

The worldwide implications of parasitic infestations for health and economic development are well appreciated. Attempts to develop effective vaccines against these infections have been actively pursued for many years. Although the progress has been slower than one would have hoped, elucidation of the fundamental mechanisms of immune responses to and immune evasion by parasites holds great promise for the future.

Strategies for Vaccine Development

The birth of immunology as a science may be dated from Edward Jenner's successful vaccination against smallpox in 1796. The importance of prophylactic immunization against infectious diseases is best illustrated by the fact that worldwide programs of vaccination have led to the complete or nearly complete eradication of many of these diseases in developed countries (see Chapter 1, Table 1–1).

Vaccines induce protection against infections by stimulating the development of long-lived effector cells and memory cells. Most vaccines in routine use today work by inducing humoral immunity, and attempts to stimulate cell-mediated immune responses by vaccination are ongoing. The success of active immunization in eradicating infectious disease is dependent on numerous factors. Vaccines are likely to be most effective against infections that are limited to human hosts and are caused by poorly infectious agents whose antigens are relatively invariant. On the other hand, the existence of animal or environmental reservoirs of infection, high infectivity of the microbes, and antigenic variation make it less likely that vaccination alone will eradicate a particular infectious disease.

In the following section, we summarize the approaches to vaccination that have been tried (Table 15–6) and their major value and limitations.

Table 15–6. Vaccine Approaches

Type of vaccine	Examples
Live attenuated or killed bacteria	BCG, cholera
Live attenuated viruses	Polio, rabies
Subunit (antigen) vaccines	Tetanus toxoid, diphtheria toxoid
Conjugate vaccines	*Haemophilus influenzae*, pneumococcus
Synthetic vaccines	Hepatitis (recombinant proteins)
Viral vectors	Clinical trials of HIV antigens in canarypox vector
DNA vaccines	Clinical trials ongoing for several infections

Abbreviations: BCG, bacillus Calmette-Guérin; HIV, human immunodeficiency virus.

Attenuated and Inactivated Bacterial and Viral Vaccines

Vaccines composed of intact nonpathogenic microbes are made by treating the microbe in such a way that it can no longer cause disease (i.e., its virulence is attenuated) or by killing the microbe while retaining its immunogenicity. The great advantage of attenuated microbial vaccines is that they elicit all the innate and adaptive immune responses that the pathogenic microbe would, and they are therefore the ideal way of inducing protective immunity. Live, attenuated bacteria were first shown by Louis Pasteur to confer specific immunity. The attenuated or killed bacterial vaccines in use today generally induce limited protection and are effective for only short periods. Live, attenuated viral vaccines are usually more effective; polio, measles, and yellow fever are three good examples. The most frequently used approach for producing such attenuated viruses is repeated passage in cell cultures. More recently, temperature-sensitive and deletion mutants are being generated with the same goal in mind. Viral vaccines often induce long-lasting specific immunity, so immunization of children is sufficient for lifelong protection. The principal limitation of these vaccines is concern about their safety because of incomplete attenuation or reversion to the wild-type pathogenic virus.

Purified Antigen (Subunit) Vaccines

Subunit vaccines are composed of antigens purified from microbes or inactivated toxins and are usually administered with an adjuvant. One effective use of purified antigens as vaccines is for the prevention of diseases caused by bacterial toxins. Toxins can be rendered harmless without loss of immunogenicity, and such "toxoids" induce strong antibody responses. Diphtheria and tetanus are two infections whose life-threatening consequences have been largely controlled because of immunization of children with toxoid preparations. Vaccines composed of bacterial polysaccharide antigens are used against pneumococcus and *H. influenzae*. Although polysaccharides are inefficient inducers of B cell memory, these vaccines often provide long-lived protective immunity, probably because the polysaccharides are not degraded easily and they persist in lymphoid tissues, where they continue to stimulate specific B lymphocytes for long periods. High-affinity antibody responses may be generated against polysaccharide antigens by coupling them to proteins to form conjugate vaccines. Such vaccines are an excellent practical application of the principle of T-B cell cooperation induced by hapten-carrier conjugates (see Chapter 9). Purified protein vaccines stimulate helper T cells and antibody responses, but they do not generate potent CTLs. The reason for poor CTL development is that exogenous proteins (and peptides) are inefficient at entering the class I MHC pathway of antigen presentation and cannot readily displace peptides from surface class I molecules. As a result, protein vaccines are not recognized efficiently by class I–restricted $CD8^+$ T cells.

Synthetic Antigen Vaccines

A current goal of vaccine research is to identify the most immunogenic microbial antigens or epitopes of the antigens, to synthesize these in the laboratory, and to use the synthetic antigens as vaccines. Early approaches for developing synthetic antigen vaccines relied on the synthesis of linear and branched polymers of three to ten amino acids based on the known sequences of microbial antigens. Such peptides are weakly immunogenic by themselves and need to be coupled to large proteins to induce antibody responses, again like generating antibody responses to hapten-carrier conjugates. Two advances may improve the efficacy of synthetic antigen vaccines. First, it is possible to deduce the protein sequences of microbial antigens from nucleotide sequence data and to prepare large quantities of proteins by recombinant DNA technology. Second, by testing overlapping peptides and by mutational analysis, it is possible to identify epitopes or even individual residues that are recognized by B or T cells or that bind to MHC molecules for presentation to MHC-restricted T lymphocytes. Empirical trial of peptides containing single or multiple amino acid substitutions has led to the construction of antigens with enhanced binding to MHC molecules or enhanced capacity to activate T cells. To date, such studies have been done largely in inbred mice. Because T cell antigen recognition is influenced by the polymorphism of MHC molecules, it is likely that in outbred human populations, it will be more difficult to "custom-design" peptides with enhanced immunogenicity. Nevertheless, this approach has the potential for creating at will vaccines that are of high potency. Vaccines made of recombinant DNA–derived antigens are now in use for hepatitis virus, herpes simplex virus, and foot-and-mouth disease virus (a major pathogen for livestock).

Live Viral Vectors

A recent approach to vaccine development is to introduce genes encoding microbial antigens into a noncytopathic virus and to infect individuals with this virus. Thus, the virus serves as a source of the antigen in an inoculated individual. The great advantage of viral vectors is that they, like other live viruses, induce the full complement of immune responses, including strong CTL responses. This technique has been used most commonly with vaccinia virus vectors, into which the gene encoding the desired antigen is inserted by the process of homologous recombination. Inoculation of such recombinant viruses into many species of animals induces both humoral and cell-mediated immunity against the antigen produced by the foreign gene (and, of course, against vaccinia virus antigens as well). A potential problem with viral vectors is that the viruses may infect various host cells, and even though they are not pathogenic, they may produce antigens that stimulate CTL responses that kill the infected host cells.

DNA Vaccines

The newest method of vaccination has been developed on the basis of an unexpected observation. Inoculation of a plasmid containing complementary DNA (cDNA) encoding a protein antigen leads to strong and long-lived humoral and cell-mediated immune responses to the antigen. It is likely that APCs, such as dendritic cells, are transfected by the plasmid and the cDNA is transcribed and translated into immunogenic protein that elicits specific responses. The unique feature of DNA vaccines is that they provide the only approach, other than live viruses, for eliciting strong CTL responses because the DNA-encoded proteins are synthesized in the cytosol of transfected cells. Furthermore, bacterial plasmids are rich in unmethylated CpG nucleotides and are recognized by a Toll-like receptor (TLR9) on macrophages and other cells, thereby eliciting an innate immune response that enhances adaptive immunity (see Chapter 12). Therefore, plasmid DNA vaccines are effective even when they are administered without adjuvants. The ease of manipulating cDNAs to express many diverse antigens, the ability to store DNA without refrigeration for use in the field, and the ability to co-express other proteins that may enhance immune responses (such as cytokines and costimulators) make this technique promising. However, the factors that determine the efficacy of DNA vaccines, especially in humans, are still not fully defined.

Adjuvants and Immunomodulators

The initiation of T cell–dependent immune responses against protein antigens requires that the antigens be administered with adjuvants. Most adjuvants elicit innate immune responses, with increased expression of costimulators and production of cytokines such as IL-12 that stimulate T cell growth and differentiation. Heat-killed bacteria are powerful adjuvants that are commonly used in experimental animals. However, the severe local inflammation that such adjuvants trigger precludes their use in humans. Much effort is currently being devoted to development of safe and effective adjuvants for use in humans. Several are in clinical practice, including aluminum hydroxide gel (which binds proteins noncovalently and induces mild inflammation) and lipid formulations that are ingested by phagocytes. An alternative to adjuvants is to administer natural substances that stimulate T cell responses together with antigens. For instance, IL-12 incorporated in vaccines promotes strong cell-mediated immunity and is being tested in early clinical trials. As mentioned, plasmid DNA has intrinsic adjuvant-like activities, and it is possible to incorporate costimulators

(B7 molecules, CD40) or cytokines into plasmid DNA vaccines.

Passive Immunization

Protective immunity can also be conferred by passive immunization, for instance, by transfer of specific antibodies. In the clinical situation, passive immunization is most commonly used for rapid treatment of potentially fatal diseases caused by toxins, such as tetanus. Antibodies against snake venom can be lifesaving treatments of poisonous snakebites. Passive immunity is short-lived because the host does not respond to the immunization and protection lasts only as long as the injected antibody persists. Moreover, passive immunization does not induce memory, so an immunized individual is not protected against subsequent exposure to the toxin or microbe.

Summary

- The interaction of the immune system with infectious organisms is a dynamic interplay of host mechanisms aimed at eliminating infections and microbial strategies designed to permit survival in the face of powerful defense mechanisms. Different types of infectious agents stimulate distinct types of immune responses and have evolved unique mechanisms for evading immunity. In some infections, the immune response is the cause of tissue injury and disease.
- Innate immunity against extracellular bacteria is mediated by phagocytes and the complement system (the alternative pathway).
- The principal adaptive immune response against extracellular bacteria consists of specific antibodies that opsonize the bacteria for phagocytosis and activate the complement system. Toxins produced by such bacteria are also neutralized by specific antibodies. Some bacterial toxins are powerful inducers of cytokine production, and cytokines account for much of the systemic disease associated with severe, disseminated infections with these microbes.
- Innate immunity against intracellular bacteria is mediated mainly by macrophages. However, intracellular bacteria are capable of surviving and replicating within host cells, including phagocytes, because they have developed mechanisms for resisting degradation within phagocytes.
- Adaptive immunity against intracellular bacteria is principally cell mediated and consists of activation of macrophages by $CD4^+$ T cells (as in DTH) as well as killing of infected cells by $CD8^+$ CTLs. The characteristic pathologic response to infection by intracellular bacteria is granulomatous inflammation.
- Protective responses to fungi consist mainly of innate immunity, mediated by neutrophils and macrophages, and adaptive cell-mediated immunity. Fungi are usually readily eliminated by phagocytes and a competent immune system, because of which disseminated fungal infections are seen mostly in immunodeficient persons.
- Innate immunity against viruses is mediated by type I IFNs and NK cells. Neutralizing antibodies protect against virus entry into cells early in the course of infection and later if the viruses are released from killed infected cells. The major defense mechanism against established infection is CTL-mediated killing of infected cells. CTLs may contribute to tissue injury even when the infectious virus is not harmful by itself. Viruses evade immune responses by antigenic variation, inhibition of antigen presentation, and production of immunosuppressive molecules.
- Animal parasites such as protozoa and helminths give rise to chronic and persistent infections because innate immunity against them is weak and parasites have evolved multiple mechanisms for evading and resisting specific immunity. The structural and antigenic diversity of pathogenic parasites is reflected in the heterogeneity of the adaptive immune responses that they elicit. Protozoa that live within host cells are destroyed by cell-mediated immunity, whereas helminths are eliminated by IgE antibody and eosinophil-mediated killing as well as by other leukocytes. Parasites evade the immune system by varying their antigens during residence in vertebrate hosts, by acquiring resistance to immune effector mechanisms, and by masking and shedding their surface antigens.

Selected Readings

Bernal A, T Proft, LD Fraser, and DN Posnett. Superantigens in human disease. Journal of Clinical Immunology 19: 149–157, 1999.

Casanova J-L, and L Abel. Genetic dissection of immunity to mycobacteria: the human model. Annual Review of Immunology 20:581–620, 2002.

Doherty PC, and JP Christensen. Accessing complexity: the dynamics of virus-specific T cell responses. Annual Review of Immunology 18:561–592, 2000.

Flynn JL, and J Chan. Immunology of tuberculosis. Annual Review of Immunology 19:93–129, 2001.

Guidotti LG, and FV Chisari. Noncytolytic control of viral infections by the innate and adaptive immune response. Annual Review of Immunology 19:65–91, 2001.

Gurunathan S, DM Klinman, and RA Seder. DNA vaccines: immunology, application, and optimization. Annual Review of Immunology 18:927–974, 2000.

Harty JT, AR Tvinnereim, and DW White. $CD8^+$ T cell effector mechanisms in resistance to infection. Annual Review of Immunology 18:275–308, 2000.

Krakauer T. Immune response to staphylococcal superantigens. Immunological Research 20:163–173, 1999.

Li H, EL Malchiodi, and RA Mariuzza. The structural basis of T cell activation by superantigens. Annual Review of Immunology 17:435–466, 1999.

Parren PW, and DR Burton. The antiviral activity of antibodies in vitro and in vivo. Advances in Immunology 77:195–262, 2001.

Pearce EJ, and AS MacDonald. The immunobiology of schistosomiasis. Nature Reviews Immunology 2:499–511, 2002.

Ploegh HL. Viral strategies of immune evasion. Science 280: 248–253, 1998.

Raupach B, and SHE Kaufmann. Immune responses to intracellular bacteria. Current Opinion in Immunology 13: 417–428, 2001.

Reiner SL, and RM Locksley. The regulation of immunity to *Leishmania major*. Annual Review of Immunology 13:151–177, 1995.

Romani L, and D Howard. Mechanisms of resistance to fungal infections. Current Opinion in Immunology 7:517–523, 1995.

Schaible UE, HL Collins, and SHE Kaufmann. Confrontation between intracellular bacteria and the immune system. Advances in Immunology 71:267–377, 1999.

Seder RA, and RT Gazzinelli. Cytokines are critical in linking the innate and adaptive immune responses to bacterial, fungal, and parasitic infection. Advances in Internal Medicine 44:144–179, 1998.

Shiloh MU, and CF Nathan. Reactive nitrogen intermediates and the pathogenesis of *Salmonella* and mycobacteria. Current Opinion in Microbiology 3:35–42, 2000.

Spriggs MK. One step ahead of the game: viral immunomodulatory molecules. Annual Review of Immunology 14: 101–130, 1996.

Tortorella D, BE Gewurz, MH Furman, DJ Schust, and HL Ploegh. Viral subversion of the immune system. Annual Review of Immunology 18:861–926, 2000.

Zinkernagel RM. Immunology taught by viruses. Science 271:173–178, 1996.

Section V

The Immune System in Disease

In this final section of the book, we apply our knowledge of the basic mechanisms of innate and adaptive immunity to understanding immunologic reactions against tumors and transplants and diseases caused by abnormal immune responses. Chapter 16 is devoted to the immunology of tissue transplantation, a promising therapy for a variety of diseases whose success is limited in large part by the immunologic rejection response. Chapter 17 describes immune responses to tumors and immunologic approaches for cancer therapy. Chapter 18 deals with the mechanisms of diseases caused by aberrant immune responses, so-called hypersensitivity diseases, and the pathogenesis of autoimmune disorders. In Chapter 19, we describe one form of hypersensitivity, immediate hypersensitivity, that represents the most common group of diseases caused by immune responses. In Chapter 20, we discuss the cellular and molecular bases of congenital and acquired immunodeficiencies, including the acquired immunodeficiency syndrome.

Chapter 16

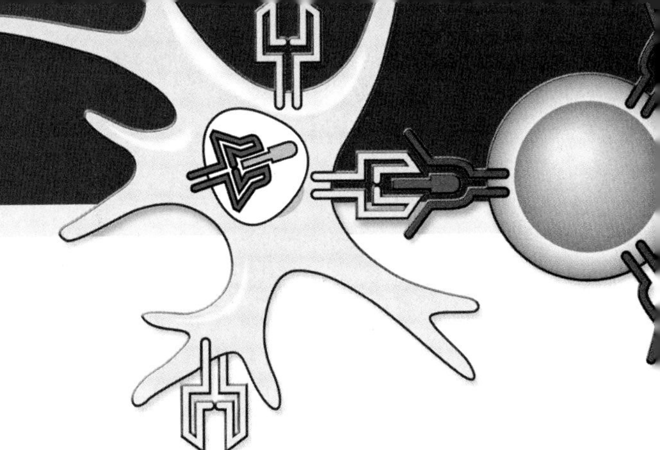

Transplantation Immunology

Transplantation is the process of taking cells, tissues, or organs, called a **graft**, from one individual and placing them into a (usually) different individual. The individual who provides the graft is called the **donor**, and the individual who receives the graft is called either the **recipient** or the host. If the graft is placed into its normal anatomic location, the procedure is called orthotopic transplantation; if the graft is placed in a different site, the procedure is called heterotopic transplantation. **Transfusion** is the transplantation of circulating blood cells or plasma from one individual to another. In clinical practice, transplantation is used to overcome a functional or anatomic deficit in the recipient. This approach to treatment of human diseases has increased steadily during the past 40 years, and transplantation of kidneys, hearts, lungs, livers, pancreas, and bone marrow is widely used today. More than 30,000 kidney, heart, lung, liver, and pancreas transplants are currently performed in the United States each year. In addition, transplantation of many other organs or cells is now being attempted.

A major limitation in the success of transplantation is the immune response of the recipient to the donor tissue. This problem was first appreciated when attempts to replace damaged skin on burn patients with skin from unrelated donors were found to be uniformly unsuccessful. During a matter of 1 to 2 weeks, the transplanted skin would undergo necrosis and fall off. The failure of the grafts led Peter Medawar and many other investigators to study skin transplantation in animal models. These experiments established that the failure of skin grafting was caused by an inflammatory reaction called **rejection**. Several lines of experimental evidence indicated that rejection is caused by an adaptive immune response (Fig. 16–1).

- A skin graft transplanted between genetically unrelated individuals, for example, from a strain A mouse to a strain B mouse, is rejected by a naive recipient in 7 to 10 days. This process is called first-set rejection and is due to a primary immune response to the graft. A subsequent skin graft transplanted from the same

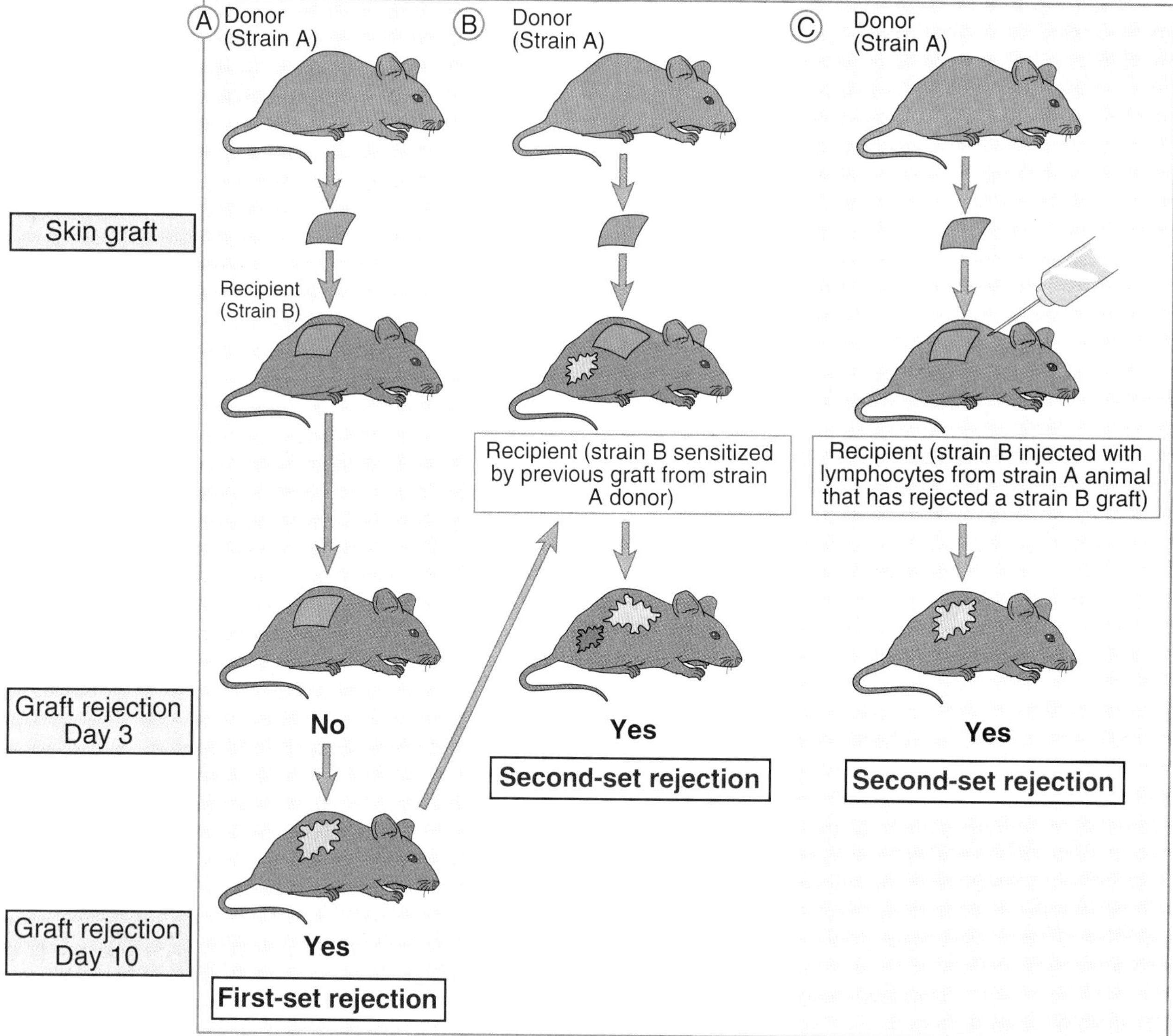

Figure 16–1 First- and second-set allograft rejection. Results of the experiments shown indicate that graft rejection displays the features of adaptive immune responses, namely, memory and mediation by lymphocytes. A strain B mouse will reject a graft from a strain A mouse with first-set kinetics *(left panel).* A strain B mouse sensitized by a previous graft from a strain A mouse will reject a second graft from a strain A mouse with second-set kinetics *(middle panel),* demonstrating memory. A strain B mouse injected with lymphocytes from another strain B mouse that has rejected a graft from a strain A mouse will reject a graft from a strain A mouse with second-set kinetics *(right panel),* demonstrating the role of lymphocytes in mediating rejection and memory. A strain B mouse sensitized by a previous graft from a strain A mouse will reject a graft from a third unrelated strain with first-set kinetics, thus demonstrating another feature of adaptive immunity, specificity (not shown). Syngeneic grafts are never rejected (not shown).

donor to the same recipient is rejected more rapidly, in only 2 or 3 days. This accelerated response, called second-set rejection, is due to a secondary immune response. Thus, grafts that are genetically disparate from the recipients induce immunologic memory, one of the cardinal features of adaptive immune responses.

- Second-set rejection ensues if the first and second skin grafts are derived from the same donor or from genetically identical donors, for example, strain A mice. However, if the second graft is derived from an individual unrelated to the donor of the first graft, for example, strain C, no second-set rejection occurs; the new graft elicits only a first-set rejection. Thus, the phenomenon of second-set rejection shows specificity, another cardinal feature of adaptive immune responses.

- The ability to mount second-set rejection against a graft from strain A mice can be adoptively transferred to a naive strain B recipient by immunocompetent lymphocytes taken from a strain B animal previously exposed to a graft from strain A mice. This experiment demonstrated that second-set rejection is mediated by sensitized lymphocytes and provided the definitive evidence that rejection is the result of an adaptive immune response.

Grafts may fail because of abnormalities other than rejection. In clinical practice, it is important to distinguish between rejection, which is immunologically mediated, and other causes of graft failure. Our discussion focuses on the immunologic basis of rejection.

Transplant immunologists have developed a special vocabulary to describe the kinds of cells and tissues encountered in the transplant setting. A graft transplanted from one individual to the same individual is called an **autologous graft** (shortened to autograft). A graft transplanted between two genetically identical or syngeneic individuals is called a **syngeneic graft**. A graft transplanted between two genetically different individuals of the same species is called an **allogeneic graft** (or **allograft**). A graft transplanted between individuals of different species is called a **xenogeneic graft** (or **xenograft**). The molecules that are recognized as foreign on allografts are called **alloantigens,** and those on xenografts are called **xenoantigens.** The lymphocytes and antibodies that react with alloantigens or xenoantigens are described as being **alloreactive** or **xenoreactive**, respectively.

The immunology of transplantation is important for two reasons. First, the immunologic rejection response is still one of the major barriers to transplantation today. Second, although an encounter with alloantigens is unlikely in the normal life of an organism, the immune response to allogeneic molecules is strong and has therefore been a useful model for studying the mechanisms of lymphocyte activation. Most of this chapter focuses on allogeneic transplantation because it is far more commonly practiced and better understood than xenogeneic transplantation, which is discussed briefly at the end of the chapter. We consider both the basic immunology and some aspects of the clinical practice of transplantation. We conclude the chapter with a discussion of allogeneic bone marrow transplantation, which raises special issues not usually encountered in solid organ transplants.

The Immunology of Allogeneic Transplantation

Alloantigens elicit both cell-mediated and humoral immune responses. In this section of the chapter, we discuss the molecular and cellular mechanisms of allorecognition, with an emphasis on the nature of graft antigens that stimulate allogeneic responses and the features of the responding lymphocytes.

Recognition of Alloantigens

Recognition of transplanted cells as self or foreign is determined by polymorphic genes that are inherited from both parents and are expressed codominantly. This conclusion is based on the results of experimental transplantation between inbred strains of mice. The basic rules of transplantation immunology are derived from such animal experiments (Fig. 16–2).

- Cells or organs transplanted between individuals of the same inbred strain of a species are never rejected.
- Cells or organs transplanted between individuals of different inbred strains of a species are almost always rejected.
- The offspring of a mating between two different inbred strains will typically not reject grafts from either parent. In other words, an $(A \times B)F_1$ animal will not reject grafts from an A or B strain animal. (This rule is violated by bone marrow transplantation, which we will discuss later in the chapter.)
- A graft derived from the offspring of a mating between two different inbred strains will almost always be rejected by either parent. In other words, a graft from an $(A \times B)F_1$ animal will be rejected by either an A or a B strain animal.

Such experimental results suggested that polymorphic, codominantly expressed molecules in the grafts were responsible for eliciting rejection. Polymorphism refers to the fact that these graft antigens differed among individuals of a species or between different inbred strains of animals, for example, between strain A and strain B mice. Codominant expression means that an $(A \times B)F_1$ animal expresses both A strain and B strain alleles. $(A \times B)F_1$ animals see both A and B tissues as self, and A or B animals see $(A \times B)F_1$ tissues as partly foreign. This is why an $(A \times B)F_1$ animal does not reject either A or B strain grafts and why both A and B strain recipients reject an $(A \times B)F_1$ graft.

Major histocompatibility complex (MHC) molecules are responsible for almost all strong (rapid) rejection reactions. George Snell and colleagues used congenic strains of inbred mice to identify the MHC complex as the locus of polymorphic genes that encode the molecular targets of allograft rejection (see Chapter 4, Fig. 4–2). Because MHC molecules, the targets of allograft rejection, are widely expressed, many different kinds of tissues evoke responses from alloreactive T cells. As discussed in Chapters 4 and 5, MHC molecules play a critical role in normal immune responses to foreign antigens, namely, the presentation of peptides derived from protein antigens in a form that can be recognized by T cells. The role of MHC molecules as alloantigens is incidental, as discussed later.

Allogeneic MHC molecules are presented for recognition by the T cells of a graft recipient in two fundamentally different ways (Fig. 16–3). The first way, called **direct presentation**, involves recognition of an intact MHC molecule displayed by donor antigen-presenting cells (APCs) in the graft and is a consequence of the similarity in structure of an intact foreign (allogeneic) MHC molecule and self MHC molecules. Therefore, direct presentation is unique to foreign MHC molecules. The second way, called **indirect presentation**, involves processing of donor MHC molecules by recipient APCs and presentation of peptides derived from the allogeneic MHC molecules in association with self MHC molecules. In this case, the foreign MHC molecule is handled as though it were any foreign protein antigen, and the mechanisms of indirect antigen presentation are indistinguishable from the mechanisms of presentation of a microbial protein antigen. Alloantigens in a graft other than MHC molecules can also

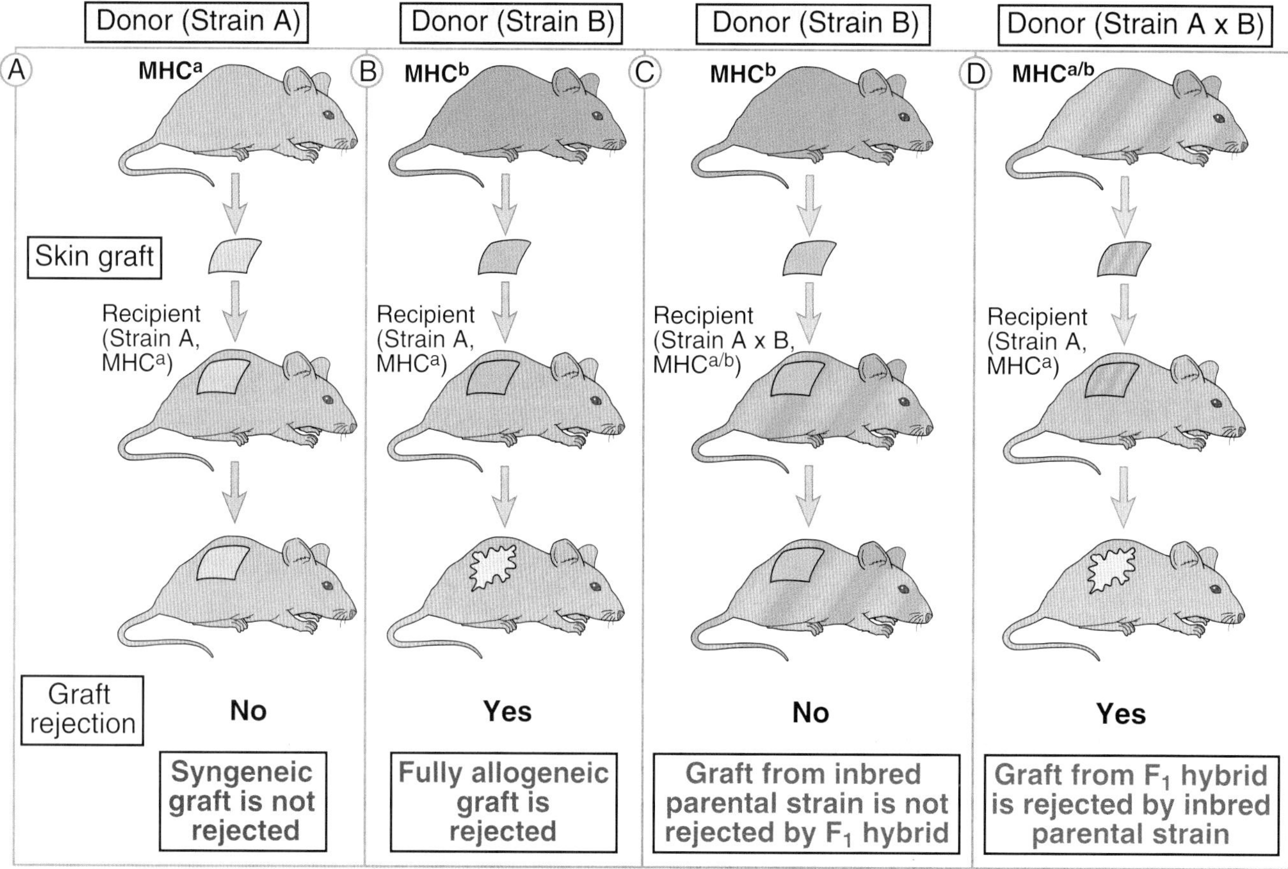

Figure 16–2 The genetics of graft rejection.
In the illustration, the two different mouse colors represent different MHC haplotypes. Inherited MHC alleles from both parents are codominantly expressed in the skin of an A × B offspring, and therefore these mice are represented by both colors. Syngeneic grafts are not rejected (A). Allografts are always rejected (B). Grafts from a parent of an A × B mating will not be rejected by the offspring (C), but grafts from the offspring will be rejected by either parent (D). These phenomena are due to the fact that MHC gene products are responsible for graft rejection; grafts are rejected only if they express an MHC type (represented by a color) that is not expressed by the recipient mouse.

be presented to host T cells by the indirect pathway. We discuss the molecular basis of direct and indirect presentation separately.

Direct Presentation of Alloantigens

Direct recognition of foreign MHC molecules is a cross-reaction of a normal T cell receptor (TCR), which was selected to recognize a self MHC molecule plus foreign peptide, with an allogeneic MHC molecule plus peptide. On face value, it seems puzzling that T cells that are normally selected to be self MHC-restricted are capable of recognizing foreign MHC molecules. The explanation for this apparent paradox came from studies with monoclonal T cell populations, which showed that the same TCR may recognize self MHC–foreign peptide complexes and allogeneic MHC molecules.

- A T cell clone that expresses a TCR specific for self MHC plus a foreign peptide may also recognize one or more allogeneic MHC molecules in the absence of that foreign peptide.
- Monoclonal antibodies specific for idiotypic determinants on the TCR molecule of such a T cell clone may inhibit the recognition of both self MHC–associated foreign peptide and allogeneic MHC molecules.
- Transfection of rearranged α and β TCR genes encoding such a TCR into another T cell confers specificity both for self MHC plus foreign peptide and for allogeneic MHC molecules.

An allogeneic MHC molecule with a bound peptide can mimic the determinant formed by a self MHC molecule plus a particular foreign peptide (Fig. 16–4). Since the same T cell can recognize self MHC–foreign peptide complexes and allogeneic MHC molecules, it follows that the determinants formed by these MHC molecules must share structural features. An allogeneic MHC molecule is sufficiently similar to self MHC plus foreign peptide that normal self MHC–restricted T cells recognize the allogeneic MHC molecules. The T cells may recognize amino acid residues of the allogeneic MHC molecule only or residues contributed by the MHC molecule and some bound peptide.

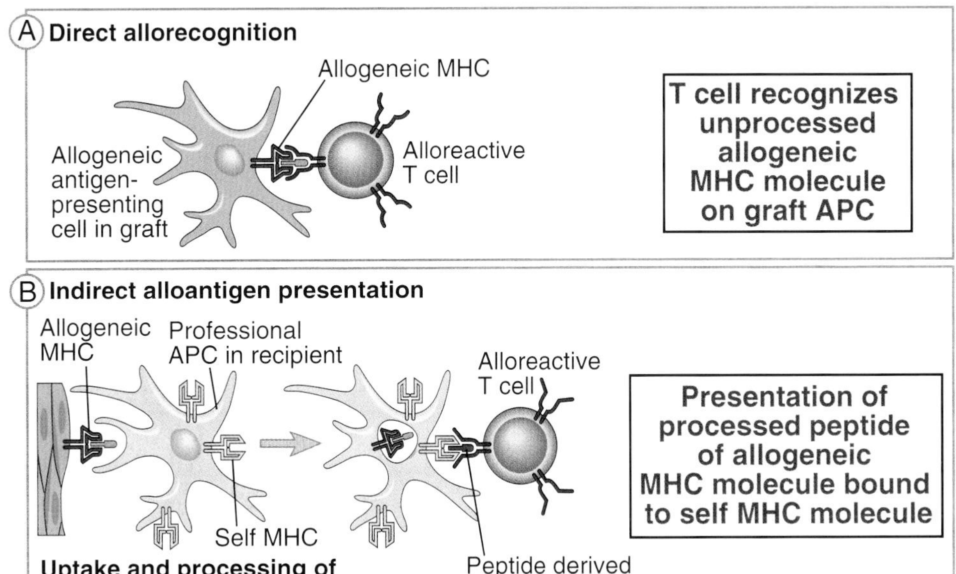

Figure 16–3 Direct and indirect alloantigen recognition.

A. Direct alloantigen recognition occurs when T cells bind directly to an intact allogeneic MHC molecule on a graft (donor) antigen-presenting cell (APC).

B. Indirect alloantigen recognition occurs when allogeneic MHC molecules from graft cells are taken up and processed by recipient APCs, and peptide fragments of the allogenic MHC molecules containing polymorphic amino acid residues are bound and presented by recipient (self) MHC molecules.

MHC molecules that are expressed on cell surfaces normally contain bound peptides. The peptides bound to allogeneic MHC molecules may play several roles in the recognition of these molecules (see Fig. 16–4). Peptides may simply be required for stable cell surface expression of the allogeneic MHC molecules. However, some alloreactive T cell clones have been shown to recognize allogeneic MHC molecules with some, but not other, bound peptides. This observation suggests that the peptide contributes to the determinant recognized by the alloreactive T cell, exactly like the role of peptides in the normal recognition of antigen by self MHC–restricted T cells. Many of the peptides associated with allogeneic MHC molecules that are involved in direct presentation are derived from proteins that are identical in the donor and recipient. In other words, they are self peptides. The mechanisms of tolerance induction, described in Chapter 10, work only to eliminate or to inactivate T cells that respond to complexes of self peptides plus self MHC molecules. Therefore, T cells specific for self peptide plus allogeneic MHC are not removed from the repertoire and are available to respond to allografts.

As many as 2% of an individual's T cells are capable of directly recognizing and responding to a single foreign MHC molecule, and this high frequency of T cells reactive with allogeneic MHC molecules is one reason that allografts elicit strong immune responses in vivo. The fact that each allogeneic MHC molecule is directly recognized by so many different TCRs, each selected for different foreign peptides, may be due to several factors.

- The highly polymorphic nature of the MHC implies that allogeneic MHC molecules will differ from self MHC molecules at multiple amino acid residues. Because many of the polymorphic residues are concentrated in the regions that bind to the TCR, each different residue may contribute to a distinct determinant recognized by a different clone of self MHC–restricted T cells. Thus, each allogeneic MHC molecule can be recognized by multiple T cell clones. In this case, the cross-reactive T cell allorecognition is entirely attributable to differences in amino acid sequences between self MHC and allogeneic MHC molecules, and bound peptide serves only to ensure stable expression of the allogeneic MHC molecule.
- Many different peptides may combine with one allogeneic MHC gene product to produce determinants that are recognized by different cross-reactive T cells. The surface of each allogeneic cell has 10^5 or more copies of each allogeneic MHC molecule, and each MHC molecule can form a complex with a different peptide. Thus, any cell in an allograft may express many distinct peptide-MHC complexes composed of different peptides bound to one or a few alleles of the foreign MHC molecules. Because only a few hundred peptide-MHC complexes are needed to activate a particular T cell clone, many different clones may be activated by the same allogeneic cell.
- All of the MHC molecules on an allogeneic APC are foreign to a recipient and can therefore be recognized by T cells. In contrast, on self APCs, most of the self MHC molecules are displaying self peptides, and any foreign peptide probably occupies 1% or less of the total MHC molecules expressed. As a result, the density of allogeneic determinants on allogeneic APCs is much higher than the density of foreign peptide–self MHC complexes on self APCs. The abundance of recognizable allogeneic MHC molecules may allow activation of T cells with low affinities for the determinant, thereby increasing the numbers of T cells that can respond.

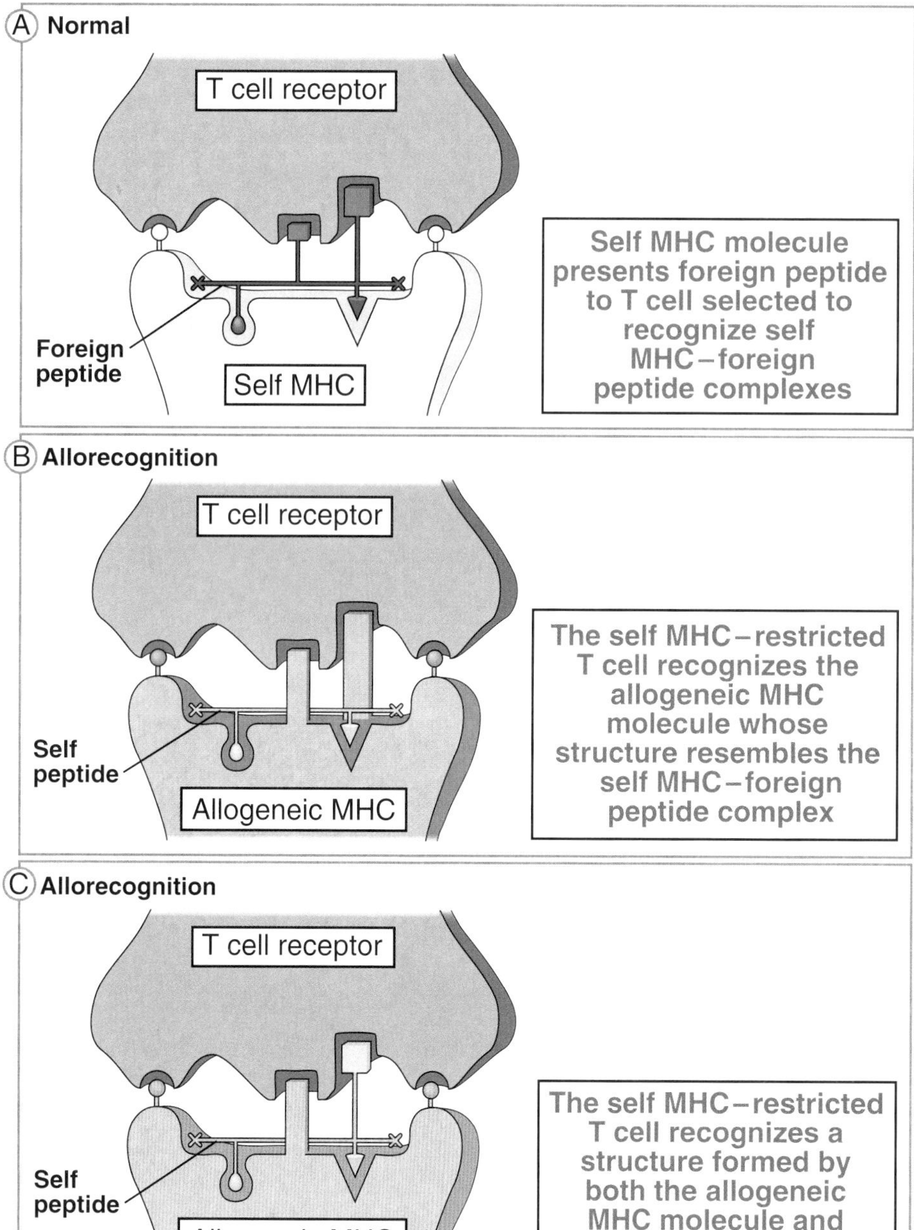

Figure 16–4 Molecular basis of direct recognition of allogeneic MHC molecules.

Direct recognition of allogeneic MHC molecules may be thought of as a cross-reaction in which a T cell specific for a self MHC molecule–foreign peptide complex (A) also recognizes an allogeneic MHC molecule (B, C). Nonpolymorphic donor peptides, labeled "self peptide," may not contribute to allorecognition (B), or they may (C).

- Many of the alloreactive T cells that respond to the first exposure to an allogeneic MHC molecule are memory T cells that were generated during previous exposure to other foreign (e.g., microbial) antigens. Thus, in contrast to the initial naive T cell response to microbial antigens, the initial response to alloantigens is mediated in part by already expanded clones of memory T cells.

Because of the high frequency of alloreactive T cells, primary responses to alloantigens are the only primary responses that can readily be detected *in vitro.*

Indirect Presentation of Alloantigens

Allogeneic MHC molecules may be processed and presented by recipient APCs that enter grafts, and the processed MHC molecules are recognized by T cells like conventional foreign protein antigens (see Fig. 16–3). Because allogeneic MHC molecules differ structurally from those of the host, they can be processed and presented in the same way that any foreign protein antigen is, generating foreign peptides associated with self MHC molecules on the surface of host APCs. This phenomenon is an example of cross-presentation or cross-priming (see Chapter 5, Fig. 5–7), in which professional APCs, usually dendritic cells, present antigens of another cell, from the graft, to activate, or "prime," T lymphocytes. Indirect presentation may result in allorecognition by $CD4^+$ T cells because alloantigen is acquired by host APCs primarily through the endosomal vesicular pathway (i.e., as a consequence of phagocytosis) and is therefore presented by class II MHC molecules. Some antigens of phagocytosed graft cells appear to enter the class I MHC pathway of antigen presentation and are indirectly recognized by $CD8^+$ T cells. Because MHC molecules are the most polymorphic proteins in the genome, each allogeneic MHC molecule may give rise to multiple foreign peptides, each recognized by different T cells.

- One of the first indications that T cell responses to allogeneic MHC molecules can occur by indirect presentation was the demonstration of cross-priming of alloreactive $CD8^+$ cytolytic T lymphocytes (CTLs) by self APCs that had been exposed to allogeneic cells.
- Evidence that indirect presentation of allogeneic MHC molecules occurs in graft rejection was obtained from studies with knockout mice lacking class II MHC expression. For example, skin grafts from donor mice lacking class II MHC are able to induce recipient $CD4^+$ (i.e., class II–restricted) T cell responses to the donor alloantigens, including peptides derived from donor class I MHC molecules. This result implies that the donor class I MHC molecules are processed and presented by class II molecules on the recipient's APCs and stimulate the recipient's helper T cells.
- More recently, evidence has been obtained from human transplant recipients that indirect antigen presentation may contribute to late rejection of allografts. For example, $CD4^+$ T cells from heart and liver allograft recipients can be activated *in vitro* by peptides derived from donor MHC and presented by host APCs.

There may be polymorphic antigens other than MHC molecules that differ between the donor and the recipient. These antigens induce weak or slower (more gradual) rejection reactions than do MHC molecules and are called **minor histocompatibility antigens**. Most minor histocompatibility antigens are proteins that are processed and presented to host T cells in association with self MHC molecules on host APCs (i.e., by the indirect pathway).

Activation of Alloreactive T Cells and Rejection of Allografts

The activation of alloreactive T cells in vivo requires presentation of alloantigens by donor-derived APCs in the graft (direct presentation of alloantigens) or by host APCs that pick up and present graft alloantigens (indirect presentation). Most organs contain resident APCs such as dendritic cells. Transplantation of these organs into an allogeneic recipient provides APCs that express donor MHC molecules as well as costimulators. Presumably, these donor APCs migrate to regional lymph nodes and are recognized by the recipient's T cells that circulate through the peripheral lymphoid organs (the direct pathway). Dendritic cells from the recipient may also migrate into the graft, or graft alloantigens may traffic into lymph nodes, where they are captured and presented by recipient APCs (the indirect pathway). Alloreactive T cells in the recipient may be activated by both pathways, and these T cells migrate into the grafts and cause graft rejection. Alloreactive $CD4^+$ helper T cells differentiate into cytokine-producing effector cells that damage grafts by reactions that resemble delayed-type hypersensitivity (DTH). Alloreactive $CD8^+$ T cells activated by the direct pathway differentiate into CTLs that kill nucleated cells in the graft, which express the allogeneic class I MHC molecules. The $CD8^+$ CTLs that are generated by the indirect pathway are self MHC-restricted, and therefore they cannot directly kill the foreign cells in the graft. Therefore, when alloreactive T cells are stimulated by the indirect pathway, the principal mechanism of rejection is probably DTH mediated by $CD4^+$ effector T cells that infiltrate the graft and recognize donor alloantigens being displayed by host APCs that have also entered the graft. The relative importance of the direct and indirect pathways in graft rejection is still unclear. It has been suggested that $CD8^+$ CTLs induced by direct recognition of alloantigens are most important for acute rejection of allografts, whereas $CD4^+$ effector T cells stimulated by the indirect pathway play a greater role in chronic rejection.

The importance of MHC molecules in the rejection of tissue allografts has been established by studies with inbred animals showing that rapid rejection usually requires class I or class II MHC differences between the graft donor and the recipient. In clinical transplantation, minimizing MHC differences between the donor and the recipient improves graft survival, as we shall discuss later.

The response of alloreactive T cells to foreign MHC molecules has also been analyzed in an *in vitro* reaction called the **mixed lymphocyte reaction** (MLR). The MLR is a model of direct T cell recognition of allogeneic MHC molecules and is used as a predictive test of T cell–mediated graft rejection. Studies of the MLR were among the first to establish the role of class I and class II MHC molecules in activating distinct populations of T cells ($CD8^+$ and $CD4^+$, respectively).

- The MLR is induced by culturing mononuclear leukocytes (which include T cells, B cells, NK cells, mononuclear phagocytes, and dendritic cells) from one individual with mononuclear leukocytes derived from another individual. In humans, these cells are typically isolated from peripheral blood; in the mouse or rat, mononuclear leukocytes are usually purified from the spleen or lymph nodes. If the two individuals have differences in the alleles of the MHC genes, a large proportion of the mononuclear cells will proliferate during a period of 4 to 7 days. This proliferative response is called the allogeneic MLR (Fig. 16–5). In this experiment, the cells from each donor react and proliferate against the other, thus resulting in a two-way MLR. To simplify the analysis, one of the two leukocyte populations can be rendered incapable of proliferation before culture, either by γ-irradiation or by treatment with the antimitotic drug mitomycin C. In this one-way MLR, the treated cells serve exclusively as stimulators and the untreated cells, still capable of proliferation, serve as the responders.
- Among the T cells that have responded in an MLR, any one cell is specific for only one allogeneic MHC

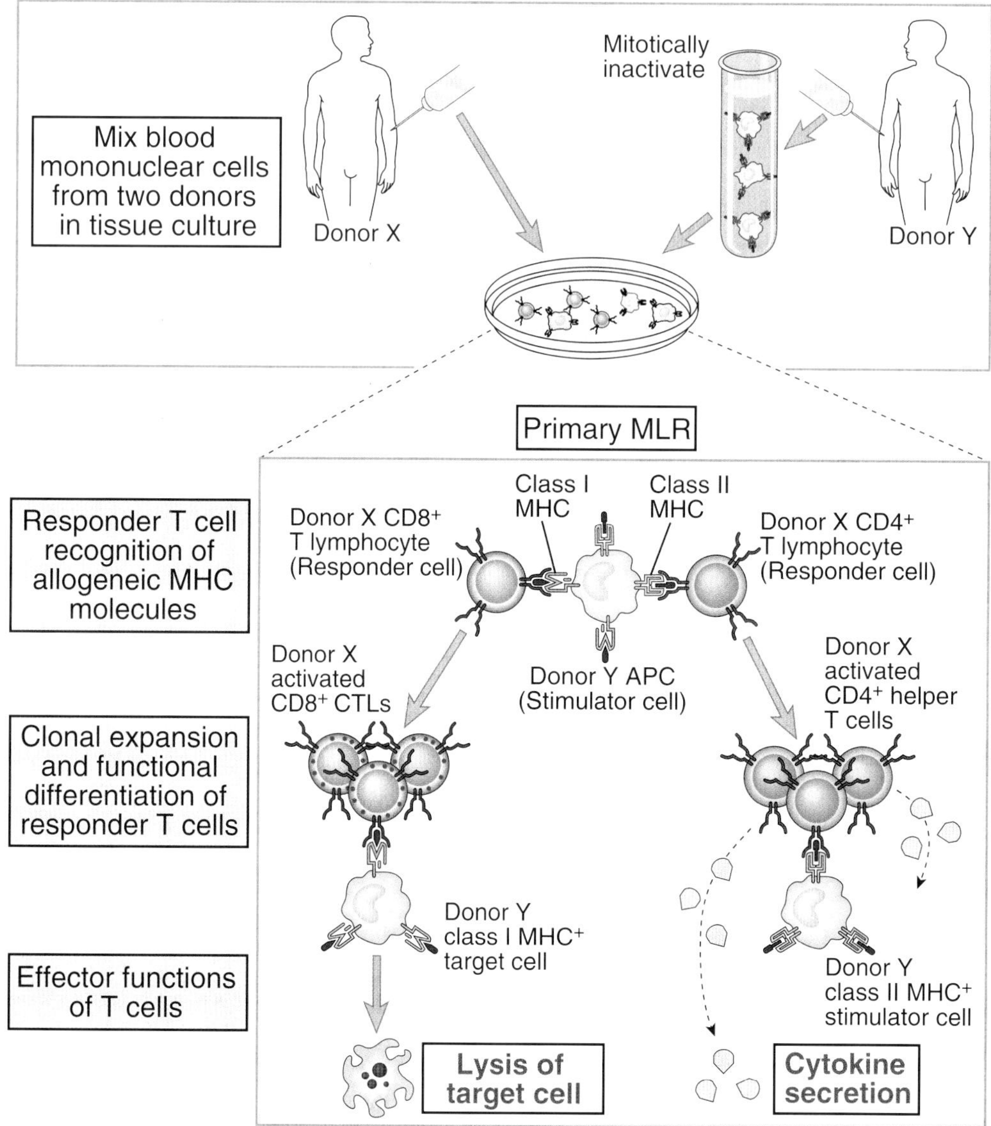

Figure 16–5 The mixed leukocyte reaction (MLR).
In a one-way primary MLR, stimulator cells (from donor Y) activate and cause the expansion of two types of responder T cells (from donor X). $CD4^+$ T cells from donor X react to donor Y class II molecules, and $CD8^+$ T lymphocytes from donor X react to donor Y class I MHC molecules. The $CD4^+$ T cells differentiate into cytokine-secreting helper T cells, and the $CD8^+$ T cells differentiate into cytolytic T lymphocytes (CTLs). APC, antigen-presenting cell.

molecule, and the entire population of activated T lymphocytes contains cells that recognize all the MHC differences between stimulators and responders. $CD8^+$ CTLs are generated only if the class I MHC alleles of the stimulators and responders are different. Similarly, $CD4^+$ effector T cells are generated only if the class II molecules are different.

- Stimulator cells lacking MHC molecules cannot activate responder cells in an MLR. Transfection of MHC genes into the stimulators makes these cells capable of inducing an MLR.

- $CD8^+$ CTLs generated in an MLR will kill cells from other donors only if these cells share some class I alleles with the original stimulators. Similarly, $CD4^+$ T cells generated in an MLR recognize APCs from other donors only if these APCs share class II alleles with the stimulators. Such experiments demonstrate that alloreactive T cells are specific for allogeneic MHC molecules, and activation of alloreactive T cells in the MLR occurs mainly by the direct pathway.

In addition to recognition of alloantigen, costimulation of T cells by B7 molecules on APCs is important for activating alloreactive T cells.

- Rejection of allografts, and stimulation of alloreactive T cells in an MLR, can be inhibited by agents that bind to and block B7 molecules. Most studies indicate that B7 antagonists are more effective at blocking acute rejection of allografts and activation of alloreactive T cells by the direct pathway. In contrast, chronic rejection and activation of alloreactive T cells by the indirect pathway are often insensitive to such agents, for unknown reasons.

Allografts survive for longer periods when they are transplanted into knockout mice lacking B7-1 (CD80) and B7-2 (CD86) compared with transplants into normal recipients. However, even in B7 knockout recipients, allografts show histologic evidence of rejection and eventually fail because of chronic rejection.

In contrast to T cell alloreactivity, much less is known about the mechanisms that lead to the production of alloantibodies against foreign MHC molecules. Presumably, B cells specific for alloantigens are stimulated by mechanisms similar to those involved in the stimulation of B cells reactive with other foreign proteins.

Many of the issues that arise in discussions of alloreactivity and graft rejection are also relevant to maternal-fetal interactions. The fetus expresses paternal MHC molecules and is therefore semiallogeneic to the mother. Nevertheless, the fetus is not rejected by the maternal immune system. Many possible mechanisms have been proposed to account for this lack of rejection, and it is not yet clear which of these mechanisms is the most significant (Box 16–1).

BOX 16–1

Immune Responses to an Allogeneic Fetus

The mammalian fetus, except in instances in which the mother and father are syngeneic, will express paternally inherited antigens that are allogeneic to the mother. In essence, the fetus is a naturally occurring allograft. Nevertheless, fetuses are not normally rejected by the mother. It is clear that the mother is exposed to fetal antigens during pregnancy since maternal antibodies against paternal MHC molecules are easily detectable. An understanding of how the fetus escapes the maternal immune system may be relevant for transplantation. Protection of the fetus against the maternal immune system probably involves several mechanisms including special molecular and barrier features of the placenta and local immunosuppression.

Several experimental observations indicate that the anatomic location of the fetus is a critical factor in the absence of rejection. For example, pregnant animals are able to recognize and reject allografts syngeneic to the fetus placed at extrauterine sites without compromising fetal survival. Wholly allogeneic fetal blastocysts that lack maternal genes can successfully develop in a pregnant or pseudopregnant mother. Thus, neither specific maternal nor paternal genes are necessary for survival of the fetus. Hyperimmunization of the mother with cells bearing paternal antigens does not compromise placental and fetal growth.

The failure to reject the fetus has focused attention on the region of physical contact between the mother and fetus. The fetal tissues of the placenta that most intimately contact the mother are composed of either vascular trophoblast, which is exposed to maternal blood for purposes of mediating nutrient exchange, or implantation site trophoblast, which diffusely infiltrates the uterine lining (decidua) for purposes of anchoring the placenta to the mother.

One simple explanation for fetal survival is that trophoblast cells fail to express paternal MHC molecules. So far, class II molecules have not been detected on trophoblast. In mice, cells of implantation trophoblast, but not of vascular trophoblast, do express paternal class I molecules. In humans, the situation may be more complex in that trophoblast cells express only a nonpolymorphic class IB molecule called HLA-G. This molecule may be involved in protecting trophoblast cells from maternal NK cell–mediated lysis. A specialized subset of NK cells called uterine NK cells are the major type of lymphocyte present at implantation sites, and IFN-γ production by these cells is essential for decidual development. The way uterine NK cells are stimulated and their role in maternal responses to fetal alloantigens are not known. Even if trophoblast cells do express classical MHC molecules, they may lack costimulator molecules and fail to act as antigen-presenting cells.

A second explanation for lack of rejection is that the uterine decidua may be an **immunologically privileged site**. These anatomic sites are tissues where immune responses generally fail to occur and include brain, eye, and testis. Several factors may contribute to immune privilege. For example, the brain vasculature limits lymphocyte access to the brain tissue, and the anterior chamber of the eye may contain high concentrations of immunosuppressive cytokines such as transforming growth factor-β (TGF-β). In support of the idea that the decidua is an immune privileged site is the observation that mouse decidua is highly susceptible to infection by *Listeria monocytogenes* and cannot support a delayed-type hypersensitivity response. The basis of immunologic privilege is clearly not a simple anatomic barrier because maternal blood is in extensive contact with trophoblast. Rather, the barrier is likely to be created by functional inhibition. Cultured decidual cells directly inhibit macrophage and T cell functions, perhaps by producing inhibitory cytokines, such as TGF-β. Some of these inhibitory decidual cells may be resident regulatory T cells, although the evidence for this proposal is limited. Some experiments have led to the suggestion that T_H2 cytokines are produced at the maternal-fetal interface and are responsible for local suppression of T_H1 responses to fetal antigens. However, this idea is not supported by the data that IL-4 and IL-10 knockout mice have normal pregnancies.

There is evidence that immune responses to the fetus may be regulated by local tryptophan concentrations in the decidua. The enzyme indolamine 2,3-dioxygenase (IDO) catabolizes tryptophan, and the IDO-inhibiting drug 1-methyl-tryptophan induces abortions in mice in a T cell–dependent manner. These observations have led to the hypothesis that T cell responses to the fetus are blocked because decidual tryptophan levels are normally maintained below the level required for T cell activation.

Trophoblast and decidua may also be relatively resistant to complement-mediated damage because they express high levels of a C3 and C4 inhibitor called Crry. Crry-deficient embryos die before birth and show evidence of complement activation on trophoblast cells. Thus, this inhibitor may block maternal alloantibody-mediated damage through the classical pathway of complement activation.

Effector Mechanisms of Allograft Rejection

Thus far, we have described the molecular basis of alloantigen recognition and the cells involved in the recognition of and responses to allografts. We now turn to a consideration of the effector mechanisms used by the immune system to reject allografts. In different experimental models in animals and in clinical transplantation, alloreactive CD4$^+$ or CD8$^+$ T cells or alloantibodies are capable of mediating allograft rejection. These different immune effectors cause graft rejection by different mechanisms.

For historical reasons, graft rejection is classified on the basis of histopathologic features or the time course of rejection after transplantation rather than immune effector mechanisms. Based on the experience of renal transplantation, the histopathologic patterns are called hyperacute, acute, and chronic (Fig. 16–6).

Hyperacute Rejection

Hyperacute rejection is characterized by thrombotic occlusion of the graft vasculature that begins within minutes to hours after host blood vessels are anastomosed to graft vessels and is mediated by preexisting antibodies in the host circulation that bind to donor endothelial antigens (Fig. 16–7). Binding of antibody to endothelium activates complement, and antibody and complement induce a number of changes in the graft endothelium that promote intravascular thrombosis. Complement activation leads to endothelial cell injury and exposure of subendothelial basement membrane proteins that activate platelets. The endothelial cells are stimulated to secrete high molecular weight forms of von Willebrand factor that mediate platelet adhesion and aggregation. Both endothelial cells and platelets undergo membrane vesiculation leading to shedding of lipid particles that promote coagulation. Endothelial cells lose the cell surface heparan sulfate proteoglycans that normally interact with antithrombin III to inhibit coagulation. These processes contribute to thrombosis and vascular occlusion, and the grafted organ suffers irreversible ischemic damage.

In the early days of transplantation, hyperacute rejection was often mediated by preexisting IgM alloantibodies, which are present at high titer before transplantation. Such "natural antibodies" are believed to arise in response to carbohydrate antigens expressed by bacteria that normally colonize the intestine. The best known examples of such alloantibodies are those directed against the ABO blood group antigens expressed on red blood cells (Box 16–2). ABO antigens are also expressed on vascular endothelial cells. Today, hyperacute rejection by anti-ABO antibodies is not a clinical problem because all donors and recipients are selected so that they have the same ABO type. However, as we shall discuss later in the chapter, hyperacute rejection caused by natural antibodies is the major barrier to xenotransplantation and limits the use of animal organs for human transplantation.

Currently, hyperacute rejection of allografts, when it occurs, is usually mediated by IgG antibodies directed against protein alloantigens, such as foreign MHC molecules, or against less well defined alloantigens expressed on vascular endothelial cells. Such antibodies generally arise as a result of previous exposure to alloantigens through blood transfusion, previous transplantation, or multiple pregnancies. If the titer of these alloreactive antibodies is low, hyperacute rejection may develop slowly, during several days. In this

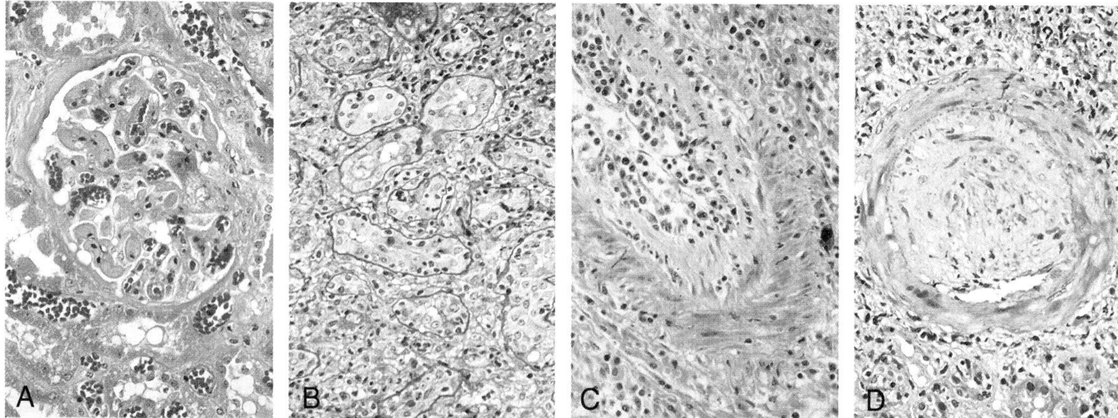

Figure 16–6 Histopathology of different forms of graft rejection.

A. Hyperacute rejection of a kidney allograft with endothelial damage, platelet and thrombin thrombi, and early neutrophil infiltration in a glomerulus.

B. Acute rejection of a kidney with inflammatory cells in the interstitium and between epithelial cells of the tubules.

C. Acute rejection of a kidney allograft with destructive inflammatory reaction destroying the endothelial layer of an artery.

D. Chronic rejection in a kidney allograft with graft arteriosclerosis. The vascular lumen is replaced by an accumulation of smooth muscle cells and connective tissue in the vessel intima. (Courtesy of Dr. Helmut Rennke, Department of Pathology, Brigham and Women's Hospital and Harvard Medical School, Boston.)

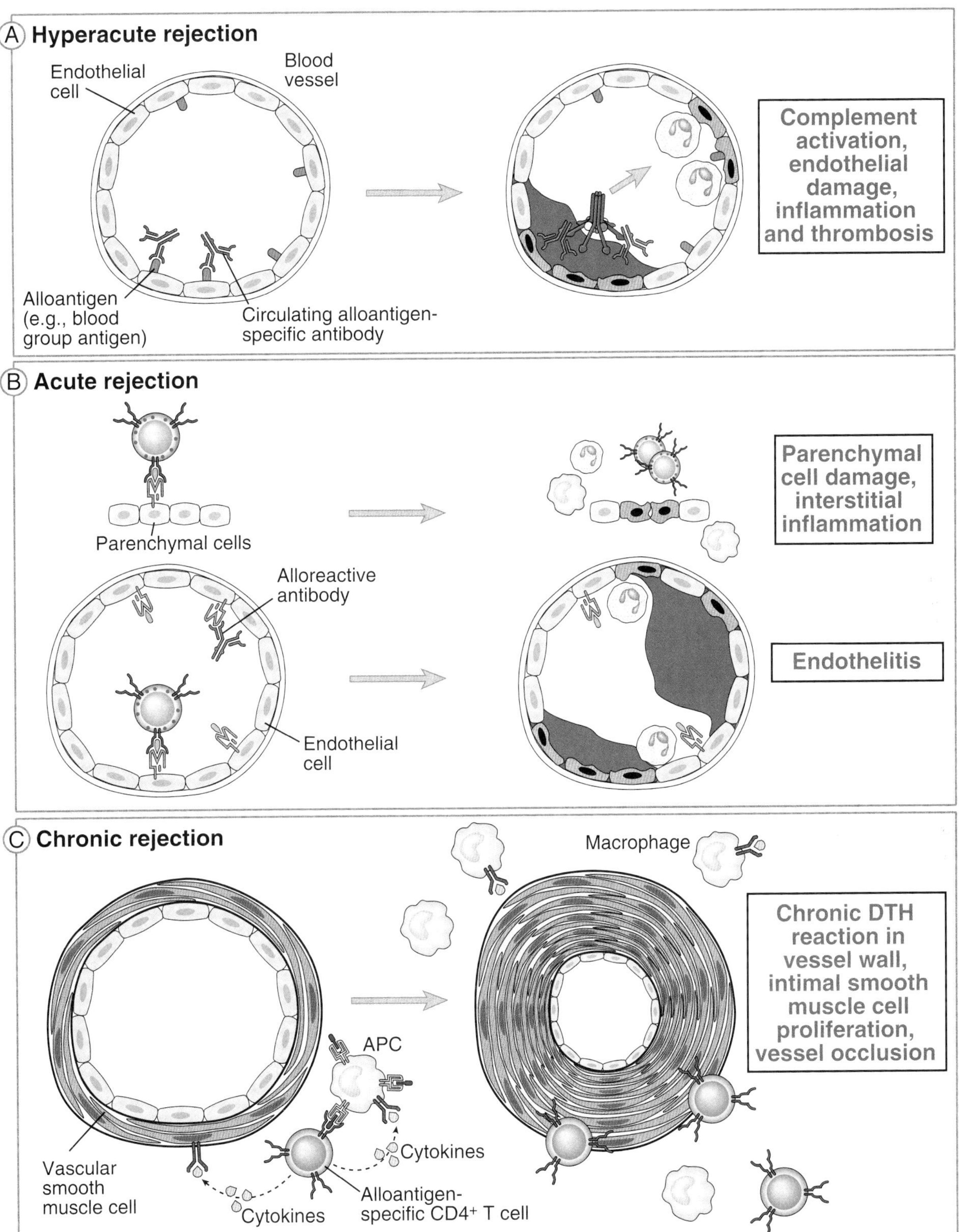

Figure 16–7 Immune mechanisms of graft rejection.

A. In hyperacute rejection, preformed antibodies reactive with vascular endothelium activate complement and trigger rapid intravascular thrombosis and necrosis of the vessel wall.

B. In acute rejection, $CD8^+$ T lymphocytes reactive with alloantigens on endothelial cells and parenchymal cells mediate damage to these cell types. Alloreactive antibodies formed after engraftment may also contribute to vascular injury.

C. In chronic rejection with graft arteriosclerosis, injury to the vessel wall leads to intimal smooth muscle cell proliferation and luminal occlusion. This lesion may be caused by a chronic delayed-type hypersensitivity (DTH) reaction to alloantigens in the vessel wall.

BOX 16–2

ABO and Rh Blood Group Antigens

The first alloantigen system to be defined in mammals was a family of red blood cell surface antigens called ABO, which are the targets of blood transfusion reactions (see text). The antigens in this system are cell surface glycosphingolipids. All normal individuals synthesize a common core glycan, called the O antigen, that is attached to a sphingolipid. Most individuals possess a fucosyltransferase that adds a fucose moiety to a side branch of the O antigen, and the fucosylated glycan is called the H antigen. (The whole antigenic system is sometimes called ABH rather than ABO.) A single gene on chromosome 9 encodes a glycosyltransferase enzyme, which further modifies the H antigen. There are three allelic variants of this gene. The O allele gene product is devoid of enzymatic activity. The A allele–encoded enzyme transfers a terminal *N*-acetylgalactosamine moiety, and the B allele gene product transfers a terminal galactose moiety. Individuals who are homozygous for the O allele cannot attach terminal sugars to the H antigen and express only the H antigen. In contrast, individuals who possess an A allele (AA homozygotes, AO heterozygotes, or AB heterozygotes) form the A antigen by adding terminal *N*-acetylgalactosamine to some of their H antigens. Similarly, individuals who express a B allele (BB homozygotes, BO heterozygotes, or AB heterozygotes) form the B antigen by adding terminal galactose to some of their H antigens. AB heterozygotes form both A and B antigens from some of their H antigens. The terminology has been simplified so that OO individuals are said to be blood type O; AA and AO individuals are blood type A; BB and BO individuals are blood type B; and AB individuals are blood type AB. Mutations in the gene encoding the fucosyltransferase that produces the H antigen are rare; people who are homozygous for such a mutation cannot produce H, A, or B antigens and are also called type O.

The same glycosphingolipid that carries the ABO determinants can be modified by other glycosyltransferases to generate minor blood group antigens that may elicit milder transfusion reactions than the ABO antigens. For example, addition of fucose moieties at other side branch positions can be catalyzed by different fucosyltransferases and results in epitopes of the Lewis antigen system. Lewis antigens have recently received much attention from immunologists because these carbohydrate groups serve as ligands for E-selectin and P-selectin.

The Rhesus (Rh) antigens, named after the monkey species in which they were originally identified, is another clinically important blood group antigen. Rh antigens are nonglycosylated, hydrophobic cell surface proteins found in the red blood cell membranes and are structurally related to other red cell membrane glycoproteins with transporter functions. Rh proteins are encoded by two tightly linked and highly homologous genes, but only one of them, called RhD, is commonly considered in clinical blood typing. This is because up to 15% of the population have a deletion or other alterations of the RhD allele. These people, called Rh negative, are not tolerant to the RhD antigen and will make antibodies to the antigen if they are exposed to Rh-positive blood cells. The clinical significance of anti-Rh antibodies is discussed in the text.

case, it is sometimes referred to as accelerated allograft rejection because the onset is still earlier than that typical for acute rejection. As we will discuss later in the chapter, patients in need of allografts are routinely screened before grafting for the presence of antibodies that bind to cells of a potential organ donor to avoid hyperacute rejection.

Acute Rejection

Acute rejection is a process of vascular and parenchymal injury mediated by T cells and antibodies that usually begins after the first week of transplantation. Effector T cells and antibodies that mediate acute rejection develop during a few days or weeks in response to the graft, accounting for the time at onset of acute rejection.

T lymphocytes play a central role in acute rejection by responding to alloantigens, including MHC molecules, present on vascular endothelial and parenchymal cells (see Fig. 16–7). The activated T cells cause direct lysis of graft cells or produce cytokines that recruit and activate inflammatory cells, which injure the graft. In vascularized grafts such as kidney grafts, endothelial cells are the earliest targets of acute rejection. Microvascular endothelitis is a frequent early finding in acute rejection episodes. Endothelitis or intimal arteritis in medium-sized arteries also occurs at an early stage of acute rejection and is indicative of severe rejection, which, left untreated, will likely result in acute graft failure.

Both CD4$^+$ T cells and CD8$^+$ T cells may contribute to acute rejection. Several lines of evidence suggest that recognition and killing of graft cells by alloreactive CD8$^+$ CTLs is an important mechanism of acute rejection.

- The cellular infiltrates present in grafts undergoing acute cellular rejection are markedly enriched for CD8$^+$ CTLs specific for graft alloantigens.
- The presence of CTLs in renal graft biopsy specimens, as indicated by sensitive reverse transcriptase–polymerase chain reaction assays for RNAs encoding CTL-specific genes (e.g., perforin and granzyme B), is a specific and sensitive indicator of clinical acute rejection.
- Alloreactive CD8$^+$ CTLs can be used to adoptively transfer acute cellular graft rejection.
- The destruction of allogeneic cells in a graft is highly specific, a hallmark of CTL killing. The best evidence for this specificity has come from mouse skin graft experiments using chimeric grafts that contain two distinct cell populations, one syngeneic to the host and

one allogeneic to the host. When these skin grafts are transplanted, the allogeneic cells are killed without injury to the "bystander" syngeneic cells.

CD4$^+$ T cells may be important in mediating acute graft rejection by secreting cytokines and inducing DTH-like reactions in grafts, and some evidence indicates that CD4$^+$ T cells are sufficient to mediate acute rejection.

- Acute rejection of allografts does occur in knockout mice lacking CD8$^+$ T cells or perforin, suggesting that other effector mechanisms also contribute.
- Adoptive transfer of alloreactive CD4$^+$ T cells into a mouse can cause rejection of an allograft.

Antibodies can also mediate acute rejection if a graft recipient mounts a humoral immune response to vessel wall antigens and the antibodies that are produced bind to the vessel wall and activate complement. The histologic pattern of this form of acute rejection is one of transmural necrosis of graft vessel walls with acute inflammation, which is different from the thrombotic occlusion without vessel wall necrosis seen in hyperacute rejection.

Chronic Rejection

Chronic rejection is characterized by fibrosis and vascular abnormalities with loss of graft function occurring during a prolonged period. As therapy for controlling acute rejection has improved, chronic rejection has emerged as the major cause of allograft loss. The pathogenesis of chronic rejection is less well understood than that of acute rejection. The fibrosis of chronic rejection may result from immune reactions and the production of cytokines that stimulate fibroblasts, or it may represent wound healing after the parenchymal cellular necrosis of acute rejection. Perhaps the major cause of chronic rejection of vascularized organ grafts is arterial occlusion as a result of the proliferation of intimal smooth muscle cells. This process is called **accelerated** (or **graft**) **arteriosclerosis** (see Fig. 16–6). Graft arteriosclerosis is frequently seen in failed cardiac and renal allografts and can develop in any vascularized organ transplant within 6 months to a year after transplantation. The lesion appears to occur without evidence of overt vascular injury, and no correlation has clearly been established between the development of graft arteriosclerosis and infection, episodes of previous acute rejection, or lipid abnormalities. The smooth muscle cell proliferation in the vascular intima may represent a specialized form of chronic DTH reaction of the organ parenchyma in which lymphocytes activated by alloantigens in the graft vessel wall induce macrophages to secrete smooth muscle cell growth factors (see Fig. 16–7).

- Knockout mice lacking different components of the adaptive immune system have been used as graft recipients and show varying resistance to graft arteriosclerosis. For instance, graft arteriosclerosis does not develop in interferon-γ (IFN-γ)–deficient recipients, consistent with the hypothesis that DTH is involved in lesion formation. Other studies with knockout mice indicate that CD4$^+$ T cells and B lymphocytes are more important for the development of graft arteriosclerosis than are CD8$^+$ T cells.

Chronic rejection of different transplanted organs is associated with distinct pathologic changes. Lung transplants undergoing chronic rejection show thickened small airways (bronchiolitis obliterans), and liver transplants show fibrotic and nonfunctional bile ducts (the vanishing bile duct syndrome).

Prevention and Treatment of Allograft Rejection

If the recipient of an allograft has a fully functional immune system, transplantation almost invariably results in some form of rejection. The strategies used in clinical practice and in experimental models to avoid or delay rejection are general immunosuppression and minimizing the strength of the specific allogeneic reaction. An important goal in transplantation is to induce donor-specific tolerance, which would allow grafts to survive without pharmacologic immunosuppression.

Immunosuppression to Prevent or to Treat Allograft Rejection

Immunosuppression is the major approach for the prevention and management of transplant rejection. Several methods of immunosuppression are commonly used (Table 16–1).

Immunosuppressive drugs that inhibit or kill T lymphocytes are the principal treatment regimen for graft rejection. The most important immunosuppressive agent in current clinical use is **cyclosporine**. Cyclosporine is a cyclic peptide made by a species of fungus. The major action of cyclosporine on T cells is to inhibit the transcription of certain genes, most notably those encoding cytokines such as interleukin (IL)-2. Cyclosporine binds with high affinity to a ubiquitous cellular protein called cyclophilin. As discussed in Chapter 8, the complex of cyclosporine and cyclophilin binds to and inhibits the enzymatic activity of the calcium/calmodulin-activated protein phosphatase calcineurin. Because calcium/calmodulin-activated calcineurin function is required to activate the transcription factor NFAT (nuclear factor of activated T cells), cyclosporine blocks NFAT activation and the transcription of IL-2 and other cytokine genes. The net result is that cyclosporine blocks the IL-2–dependent growth and differentiation of T cells.

The introduction of cyclosporine into clinical practice ushered in the modern era of transplantation. Before the use of cyclosporine, the majority of transplanted hearts and livers were rejected. Now the majority of these allografts survive for more than 5 years (Fig. 16–8). Nevertheless, cyclosporine is not a panacea for transplantation. Drug levels needed for optimal immunosuppression cause kidney damage, and some

Table 16–1. Methods of Immunosuppression in Clinical Use

Drug	Mechanism of action
Cyclosporine and FK-506	Block T cell cytokine production by inhibiting activation of the NFAT transcription factor
Azathioprine	Blocks proliferation of lymphocyte precursors
Mycophenolate mofetil	Blocks lymphocyte proliferation by inhibiting guanine nucleotide synthesis in lymphocytes
Rapamycin	Blocks lymphocyte proliferation by inhibiting IL-2 signaling
Corticosteroids	Reduce inflammation by inhibiting macrophage cytokine secretion
Anti-CD3 monoclonal antibody	Depletes T cells by binding to CD3 and promoting phagocytosis or complement-mediated lysis (used to treat acute rejection)
Anti–IL-2 receptor antibody	Inhibits T cell proliferation by blocking IL-2 binding
CTLA4-Ig	Inhibits T cell activation by blocking B7 costimulator binding to T cell CD28; used to induce tolerance (experimental)
Anti–CD40 ligand	Inhibits macrophage and endothelial activation by blocking T cell CD40 ligand binding to macrophage CD40 (experimental)

rejection episodes are refractory to cyclosporine treatment. Another immunosuppressive fungal metabolite in clinical use is called FK-506, and it functions like cyclosporine. FK-506 and its binding protein (called FKBP) share with the cyclosporine-cyclophilin complex the ability to bind calcineurin and inhibit its activity. FK-506 has been used most frequently in liver transplant recipients and in cases of kidney allograft rejection that are not adequately controlled by cyclosporine.

An immunosuppressive agent with a different mechanism of action is the antibiotic rapamycin, whose principal effect is to inhibit T cell proliferation. Like FK-506, rapamycin also binds to FKBP, but the rapamycin-FKBP complex does not inhibit calcineurin. Instead, this complex binds to another cellular protein called the mammalian target of rapamycin (MTOR). The mechanism by which rapamycin inhibits T cell growth is not known. Rapamycin-treated T cells display abnormalities in the levels of certain cyclin/cyclin-dependent kinase complexes, suggesting that MTOR may be a regulator of a protein kinase that participates in cell cycle control. Combinations of cyclosporine (which blocks IL-2 synthesis) and rapamycin (which blocks IL-2–driven proliferation) are potent inhibitors of T cell responses.

Metabolic toxins that kill proliferating T cells are also used to treat graft rejection. These agents inhibit the maturation of lymphocytes from immature precursors and also kill proliferating mature T cells that have been stimulated by alloantigens. The first such drug to be developed for prevention and treatment of rejection was azathioprine. This drug is still used, but it is toxic to precursors of leukocytes in the bone marrow and enterocytes in the gut. The newest and most widely used drug in this class is mycophenolate mofetil (MMF). MMF is metabolized to mycophenolic acid, which blocks a lymphocyte-specific isoform of inosine monophosphate dehydroxygenase, an enzyme required for *de novo* synthesis of guanine nucleotides. Because MMF selectively inhibits the lymphocyte-specific isoform of this enzyme, it has relatively few toxic effects. MMF is now routinely used in combination with cyclosporine to prevent acute allograft rejection.

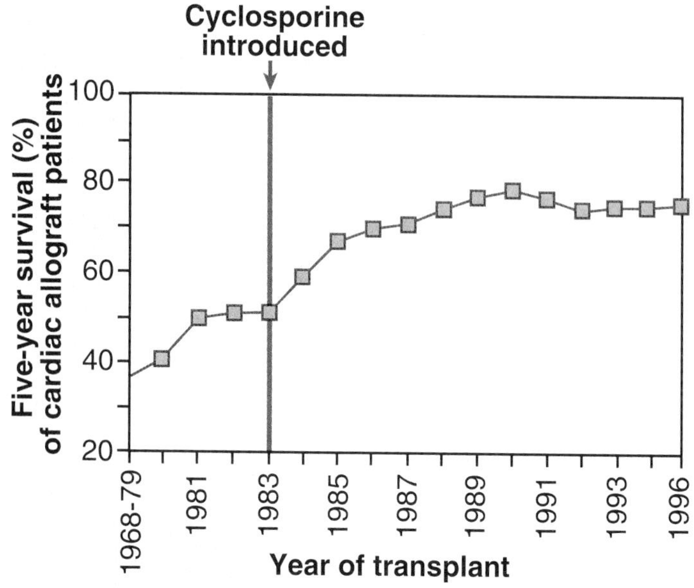

Figure 16–8 Influence of cyclosporine on graft survival.
Five-year survival rates for patients receiving cardiac allografts are seen to have increased significantly beginning when cyclosporine was introduced in 1983. (Data from Transplant Patient DataSource, United Network for Organ Sharing, Richmond, Va. Retrieved February 16, 2000, from the World Wide Web: http://207.239.150.13/tpd/.)

Antibodies that react with T cell surface structures and deplete or inhibit T cells are used to treat acute rejection episodes. The most widely used antibody is a mouse monoclonal antibody called OKT3 that is specific for human CD3. It may seem surprising that one would use a potential polyclonal activator such as anti-CD3 antibody to reduce T cell reactivity. *In vivo,* however, OKT3 either acts as a lytic antibody by activating the complement system to eliminate T cells or opsonizes T cells for phagocytosis. T cells that escape probably do so by capping and endocytosing ("modulating") CD3 off their surface, but such cells may be rendered transiently nonfunctional. Another antibody now in clinical use is specific for CD25, the α-subunit of the IL-2 receptor. This reagent, which is administered at the time of transplantation, may prevent T cell activation by blocking IL-2 binding to activated T cells, or it may deplete CD25-expressing activated T cells by mechanisms similar to those described for OKT3. The major limitation on the use of mouse monoclonal antibodies is that humans given these agents produce anti-mouse immunoglobulin (Ig) antibodies that eliminate the injected mouse Ig. For this reason, human-mouse chimeric ("humanized") antibodies to CD3 and CD25 that may be less immunogenic have been developed.

Acute rejection mediated by antibodies can be treated with drugs that inhibit antibody production. Several new immunosuppressive agents, including rapamycin and brequinar, inhibit antibody synthesis and are therefore potentially useful in preventing acute vascular rejection.

Anti-inflammatory agents are also routinely used for the prevention and treatment of graft rejection. The most potent anti-inflammatory agents available are corticosteroids. The proposed mechanism of action for these natural hormones and their synthetic analogues is to block the synthesis and secretion of cytokines, including tumor necrosis factor (TNF) and IL-1, by macrophages. Lack of TNF and IL-1 synthesis reduces graft endothelial cell activation and recruitment of inflammatory leukocytes (see Chapters 12 and 13). Corticosteroids may also block other effector mechanisms of macrophages, such as the generation of prostaglandins, reactive oxygen intermediates, and nitric oxide. Very high doses of corticosteroids may inhibit T cell secretion of cytokines or even kill T cells, but it is unlikely that the levels of corticosteroids achieved *in vivo* act in this way. Newer anti-inflammatory agents are in clinical trials, including soluble cytokine receptors, anticytokine antibodies, and antibodies that block leukocyte-endothelial adhesion (e.g., anti–intercellular adhesion molecule-1 [anti–ICAM-1]).

Current immunosuppressive protocols have dramatically improved graft survival. Before the use of cyclosporine, the 1-year survival rate of unrelated cadaveric kidney grafts was between 50% and 60%, with a 90% rate for grafts from living related donors (which are better matched with the recipients). Since cyclosporine and MMF have been introduced, the survival rate of unrelated cadaveric kidney grafts has approached about 90% at 1 year. The use of rapamycin promises to improve early survival of grafts even more. Heart transplantation, for which HLA matching (discussed later) is not practical, has significantly improved with the use of cyclosporine and now has a similar 90% 1-year survival rate. Experience with other organs is more limited, but survival rates for liver and lung transplants have also benefited from modern immunosuppressive therapy.

Acute rejection, when it occurs, is managed by rapidly intensifying immunosuppressive therapy. In modern transplantation, chronic rejection has become a more common cause of allograft failure, especially in cardiac transplantation. Chronic rejection is more insidious than acute rejection, and it is much less reversible by immunosuppression. It is likely that prevention rather than treatment will be the best approach to this problem, but successful intervention will require a better understanding of its pathogenesis.

Sustained immunosuppression required for prolonged graft survival leads to increased susceptibility to viral infections and virus-associated malignant tumors. The major thrust of transplant-related immunosuppression is to reduce the generation and function of helper T cells and CTLs, which mediate acute cellular rejection. It is therefore not surprising that defense against viruses, the physiologic function of CTLs, is also undermined in immunosuppressed transplant recipients. Reactivation of latent cytomegalovirus, a herpesvirus, is particularly common in immunosuppressed patients. For this reason, transplant recipients are now given prophylactic antiviral therapy for cytomegalovirus infections. Two malignant tumors commonly seen in allograft patients are B cell lymphomas and squamous cell carcinoma of the skin. The B cell lymphomas are thought to be sequelae of unchecked infection by Epstein-Barr virus, another herpesvirus (see Chapter 17, Box 17–2). The squamous cell carcinomas of the skin are associated with human papillomavirus.

Methods to Reduce the Immunogenicity of Allografts

In human transplantation, the major strategy to reduce graft immunogenicity has been to minimize alloantigenic differences between the donor and recipient by donor selection. To avoid hyperacute rejection, the ABO blood group antigens of the graft donor are selected to be identical to those of the recipient. Patients in need of allografts are also tested for the presence of preformed antibodies against donor cells. This type of testing is called crossmatching and involves mixing recipient serum with leukocytes from potential donors. Complement is added to promote classical pathway–mediated lysis of donor cells. If preformed antibodies, usually against donor MHC molecules, are present in the recipient's serum, the donor cells are lysed (a positive crossmatch), and such lysis indicates that the donor is not suitable for that recipient. For kidney transplantation from living related donors, attempts are made to minimize both class I and class II MHC allelic differences between the donor and recipient. All potential kidney donors and recipients are

BOX 16–3

Testing for Donor-Recipient Compatibility in Transplantation

Several clinical laboratory tests are routinely performed to reduce the risk of immunologic rejection in transplantation. These include ABO blood typing; the determination of HLA alleles expressed on donor and recipient cells, called tissue typing; the detection of preformed antibodies in the recipient that recognize HLA and other antigens representative of the donor population; and the detection of preformed antibodies in the recipient that bind to antigens of an identified donor's leukocytes, called crossmatching. Not all of these tests are done in all types of transplantation.

ABO BLOOD TYPING This test is uniformly used in all transplantation because no type of graft will survive if there are ABO incompatibilities between the donor and recipient. Natural IgM antibodies specific for allogeneic ABO blood group antigens (see Box 16–2) will cause hyperacute rejection. Blood typing is performed by mixing a patient's red blood cells with standardized sera containing anti-A or anti-B antibodies. If the patient expresses either blood group antigen, the serum specific for that antigen will agglutinate the red cells.

TISSUE TYPING: HLA MATCHING For living related kidney transplantation, attempts are made to reduce the number of differences in HLA alleles expressed on donor and recipient cells, which will have a modest effect in reducing the chance of rejection. In bone marrow transplantation, HLA matching is essential to reduce the risk of GVHD. Routine HLA typing focuses only on HLA-A, HLA-B, and HLA-DR because these are the only loci that appear to predict the likelihood of rejection or GVHD. Until recently, most HLA haplotype determinations were performed by serologic testing. This procedure relies on standardized collections of sera from multiple donors previously sensitized to different HLA molecules by pregnancy or transfusions. Each of these sera is mixed with a person's lymphocytes in separate wells of a tissue culture plate. A source of complement is added to the wells, as is a fluorescent dye that will enter only dead cells. After an incubation time, the wells are examined under a fluorescent microscope for the presence of dead cells. B lymphocytes are used as target cells because they normally express both class I and class II MHC molecules. On the basis of which antisera cause lysis, the HLA haplotype of the individual can be determined. Since the typing sera may not be absolutely specific for a single allelic product, serologic typing cannot always resolve exactly which alleles are present.

The polymerase chain reaction (PCR) has recently been used to permit more complete typing of the class II loci, replacing serologic methods. The polymorphic residues of class II MHC molecules are largely encoded within exon 2 of both the α and β chains (i.e., within the α1 and β1 polypeptide regions). This entire region of the gene can be amplified by PCR methods with use of primers that bind to conserved sequences within the 5′ and 3′ ends of these exons. The amplified segment of DNA can then readily be sequenced. Thus, the actual nucleotide sequence, and therefore the predicted amino acid sequence, can be directly determined for the HLA-DR, -DQ, and -DP alleles of any cell, providing precise molecular tissue typing.

SCREENING FOR THE PRESENCE OF PREFORMED ANTIBODIES Patients waiting for organ transplants are screened for the presence of preformed antibodies reactive with allogeneic HLA molecules. These antibodies, which may be produced as a result of previous pregnancies, transfusions, or transplantation, can identify risk of hyperacute or acute vascular rejection. Small amounts of the patient's serum are mixed, in separate wells, with cells from a panel of 40–60 different donors representative of the organ donor population. Binding of the patient's antibodies to cells of each donor of the panel is determined by complement-mediated lysis, as described before, or by flow cytometry with use of fluorescent-labeled secondary antibodies to human IgG. The results are reported as PRA (percent reactive antibody), which is the percentage of the donor cell pool with which the patient's serum reacts. The PRA is determined on multiple occasions while a patient waits for an organ allograft. This is because the PRA can vary, since each panel is chosen at random, and the patient's serum antibody titers may change over time.

CROSSMATCHING If a potential donor is identified, the crossmatching test will determine whether the patient has antibodies that react specifically with the donor cells. The test is performed in a way similar to the antibody screening assays, but in this case, the recipient's serum is tested for reactivity against only the particular donor's cells (typically lymphocytes). Cytotoxic and flow cytometric assays can be used.

"tissue-typed" to determine the identity of the HLA molecules that are expressed (Box 16–3).

In kidney transplantation, the larger the number of MHC alleles that are matched between the donor and recipient, the better the graft survival, especially in the first year after transplantation (Fig. 16–9). MHC matching had a more profound influence on graft survival before modern immunosuppressive drugs were routinely used. Clinical experience has shown that of all the class I and class II loci, matching only HLA-A, HLA-B, and HLA-DR is important for predicting outcome. (HLA-C is not as polymorphic as HLA-A or HLA-B, and HLA-DR and HLA-DQ are in strong linkage disequilibrium, so matching at the DR locus often also matches at the DQ locus. DP typing is not in common use, and its importance is unknown.) Because two codominantly expressed alleles are inherited for each of these MHC genes, it is possible to have zero to six MHC antigen mismatches between the donor and recipient. Zero-antigen mismatches predict the best living donor graft survival, and one-antigen–matched grafts do slightly worse. The survival of grafts with two to six MHC mismatches all are significantly worse than zero- or one-antigen mismatches.

HLA matching in renal transplantation is possible because donor kidneys can be stored in organ banks

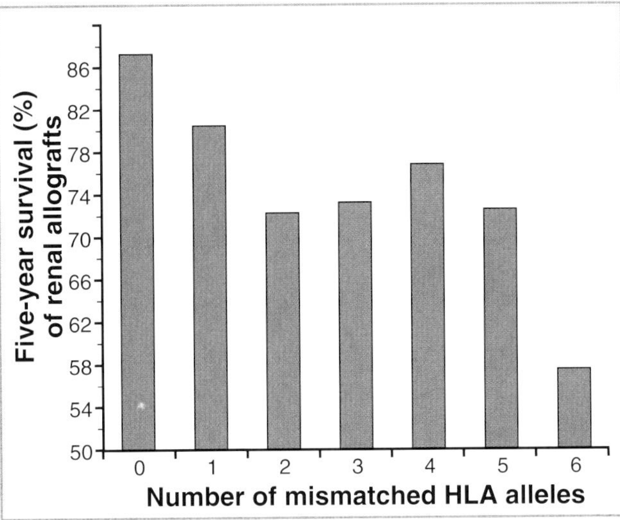

Figure 16–9 Influence of MHC matching on graft survival. Matching of MHC alleles between the donor and recipient significantly improved living donor renal allograft survival. HLA matching has more of an impact on survival of renal allografts from cadaver donors than from living donors, and some MHC alleles are more important than others in determining outcome. (Data from Organ Procurement and Transplantation Network/Scientific Registry annual report, 1999.)

before transplantation until a well-matched recipient can be identified and because patients needing a kidney allograft can be maintained with dialysis until a well-matched organ is available. In the case of heart and liver transplantation, organ preservation is more difficult, and potential recipients are often in critical condition. For these reasons, HLA typing is simply not considered in pairing of potential donors and recipients, and the choice of donor and recipient is based only on ABO blood group matching and anatomic compatibility.

Methods to Induce Donor-Specific Tolerance or Suppression

Allograft rejection may be prevented by making the host tolerant to the alloantigens of the graft. Tolerance in this setting means that the host does not injure the graft despite the absence or withdrawal of immunosuppressive and anti-inflammatory agents. It is presumed that tolerance to an allograft will involve the same mechanisms that are involved in tolerance to self antigens (see Chapter 10), namely, central deletion of alloreactive T cells, peripheral anergy or deletion of alloreactive T cells, and active suppression of alloreactive T cells. Tolerance is desirable in transplantation because it is alloantigen specific and will therefore avoid the major problem associated with nonspecific immunosuppression, namely, increased susceptibility to infection and to virus-induced tumors. In addition, achieving graft tolerance may reduce chronic rejection, which has to date been unaffected by the commonly used immunosuppressive agents that prevent and reverse acute rejection episodes.

Several experimental approaches and clinical observations have suggested that it should be possible to achieve tolerance to allografts.

- In experiments with skin grafts in mice, Medawar and colleagues showed that if neonatal mice of one strain (the recipient) are given spleen cells of another strain (the donor), the recipients will subsequently accept grafts from the donor. Such tolerance is alloantigen specific because the recipients will reject grafts from mouse strains that express MHC alleles that differ from the donor's (see Chapter 10, Fig. 10–2).
- Renal transplant patients who have received blood transfusions containing allogeneic leukocytes have a lower incidence of acute rejection episodes than do those who have not been transfused. The postulated explanation for this effect is that the introduction of allogeneic leukocytes by transfusion produces tolerance to alloantigens. Indeed, pretreatment of potential recipients with blood transfusions is now widely used as prophylactic therapy to reduce rejection.
- Animals given bone marrow transplants who subsequently contain both donor and recipient cells in the circulation (called mixed chimerism) are tolerant to organ allografts derived from the same donor as the bone marrow graft. Human allogeneic bone marrow transplantation to establish mixed chimerism has been tried in a small number of patients before solid organ transplantation, but this approach may be limited by the problem of graft-versus-host disease, which is discussed later in this chapter. More benign methods to establish mixed chimerism in humans are under investigation.
- Experimentally, graft rejection is reduced or delayed by blocking costimulatory signals, such as with a soluble form of CTLA-4 that prevents the B7 molecules on APCs from interacting with T cell CD28 or with an antibody that binds to T cell CD40 ligand and prevents its interactions with CD40 on APCs (see Chapters 6 and 8). In some experimental protocols, simultaneous blockade of both B7 and CD40 appears to be more effective than either alone in promoting graft survival. Antibody to CD40 ligand also delays the rejection of kidney and pancreatic islet allografts in primates. It is not established whether these treatments inhibit the activation of alloreactive T cells or actually induce long-lived tolerance in these cells. Clinical trials of costimulator blockade in transplantation are ongoing, but the initial results are not encouraging.
- The potentially important role of indirect presentation of allogeneic MHC antigens in graft rejection raises the possibility of another approach for inducing tolerance, namely, the use of peptides derived from donor MHC molecules as tolerogens. In this approach, immunodominant peptides derived from donor MHC molecules would be administered to future recipients of a graft in a manner that would favor tolerance induction, such as high-dose intravenous injection (see Chapter 10).

Although the best approaches for inducing tolerance need to be established in clinical trials, it is hoped that tolerance induction will become a standard part of transplantation therapy in the near future.

Xenogeneic Transplantation

The use of solid organ transplantation as a clinical therapy is greatly limited by the lack of availability of donor organs. For this reason, the possibility of transplantation of organs from other mammals, such as pigs, into human recipients has kindled great interest.

A major immunologic barrier to xenogeneic transplantation is the presence of natural antibodies that cause hyperacute rejection. More than 95% of primates have natural IgM antibodies that are reactive with the carbohydrate determinants expressed by the cells of members of species that are evolutionarily distant, such as the pig. The vast majority of human anti-pig natural antibodies are directed at one particular carbohydrate determinant formed by the action of a pig α-galactosyltransferase enzyme. This enzyme places an α-linked galactose moiety on the same substrate that in human and other primate cells is fucosylated to form the blood group H antigen (see Box 16–2). Species combinations that give rise to natural antibodies against each other are said to be discordant. Natural antibodies are rarely produced against carbohydrate determinants of closely related, concordant species, such as human and chimpanzee. Thus, chimpanzees or other higher primates technically can and have been used as organ donors to humans. However, both ethical and logistic concerns have limited such procedures. For reasons of anatomic compatibility, pigs are the preferred xenogeneic species for organ donation to humans.

Natural antibodies against xenografts induce hyperacute rejection by the same mechanisms as those seen in hyperacute allograft rejection. These mechanisms include the generation of endothelial cell procoagulants and platelet aggregating substances, coupled with the loss of endothelial anticoagulant mechanisms. However, the consequences of activating human complement on pig cells are typically more severe than the consequences of activation of complement by natural antibodies on human allogeneic cells, possibly because some of the complement regulatory proteins made by pig cells, such as decay accelerating factor, are not able to interact with human complement proteins and thus cannot limit the extent of complement-induced injury (see Chapter 14). A strategy under exploration for reducing hyperacute rejection in xenotransplantation is to construct and breed transgenic pigs expressing human proteins that inhibit complement activation or fail to express enzymes that synthesize pig antigens. Such pigs could, for example, overexpress human H group fucosyltransferase and overexpress human complement regulatory proteins such as decay accelerating factor.

Even when hyperacute rejection is prevented, xenografts are often damaged by a form of acute vascular rejection that occurs within 2 to 3 days of transplantation. This form of rejection has been called delayed xenograft rejection, accelerated acute rejection, or acute vascular rejection and is characterized by intravascular thrombosis and fibrinoid necrosis of vessel walls. The mechanisms of delayed xenograft rejection are incompletely understood, but it is likely to be caused by natural antibodies to various endothelial antigens and by T cell activation and cytokine-mediated endothelial damage.

Xenografts can also be rejected by T cell–mediated immune responses to xenoantigens. The mechanisms of cell-mediated rejection of xenografts are believed to be similar to those that we have described for allograft rejection, and T cell responses to xenoantigens can be as strong as or even stronger than responses to alloantigens. Human T cell recognition of pig MHC molecules may involve both direct and indirect pathways. Furthermore, several intercellular molecular interactions required for T cell responses, such as CD4/class II MHC, CD8/class I MHC, CD2/LFA-3, CD28/B7, CD40L/CD40, and VLA-4/vascular cell adhesion molecule-1 (VCAM-1), are functional even when one member of these pairs is from a pig and the other from a human.

Cell-mediated responses to xenografts may be too strong to be adequately controlled by the immunosuppressive protocols used for allograft rejection, and research is therefore focused on inducing specific tolerance to xenografts. The methods of tolerance induction that are being considered include those we have discussed for allografts, such as blocking costimulation when the recipient is first exposed to the donor tissue, administration of peptides from xenogeneic MHC molecules, and establishment of xenogeneic mixed lymphohematopoietic chimerism.

Blood Transfusion

Blood transfusion is a form of transplantation in which whole blood or blood cells from one or more individuals are transferred intravenously into the circulation of a host. Blood transfusions are performed to replace blood lost by hemorrhage or to correct defects caused by inadequate production of blood cells, which may occur in a variety of diseases. The major barrier to successful blood transfusions is the immune response to cell surface molecules that differ between individuals. The most important alloantigen system in blood transfusion is the ABO system (see Box 16–2). ABO antigens are expressed on all cells, including red blood cells. Individuals lacking a particular blood group antigen may produce natural IgM antibodies against that antigen, probably as a result of responses to cross-reactive antigens expressed on bacteria that colonize the gut. If such individuals are given blood cells expressing the missing antigen, the preexisting antibodies bind to the transfused cells, activate complement, and lyse the transfused cells. Lysis of the foreign red blood cells results in **transfusion reactions**, which can be life-threatening. Transfusion across an ABO barrier may trigger an immediate hemolytic reaction, resulting in both intravascular lysis of red blood cells, probably mediated by the complement system, and extensive phagocytosis of antibody- and complement-coated erythrocytes by macrophages of the liver and spleen. Hemoglobin is liberated from the lysed red cells in quantities that may be toxic for kidney cells, producing acute renal tubular cell necrosis and kidney failure. High fevers, shock, and disseminated intravascular coagulation may also develop, suggestive of massive cytokine release (e.g., of TNF or IL-1; see Chapter 12, Box 12–2). The disseminated intravascular coagulation consumes clotting factors faster than they can be synthesized, and the patient may paradoxically die of bleeding in the presence of widespread clotting. More delayed hemolytic reactions may result from incompatibilities of minor blood group antigens. These result in progressive loss of the transfused red cells, leading to anemia, and jaundice, a consequence of overloading the liver with hemoglobin-derived pigments.

The choice of blood donors for a particular recipient is based on our understanding of blood group antigens. Virtually all individuals express the H antigen, and therefore they are tolerant to this antigen and do not produce anti-H antibodies. Individuals who express A or B antigens are tolerant to these molecules and do not produce anti-A or anti-B antibodies, respectively. However, OO and AO individuals (see Box 16–2) produce anti-B IgM antibodies, whereas OO and BO individuals produce anti-A IgM antibodies. If a patient receives a transfusion of red blood cells from a donor who expresses a form of the antigen not expressed on self red blood cells, a transfusion reaction may result (described above). It follows that AB individuals can tolerate transfusions from all potential donors and are therefore called universal recipients; similarly, OO individuals can tolerate transfusions only from OO donors but can provide blood to all recipients and are therefore called universal donors. In general, differences in minor blood groups lead to red cell lysis only after repeated transfusions produce a secondary antibody response.

ABO antigens are expressed on many other cell types in addition to blood cells, including endothelial cells. For this reason, ABO typing is critical to avoid hyperacute rejection of solid organ allografts, as discussed earlier in the chapter.

Rh antigen is another important red blood cell antigen that may be responsible for transfusion reactions (see Box 16–2). Although there are no natural antibodies to Rh antigens, individuals who do not express Rhesus D (Rh) antigen (approximately 15% of the population) can be sensitized to this antigen and produce anti-Rh antibodies if they receive blood transfusions from an RhD-expressing donor. Transfusion reactions can arise after a second transfusion of Rh-positive blood. In addition, Rh-negative mothers carrying an Rh-positive fetus can be sensitized by fetal red blood cells that enter the maternal circulation, usually during childbirth. Subsequent pregnancies in which the fetus is Rh positive are at risk because the maternal anti-Rh antibodies can cross the placenta and mediate the destruction of the fetal red blood cells. This causes **erythroblastosis fetalis** (hemolytic disease of the newborn) and can be lethal for the fetus. This disease can be prevented by administration of anti-RhD antibodies to the mother within 72 hours of birth of the first Rh-positive baby. The treatment kills the baby's Rh-positive red blood cells that entered the mother's circulation and prevents sensitization and production of anti-Rh antibodies in the mother.

Bone Marrow Transplantation

Bone marrow transplantation is the transplantation of pluripotent hematopoietic stem cells, most commonly in an inoculum of bone marrow cells collected by aspiration. Hematopoietic stem cells can also be purified from the blood of donors, especially after treatment with colony-stimulating factors, which mobilize stem cells from the bone marrow. After transplantation, stem cells repopulate the recipient's bone marrow with their differentiating progeny. We consider bone marrow transplantation separately in this chapter because several unique features of this type of grafting are not encountered with solid organ transplantation.

Bone marrow transplantation may be used clinically to remedy acquired defects in the hematopoietic system or in the immune system because blood cells and lymphocytes develop from a common stem cell. It has also been proposed as a means of correcting inherited deficiencies or abnormalities of enzymes or other proteins (e.g., abnormal hemoglobin) by providing a self-renewing source of normal stem cells. In addition, allogeneic bone marrow transplantation may be used as part of the treatment of bone marrow malignant disease (i.e., leukemias) and disseminated solid tumors. In this case, the chemotherapeutic agents needed to destroy cancer cells also destroy normal marrow elements, and bone marrow transplantation is used to "rescue" the patient from the side effects of chemotherapy. In addition, in some forms of leukemia, the grafted cells can be effective in destroying residual leukemia cells by a process analogous to the graft-versus-host responses discussed later. For other malignant tumors, when the marrow is not involved by tumor or when it can be purged of tumor cells, the patient's own bone marrow may be harvested and reinfused after chemotherapy. This procedure, called autologous bone marrow transplantation, does not elicit the immune responses associated with allogeneic bone marrow transplantation and will not be discussed further.

Before bone marrow is transplanted, recipients must often be "prepared" with radiation and chemotherapy to deplete their own marrow cells and vacate these sites to allow the transplanted stem cells to "home" to the marrow and establish themselves in the appropriate environment. Allogeneic stem cells are readily rejected by even a minimally immunocompetent host, and therefore the donor and recipient must be carefully matched at all polymorphic MHC loci. In addition, it is often necessary to greatly suppress the recipient's immune system to permit successful bone marrow transplantation. Such suppression is accomplished by radiation and chemotherapy. The mechanisms of rejection of bone marrow cells are not completely known, but in addition to adaptive immune mechanisms, hematopoietic stem cells may also be rejected by NK cells. The role of NK cells in bone marrow rejection has been studied in experimental animals.

- Irradiated F_1 hybrid mice reject bone marrow donated by either inbred parent. This phenomenon, called hybrid resistance, is in distinction to the classical laws of solid tissue transplantation (see Fig. 16–2). Hybrid resistance is seen in T cell–deficient mice, and depletion of recipient NK cells with anti–NK cell antibodies prevents the rejection of parental bone marrow. Hybrid resistance is probably due to host NK cells reacting against bone marrow precursors that lack class I MHC molecules expressed by the host.

Even after successful engraftment, two additional problems are frequently associated with bone marrow transplantation, namely, graft-versus-host disease and immunodeficiency. These complications are discussed in the following.

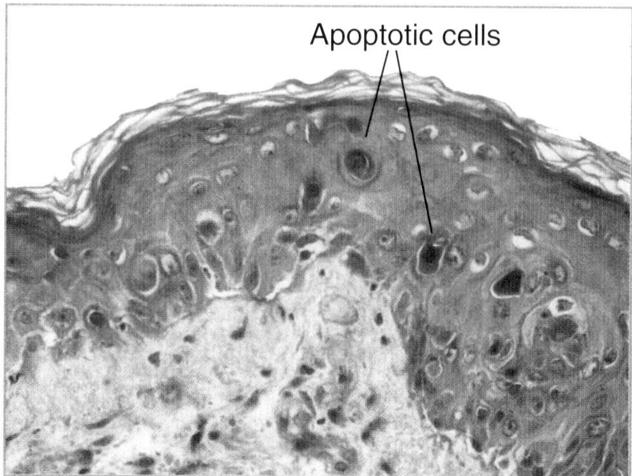

Figure 16–10 Histopathology of acute graft-versus-host disease in the skin.

A sparse lymphocytic infiltrate can be seen at the dermal-epidermal junction, and damage to the epithelial layer is evident as vacuolization at the dermal-epidermal junction, cells with abnormal keratin staining (dyskeratosis), and disorganization of maturation of keratinocytes from the basal layer to the surface. (Courtesy of Dr. Scott Grantor, Department of Pathology, Brigham and Women's Hospital and Harvard Medical School, Boston.)

Graft-Versus-Host Disease

Graft-versus-host disease (GVHD) is caused by the reaction of grafted mature T cells in the marrow inoculum with alloantigens of the host. It occurs when the host is immunocompromised and therefore unable to reject the allogeneic cells in the graft. In most cases, the reaction is directed against minor histocompatibility antigens of the host because bone marrow transplantation is not commonly performed when the donor and recipient have differences in MHC molecules. GVHD may also develop when solid organs that contain significant numbers of T cells are transplanted, such as the small bowel, lung, or liver.

GVHD is the principal limitation to the success of bone marrow transplantation. As in solid organ transplantation, GVHD may be classified on the basis of histologic patterns into acute and chronic forms.

Acute GVHD is characterized by epithelial cell death in the skin, liver (biliary epithelium), and gastrointestinal tract (Fig. 16–10). Acute GVHD is manifested clinically by rash, jaundice, diarrhea, and gastrointestinal hemorrhage. When the epithelial cell death is extensive, the skin or lining of the gut may simply slough off. In this circumstance, acute GVHD may be fatal.

Chronic GVHD is characterized by fibrosis and atrophy of one or more of the same organs, without evidence of acute cell death. Chronic GVHD may also involve the lungs and produce obliteration of small airways. When it is severe, chronic GVHD leads to complete dysfunction of the affected organ and may be fatal.

In animal models, acute GVHD is initiated by mature T cells present in the bone marrow inoculum, and elimination of mature donor T cells from the graft can prevent the development of GVHD. Efforts to eliminate T cells from the marrow inoculum have reduced the incidence of GVHD but also appear to reduce the efficiency of engraftment, probably because mature T cells produce colony-stimulating factors that aid in stem cell repopulation. A current approach is to combine removal of T cells with supplemental granulocyte-macrophage colony-stimulating factor to promote engraftment. Elimination of T cells from the donor marrow also decreases the graft-versus-leukemia effect that is often critical in treating leukemias by bone marrow transplantation.

Although GVHD is initiated by grafted T cells recognizing host alloantigens, the effector cells that cause epithelial cell injury are less well defined. On histologic examination, NK cells are often attached to the dying epithelial cells, suggesting that NK cells are important effector cells of acute GVHD. $CD8^+$ CTLs and cytokines also appear to be involved in tissue injury in acute GVHD.

The relationship of chronic GVHD to acute GVHD is not known and raises issues similar to those of relating chronic allograft rejection to acute allograft rejection. For example, chronic GVHD may represent the fibrosis of wound healing secondary to loss of epithelial cells. However, chronic GVHD can arise without evidence of prior acute GVHD. An alternative explanation is that chronic GVHD represents a response to ischemia caused by vascular injury.

Both acute and chronic GVHD are commonly treated with intense immunosuppression. It is not clear that either condition responds very well. A possible explanation for this therapeutic failure is that conventional immunosuppression is targeted against T lymphocytes, especially CTLs, but is less efficacious for NK cell–mediated responses. Agents that suppress cytokine production, such as the drug thalidomide, or that antagonize cytokine action have been effective in treating GVHD in clinical trials. Much effort has focused on prevention of GVHD, and HLA typing is important in this regard. Indeed, most human bone marrow transplants are performed between siblings who are completely identical at all HLA loci, and clinical GVHD is due to differences at minor histocompatibility loci.

Cyclosporine and the metabolic toxin methotrexate are also used for prophylaxis against GVHD.

Immunodeficiency After Bone Marrow Transplantation

Bone marrow transplantation is often accompanied by clinical immunodeficiency. Several factors may contribute to defective immune responses in recipients. Bone marrow transplant recipients may be unable to regenerate a complete new lymphocyte repertoire. The transplanted bone marrow may not contain a sufficient number and variety of self-renewing lymphoid progenitors, and the thymus gland of the recipient may have involuted so that T cell maturation does not occur. Studies in mice suggest that irradiation may unmask a population of "natural suppressor" cells that inhibit immune responses.

The consequence of immunodeficiency is that bone marrow transplant recipients are susceptible to viral infections, especially cytomegalovirus infection, and to many bacterial infections. They are also susceptible to Epstein-Barr virus–provoked B cell lymphomas. The immunodeficiencies of bone marrow transplant recipients can be more severe than those of conventionally immunosuppressed patients. Therefore, bone marrow transplant recipients commonly receive prophylactic antibiotics and anticytomegalovirus therapy and are often actively immunized against capsular bacteria such as pneumococcus.

Summary

- Transplantation of tissues from one individual to a genetically nonidentical recipient leads to a specific immune response called rejection that can destroy the graft. The major molecular targets in transplant rejection are allogeneic class I and class II MHC molecules.
- Many different, normally present T cell clones specific for different foreign peptides plus self MHC molecules may cross-react with an individual allogeneic MHC molecule. This high frequency of T cells capable of directly recognizing allogeneic MHC molecules explains why the response to alloantigens is much stronger than the response to conventional foreign antigens.
- Allogeneic MHC molecules may be presented on donor APCs to recipient T cells (the direct pathway), or the alloantigens may be picked up by host APCs that enter the graft or reside in draining lymphoid organs and be processed and presented to T cells as peptides associated with self MHC molecules (the indirect pathway).
- Graft rejection is mediated by T cells, including CTLs that kill graft cells and helper T cells that cause DTH reactions, and by antibodies.
- Several effector mechanisms cause rejection of solid organ grafts, and each mechanism may lead to a histologically characteristic reaction. Preexisting antibodies cause hyperacute rejection characterized by thrombosis of graft vessels. Alloreactive T cells and antibodies produced in response to the graft cause blood vessel wall damage and parenchymal cell death, called acute rejection. Chronic rejection is characterized by fibrosis and vascular abnormalities (accelerated arteriosclerosis), which may represent a chronic DTH reaction in the walls of arteries.
- Rejection may be prevented or treated by immunosuppression of the host, by minimizing the immunogenicity of the graft (e.g., by limiting MHC allelic differences), or by induction of tolerance. Most immunosuppression is directed at T cell responses and entails the use of cytotoxic drugs, specific immunosuppressive agents, or anti–T cell antibodies. The most widely used immunosuppressive agent is cyclosporine, which blocks T cell cytokine synthesis. Immunosuppression is often combined with anti-inflammatory drugs such as corticosteroids that inhibit cytokine synthesis by macrophages.
- Patients receiving solid organ transplants may become immunodeficient because of their therapy and are susceptible to viral infections and virus-related malignant tumors.
- Xenogeneic transplantation of solid organs is limited by the presence of natural antibodies to carbohydrate antigens on the cells of discordant species that cause hyperacute rejection, antibody-mediated acute vascular rejection, and a strong T cell–mediated immune response to xenogeneic MHC molecules.
- Bone marrow transplants are susceptible to rejection, and recipients require intense preparatory immunosuppression. In addition, T lymphocytes in the bone marrow graft may respond to alloantigens of the host and produce GVHD. Acute GVHD is characterized by epithelial cell death in the skin, intestinal tract, and liver; it may be fatal. Chronic GVHD is characterized by fibrosis and atrophy of one or more of these same target organs as well as the lungs and may also be fatal. Bone marrow transplant recipients also often develop severe immunodeficiency, rendering them susceptible to infections.

Selected Readings

The April 2001 issue of *Immunity* (14:345–446, 2001) has a collection of review articles on immunological issues in transplantation; these are not included in this list.

Cascalho M, and JL Platt. Xenotransplantation and other means of organ replacement. Nature Reviews Immunology 1:154–160, 2001.

Erlebacher A. Why isn't the fetus rejected? Current Opinion in Immunology 13:590–593, 2001.

Gould DS, and H Auchincloss Jr. Direct and indirect recognition: the role of MHC antigens in graft rejection. Immunology Today 20:77–82, 1999.

Mellor AL, and DH Munn. Immunology at the maternal–fetal interface: lessons for T cell tolerance and suppression. Annual Review of Immunology 18:367–392, 2000.

Pascual M, T Theruvath, T Kawai, N Tolkoff-Rubin, and AB Cosimi. Strategies to improve long-term outcomes after renal transplantation. New England Journal of Medicine 346:580–590, 2002.

Salama AD, G Remuzzi, WE Harmon, and MH Sayegh. Challenges to achieving clinical transplantation tolerance. Journal of Clinical Investigation 108:943–948, 2001.

Wekerle T, and M Sykes. Mixed chimerism and transplantation tolerance. Annual Review of Medicine 52:353–370, 2001.

Yamada A, AD Salama, and MH Sayegh. The role of novel costimulatory pathways in autoimmunity and transplantation. Journal of the American Society of Nephrology 13: 559–575, 2002.

Chapter 17

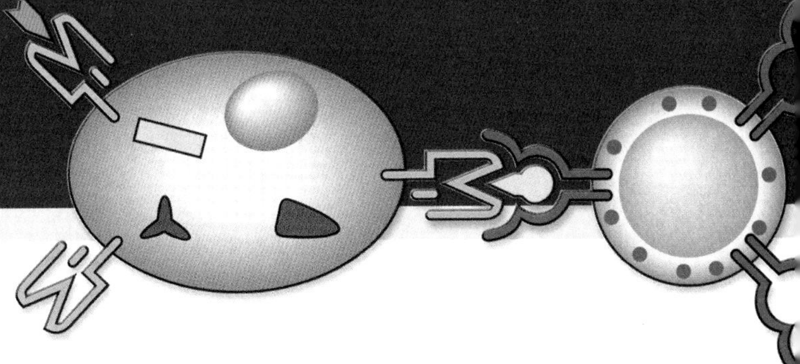

Immunity to Tumors

Cancer is a major health problem worldwide and one of the most important causes of morbidity and mortality in children and adults. Cancers arise from the uncontrolled proliferation and spread of clones of transformed cells. The growth of malignant tumors is determined in large part by the proliferative capacity of the tumor cells and by the ability of these cells to invade host tissues and metastasize to distant sites. The possibility that cancers can be eradicated by specific immune responses has been the impetus for a large body of work in the field of tumor immunology. The concept of **immune surveillance**, which was proposed by Macfarlane Burnet in the 1950s, states that a physiologic function of the immune system is to recognize and destroy clones of transformed cells before they grow into tumors and to kill tumors after they are formed. The importance and even the existence of immune surveillance have been questioned by the results of some experiments, and the role of immune surveillance may vary in different types of tumors. Nevertheless, it is now clear that the immune system does react against many tumors, and exploiting these reactions to specifically destroy tumors remains an important goal of tumor immunologists. In addition, one of the factors in the growth of malignant tumors is the ability of these cancers to evade or overcome the mechanisms of host defense. In this chapter, we describe the types of antigens that are expressed by malignant tumors, how the immune system recognizes and responds to these antigens, and the application of immunologic approaches to the treatment of cancer.

General Features of Tumor Immunity

Several characteristics of tumor antigens and immune responses to tumors are fundamental to understanding tumor immunity and developing strategies for cancer immunotherapy.

- ***Tumors express antigens that are recognized as foreign by the immune system of the tumor-bearing host.*** Clinical observations and animal experiments have established that although tumor cells are derived from host cells, the tumors elicit immune responses.

- Histopathologic studies show that many tumors are surrounded by mononuclear cell infiltrates composed of T lymphocytes, NK (natural killer) cells, and macrophages, and activated lymphocytes and macrophages are present in lymph nodes draining the sites of tumor growth. The presence of lymphocytic infiltrates in some types of melanoma and breast cancer is predictive of a better prognosis.
- The first experimental demonstration that tumors can induce protective immune responses came from studies of transplanted tumors performed in the 1950s (Fig. 17–1). A sarcoma may be induced in an inbred mouse by painting its skin with the chemical carcinogen methylcholanthrene (MCA). If the MCA-induced tumor is excised and transplanted into other syngeneic mice, the tumor grows. In contrast, if the tumor is transplanted back into the original host, the mouse rejects the tumor. The same mouse that had become immune to its tumor is incapable of rejecting MCA-induced tumors produced in other mice. Furthermore, T cells from the tumor-bearing animal can transfer protective immunity to the tumor to another tumor-free animal. Thus, immune responses to tumors exhibit the defining characteristics of adaptive immunity, namely, specificity and memory, and are mediated by lymphocytes.

The immunogenicity of tumors implies that tumor cells express antigens that are recognized as foreign by the adaptive immune system. As predicted from the transplantation experiments, defense against tumors is mediated mainly by T lymphocytes.

- ***Immune responses frequently fail to prevent the growth of tumors.*** There may be several reasons that anti-tumor immunity is unable to eradicate transformed cells. First, tumor cells are derived from host cells and therefore resemble normal cells in many respects. In other words, most tumors express only a few antigens that may be recognized as nonself, and as a result, most tumors tend to be weakly immunogenic. Tumors that elicit strong immune responses include those induced by oncogenic viruses, in which the viral proteins are foreign antigens, and

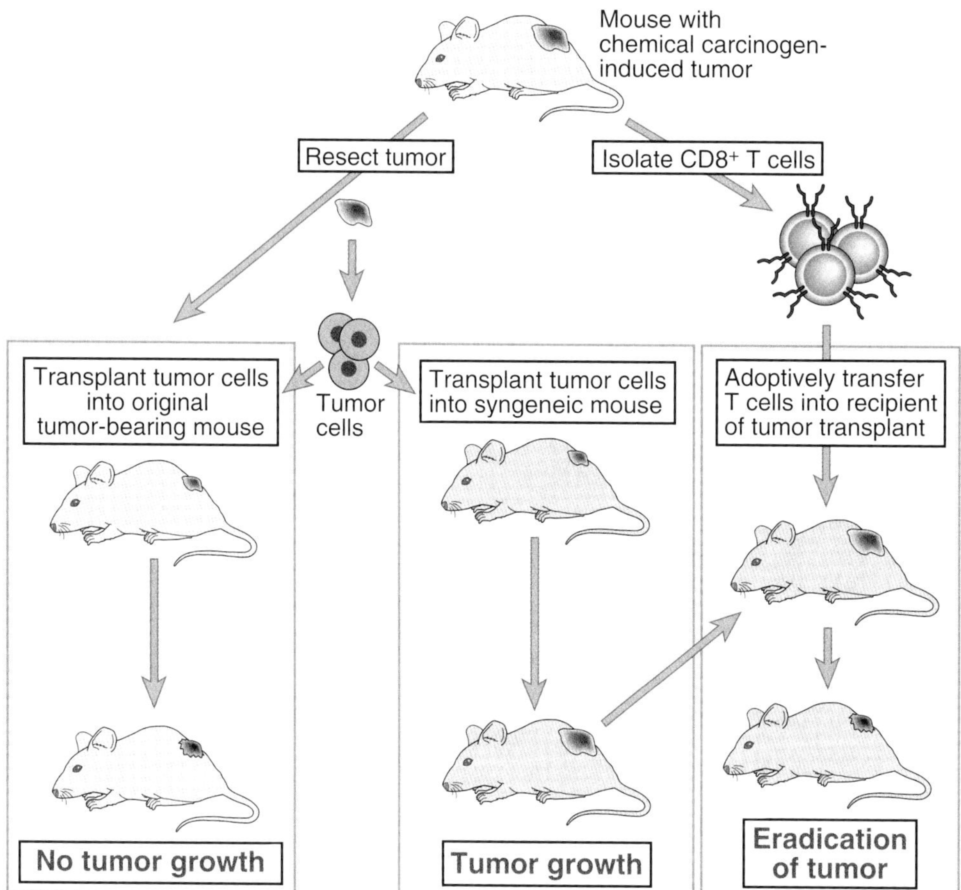

Figure 17–1 Experimental demonstration of tumor immunity.
Mice that have been surgically cured of a chemical carcinogen (methylcholanthrene)–induced tumor reject subsequent transplants of the same tumor, whereas the transplanted tumor grows in normal syngeneic mice. The tumor is also rejected in normal mice that are given adoptive transfer of T lymphocytes from the original tumor-bearing animal.

tumors induced in animals by potent carcinogens, which often cause mutations in normal cellular genes. Many spontaneous tumors induce weak or even undetectable immunity, and studies of such tumors led to considerable skepticism about the concept of immune surveillance. In fact, as we stated earlier, the importance of immune surveillance and tumor immunity is likely to vary with the type of tumor. Second, the rapid growth and spread of tumors may overwhelm the capacity of the immune system to eradicate tumor cells, and control of a tumor requires that all the malignant cells be eliminated. Third, many tumors have specialized mechanisms for evading host immune responses. We will return to these mechanisms later in the chapter.

- ***The immune system can be activated by external stimuli to effectively kill tumor cells and eradicate tumors.*** As we shall see at the end of the chapter, this realization has spurred new directions in tumor immunotherapy in which augmentation of the host anti-tumor response is the goal of treatment.

Tumor Antigens

A variety of tumor antigens that may be recognized by T and B lymphocytes have been identified in human and animal cancers. In the experimental situation, as in MCA-induced mouse sarcomas, it is often possible to demonstrate that these antigens elicit adaptive immune responses and are the targets of such responses. Tumor antigens have also been identified in humans, but the methods used in this case are generally not suitable for proving that these antigens can elicit protective immunity to tumors. Nevertheless, it is important to identify tumor antigens in humans because they may be used as components of tumor vaccines, and antibodies and effector T cells generated against these antigens may be used for immunotherapy.

The earliest classification of tumor antigens was based on their patterns of expression. Antigens that are expressed on tumor cells but not on normal cells were called tumor-specific antigens; some of these antigens are unique to individual tumors, whereas others are shared among tumors of the same type. Tumor antigens that are also expressed on normal cells were called tumor-associated antigens; in most cases, these antigens are normal cellular constituents whose expression is aberrant or dysregulated in tumors. The modern classification of tumor antigens relies on the molecular structure and source of the antigens, which is how we will discuss tumor antigens.

The existence of tumor antigens was first established by transplantation experiments in animals, as described earlier. The initial attempts to purify and characterize these antigens were based on producing monoclonal antibodies specific for tumor cells and defining the antigens that these antibodies recognized. The antibodies were made by immunizing mice with tumors from other species, and most of the anti-tumor antibodies recognized antigens that are shared by different tumors arising from the same types of cells and that are also found on some normal cells and benign tumor cells. Anti-tumor antibodies also do not recognize the major histocompatibility complex (MHC)–associated peptides that are the targets of T cells. Tumor antigens that are recognized by T cells are likely to be the major inducers of tumor immunity and the most promising candidates for tumor vaccines. An important breakthrough in tumor immunology was the development of techniques for identifying antigens that are recognized by tumor-specific T lymphocytes (Box 17–1). Much of our knowledge of these antigens is limited to antigens recognized by $CD8^+$ cytolytic T lymphocytes (CTLs), and only recently have attempts been made to identify antigens that are recognized by $CD4^+$ helper cells. Tumor antigens that are recognized by $CD8^+$ T cells are peptides derived from proteins processed in the cytosol and displayed on the tumor cell surface bound to class I MHC molecules (see Chapter 5). In the following section, we describe the main classes of tumor antigens (Fig. 17–2 and Table 17–1) and use selected examples of human and animal tumors to illustrate the importance of these antigens in tumor immunity and their potential as therapeutic targets.

Products of Mutated Oncogenes and Tumor Suppressor Genes

Some tumor antigens are produced by oncogenic mutants of normal cellular genes. Many tumors express genes whose products are required for malignant transformation or for maintenance of the malignant phenotype. Often, these genes are produced by point mutations, deletions, chromosomal translocations, or viral gene insertions involving cellular proto-oncogenes or tumor suppressor genes. The products of these altered proto-oncogenes and tumor suppressor genes are synthesized in the cytoplasm of the tumor cells, and like any cytosolic protein, they may enter the class I antigen-processing pathway. In addition, these proteins may enter the class II antigen-processing pathway in antigen-presenting cells (APCs) that have phagocytosed dead tumor cells. Because these altered genes are not present in normal cells, they do not induce self-tolerance, and peptides derived from them may stimulate T cell responses in the host. Some patients with cancer have circulating $CD4^+$ and $CD8^+$ T cells that can respond to the products of mutated oncogenes such as Ras, p53, and Bcr-Abl proteins. Furthermore, in animals, immunization with mutated Ras or p53 proteins induces CTLs and rejection responses against tumors expressing these mutants. However, these proteins do not appear to be major targets of tumor-specific CTLs in most patients with a variety of tumors.

Products of Other Mutated Genes

Tumor antigens may be produced by mutated genes whose products are not related to the transformed phenotype and have no known function. Tumor antigens that were defined by the transplantation of carcinogen-induced tumors in animals, called

BOX 17–1

Identification of Tumor Antigens Recognized by T Lymphocytes

Tumor antigens recognized by T cells have been identified by two main approaches—transplantation of tumors in rodents and the identification of peptides recognized by tumor-specific CTLs or identification of the genes encoding these peptides.

TUMOR TRANSPLANTATION Studies of transplanted tumors in rodents were the first experiments to indicate the existence of tumor antigens recognized by T cells. Initial studies of this type used chemically induced rodent sarcomas (see Fig. 17–1 and the text), and they demonstrated the existence of tumor-specific transplantation antigens (TSTAs) that elicited highly specific immune responses. Another, more recent approach to characterize antigens that stimulate tumor rejection by CTLs relies on the *in vitro* mutagenesis of an established tumorigenic mouse cell line and isolation of non-tumorigenic variants that are rejected on transplantation into syngeneic mice. In this system, the tumorigenic cell line does not express TSTAs and therefore grows unchecked when it is injected into a host animal, but the mutagenized cell line does express mutant protein antigens that induce its rejection. The role of CTLs in the rejection process in this model has been established by adoptive transfer experiments and by the propagation of CTL clones that recognize the tumor, as discussed below. The actual genes encoding the rejection antigens in a few of these tumor variants have been cloned, by methods described here.

GENERATION OF TUMOR-SPECIFIC CTL CLONES The establishment of cloned CTL lines that recognize tumor antigens has been a key advance in the identification of tumor antigens because such clones provide sensitive probes for identifying tumor antigens that are likely to be important targets of host anti-tumor immune responses. This approach is particularly valuable for human tumors, whose immunogenicity cannot easily be studied by transplantation in animals. Many cloned CTL lines specific for human tumors, particularly melanomas, have been generated from the T cells of patients. Melanomas, which are malignant tumors of melanocytes, are often readily accessible, surgically resectable tumors that may be grown in tissue culture. CTLs specific for these tumors may be propagated and subsequently cloned by culturing T cells from a melanoma patient with cells derived from the patient's melanoma. The T cells can be isolated from peripheral blood, lymph nodes draining the tumor, or cells that have actually infiltrated the tumor *in vivo.* Because the T cells and the tumor are from the same individual, the MHC restriction of the T cells matches the MHC alleles expressed by the tumor. In these cocultures, CTLs that recognize peptide antigens displayed by the tumor cells are stimulated to grow, and single-cell clones are propagated in IL-2 by limiting dilution techniques (see Figure).

IDENTIFICATION OF TUMOR ANTIGENS RECOGNIZED BY T CELLS Identification of the peptide antigens that induce CTL responses in patients with tumors and identification of the genes encoding the proteins from which the peptides are derived have relied on cloned tumor-specific CTL lines. These tumor antigens have been identified by two methods. First, a direct biochemical approach is used in which peptides bound to tumor cell class I MHC molecules are eluted by acid treatment and fractionated by reverse-phase high-performance liquid chromatography (HPLC). The fractions are tested for their ability to sensitize MHC-matched non-tumor target cells for lysis by a tumor-specific CTL clone. This strategy relies on having a target cell that expresses the class I MHC molecules for which the CTL clone is specific but does not normally express the tumor antigen and on the ability to load these cell surface MHC molecules with the exogenous HPLC-purified peptides. Peptide fractions that do sensitize the target cells are then analyzed by mass spectroscopy to determine their amino acid sequences. Once the peptide sequence is known, it may be possible to compare it with databases of protein sequences to see whether it matches with any previously characterized protein and to determine whether any point mutations are present in the normal sequences.

The second method of identifying tumor antigens is molecular cloning of the genes encoding these antigens (see Figure). This method relies on preparing a cDNA library from a tumor cell line that contains genes encoding all the tumor proteins. The library is prepared in molecular constructs that will allow constitutive expression of the genes when they are introduced into cell lines. Pools of DNA from such a library are transfected into a cell line expressing the same class I MHC allele as the tumor, and the transfected cells are tested for sensitivity to lysis by an anti-tumor CTL clone. The DNA pools that sensitize the target cell line contain the gene that encodes the protein antigen recognized by the CTL clone. Multiple rounds of transfections using smaller and smaller subfractions of the DNA pool can lead to isolation of the single relevant gene. The sequence of the gene can then be determined, and comparisons can be made with known genes. Synthetic peptides corresponding to different regions of the encoded protein can be tested for their ability to sensitize target cells in much the same way as in the peptide elution approach. Both the biochemical and genetic approaches have been used successfully to identify human melanoma antigens that stimulate CTL responses in the patients with melanoma.

Continued on following page

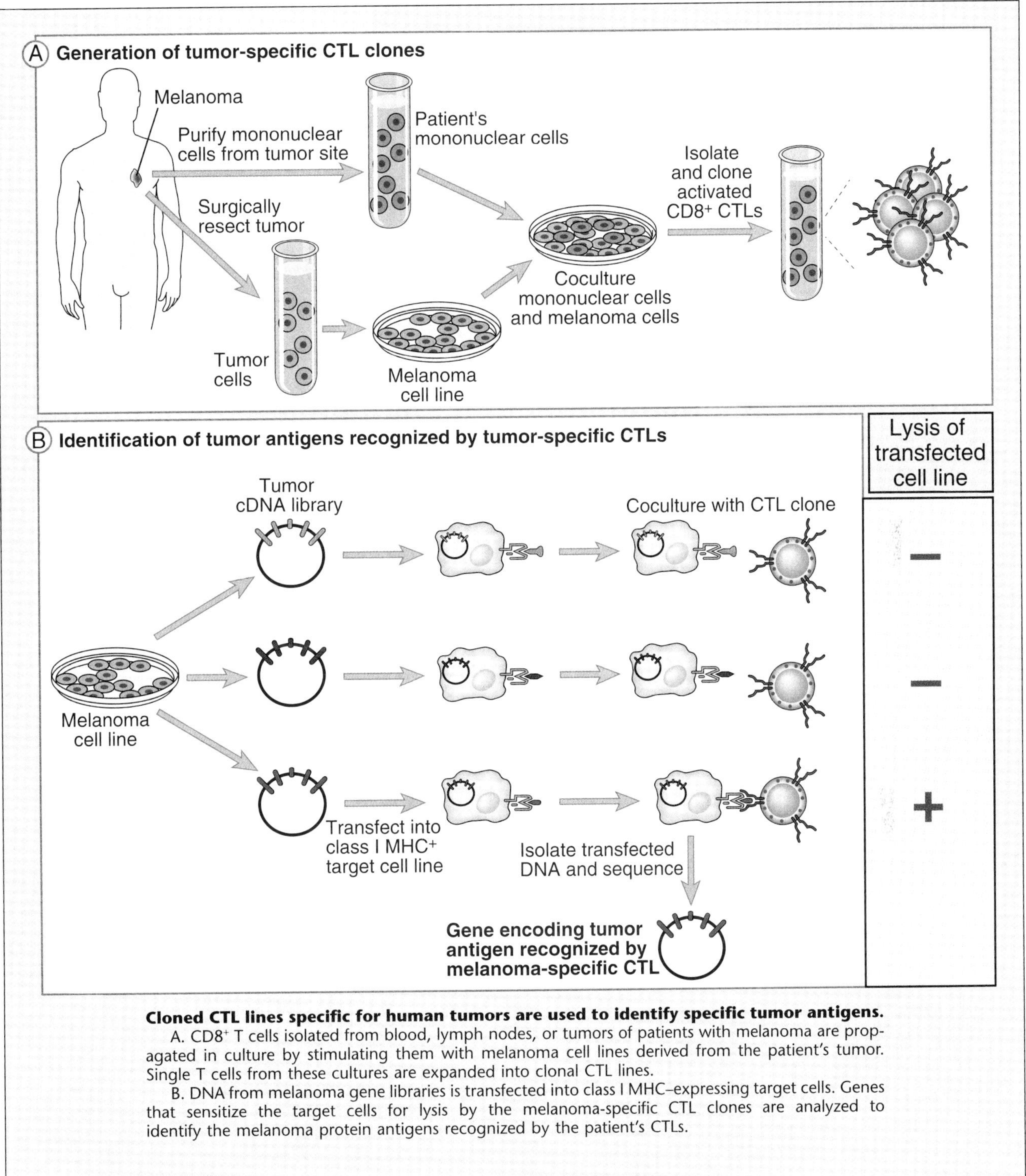

Cloned CTL lines specific for human tumors are used to identify specific tumor antigens. A. CD8+ T cells isolated from blood, lymph nodes, or tumors of patients with melanoma are propagated in culture by stimulating them with melanoma cell lines derived from the patient's tumor. Single T cells from these cultures are expanded into clonal CTL lines.

B. DNA from melanoma gene libraries is transfected into class I MHC–expressing target cells. Genes that sensitize the target cells for lysis by the melanoma-specific CTL clones are analyzed to identify the melanoma protein antigens recognized by the patient's CTLs.

tumor-specific transplantation antigens (TSTAs), are mutants of various host cellular proteins. Studies with chemically induced rodent sarcomas, such as those illustrated in Figure 17–1, established that different rodent tumors, all induced by the same carcinogen, expressed different transplantation antigens. For example, one MCA-induced sarcoma will induce protective immunity against itself but not against another MCA-induced sarcoma, even if both tumors are derived from the same normal cell type and in the same mouse. We now know that the tumor antigens identified by such experiments are peptides derived from mutated self proteins and presented in the form of peptide–class I MHC complexes capable of stimulating CTLs. These antigens are extremely diverse because the carcinogens that induce the tumors may randomly mutagenize virtually any host gene, and the class I MHC antigen-presenting pathway can display peptides from

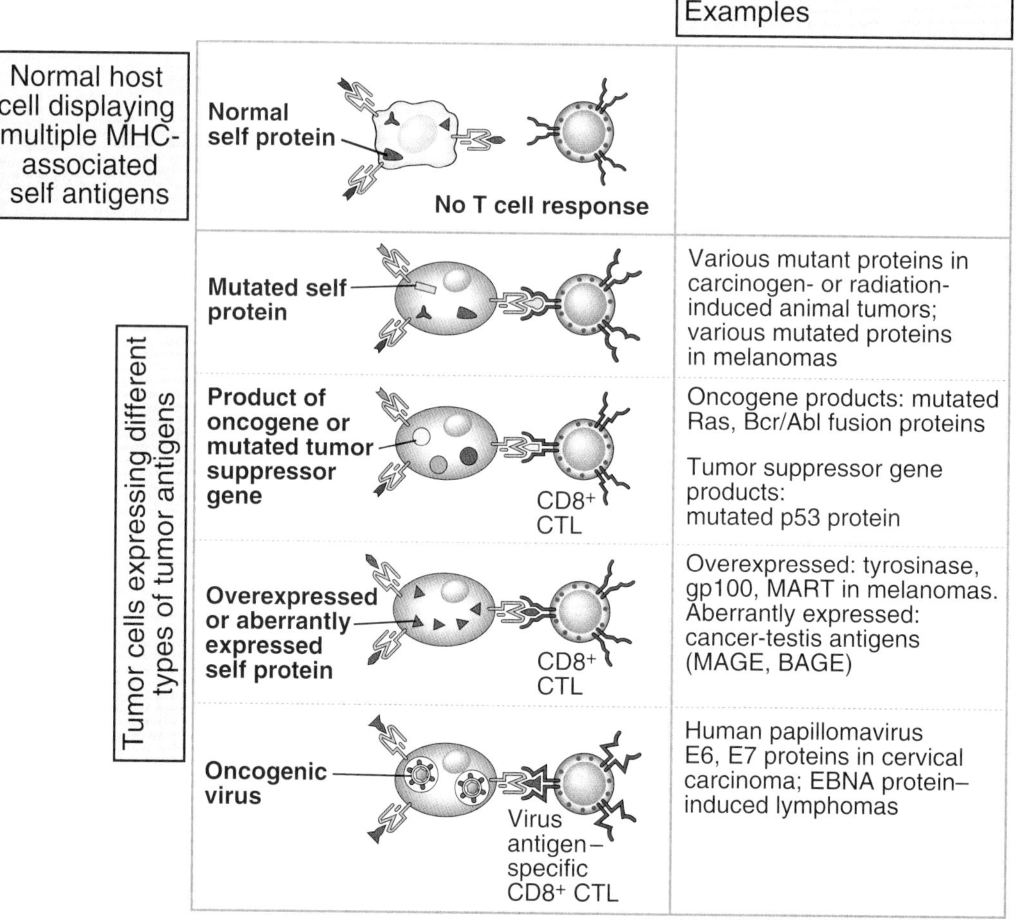

Figure 17–2 Types of tumor antigens recognized by T cells. Tumor antigens that are recognized by tumor-specific $CD8^+$ T cells may be mutated forms of normal self proteins, products of oncogenes, overexpressed or aberrantly expressed self proteins, or products of oncogenic viruses.

any mutated cytosolic protein in each tumor. Mutated cellular proteins are found more frequently in chemical carcinogen– or radiation-induced animal tumors than in spontaneous human cancers, probably because chemical carcinogens and radiation mutagenize many cellular genes. Nevertheless, TSTAs of experimental animal tumors are relevant to the study of human cancers in two ways. First, the finding of TSTAs was the first result to prove that adaptive immune responses may be able to control tumors. Second, the general principle that mutated host proteins can function as tumor antigens, which also came from studies of animal TSTAs, has been demonstrated in human cancers as well.

Overexpressed and Abnormally Expressed Cellular Proteins

Tumor antigens may be normal cellular proteins that are abnormally expressed in tumor cells and elicit immune responses. Many such antigens have been identified in human tumors, such as melanomas, by the molecular cloning of antigens that are recognized by T cells from tumor-bearing patients (see Box 17–1). One of the surprises that emerged from these studies was that some tumor antigens are normal proteins that are produced at low levels in normal cells and overexpressed in tumor cells (see Table 17–1). One such antigen is tyrosinase, an enzyme involved in melanin biosynthesis that is expressed only in normal melanocytes and melanomas. Both class I MHC–restricted $CD8^+$ CTL clones and class II MHC–restricted $CD4^+$ T cell clones from melanoma patients recognize peptides derived from tyrosinase. On face value, it is surprising that these patients are able to respond to a normal self antigen. The likely explanation is that tyrosinase is normally produced in such small amounts and in so few cells that it is not recognized by the immune system and fails to induce tolerance. The finding of tyrosinase-specific T cell responses in patients raises the possibility that tyrosinase vaccines may stimulate such responses to melanomas; clinical trials with these vaccines are ongoing.

Other tumor antigens may be derived from genes that are not expressed in normal tissues or are expressed only early during development and are dysregulated as a consequence of malignant transformation of a cell. Transformation may result in

Table 17–1. Tumor Antigens

Type of antigen	Examples of human tumor antigens
Products of oncogenes, tumor suppressor genes	Oncogenes: Ras mutations (~10% of human carcinomas), p210 product of Bcr/Abl rearrangements (CML), overexpressed Her-2/neu (breast and other carcinomas)
	Tumor suppressor genes: mutated p53 (present in ~50% of human tumors)
Mutants of cellular genes not involved in tumorigenesis	p91A mutation in mutagenized murine mastocytoma; various mutated proteins in melanomas recognized by CTLs
Products of genes that are silent in most normal tissues	MAGE, BAGE, GAGE proteins expressed in melanomas and many carcinomas; normally expressed mainly in the testis and placenta
Products of overexpressed genes	Tyrosinase, gp100, MART in melanomas (normally expressed in melanocytes)
Products of oncogenic viruses	Papillomavirus E6 and E7 proteins (cervical carcinomas)
	EBNA-1 protein of EBV (EBV-associated lymphomas, nasopharyngeal carcinoma)
	SV40 T antigen (SV40-induced rodent tumors)
Oncofetal antigens	Carcinoembryonic antigen on many tumors, also expressed in liver and other tissues during inflammation
	Alpha-fetoprotein
Glycolipids and glycoproteins	GM_2, GD_2 on melanomas
Differentiation antigens normally present in tissue of origin	Prostate-specific antigen
	Markers of lymphocytes: CD10, CD20, Ig idiotypes on B cells

Abbreviations: CML, chronic myelogenous leukemia; CTL, cytolytic T lymphocyte; EBNA, Epstein-Barr nuclear antigen; EBV, Epstein-Barr virus; Ig, immunoglobulin; MAGE, melanoma antigen (BAGE and GAGE are structurally unrelated melanoma proteins named after MAGE); MART, melanoma antigen recognized by T cells.

inappropriate expression of the normal genes in the wrong tissues or at the wrong time, and the proteins produced may behave like tumor antigens and evoke immune responses. The functions of the proteins encoded by these genes may be unknown, but they are not required for the malignant phenotype of the cells, and their sequences are identical to the corresponding genes in normal cells, that is, they are not mutated. Melanoma antigen (MAGE) genes, first isolated from human melanoma cells, encode cellular protein antigens recognized by melanoma-specific CTL clones derived from different melanoma-bearing patients. MAGE proteins are expressed on tumors in addition to melanomas, including carcinomas of the bladder, breast, skin, lung, and prostate and some sarcomas. In normal tissues, MAGE expression is restricted to the testis. Subsequent to identification of the MAGE genes, several other unrelated gene families have been identified that encode melanoma antigens recognized by CTL clones derived from melanoma patients. Like the MAGE proteins, these other melanoma antigens are silent in most normal tissues, except the testis, but they are expressed in a variety of malignant tumors. Because of the expression on cancers and in the testis, all these tumor antigens are now classified in the cancer-testis (CT) antigen family.

Tumor Antigens Encoded by Genomes of Oncogenic Viruses

The products of oncogenic viruses function as tumor antigens and elicit specific T cell responses that may serve to eradicate the tumors. DNA viruses are implicated in the development of a variety of tumors in humans and experimental animals. Examples in humans include the Epstein-Barr virus (EBV), which is associated with B cell lymphomas and nasopharyngeal carcinoma (Box 17–2), and human papillomavirus (HPV), which is associated with cervical carcinoma. Papovaviruses, including polyomavirus and simian virus 40 (SV40), and adenoviruses induce malignant tumors in neonatal or immunodeficient adult rodents. In most of these DNA virus–induced tumors, virus-encoded protein antigens are found in the nucleus, cytoplasm, or plasma membrane of the tumor cells. These endogenously synthesized proteins can be processed, and complexes of processed viral peptides with class I MHC molecules may be expressed on the tumor cell

BOX 17–2

The Relationships Between Epstein-Barr Virus, Malignancy, and Immunodeficiency

Epstein-Barr virus (EBV) is a double-stranded DNA virus of the herpesvirus family. The virus is transmitted by saliva, infects nasopharyngeal epithelial cells and B lymphocytes, and is ubiquitous in human populations worldwide. It infects human B cells by binding specifically to complement receptor type 2 (CR2, or CD21), followed by receptor-mediated endocytosis. Two types of cellular infections can occur. In a lytic infection, viral DNA, RNA, and protein are synthesized, followed by assembly of viral particles and lysis of the infected cell. Alternatively, a latent nonlytic infection can occur in which the viral DNA is maintained as an episome in infected cells. Various virally encoded antigens are detectable in infected cells. At least six Epstein-Barr nuclear antigens (EBNAs) are expressed early in lytic infections and may also be expressed by some latently infected cells. Two other proteins, called latent membrane proteins (LMPs), are expressed on the surface of latently infected cells. Other viral structural protein antigens, including viral capsid antigens (VCAs), are expressed within infected cells and on released viral particles during lytic infections. Antibodies specific for VCAs are first produced during acute infections and persist for many years thereafter.

EBV has profound effects on B lymphocyte growth *in vitro.* The virus is a T cell–independent polyclonal activator of B cell proliferation. EBV immortalizes human B cells so that they proliferate in culture indefinitely. The resulting long-term B lymphoblastoid cell lines are latently infected with the virus, express EBNAs and LMPs, and have a malignant phenotype as demonstrated by transplantation into immunodeficient mice. Five EBNAs and LMP-1 have been shown to be critical for transforming B lymphocytes into immortal cells. The cytoplasmic tail of LMP-1 binds the physiologic signaling molecules TRAF-1 and TRAF-2, which normally transduce signals resulting from engagement of TNF receptors and the important B cell activation molecule CD40 (see Chapter 11, Box 11–1). By this mechanism, EBV appears to have co-opted a normal B cell activation pathway to promote proliferation of the cells that the virus infects and lives in.

The spectrum of clinical sequelae to EBV infection is wide. Most people are infected during childhood; they do not experience any symptoms, and viral replication is apparently controlled by humoral and T cell–mediated immune responses. In previously uninfected young adults, infectious mononucleosis typically develops during EBV infection. This disease is characterized by sore throat, fever, and generalized lymphadenopathy. Large morphologically atypical lymphocytes are abundant in the peripheral blood of patients with infectious mononucleosis. Most of these cells are CTLs; in fact, in acute infections, up to 10% of all the $CD8^+$ T cells in the blood may be EBV specific, and small numbers of these CTLs may persist for life. Previously infected, healthy individuals harbor the virus for the rest of their lives in latently infected B cells and often in nasopharyngeal epithelium. An estimated one of every million B cells in a previously infected individual is latently infected. Importantly, EBV infection is one of the etiologic factors for the development of certain malignant tumors, including nasopharyngeal carcinoma in Chinese populations, Burkitt's lymphoma in equatorial Africa, and B cell lymphomas in immunosuppressed patients.

The evidence is compelling that T cell–mediated immunity is required for control of EBV infections and, in particular, for killing of EBV-infected B cells. First, individuals with deficiencies in T cell–mediated immunity are susceptible to uncontrolled, widely disseminated, and lethal acute EBV infections. Second, EBV-infected B cells isolated from patients with infectious mononucleosis can be propagated *in vitro* indefinitely, but only if the patient's T cells are removed or inactivated by drugs such as cyclosporine. In fact, immortalization of normal peripheral blood B cells by *in vitro* infection with EBV is successful only if the donor's T cells are removed or inactivated. Third, CTLs specific for EBV-encoded antigens, including EBNAs and LMP, are present in patients suffering from acute infectious mononucleosis and recovered patients. Cloned CTL lines have been established *in vitro* that specifically lyse EBV-infected B cells, and these CTLs most often recognize peptide fragments of EBNA or LMP proteins in association with class I MHC molecules. EBV-specific T cells are required *in vivo* to limit the polyclonal proliferation of infected B cells as well as to kill potentially immortalized clones of latently infected B cells. A loss of normal T cell–mediated immunity allows latently infected B cells to progress toward malignant transformation. Infusion of EBV-specific CTLs restores the normal balance and provides protection against the growth of malignant B cell tumors.

The epidemiology and molecular genetics of Burkitt's lymphoma and other EBV-associated lymphomas have been the subject of intense investigation, and they offer fascinating insight into various aspects of viral oncogenesis and tumor immunity. Burkitt's lymphoma is a histologic type of malignant B cell tumor composed of monotonous small malignant B cells. The African form of the disease is endemic in regions where both EBV and malaria infection are common. In these regions, the tumor occurs frequently in young children, often beginning in the jaw. Virtually 100% of patients with African Burkitt's lymphoma have evidence of previous EBV infection, and their tumors usually carry the EBV genome and express EBV-encoded antigens. Malarial infections in this population are known to cause T cell immunodeficiencies, and this association may be the link between EBV infection and the development of lymphoma. Sporadic Burkitt's lymphoma occurs less frequently in other parts of the world, and although these B cell tumors are histologically similar to the endemic form, only about 20% carry the EBV genome. Both endemic and sporadic Burkitt's lymphoma cells have reciprocal chromosomal translocations involving Ig gene loci and the cellular *myc* gene on chromosome 8.

B cell lymphomas occur at a high frequency in T cell–immunodeficient individuals, including individuals with congenital immunodeficiencies, patients with AIDS, and kidney or heart allograft recipients receiving immunosuppressive drugs. Only some of these tumors can be called Burkitt's lymphomas on the basis of histology. Regardless of their histologic appearance, many of these tumors are latently infected with EBV, like Burkitt's lymphoma. A smaller subset also contains *myc* translocations to Ig loci.

Continued on following page

These observations can be synthesized into a hypothesis about the pathogenesis of EBV-associated B cell tumors. African children with malaria, allograft recipients, congenitally immunodeficient children, and AIDS patients all have abnormalities in T cell function. Because of a deficiency of EBV-specific T cells, EBV-induced polyclonal proliferation of B cells is uncontrolled. This exuberant proliferation of B cells increases the chances of errors made during DNA replication, including translocations of oncogenes. The Ig loci are accessible sites for translocations compared with other loci in B cells. Translocation of the *myc* gene to the Ig locus leads to transcriptional deregulation and abnormal expression of Myc, and this alteration appears to be causally related to malignant transformation and outgrowth of a neoplastic clone of cells. Many EBV-positive tumors in immunosuppressed patients do not have *myc* translocations, and the proteins encoded by the integrated EBV genome may be sufficient to cause lymphomas. This proposed scheme predicts that early in their course, EBV-associated B cell tumors may be polyclonal because they arise from a polyclonally stimulated population of normal B cells. Later, one or a few clones may obtain selective growth advantages, perhaps because of deregulation of *myc* or other cellular or viral genes. As a result, the polyclonal proliferation evolves into a monoclonal or oligoclonal tumor. In fact, such has been shown to be the case by Southern blot analysis of Ig gene rearrangements in some EBV-positive B cell tumors from immunosuppressed patients.

surface. Because the viral peptides are foreign antigens, DNA virus–induced tumors are among the most immunogenic tumors known.

The ability of adaptive immunity to prevent the growth of DNA virus–induced tumors has been established by many observations.

- EBV-associated lymphomas and HPV-associated skin cancers arise more frequently in immunosuppressed individuals, such as allograft recipients receiving immunosuppressive therapy and patients with acquired immunodeficiency syndrome (AIDS), than in normal individuals.
- Adenovirus infection induces tumors much more frequently in neonatal or T cell–deficient mice than in normal adult mice.
- Tumor transplantation experiments of the kind illustrated in Figure 17–1 have shown that animals may be specifically immunized against DNA virus–induced tumors and will reject transplants of these tumors. Unlike MCA-induced tumor antigens, which are the products of randomly mutated cellular genes, virus-encoded tumor antigens are not unique for each tumor but are shared by all tumors induced by the same type of virus.
- Immunization of experimental animals with SV40 virus and adenovirus produces protective immunity against the development of tumors induced by each virus, and immunity is mediated by class I MHC–restricted CTLs specific for the antigens of that virus.

Thus, a competent immune system may play a role in surveillance against virus-induced tumors because of its ability to recognize and kill virus-infected cells. In fact, the concept of immune surveillance against tumors is better established for DNA virus–induced tumors than for any other type of tumor.

RNA tumor viruses (retroviruses) are important causes of tumors in animals. Retroviral oncogene products theoretically have the same potential antigenic properties as mutated cellular oncogenes, and humoral and cell-mediated immune responses to retroviral gene products on tumor cells can be observed experimentally. The only well-defined human retrovirus that is known to cause tumors is human T cell lymphotropic virus 1 (HTLV-1), the etiologic agent for adult T cell leukemia/lymphoma (ATL), a malignant tumor of CD4$^+$ T cells. Although immune responses specific for HTLV-1–encoded antigens have been demonstrated in individuals infected with the virus, it is not clear whether they play any role in protective immunity against the development of tumors. Furthermore, patients with ATL are often profoundly immunosuppressed, probably because the virus infects CD4$^+$ T cells and induces functional abnormalities in these cells.

Oncofetal Antigens

Oncofetal antigens are proteins that are expressed at high levels on cancer cells and in normal developing fetal but not adult tissues. It is believed that the genes encoding these proteins are silenced during development and are derepressed on malignant transformation. Oncofetal antigens were identified with antibodies raised in other species, and their main importance is that they provide markers that aid in tumor diagnosis. As techniques for detecting these antigens have improved, it has become clear that their expression in adults is not limited to tumors. The proteins are increased in tissues and in the circulation in various inflammatory conditions and are found in small quantities even in normal tissues. There is no evidence that oncofetal antigens are important inducers or targets of anti-tumor immunity. The two most thoroughly characterized oncofetal antigens are carcinoembryonic antigen (CEA) and alpha-fetoprotein (AFP).

CEA (CD66) is a highly glycosylated integral membrane protein that is a member of the immunoglobulin (Ig) superfamily. It is an intercellular adhesion molecule that functions to promote the binding of tumor cells to one another. High CEA expression is normally restricted to cells in the gut, pancreas, and liver during the first two trimesters of gestation, and low expression is seen in normal adult colonic mucosa and lactating breast. CEA expression is increased in many carcinomas of the colon, pancreas, stomach, and breast, and serum levels are increased in these patients. The level of serum CEA is used to monitor the persistence or recurrence of the tumors after treatment. The usefulness of CEA as a diagnostic marker for cancer is limited by the fact that serum CEA can also be elevated in the setting of non-neoplastic diseases, such as chronic inflammatory conditions of the bowel or liver.

AFP is a circulating glycoprotein normally synthesized and secreted in fetal life by the yolk sac and liver. Fetal serum concentrations can be as high as 2 to 3 mg/mL, but in adult life, the protein is replaced by albumin, and only low levels are present in serum. Serum levels of AFP can be significantly elevated in patients with hepatocellular carcinoma, germ cell tumors, and, occasionally, gastric and pancreatic cancers. An elevated serum AFP level is a useful indicator of advanced liver or germ cell tumors or of recurrence of these tumors after treatment. Furthermore, the detection of AFP in tissue sections by immunohistochemical techniques can help in the pathologic identification of tumor cells. The diagnostic value of AFP as a tumor marker is limited by the fact that elevated serum levels are also found in non-neoplastic diseases, such as cirrhosis of the liver.

Altered Glycolipid and Glycoprotein Antigens

Most human and experimental tumors express higher than normal levels or abnormal forms of surface glycoproteins and glycolipids, which may be diagnostic markers and targets for therapy. These altered molecules include gangliosides, blood group antigens, and mucins. Some aspects of the malignant phenotype of tumors, including tissue invasion and metastatic behavior, may reflect altered cell surface properties that result from abnormal glycolipid and glycoprotein synthesis. Many antibodies have been raised in animals that recognize the carbohydrate groups or peptide cores of these molecules. Although most of the epitopes recognized by these antibodies are not specifically expressed on tumors, they are present at higher levels on cancer cells than on normal cells. This class of tumor-associated antigen is a target for cancer therapy with specific antibodies.

Among the glycolipids expressed at high levels in melanomas are the gangliosides GM_2, GD_2, and GD_3. Clinical trials of anti-GM_2 and anti-GD_3 antibodies and immunization with vaccines containing GM_2 are under way in patients with melanoma. Mucins are high molecular weight glycoproteins containing numerous O-linked carbohydrate side chains on a core polypeptide. Tumors often have dysregulated expression of the enzymes that synthesize these carbohydrate side chains, which leads to the appearance of tumor-specific epitopes on the carbohydrate side chains or on the abnormally exposed polypeptide core. Several mucins have been the focus of diagnostic and therapeutic studies, including CA-125 and CA-19-9, expressed on ovarian carcinomas, and MUC-1, expressed on breast carcinomas. Unlike many mucins, MUC-1 is an integral membrane protein that is normally expressed only on the apical surface of breast ductal epithelium, a site that is relatively sequestered from the immune system. In ductal carcinomas of the breast, however, the molecule is expressed in an unpolarized fashion and contains new, tumor-specific carbohydrate and peptide epitopes detectable by mouse monoclonal antibodies. The peptide epitopes induce both antibody and T cell responses in cancer patients and are therefore being considered as candidates for tumor vaccines.

Tissue-Specific Differentiation Antigens

Tumors express molecules that are normally present on the cells of origin. These antigens are called differentiation antigens because they are specific for particular lineages or differentiation stages of various cell types. Their importance is as potential targets for immunotherapy and for identifying the tissue of origin of tumors. For example, several melanoma antigens that are targets of CTLs in patients are melanocyte differentiation antigens, such as tyrosinase mentioned earlier. Lymphomas may be diagnosed as B cell–derived tumors by the detection of surface markers characteristic of this lineage, such as CD10 (previously called common acute lymphoblastic leukemia antigen, or CALLA) and CD20. Antibodies against these molecules are also used for tumor immunotherapy. The idiotypic determinants of the surface Ig of a clonal B cell population are markers for that B cell clone because all other B cells express different idiotypes. Therefore, the Ig idiotype is a highly specific tumor antigen for B cell lymphomas and leukemias. These differentiation antigens are normal self molecules, and therefore they do not usually induce strong immune responses in tumor-bearing hosts.

Immune Responses to Tumors

The effector mechanisms of both cell-mediated immunity and humoral immunity have been shown to kill tumor cells *in vitro*. The challenge for tumor immunologists is to determine which of these mechanisms may contribute to protective immune responses against tumors and to enhance these effector mechanisms in ways that are tumor specific. In this section, we review the evidence for tumor killing by various immune effector mechanisms and discuss which are the most likely to be relevant to human tumors.

T Lymphocytes

The principal mechanism of tumor immunity is killing of tumor cells by CD8⁺ CTLs. The ability of CTLs to provide effective anti-tumor immunity *in vivo* is most clearly seen in animal experiments using carcinogen-induced and DNA virus–induced tumors. As discussed previously, CTLs may perform a surveillance function by recognizing and killing potentially malignant cells that express peptides derived from mutant cellular proteins or oncogenic viral proteins and presented in association with class I MHC molecules. The role of immune surveillance in preventing common, non–virally induced tumors has been questioned because such tumors do not arise more frequently in T cell–deficient animals or people. However, tumor-specific

CTLs can be isolated from animals and humans with established tumors, such as melanomas. Furthermore, mononuclear cells derived from the inflammatory infiltrate in human solid tumors, called tumor-infiltrating lymphocytes (TILs), also include CTLs with the capacity to kill the tumor from which they were derived.

There has been great interest in the mechanisms by which tumors stimulate CD8$^+$ T cell responses specific for tumor antigens. Most tumor cells are not derived from APCs and therefore do not express the costimulators needed to initiate primary T cell responses or the class II MHC molecules needed to stimulate helper T cells that promote the differentiation of CD8$^+$ T cells. A likely possibility is that tumor cells or their antigens are ingested by host APCs, particularly dendritic cells; the tumor antigens are then processed inside the APCs, and peptides derived from these antigens are displayed bound to class I MHC molecules for recognition by CD8$^+$ T cells. The APCs express costimulators that may provide the signals needed for differentiation of CD8$^+$ T cells into anti-tumor CTLs, and the APCs express class II MHC molecules that may present internalized tumor antigens and activate CD4$^+$ helper T cells as well (Fig. 17–3). This process of cross-presentation, or cross-priming, has been described in earlier chapters as a general mechanism for inducing CTL responses against cells other than professional APCs (see Chapter 5, Fig. 5–7). Once effector CTLs are generated, they are able to recognize and kill the tumor cells without a requirement for costimulation. A practical application of the concept of cross-priming is to grow dendritic cells from a patient with cancer, incubate the APCs with the cells or antigens from that patient's tumor, and use these antigen-pulsed APCs as vaccines to stimulate anti-tumor T cell responses.

The importance of CD4$^+$ helper T cells in tumor immunity is less clear. CD4$^+$ cells may play a role in anti-tumor immune responses by providing cytokines for effective CTL development (see Chapter 13). In addition, helper T cells specific for tumor antigens may secrete cytokines, such as tumor necrosis factor (TNF) and interferon-γ (IFN-γ), that can increase tumor cell class I MHC expression and sensitivity to lysis by CTLs. IFN-γ may also activate macrophages to kill tumor cells. The importance of IFN-γ in tumor immunity is demonstrated by the finding of increased incidence of tumors in knockout mice lacking this cytokine.

Antibodies

Tumor-bearing hosts may produce antibodies against various tumor antigens. For example, patients with EBV-associated lymphomas have serum antibodies against EBV-encoded antigens expressed on the surface of the lymphoma cells. Antibodies may kill tumor cells by activating complement or by antibody-dependent cell-mediated cytotoxicity, in which Fc receptor–bearing macrophages or NK cells mediate the killing. However, the ability of antibodies to eliminate tumor cells has been demonstrated largely *in vitro*, and there is little evidence for effective humoral immunity against tumors.

NK Cells

NK cells kill many types of tumor cells, especially cells that have reduced class I MHC expression and can escape killing by CTLs. *In vitro*, NK cells can kill virally infected cells and certain tumor cell lines, especially hematopoietic tumors. NK cells also respond to the absence of class I MHC molecules because the

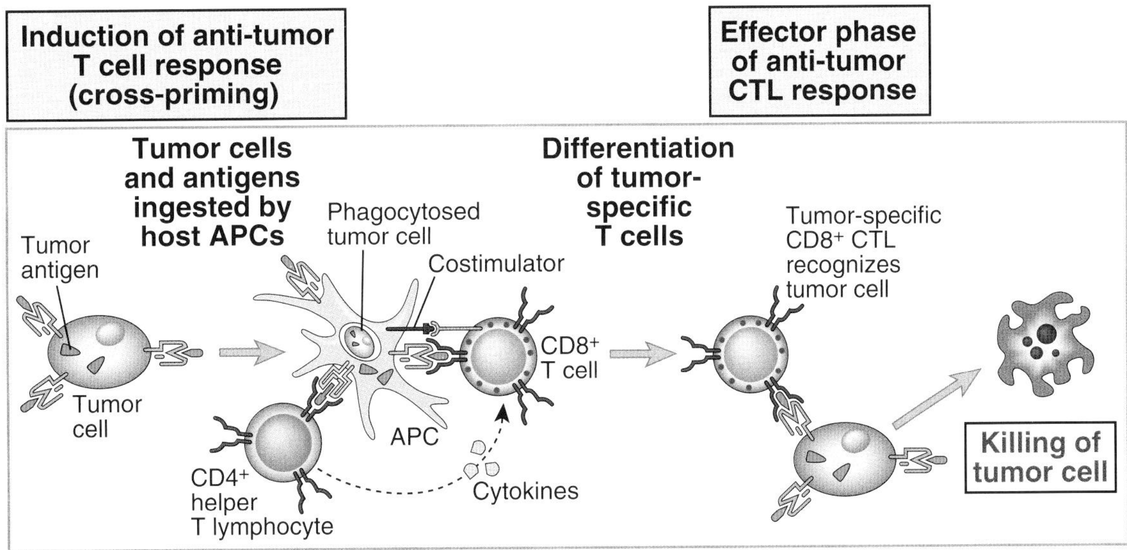

Figure 17–3 Induction of T cell responses to tumors.
CD8$^+$ T cell responses to tumors may be induced by cross-priming, in which the tumor cells or tumor antigens are taken up, processed, and presented to T cells by professional antigen-presenting cells (APCs). In some cases, B7 costimulators expressed by the APCs provide the second signals for differentiation of CD8$^+$ T cells. The APCs may also stimulate CD4$^+$ helper T cells, which provide the second signals for cytolytic T lymphocyte (CTL) development (see Chapter 13, Fig. 13–4). Differentiated CTLs kill tumor cells without a requirement for costimulation or T cell help.

recognition of class I MHC molecules delivers inhibitory signals to NK cells (see Chapter 12, Fig. 12–7). As we shall see later, some tumors lose expression of class I MHC molecules, perhaps as a result of selection against class I MHC–expressing cells by CTLs. This loss of class I MHC molecules makes the tumors particularly good targets for NK cells. In addition, NK cells can be targeted to IgG antibody–coated cells by Fc receptors (FcγRIII or CD16). The tumoricidal capacity of NK cells is increased by cytokines, including interferons and interleukins (IL-2 and IL-12), and the anti-tumor effects of these cytokines are partly attributable to stimulation of NK cell activity. IL-2–activated NK cells, called lymphokine-activated killer (LAK) cells, are derived by culturing peripheral blood cells or TILs from tumor patients with high doses of IL-2. The use of LAK cells in adoptive immunotherapy for tumors is discussed later.

The role of NK cells in tumor immunity *in vivo* is unclear. It has been suggested that T cell–deficient mice do not have a high incidence of spontaneous tumors because they have normal numbers of NK cells that serve an immune surveillance function. A few patients have been described with deficiencies of NK cells and an increased incidence of EBV-associated lymphomas.

Macrophages

The role of macrophages in anti-tumor immunity is largely inferred from the demonstration that *in vitro*, activated macrophages can kill many tumor cells more efficiently than they can kill normal cells. How macrophages are activated by tumors is not known. Possible mechanisms include direct recognition of some surface antigens of tumor cells and activation of macrophages by IFN-γ produced by tumor-specific T cells. Macrophages can kill tumor cells by several mechanisms, probably the same as the mechanisms of macrophage killing of infectious organisms. These mechanisms include the release of lysosomal enzymes, reactive oxygen intermediates, and nitric oxide. Activated macrophages also produce the cytokine TNF, which was first characterized, as its name implies, as an agent that can kill tumors mainly by inducing thrombosis in tumor blood vessels.

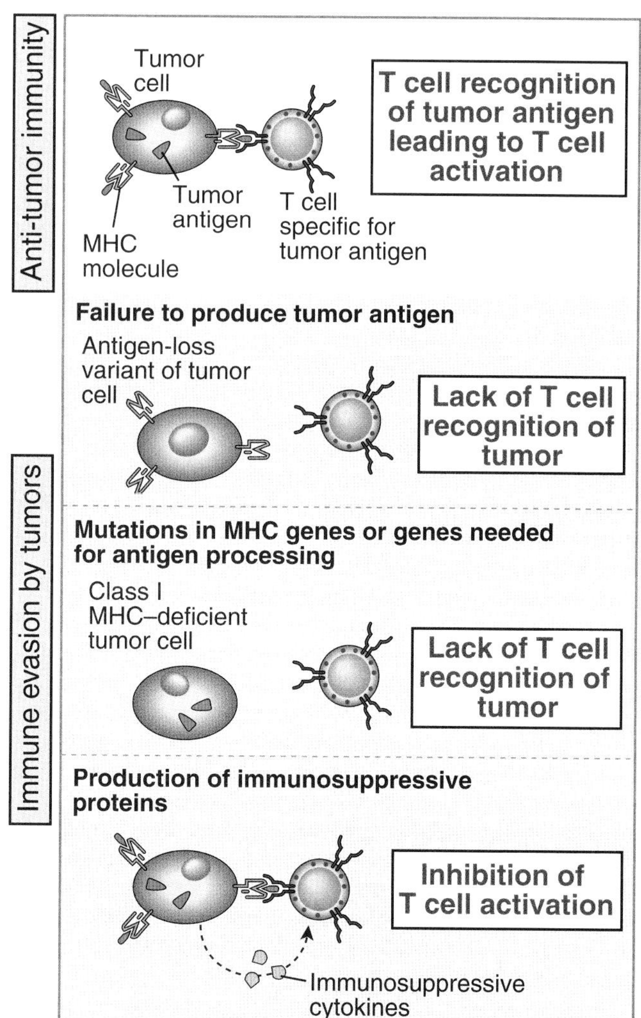

Figure 17–4 Mechanisms by which tumors escape immune defenses.
Anti-tumor immunity develops when T cells recognize tumor antigens and are activated. Tumor cells may evade immune responses by losing expression of antigens or MHC molecules or by producing immunosuppressive cytokines.

Evasion of Immune Responses by Tumors

Many malignant tumors possess mechanisms that enable them to evade or resist host immune responses (Fig. 17–4). A major focus of tumor immunology is to understand the ways in which tumor cells evade immune destruction, with the hope that interventions can be designed to increase the immunogenicity of tumors and the responses of the host. The process of evasion, often called tumor escape, may be a result of several mechanisms.

- ***Class I MHC expression may be down-regulated on tumor cells so that they cannot be recognized by CTLs.*** In experimental models, increasing class I MHC expression on tumor cells by treatment with cytokines such as IFN-γ or by gene transfection results in increased susceptibility of these cells to CTL lysis *in vitro* and decreased tumorigenicity *in vivo*. Various tumors show decreased synthesis of class I MHC molecules, β_2-microglobulin, or components of the antigen-processing machinery, including the transporter associated with antigen processing and some subunits of the proteasome. These mechanisms are presumably adaptations of the tumors that arise in response to the selection pressures of host immunity, and they may allow tumor cells to evade immune responses. However, when the level of MHC expression on a broad range of experimental or human tumor cells is compared with the *in vivo* growth of these cells, there is no clear correlation. Furthermore, metastatic tumors, which presumably have evaded immune attack, do not express fewer MHC molecules than nonmetastatic tumors do.

- ***Tumors lose expression of antigens that elicit immune responses.*** Such "antigen loss variants" are common in rapidly growing tumors and can readily be induced in tumor cell lines by culture with tumor-specific antibodies or CTLs. Given the high mitotic rate of tumor cells and their genetic instability, mutations or deletions in genes encoding tumor antigens are common. If these antigens are not required for growth of the tumors or maintenance of the transformed phenotype, the antigen-negative tumor cells have a growth advantage in the host. Analysis of tumors that are serially transplanted from one animal to another has shown that the loss of antigens recognized by tumor-specific CTLs correlates with increased growth and metastatic potential.

- ***Tumors may fail to induce CTLs because most tumor cells do not express costimulators or class II MHC molecules.*** Costimulators are required for initiating T cell responses, and class II molecules are needed for the activation of helper T cells, which stimulate the differentiation of CTLs. Therefore, the induction of tumor-specific T cell responses often requires cross-priming by professional APCs, which express costimulators and class II molecules. If such APCs do not adequately take up and present tumor antigens and activate helper T cells, CTLs specific for the tumor cells may not develop. Tumor cells transfected with genes encoding the costimulators B7-1 (CD80) and B7-2 (CD86) are able to elicit strong cell-mediated immune responses. Predictably, CTLs induced by B7-transfected tumors are effective against the parent (B7-negative) tumor as well because the effector phase of CTL-mediated killing does not require costimulation (see Fig. 17–3). As we shall see later, these experimental results are being extended to the clinical situation as immunotherapy for tumors.

- ***The products of tumor cells may suppress antitumor immune responses.*** An example of an immunosuppressive tumor product is transforming growth factor-β, which is secreted in large quantities by many tumors and inhibits the proliferation and effector functions of lymphocytes and macrophages (see Chapter 11). Some tumors express Fas ligand (FasL), which recognizes the death receptor Fas on leukocytes that attempt to attack the tumor; engagement of Fas by FasL results in apoptotic death of the leukocytes. The importance of this mechanism of tumor escape is not established because FasL has been detected on only a few spontaneous tumors, and when it is expressed in tumors by gene transfection, it is not always protective.

- ***Tumor antigens may induce specific immunologic tolerance.*** Tolerance may occur because tumor antigens are self antigens encountered by the developing immune system or because the tumor cells present their antigens in a tolerogenic form to mature lymphocytes. Several experimental studies have shown that tolerance to tumor antigens promotes the outgrowth of tumors expressing these antigens.

  - Neonatal mice may acquire the mouse mammary tumor virus from their mothers during nursing. The mice become tolerant to the virus and carry it for life. When these mice become adults, mammary cancers induced by the virus often develop, and the tumors do not elicit immune responses. However, the tumors are immunogenic because they are rejected when they are transplanted into syngeneic, virus-free (uninfected) adult mice.

  - Transgenic mice expressing the SV40 T antigen throughout their lives develop tumors when they are infected with the SV40 virus, and the high incidence of these tumors correlates with tolerance to the SV40 T antigen. In contrast, other SV40 T antigen transgenic mice in which expression of the transgene is delayed until later in life are not tolerant to the T antigen and have a low incidence of tumors.

  - In some experimental models, tumor cells transplanted into adult mice induce anergy in T cells specific for antigens expressed in these tumors. Immunity against the tumors may be stimulated by blocking CTLA-4, the inhibitory T cell receptor for B7 molecules. This result suggests that the tumor antigens may be presented to host T cells by APCs that induce T cell tolerance, in part as a result of B7:CTLA-4 interactions (see Chapter 10).

- The cell surface antigens of tumors may be hidden from the immune system by glycocalyx molecules, such as sialic acid–containing mucopolysaccharides. This process is called antigen masking and may be a consequence of the fact that tumor cells often express more of these glycocalyx molecules than normal cells do.

Immunotherapy for Tumors

The potential for treatment of patients with cancer by immunologic approaches has held great promise for immunologists and cancer biologists for many years. The main reason for interest in an immunologic approach is that current therapies for cancer rely on drugs that kill dividing cells or block cell division, and these treatments have severe effects on normal proliferating cells in patients with cancer. As a result, the treatment of cancers causes significant morbidity and mortality. Immune responses to tumors may be specific for tumor antigens and will not injure most normal cells. Therefore, immunotherapy has the potential of being the most tumor-specific treatment that can be devised. Advances in our understanding of the immune system and in defining antigens on tumor cells have encouraged many new strategies. Immunotherapy for tumors aims to augment the weak host immune response to the tumors (active immunity) or to administer tumor-specific antibodies or T cells, a form of passive immunity. In this section, we describe some of the modes of tumor immunotherapy that have been tried in the past or are currently being investigated.

Stimulation of Active Host Immune Responses to Tumors

The earliest attempts to boost anti-tumor immunity relied on nonspecific immune stimulation. More recently, vaccines composed of killed tumor cells or tumor antigens have been administered to patients, and strategies for enhancing immune responses against the tumor are being developed.

Vaccination with Tumor Cells and Tumor Antigens

Immunization of tumor-bearing individuals with killed tumor cells or tumor antigens may result in enhanced immune responses against the tumor (Table 17–2 and Fig. 17–5). The identification of peptides recognized by tumor-specific CTLs and the cloning of genes that encode tumor-specific antigens recognized by CTLs have provided many candidates for tumor vaccines. One of the earliest vaccine approaches, immunization with purified tumor antigens plus adjuvants, is still being tried. More recently, attempts to immunize patients with cancer have been made with dendritic cells purified from the patients and either incubated with tumor antigens or transfected with genes encoding these antigens and by injection of plasmids containing complementary DNAs (cDNAs) encoding tumor antigens (DNA vaccines). The cell-based and DNA vaccines may be the best ways to induce CTL responses because the encoded antigens are synthesized in the cytoplasm and enter the class I MHC pathway of antigen presentation. For antigens that are unique to individual tumors, such as antigens produced by random point mutations in cellular genes, these vaccination methods are impractical because they would require identification of the antigens from every tumor. On the other hand, tumor antigens shared by many tumors, such as the MAGE, tyrosinase, and gp100 antigens on melanomas and mutated Ras and p53 proteins in various tumors, are potentially useful immunogens for all patients with certain types of cancer. In fact, clinical trials of such cancer vaccines are under way for a variety of tumors. A limitation of treating established tumors with vaccines is that these vaccines need to be therapeutic and not simply preventive, and it is often difficult to induce a strong enough immune response that will eradicate all the cells of growing tumors.

The development of virally induced tumors can be blocked by preventive vaccination with viral antigens or attenuated live viruses. This approach is successful in reducing the incidence of feline leukemia virus–induced hematologic malignant tumors in cats and

Table 17–2. Tumor Vaccines

Type of vaccine	Vaccine preparation	Animal models	Clinical trials
Killed tumor vaccine	Killed tumor cells + adjuvants	Melanoma, colon cancer, others	Melanoma, colon cancer
	Tumor cell lysates + adjuvants	Sarcoma	Melanoma
Purified tumor antigens	Melanoma antigens	Melanoma	Melanoma
	Heat shock proteins	Various	Melanoma, renal cancer, sarcoma
Professional APC-based vaccines	Dendritic cells pulsed with tumor antigens	Melanoma, B cell lymphoma, sarcoma	Melanoma, non-Hodgkin's lymphoma, prostate cancer, others
	Dendritic cells transfected with genes encoding tumor antigens	Melanoma, colon cancer	Various carcinomas
Cytokine- and costimulator-enhanced vaccines	Tumor cells transfected with cytokine or B7 genes	Renal cancer, sarcoma, B cell leukemia, lung cancer	Melanoma, sarcoma, others
	APCs transfected with cytokine genes and pulsed with tumor antigens		Melanoma, renal cancer, others
DNA vaccines	Immunization with plasmids encoding tumor antigens	Melanoma	Melanoma
Viral vectors	Adenovirus, vaccinia virus encoding tumor antigen ± cytokines	Melanoma, sarcoma	Melanoma

Abbreviation: APC, antigen-presenting cell.

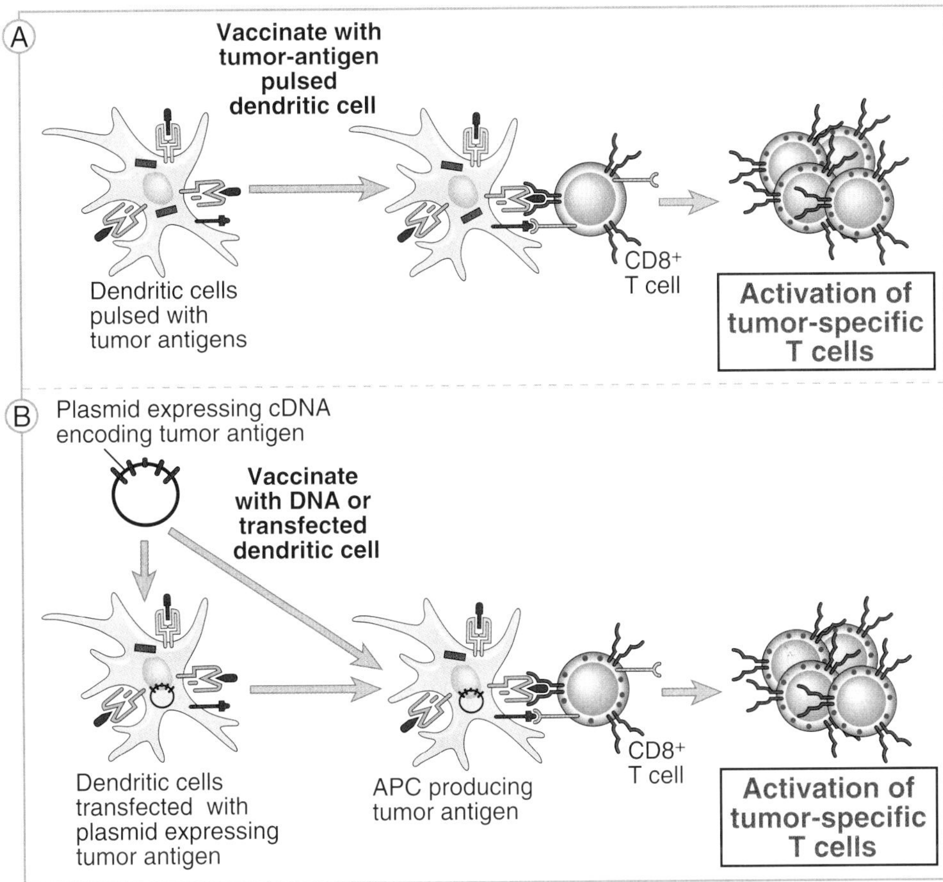

Figure 17–5 Tumor vaccines. The types of tumor vaccines that have shown efficacy in animal models are illustrated. Many vaccine approaches are undergoing clinical testing.

in preventing the herpesvirus-induced lymphoma called Marek's disease in chickens. In humans, the ongoing vaccination program against hepatitis B virus may reduce the incidence of hepatocellular carcinoma, a liver cancer associated with hepatitis B virus infection.

Augmentation of Host Immunity to Tumors with Cytokines and Costimulators

Cell-mediated immunity to tumors may be enhanced by expressing costimulators and cytokines in tumor cells and by treating tumor-bearing individuals with cytokines that stimulate the proliferation and differentiation of T lymphocytes and NK cells. As discussed earlier in this chapter, tumor cells may induce weak immune responses because they lack costimulators and usually do not express class II MHC molecules, so they do not activate helper T cells. Two potential approaches for boosting host responses to tumors are to artificially provide costimulation for tumor-specific T cells and to provide cytokines that can enhance the activation of tumor-specific T cells, particularly CD8⁺ CTLs (Fig. 17–6). Many cytokines also have the potential to induce nonspecific inflammatory responses, which by themselves may have anti-tumor activity.

The efficacy of enhancing T cell costimulation for anti-tumor immunotherapy has been demonstrated by animal experiments in which tumor cells were transfected with genes that encode B7 costimulatory molecules and used to vaccinate animals. These B7-expressing tumor cells induce protective immunity against unmodified tumor cells injected at a distant site. These successes with experimental tumor models have led to therapeutic trials in which a sample of a patient's tumor is propagated *in vitro*, transfected with costimulator genes, irradiated, and reintroduced into the patient. Such approaches may succeed even if the immunogenic antigens expressed on tumors are not known. Another strategy that exploits the role of costimulators is based on the idea that T cells use the inhibitory receptor for B7, called CTLA-4, to shut off responses (see Chapter 10). If tumor-bearing mice are vaccinated with the tumor and also treated with an antibody that blocks CTLA-4, the mice develop strong anti-tumor T cell responses and destroy the tumor. The potential of such approaches for tumor immunotherapy in humans is being evaluated.

It is possible to use cytokines to enhance adaptive and innate immune responses against tumors. Tumor cells may be transfected with cytokine genes to localize the cytokine effects to where they are needed (Table 17–3). For instance, when rodent tumors transfected with IL-2, IL-4, IFN-γ, or granulocyte-macrophage colony-stimulating factor (GM-CSF) genes are injected into animals, the tumors are rejected or begin to grow and then regress. In some cases, intense inflammatory infiltrates accumulate around the cytokine-secreting tumors, and the nature of the infiltrate varies with the cytokine. Different cytokines may stimulate anti-tumor immunity by different mechanisms (see Fig. 17–6).

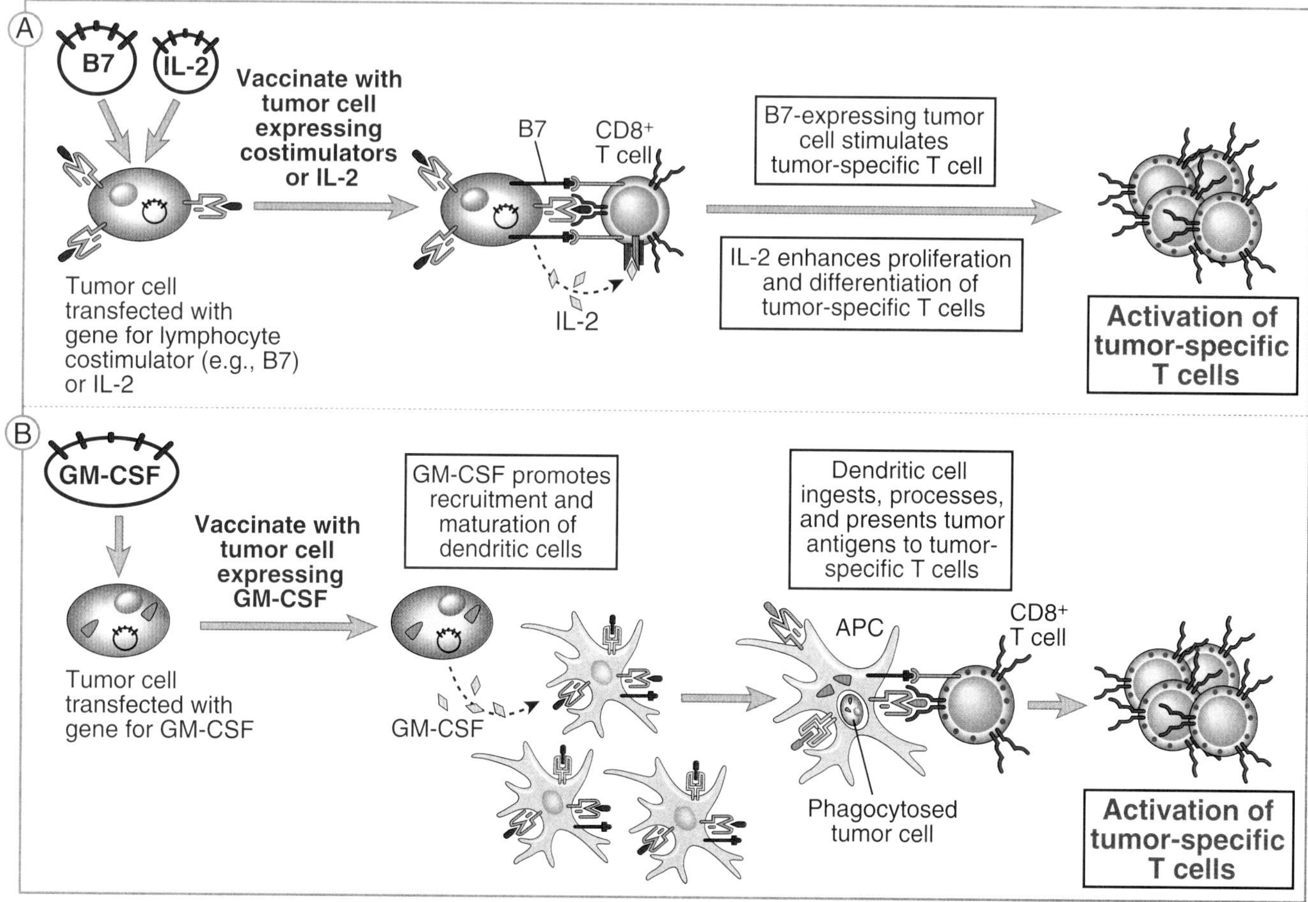

Figure 17–6 Enhancement of tumor cell immunogenicity by transfection of costimulator and cytokine genes.
Tumor cells that do not adequately stimulate T cells on transplantation into an animal will not be rejected and will therefore grow into tumors. Vaccination with tumor cells transfected with genes encoding costimulators or IL-2 (A) can lead to enhanced activation of T cells, and tumors transfected with GM-CSF (B) activate professional APCs, notably dendritic cells. These transfected tumor cell vaccines stimulate tumor-specific T cells, leading to T cell–mediated rejection of the tumor (even untransfected tumor cells).

Importantly, in several of these studies, the injection of cytokine-secreting tumors induced specific, T cell–mediated immunity to subsequent challenges by unmodified tumor cells. Thus, the local production of cytokines may augment T cell responses to tumor antigens, and cytokine-expressing tumors may act as effective tumor vaccines. Several clinical trials with cytokine gene–transfected tumors are under way in patients with advanced cancer.

Cytokines may also be administered systemically for the treatment of various human tumors (Table 17–4). This type of experimental therapy became feasible when pure preparations of cytokines became available in sufficient quantities. The largest clinical experience is with IL-2 administered in high doses alone or in combination with adoptive cellular immunotherapy (discussed later). After the administration of IL-2, numbers of blood T and B lymphocytes and NK cells are increased, NK cell activity is increased, and serum concentrations of TNF, IL-1, and IFN-γ are elevated. IL-2 presumably works by stimulating the proliferation and anti-tumor activity of NK cells and CTLs. The limitation of this treatment is that it can be highly toxic and induces fever, pulmonary edema, and vascular shock. These side effects occur because IL-2 stimulates the production of other cytokines by T cells, such as TNF and IFN-γ, and these cytokines act on vascular endothelium and other cell types. IL-2 has been effective in inducing measurable tumor regression responses in about 10% of patients with advanced melanoma and renal cell carcinoma and is currently an approved therapy for these cancers. IFN-α may be effective against tumors because it increases the cytolytic activity of NK cells and increases class I MHC expression on various cell types (see Chapter 11). Clinical trials of this cytokine indicate that it can induce the regression of renal carcinomas, melanomas, Kaposi's sarcoma, various lymphomas, and hairy cell leukemia (a B cell lineage tumor). IFN-α is currently used in combination with chemotherapy for the treatment of melanoma. Other cytokines, such as TNF and IFN-γ, are effective anti-tumor agents in animal models, but their use in patients is limited by serious toxic side effects. In some clinical trials, TNF is administered by isolated limb perfusion to patients with

Table 17–3. Immunotherapy with Cytokine Gene–Transfected Tumor Cells

Cytokine	Tumor rejection in animals	Inflammatory infiltrate	Immunity against parental tumor (animal models)	Clinical trials
Interleukin-2	Yes; mediated by T cells	Lymphocytes, neutrophils	In some cases of renal cancer, melanoma	Renal cancer, melanoma
Interleukin-4	Yes	Eosinophils, macrophages	No long-lasting immunity in human trials	Melanoma, renal cancer
Interferon-γ	Variable	Macrophages, other cells	Sometimes	
TNF	Variable	Neutrophils and lymphocytes	No	
GM-CSF	Yes	Macrophages, other cells	Yes (long-lived T cell immunity)	Renal cancer
Interleukin-3	Sometimes	Macrophages, other cells	Sometimes	

Abbreviations: GM-CSF, granulocyte-macrophage colony-stimulating factor; TNF, tumor necrosis factor.

melanomas or sarcomas limited to that limb. The potential of IL-12 to enhance anti-tumor T cell– and NK cell–mediated immune responses has aroused great interest, and early trials in patients with advanced cancer are now under way. Hematopoietic growth factors, including GM-CSF, G-CSF, and IL-11, are used in cancer treatment protocols to shorten periods of neutropenia and thrombocytopenia after chemotherapy or autologous bone marrow transplantation.

Nonspecific Stimulation of the Immune System

Immune responses to tumors may be stimulated by the local administration of inflammatory substances or by systemic treatment with agents that function as polyclonal activators of lymphocytes. Nonspecific immune stimulation of patients with tumors by injection of inflammatory substances such as bacillus Calmette-Guérin (BCG) at the sites of tumor growth has been tried for many years. The BCG mycobacteria activate macrophages and thereby promote macrophage-mediated killing of the tumor cells. In addition, the bacteria function as adjuvants and may stimulate T cell responses to tumor antigens. Another approach for immune stimulation is to administer low doses of activating anti-CD3 antibodies. In animal studies of transplantable tumors, this treatment results in polyclonal activation of T cells and, concomitantly, prevention of tumor growth. Early clinical trials with anti-CD3 antibody in patients with disseminated tumors are ongoing.

Table 17–4. Systemic Cytokine Therapy for Tumors

Cytokine	Tumor rejection in animals	Clinical trials	Toxicity
Interleukin-2	Yes	Melanoma, renal cancer, colon cancer; limited success (<15% response rate)	Vascular leak, shock, pulmonary edema
TNF	Only with local administration	Sarcoma, melanoma (isolated limb perfusion)	Septic shock syndrome
Interleukin-12	Variable	Toxicity trials (phase I) in melanoma, others	Abnormal liver function
Interleukin-6	Melanoma	Renal cancer (no benefit seen)	Fever, abnormal liver functions, CNS toxicity, hypotension
GM-CSF	No	In routine use to promote bone marrow recovery	Bone pain

Abbreviations: CNS, central nervous system; GM-CSF, granulocyte-macrophage colony-stimulating factor; TNF, tumor necrosis factor.

Cytokine therapies, discussed before, represent another method of enhancing immune responses in a non-specific manner.

Passive Immunotherapy for Tumors with T Cells and Antibodies

Passive immunotherapy involves the transfer of immune effectors, including tumor-specific T cells and antibodies, into patients. Passive immunization against tumors is rapid but does not lead to long-lived immunity. Several approaches to passive immunotherapy are being tried, with variable success.

Adoptive Cellular Therapy

Adoptive cellular immunotherapy is the transfer of cultured immune cells that have anti-tumor reactivity into a tumor-bearing host. The cells to be transferred are expanded from the lymphocytes of patients with the tumor. One protocol for adoptive cellular immunotherapy is to generate lymphokine-activated killer (LAK) cells by removing peripheral blood leukocytes from patients with the tumor, culturing the cells in high concentrations of IL-2, and injecting the LAK cells back into the patients (Fig. 17–7). As discussed previously, LAK cells are derived mainly from NK cells. Adoptive therapy with autologous LAK cells, in conjunction with *in vivo* administration of IL-2 or chemotherapeutic drugs, has yielded impressive results in mice, with regression of solid tumors. Human LAK cell therapy trials have thus far been largely restricted to advanced cases of metastatic tumors, and the efficacy of this approach appears to vary from patient to patient. A variation of this approach is to isolate tumor-infiltrating lymphocytes (TILs) from the inflammatory infiltrate present in and around solid tumors, obtained from surgical resection specimens, and to expand the TILs by culture in IL-2. The rationale for this approach is that TILs may be enriched for tumor-specific CTLs and for activated NK cells. Human trials with TIL therapy are ongoing.

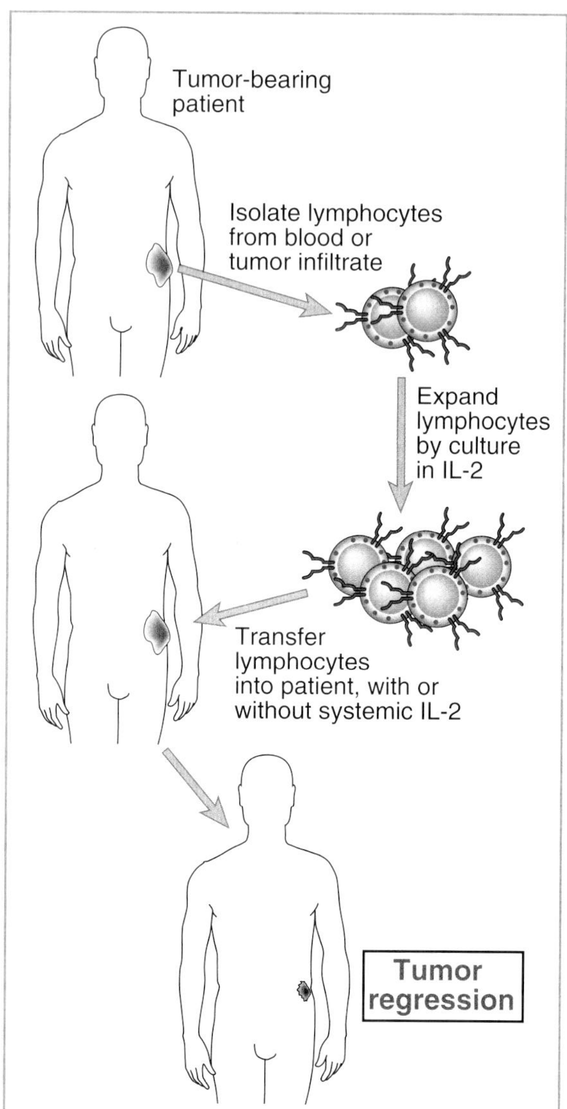

Figure 17–7 Adoptive cellular therapy. In a commonly used approach for adoptive cellular therapy, lymphocytes isolated from the blood or tumor infiltrate of a patient are expanded by culture in IL-2 and are infused back into the patient. This treatment, often combined with systemic IL-2 administration, leads to tumor regression in some patients.

Therapy with Anti-tumor Antibodies

Tumor-specific monoclonal antibodies may be useful for specific immunotherapy for tumors. The potential of using antibodies as "magic bullets" has been alluring to investigators for many years and is still an active area of research (Table 17–5). Anti-tumor antibodies eradicate tumors by the same effector mechanisms that are used to eliminate microbes, including opsonization and phagocytosis and activation of the complement system (see Chapter 14). A monoclonal antibody specific for the oncogene product Her-2/Neu, which is expressed at high levels in some tumors, has shown success in patients with breast cancer and is now approved for clinical use. In addition to eliciting immune effector mechanisms, the anti–Her-2/Neu antibody interferes with growth-signaling functions of the Her-2/Neu molecule. Because the anti-tumor antibodies used in the early human trials were mouse monoclonal antibodies, an immune response frequently occurred against the mouse Ig, resulting in anti-mouse Ig antibodies that caused increased clearance of the anti-tumor antibodies or blocked binding of the therapeutic agent to its target. This problem has been diminished by use of "humanized" antibodies consisting of the variable regions of a mouse monoclonal antibody specific for the tumor antigen combined with human Fc portions. One of the most difficult problems with the use of anti-tumor antibodies is the outgrowth of antigen loss variants of the tumor cells that no longer express the antigens that the antibodies recognize. One way to avoid this problem may be to use cocktails of antibodies specific for different antigens expressed on the same tumor.

Many variations on anti-tumor antibodies have been tried in attempts to improve their effectiveness. Tumor-

Table 17–5. Anti-tumor Antibodies for Immunotherapy

Specificity of antibody	Form of antibody used	Clinical trials
Her-2/Neu	Humanized mouse monoclonal	Breast cancer (approved for clinical use)
CD20 (B cell marker)	Humanized mouse monoclonal	B cell lymphoma
CD10	Humanized mouse monoclonal, immunotoxin	B cell lymphoma; in routine use to purge bone marrow of residual tumor cells
CEA	Humanized mouse monoclonal	Gastrointestinal cancers, lung cancer
CA-125	Mouse monoclonal	Ovarian cancer
GD3 ganglioside	Humanized mouse monoclonal	Melanoma

Abbreviation: CEA, carcinoembryonic antigen.

specific antibodies may be coupled to toxic molecules, radioisotopes, and anti-tumor drugs to promote the delivery of these cytotoxic agents specifically to the tumor. Toxins such as ricin and diphtheria toxin are potent inhibitors of protein synthesis and can be effective at extremely low doses if they are carried to tumors attached to anti-tumor antibodies; such conjugates are called **immunotoxins**. This approach requires covalent coupling of the toxin (lacking its cell-binding component) to an anti-tumor antibody molecule without loss of toxicity or antibody specificity. The systemically injected immunotoxin is endocytosed by tumor cells, and the toxin part is delivered to its intracellular site of action. Several practical difficulties must be overcome for this technique to be successful. The specificity of the antibody must be such that it does not bind to non-tumor cells. A sufficient amount of antibody must reach the appropriate tumor target before it is cleared from the blood by Fc receptor–bearing phagocytic cells. The toxins, drugs, or radioisotopes attached to the antibody may have systemic effects as a result of circulation through normal tissues. For example, hepatotoxicity and vascular leak syndromes are common problems with immunotoxin therapy. Administration of immunotoxins may result in antibody responses against the toxins and the injected antibodies. Because of these practical difficulties, clinical trials of immunotoxins have had variable and modest success.

Anti-idiotypic antibodies have been used to treat B cell lymphomas that express surface Ig with particular idiotypes. The idiotype is a highly specific tumor antigen because it is expressed only on the neoplastic clone of B cells, and it was once hoped that anti-idiotypic antibodies would be effective therapeutic reagents with absolute tumor specificity. (Anti-idiotypic antibodies are raised by immunizing rabbits with a patient's B cell tumor and depleting the serum of reactivity against all other human immunoglobulins.) The approach has not proved generally successful, largely because of the selective outgrowth of tumor cells with altered idiotypes that do not bind the anti-idiotypic antibody. In part, this result may reflect the high rate of somatic mutation in Ig genes and the fact that the surface Ig is dispensable for tumor growth.

Anti-tumor antibodies are also used to remove cancer cells from the bone marrow before autologous marrow transplantation. In this protocol, some of the patient's bone marrow is removed, and the patient is given doses of radiation and chemotherapy lethal enough to destroy tumor cells as well as the remaining normal marrow cells. The bone marrow cells removed from the patient are treated with antibodies or immunotoxins specific for tumor antigens to kill any tumor cells. The treated marrow, having been purged of tumor cells, is transplanted back into the patient to reconstitute the hematopoietic system destroyed by irradiation and chemotherapy.

Summary

- Tumors express antigens that are recognized by the immune system, but most tumors are weakly immunogenic, and immune responses often fail to prevent the growth of tumors. The immune system can be stimulated to effectively kill tumors.
- Tumor antigens recognized by CTLs are the principal inducers of and targets for antitumor immunity. These antigens include mutants of oncogenes and other cellular proteins, normal proteins whose expression is dysregulated or increased in tumors, and products of oncogenic viruses.
- Antibodies specific for tumor cells recognize antigens that are used for diagnosis and are potential

targets for antibody therapy. These antigens include oncofetal antigens, which are expressed normally during fetal life and whose expression is dysregulated in some tumors; altered surface glycoproteins and glycolipids; and molecules that are normally expressed on the cells from which the tumors arise and are thus differentiation antigens for particular cell types.

- Immune responses that are capable of killing tumor cells consist of CTLs, NK cells, and activated macrophages. The role of these immune effector mechanisms in protecting individuals from tumors is not well defined.

- Tumors evade immune responses by several mechanisms, including down-regulating the expression of MHC molecules, selecting cells that do not express tumor antigens, producing immunosuppressive substances, and inducing tolerance to tumor antigens.

- Immunotherapy for tumors is designed to augment active immune responses against these tumors or to administer tumor-specific immune effectors to patients. Immune responses may be actively enhanced by vaccination with tumor cells or antigens, administration of tumors modified to express high levels of costimulators or cytokines that stimulate T cell proliferation and differentiation, and systemic administration of cytokines. Approaches for passive immunotherapy include the administration of antitumor antibodies, antibodies conjugated with toxic drugs (immunotoxins), and tumor-reactive T cells and NK cells isolated from patients and expanded by culture with growth factors.

Selected Readings

Burnet FM. The concept of immunological surveillance. Progress in Experimental Tumor Research 13:1–27, 1970.

Carter P. Improving the efficacy of antibody-based cancer therapies. Nature Reviews Cancer 1:118–129, 2001.

Coulie PG, T Hanagiri, and M Takenoyama. From tumor antigens to immunotherapy. International Journal of Clinical Oncology 6:163–170, 2001.

Fong L, and EG Engelman. Dendritic cells in cancer immunotherapy. Annual Review of Immunology 18:245–273, 2000.

Herberman RB. Cancer immunotherapy with natural killer cells. Seminars in Oncology 29:27–30, 2002.

Jager D, E Jager, and A Knuth. Immune responses to tumor antigens: implications for antigen specific immunotherapy of cancer. Journal of Clinical Pathology 54:669–674, 2001.

Kreitman RJ. Immunotoxins in cancer therapy. Current Opinion in Immunology 11:570–578, 1999.

Pardoll DM. Spinning molecular immunology into successful immunotherapy. Nature Reviews Immunology 2:227–238, 2002.

Reiter Y. Recombinant immunotoxins in targeted cancer cell therapy. Advances in Cancer Research 81:93–124, 2001.

Rosenberg SA. Progress in human tumor immunology and immunotherapy. Nature 411:380–384, 2001.

Smyth MJ, DI Godfrey, and JA Trapani. A fresh look at tumor immunosurveillance and immunotherapy. Nature Immunology 2:293–299, 2001.

Stevanovic S. Identification of tumour-associated T-cell epitopes for vaccine development. Nature Reviews Cancer 2:514–520, 2002.

Yee C, SR Riddell, and PD Greenberg. Prospects for adoptive T cell therapy. Current Opinion in Immunology 9:702–708, 1997.

Yee C, and P Greenberg. Modulating T-cell immunity to tumours: new strategies for monitoring T-cell responses. Nature Reviews Cancer 2:409–419, 2002.

Chapter 18

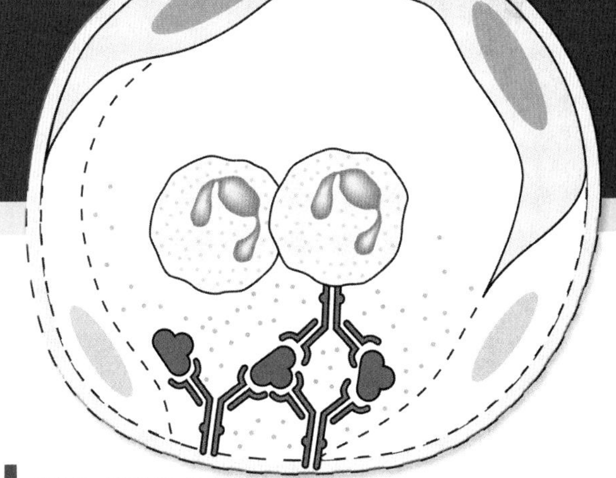

Diseases Caused by Immune Responses: Hypersensitivity and Autoimmunity

Adaptive immunity serves the important function of host defense against microbial infections, but immune responses are also capable of causing tissue injury and disease. Disorders caused by immune responses are called **hypersensitivity diseases.** This term arose from the clinical definition of immunity as "sensitivity," which is based on the observation that an individual who has been exposed to an antigen exhibits a detectable reaction, or is "sensitive," to subsequent encounters with that antigen. A common cause of hypersensitivity diseases is failure of self-tolerance, which is the property of the immune system that ensures that individuals normally do not respond to their own antigens. Diseases caused by failure of self-tolerance and subsequent immune responses against self, or autologous, antigens are called **autoimmune diseases.** Hypersensitivity diseases may also result from uncontrolled or excessive responses against foreign antigens, such as microbes and noninfectious environmental antigens.

In this chapter, we describe the pathogenesis of different types of hypersensitivity diseases, with an emphasis on the effector mechanisms that cause tissue injury and on the mechanisms of autoimmunity. Throughout the chapter, we use examples of clinical and experimental diseases to illustrate important principles. We conclude with a brief consideration of the treatment of immunologic diseases.

Types of Hypersensitivity Diseases

Hypersensitivity diseases represent a clinically heterogeneous group of disorders. The two principal factors that determine the clinical and pathologic manifestations of such diseases are the type of immune response that causes tissue injury and the nature and location of the antigen that is the target of this response.

Hypersensitivity diseases are commonly classified according to the type of immune response and the

effector mechanism responsible for cell and tissue injury (Table 18–1). Immediate hypersensitivity caused by IgE antibodies and mast cells, which is also called type I hypersensitivity, is the most prevalent type of hypersensitivity disease and will be described separately in Chapter 19. Antibodies other than IgE can cause tissue injury by recruiting and activating inflammatory cells and by interfering with normal cellular functions. Some of these antibodies are specific for antigens of particular cells or the extracellular matrix and are found either attached to these cells or tissues or as unbound antibodies in the circulation; the diseases induced by such antibodies are called type II hypersensitivity disorders. Other antibodies may form immune complexes in the circulation, and the complexes are subsequently deposited in tissues, particularly in blood vessels, and cause injury. Immune complex diseases are also called type III hypersensitivity. Finally, tissue injury may be due to T lymphocytes that activate the effector mechanisms of delayed-type hypersensitivity (DTH) or directly kill target cells; such conditions are called type IV hypersensitivity disorders.

In our discussion, we use descriptions that identify the pathogenic mechanisms rather than the less informative numerical designations. This classification is useful because distinct types of pathogenic immune responses show different patterns of tissue injury and may vary in their tissue specificity. As a result, they produce disorders with distinct clinical and pathologic features. However, immunologic diseases in the clinical situation are often complex and due to combinations of humoral and cell-mediated immune responses and multiple effector mechanisms. This complexity is not surprising given that a single antigen may normally stimulate both humoral and cell-mediated immune responses.

Effector Mechanisms of Immunologic Tissue Injury and Disease

The effector mechanisms of immunologic diseases are the same as the mechanisms of humoral and cell-mediated immunity against microbes and other foreign antigens. Immune responses cause disease when these responses are directed against self antigens, as in autoimmune disorders, or when they are against foreign antigens but are uncontrolled. The first immunologic diseases in which the pathogenic mechanisms were defined were diseases caused by the deposition of antibodies in tissues. These types of diseases were identified before T cell–mediated diseases largely because techniques for detecting circulating autoantibodies and immunoglobulin deposited in diseased tissues were developed well before methods for identifying and isolating T cells from lesions or from the blood of patients. The importance of T lymphocytes as mediators of human immunologic diseases was increasingly recognized in the 1980s. This insight was largely due to two technological advances—the production of monoclonal antibodies that identify phenotypically and functionally distinct subsets of T cells, and methods for isolating and propagating T cells from lymphoid tissues and lesions. Moreover, the realization that T lymphocytes are critical for maintaining self-tolerance to many protein antigens has led to increasing interest in their role in autoimmune disorders.

Table 18–1. Classification of Immunologic Diseases

Type of hypersensitivity	Pathologic immune mechanisms	Mechanisms of tissue injury and disease
Immediate hypersensitivity: Type I	IgE antibody	Mast cells and their mediators (vasoactive amines, lipid mediators, cytokines)
Antibody mediated: Type II	IgM, IgG antibodies against cell surface or extracellular matrix antigens	Opsonization and phagocytosis of cells Complement- and Fc receptor–mediated recruitment and activation of leukocytes (neutrophils, macrophages) Abnormalities in cellular functions, e.g., hormone receptor signaling
Immune complex mediated: Type III	Immune complexes of circulating antigens and IgM or IgG antibodies	Complement- and Fc receptor–mediated recruitment and activation of leukocytes
T cell mediated: Type IV	1. $CD4^+$ T cells (delayed-type hypersensitivity) 2. $CD8^+$ CTLs (T cell–mediated cytolysis)	1. Macrophage activation, cytokine-mediated inflammation 2. Direct target cell killing, cytokine-mediated inflammation

Diseases Caused by Antibodies

Antibody-mediated diseases are produced either by antibodies that bind to antigens in particular cells or extracellular tissues or by antigen-antibody complexes that form in the circulation and are deposited in vessel walls (Fig. 18–1). To prove that a particular disease is caused by antibodies, one would need to demonstrate that the lesions can be induced in a normal animal by the adoptive transfer of immunoglobulin purified from the blood or affected tissues of individuals with the disease. An experiment of nature is occasionally seen in children of mothers suffering from antibody-mediated diseases. These infants may be born with transient expression of such diseases because of transplacental passage of antibodies. However, in clinical situations, the diagnosis of diseases caused by antibodies or immune complexes is usually based on the demonstration of antibodies or immune complexes in the circulation or deposited in tissues as well as clinicopathologic similarities with experimental diseases that are proved to be antibody mediated by adoptive transfer.

Diseases Caused by Antibodies Against Fixed Cell and Tissue Antigens

Antibodies against cellular or matrix antigens cause diseases that specifically affect the cells or tissues where these antigens are present, and these diseases are often not systemic. In most cases, such antibodies are autoantibodies, but they may occasionally be produced against a foreign antigen that is immunologically cross-reactive with a component of self tissues. Antibodies against tissue antigens cause disease by three main mechanisms (Fig. 18–2). First, antibodies may opsonize cells or activate the complement system, resulting in the production of complement proteins that opsonize cells. These cells are phagocytosed and destroyed by phagocytes that express receptors for the Fc portions of antibodies and receptors for complement proteins. This is the principal mechanism of cell destruction in autoimmune hemolytic anemia and autoimmune thrombocytopenic purpura. The same mechanism is responsible for hemolysis in transfusion reactions. Second, antibodies deposited in tissues recruit neutrophils and macrophages, which bind to the antibodies or attached

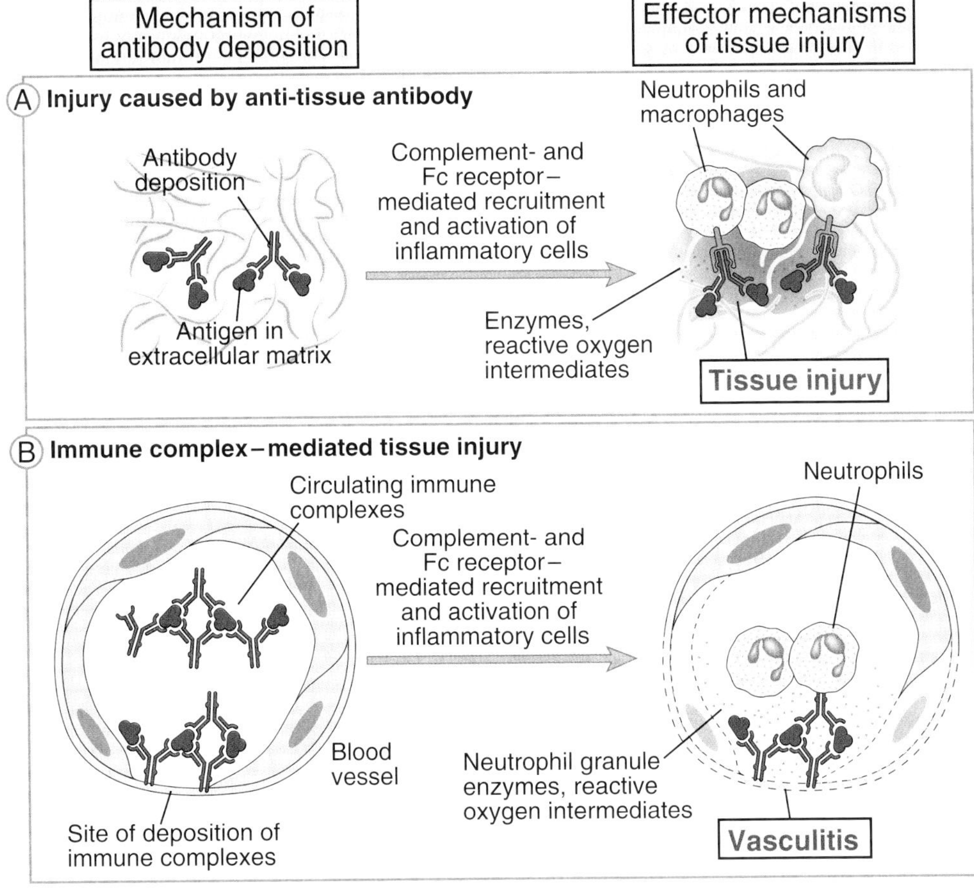

Figure 18–1 Types of antibody-mediated diseases.
Antibodies may bind specifically to tissue antigens (A), or they may be deposited as immune complexes that are formed in the circulation (B). In both cases, the deposited antibodies induce inflammation, leading to tissue injury.

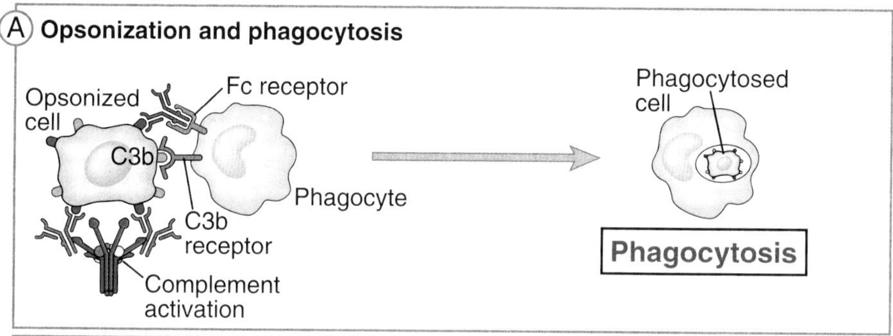

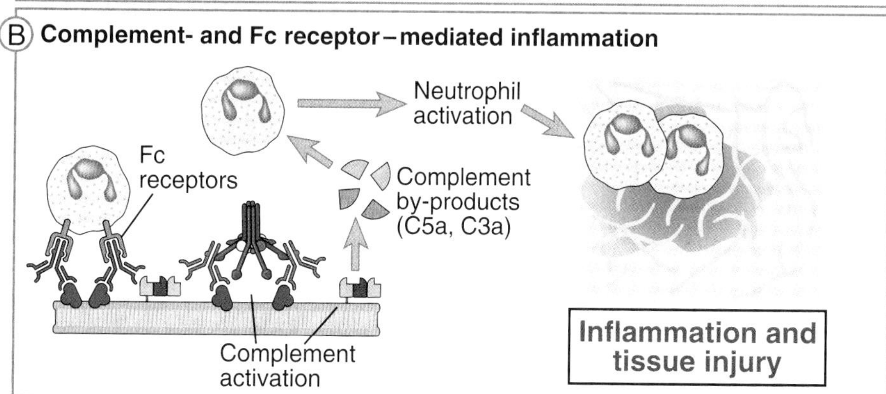

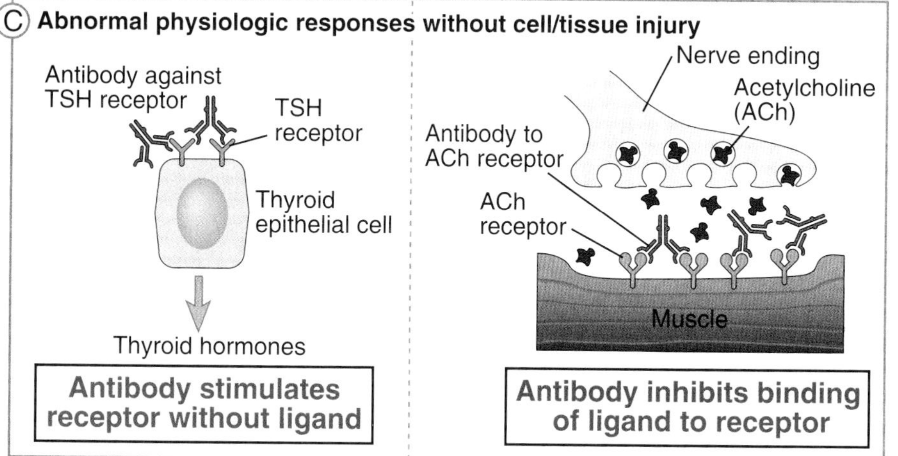

Figure 18–2 Effector mechanisms of antibody-mediated disease.

A. Antibodies opsonize cells and may activate complement, generating complement products that also opsonize cells, leading to phagocytosis of the cells through phagocyte Fc receptors or C3 receptors.

B. Antibodies recruit leukocytes by binding to Fc receptors or by activating complement and thereby releasing by-products that are chemotactic for leukocytes.

C. Antibodies specific for cell surface receptors for hormones or neurotransmitters may stimulate the activity of the receptors even in the absence of the hormone *(left panel)* or may inhibit binding of the neurotransmitter to its receptor *(right panel)*. TSH, thyroid-stimulating hormone.

complement proteins by Fc and complement receptors. These leukocytes are activated and their products induce tissue injury. This is the mechanism of injury in antibody-mediated glomerulonephritis and many other diseases. Third, antibodies that bind to normal cellular receptors or other proteins may interfere with the functions of these receptors or proteins and cause disease without actual tissue damage. Antibody-mediated functional abnormalities are the cause of Graves' disease (hyperthyroidism) and myasthenia gravis. Examples of hypersensitivity diseases in humans that are caused by autoantibodies against self antigens are listed in Table 18–2. Tissue deposits of antibodies may be detected by morphologic examination in some of these diseases, and the deposition of antibody is often associated with local complement activation, inflammation, and tissue injury (Fig. 18–3).

Immune Complex–Mediated Diseases

Immune complexes that cause disease may be composed of either self antigens or foreign antigens with bound antibodies. The pathologic features of diseases caused by immune complexes reflect the site of immune complex deposition and are not determined by the cellular source of the antigen. Therefore, immune complex–mediated diseases tend to be systemic, with little or no specificity for a particular tissue or organ.

The occurrence of diseases caused by immune complexes was suspected as early as 1911 by an astute physician named Clemens von Pirquet. At that time, diphtheria infections were being treated with serum from horses immunized with the diphtheria toxin, which is an example of passive immunization against

Table 18–2. Examples of Diseases Caused by Cell- or Tissue-Specific Antibodies

Disease	Target antigen	Mechanisms of disease	Clinicopathologic manifestations
Autoimmune hemolytic anemia	Erythrocyte membrane proteins (Rh blood group antigens, I antigen)	Opsonization and phagocytosis of erythrocytes	Hemolysis, anemia
Autoimmune thrombocytopenic purpura	Platelet membrane proteins (gpIIb:IIIa integrin)	Opsonization and phagocytosis of platelets	Bleeding
Pemphigus vulgaris	Proteins in intercellular junctions of epidermal cells (epidermal cadherin)	Antibody-mediated activation of proteases, disruption of intercellular adhesions	Skin vesicles (bullae)
Vasculitis caused by ANCA	Neutrophil granule proteins, presumably released from activated neutrophils	Neutrophil degranulation and inflammation	Vasculitis
Goodpasture's syndrome	Noncollagenous protein in basement membranes of kidney glomeruli and lung alveoli	Complement- and Fc receptor–mediated inflammation	Nephritis, lung hemorrhage
Acute rheumatic fever	Streptococcal cell wall antigen; antibody cross-reacts with myocardial antigen	Inflammation, macrophage activation	Myocarditis, arthritis
Myasthenia gravis	Acetylcholine receptor	Antibody inhibits acetylcholine binding, down-modulates receptors	Muscle weakness, paralysis
Graves' disease (hyperthyroidism)	TSH receptor	Antibody-mediated stimulation of TSH receptors	Hyperthyroidism
Insulin-resistant diabetes	Insulin receptor	Antibody inhibits binding of insulin	Hyperglycemia, ketoacidosis
Pernicious anemia	Intrinsic factor of gastric parietal cells	Neutralization of intrinsic factor, decreased absorption of vitamin B_{12}	Abnormal erythropoiesis, anemia

Abbreviations: ANCA, antineutrophil cytoplasmic antibodies; TSH, thyroid-stimulating hormone.

the toxin by the transfer of serum containing antitoxin antibodies. von Pirquet noted that joint inflammation (arthritis), rash, and fever developed in patients injected with the antitoxin-containing horse serum. Two clinical features of this reaction suggested that it was not due to the infection or a toxic component of the serum itself. First, these symptoms appeared even after the injection of horse serum not containing the antitoxin, so the lesions could not be attributed to the anti-diphtheria antibody. Second, the symptoms appeared at least a week after the first injection of horse serum and more rapidly with each repeated injection. von Pirquet concluded that this disease was due to a host response to some component of the serum. He suggested that the host made antibodies to horse serum proteins, these antibodies formed complexes with the injected proteins, and the disease was due to the antibodies or immune complexes. We now know that his conclusions were entirely accurate. He called this disease serum disease; it is now more commonly known as **serum sickness** and is the prototype for systemic immune complex–mediated disorders.

Much of our current knowledge of immune complex diseases is based on analyses of experimental models of serum sickness. Immunization of an animal such as a rabbit with a large dose of a foreign protein antigen leads to the formation of antibodies against the antigen (Fig. 18–4). These antibodies complex with circulating antigen and initially lead to enhanced phagocytosis and clearance of the antigen by macrophages in the liver and spleen. As more and more antigen-antibody complexes are formed, some of them are deposited in vascular beds. In these tissues, the antibodies in the complexes may activate complement, with a concomitant fall in serum complement levels.

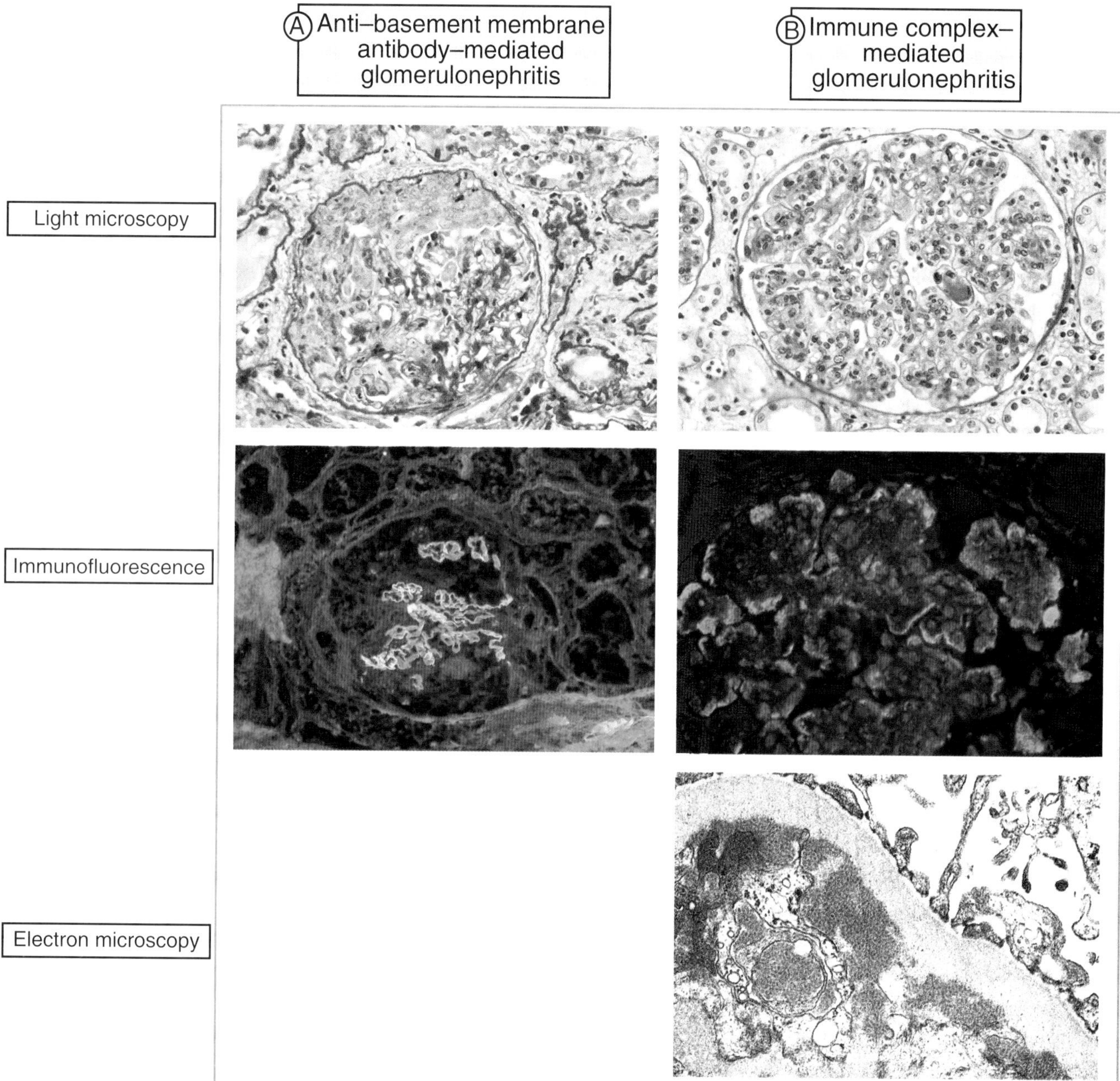

Figure 18–3 Pathologic features of antibody-mediated glomerulonephritis.
A. Glomerulonephritis induced by an antibody against the glomerular basement membrane (Goodpasture's syndrome): the light micrograph shows glomerular inflammation and severe damage, and immunofluorescence shows smooth (linear) deposits of antibody along the basement membrane.
B. Glomerulonephritis induced by the deposition of immune complexes (systemic lupus erythematosus): the light micrograph shows neutrophilic inflammation, and the immunofluorescence and electron micrograph show coarse (granular) deposits of antigen-antibody complexes along the basement membrane. (Courtesy of Dr. Helmut Rennke, Department of Pathology, Brigham and Women's Hospital, Boston.)

Complement activation leads to recruitment and activation of inflammatory cells, predominantly neutrophils, at the sites of immune complex deposition, and the neutrophils cause tissue injury. Neutrophils also bind to the immune complexes by their Fcγ receptors. Because the complexes are deposited mainly in small arteries, renal glomeruli, and the synovia of joints, the clinical and pathologic manifestations are vasculitis, nephritis, and arthritis. The clinical symptoms are usually short-lived, and the lesions heal unless the antigen is injected again. This type of disease is an example of acute serum sickness. A more indolent and prolonged disease, called chronic serum sickness, is produced by multiple injections of antigen, which

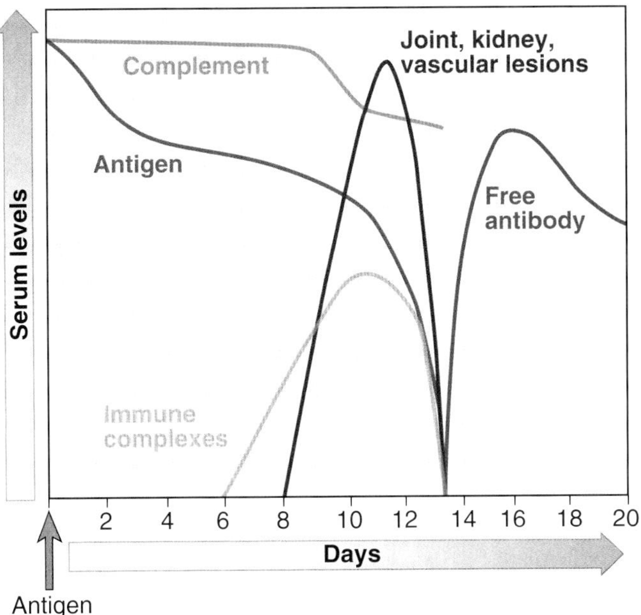

Figure 18–4 Sequence of immunologic responses in experimental acute serum sickness.
Injection of bovine serum albumin into a rabbit leads to the production of specific antibody and the formation of immune complexes. These complexes are deposited in multiple tissues, activate complement (leading to a fall in serum complement levels), and cause inflammatory lesions, which resolve as the complexes and the remaining antigen are removed. (Adapted from Cochrane CG. Immune complex–mediated tissue injury. *In* Cohen S, PA Ward, and RT McCluskey [eds]. Mechanisms of Immunopathology. Werbel & Peck, New York, 1979, pp 29–48. Copyright 1979, Wiley-Liss, Inc.)

lead to the formation of smaller complexes that are deposited most often in the kidneys, arteries, and lungs.

- A localized form of experimental immune complex–mediated vasculitis is called the **Arthus reaction.** It is induced by injecting an antigen subcutaneously into a previously immunized animal or an animal that has been given intravenous antibody specific for the antigen. Circulating antibodies rapidly bind to the injected antigen and form immune complexes that are deposited in the walls of small arteries at the injection site. This deposition gives rise to a local cutaneous vasculitis with necrosis.

Antigen-antibody complexes are produced during normal immune responses, but they cause disease only when they are produced in excessive amounts, are not efficiently cleared, and become deposited in tissues. The amount of immune complex deposition in tissues is determined by the nature of the complexes and the characteristics of the blood vessels. Small complexes are often not phagocytosed and tend to be deposited in vessels more than large complexes, which are usually cleared by phagocytes. Complexes containing cationic antigens bind avidly to negatively charged components of the basement membranes of blood vessels and kidney glomeruli. Such complexes typically produce severe and long-lasting tissue injury. Capillaries in the renal glomeruli and synovia are vessels in which plasma is ultrafiltered (to form urine and synovial fluid, respectively) by passing through the capillary wall at high hydrostatic pressure, and these locations are among the most common sites of immune complex deposition. Immune complexes may also activate inflammatory cells and mast cells to secrete cytokines and vasoactive mediators, which cause increased adhesion of leukocytes to the endothelium, increased vascular permeability, and enhanced deposition of immune complexes in vessel walls by enlarging the interendothelial spaces.

The deposition of immune complexes in vessel walls leads to complement- and Fc receptor–mediated inflammation and injury to the vessels and adjacent tissues. Deposits of antibody and complement may be detected in the vessels, and if the antigen is known, it is possible to identify antigen molecules in the deposits as well (see Fig. 18–3). Many systemic immunologic diseases in humans are caused by the deposition of immune complexes in blood vessels (Table 18–3). A prototype of such diseases is **systemic lupus erythematosus** (SLE), an autoimmune disease in which numerous autoantibodies are produced. Its clinical manifestations include glomerulonephritis and arthritis, which are attributed to the deposition of immune complexes composed of self DNA or nucleoprotein antigens and specific antibodies (Box 18–1).

Table 18–3. Examples of Human Immune Complex–Mediated Diseases

Disease	Antigen involved	Clinicopathologic manifestations
Systemic lupus erythematosus	DNA, nucleoproteins, others	Nephritis, arthritis, vasculitis
Polyarteritis nodosa	Hepatitis B virus surface antigen	Vasculitis
Poststreptococcal glomerulonephritis	Streptococcal cell wall antigen(s); may be "planted" in glomerular basement membrane	Nephritis
Serum sickness	Various proteins	Arthritis,vasculitis, nephritis

BOX 18–1

Systemic Lupus Erythematosus

CLINICAL FEATURES Systemic lupus erythematosus (SLE) is a chronic, remitting and relapsing, multisystem autoimmune disease that affects predominantly women, with an incidence of 1 in 700 among women between the ages of 20 and 60 years (about 1 in 250 among black women) and a female-to-male ratio of 10:1. The principal clinical manifestations are rashes, arthritis, and glomerulonephritis, but hemolytic anemia, thrombocytopenia, and central nervous system involvement are also common. Many different autoantibodies are found in patients with SLE. The most frequent are antinuclear, particularly anti-DNA, antibodies; others include antibodies against ribonucleoproteins, histones, and nucleolar antigens. Immune complexes formed from these autoantibodies and their specific antigens are responsible for glomerulonephritis, arthritis, and vasculitis involving small arteries throughout the body. Hemolytic anemia and thrombocytopenia are due to autoantibodies against erythrocytes and platelets, respectively. The principal diagnostic test for the disease is the presence of antinuclear antibodies; antibodies against double-stranded native DNA are specific for SLE.

PATHOGENESIS In animal models of SLE, the production of high-affinity antinuclear antibodies has been shown to depend on helper T cells. Pathogenic helper T cells are specific mainly for peptides derived from nucleosomal proteins. Presumably, B cells specific for self DNA bind nucleosomal protein-DNA complexes, process the proteins, and present peptide epitopes to helper T cells, with the subsequent production of anti-DNA autoantibodies. It is not known whether the primary pathogenic defect (failure of central or peripheral tolerance) is in B lymphocytes, in helper T cells, or in both. It is thought that the antigens that elicit autoantibody production are released from apoptotic cells, which is one reason that exposure to ultraviolet light (which promotes apoptosis) exacerbates disease. Genetic factors also contribute to the disease. The relative risk for individuals with HLA-DR2 or HLA-DR3 is 2 to 3, and if both haplotypes are present, the relative risk is about 5. Deficiencies of classical pathway complement proteins, especially C2 or C4, are seen in about 10% of patients with SLE. The complement deficiencies may result in defective clearance of immune complexes. Studies with mice also suggest a role of complement proteins in displaying self antigens and maintaining B cell tolerance.

ANIMAL MODELS Several inbred mouse strains in which lupus-like autoimmune diseases spontaneously develop have provided valuable experimental systems for analyzing the pathogenesis of this disorder. The first to be described and the ones most like SLE are the NZB strain and the (NZB × NZW)F_1. Kidney lesions and hemolytic anemia develop in female mice, and anti-DNA autoantibodies are produced spontaneously. The B cells of (NZB × NZW)F_1 mice are hyperresponsive to foreign antigens as well as to polyclonal activators and cytokines, and autoantibody production is dependent on pathogenic helper T cells reactive with nucleosomal peptides. Extensive breeding studies have shown that MHC genes from the NZW parent and non-MHC genes inherited from both parental strains contribute to development of the disease. Attempts are being made to introduce the susceptibility genes from these mice individually into normal mice and to examine the immunologic abnormalities induced by the presence of each of these genes. Such approaches hold great promise for elucidating the genetic basis of autoimmunity.

Mice with mutations in either the Fas or Fas ligand genes develop an autoimmune disease with some resemblance to SLE. The *lpr* (for *lympho**pr**oliferation*) and *gld* (for *g*eneralized *l*ymphoproliferative *d*isease) genes are mutant alleles of the Fas and Fas ligand genes, respectively, and the mouse strains that are homozygous for these mutant alleles have greatly reduced expression of Fas or nonfunctional Fas ligand. Both lpr and gld mice produce multiple autoantibodies, especially anti-DNA antibodies, and develop immune complex nephritis. Severe lymphadenopathy also develops in these inbred strains because of the accumulation of an unusual population of functionally inert, $CD3^+CD4^-CD8^-$ T cells that also express a CD45 isoform called B220 that is normally found on B cells. Because of the defect in Fas or Fas ligand in these mice, activation-induced cell death of mature $CD4^+$ T lymphocytes is defective, and this defect apparently results in the accumulation of self-reactive helper T cells. In addition, anergic B cells cannot be eliminated by Fas-mediated killing. Both functional abnormalities contribute to autoantibody production. The lymphadenopathy can be segregated from and appears to be unrelated to the autoimmune disease. The disease of lpr and gld mice is also influenced by background genes in that it is more severe in an inbred strain called MRL than in any other. A phenotypically similar human disease called the autoimmune lymphoproliferative syndrome is caused by mutations in the gene encoding Fas that abolish the ability of this death receptor to deliver apoptotic signals. No evidence for Fas or Fas ligand abnormalities has been demonstrated in typical SLE, and by this criterion, these inbred mouse strains are not true animal models of human SLE.

A third inbred strain in which a lupus-like disease develops is a recombinant strain called BXSB; disease susceptibility in this strain is linked to the Y chromosome, and only males are affected. These mice produce anti-DNA antibodies, and severe nephritis and vasculitis develop.

Another mutant mouse strain, called the viable moth-eaten mouse (because of skin lesions), also produces high levels of autoantibodies. The moth-eaten mouse carries a mutation of the tyrosine phosphatase SHP-1, which associates with several receptors that serve negative regulatory functions in cells of the immune system. The signal transduction abnormalities caused by the phosphatase mutation and the mechanism of autoantibody production in moth-eaten mice are not well defined.

Transgenic mouse models of lupus have been created in which an antibody against self DNA is expressed in B cells as a transgene. How these B cells are normally regulated and how the controls may fail and give rise to anti-DNA antibody production are important questions that are being addressed.

Diseases Caused by T Lymphocytes

T lymphocytes cause tissue injury either by triggering delayed-type hypersensitivity (DTH) reactions or by directly killing target cells (Fig. 18–5). DTH reactions are elicited by CD4$^+$ T cells of the T_H1 subset and CD8$^+$ cells, both of which secrete cytokines that activate macrophages (interferon-γ [IFN-γ]) and induce inflammation (such as tumor necrosis factor [TNF]). In some T cell–mediated disorders, CD8$^+$ cytolytic T lymphocytes (CTLs) directly kill target cells bearing class I major histocompatibility complex (MHC)–associated antigens. The T cells that cause tissue injury may be autoreactive, or they may be specific for foreign protein antigens that are present in or bound to cells or tissues. T lymphocyte–mediated tissue injury may also accompany strong protective immune responses against persistent microbes, especially intracellular microbes that resist eradication by phagocytes and antibodies.

A role for T cells in causing a particular immunologic disease is suspected largely because of the demonstration of T cells in lesions and the isolation of T cells specific for self antigens from the tissues or blood of patients. Furthermore, cytokines secreted by activated T cells induce alterations in adjacent tissues that are used as indicators of local T cell stimulation. For instance, IFN-γ induces the expression of class II MHC molecules on cells that do not express these molecules constitutively. Abnormal expression of class II MHC molecules in a tissue suggests that T cells have been activated in the immediate environment.

Diseases Caused by Delayed-type Hypersensitivity

In DTH reactions, tissue injury results from the products of activated macrophages, such as hydrolytic enzymes, reactive oxygen intermediates, nitric oxide, and proinflammatory cytokines (see Chapter 13). Vascular endothelial cells in the lesions may express enhanced levels of cytokine-regulated surface proteins such as adhesion molecules and class II MHC molecules. Chronic DTH reactions often produce fibrosis as a result of the secretion of cytokines and growth factors by the macrophages.

Many organ-specific autoimmune diseases are caused by DTH reactions induced by autoreactive T cells (Table 18–4). In **insulin-dependent diabetes mellitus** (IDDM) (Box 18–2), infiltrates of lymphocytes and macrophages are found around the islets of Langerhans in the pancreas, with destruction of insulin-producing β cells in the islets and a resultant deficiency in insulin production. In animal models of IDDM, the disease can be transferred to young, prediseased animals by injecting T cells from older diseased animals. **Multiple sclerosis** (MS) is an autoimmune disease of the central nervous system in which CD4$^+$ T

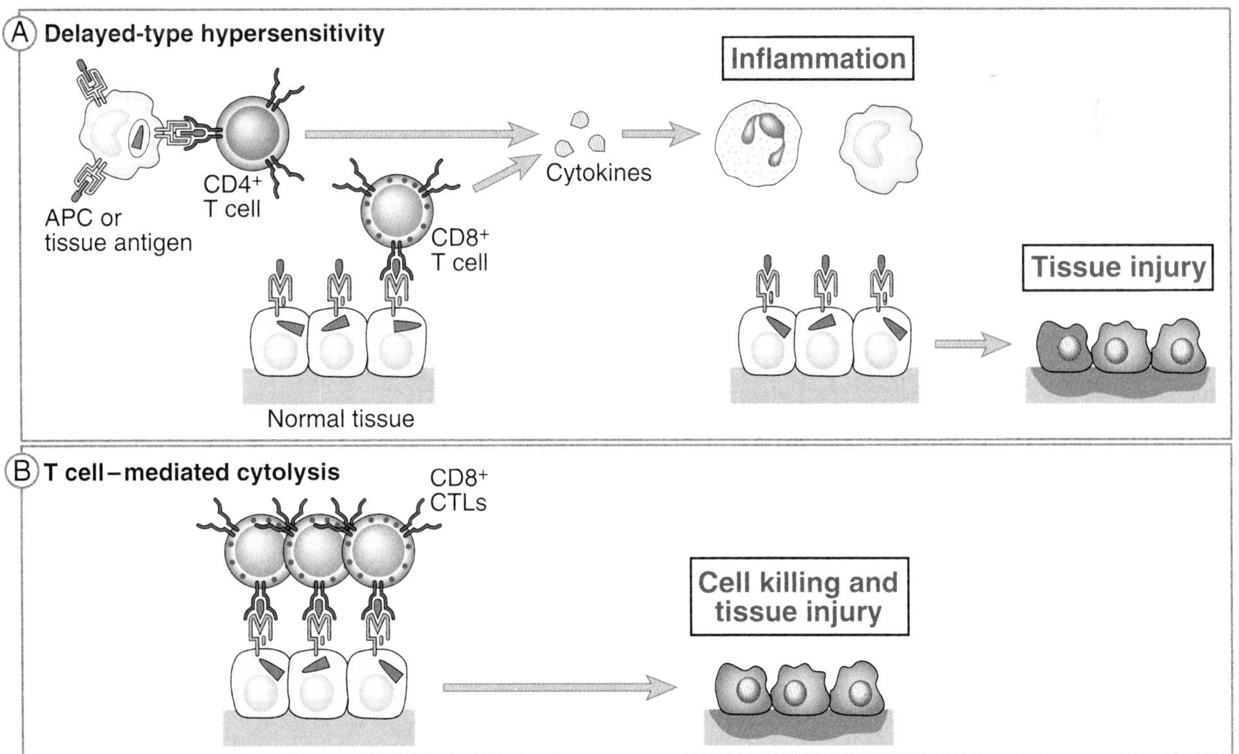

Figure 18–5 Mechanisms of T cell–mediated diseases.
A. In delayed-type hypersensitivity reactions, CD4$^+$ T cells (and sometimes CD8$^+$ cells) respond to tissue antigens by secreting cytokines that stimulate inflammation and activate phagocytes, leading to tissue injury. APC, antigen-presenting cell.
B. In some diseases, CD8$^+$ cytolytic T lymphocytes (CTLs) directly kill tissue cells.

Table 18–4. Examples of T Cell–Mediated Immunologic Diseases

Disease	Specificity of pathogenic T cells	Human disease	Animal models
Insulin-dependent (type I) diabetes mellitus	Islet cell antigens (insulin, glutamic acid decarboxylase, others)	Yes; specificity of T cells not established	NOD mouse, BB rat, transgenic mouse models
Rheumatoid arthritis	Unknown antigen in joint synovium	Yes; specificity of T cells and role of antibody not established	Collagen-induced arthritis, others
Multiple sclerosis, experimental autoimmune encephalomyelitis (EAE)	Myelin basic protein, proteolipid protein	Yes; T cells recognize myelin antigens	EAE is induced by immunization with CNS myelin antigens; TCR transgenic models
Peripheral neuritis	P2 protein of peripheral nerve myelin	Guillain-Barré syndrome	Induced by immunization with peripheral nerve myelin antigens
Experimental autoimmune myocarditis	Myosin	?	Induced by immunization with myosin

Abbreviations: CNS, central nervous system; NOD nonobese diabetic; TCR, T cell receptor.

In some autoimmune diseases such as myasthenia gravis, the lesions are caused by autoantibodies but the disease may be transferred in experimental models by helper T cells specific for self antigens. In such disorders, the function of the T cells is to stimulate the production of autoantibodies.

cells of the T_H1 subset react against self myelin antigens (Box 18–3). The DTH reaction results in the activation of macrophages around nerves in the brain and spinal cord, destruction of the myelin, abnormalities in nerve conduction, and neurologic deficits. An animal model of MS is **experimental autoimmune encephalomyelitis** (EAE), induced by immunization with protein antigens of central nervous system myelin in adjuvant. Such immunization leads to an autoimmune T cell response against myelin. EAE can be transferred to naive animals with myelin antigen–specific $CD4^+$ T_H1 cells, and the disease can be prevented by treating immunized animals with antibodies specific for class II MHC or for CD4 molecules, indicating that $CD4^+$ class II MHC–restricted T cells play an obligatory role in this disorder. **Rheumatoid arthritis** (Box 18–4) is a systemic disease affecting the small joints and many other tissues. A role for T cell–mediated inflammation is suspected in this disease because of its similarity to animal models in which arthritis is known to be caused by T cells specific for joint collagen. Antibodies may also contribute to joint inflammation in this disease. Antagonists against the inflammatory cytokine TNF have a beneficial effect in rheumatoid arthritis.

Cell-mediated immune responses to microbes and other foreign antigens may also lead to tissue injury at the sites of infection or antigen exposure. Intracellular bacteria such as *Mycobacterium tuberculosis* induce strong T cell and macrophage responses that result in granulomatous inflammation and fibrosis; the inflammation and fibrosis may cause extensive tissue destruction and functional impairment, in this case in the lungs. Tuberculosis is a good example of an infectious disease in which tissue injury is mainly due to the host immune response (see Chapter 15). A variety of skin diseases that result from topical exposure to chemicals and environmental antigens, called **contact sensitivity,** are due to DTH reactions, presumably against neoantigens formed by the binding of the chemicals to self proteins.

Some immunologic diseases are associated with abnormal production of cytokines. **Inflammatory bowel disease** (IBD) consists of a heterogeneous group of disorders, including Crohn's disease and ulcerative colitis, in which an immunologic etiology has been suspected for many years. Several knockout mouse models of IBD illustrate the roles of cytokines in immune inflammation in these diseases. Severe IBD develops in mice in which the genes for the cytokines IL-10 or IL-2 are knocked out. It is thought that in IL-10 knockouts, the mechanism of the lesions is unregulated macrophage responses to enteric bacteria, because the disease does not develop in germ-free knockout mice. Autoimmunity may develop in IL-2 knockouts because of defective

BOX 18–2

Insulin-Dependent Diabetes Mellitus

Insulin-dependent (type I) diabetes mellitus (IDDM) is a multisystem metabolic disease resulting from impaired insulin production or function. The disease is characterized by hyperglycemia and ketoacidosis. Chronic complications of IDDM include progressive atherosclerosis of arteries, which can lead to ischemic necrosis of limbs and internal organs, and microvascular obstruction causing damage to the retina, renal glomeruli, and peripheral nerves. The relationship of abnormal glucose metabolism and vascular lesions is not known. IDDM (also called juvenile or type I diabetes) affects about 0.2% of the U.S. population, with a peak age at onset of 11 to 12 years. These patients have a deficiency of insulin resulting from destruction of the insulin-producing β cells of the islets of Langerhans in the pancreas, and continuous hormone replacement therapy is needed.

Several mechanisms may contribute to β cell destruction, including DTH reactions mediated by $CD4^+$ T_H1 cells reactive with islet antigens, CTL-mediated lysis of islet cells, local production of cytokines (TNF and IL-1) that damage islet cells, and autoantibodies against islet cells. In the rare cases in which the pancreatic lesions have been examined at the early active stages of the disease, the islets show cellular necrosis and lymphocytic infiltration. This lesion is called insulitis. The infiltrates consist of both $CD4^+$ and $CD8^+$ T cells. Surviving islet cells often express class II MHC molecules, probably an effect of local production of IFN-γ by the T cells. Autoantibodies against islet cells and insulin are also detected in the blood of these patients. These antibodies may participate in causing the disease or may be a result of T cell–mediated injury and release of normally sequestered antigens. In susceptible children who have not developed diabetes (such as relatives of patients), the presence of antibodies against islet cells is predictive of the development of IDDM. This suggests that the anti–islet cell antibodies contribute to injury to the islets.

Multiple genes are involved in IDDM (see text, Table 18–5). A great deal of attention has been devoted to the role of HLA genes. Ninety percent to 95% of whites with IDDM have HLA-DR3, or DR4, or both, in contrast to about 40% of normal subjects, and 40% to 50% of patients are DR3/DR4 heterozygotes, in contrast to 5% of normal subjects. Interestingly, susceptibility to IDDM is actually associated with a linked DQ allele called DQ3.2 that is often in linkage disequilibrium with DR4. Sequencing of DQ molecules associated with diabetes, both in humans and in the IDDM-susceptible NOD mouse strain, suggests that an asparagine at position 57 in the DQβ chain (I-A in the mouse) protects against IDDM, and its absence increases susceptibility. Although there are many exceptions to this finding, a general hypothesis is that development of IDDM is influenced by the structure of the entire DQ peptide-binding cleft, with residue 57 playing a significant but not exclusive role. Despite the high relative risk of IDDM in individuals with particular class II alleles, most persons who inherit these alleles do not develop the disease. For instance, the frequency of DQ3.2 in the general population is approximately 27%, but only a small fraction of these individuals develop IDDM.

Non-HLA genes also contribute to the disease. The first of these to be identified is insulin, with tandem repeats in the promoter region being associated with disease susceptibility. The mechanism of this association is unknown. In the NOD mouse model, another polymorphism associated with the disease is believed to be in the IL-2 gene. The functional consequences of this polymorphism are not known, but it is intriguing that IL-2 knockout mice develop autoimmunity. Furthermore, some studies have suggested that viral infections (e.g., with coxsackievirus B4) may precede the onset of IDDM, perhaps by initiating cell injury, inducing inflammation and the expression of costimulators, and triggering an autoimmune response. However, epidemiological data suggest that repeated infections protect against IDDM, and this is similar to the NOD model. In fact, it has been postulated that one reason for the increased incidence of IDDM in developed countries is the control of infectious diseases.

ANIMAL MODELS OF SPONTANEOUS IDDM The NOD mouse strain develops a spontaneous T cell–mediated insulitis, which is followed by overt diabetes. Disease can be transferred to young NOD mice with T cells from older, affected animals. As mentioned earlier, the linkage of this disease with the MHC is remarkably similar to the HLA linkage of IDDM in humans. In NOD mice, disease is induced by diabetogenic T cells that may recognize various islet antigens, including insulin and an islet cell enzyme called glutamic acid decarboxylase. Induction of T cell tolerance to these antigens retards the onset of diabetes in NOD mice. Another animal model of the disease is the BB rat, in which insulitis and diabetes are associated with lymphopenia.

TRANSGENIC MOUSE MODELS OF IDDM Several different transgenic models have been created by expressing transgenes in pancreatic islet β cells by introducing these genes into mice under the control of insulin promoters. Allogeneic class I and class II MHC molecules can be expressed in islet cells to test the hypothesis that this will create an endogenous "allograft" that should be attacked by the immune system. Insulitis does not develop in these mice because T cells specific for the allogeneic MHC molecules become tolerant, in part because the insulin promoter is leaky and the alloantigens are expressed in the thymus. Expression of the costimulator B7-1 in islet cells increases susceptibility to insulitis (see text). In some models, if both allogeneic MHC molecules and IL-2 are expressed in islets, insulitis does develop, probably because local IL-2 production breaks T cell anergy and initiates an allogeneic reaction against the islets. Other model protein antigens have also been expressed in islet β cells, and the reaction of T cells to these antigens has been studied as a model for IDDM.

A different transgenic model involves expressing in T cells a T cell receptor (TCR) specific for an islet cell antigen in T cells. As these mice age, they develop insulitis and diabetes. Interestingly, the TCR transgene-expressing T cells are not deleted in the thymus, indicating that islet antigens do not cause central tolerance. In addition, insulitis develops many weeks before overt diabetes, but the factors responsible for stepwise disease progression are not known. A variation of this approach is to express a model protein antigen in the islets and introduce into these antigen-expressing mice T cells from TCR transgenic mice expressing receptors specific for that antigen. These models are valuable for studying T cell tolerance and responses to tissue antigens.

BOX 18–3

Multiple Sclerosis and Experimental Autoimmune Encephalomyelitis

Multiple sclerosis (MS) is the most common neurologic disease of young adults. On pathologic examination, there is inflammation in the central nervous system (CNS) white matter with secondary demyelination. The disease is characterized clinically by weakness, paralysis, and ocular symptoms with exacerbations and remissions; CNS imaging suggests that in patients with active disease, there is frequent new lesion formation. The disease is modeled by experimental autoimmune encephalomyelitis (EAE) in mice, rats, guinea pigs, and nonhuman primates, and this is probably the best characterized experimental model of an organ-specific autoimmune disease mediated exclusively by T lymphocytes. EAE is induced by immunizing animals with antigens normally present in CNS myelin, such as myelin basic protein (MBP), proteolipid protein (PLP), and myelin oligodendrocyte glycoprotein (MOG), with an adjuvant containing heat-killed mycobacterium, which is necessary for stimulating the innate immune system. About 1 to 2 weeks after immunization, animals develop an encephalomyelitis, characterized by perivascular infiltrates composed of lymphocytes and macrophages in the CNS white matter, followed by demyelination. The severity of the lesions depends on the animal species, antigen, and adjuvant. The neurologic lesions can be mild and self-limited or chronic and relapsing.

In mice, EAE is caused by activated, $CD4^+$ T_H1 cells specific for MBP, PLP, or MOG. This has been established by many lines of experimental evidence. Mice immunized with MBP or PLP contain $CD4^+$ T cells that secrete IL-2 and IFN-γ and proliferate in response to that antigen *in vitro.* The disease can be transferred to naive animals by $CD4^+$ T cells from MBP- or PLP-immunized syngeneic animals or with MBP- or PLP-specific cloned $CD4^+$ T cell lines. All disease-producing clones have a T_H1 phenotype, and the lesions of EAE usually have the characteristics of delayed-type hypersensitivity reactions. In humans, T cells specific for myelin proteins can be isolated from the peripheral blood of normal subjects as well as from patients with MS; however, as predicted by the EAE model, the myelin-reactive T cells derived from patients with MS are in an activated state compared with those from normal subjects, which appear to be naive.

Disease-causing T cells in EAE express high levels of the β_1 integrin VLA-4. The infiltration of T cells into the CNS is thought to depend on the binding of VLA-4 to its ligand, VCAM-1, on microvascular endothelium. Studies in EAE have demonstrated that monoclonal antibodies blocking the VLA-4–VCAM interaction block the onset of EAE. Similarly, data from early clinical trials indicate that blocking VLA-4 can significantly prevent the onset of new lesions as measured by magnetic resonance imaging of the brain. Whether this will translate into an acceptable, long-lasting therapy for the disease is not yet known.

The sequence of events in the development of EAE, and by analogy MS, is thought to be the following. Potentially autoreactive T cells specific for myelin proteins are present in the circulation of normal individuals. Immunization with a myelin antigen together with an adjuvant leads to T cell activation against epitopes of autologous myelin proteins. Activated T cells traffic into the CNS more readily than do naive cells. In the CNS, the activated T cells encounter myelin proteins and release cytokines that recruit and activate macrophages and other T cells, leading to myelin destruction. Microbes potentiate disease by stimulating the expression of costimulators and cytokines and the "bystander activation" of autoreactive T cells and perhaps by expressing antigenic epitopes that cross-react with self myelin antigens. The disease is propagated by the process known as epitope spreading. Within weeks after the onset of EAE, there is tissue breakdown with release of new protein epitopes; local antigen-presenting cells in the CNS itself express high levels of class II MHC and costimulatory molecules. Thus, the immunologically activated brain tissue induces the activation of autoreactive T cells recognizing many myelin proteins other than the antigen that triggered the disease. The clinical relevance of the phenomenon is that by the time patients present to the clinic, there is unlikely to be a single antigen driving the disease.

EAE has been used to analyze the fine specificity of myelin-reactive encephalitogenic T cells and to help define immunodominant regions of myelin proteins that may be relevant to MS in humans. Mutational analysis of various MBP and PLP peptides has shown that some amino acid residues are critical for binding to MHC molecules and others for recognition by T cells. Altered peptide ligands (APLs, see Chapter 8) may be produced by introducing conservative substitutions in the TCR contact residues of MBP or PLP. Administration of such mutant peptides blocks the induction of EAE. It is thought that the altered peptide ligands induce anergy in T_H1 cells specific for native MBP or PLP or stimulate the development of anti-inflammatory T_H2 cells specific for these myelin antigens. This approach has recently been tried in patients with MS. TCR contact residues identified in an immunodominant MBP peptide were modified to produce an APL, and the APL was injected into patients. At high antigen doses, a subset of patients experienced a flare-up of the disease associated with very high frequencies of APL-reactive T cells that were cross-reactive with the native self antigen. These unfortunate results provide strong evidence that flare-ups of MS are related to T cell responses to myelin proteins.

Both EAE and MS have strong genetic components and occur only in genetically susceptible hosts. Identical twins have a 25% to 40% concordance rate for development of MS, whereas nonidentical twins have a 1% concordance rate. In both mice and humans, certain MHC haplotypes have been linked to the disease.

BOX 18–4

Rheumatoid Arthritis

Rheumatoid arthritis is an inflammatory disease involving small joints of the extremities, particularly of the fingers, as well as larger joints including shoulders, elbows, knees, and ankles. Rheumatoid arthritis is characterized by inflammation of the synovium associated with destruction of the joint cartilage and bone, with a morphologic picture suggestive of a local immune response. Both cell-mediated and humoral immune responses may contribute to development of synovitis. $CD4^+$ T cells, activated B lymphocytes, plasma cells, and macrophages as well as other inflammatory cell types are found in the inflamed synovium, and in severe cases, well-formed lymphoid follicles with germinal centers may be present. Numerous cytokines, including IL-1, IL-8, TNF, and IFN-γ, have been detected in the synovial (joint) fluid. Cytokines are believed to activate resident synovial cells to produce proteolytic enzymes, such as collagenase, that mediate destruction of the cartilage, ligaments, and tendons of the joints. Many of the cytokines thought to play a role in initiating joint destruction are probably produced as a result of local T cell and macrophage activation. Antagonists against TNF have proved to be of benefit in patients, and soluble TNF receptor as well as anti-TNF antibody are now approved for treatment of the disease. The bone destruction in rheumatoid arthritis is due to increased osteoclast activity in the joints, and this may be related to the production of the TNF family cytokine RANK ligand (osteoprotegerin ligand) by activated T cells. RANK ligand binds to RANK, a member of the TNF receptor family that is on osteoclast precursors, and induces their differentiation and activation. The specificity of the T cells that may be involved in the pathogenesis of arthritis and the nature of the initiating antigen are not known. Significant numbers of T cells expressing the γδ antigen receptor have also been detected in the synovial fluid of some patients with rheumatoid arthritis. However, the pathogenic role of this subset of T cells, like their physiologic function, is obscure.

Systemic complications of rheumatoid arthritis include vasculitis, presumably caused by immune complexes, and lung injury. The nature of the antigen or the antibodies in these complexes is not known. Patients with the adult form of rheumatoid arthritis frequently have circulating antibodies, which may be IgM or IgG, reactive with the Fc (and rarely Fab) portions of their own IgG molecules. These autoantibodies are called rheumatoid factors, and their presence is used as a diagnostic test for rheumatoid arthritis. Rheumatoid factors may participate in the formation of injurious immune complexes, but their pathogenic role is not established. Although activated B cells and plasma cells are often present in the synovia of affected joints, the specificities of the antibodies produced by these cells or their roles in causing joint lesions are not known. Susceptibility to rheumatoid arthritis is linked to the HLA-DR4 haplotype and less so to DR1 and DRW1D. In all these alleles, the amino acid sequences from positions 65 to 75 of the β chain are nearly identical. These residues are located in or close to the peptide-binding clefts of the HLA molecules, suggesting that they influence antigen presentation or T cell recognition.

There are several experimental models of arthritis. MRL/lpr mice develop spontaneous arthritis and have high serum levels of rheumatoid factors. The immune mechanisms of joint disease in MRL/lpr mice are not known. T cell–mediated arthritis can be induced in susceptible strains of mice and rats by immunization with type II collagen (the type found in cartilage), and the disease can be adoptively transferred to unimmunized animals with collagen-specific T cells. However, in the human disease, there is no convincing evidence for collagen-specific autoimmunity. An antibody-mediated arthritis closely resembling rheumatoid arthritis is seen in a TCR transgenic strain of mice called K/B × N. In this model, autoantibodies that recognize the ubiquitous cytoplasmic enzyme glucose-6-phosphate isomerase mediate inflammation specifically on articular surfaces. The relevance of this mechanism to human disease is not yet known. Experimental arthritis can also be produced by immunization with various bacterial antigens, including mycobacterial and streptococcal cell wall proteins. However, such diseases bear little resemblance to human rheumatoid arthritis.

deletion of autoreactive T cells and deficiency of regulatory cells (see Chapter 10). These findings have spurred considerable interest in defining the roles of T cells and cytokines in human IBD and in trying cytokine (e.g., IL-10) therapy for the human disease.

Diseases Caused by Cytolytic T Lymphocytes

CTL responses to viral infection can lead to tissue injury by killing infected cells, even if the virus itself has no cytopathic effects. The principal physiologic function of CTLs is to eliminate intracellular microbes, primarily viruses, by killing infected cells. Some viruses directly injure infected cells and are said to be cytopathic, whereas others are not. Because CTLs cannot *a priori* distinguish between cytopathic and noncytopathic viruses, they kill virally infected cells regardless of whether the infection itself is harmful to the host. Examples of viral infections in which the lesions are due to the host CTL response and not the virus itself include lymphocytic choriomeningitis in mice and certain forms of viral hepatitis in humans (see Chapter 15).

Few examples of autoimmune diseases mediated by CTLs have been documented. Myocarditis with infiltration of the heart by $CD8^+$ T cells develops in mice, and sometimes in humans, infected with coxsackievirus B. The infected animals contain virus-specific, class I MHC–restricted CTLs as well as CTLs that kill uninfected myocardial cells. It is postulated that the heart lesions are initiated by the virus infection and virus-specific CTLs, and myocardial injury leads to the exposure or alteration of self antigens and the subsequent development of autoreactive CTLs. CTLs may also contribute to tissue injury in disorders that are caused primarily by CD4$^+$ T cells, such as IDDM.

Pathogenesis of Autoimmunity

The possibility that an individual's immune system may react against autologous antigens and cause tissue injury was appreciated by immunologists from the time that the specificity of the immune system for foreign antigens was recognized. In the early 1900s, Paul Ehrlich coined the rather melodramatic phrase "horror autotoxicus" for harmful ("toxic") immune reactions against self. When Macfarlane Burnet proposed the clonal selection hypothesis about 50 years later, he added the corollary that clones of autoreactive lymphocytes were deleted during development to prevent autoimmune reactions. We now know that the key events in the development of autoimmunity are the recognition of self antigens by autoreactive lymphocytes, the activation of these cells to proliferate and differentiate into effector cells, and the tissue injury caused by the effector cells and their products. How self-tolerance fails and self-reactive lymphocytes are activated are the fundamental issues in autoimmunity and likely to be the basis for understanding the pathogenesis of these diseases.

Autoimmunity is an important cause of disease in humans and is estimated to affect at least 1% to 2% of the U.S. population. The term *autoimmunity* is often erroneously used for any disease in which immune reactions accompany tissue injury, even though it may be difficult or impossible to establish a role for immune responses to self antigens in causing these disorders. Our understanding of autoimmunity has improved greatly during the last two decades, mainly because of the development of a variety of animal models of these diseases and the identification of genes that may predispose to autoimmunity. Nevertheless, the etiology of most human autoimmune diseases remains obscure, and understanding these disorders is a major challenge in immunology.

Several important general concepts have emerged from analyses of autoimmunity.

- ***Autoimmunity results from a failure or breakdown of the mechanisms normally responsible for maintaining self-tolerance in B cells, T cells, or both.*** The potential for autoimmunity exists in all individuals because during their development, lymphocytes may express receptors specific for self antigens, and many self antigens are readily accessible to the immune system. As discussed in Chapter 10, tolerance to self antigens is normally maintained by selection processes that prevent the maturation of some self antigen–specific lymphocytes and by mechanisms that inactivate or delete self-reactive lymphocytes that do mature. Loss of self-tolerance may result from abnormal selection or regulation of self-reactive lymphocytes and by abnormalities in the way that self antigens are presented to the immune system.

  Much recent attention has focused on the role of T cells in autoimmunity, for two main reasons. First, helper T cells are the key regulators of all immune responses to proteins. Second, several autoimmune diseases are genetically linked to the MHC (the HLA complex in humans), and the function of MHC molecules is to present peptide antigens to T cells. Therefore, it is believed that failure of T cell tolerance is an important mechanism of autoimmune diseases. Failure of self-tolerance in T lymphocytes may result in autoimmune diseases in which the lesions are caused by cell-mediated immune reactions. Helper T cell abnormalities may also lead to autoantibody production because helper T cells are necessary for the production of high-affinity antibodies against protein antigens.

- ***The major factors that contribute to the development of autoimmunity are genetic susceptibility and environmental triggers, such as infections.*** Susceptibility genes and infections both contribute to the breakdown of self-tolerance, and infections in tissues promote the influx of autoreactive lymphocytes and activation of these cells, resulting in tissue injury (Fig. 18–6). Infections and tissue injury may also alter the way in which self antigens are displayed to the immune system, leading to failure of self-tolerance. The roles of these factors in the development of autoimmunity are discussed later.

- ***Autoimmune diseases may be either systemic or organ specific.*** For instance, the formation of circulating immune complexes composed of self antigens and specific antibodies typically produces systemic diseases, such as SLE. In contrast, autoantibody or T cell responses against self antigens with restricted tissue distribution lead to organ-specific diseases, such as myasthenia gravis, type I diabetes mellitus, and multiple sclerosis.

- ***Various effector mechanisms are responsible for tissue injury in different autoimmune diseases.*** These mechanisms include immune complexes, circulating autoantibodies, and autoreactive T lymphocytes and are discussed earlier in the chapter.

- Autoimmune reactions initiated against one self antigen may injure tissues, resulting in the release and alterations of other tissue antigens, activation of lymphocytes specific for these other antigens, and exacerbation of the disease. This phenomenon is called **epitope spreading,** and it may explain why once an autoimmune disease has developed, it tends to be chronic and often progressive.

In the following section, we describe the general principles of the pathogenesis of autoimmune diseases, with an emphasis on susceptibility genes, infections, and other factors that contribute to the development of autoimmunity.

Genetic Susceptibility to Autoimmunity

From the earliest studies of autoimmune diseases in patients and experimental animals, it has been appre-

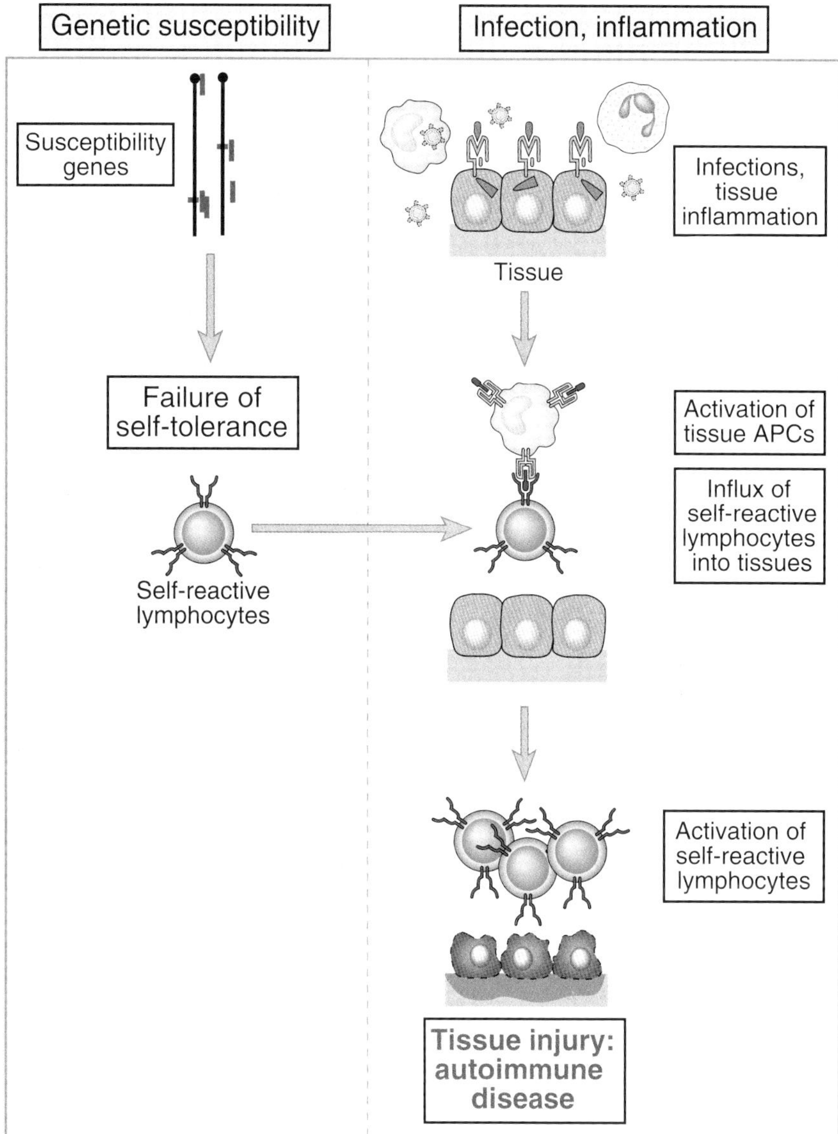

Figure 18–6 Postulated mechanisms of autoimmunity.

In this proposed model of an organ-specific T cell–mediated autoimmune disease, various genetic loci may confer susceptibility to autoimmunity, in part by influencing the maintenance of self-tolerance. Environmental triggers, such as infections and other inflammatory stimuli, promote the influx of lymphocytes into tissues and the activation of self-reactive T cells, resulting in tissue injury.

ciated that these diseases have a strong genetic component. For instance, IDDM (see Box 18–2) shows a concordance of 35% to 50% in monozygotic twins and 5% to 6% in dizygotic twins. Much more has been learned about the genes involved in autoimmune diseases by linkage analyses in families, breeding studies in animal models, and genome scanning methods exploiting the large amount of information that has been developed about human and mouse genome sequences.

Most autoimmune diseases are polygenic, and affected individuals inherit multiple genetic polymorphisms that contribute to disease susceptibility. Most of these genes are not disease specific, and an individual susceptibility gene may contribute to different autoimmune diseases (Fig. 18–7). It is believed that the products of many of these polymorphic genes influence the development of self-tolerance, and affected individuals express products of the genes that are defective in the maintenance of tolerance. However, most of the susceptibility loci identified to date span large chromosomal segments that have been shown to be disease associated by family and linkage studies. These loci may contain tens or hundreds of genes, and the actual disease-associated genes or their causal associations with the disease are often not known. An illustrative example is IDDM (see Box 18–2). In both the human disease and the mouse model, the nonobese diabetic (NOD) strain, more than 20 susceptibility loci have been identified; several of these are also susceptibility loci for other autoimmune diseases. The first disease-associated gene to be identified in this disease, and the only one that is common to both humans and mice, is a class II MHC gene, consistent with the fact that the disease is caused by class II–restricted $CD4^+$ T lymphocytes. The functional significance of the various susceptibility loci has been analyzed mainly in the mouse model. Some are believed to influence negative selection of self-reactive T cells (central tolerance, see Chapter 10), and others control T cell anergy to self antigens (one of the mechanisms of peripheral toler-

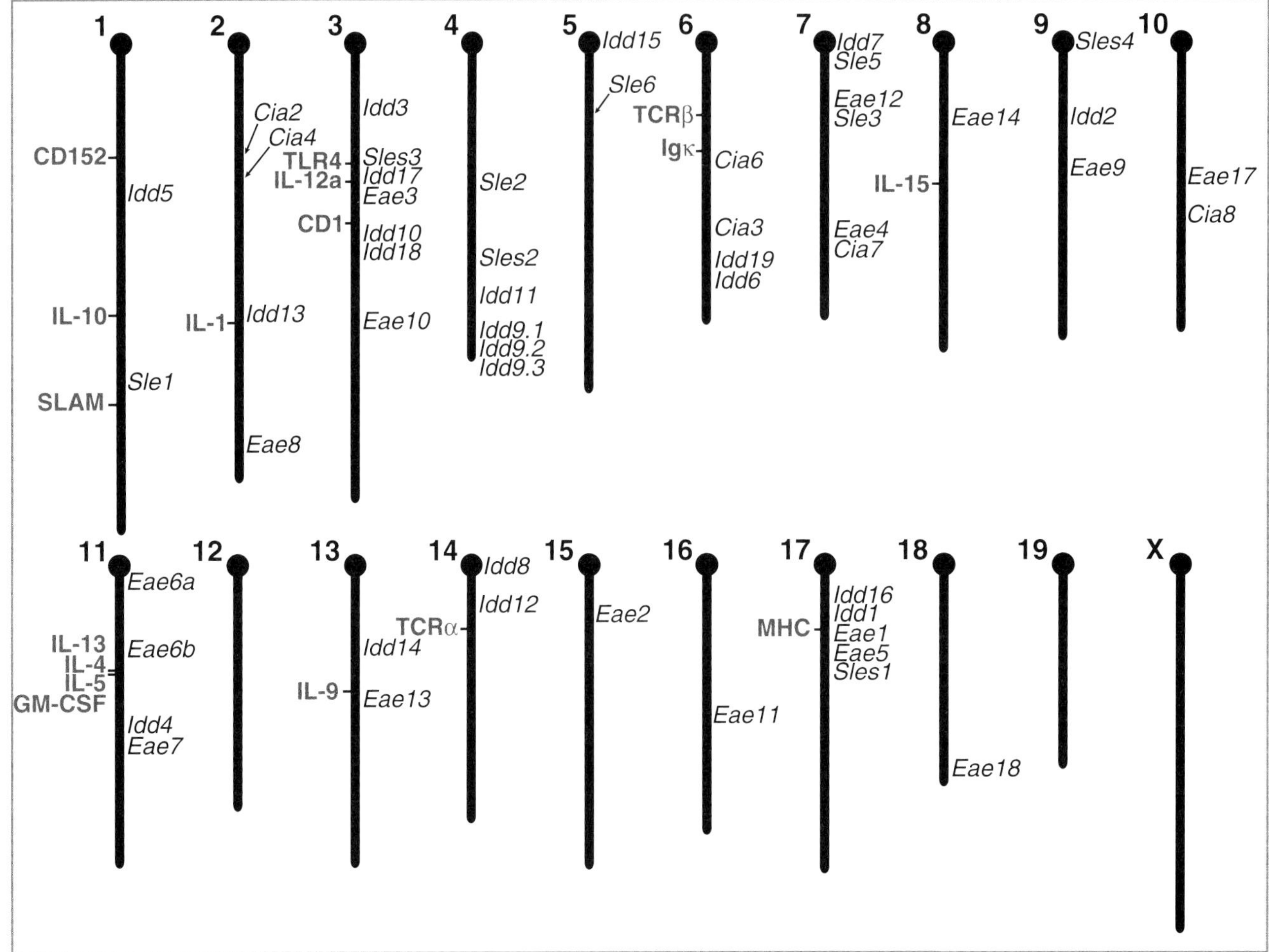

Figure 18–7 Susceptibility loci for autoimmune diseases.
The chromosomal locations of susceptibility loci for several autoimmune diseases in inbred mice are shown as follows: *Cia*, collagen-induced arthritis; *Eae*, experimental autoimmune encephalomyelitis; *Idd*, insulin-dependent (type I) diabetes; *Sle*, systemic lupus erythematosus (*Sles* refers to loci that suppress SLE). Also shown in red are the locations of genes of immunologic interest, such as the MHC, cytokines (interleukins, ILs), and some CD molecules. (Courtesy of Dr. Vijay Kuchroo, Department of Neurology, Harvard Medical School, and Dr. Jeffrey Encinas, Bayer.)

ance, see Chapter 10). Similarly, multiple genetic loci are involved in SLE (see Box 18–1). In a mouse model of SLE, different loci contribute to unregulated B cell activation, autoantibody production, or manifestations of kidney disease. The mechanistic links between susceptibility genes and failure of self-tolerance are not yet established. However, it is likely that as the mapping of susceptibility genes becomes more sophisticated, we will be able to identify the combinations of genes associated with different autoimmune diseases, and the mechanisms by which these genes affect self-tolerance will become clearer.

Among the genes that are associated with autoimmunity, the strongest associations are with MHC genes, especially class II MHC genes. HLA typing of large groups of patients with various autoimmune diseases has shown that some HLA alleles occur at higher frequency in these patients than in the general population. From such studies, one can calculate the relative risk for development of a disease in individuals who inherit various HLA alleles (Table 18–5). The strongest such association is between ankylosing spondylitis, an inflammatory, presumably autoimmune, disease of vertebral joints, and the class I HLA allele B27. Individuals who are HLA-B27 positive have a 90- to 100-fold greater chance for development of ankylosing spondylitis than do individuals lacking B27. Neither the mechanism of this disease nor the basis of its association with HLA-B27 is known. Much more work has been done recently on the association of class II HLA-DR and HLA-DQ alleles with autoimmune diseases, mainly because class II MHC molecules are involved in the selection and activation of $CD4^+$ T cells, and $CD4^+$ T cells regulate both humoral and cell-mediated immune responses to protein antigens.

Several features of the association of HLA alleles with autoimmune diseases are noteworthy. First, an HLA-disease association may be identified by serologic typing of one HLA locus, but the actual association may be with other alleles that are linked to the typed allele and

Table 18–5. Examples of HLA-Linked Immunologic Diseases

Disease	HLA allele	Relative risk*
Rheumatoid arthritis	DR4	4
Insulin-dependent diabetes mellitus	DR3	5
	DR4	5–6
	DR3/DR4 heterozygote	25
Multiple sclerosis	DR2	4
Systemic lupus erythematosus	DR2/DR3	5
Pemphigus vulgaris	DR4	14
Ankylosing spondylitis	B27	90–100

*Relative risk is defined as the probability of development of a disease in individuals with a particular HLA allele versus individuals lacking that HLA allele. The numbers given are approximations.

inherited together. For instance, individuals with a particular HLA-DR allele (hypothetically, DR1) may show a higher probability of inheriting a particular HLA-DQ allele, hypothetically DQ2, than the probability of inheriting these alleles separately and randomly (i.e., at equilibrium) in the population. Such inheritance is an example of linkage disequilibrium. A disease may be found to be DR1 associated by HLA typing, but the causal association may actually be with the co-inherited DQ2. This realization has emphasized the concept of "extended HLA haplotypes," which refers to sets of linked genes, both classical HLA and adjacent non-HLA genes, that tend to be inherited together as a single unit. Second, in many autoimmune diseases, the disease-associated HLA molecules differ from HLA molecules that are not disease associated in their peptide-binding clefts. This finding is not surprising because polymorphic residues of MHC molecules are located within and adjacent to the clefts, and the structure of the clefts is the key determinant of both functions of MHC molecules, namely, antigen presentation and recognition by T cells (see Chapters 4 and 5). These results support the general concept that MHC molecules influence the development of autoimmunity by controlling T cell selection and activation. Third, disease-associated HLA sequences are found in healthy individuals. In fact, if all individuals bearing a particular disease-associated HLA allele are monitored prospectively, most will never acquire the disease. Therefore, expression of a particular HLA gene is not by itself the cause of any autoimmune disease, but it may be one of several factors that contribute to autoimmunity.

It is still not known why particular autoimmune diseases are associated with the inheritance of particular MHC alleles. One possibility is that the structures of MHC molecules determine which clones of T lymphocytes are negatively selected during their maturation. For instance, if the MHC molecules in the thymus of an individual cannot bind a self protein with high affinity, immature T cells reactive with this self antigen may escape negative selection and mature to functional competence. Such a mechanism has been suggested as the reason for the failure of central T cell tolerance in the NOD mouse model of diabetes mentioned earlier. It is also possible that class II MHC molecules influence the activation of regulatory T cells whose normal function is to prevent autoimmunity. However, no evidence exists to support this hypothesis.

Studies with knockout mice and patients have identified several genes that influence the maintenance of tolerance to self antigens. Many of these genes were mentioned in Chapter 10, when we discussed the molecular pathways of different mechanisms of peripheral T cell tolerance. Several of the known mutations that predispose to autoimmunity have provided valuable information about the importance of various mechanisms of self-tolerance (Table 18–6).

- Knockout of the gene encoding CTLA-4, the inhibitory T cell receptor for B7 molecules, results in fatal autoimmunity with T cell infiltrates and tissue destruction involving the heart, pancreas, and other organs. Blocking CTLA-4 with specific antibodies also greatly exacerbates the severity of autoimmune tissue injury in mouse models of encephalomyelitis and diabetes. Because CTLA-4 may function normally to induce and maintain T cell anergy to self antigens, eliminating this function leads to autoimmunity.

- The first clear evidence demonstrating that failure of activation-induced apoptotic cell death results in autoimmunity came from studies of two homozygous inbred mouse mutants called lpr/lpr (for lymphoproliferation) and gld/gld (for generalized lymphoproliferative disease) (see Box 18–1). These mice die by the age of 6 months of a systemic autoimmune disease with multiple autoantibodies and nephritis. The lpr defect is due to an abnormality in the gene encoding the death receptor Fas that reduces expression of this protein, and the gld defect is due to a point mutation in Fas ligand that abolishes the signaling capacity of this molecule. Defects in Fas or Fas ligand result in an inability to delete mature $CD4^+$ T cells by activation-induced cell death. This failure of apoptosis results in the survival and persistence of helper T cells specific for some as yet unidentified self antigens. Functional B cell abnormalities also contribute to autoimmunity in Fas- or Fas ligand–defective mice because some anergic B cells are normally eliminated by Fas-dependent death resulting from interactions with T cells, and this pathway of B cell deletion is defective in lpr and gld mice. Children with a phenotypically similar disease have been identified and shown to carry mutations in the gene encoding Fas or in genes in the Fas-mediated death pathway that result in a failure of activation-induced cell death. These diseases are the only ones known in which genetic abnormalities in one

Table 18–6. Examples of Gene Mutations That Result in Autoimmunity

Gene	Phenotype of knockout mouse	Mechanism of failure of tolerance	Human disease?
CTLA-4	Lymphoproliferation; T cell infiltrates in multiple organs, especially heart; lethal by 3-4 weeks	Failure of anergy in CD4+ T cells	CTLA-4 polymorphisms associated with several autoimmune diseases
Fas/FasL	Anti-DNA and other autoantibodies; immune complex nephritis; arthritis; lymphoproliferation	Defective AICD in CD4+ T cells and deletion of anergic self-reactive B cells	Autoimmune lymphoproliferative syndrome (ALPS)
IL-2; IL-2Rα/β	Inflammatory bowel disease; antierythrocyte and anti-DNA autoantibodies	Defective development or function of regulatory T cells; defective AICD of CD4+ T cells	None known
SHP-1	Multiple autoantibodies	Failure of negative regulation of B cells	None known
PD-1	Antibody-mediated dilated cardiomyopathy (on some genetic backgrounds, there is SLE-like disease)	? Failure of T cell anergy	None known
C4	SLE	Defective clearance of immune complexes; ?Failure of B cell tolerance	SLE

Abbreviations: AICD, activation-induced cell death; IL-2, interleukin-2; PD-1, programmed death gene-1 (an inhibitory receptor that is homologous to CD28); SHP-1, SH2-containing phosphatase-1.

Most of the examples refer to knockout mice; mutations of the complement protein C4 are seen in systemic lupus erythematosus (SLE) in humans.

apoptosis-inducing ligand-receptor pair lead to phenotypically complex autoimmune diseases.

- Severe splenomegaly and lymphadenopathy and an autoimmune syndrome characterized by autoimmune hemolytic anemia and, occasionally, anti-DNA autoantibodies develop in mice lacking IL-2 or the α or β chain of the IL-2 receptor; IBD also develops in some of these knockout mice. (Mutations in the IL-2 receptor γ chain lead to immunodeficiency, mainly because of loss of the lymphopoietic activity of IL-7, a cytokine whose receptor uses the same γ chain as IL-2.) The pathogenesis of this autoimmune disease is not known. It may result from failure of Fas-dependent cell death because IL-2 potentiates Fas-mediated apoptotic signals. Defective activation of regulatory T cells in the absence of IL-2 or IL-2–mediated signals may also be involved. Further supporting the importance of IL-2 as a susceptibility gene for autoimmunity is the finding that a polymorphism in IL-2 that may reduce the half-life of the cytokine is associated with the NOD mouse model of diabetes and susceptibility of mice to EAE.
- Genetic deficiencies of several complement proteins, including C2 and C4 (see Chapter 14, Box 14–2), are associated with lupus-like autoimmune diseases. The postulated mechanism of this association is that complement activation promotes the clearance of circulating immune complexes, and in the absence of complement proteins, these complexes accumulate in the blood and are deposited in tissues.

Role of Infections in Autoimmunity

Viral and bacterial infections may contribute to the development and exacerbation of autoimmunity. In patients, the onset of autoimmune diseases is often associated with or preceded by infections, and in several animal models, autoimmune tissue injury is reduced when the animals are free of infections. (One notable and unexplained exception is the NOD mouse, in which infections tend to ameliorate insulitis and diabetes.) In most of these cases, the infectious microorganism is not present in lesions and is not even detectable in the individual when autoimmunity develops. Therefore, the lesions of autoimmunity are not due to the infectious agent itself but result from host immune responses that may be triggered or dysregulated by the microbe.

Infections may promote the development of autoimmunity by two principal mechanisms (Fig. 18–8).

- Infections of particular tissues may induce local innate immune responses that recruit leukocytes into the tissues and result in the expression of costimulators on tissue APCs and the breakdown of T cell tolerance to self antigens. Thus, the infection

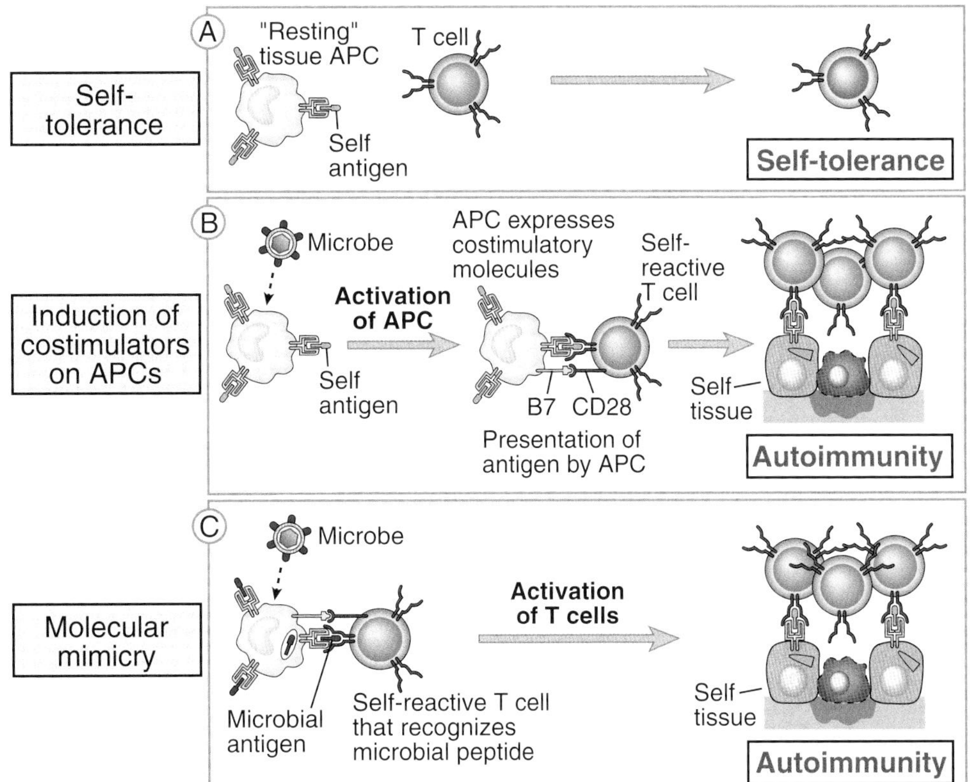

Figure 18–8 Role of infections in the development of autoimmunity.

A. Normally, encounter of a mature self-reactive T cell with a self antigen presented by a costimulator-deficient resting tissue antigen-presenting cell (APC) results in peripheral tolerance by anergy. (Other possible mechanisms of self-tolerance are not shown.)

B. Microbes may activate the APCs to express costimulators, and when these APCs present self antigens, the self-reactive T cells are activated rather than rendered tolerant.

C. Some microbial antigens may cross-react with self antigens (molecular mimicry). Therefore, immune responses initiated by the microbes may activate T cells specific for self antigens.

results in the activation of T cells that are not specific for the infectious pathogen; this type of response is called bystander activation. The importance of aberrant expression of costimulators has been demonstrated by several types of experiments.

- Experimental T cell–mediated autoimmune diseases, such as encephalomyelitis (see Box 18–3) and thyroiditis, develop only if the self antigens (myelin proteins and thyroglobulin, respectively) are administered with strong adjuvants. Such adjuvants may function like infectious agents to activate tissue dendritic cells and macrophages, leading to the expression of the costimulators B7-1 and B7-2, the breakdown of T cell anergy, and the development of effector T cells reactive with the self antigen.

- More formal demonstration of autoimmune tissue injury resulting from the abnormal expression of costimulators and breakdown of T cell anergy has come from transgenic mouse models of IDDM (see Box 18–1). Various genes can be expressed selectively in pancreatic islet β cells as transgenes under the control of insulin promoters. If a foreign antigen such as a viral protein is expressed as a transgene in islet β cells, this antigen effectively becomes "self" and does not elicit an autoimmune reaction. However, coexpression of the viral antigen and B7-1 breaks peripheral tolerance in viral antigen–specific T cells, triggers a response to the antigen in the islets, and results in insulitis and diabetes. In this model, transgene-encoded expression of the costimulator is equivalent to converting resting tissue APCs to activated APCs, much like what happens in infections.

- Infectious microbes may contain antigens that cross-react with self antigens, so immune responses to the microbes may result in reactions against self antigens. This phenomenon is called **molecular mimicry,** because the antigens of the microbe cross-react with, or mimic, self antigens.

  - One example of an immunologic cross-reaction between microbial and self antigens is rheumatic fever, which develops after streptococcal infections and is caused by antistreptococcal antibodies that cross-react with myocardial proteins. These antibodies are deposited in the heart and cause myocarditis. Molecular sequencing has revealed numerous short stretches of homologies between myocardial proteins and streptococcal protein.

  - Homologies have also been detected between myocardial protein antigens and the antigens of *Chlamydia* and *Trypanosoma cruzi*, both of which are associated with myocarditis. In these infections, the myocarditis develops after the infectious microbes have been eliminated, suggesting that the disease is due to an immune response and not the infection itself.

The significance of such limited homologies between microbial and self antigens remains to be established, and it has been difficult to prove that a microbial protein can actually cause a disease that resembles a spontaneous autoimmune disease. On the basis of transgenic mouse models, it has been suggested that molecular mimicry is involved in triggering autoimmunity when the frequency of autoreactive lymphocytes is low; in this situation, the microbial mimic of the self antigen serves to expand the number of self-reactive lymphocytes above some pathogenic threshold. When the frequency of self-reactive lymphocytes is high, the role of microbes may be to induce tissue inflammation, to recruit self-reactive lymphocytes into the tissue, and to provide second signals for the activation of these bystander lymphocytes.

Other Factors in Autoimmunity

The development of autoimmunity is related to several factors in addition to susceptibility genes and infections.

Anatomic alterations in tissues, such as inflammation (possibly secondary to infections), ischemic injury, or trauma, may lead to the exposure of self antigens that are normally concealed from the immune system. Such sequestered antigens may not have induced self-tolerance. Therefore, if previously sequestered self antigens are released, they can interact with immunocompetent lymphocytes and induce specific immune responses. Examples of anatomically sequestered antigens include intraocular proteins and sperm. Post-traumatic uveitis and orchitis after vasectomy are thought to be due to autoimmune responses to self antigens that are released from their normal locations. Tissue inflammation may also cause structural alterations in self antigens and the formation of new determinants capable of inducing autoimmune reactions.

Hormonal influences play a role in some human and experimental autoimmune diseases. Many autoimmune diseases have a higher incidence in females than in males. For instance, SLE affects women about 10 times as frequently as men. The SLE-like disease of (NZB × NZW)F_1 mice develops only in females and is retarded by androgen treatment. Whether this predominance results from the influence of sex hormones or other gender-related factors is not known.

Autoimmune diseases are among the most challenging scientific and clinical problems in immunology. The current knowledge of pathogenetic mechanisms remains incomplete, so theories and hypotheses continue to outnumber facts. The application of new technical advances and the rapidly improving understanding of self-tolerance will, it is hoped, lead to clearer and more definitive answers to the enigmas of autoimmunity.

Therapeutic Approaches for Immunologic Diseases

Strategies for treatment of immune-mediated diseases are similar to the approaches used to prevent graft rejection, another form of injurious immune response (see Chapter 16). The mainstay of therapy for hypersensitivity diseases is anti-inflammatory drugs, particularly corticosteroids. Such drugs are targeted at reducing tissue injury, specifically, the effector phases of the pathologic immune responses. Antagonists of proinflammatory cytokines, such as IL-1 and TNF, and agents that block leukocyte emigration into tissues, such as antibodies against integrins, are also being tested for their anti-inflammatory effects. A soluble form of the TNF receptor and an anti-TNF antibody that bind to and neutralize TNF are now approved for treatment of rheumatoid arthritis and IBD. Other approaches to inhibit pathologic immune reactions include antagonists against costimulators, such as B7 molecules, and against T cell effector molecules, such as CD40 ligand. These antagonists are now in clinical trials for SLE, psoriasis, and other diseases. In severe cases, immunosuppressive drugs such as cyclosporine are used to block T cell activation. Plasmapheresis has been used during exacerbations of antibody-mediated diseases to reduce circulating levels of antibodies or immune complexes. Large doses of intravenous IgG have beneficial effects in some hypersensitivity diseases. It is not clear how this agent suppresses immune inflammation; one possibility is that the IgG binds to inhibitory Fc receptors on B lymphocytes and shuts off antibody production, similar to the phenomenon of antibody feedback (see Fig. 9–19, Chapter 9). More specific treatment aimed at disease-producing lymphocyte clones or at the antigen that initiates the disease requires accurate identification of the antigen. Approaches include attempts to induce tolerance, such as by oral administration of antigens that cause autoimmunity (for treatment of multiple sclerosis and rheumatoid arthritis), and administration of altered forms of self antigens (for multiple sclerosis). Although the value of such therapies has been demonstrated in various animal models, their application to clinical disease has not been established.

Summary

- Disorders caused by abnormal immune responses are called hypersensitivity diseases. Pathologic immune responses may be autoimmune responses directed against self antigens or uncontrolled and excessive responses to foreign antigens.
- Hypersensitivity diseases may result from antibodies that bind to cells or tissues, circulating immune complexes that are deposited in tissues, or T lymphocytes reactive with antigens in tissues.
- The effector mechanisms of antibody-mediated tissue injury are complement activation and Fc receptor–mediated inflammation. Some antibodies cause disease by interfering with normal cellular functions without producing tissue injury. The effector mechanisms of T cell–mediated tissue injury are DTH reactions and cell lysis by CTLs.

- Autoimmunity results from a failure of self-tolerance. Autoimmune reactions may be triggered by environmental stimuli, such as infections, in genetically susceptible individuals.
- Most autoimmune diseases are polygenic, and numerous susceptibility genes contribute to disease development. The greatest contribution is from MHC genes; other genes are believed to influence the selection of self-reactive lymphocytes and the development of self-tolerance.
- Infections may predispose to autoimmunity by several mechanisms, including enhanced expression of costimulators in tissues and cross-reactions between microbial antigens and self antigens.
- The current treatment of autoimmune diseases is targeted at minimizing the injurious consequences of the autoimmune reaction. A future goal of therapy is to inhibit the responses of lymphocytes specific for self antigens and to induce tolerance in these cells.

Selected Readings

Dorner T, and PE Lipsky. Immunoglobulin variable region gene usage in systemic autoimmune diseases. Arthritis and Rheumatism 44:2715–2727, 2001.

Encinas J, and VK Kuchroo. Mapping and identification of autoimmunity genes. Current Opinion in Immunology 12:691–697, 2000.

Falcone M, and N Sarvetnick. Cytokines that regulate autoimmune responses. Current Opinion in Immunology 11: 670–676, 1999.

Feldmann M, FM Brennan, and R Maini. Cytokines in autoimmune disorders. International Review of Immunology 17:217–228, 1998.

Hammer J, T Sturniolo, and F Sinigaglia. HLA class II peptide binding specificity and autoimmunity. Advances in Immunology 66:67–100, 1997.

Horwitz MS, and N Sarvetnick. Viruses, host responses, and autoimmunity. Immunological Reviews 169:241–253, 1999.

Kalden JR, FC Breedveld, H Burkhardt, and GR Burmester. Immunological treatment of autoimmune diseases. Advances in Immunology 68:333–418, 1998.

Kuchroo VK, AC Anderson, H Waldner, E Bettelli, and LB Nicholson. T cell response in experimental autoimmune encephalomyelitis (EAE): role of self and cross-reactive antigens in shaping, tuning, and regulating the autopathogenic T cell repertoire. Annual Review of Immunology 20:101–123, 2002.

Marrack P, J Kappler, and BL Kotzin. Autoimmune disease: why and where it occurs. Nature Medicine 7:899–905, 2001.

O'Shea JJ, A Ma, and P Lipsky. Cytokines and autoimmunity. Nature Reviews Immunology 2:37–45, 2002.

Refaeli Y, L van Parijs, and AK Abbas. Genetic models of abnormal apoptosis in lymphocytes. Immunological Reviews 169:273–282, 1999.

Rose NR, and C Bona. Defining criteria for autoimmune diseases (Witebsky's postulates revisited). Immunology Today 14:426–430, 1993.

Siegel RM, FK-M Chan, and MJ Lenardo. The multifaceted role of Fas signaling in immune cell homeostasis and autoimmunity. Nature Immunology 1:469–474, 2000.

Todd JA, and LS Wicker. Genetic protection from the inflammatory disease type 1 diabetes in humans and animal models. Immunity 15:387–395, 2001.

Vanderlugt CL, and SD Miller. Epitope spreading in immune-mediated diseases: implications for immunotherapy. Nature Reviews Immunology 2:85–95, 2002.

Vyse TJ, and BL Kotzin. Genetic susceptibility to systemic lupus erythematosus. Annual Review of Immunology 16: 261–292, 1998.

Wucherpfennig KW. Mechanisms for the induction of autoimmunity by infectious agents. Journal of Clinical Investigation 108:1097–1104, 2001.

Chapter 19

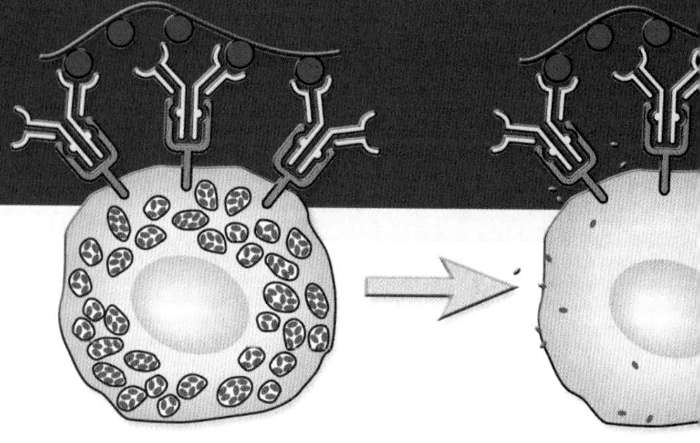

Immediate Hypersensitivity

One of the most powerful pathologic reactions of the immune system is elicited by immunoglobulin E (IgE)–mediated stimulation of tissue mast cells. IgE antibodies that are produced in response to an antigen bind to Fc receptors on mast cells. When these cell-associated antibodies are cross-linked by the antigen, the cells are activated to rapidly release a variety of mediators. These mediators collectively cause increased vascular permeability, vasodilation, bronchial and visceral smooth muscle contraction, and local inflammation. This reaction is called **immediate hypersensitivity** because it begins rapidly, within minutes of antigen challenge (immediate), and has major pathologic consequences (hypersensitivity). In clinical medicine, these reactions are commonly called **allergy** or **atopy**. Although atopy originally meant "unusual," we now realize that allergy is the most common disorder of immunity and affects 20% of all individuals in the United States. This chapter focuses on immune reactions mediated by IgE. We begin by summarizing some important general features of immediate hypersensitivity and proceed to describe the production of IgE, the structure and functions of IgE-specific Fc receptors, and the cellular components of immediate hypersensitivity, including mast cells, basophils, and eosinophils. We then describe selected clinical syndromes associated with immediate hypersensitivity and the principles of therapy for these diseases. We conclude with a discussion of the physiologic role of IgE-mediated immune reactions in host defense.

General Features of Immediate Hypersensitivity Reactions

All immediate hypersensitivity reactions share common features, although they differ greatly in the types of antigens that elicit these reactions and their clinical and pathologic manifestations.

- ***The typical sequence of events in immediate hypersensitivity consists of exposure to an antigen, activation of T_H2 cells specific for the antigen, production of IgE antibody, binding of the antibody to Fc receptors of mast cells, and triggering of the***

mast cells by re-exposure to the antigen, resulting in the release of mediators from the mast cells and the subsequent pathologic reaction (Fig. 19–1). Binding of IgE to mast cells is also called **sensitization** because IgE-coated mast cells are ready to be activated on antigen encounter. We describe each of these steps in the following sections.

- ***There is a strong genetic predisposition for the development of immediate hypersensitivity.*** Many susceptibility genes are associated with atopy. These genes are thought to influence different steps in the development and reactions of immediate hypersensitivity. We will discuss some of the major known susceptibility genes and their likely roles later in the chapter.

- ***The antigens that elicit immediate hypersensitivity, also called allergens, are usually common environmental proteins and chemicals.*** Most individuals who encounter these antigens do not produce specific IgE or develop potentially harmful reactions, whereas such reactions develop in genetically susceptible individuals.

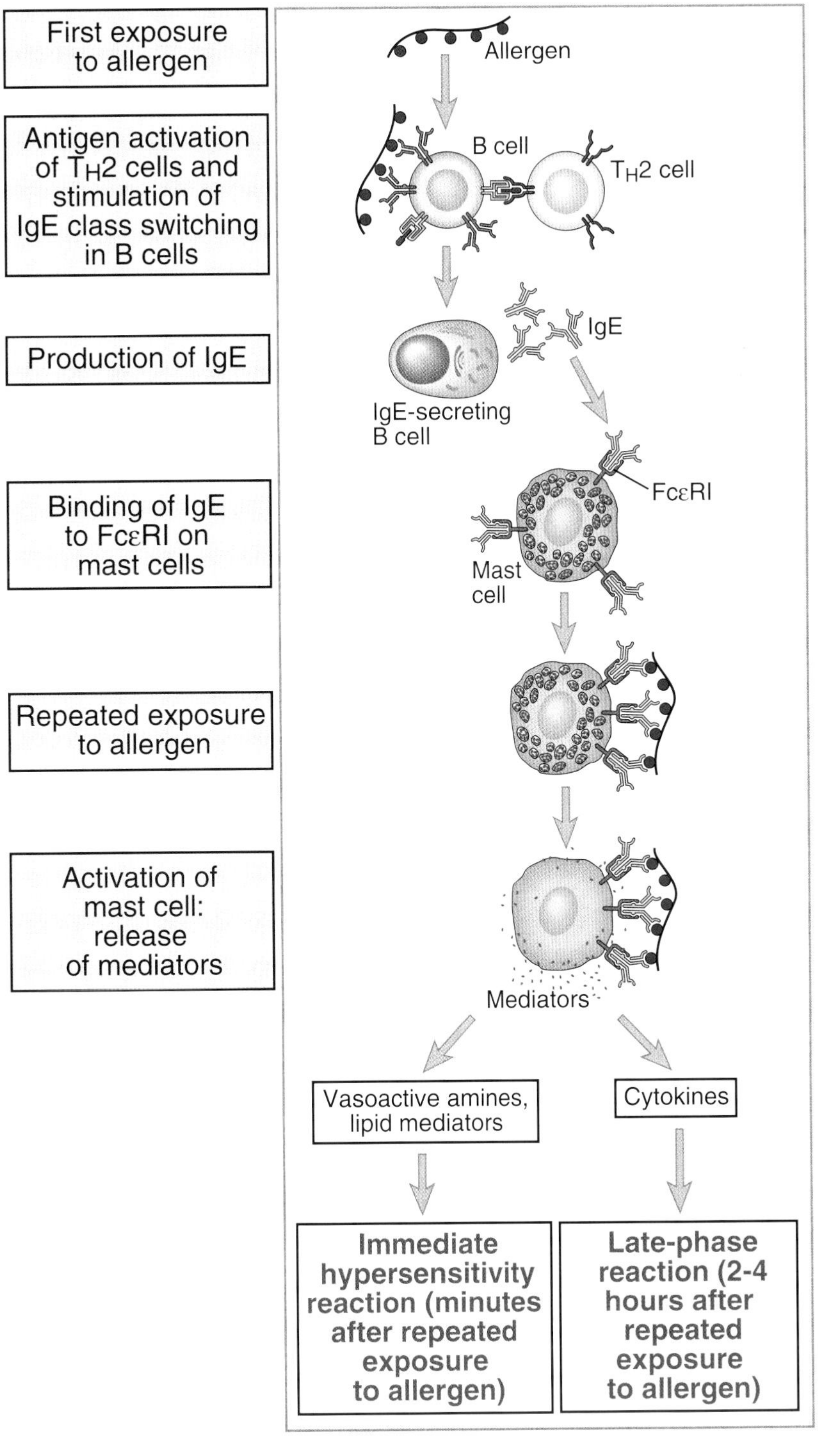

Figure 19–1 Sequence of events in immediate hypersensitivity reactions. Immediate hypersensitivity diseases are initiated by the introduction of an allergen, which stimulates T_H2 reactions and IgE production. IgE sensitizes mast cells by binding to FcεRI, and subsequent exposure to the allergen activates the mast cells to secrete the mediators that are responsible for the pathologic reactions of immediate hypersensitivity.

- ***Immediate hypersensitivity reactions are dependent on the activation of T_H2 cells.*** The cytokines produced by T_H2 cells are responsible for many of the features of immediate hypersensitivity. Thus, immediate hypersensitivity is a T_H2-mediated disorder, in contrast to delayed-type hypersensitivity, which is the classical T_H1-mediated immune reaction.
- ***The clinical and pathologic manifestations of immediate hypersensitivity consist of the vascular and smooth muscle reaction that develops rapidly after repeated exposure to the allergen (the immediate reaction) and a delayed late-phase reaction consisting mainly of inflammation.*** These reactions may be triggered by IgE-mediated mast cell activation, but different mediators are responsible for different components of the immediate and late-phase reactions. Since mast cells are present in all connective tissues and under all epithelia, these are the most common sites of immediate hypersensitivity reactions. Some allergic reactions may be triggered by nonimmunologic stimuli, such as exercise and exposure to cold. Such stimuli presumably induce mast cell degranulation and the release of mediators without antigen exposure or IgE production. Such reactions are said to be nonatopic.
- ***Immediate hypersensitivity reactions are manifested in different ways, including skin and mucosal allergies, food allergies, asthma, and systemic anaphylaxis.*** In the most extreme systemic form, called anaphylaxis, mast cell–derived mediators can restrict airways to the point of asphyxiation and produce cardiovascular collapse leading to death. (The term *anaphylaxis* was coined to indicate that antibodies, especially IgE antibodies, could confer the opposite of protection [prophylaxis] on an unfortunate individual.) We will return to the pathogenesis of these reactions later in the chapter.

With this introduction, we proceed to a description of the steps in the development and reactions of immediate hypersensitivity.

Production of IgE

IgE antibody is responsible for sensitizing mast cells and provides recognition of antigen for immediate hypersensitivity reactions. IgE is the antibody isotype that contains the ε heavy chain (see Chapter 3). IgE sensitizes mast cells by binding to ε heavy chain–specific Fc receptors on these cells. We will describe the experimental evidence demonstrating the essential role of IgE in immediate hypersensitivity later in the chapter.

Atopic individuals produce high levels of IgE in response to environmental allergens, whereas normal individuals generally synthesize other Ig isotypes, such as IgM and IgG, and only small amounts of IgE. Regulation of IgE synthesis depends on the propensity of an individual to mount a T_H2 response to allergens because T_H2 cell–derived cytokines stimulate heavy chain isotype switching to the IgE class in B cells. This propensity toward T_H2 responses against particular antigens may be influenced by a variety of factors, including inherited genes, the nature of the antigens, and the history of antigen exposure.

The Nature of Allergens

Antigens that elicit immediate hypersensitivity reactions (allergens) are proteins or chemicals bound to proteins to which the atopic individual is chronically exposed. Typical allergens include proteins in pollen, house dust mites, animal dander, and foods and chemicals like the antibiotic penicillin. It is not known why some antigens induce strong T_H2 responses and allergic responses whereas others do not. Two important characteristics of allergens are that individuals are exposed to them repeatedly and, unlike microbes, they do not stimulate the innate immune responses that would promote macrophage activation and secretion of the T_H1-inducing cytokines IL-12 and IL-18. Chronic or repeated T cell activation in the absence of innate immunity may drive $CD4^+$ T cells toward the T_H2 pathway, as the T cells themselves make IL-4, the major T_H2-inducing cytokine (see Chapter 13). The property of being allergenic may also reside in the chemical nature of the antigen itself. Although no structural characteristics of proteins can definitively predict whether they will be allergenic, some features are typical of many common allergens. These features include low molecular weight, glycosylation, and high solubility in body fluids. Anaphylactic responses to foods typically involve highly glycosylated small proteins. These structural features probably protect the antigens from denaturation and degradation in the gastrointestinal tract and allow them to be absorbed intact. Curiously, many allergens, such as the cysteine protease of the house dust mite *Dermatophagoides pteronyssinus* and phospholipase A_2 in bee venom, are enzymes, but the importance of the enzymatic activity in triggering immediate hypersensitivity reactions is not known.

Because immediate hypersensitivity reactions are dependent on T cells, T cell–independent antigens such as polysaccharides cannot elicit such reactions unless they become attached to proteins. Some drugs such as penicillin often do elicit strong IgE responses. These drugs react chemically with amino acid residues in self proteins to form hapten-carrier conjugates, which stimulate IgE production and mast cell activation.

The natural history of antigen exposure is an important determinant of the level of specific IgE antibodies. Repeated exposure to a particular antigen is necessary for development of an allergic reaction to that antigen because IgE isotype switching and sensitization of mast cells with IgE must happen before a hypersensitivity reaction to an antigen can occur. Individuals with allergic rhinitis or asthma often benefit from a geographic change of residence with a change in indigenous plant pollen, although local antigens in the new residence may trigger an eventual return of the symptoms. The most dramatic examples of the importance of repeated exposure to antigen in allergic disease are seen in cases of bee stings. The protein toxins in the insect venoms are not usually of concern on the first encounter because an atopic individual has no preexisting specific IgE antibodies. However, an IgE response may occur after a single encounter with antigen, and a second sting by an insect of the same species may induce fatal anaphylaxis!

Activation of T_H2 Cells

IgE synthesis is dependent on the activation of $CD4^+$ helper T cells of the T_H2 subset and their secretion of IL-4. It is likely that dendritic cells in epithelia through which allergens enter capture the antigens, transport them to draining lymph nodes, process them, and present peptides to T cells. The T cells then differentiate into the T_H2 subset of effector cells. Differentiated T_H2 cells promote switching to IgE mainly through the secretion of IL-4. T_H2 cells are involved in other components of the immediate hypersensitivity reaction in addition to promoting switching to IgE. IL-5 secreted by T_H2 cells activates eosinophils, a cell type that is abundant in many immediate hypersensitivity reactions. IL-13 stimulates epithelial cells (e.g., in the airways) to secrete increased amounts of mucus, and excessive mucus production is also a common feature of these reactions. Consistent with a central role of T_H2 cells in immediate hypersensitivity, atopic individuals contain larger numbers of allergen-specific IL-4–secreting T cells in their circulation than do nonatopic persons. In atopic patients, the allergen-specific T cells also produce more IL-4 per cell than in normal individuals.

- The central role of T_H2 cells in allergic reactions is demonstrated by experiments in which mice are made to inhale a model protein antigen, such as chicken egg albumin, and are injected with T cells specific for the antigen. The adoptive transfer of T_H2 cells induces airway hyperresponsiveness, resembling asthma.
- Knockout mice lacking the T_H1 transcription factor T-bet (see Chapter 13) show defective T_H1 responses and a compensatory increase in T_H2 responses. Such mice develop spontaneous airway allergic reactions.

In addition to stimulating IgE production, T_H2 cells contribute to the inflammation of the late-phase reaction. Accumulations of T_H2 cells are found at sites of immediate hypersensitivity reactions in the skin and bronchial mucosa. These T cells are recruited to sites of immediate hypersensitivity mainly in response to chemokines. T_H2 cells express the chemokine receptors CCR4 and CCR8, and the chemokines that bind to these receptors are produced by many cell types at sites of immediate hypersensitivity reactions, including epithelial cells.

Activation of B Cells and Switching to IgE

B cells specific for allergens are activated by T_H2 cells, as in other T-dependent B cell responses (see Chapter 9). Under the influence of CD40 ligand and cytokines, mainly IL-4, produced by the T_H2 cells, the B cells undergo heavy chain isotype switching and produce IgE. IgE circulates as a bivalent antibody and is normally present in plasma at a concentration of less than 1 μg/mL. In pathologic conditions such as helminthic infections and severe atopy, this level can rise to more than 1000 μg/mL. Allergen-specific IgE produced by B cells enters the circulation and binds to Fc receptors on tissue mast cells, so that these cells are sensitized and poised to react to a subsequent encounter with the allergen. Circulating basophils and eosinophils are also capable of binding IgE. We will first describe the Fc receptors used by these cell types to bind IgE and then the properties and reactions of the cells.

Binding of IgE to Mast Cells and Basophils

IgE antibodies bind to a high-affinity Fc receptor specific for ε heavy chains, called FcεRI, that is expressed on mast cells, basophils, and eosinophils. IgE, like all other antibody molecules, is made exclusively by B cells, yet IgE functions as an antigen receptor on the surface of the cells of immediate hypersensitivity. This function is accomplished by IgE binding to FcεRI on these cells. The affinity of FcεRI for IgE is very high (dissociation constant [K_d] of about 1×10^{-10} M); this binding is much stronger than that of any other Fc receptor for its ligand (see Chapter 14, Box 14–1). Therefore, the normal serum concentration of IgE, although low in comparison to other Ig isotypes (less than 5×10^{-10} M), is sufficiently high to allow occupancy of FcεRI receptors. Tissue mast cells in all individuals are normally coated with IgE, which is bound to the FcεRI. In atopic individuals, enough of this bound IgE is specific for one or a few antigens that exposure to that antigen or antigens is able to cross-link the Fc receptors and activate the cells (discussed later). In addition to mast cells, basophils, and eosinophils, FcεRI, usually lacking the β chain, has been detected on epidermal Langerhans cells, some dermal macrophages, and activated monocytes; its function on these cells is not known.

Structure and Function of the Fc Receptor for IgE

Each FcεRI molecule is composed of one α chain that mediates ligand binding and a β chain and two γ chains that are responsible for signaling (Fig. 19–2). The amino terminal extracellular portion of the α chain includes two Ig-like domains that form the binding site for IgE. The β chain of FcεRI, which crosses the membrane four times, contains a single immunoreceptor tyrosine-based activation motif (ITAM) in the cytoplasmic carboxyl terminus. The two identical γ chain polypeptides are linked by a disulfide bond and are homologous to the ζ chain of the T cell antigen receptor complex (see Chapter 6). The cytoplasmic portion of each γ chain contains one ITAM. The γ chain of FcεRI serves as the signaling subunit for FcγRI, FcγRIIIA, and FcαR and is called the FcR γ chain (see Chapter 14, Box14–1). Tyrosine phosphorylation of the

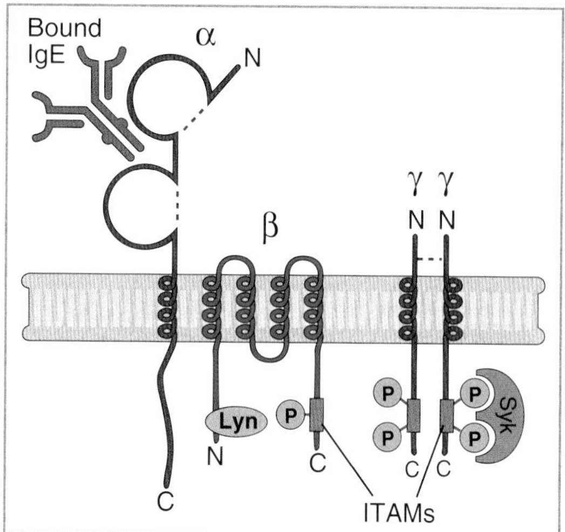

Figure 19–2 Polypeptide chain structure of the high-affinity IgE Fc receptor (FcεRI).
IgE binds to the Ig-like domains of the α chain. The β chain and the γ chains mediate signal transduction. The boxes in the cytoplasmic region of the β and γ chains are immunoreceptor tyrosine activation motifs (ITAMs), similar to those found in the T cell receptor complex (see Fig. 6–5). A model structure of FcεRI is shown in Chapter 14, Box 14–1.

ITAMs of the β and γ chains initiates the signals from the receptor that are required for mast cell activation. We will return to the nature of these signals when we discuss mast cells later in the chapter.

- The importance of FcεRI in IgE-mediated immediate hypersensitivity reactions has been demonstrated in FcεRI α chain knockout mice. When these mice are given intravenous injections of IgE specific for a known antigen followed by that antigen, anaphylaxis does not develop, whereas it does in wild-type mice treated in the same way.

FcεRI expression on mast cells and basophils is upregulated by IgE, thereby providing a mechanism for the amplification of IgE-mediated reactions. The relationship between the levels of IgE and FcεRI expression is supported by several observations.

- A positive correlation between FcεRI expression on human blood basophils and circulating IgE levels has been observed.
- Treatment of mast cells *in vitro* with IgE induces increased expression of FcεRI.
- Mast cells from knockout mice lacking IgE have very low levels of FcεRI.

Another IgE receptor is FcεRII, a protein related to C-type mammalian lectins, whose affinity for IgE is much lower than that of FcεRI. Two different isoforms of FcεRII have been identified, one called FcεRIIA, which is B cell specific, and the other called FcεRIIB or CD23, whose expression is induced on B cells, monocytes, and eosinophils in response to IL-4. The biologic roles of FcεRII are not known.

Role of Mast Cells, Basophils, and Eosinophils in Immediate Hypersensitivity

Mast cells, basophils, and eosinophils are the effector cells of immediate hypersensitivity reactions and allergic disease. Although each of these cell types has unique characteristics, all three contain cytoplasmic granules whose contents are the major mediators of allergic reactions, and all three cell types produce lipid mediators and cytokines that induce inflammation. In this section of the chapter, we discuss the properties and functions of each of these effector cell types (Table 19–1). Because mast cells are the major cell type responsible for immediate hypersensitivity reactions in tissues, much of our subsequent discussion focuses on mast cells.

Properties of Mast Cells and Basophils

All mast cells are derived from progenitors in the bone marrow. Normally, mature mast cells are not found in the circulation. Progenitors migrate to the peripheral tissues as immature cells and undergo differentiation *in situ*. Mature mast cells are found throughout the body, predominantly near blood vessels and nerves and beneath epithelia. They are also present in lymphoid organs. By microscopy, human mast cells vary in shape and have round nuclei, and the cytoplasm contains membrane-bound granules and lipid bodies (Fig. 19–3). The granules contain acidic proteoglycans that bind basic dyes.

There are two major subsets of mast cells that differ in their anatomic locations, granule contents, and activities (Table 19–2). In rodents, one subset of mast cells is found in the mucosa of the gastrointestinal tract. These mucosal mast cells have abundant chondroitin sulfate and little histamine in their granules. The presence of mucosal mast cells *in vivo* depends on T cells as indicated by the lack of these mast cells in athymic mice. Mast cells may be cultured from rodent bone marrow in the presence of IL-3, and such cultured mast cells resemble mucosal mast cells on the basis of the high granule content of chondroitin sulfate and low histamine concentration. It is likely that T cell dependence of mucosal mast cell development *in vivo* reflects the dependence on IL-3 produced by helper T cells. The human counterpart to this subset is most often identified by the presence of tryptase and not other neutral proteases in the granules. Human mucosal mast cells predominate in intestinal mucosa and alveolar spaces in the lung, and their presence is also T cell dependent. A second subset of rodent mast cells is found in the lung and in the serosa of body cavities, and these cells are called connective tissue mast cells. Their major granule proteoglycan is heparin, and they also produce large quantities of histamine. Unlike mucosal mast cells, connective tissue mast cells show little T cell dependence. In humans, the corresponding subset is identified by the presence of several neutral proteases in the granules, including tryptase, chymase, cathepsin G–like protease, and carboxypeptidase. Human con-

Table 19–1. Properties of Mast Cells, Basophils, and Eosinophils

Characteristic	Mast cells	Basophils	Eosinophils
Origin of precursor	CD34+ hematopoietic progenitor cells	CD34+ hematopoietic progenitor cells	CD34+ hematopoietic progenitor cells
Major site of maturation	Connective tissue	Bone marrow	Bone marrow
Cells in circulation	No	Yes (0.5% of blood leukocytes)	Yes (2.7% of blood leukocytes)
Mature cells recruited into tissues from circulation	No	Yes	Yes
Mature cells residing in connective tissue	Yes	No	Yes
Proliferative ability of mature cells	Yes	No	No
Life span	Weeks to months	Days	Days to weeks
Major development factor (cytokine)	Stem cell factor	IL-3	IL-5
Expression of FcεRI	High levels	High levels	Low levels
Major granule contents	Histamine, heparin and/or chondroitin sulfate, proteases	Histamine, chondroitin sulfate, protease	Major basic protein, eosinophil cationic protein, peroxidases, hydrolases, lysophospholipase

Modified from Costa JJ, PW Weller, and SJ Galli. The cells of the allergic response. JAMA 178:1815–1822, 1994. Copyright American Medical Association.

nective tissue mast cells are found in the skin and intestinal submucosa.

Although we do not know if these mast cell subsets serve distinct functions, their locations, granule contents, and relative T cell dependence suggest that each subset may be important in a different set of disease processes. It is likely that mucosal mast cells are involved in T cell– and IgE-dependent immediate hypersensitivity diseases involving the airways, such as bronchial asthma, and other mucosal tissues. Conversely, connective tissue mast cells mediate immediate hypersensitivity reactions in the skin. The phenotype of a mast cell is not fixed and may vary in response to cytokines and growth factors. For example, bone marrow–derived mucosal mast cells can be changed to a connective tissue mast cell phenotype by coculture with fibroblasts or incubation with c-Kit ligand (stem cell factor) (see Chapter 11). Repopulation experiments in mast cell–deficient mice further suggest that the mucosal and connective tissue phenotypes are not distinct lineages and that bidirectional changes occur in different microenvironments.

Table 19–2. Mast Cell Subunits

Characteristic	Connective tissue mast cells		Mucosal mast cells	
	Rodent	Human	Rodent	Human
Location	Peritoneal cavity	Skin, intestinal submucosa	Intestinal mucosa	Alveoli, intestinal mucosa
T cell dependence for development of phenotype in tissues	No	No	Yes	Yes
Granule contents	High levels of histamine, heparin	Major neutral proteases: tryptase, chymase, carboxypeptidase, cathepsin G	Low levels of histamine; high levels of chondroitin sulfate	Major neutral protease: tryptase

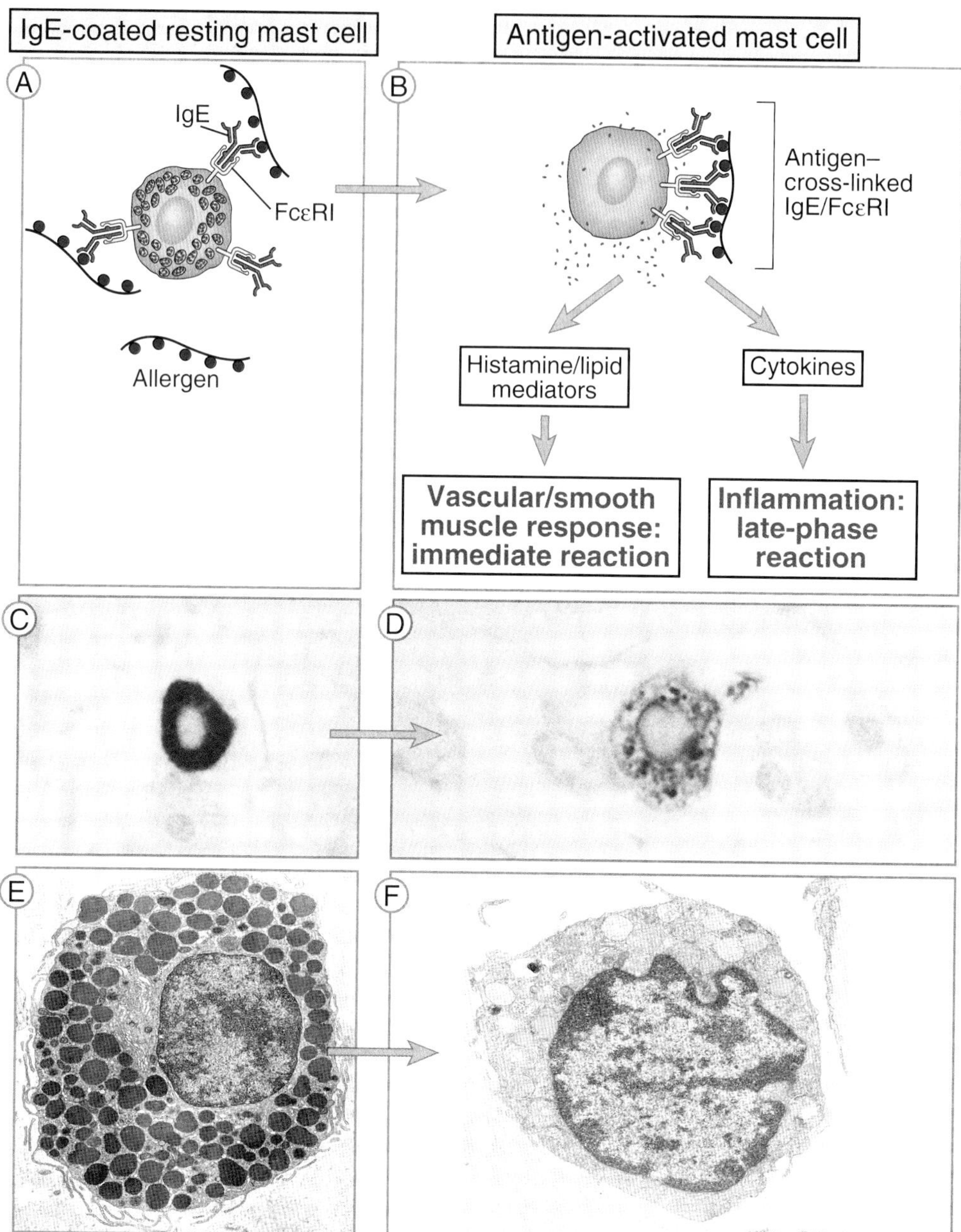

Figure 19–3 Mast cell activation.
Antigen binding to IgE cross-links FcεRI molecules on mast cells, which induces the release of mediators that cause the hypersensitivity reaction (A, B). Other stimuli, including the complement fragment C5a, can also activate mast cells. A light photomicrograph of a resting mast cell with abundant purple-staining cytoplasmic granules is shown in C. These granules are also seen in the electron micrograph of a resting mast cell shown in E. In contrast, the depleted granules of an activated mast cell are shown in the light photomicrograph (D) and electron micrograph (F). (Courtesy of Dr. Daniel Friend, Department of Pathology, Brigham and Women's Hospital and Harvard Medical School, Boston.)

Basophils are blood granulocytes with structural and functional similarities to mast cells. Like other granulocytes, basophils are derived from bone marrow progenitors (a lineage different from that of mast cells), mature in the bone marrow, and circulate in the blood (Fig. 19–4). Basophils constitute less than 1% of the total blood leukocytes. Although they are normally not present in tissues, basophils may be recruited to some inflammatory sites, usually together with eosinophils. Basophils contain granules that bind basic dyes, and they are capable of synthesizing many of the same mediators as mast cells (see Table 19–2). Like mast cells, basophils express FcεRI, bind IgE, and can be triggered by antigen binding to the IgE. Therefore, basophils that are recruited into tissue sites where antigen is present may contribute to immediate hypersensitivity reactions.

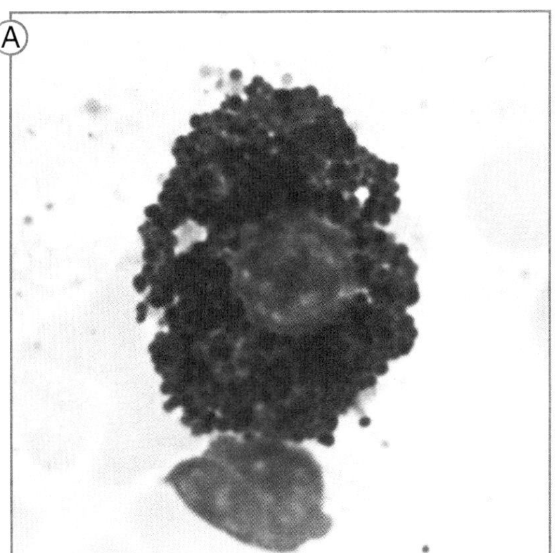

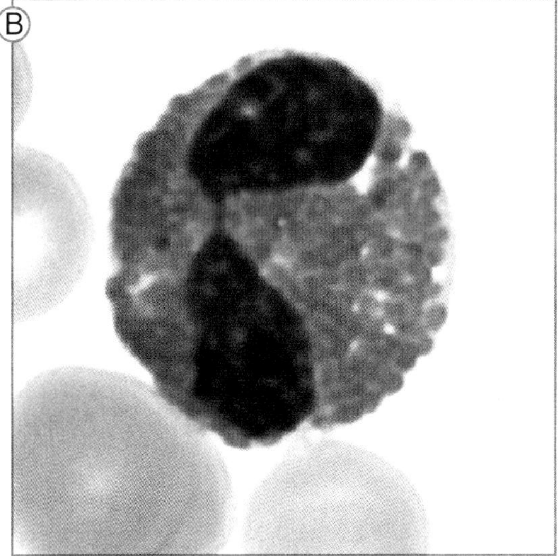

Figure 19–4 Morphology of basophils and eosinophils.
Photomicrographs of a Wright-Giemsa–stained peripheral blood basophil (A) and eosinophil (B) are presented. Note the characteristic red staining of the cytoplasmic granules in the eosinophil and blue-staining cytoplasmic granules of the basophil. (Courtesy of Dr. Jonathan Hecht, Department of Pathology, Brigham and Women's Hospital, Boston.)

Activation of Mast Cells

Mast cells are activated by cross-linking of FcεRI molecules, which occurs by binding of multivalent antigens to the attached IgE molecules (see Fig. 19–3). In an individual allergic to a particular antigen, a large proportion of the IgE bound to mast cells is specific for that antigen. Exposure to the antigen will cross-link sufficient IgE molecules to trigger mast cell activation. In contrast, in nonatopic individuals, the mast cell–associated IgE is specific for many different antigens, all of which may have induced low levels of IgE production. Therefore, no single antigen will cross-link enough of the IgE molecules to cause mast cell activation. Experimentally, antigen binding can be mimicked by polyvalent anti-IgE or by anti-FcεRI antibodies. In fact, anti-IgE antibodies can cross-link IgE molecules regardless of antigen specificity and lead to comparable triggering of mast cells from both atopic and nonatopic individuals.

Activation of mast cells results in three types of biologic response: secretion of the preformed contents of their granules by a regulated process of exocytosis, synthesis and secretion of lipid mediators, and synthesis and secretion of cytokines. These responses result from the cross-linking of FcεRI, which initiates a signaling cascade in mast cells involving protein tyrosine kinases (Fig. 19–5). The signaling cascade is similar to the proximal signaling events initiated by antigen binding to lymphocytes (see Chapters 8 and 9). The Lyn tyrosine kinase is constitutively associated with the cytoplasmic tail of the FcεRI β chain. On cross-linking of FcεRI molecules by antigen, Lyn tyrosine kinase phosphorylates the ITAMs in the cytoplasmic domains of FcεRI β and γ chains. The Syk tyrosine kinase is then recruited to the ITAMs of the γ chain, becomes activated, and phosphorylates and activates other proteins in the signaling cascade, including several adapter molecules and enzymes that participate in the formation of a multicomponent signaling complex, as described in T cells. One of the enzymes recruited to this complex and phosphorylated is the γ isoform of a phosphatidylinositol-specific phospholipase C (PLCγ), which catalyzes phosphatidylinositol bisphosphate breakdown to inositol triphosphate (IP_3) and diacylglycerol (DAG) (see Chapter 8). IP_3 causes elevation of cytoplasmic calcium levels, and DAG activates protein kinase C. Phosphorylation of the myosin light chains by activated protein kinase C leads to disassembly of the actin-myosin complexes beneath the plasma membrane, thereby allowing granules to come in contact with the plasma membrane. Fusion of the granule membrane and the plasma membrane is mediated by interactions between proteins associated with the granule membrane and proteins associated with the plasma membrane; these events are apparently regulated by the guanosine triphosphate (GTP)–binding (activated) form of Ras-related Rab proteins.

Cross-linking of FcεRI also activates the enzyme adenylate cyclase through a heterotrimeric GTP-binding protein. Activated adenylate cyclase in turn elevates cyclic adenosine monophosphate (cAMP) levels, and cAMP activates protein kinase A. Protein kinase A inhibits degranulation, thus suggesting that this pathway is a negative feedback loop. Certain pharmacologic approaches to treatment of allergic disease take advantage of cAMP-mediated inhibition of mast cell degranulation (discussed later).

Synthesis of lipid mediators is controlled by activation of the cytosolic enzyme phospholipase A_2 (PLA_2) (see Fig. 19–5). This enzyme is activated by two signals: elevated cytoplasmic calcium and phosphorylation catalyzed by a mitogen-activated protein (MAP) kinase such as extracellular receptor-activated kinase (ERK).

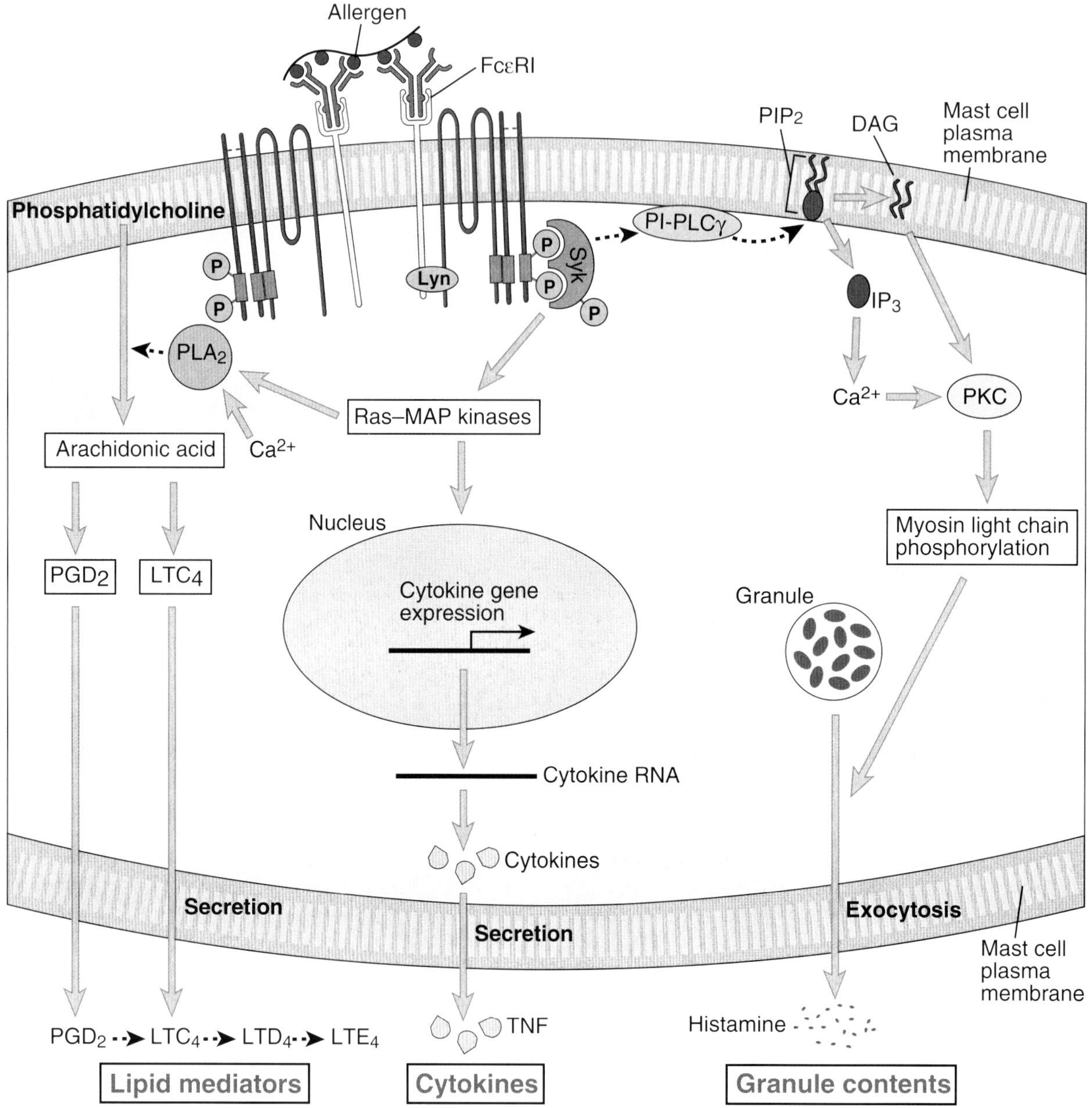

Figure 19–5 Biochemical events of mast cell activation.
Cross-linking of bound IgE by antigen is thought to activate protein tyrosine kinases (Syk and Lyn), which in turn cause activation of a mitogen-activated protein (MAP) kinase cascade and a phosphatidylinositol-specific phospholipase C (PI-PLCγ). PI-PLCγ catalyzes the release of inositol triphosphate (IP_3) and diacylglycerol (DAG) from membrane PIP_2. IP_3 causes release of intracellular calcium from the endoplasmic reticulum. Calcium and DAG activate protein kinase C (PKC), which phosphorylates substrates such as myosin light chain protein and thereby leads to the degradation and release of preformed mediators. Calcium and MAP kinases combine to activate the enzyme cytosolic phospholipase A_2 ($cPLA_2$), which initiates the synthesis of lipid mediators.

ERK is activated as a consequence of a kinase cascade initiated through the receptor ITAMs, probably using the same intermediates as in T cells (see Chapter 8). Once activated, PLA_2 hydrolyzes membrane phospholipids to release substrates, which are then converted by enzyme cascades into the ultimate mediators. The major substrate is arachidonic acid, which is converted by cyclooxygenase or lipoxygenase into different mediators (discussed later).

Cytokine production by activated mast cells is a consequence of newly induced cytokine gene transcription. The biochemical events that regulate cytokine gene transcription in mast cells appear to be similar to the events that occur in T cells. Recruitment and activation of various adapter molecules and kinases in response to FcεRI cross-linking lead to nuclear translocation of NFAT (nuclear factor of activated T cells) and NF-κB as well as activation of AP-1 by protein kinases such as c-Jun N-terminal kinase. These transcription factors stimulate transcription of several cytokines (IL-4, IL-5, IL-6, and tumor necrosis factor [TNF], among others) but, in contrast to T cells, not IL-2.

Mast cell activation through the FcεRI pathway is regulated by the inhibitory Fc receptor FcγRIIb, which contains a single immunoreceptor tyrosine-based inhibition motif (ITIM) within its cytoplasmic tail. FcγRIIb appears to coaggregate with FcεRI during mast cell activation, and the ITIM is phosphorylated by Lyn. This leads to recruitment of the tyrosine phosphatase SH2 domain–containing inositol 5-phosphatase (SHIP) and inhibition of FcεRI signaling.

Mast cells can be directly activated by a variety of biologic substances independent of allergen-mediated cross-linking of FcεRI, including polybasic compounds, peptides, chemokines, and complement-derived anaphylatoxins. These additional modes of mast cell activation may be important in non–immune-mediated immediate hypersensitivity reactions, or they may amplify IgE-mediated reactions. Certain types of mast cells or basophils may respond to mononuclear phagocyte–derived chemokines, such as macrophage inflammatory protein-1α (MIP-1α), produced as part of innate immunity, and to T cell–derived chemokines, produced as part of adaptive cell-mediated immunity. The complement-derived anaphylatoxins, especially C5a, bind to specific receptors on mast cells and stimulate degranulation. In humans, skin mast cells but not lung mast cells are sensitive to C5a. These chemokines and complement fragments are likely to be produced at sites of inflammation. Therefore, mast cell activation and release of mediators may amplify even IgE-independent reactions. Polybasic compounds, such as compound 48/40 and mastoparan, are used as pharmacologic triggers for mast cells. These agents contain a cationic region adjacent to a hydrophobic moiety, and they work by activating G proteins.

Many neuropeptides, including substance P, somatostatin, and vasoactive intestinal peptide, induce mast cell histamine release and may mediate neuroendocrine-linked mast cell activation. The nervous system is known to affect immediate hypersensitivity reactions, and neuropeptides may be involved. The flare produced at the edge of the wheal in elicited immediate hypersensitivity reactions is in part mediated by the nervous system, as shown by the observation that it is markedly diminished in skin sites lacking innervation. Cold temperatures and intense exercise may also trigger mast cell degranulation, but the mechanisms involved are not known.

Mast cells also express Fc receptors for IgG heavy chains, and these cells can be activated by cross-linking bound IgG. This IgG-mediated reaction is the likely explanation for the finding that ε chain knockout mice remain susceptible to antigen-induced mast cell–mediated anaphylaxis. However, IgE is by far the major antibody isotype involved in most immediate hypersensitivity reactions.

Mediators Derived from Mast Cells

The effector functions of mast cells are mediated by soluble molecules released from the cells on activation (Fig. 19–6 and Table 19–3). These mediators may be divided into preformed mediators, which include biogenic amines and granule macromolecules, and newly synthesized mediators, which include lipid-derived mediators and cytokines.

Biogenic Amines

Many of the biologic effects of mast cell activation are mediated by biogenic amines that are stored in and released from cytoplasmic granules. Biogenic amines, sometimes called vasoactive amines, are low molecular weight compounds that share the structural feature of an amine group. In human mast cells, the only mediator of this class that is present in significant quantities is **histamine,** but in some rodents, serotonin may be of equal or greater import. Histamine acts by binding to target cell receptors, and different cell types express distinct classes of histamine receptors (e.g., H_1, H_2, H_3) that can be distinguished by pharmacologic inhibitors. The actions of histamine are short-lived because histamine is rapidly removed from the extracellular milieu by amine-specific transport systems. On binding to cellular receptors, histamine initiates intracellular events, such as phosphatidylinositol breakdown to IP_3 and DAG, that cause different changes in different cell types. Binding of histamine to endothelium causes cell contraction leading to leakage of plasma into the tissues. Histamine also stimulates endothelial cells to synthesize vascular smooth muscle cell relaxants, such as prostacyclin (PGI_2) and nitric oxide, which cause vasodilation. These actions of histamine produce the wheal and flare response of immediate hypersensitivity (described later). H_1 histamine receptor antagonists (commonly called antihistamines) can inhibit the wheal and flare response to intradermal allergen or anti-IgE antibody. Histamine also causes constriction of intestinal and bronchial smooth muscle. Thus, histamine may contribute to the increased peristalsis and bronchospasm associated with ingested allergens and asthma, respectively. However, in these instances, especially in asthma, antihistamines are not effective at blocking the reaction. Moreover, bronchoconstriction in asthma is more prolonged than are the effects of histamine, suggesting that other mast cell–derived mediators are important in some forms of immediate hypersensitivity.

Granule Proteins and Proteoglycans

Neutral serine proteases, including tryptase and chymase, are the most abundant protein constituents of mast cell secretory granules and contribute to tissue damage in immediate hypersensitivity reactions. Tryptase is present in all human mast cells and is not known to be present in any other cell type. Consequently, the presence of tryptase in human biologic fluids is interpreted as a marker of mast cell activation. Chymase is found in some human mast cells, and its presence or absence is one criterion for characterizing human mast cell subsets, as discussed earlier. The functions of these enzymes *in vivo* are not known; however, several activities demonstrated *in vitro* suggest important biologic effects. For example, tryptase cleaves

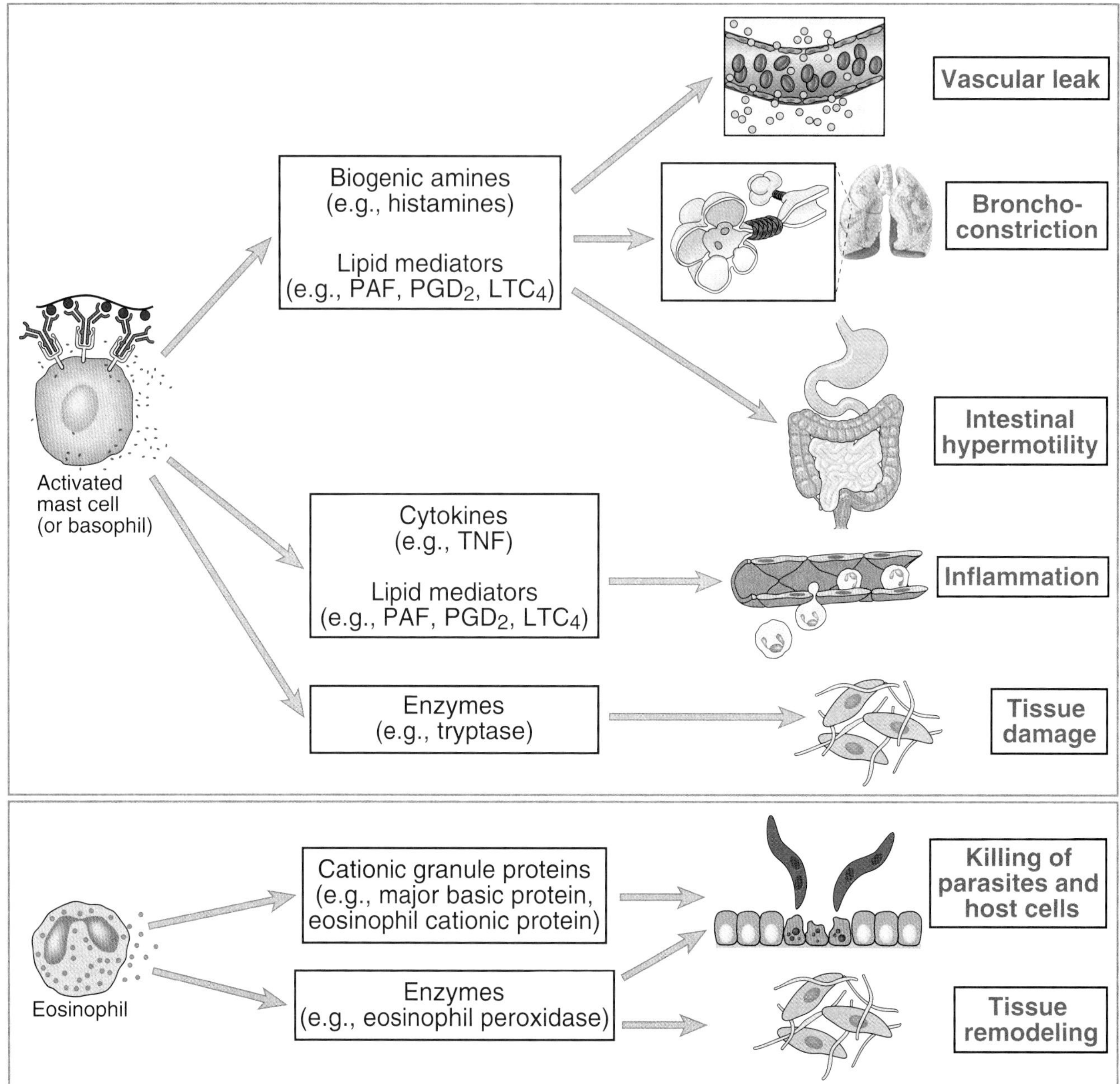

Figure 19–6 Biologic effects of mediators of immediate hypersensitivity. Mast cells and basophil mediators include biogenic amines and enzymes stored preformed in granules as well as cytokines and lipid mediators, which are largely newly synthesized on cell activation. The biogenic amines and lipid mediators induce vascular leakage, bronchoconstriction, and intestinal hypermotility, all components of the immediate response. Cytokines and lipid mediators contribute to inflammation, which is part of the late-phase reaction. Enzymes probably contribute to tissue remodeling. Activated mast cells release preformed cationic proteins as well as enzymes that are toxic to parasites and host cells. Some eosinophil granule enzymes probably contribute to tissue remodeling in chronic allergic diseases.

fibrinogen and activates collagenase, thereby causing tissue damage, whereas chymase can convert angiotensin I to angiotensin II, degrade epidermal basement membrane, and stimulate mucus secretion. Other enzymes found within mast cell granules include carboxypeptidase A and cathepsin G. Basophil granules also contain several enzymes, some of which are the same as those in mast cell granules, such as neutral proteases; others are found in eosinophil granules, such as major basic protein and lysophospholipase.

Proteoglycans, including heparin and chondroitin sulfate, are also major constituents of both mast cell and basophil granules. These molecules are composed of a polypeptide core and multiple unbranched glycosaminoglycan side chains that impart a strong net negative charge to the molecules. Within the granules,

Table 19–3. Mediators Produced by Mast Cells, Basophils, and Eosinophils

Cell type	Mediator category	Mediator	Function/pathologic effects
Mast cells and basophils			
	Stored preformed in cytoplasmic granules	Histamine	Increases vascular permeability; stimulates smooth muscle cell contraction
		Enzymes: neutral proteases (tryptase and/or chymase), acid hydrolases, cathepsin G, carboxypeptidase	Degrade microbial structures; tissue damage/remodeling
	Major lipid mediators produced on activation	Prostaglandin D_2	Vasodilation, bronchoconstriction, neutrophil chemotaxis
		Leukotriene C_4, D_4, E_4	Prolonged bronchoconstriction, mucus secretion, increased vascular permeability
		Platelet-activating factor	Chemotaxis and activation of leukocytes, bronchoconstriction, increased vascular permeability
	Cytokines produced on activation	IL-3	Promotes mast cell proliferation
		TNF-α, MIP-1α	Promote inflammation/late-phase reaction
		IL-4, IL-13	Promote T_H2 differentiation
		IL-5	Promotes eosinophil production and activation
Eosinophils			
	Stored preformed in cytoplasmic granules	Major basic protein, eosinophil cationic protein	Toxic to helminths, bacteria, host cells
		Eosinophil peroxidase, lysosomal hydrolases, lysophospholipase	Degrade helminthic and protozoan cell walls; tissue damage/remodeling
	Major lipid mediators produced on activation	Leukotriene C_4, D_4, E_4	Prolonged bronchoconstriction; mucus secretion, increased vascular permeability
		Lipoxins	Promote inflammation
	Cytokines produced on activation	IL-3, IL-5, GM-CSF	Promote eosinophil production and activation
		IL-8, IL-10, RANTES, MIP-1α, eotaxin	Chemotaxis of leukocytes

Modified from Costa JJ, PW Weller, and SJ Galli. The cells of the allergic response. JAMA 178:1815–1822, 1994. Copyright American Medical Association.

proteoglycans serve as storage matrices for positively charged biogenic amines, proteases, and other mediators and prevent their accessibility to the rest of the cell. The mediators are released from the proteoglycans at different rates after granule exocytosis, biogenic amines dissociating much more rapidly than tryptase or chymase. In this way, the proteoglycans may control the kinetics of immediate hypersensitivity reactions.

Lipid Mediators

Mast cell activation results in the rapid de novo ***synthesis and release of lipid-derived mediators that have a variety of effects on blood vessels, bronchial smooth muscle, and leukocytes.*** The most important of these mediators are cyclooxygenase and lipoxygenase metabolites of arachidonic acid.

The major arachidonic acid–derived mediator produced by the cyclooxygenase pathway in mast cells is **prostaglandin D_2** (PGD_2). Released PGD_2 binds to receptors on smooth muscle cells and acts as a vasodilator and as a bronchoconstrictor. PGD_2 also promotes neutrophil chemotaxis and accumulation at inflammatory sites. PGD_2 synthesis can be prevented by inhibitors of cyclooxygenase, such as aspirin and nonsteroidal anti-inflammatory agents. These drugs may paradoxically exacerbate asthmatic bronchoconstriction, because they shunt arachidonic acid toward production of leukotrienes, discussed next.

The most important arachidonic acid–derived mediators produced by the lipoxygenase pathway are the **leukotrienes**, especially LTC_4 and its degradation products LTD_4 and LTE_4. LTC_4 is made by mucosal mast cells and basophils, but not by connective tissue mast cells.

Mast cell–derived leukotrienes bind to specific receptors on smooth muscle cells, different from the receptors for PGD_2, and cause prolonged bronchoconstriction. When injected into the skin, these leukotrienes produce a characteristic long-lived wheal and flare reaction. Collectively, LTC_4, LTD_4, and LTE_4 constitute what was once called slow-reacting substance of anaphylaxis (SRS-A) and are thought to be major mediators of asthmatic bronchoconstriction. Pharmacologic inhibitors of 5-lipoxygenase also block anaphylactic reactions in experimental systems.

A third type of lipid mediator produced by mast cells is called **platelet-activating factor** (PAF) for its original bioassay as an inducer of rabbit platelet aggregation. In mast cells and basophils, PAF is synthesized by acylation of lysoglyceryl ether phosphorylcholine, a derivative of PLA_2-mediated hydrolysis of membrane phospholipids. PAF has direct bronchoconstricting actions. It also causes retraction of endothelial cells and can relax vascular smooth muscle. However, PAF is hydrophobic and is rapidly destroyed by a plasma enzyme called PAF hydrolase, which limits its biologic actions. Pharmacologic inhibitors of PAF receptors ameliorate some aspects of immediate hypersensitivity in the rabbit lung. Recent genetic evidence has pointed to PAF as a mediator of asthma. Asthma develops in early childhood in individuals with a genetic deficiency of PAF hydrolase. PAF may also be important in late-phase reactions, in which it can activate inflammatory leukocytes. In this situation, the major source of PAF may be basophils or vascular endothelial cells (stimulated by histamine or leukotrienes) rather than mast cells.

Cytokines

Mast cells (and basophils) produce many different cytokines that may contribute to allergic inflammation. These cytokines include TNF, IL-1, IL-4, IL-5, IL-6, IL-13, MIP-1α, MIP-1β, and various colony-stimulating factors such as IL-3 and granulocyte-monocyte colony-stimulating factor (GM-CSF). As mentioned before, mast cell activation induces transcription and *de novo* synthesis of these cytokines, but preformed TNF may also be stored in granules and rapidly released on FcεRI cross-linking. T_H2 cells that are recruited into the sites of allergic reactions also produce some of these cytokines. The cytokines that are released on IgE-mediated mast cell or basophil activation or on T_H2 cell activation are mainly responsible for the late-phase reaction. TNF, in particular, activates endothelial expression of the adhesion molecules that account for sequential polymorphonuclear and mononuclear cell infiltrates by the same mechanisms described in Chapter 12. In addition to allergic inflammation, mast cell cytokines also apparently contribute to the innate immune responses to infections. For example, as we will discuss later, mouse models indicate that mast cells are required for effective defense against some bacterial infections, and this effector function is mediated largely by TNF.

Properties of Eosinophils

Eosinophils are bone marrow–derived granulocytes that are abundant in the inflammatory infiltrates of late-phase reactions and contribute to many of the pathologic processes in allergic diseases. Eosinophils develop in the bone marrow, and after maturation, they circulate in the blood. GM-CSF, IL-3, and IL-5 promote eosinophil maturation from myeloid precursors. Eosinophils are normally present in peripheral tissues, especially in mucosal linings of the respiratory, gastrointestinal, and genitourinary tracts, and their numbers can increase by recruitment in the setting of inflammation. The granules of eosinophils contain basic proteins that bind acidic dyes such as eosin (see Fig. 19–5).

Cytokines produced by T_H2 cells promote the activation of eosinophils and their recruitment to late-phase reaction inflammatory sites. IL-5 is a potent eosinophil-activating cytokine. It enhances the ability of eosinophils to release granule contents on cross-linking of FcεRI. IL-5 also increases maturation of eosinophils from bone marrow precursors, and in the absence of this cytokine (e.g., in IL-5 knockout mice), there is a deficiency of eosinophil numbers and functions. Eosinophils are recruited into late-phase reaction sites as well as sites of helminthic infection, and their recruitment is mediated by a combination of adhesion molecule interactions and chemokines. Eosinophils bind to endothelial cells expressing E-selectin and the ligand for the VLA-4 integrin. Eosinophil recruitment and infiltration into tissues also depend on various chemokines such as eotaxin and monocyte chemotactic protein-5, which are produced by epithelial cells at sites of allergic reactions. In addition, the complement product C5a and the lipid mediators PAF and LTB_4, which are produced by mast cells, also function as chemoattractants for eosinophils.

Eosinophils release granule proteins that are toxic to parasitic organisms and may injure normal tissue. Little is known about the mechanisms involved in eosinophil degranulation and mediator production. Although eosinophils express Fc receptors for IgG, IgA, and IgE, they do not appear to be as sensitive to activation by antigen-mediated cross-linking of these receptors as are mast cells and basophils. Nonetheless, eosinophils can kill microorganisms by antibody-dependent cell-mediated cytotoxicity (ADCC) with the use of FcεRI and perhaps FcαR. During this process, eosinophils bind to microorganisms coated with IgE (or IgA) antibody, and their granule contents are released onto the microbes. The granule contents of eosinophils include lysosomal hydrolases found in other granulocytes as well as eosinophil-specific proteins that are particularly toxic to helminthic organisms, including major basic protein and eosinophil cationic protein. These two cationic polypeptides have no known enzymatic activities, but they are toxic to helminths, bacteria, and normal tissue. In addition, eosinophilic granules contain eosinophil peroxidase, which is distinct from the myeloperoxidase found in neutrophils and catalyzes the production of hypochlorous or hypobromous acid. These products are also toxic to helminths, protozoa, and host cells.

Activated eosinophils, like mast cells and basophils, produce and release lipid mediators, including PAF, prostaglandins, and leukotrienes (LTC_4 and its derivatives LTD_4 and LTE_4). The importance of eosinophil-derived lipid mediators in immediate hypersensitivity is not completely known, but it is likely that they contribute to the pathologic processes of allergic diseases. Eosinophils also produce a variety of cytokines that may promote inflammatory responses, but the biologic significance of eosinophil cytokine production is not known.

Reactions of Immediate Hypersensitivity

The IgE- and mast cell–mediated reactions of immediate hypersensitivity consist of the immediate reaction, in which vascular and smooth muscle responses to mediators are dominant, and the late-phase reaction, characterized by leukocyte recruitment and inflammation (Fig. 19–7).

The Immediate Reaction

The early vascular changes that occur during immediate hypersensitivity reactions are demonstrated by the wheal and flare reaction to the intradermal injection of an allergen (Fig. 19–8). When an individual who has previously encountered an allergen and produced IgE antibody is challenged by intradermal injection of the same antigen, the injection site becomes red from locally dilated blood vessels engorged with red blood cells. The site then rapidly swells as a result of leakage of plasma from the venules. This soft swelling is called a wheal and can involve an area of skin as large as several centimeters in diameter. Subsequently, blood vessels at the margins of the wheal dilate and become engorged with red blood cells and produce a characteristic red rim called a flare. The full wheal and flare reaction can appear within 5 to 10 minutes after administration of antigen and usually subsides in less than an hour. By electron microscopy, the venules in the area of the wheal show slight separation of the endothelial cells, which accounts for the escape of macromolecules and fluid, but not cells, from the vascular lumen.

The wheal and flare reaction is dependent on IgE and mast cells. Histologic examination shows that mast

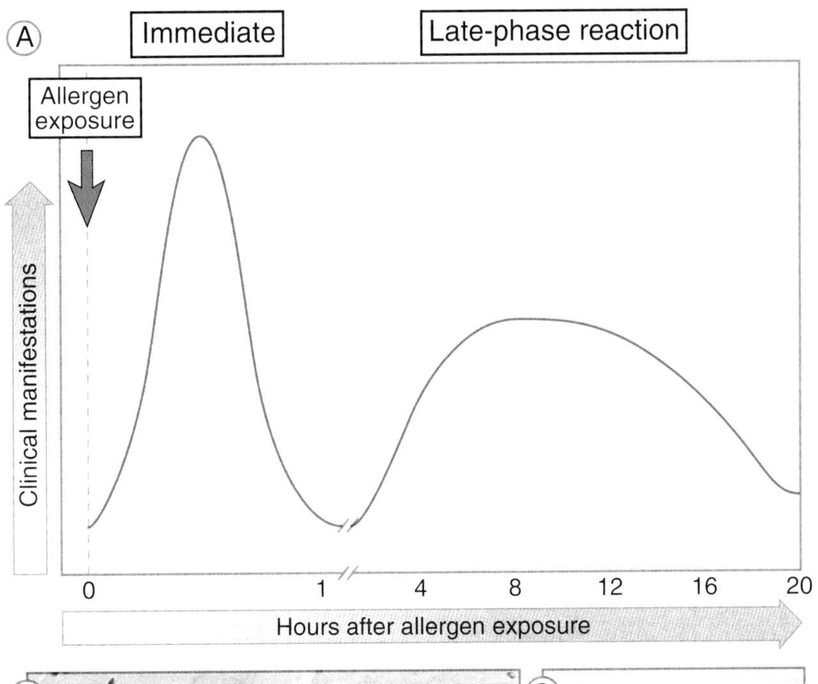

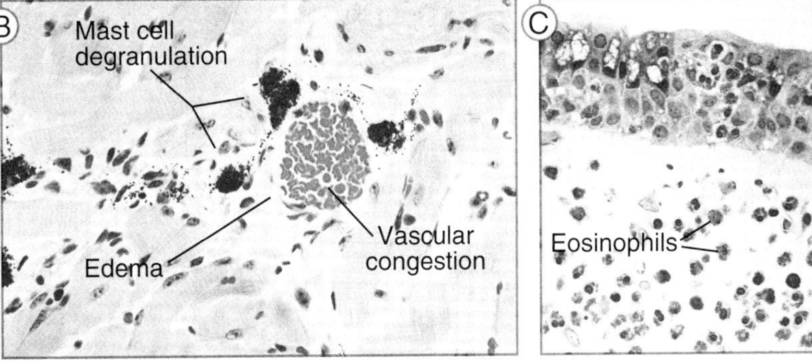

Figure 19–7 The immediate and late-phase reactions.

A. Kinetics: The immediate vascular and smooth muscle reaction to allergen develops within minutes after challenge (allergen exposure in a previously sensitized individual), and the late-phase reaction develops 2 to 24 hours later.

B, C. Morphology: The immediate reaction (B) is characterized by vasodilation, congestion, and edema, and the late-phase reaction (C) is characterized by an inflammatory infiltrate rich in eosinophils, neutrophils, and T cells. (Courtesy of Dr. Daniel Friend, Department of Pathology, Brigham and Women's Hospital, Boston.)

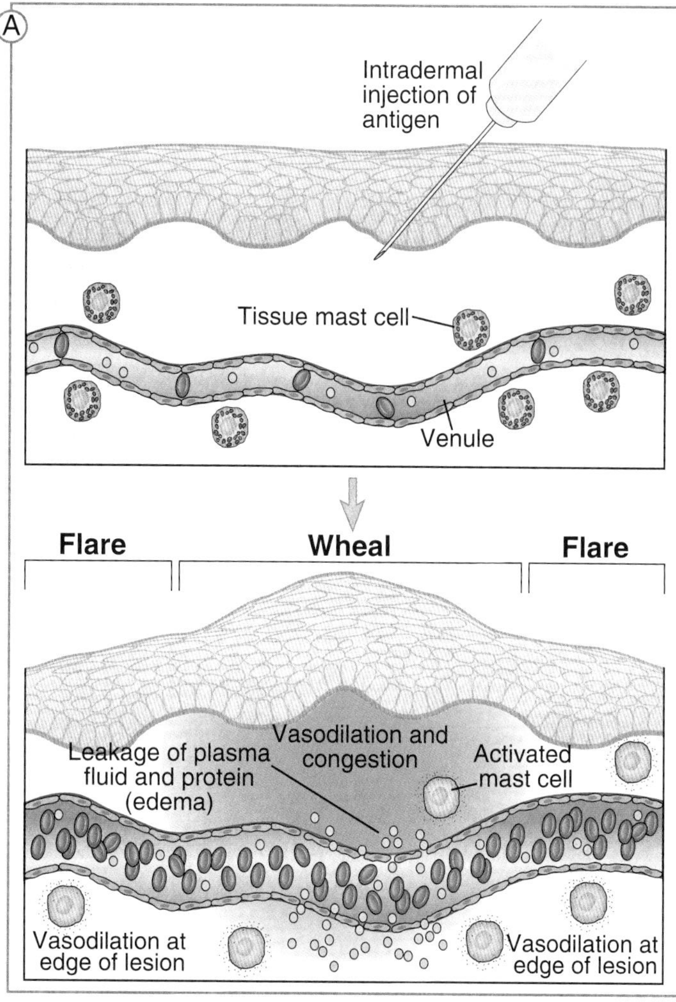

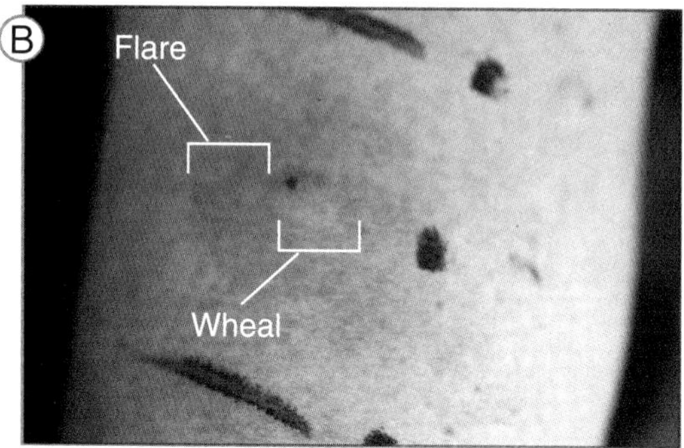

Figure 19–8 The wheal and flare reaction in the skin. A. In response to antigen-stimulated release of mast cell mediators, local blood vessels first dilate and then become leaky to fluid and macromolecules, which produces redness and local swelling (a wheal). Subsequent dilation of vessels on the edge of the swelling produces the appearance of a red rim (the flare).

B. Photograph of a typical wheal and flare reaction in the skin in response to injection of an allergen. (Courtesy of Dr. James D. Faix, Department of Pathology, Stanford University School of Medicine, Palo Alto, Calif.)

cells in the area of the wheal and flare have released preformed mediators; that is, their cytoplasmic granules have been discharged. A causal association of IgE and mast cells with immediate hypersensitivity was deduced from three kinds of experiments.

- Immediate hypersensitivity reactions against an allergen can be elicited in unresponsive individuals if the local skin site is first injected with IgE from a responsive individual. Thus, IgE is responsible for specific recognition of antigen and can be used to adoptively transfer immediate hypersensitivity. Such adoptive transfer experiments were first performed with serum from immunized individuals, and the serum factor responsible for the reaction was originally called reagin. For this reason, IgE molecules are still sometimes called reaginic antibodies. The antigen-initiated skin reaction that follows adoptive transfer of IgE is called passive cutaneous anaphylaxis.

- Immediate hypersensitivity reactions can be mimicked by injecting anti-IgE antibody instead of antigen. Anti-IgE antibodies act as an analogue of antigen and directly activate mast cells that have bound IgE on their surface. This use of anti-IgE to activate mast cells is similar to the use of anti-IgM antibodies as analogues of antigen to activate B cells (see Chapter 9), except that in the case of mast cells, secreted IgE, made by B cells, is bound to high-affinity Fc receptors on the cell surface rather than being synthesized as membrane IgE. Anti-IgE antibodies activate mast cells even in normal (nonatopic) individuals because, as mentioned earlier, mast cells are normally coated with IgE by virtue of the high-affinity FcεRI. In contrast, any antigen will activate mast cells only in individuals who are allergic to that antigen because only these individuals will produce enough specific IgE to sensitize mast cells for antigen-induced responses.

- Immediate hypersensitivity reactions can be mimicked by the injection of other agents that directly activate mast cells, such as the complement fragments C5a, C4a, and C3a, called anaphylatoxins, or by local trauma, which also causes degranulation of mast cells. Conversely, these reactions can be inhibited by agents that prevent mast cell activation.

The wheal and flare reaction results from sensitization of dermal mast cells by IgE bound to FcεRI, cross-linking of the IgE by the antigen, and activation of mast cells with release of mediators, notably histamine. Histamine binds to histamine receptors on venular endothelial cells; the endothelial cells synthesize and release PGI_2, nitric oxide, and PAF; and these mediators cause vasodilation and vascular leak, as described earlier in the chapter. Skin mast cells appear to produce only small amounts of long-acting mediators such as leukotrienes, and the wheal and flare response typically subsides after about 15 to 20 minutes. Allergists often test patients for allergies to different antigens by examining the ability of these antigens applied in skin patches to elicit wheal and flare reactions.

The Late-Phase Reaction

The immediate wheal and flare reaction is followed 2 to 4 hours later by a late-phase reaction consisting of the accumulation of inflammatory leukocytes, including neutrophils, eosinophils, basophils, and T_H2 cells (see Fig. 19–7). The inflammation is maximal by about 24 hours and then gradually subsides. The capacity to mount a late-phase reaction can be adoptively transferred with IgE, and the reaction can be mimicked by anti-IgE antibodies or mast cell–activating agents, like the wheal and flare reaction. Mast cell granules contain cytokines, including TNF, that can up-regulate endothelial expression of leukocyte adhesion molecules, such as E-selectin and intercellular adhesion molecule-1 (ICAM-1). Thus, mast cell degranulation can lead to the induction of adhesion molecules on vascular endothelial cells that promote the recruitment of leukocytes into tissues. The types of leukocytes that are typical of late-phase reactions are eosinophils and T_H2 cells; in addition, neutrophils are often present in these reactions. Eosinophils and T_H2 cells express receptors for many of the same chemokines, such as eotaxin and MCP-5, and this is why both cell types are recruited to sites of production of these chemokines. The late-phase reaction differs from delayed-type hypersensitivity reactions, in which macrophages and T_H1 cells are abundant.

The late-phase reaction may occur without a detectable preceding immediate hypersensitivity reaction. Bronchial asthma and eczema are diseases in which there is chronic inflammation with accumulations of eosinophils and T_H2 cells without the vascular changes that are characteristic of the wheal and flare response. It is believed that in such disorders, the cytokines that induce the chronic late-phase reaction are derived from T_H2 cells.

Genetic Susceptibility to Immediate Hypersensitivity

The propensity to produce IgE is influenced by the inheritance of several genes. Abnormally high levels of IgE synthesis and associated atopy often run in families. Family studies have shown clear autosomal transmission of atopy, although the full inheritance pattern is probably multigenic. Within the same family, the target organ of atopic disease is variable. Thus, hay fever, asthma, and eczema can be present to various degrees in different members of the same kindred. All these individuals, however, will show higher than average plasma IgE levels.

A variety of studies have identified candidate genes or loci that may be involved in allergy (Table 19–4). One of these susceptibility loci for atopy is on chromosome 5q, near the site of the gene cluster encoding the cytokines IL-3, IL-4, IL-5, IL-9, and IL-13 and the IL-4 receptor. This region is of great interest because of the connection between several of the genes located here and the mechanisms of IgE regulation and mast cell and eosinophil growth and differentiation. In addition, polymorphisms of the IL-9 gene have been associated with human bronchial asthma, and this cytokine can induce airway inflammation in experimental models of asthma. Furthermore, the homologous chromosomal region in mice has been linked to a propensity for $CD4^+$ T cells in some inbred strains of mice to differentiate into T_H2 cells in response to model protein antigens. Another atopy/asthma-associated locus is on chromosome 11q13, the location of the gene encoding the β chain of the high-affinity IgE receptor. Some studies have shown that a polymorphism in this receptor is associated with atopy, but many other studies have failed to establish a linkage of atopy with the FcεRI β chain or even this chromosomal region. A polymorphism in the IL-4 receptor α chain has been associated with atopic asthma in some families. Several other chromosomal regions have been shown to be associated with high serum IgE levels, atopy, and asthma, but the studies are preliminary and candidate genes have not been identified. Finally, the tendency to produce IgE antibodies against some but not all antigens, such as ragweed pollen, may be linked to particular class II major histocompatibility complex (MHC) alleles. This linkage may be an example of an immune response gene (Ir gene) effect in which atopic individuals inherit class II MHC alleles that can bind and display dominant epitopes of certain allergens (see Chapter 4).

Table 19–4. Candidate Genes Associated with Atopy and Asthma

Chromosomal location	Candidate genes	Role of gene products in immediate hypersensitivity
5q31	IL-4, IL-5, IL-9, IL-13, GM-CSF	IL-4 and IL-13 promote IgE switching, and IL-5 promotes eosinophil growth and activation
5q32	β_2-Adrenergic receptor	Regulates arterial and bronchial smooth muscle contraction
6p	Class II MHC	Some alleles may regulate T cell responsiveness to allergens
6p21.3	TNF-α	Mast cell inflammatory mediator
11q13	FcεRI β chain	Mast cell IgE receptor
12q	Interferon-γ	Opposes actions of IL-4
14q	TCR α	??

Adapted from Leung DYM. Molecular basis of allergic diseases. Molecular Genetics and Metabolism 63:157–167, 1998.

Allergic Diseases in Humans: Pathogenesis and Therapy

Mast cell degranulation is a central component of all allergic diseases, and the clinical and pathologic manifestations of the diseases depend on the tissues in which the mast cell mediators have effects as well as the chronicity of the resulting inflammatory process. Atopic individuals may have one or more manifestations of atopic disease. The most common forms of atopic disease are allergic rhinitis (hay fever), bronchial asthma, atopic dermatitis (eczema), and food allergies. The clinical and pathologic features of allergic reactions vary with the anatomic site of the reaction, for several reasons. The point of contact with the allergen determines the organs or tissues that are involved. For example, inhaled antigens cause rhinitis or asthma, ingested antigens often cause vomiting and diarrhea, and injected antigens cause systemic effects on the circulation. The concentrations of mast cells in various target organs influence the severity of responses. Mast cells are particularly abundant in the skin and the mucosa of the respiratory and gastrointestinal tracts, and these tissues frequently suffer the most injury in immediate hypersensitivity reactions. The local mast cell phenotype may influence the characteristics of the immediate hypersensitivity reaction. For example, connective tissue mast cells with abundant histamine are responsible for wheal and flare reactions in the skin. In the following section, we discuss the major features of allergic diseases manifested in different tissues.

Systemic Anaphylaxis

Anaphylaxis is a systemic immediate hypersensitivity reaction characterized by edema in many tissues and fall in blood pressure, secondary to vasodilation. These effects usually result from the systemic presence of antigen introduced by injection, an insect sting, or absorption across an epithelial surface such as the skin or gut mucosa. The allergen activates mast cells in many tissues, resulting in the release of mediators that gain access to vascular beds throughout the body. The decrease in vascular tone and leakage of plasma caused by the released mediators can lead to a fall in blood pressure or shock, called **anaphylactic shock,** which is often fatal. The cardiovascular effects are accompanied by constriction of the upper and lower airways, hypersensitivity of the gut, outpouring of mucus in the gut and respiratory tree, and urticarial lesions (hives) in the skin. It is not known which mast cell mediators are the most important in anaphylactic shock. The mainstay of treatment is systemic epinephrine, which can be lifesaving by reversing the bronchoconstrictive and vasodilatory effects of the various mast cell mediators. Epinephrine also improves cardiac output, further aiding survival from threatened circulatory collapse. Antihistamines may also be beneficial in anaphylaxis, suggesting a role for histamine in this reaction. In some animal models, PAF receptor antagonists offer partial protection.

Bronchial Asthma

Asthma is an inflammatory disease caused by repeated immediate hypersensitivity and late-phase reactions in the lung leading to the clinicopathologic triad of intermittent and reversible airway obstruction, chronic bronchial inflammation with eosinophils, and bronchial smooth muscle cell hypertrophy and hyperreactivity to bronchoconstrictors (Fig. 19–9). Patients suffer paroxysms of bronchial constriction and increased production of thick mucus, which leads to bronchial obstruction and exacerbates respiratory diffi-

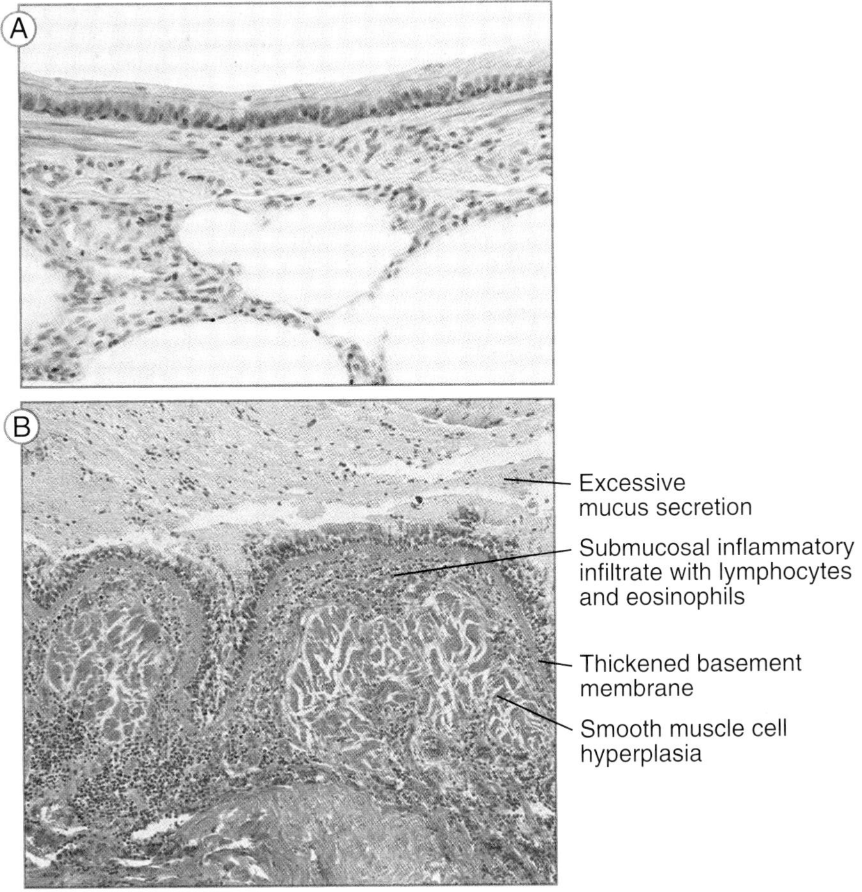

Figure 19–9 Histopathologic features of bronchial asthma.
Atopic bronchial asthma results from repeated immediate hypersensitivity reactions in the lungs with chronic late-phase reactions. A cross-section of a normal bronchus is shown in A; a bronchus from a patient with asthma is shown in B. The diseased bronchus has excessive mucus production, many submucosal inflammatory cells (including eosinophils), and smooth muscle hypertrophy. (Courtesy of Dr. James D. Faix, Department of Pathology, Stanford University School of Medicine, Palo Alto, Calif.)

culties. Asthma frequently coexists with bronchitis or emphysema, and the combination of diseases can cause severe tissue destruction. Asthma affects about 10 million people in the United States, and the frequency of this disease has increased significantly in recent years. The prevalence rate is similar to that in other industrialized countries, but it may be lower in less developed areas of the world. Affected individuals may suffer considerable morbidity, and asthma causes death in some patients.

About 70% of cases of asthma are due to IgE-mediated immediate hypersensitivity. In the remaining 30% of patients, asthma may not be associated with atopy and may be triggered by nonimmune stimuli such as drugs, cold, and exercise. Even among nonatopic asthmatics, the pathophysiologic process of airway constriction is similar, which suggests that alternative mechanisms of mast cell degranulation (e.g., by locally produced neurotransmitters) may underlie the disease.

The pathophysiologic sequence in atopic asthma is initiated by mast cell activation in response to allergen binding to IgE as well as by T_H2 cells reacting to allergens (Fig. 19–10). Cytokines produced by the mast cells and T cells lead to the recruitment of eosinophils, basophils, and more T_H2 cells. The chronic inflammation in this disease may continue without mast cell activation. Smooth muscle cell hypertrophy and hyperreactivity are thought to result from leukocyte-derived mediators and cytokines. Mast cells, basophils, and eosinophils all produce mediators that constrict airway smooth muscle. The most important of the bronchoconstricting mediators are LTC_4, its breakdown products LTD_4 and LTE_4, and PAF. In clinical experiments, antagonists of LTC_4 synthesis or leukotriene receptor antagonists prevent allergen-induced airway constriction.

Current therapy for asthma has two major targets: prevention and reversal of inflammation and relaxation of airway smooth muscle. In recent years, the balance of therapy has shifted toward anti-inflammatory agents as the primary mode of treatment. Two major classes of drugs are in current use: corticosteroids, which block the production of inflammatory cytokines, and sodium cromolyn. The mechanism of action of sodium cromolyn is not clear, but it appears to antagonize IgE-induced release of mediators. Both agents can be used prophylactically as inhalants. Corticosteroids may also be given systemically, especially once an attack is under way, to reduce inflammation. Newer anti-inflammatory therapies are in preclinical and clinical trials. For example, leukotriene receptor antagonists and 5-lipoxygenase inhibitors are proving to be effective asthma treatments. Other experimental drugs include inhibitors of leukocyte adhesion to endothelial cells (e.g., antibodies to VCAM-1, ICAM-1, or E-selectin) and PAF receptor antagonists. It remains to be seen whether these agents are effective in treating asthma. Because histamine has little role in airway constriction, antihis-

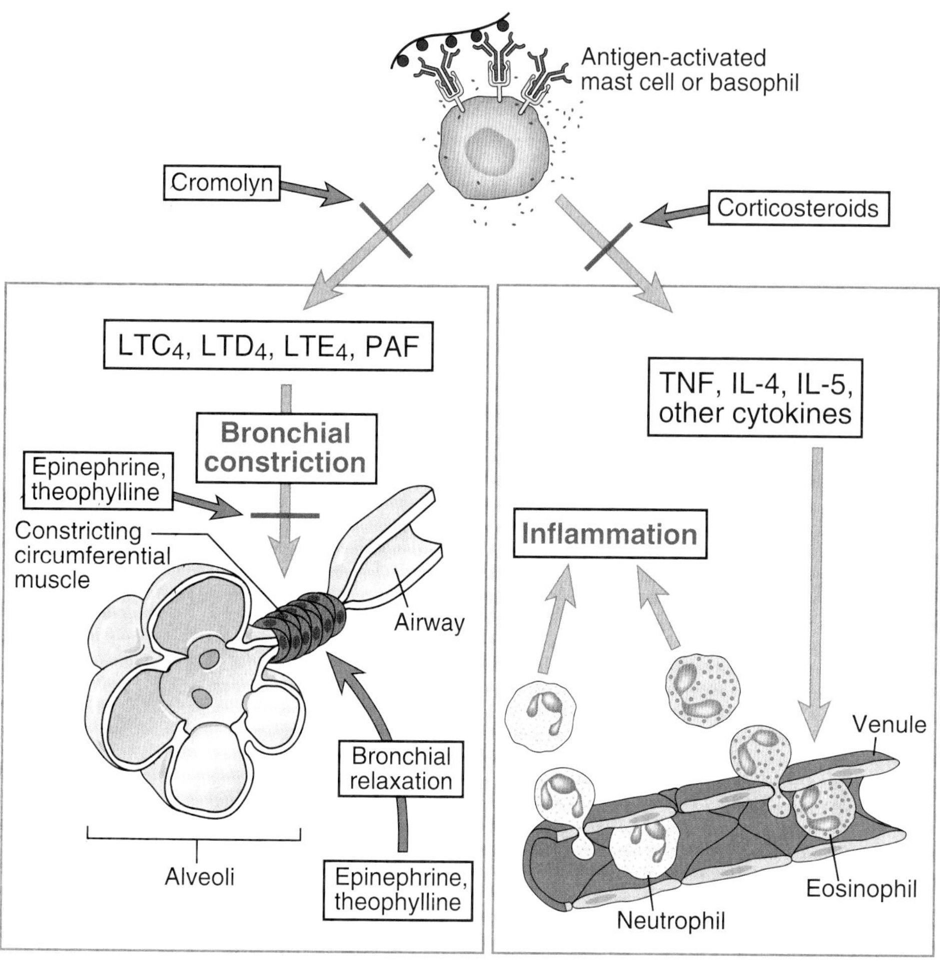

Figure 19–10 Mediators and treatment of asthma. Mast cell–derived leukotrienes and platelet-activating factor (PAF) are thought to be the major mediators of acute bronchoconstriction. Therapy is targeted both at reducing mast cell activation with inhibitors such as cromolyn and at countering mediator actions on bronchial smooth muscle by bronchodilators such as epinephrine and theophylline. These drugs also inhibit mast cell activation. Mast cell–derived cytokines are thought to be the major mediators of sustained airway inflammation, which is an example of a late-phase reaction, and corticosteroid therapy is used to inhibit cytokine synthesis.

tamines (H_1 receptor antagonists) are not useful in the treatment of asthma. Indeed, because many antihistamines are also anticholinergics, these drugs may worsen airway obstruction by causing thickening of mucus secretions.

Bronchial smooth muscle cell relaxation has principally been achieved by elevating intracellular cAMP levels in smooth muscle cells, which inhibits contraction. The major drugs used are activators of adenylate cyclase, such as epinephrine and related β_2-adrenergic agents, and inhibitors of the phosphodiesterase enzymes that degrade cAMP, such as theophylline. These drugs also raise cAMP levels in mast cells and act to inhibit mast cell degranulation.

Immediate Hypersensitivity Reactions in the Upper Respiratory Tract, Gastrointestinal Tract, and Skin

Allergic rhinitis, also called hay fever, is perhaps the most common allergic disease and is a consequence of immediate hypersensitivity reactions to common allergens such as plant pollen or house dust mites localized to the upper respiratory tract by inhalation. The pathologic and clinical manifestations include mucosal edema, leukocyte infiltration with abundant eosinophils, mucus secretion, coughing, sneezing, and difficulty breathing. Allergic conjunctivitis with itchy eyes is commonly associated with the rhinitis. Focal protrusions of the nasal mucosa, called nasal polyps, filled with edema fluid and eosinophils may develop in patients who suffer frequent repetitive bouts of allergic rhinitis. Antihistamines are the most common drugs used to treat allergic rhinitis.

Food allergies are immediate hypersensitivity reactions to ingested foods that lead to the release of mediators from intestinal mucosal and submucosal mast cells. Clinical manifestations include enhanced peristalsis, increased fluid secretion from intestinal lining cells, and associated vomiting and diarrhea. Urticaria is often associated with allergic reactions to food, and systemic anaphylaxis may occasionally ensue. Allergic reactions to many different types of food have been described, but some of the most common are peanuts and shellfish. Individuals may be so sensitive to these allergens that severe systemic reactions can occur in response to minute contaminants of the allergen introduced accidentally during food preparation.

Allergic reactions in the skin are manifested as **urticaria** and **eczema.** Urticaria, which is essentially an acute wheal and flare reaction induced by mast cell mediators, occurs in response to direct contact with the allergen or after an allergen enters the circulation through the intestinal tract or by injection. Because the reaction that ensues is mediated largely by histamine, antihistamines (H_1 receptor antagonists) can block this response almost completely. The urticaria may persist for several hours, probably because antigen persists in the plasma. Chronic eczema is a common skin disorder that may be caused by a late-phase reaction to an allergen in the skin. In the cutaneous late-phase reaction, TNF, IL-4, and other cytokines, probably derived from T_H2 cells and mast cells, act on the venular endothelial cells to promote inflammation. As may be expected for a cytokine-mediated response, the late-phase inflammatory reaction is not inhibited by antihistamines. It can be blocked by treatment with corticosteroids, which inhibit cytokine synthesis.

Immunotherapy for Allergic Diseases

In addition to therapy aimed at the consequences of immediate hypersensitivity, clinical immunologists often try to limit the onset of allergic reactions by treatments aimed at reducing the quantity of IgE present in the individual. Several empirical protocols have been developed to diminish specific IgE synthesis. In one approach, called **desensitization,** small but increasing quantities of antigen are administered subcutaneously during a period of hours or more gradually during weeks or months. As a result of this treatment, specific IgE levels decrease and IgG titers often rise, perhaps further inhibiting IgE production by neutralizing the antigen and by antibody feedback (see Chapter 9). It is also possible that desensitization may work by inducing specific T cell tolerance or by changing the predominant phenotype of antigen-specific T cells from T_H2 to T_H1; however, few direct data support these hypotheses. The beneficial effects of desensitization may occur in a matter of hours, much earlier than changes in IgE levels. Although the precise mechanism is unknown, this approach has been successful in preventing acute anaphylactic responses to protein antigens (e.g., insect venom) or vital drugs (e.g., penicillin). It is more variable in its effectiveness for chronic atopic conditions such as hay fever and asthma.

Other approaches being tried to reduce IgE levels include systemic administration of humanized monoclonal anti-IgE antibodies. Antagonists against the cytokines IL-4 and IL-5 are also in clinical trials.

The Protective Roles of IgE- and Mast Cell–Mediated Immune Reactions

Although most of our understanding of mast cell– and basophil-mediated responses comes from analysis of hypersensitivity or disease, it is logical to assume that these responses have evolved because they provide protective functions. In fact, some evidence shows that IgE- and mast cell–mediated responses are important for defense against certain types of infection.

A major protective function of IgE-initiated immune reactions is the eradication of parasites. Eosinophil-mediated killing of IgE-coated helminths by the process of ADCC is an effective defense against these organisms (see Chapter 14, Fig. 14–4). Thus, the activities of IL-4, IL-5, and IL-13 in IgE production and eosinophil activation contribute to a coordinated defense against helminths. It has also been speculated that IgE-dependent mast cell activation in the gastrointestinal tract promotes the expulsion of parasites by increasing peristalsis and by an outpouring of mucus. Studies in mice have highlighted the beneficial roles of IgE and mast cells.

- Mice treated with anti–IL-4 antibody and IL-4 knockout mice do not make IgE and appear to be less resistant than normal animals to some helminthic infections. IL-5 knockout mice, which are unable to activate eosinophils, also show increased susceptibility to some helminths.
- Genetically mast cell–deficient mice show increased susceptibility to infection by tick larvae, and immunity can be provided to these mice by adoptive transfer of specific IgE and mast cells (but not by either component alone). The larvae are eradicated by the late-phase reaction.

Mast cells play an important protective role as part of the innate immune response to bacterial infections. Studies in mice have indicated that mast cells can be activated by IgE-independent mechanisms in the course of an acute bacterial infection and that the mediators they release are critical for clearing the infection.

- Mast cell–deficient mice are less capable of clearing and are more likely to die of acute bacterial infection of the peritoneum than are normal mice. The protective role of mast cells in this setting is mediated by TNF and depends on TNF-stimulated influx of neutrophils to the peritoneum, specifically, the late-phase reaction. The mechanisms by which mast cells are activated during innate immune responses to bacterial infection are not known but may involve complement activation and the release of C5a, which directly triggers mast cell degranulation. The alternative pathway of complement can be activated directly by microbial products. It is also possible that the classical pathway of complement could be activated by natural antibodies that are produced by B-1 B cells and that recognize common microbial pathogens.

Summary

- Immediate hypersensitivity is an immune reaction that is triggered by antigen binding to IgE preattached to mast cells and that leads to inflammatory mediator release.
- The steps in the development of immediate hypersensitivity are exposure to an antigen (allergen) that stimulates T_H2 responses and IgE production, binding of the IgE to Fcε receptors on mast cells, cross-linking of the IgE and the Fcε receptors by the allergen, activation of mast cells, and release of mediators.

- Individuals susceptible to immediate hypersensitivity reactions are called atopic and often have more IgE in the blood and more IgE-specific Fc receptors per mast cell than do nonatopic individuals. IgE synthesis is induced by exposure to antigen and T_H2 cytokines, particularly IL-4.
- Mast cells are derived from the bone marrow and mature in the tissues. They express high-affinity receptors for IgE (FcεRI) and contain cytoplasmic granules in which are stored various inflammatory mediators. Subsets of mast cells, including mucosal and connective tissue mast cells, may produce different mediators. Basophils are a type of circulating granulocyte that expresses high-affinity Fcε receptors and contains granules with contents similar to mast cells.
- Eosinophils are a special class of granulocyte; they are recruited into inflammatory reactions by chemokines and IL-4 and are activated by IL-5. Eosinophils are effector cells of IgE-initiated reactions. They mediate IgE-directed ADCC to eradicate parasites. In allergic reactions, eosinophils contribute to tissue injury.
- On binding of antigen to IgE on the surface of mast cells or basophils, the high-affinity Fcε receptors become cross-linked and activate intracellular second messengers that lead to granule release and new synthesis of mediators. Activated mast cells and basophils produce three important classes of mediators: biogenic amines, such as histamine; lipid mediators, such as prostaglandins, leukotrienes, and PAF; and cytokines, such as TNF, IL-4, and IL-5.
- Biogenic amines and lipid mediators cause the rapid vascular and smooth muscle reactions of immediate hypersensitivity, such as vascular leakage, vasodilation, and bronchoconstriction. Cytokines mediate the late-phase reaction.
- Various organs show distinct forms of immediate hypersensitivity involving different mediators and target cell types. Any allergen may lead to a systemic reaction called anaphylactic shock. Asthma is a manifestation of immediate hypersensitivity and late-phase reactions in the lung. Allergic rhinitis (hay fever) is the most common allergic disease of the upper respiratory tract. Food allergens can cause diarrhea and vomiting. In the skin, immediate hypersensitivity is manifested as wheal and flare and late-phase reactions and may lead to chronic eczema.
- Drug therapy is aimed at inhibiting mast cell mediator production and at blocking or counteracting the effects of released mediators on target organs. The goal of immunotherapy is to prevent or to reduce T_H2 cell responses to specific allergens and the production of IgE.
- Immediate hypersensitivity reactions provide protection against helminthic infections by promoting IgE- and eosinophil-mediated ADCC and gut peristalsis. Furthermore, mast cells may play an important role in innate immune responses to bacterial infections.

Selected Readings

Costa JJ, PF Weller, and SJ Galli. The cells of the allergic response. JAMA 278:1815–1822, 1997.

Galli SJ, M Maurer, and CS Lantz. Mast cells as sentinels of innate immunity. Current Opinion in Immunology 11: 53–59, 1999.

Kay AB. Allergy and allergic diseases. New England Journal of Medicine 344:30–37, 109–113, 2001.

Maddox L, and DA Schwartz. The pathophysiology of asthma. Annual Review of Medicine 53:477–498, 2002.

Marsh KC, and DG Marsh. The genetics and complexity of asthma. Immunology Today 19:325–332, 1998.

Nadler MJ, SA Matthews, H Turner, and J-P Kinet. Signal transduction by the high affinity immunoglobulin E receptor FcεRI: coupling form to function. Advances in Immunology 76:325–355, 2000.

Ono SJ. Molecular genetics of allergic diseases. Annual Review of Immunology 18:347–365, 2000.

Paul WE, RA Seder, and M Plaut. Lymphokine and cytokine production by FcεRI cells. Advances in Immunology 53:1–29, 1993.

Piccini MP, E Maggi, and S Romagnani. Environmental factors favoring the allergen-specific Th2 response in allergic subjects. Annals of the New York Academy of Sciences 917:844–852, 2000.

Robinson DS, AB Kay, and AJ Wardlaw. Eosinophils. Clinical Allergy and Immunology 16:43–75, 2002.

Wedemeyer J, M Tsai, and SJ Galli. Roles of mast cells and basophils in innate and acquired immunity. Current Opinion in Immunology 12:624–631, 2000.

Wurtzburg BA, and TS Jardetzky. Structural insights into the interactions between IgE and its high affinity receptor FcεRI. Molecular Immunology 38:1063–1072, 2001.

Chapter 20

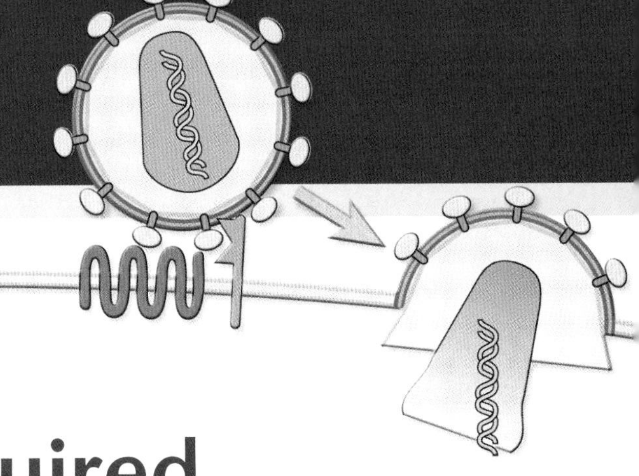

Congenital and Acquired Immunodeficiencies

Integrity of the immune system is essential for defense against infectious organisms and their toxic products and therefore for the survival of all individuals. Defects in one or more components of the immune system can lead to serious and often fatal disorders, which are collectively called immunodeficiency diseases. These diseases are broadly classified into two groups. The **congenital** or **primary immunodeficiencies** are genetic defects that result in an increased susceptibility to infection that is frequently manifested early in infancy and childhood but is sometimes clinically detected later in life. It is estimated that in the United States, approximately 1 in 500 individuals is born with a defect in some component of the immune system, although only a small proportion are affected severely enough for development of life-threatening complications. **Acquired** or **secondary immunodeficiencies** develop as a consequence of malnutrition, disseminated cancer, treatment with immunosuppressive drugs, or infection of cells of the immune system, most notably with the human immunodeficiency virus (HIV), the etiologic agent of acquired immunodeficiency syndrome (AIDS). This chapter describes the major types of congenital and acquired immunodeficiencies, with an emphasis on their pathogenesis and the components of the immune system that are involved in each.

General Features of Immunodeficiency Diseases

Before beginning our discussion of individual diseases, it is important to summarize some general features of immunodeficiencies.

- ***The principal consequence of immunodeficiency is an increased susceptibility to infection.*** The nature of the infection in a particular patient depends largely on the component of the immune system that is defective (Table 20–1). Deficient humoral immunity usually results in increased susceptibility to infection by pyogenic bacteria, whereas defects in cell-mediated immunity lead to infection by viruses

Table 20–1. Features of Immunodeficiencies Affecting T or B Lymphocytes

Feature	B cell deficiency	T cell deficiency
Diagnosis		
Serum Ig levels	Reduced	Normal or reduced
DTH reactions to common antigens	Normal	Reduced
Morphology of lymphoid tissues	Absent or reduced follicles and germinal centers (B cell zones)	Usually normal follicles, may be reduced parafollicular cortical regions (T cell zones)
Susceptibility to infection	Pyogenic bacteria (otitis, pneumonia, meningitis, osteomyelitis), enteric bacteria and viruses, some parasites	*Pneumocystis carinii*, many viruses, atypical mycobacteria, fungi

Abbreviation: DTH, delayed-type hypersensitivity.

and other intracellular microbes. Combined deficiencies in both humoral and cell-mediated immunity make patients susceptible to infection by all classes of microorganisms.

- ***Patients with immunodeficiencies are also susceptible to certain types of cancer.*** Many of these cancers appear to be caused by oncogenic viruses, such as the Epstein-Barr virus (EBV). An increased incidence of cancer is most often seen in T cell immunodeficiencies because, as discussed in Chapter 17, T cells play an important role in surveillance against oncogenic viruses and the tumors they cause. In addition, paradoxically, certain immunodeficiencies are associated with an increased incidence of autoimmunity. The mechanism underlying this association is not known; it may reflect a deficiency of regulatory T lymphocytes that normally serve to maintain self-tolerance.
- ***Immunodeficiency may result from defects in lymphocyte maturation or activation or from defects in the effector mechanisms of innate and adaptive immunity.*** Immunodeficiency diseases are clinically and pathologically heterogeneous, in part because different diseases involve different components of the immune system.

In this chapter, we first describe congenital immunodeficiencies, including defects in the humoral and cell-mediated arms of the adaptive immune system and defects in components of the innate immune system. We conclude with a discussion of acquired immunodeficiencies, with an emphasis on AIDS.

Congenital (Primary) Immunodeficiencies

The first inherited immunodeficiency to be described, in 1952, was a disease called X-linked agammaglobulinemia that affected boys and is now known to be caused by a defect in B lymphocyte maturation. Since then, a large number of other congenital immunodeficiencies have been described, and the genetic bases of many of these disorders are now known. This understanding has led to an increased hope for gene replacement as therapy for the diseases.

In different immunodeficiencies, the primary abnormality may be at different stages of lymphocyte maturation or in the responses of mature lymphocytes to antigenic stimulation. Abnormalities in B lymphocyte development and function result in deficient antibody production and increased susceptibility to infection by extracellular microbes. B cell immunodeficiencies are diagnosed by reduced levels of serum immunoglobulin (Ig), defective antibody responses to vaccination, and, in some cases, reduced numbers of B cells in the circulation or lymphoid tissues or absent plasma cells in tissues (see Table 20–1). Abnormalities in T lymphocyte maturation and function lead to deficient cell-mediated immunity and an increased incidence of infection with intracellular microbes. Deficiencies of helper T cells may also result in reduced antibody production. Primary T cell immunodeficiencies are diagnosed by reduced numbers of peripheral blood T cells; low proliferative responses of blood lymphocytes to polyclonal T cell activators, such as phytohemagglutinin; and deficient cutaneous delayed-type hypersensitivity (DTH) reactions to ubiquitous microbial antigens, such as *Candida* antigens. In the following sections, we describe immunodeficiencies caused by different defects in lymphocyte maturation or activation and in innate immunity and conclude with a brief discussion of therapeutic strategies for these diseases.

Defects in Lymphocyte Maturation

The process of lymphocyte maturation from stem cells to functionally competent mature lymphocytes involves cell proliferation, expression of antigen receptors, selection of cells with useful specificities, and changes in the expression of numerous genes (see Chapter 7).

Genetic defects in many of these stages have been described in experimental models and humans. In fact, the abnormalities in lymphocyte development caused by inherited mutations and targeted disruption of genes encoding a variety of molecules, including enzymes and transcription factors, have been useful in elucidating the mechanisms of lymphocyte maturation (see Chapter 7, Box 7–1). In the following section, we focus on congenital immunodeficiencies in humans that are known to result from blocks at various stages of lymphocyte maturation (Fig. 20–1 and Table 20–2). Disorders that affect both B and T lymphocytes, with resultant defects in humoral and cell-mediated immunity, are called **severe combined immunodeficiencies** (SCIDs). Children with SCID usually have infections during the first year of life and succumb to these infections unless they are treated. Other diseases affect either the B or T cell lineage and are given specific names for the clinicopathologic condition.

X-Linked Severe Combined Immunodeficiency Caused by Mutations in the Cytokine Receptor Common γ Chain

Approximately 50% of SCID cases are X-linked and due to mutations in the gene encoding the **common γ chain** (γ_C) shared by the receptors for the interleukins IL-2, IL-4, IL-7, IL-9, and IL-15 (see Chapter 11). These mutations are recessive, so heterozygous females are usually phenotypically normal carriers, whereas males who inherit the abnormal X chromosome manifest the disease. Because developing cells in females randomly inactivate one of the two X chromosomes, the normal allele encoding a functional γ_C protein will not be expressed in half the lymphocyte precursors in a female carrier. These cells will fail to mature, and consequently, all the mature lymphocytes in a female carrier will have inactivated the same X chromosome (carrying the mutant allele). In contrast, half of all nonlymphoid cells

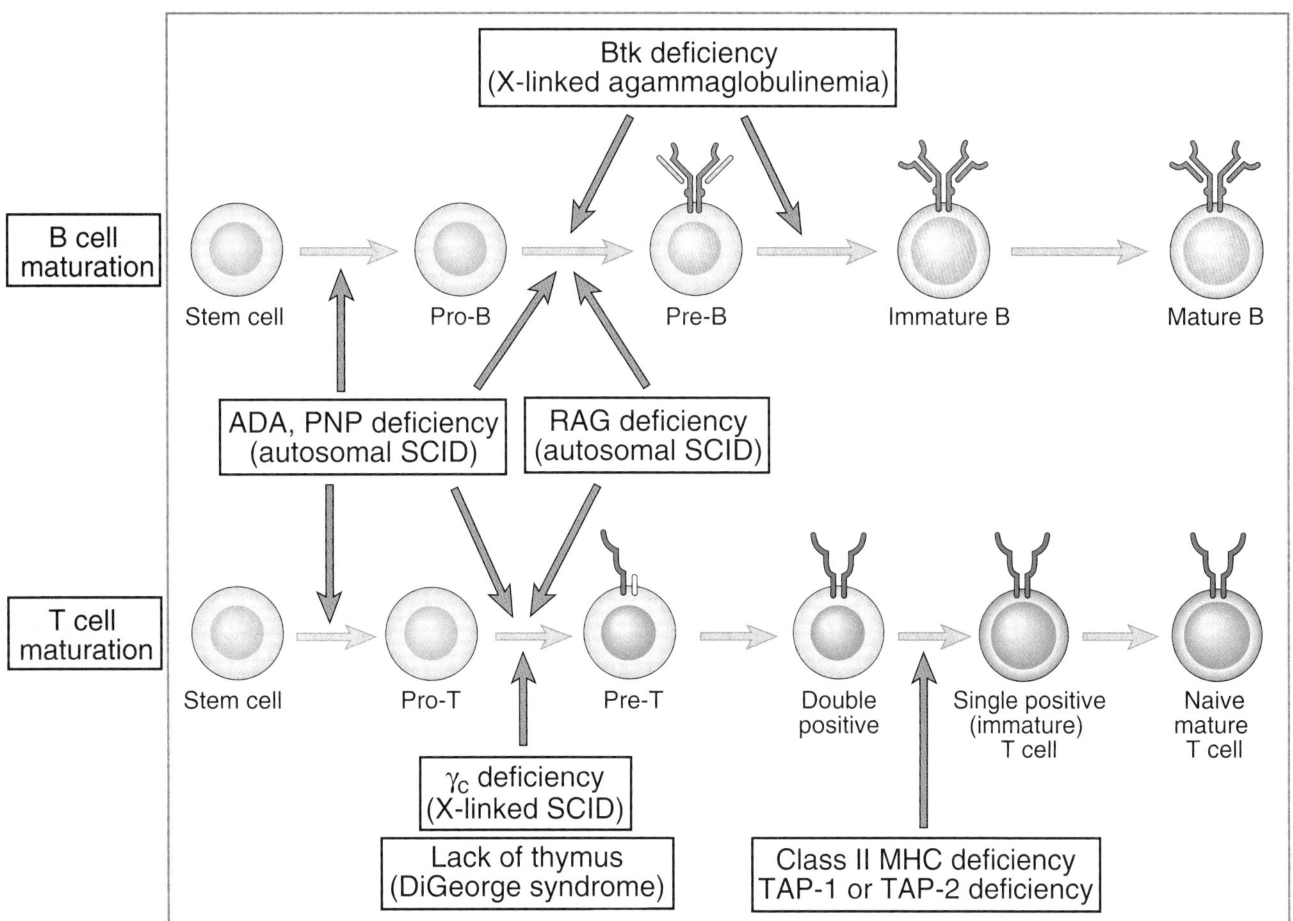

Figure 20–1 Immunodeficiency caused by defects in B and T cell maturation. Primary immunodeficiencies caused by genetic defects in lymphocyte maturation are shown. These defects may affect B cell maturation alone, T cell maturation alone, or both. Lymphocyte maturation pathways are described in detail in Chapter 7. ADA, adenosine deaminase; Btk, B cell tyrosine kinase; MHC, major histocompatibility complex; PNP, purine nucleoside phosphorylase; RAG, recombinase-activating gene; SCID, severe combined immunodeficiency disease; TAP, transporter associated with antigen processing.

Table 20–2. Defects of Lymphocyte Maturation

Disease	Functional deficiencies	Presumed mechanism of defect
Severe combined immunodeficiency		
X-linked	Markedly decreased T cells, normal or increased B cells, reduced serum Ig	Cytokine receptor common γ chain gene mutations, defective T cell maturation from lack of IL-7 signals
ADA, PNP deficiency (autosomal recessive)	Progressive decrease in T and B cells (mostly T); reduced serum Ig in ADA deficiency, normal B cells and serum Ig in PNP deficiency	ADA or PNP deficiency leading to accumulation of toxic metabolites in lymphocytes
Other autosomal recessive	Decreased T and B cells, reduced serum Ig	Defective maturation of T and B cells; genetic basis unknown in most cases, may be mutations in *RAG* genes
B cell immunodeficiencies		
X-linked agammaglobulinemia	Decrease in all serum Ig isotypes, reduced B cell numbers	Block in maturation beyond pre-B cells because of mutation in B cell tyrosine kinase
Ig heavy chain deletions	IgG1, IgG2, or IgG4 absent; sometimes associated with absent IgA or IgE	Chromosomal deletion at 14q32 (Ig heavy chain locus)
T cell immunodeficiencies		
DiGeorge syndrome	Decreased T cells, normal B cells, normal or decreased serum Ig	Anomalous development of 3rd and 4th branchial pouches leading to thymic hypoplasia

Abbreviations: ADA, adenosine deaminase; PNP, purine nucleoside phosphorylase; RAG, recombinase-activating gene.

will have inactivated one X chromosome, and half the other. A comparison of X chromosome inactivation in lymphoid cells versus nonlymphoid cells may be used to identify carriers of the mutant allele. The nonrandom use of X chromosomes in mature lymphocytes is also characteristic of female carriers of other X-linked mutations of genes that affect lymphocyte development, as discussed later.

X-linked SCID is characterized by impaired maturation of T cells and NK (natural killer) cells and greatly reduced numbers of mature T cells and NK cells, but the number of B cells is usually normal or increased. The humoral immunodeficiency in this disease is due to a lack of T cell help for antibody production. This disease is a result of the inability of the lymphopoietic cytokine IL-7, whose receptor uses the γ_C chain for signaling, to stimulate the growth of immature thymocytes. In addition, the receptor for IL-15, which is a potent stimulus for the proliferation of NK cells, also uses the γ_C signaling chain, and the failure of IL-15 function accounts for the deficiency of NK cells.

Some patients with a disease identical to X-linked SCID show an autosomal recessive inheritance pattern. These patients have mutations in the JAK3 kinase, which associates with the γ_C chain and is required for signaling by this protein (see Chapter 11, Box 11–2). Knockout mice lacking the γ_C chain, IL-7, the cytokine-binding chain of the IL-7 receptor, or JAK3 develop a disease similar to human X-linked SCID, although B cell maturation in mice is decreased more than in humans.

Severe Combined Immunodeficiency Caused by Adenosine Deaminase Deficiency

About 50% of patients with SCID show an autosomal recessive pattern of inheritance, and half of these cases are due to deficiency of an enzyme called **adenosine deaminase** (ADA). ADA functions in the salvage pathway of purine degradation and catalyzes the irreversible deamination of adenosine and 2′-deoxyadenosine to inosine and 2′-deoxyinosine, respectively. Deficiency of the enzyme leads to the accumulation of deoxyadenosine and its precursors *S*-adenosylhomocysteine and deoxyadenosine triphosphate (dATP). These by-products have many toxic effects, including inhibition of DNA synthesis. Although ADA is present in most cells, developing lymphocytes are less efficient than most other cell types at degrading dATP into 2′-deoxyadenosine, and therefore lymphocyte maturation is particularly sensitive to ADA deficiency. ADA deficiency leads to reduced numbers of B and T cells; lymphocyte cell numbers are usually normal at birth but fall off precipitously during the first year of life. A few patients may have nearly normal numbers of T cells, but these cells do not proliferate in response to antigenic stimulation. A rarer autosomal recessive form of SCID is due to the deficiency of another enzyme, called purine nucleoside phosphorylase (PNP), that is also involved in purine catabolism. PNP catalyzes the conversion of inosine to hypoxanthine and guanosine to guanine, and deficiency of PNP leads to the accumulation of deoxyguanosine and deoxyguanosine triphosphate, with toxic effects on immature lymphocytes, mainly T cells.

Other Causes of Severe Combined Immunodeficiency

About half the cases of autosomal recessive SCID are caused by mutations in various genes involved in lymphocyte maturation or genetic defects that are not yet known. Mutations in *RAG1* or *RAG2* genes, or genes encoding other components of the recombinase enzyme, cause a defect in antigen receptor gene recombination leading to an absence of mature B and T lymphocytes, similar to knockout mice lacking RAG-1 or RAG-2. A severe form of SCID is seen in a disease called **reticular dysgenesis.** This disorder is characterized by the absence of T and B lymphocytes and myeloid cells, such as granulocytes, and is presumably due to a defect at the level of the hematopoietic stem cell. This disease is rare, and neither its molecular basis nor its mode of inheritance is known. An instructive experimental model is the **SCID mouse,** in which B and T cells are absent because of an early block in maturation from bone marrow precursors. The defect in SCID mice is a mutation in a component of the enzyme DNA-dependent protein kinase, which is required for double-stranded DNA break repair. This defect results in abnormal joining of Ig and T cell receptor (TCR) gene segments during recombination and therefore failure to express antigen receptors.

Defect in B Cell Maturation: X-Linked Agammaglobulinemia

X-linked agammaglobulinemia, also called Bruton's agammaglobulinemia, is characterized by the absence of gamma globulin in the blood, as the name implies. It is one of the most common congenital immunodeficiencies and the prototype of a failure of B cell maturation. The defect in X-linked agammaglobulinemia is a failure of B cells to mature beyond the pre-B cell stage in the bone marrow (see Fig. 20–1). This failure is caused by mutations or deletions in the gene encoding an enzyme called **B cell tyrosine kinase** (Btk). Btk is involved in transducing signals from the pre-B cell receptor that are required for continued maturation of the cells. In female carriers of this disease, only B cells that have inactivated the X chromosome carrying the mutant allele mature. Unlike the case with X-linked SCID, described earlier, this nonrandom X chromosome inactivation is not seen in T cells. Patients with X-linked agammaglobulinemia usually have low or undetectable serum Ig, reduced or absent B cells in peripheral blood and lymphoid tissues, no germinal centers in lymph nodes, and no plasma cells in tissues. The maturation, numbers, and functions of T cells are generally normal. Some studies have revealed reduced numbers of activated T cells in patients, which may be a consequence of reduced antigen presentation caused by the lack of B cells. Autoimmune disorders develop in almost 20% of patients, for unknown reasons. The infectious complications of X-linked agammaglobulinemia are greatly reduced by periodic (e.g., weekly or monthly) injections of pooled gamma globulin preparations. Such preparations contain preformed antibodies against common pathogens and provide effective passive immunity.

Knockout mice lacking Btk show a much less severe defect in B cell maturation than humans do, which suggests the existence of other compensatory signaling mechanisms. An inbred mouse strain called **CBA/N** has an X-linked defect in B cell maturation that is a result of a point mutation in the *btk* gene. The major abnormality in the CBA/N mouse is defective antibody responses to some polysaccharide antigens, but the numbers of B cells in lymphoid tissues are nearly normal.

Defect in T Cell Maturation: The DiGeorge Syndrome

This selective T cell deficiency is due to a congenital malformation that results in defective development of the thymus and the parathyroid glands as well as other structures that develop from the third and fourth pharyngeal pouches during fetal life. The congenital defect is manifested by hypoplasia or agenesis of the thymus leading to deficient T cell maturation, absent parathyroid glands causing abnormal calcium homeostasis and muscle twitching (tetany), abnormal development of the great vessels, and facial deformities. Different patients may show varying degrees of these abnormalities. The disease is caused by a deletion in chromosome 22q11.2, but the responsible gene has not been identified. Peripheral blood T lymphocytes are absent or greatly reduced in number, and the cells do not respond to polyclonal T cell activators or in mixed leukocyte reactions. Antibody levels are usually normal but may be reduced in severely affected patients. As in other severe T cell deficiencies, patients are susceptible to mycobacterial, viral, and fungal infections.

The immunodeficiency associated with DiGeorge syndrome can be corrected by fetal thymic transplantation or by HLA-identical bone marrow transplantation. Such treatment is not usually necessary, however, because T cell function tends to improve with age and is often normal by 5 years. Improvement with age probably occurs because of the presence of some thymic tissue or because some as yet undefined extrathymic sites assume the function of T cell maturation. It is also possible that as these patients grow older, typical thymus tissue develops at ectopic sites (i.e., other than the normal location).

An animal model of T cell immunodeficiency resulting from abnormal development of the thymus is the

nude (athymic) mouse. These mice have an inherited defect of epithelial cells in the skin leading to hairlessness and in the lining of the third and fourth pharyngeal pouches causing thymic hypoplasia. The disorder is due to a mutation in a gene encoding a transcription factor that is believed to be required for normal development of certain epidermal cells. Affected mice have rudimentary thymuses in which T cell maturation cannot occur normally. As a result, few or no mature T cells are present in peripheral lymphoid tissues, and cell-mediated immune reactions cannot occur. Several knockout mouse strains have been developed with targeted disruption of the genes required for T cell development (see Chapter 7, Box 7–1), and these mice are useful models for studying T cell maturation.

Defects in Lymphocyte Activation and Function

Congenital abnormalities in immune responses despite the presence of mature T and B lymphocytes are being increasingly recognized as our understanding of the molecular basis of lymphocyte activation has improved. These diseases may affect either B or T lymphocytes and are associated with deficient humoral or cell-mediated immunity, respectively (Fig. 20–2 and Table 20–3).

Selective Immunoglobulin Isotype Deficiencies

Many immunodeficiencies that selectively involve one or a few Ig isotypes have been described. The most common is **selective IgA deficiency,** which affects about 1 in 700 white individuals and is thus the most common primary immunodeficiency known. IgA deficiency usually occurs sporadically, but many familial cases with either autosomal dominant or recessive patterns of inheritance are also known. The clinical features are variable. Many patients are entirely normal; others have occasional respiratory infections and diarrhea; and rarely, patients have severe, recurrent infections leading to permanent intestinal and airway damage, with associated autoimmune disorders. IgA deficiency is characterized by low serum IgA, usually less than 50 μg/mL (normal, 2 to 4 mg/mL), with normal or elevated levels of IgM and IgG. The defect in these patients is a block in the differentiation of B cells to IgA antibody–secreting plasma cells. The α heavy chain genes and the expression of membrane-associated IgA are normal. It is not known whether the block in B cell differentiation is due to an intrinsic B cell defect or to an abnormality in T cell help such as the production of cytokines that enhance IgA secretion (e.g., transforming growth factor-β and IL-5) or in B cell responses to these

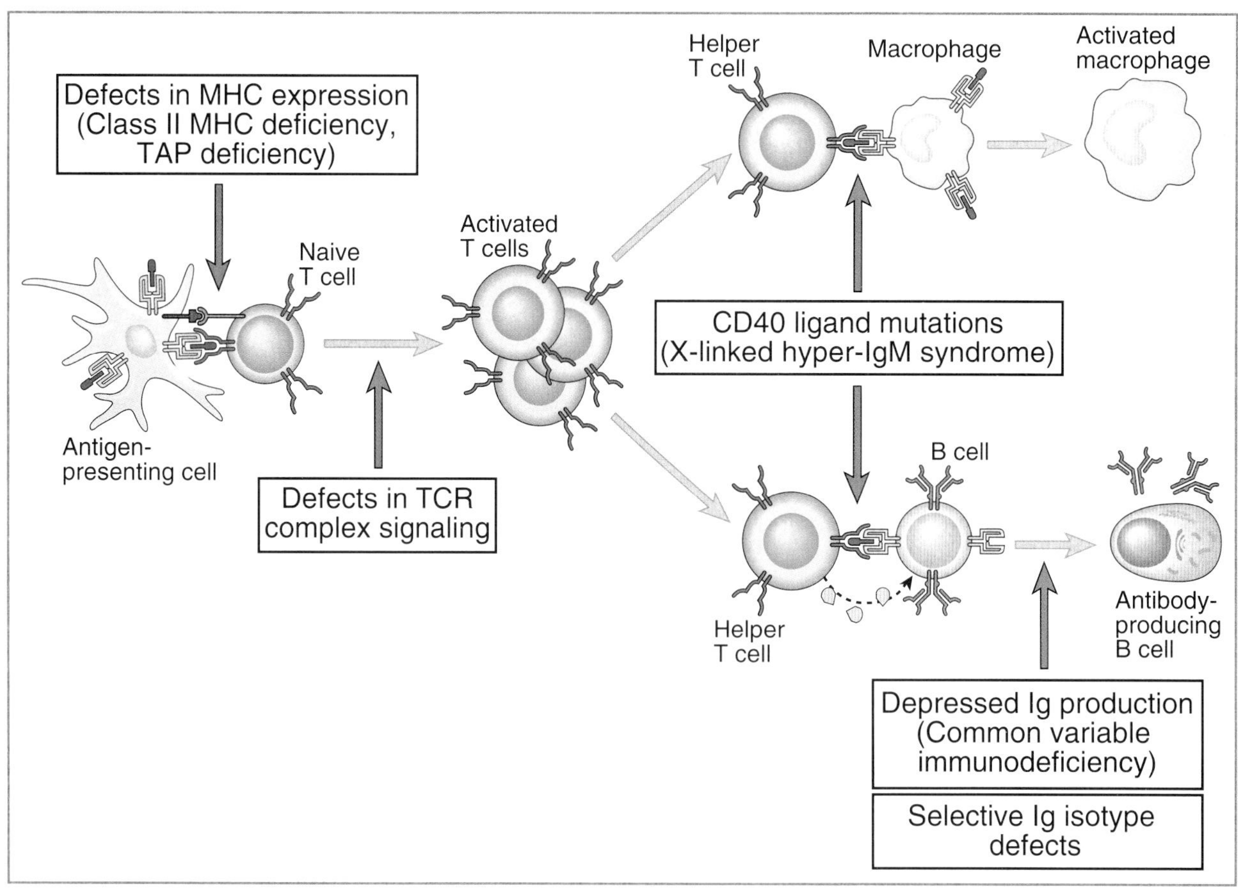

Figure 20–2 Immunodeficiency caused by defects in B and T cell activation. Primary immunodeficiencies may be caused by genetic defects in the expression of molecules required for antigen presentation to T cells, T or B lymphocyte antigen receptor signaling, helper T cell activation of B cells or macrophages, or differentiation of antibody-producing B cells.

Table 20–3. Defects in Lymphocyte Activation

Disease	Functional deficiencies	Mechanisms of defect
Selective Ig isotype deficiencies	Reduced or no production of selective isotypes or subtypes of Ig (IgA deficiency most common isotype deficiency, IgG3 deficiency most common subtype deficiency); susceptibility to bacterial infections or no clinical problems	Defect in B cell differentiation or T cell help; rare cases of homozygous deletions/mutations of Ig constant region genes
X-linked hyper-IgM syndrome	Defects in helper T cell–dependent B cell and macrophage activation	Mutation in CD40 ligand
Common variable immunodeficiency	Variable reductions in multiple Ig isotypes; normal or decreasd B cells	Defect in B cell activation, usually caused by intrinsic B cell abnormality (nature unknown)
T cell receptor complex expression or signaling defects	Decreased T cells or abnormal ratios of CD4+ and CD8+ subsets; decreased cell-mediated immunity	Rare cases caused by mutations or deletions in genes encoding CD3 proteins, ZAP-70
X-linked lympho-proliferative syndrome	Uncontrolled B cell proliferation in the setting of Epstein-Barr virus infection leading to B cell lymphomas and hypogammaglobulinemia	Mutation in the gene encoding the SAP adapter protein, which is normally required for inhibiting signaling by the SLAM molecule
Defective class II MHC expression: the bare lymphocyte syndrome	Lack of class II expression and impaired CD4+ T cell development and activation; defective cell-mediated immunity and T cell–dependent humoral immunity	Mutation in genes encoding transcription factors required for class II MHC gene expression
TAP deficiency	Lack of class I MHC molecule expression, decreased number of CD8+ T cells; susceptibility to bacterial infections	Mutation in the *TAP* genes preventing peptide loading of class I MHC molecules

Abbreviations: SAP, SLAM-associated protein; SLAM, signaling lymphocyte activation molecule; TAP, transporter associated with antigen processing; ZAP-70, zeta-associated protein of 70-kD.

cytokines. No gross abnormalities in the numbers, phenotypes, or functional responses of T cells have been noted in these patients.

Selective IgG subclass deficiencies have been described in which total serum IgG levels are normal but concentrations of one or more subclasses are below normal. Deficiency of IgG3 is the most common subclass deficiency in adults, and IgG2 deficiency, associated with IgA deficiency, is the most common in children. Some individuals with these deficiencies have recurrent bacterial infections, but many do not have any clinical problems. Selective IgG subclass deficiencies are usually due to abnormal B cell differentiation and rarely to homozygous deletions of various constant region (C_γ) genes.

Defect in T Cell–Dependent B Cell Activation: The X-Linked Hyper-IgM Syndrome

The X-linked hyper-IgM syndrome is a rare disorder associated with defective switching of B cells to the IgG and IgA isotypes; these antibodies are therefore absent, and a compensatory increase in IgM in the blood occurs. The defect is caused by mutations in the gene encoding the T cell effector molecule CD40 ligand. The mutant forms of CD40 ligand produced in these patients do not bind to or transduce signals through CD40 and therefore do not stimulate B cells to undergo heavy chain isotype switching, which requires T cell help (see Chapter 9). Patients suffer from infections similar to those seen in other hypogammaglobulinemias. Patients with X-linked hyper-IgM syndrome show defects in cell-mediated immunity (see Chapter 13), with a striking susceptibility to infection by the intracellular microbe *Pneumocystis carinii.* Defective cell-mediated immunity occurs because CD40 ligand is also involved in T cell–dependent activation of macrophages (see Chapter 13). Knockout mice lacking CD40 or CD40 ligand have a phenotype similar to that of the human disease.

There are rare cases of hyper-IgM syndrome that show an autosomal recessive inheritance pattern. In these patients, the genetic defects are in CD40 or in the enzyme activation-induced deaminase that is involved in heavy chain isotype switching and affinity maturation (see Chapter 9).

Defects in B Cell Differentiation: Common Variable Immunodeficiency

Common variable immunodeficiency is a group of heterogeneous disorders defined by reduced levels of serum Ig, impaired antibody responses to infection or vaccines, and increased incidence of infections. The diagnosis is usually one of exclusion when other primary immunodeficiency diseases are ruled out. The presentation and pathogenesis are, as the name implies, highly variable. Although Ig deficiency and associated pyogenic infections are major components of these disorders, autoimmune diseases, including pernicious anemia, hemolytic anemia, and rheumatoid arthritis, may be just as significant. A high incidence of malignant tumors is also associated with common variable immunodeficiency. These disorders may be diagnosed early in childhood or late in life. Both sporadic and familial cases occur, the latter with both autosomal dominant and recessive inheritance patterns. Mature B lymphocytes are present in these patients, but plasma cells are absent in lymphoid tissues, which suggests a block in B cell differentiation to antibody-producing cells. The defective antibody production has been attributed to multiple abnormalities, including intrinsic B cell defects, deficient T cell help, and excessive "suppressor cell" activity. The genetic basis of the disease is not known.

Defects in T Lymphocyte Activation and Function

Many examples of rare immunodeficiency diseases caused by defects in the expression of molecules required for T cell activation and function have been identified. Modern biochemical and molecular analyses of affected individuals have revealed mutations in the genes encoding various T cell proteins. Examples include impaired TCR complex expression or function caused by mutations in the CD3 ε or γ genes, defective TCR-mediated signaling caused by mutations in the ZAP-70 gene, reduced synthesis of cytokines such as IL-2 and interferon-γ (IFN-γ) (in some cases caused by defects in transcription factors), and lack of expression of IL-2 receptors. These defects are often found in only a few isolated cases or in a few families, and the clinical features and severity vary widely. Patients with these abnormalities may have deficiencies predominantly in T cell function or have mixed T cell and B cell immunodeficiencies despite normal or even elevated numbers of blood lymphocytes. Some of these defects are associated with abnormal ratios of $CD4^+$ and $CD8^+$ T cell subsets, which may reflect impaired development of one subset in the thymus or impaired expansion of one subset in the peripheral immune system. For example, patients with ZAP-70 deficiency have more $CD8^+$ than $CD4^+$ T cells, although the reason for the abnormal ratio is not clear.

X-linked lymphoproliferative disease is a disorder characterized by an inability to eliminate EBV, eventually leading to fulminant infectious mononucleosis and the development of B cell tumors and associated hypogammaglobulinemia. The disease is due to mutations in the gene encoding an adapter molecule that binds to a cell surface molecule involved in activation of T and B lymphocytes, called signaling lymphocyte activation molecule (SLAM). The role of SLAM and the associated adapter protein in immune responses is not well understood. However, defects in the SLAM-associated adapter protein result in increased susceptibility to viral infections, which is most commonly manifested by severe EBV infections, probably because of the ubiquitous nature of EBV.

Defective Class II MHC Expression: The Bare Lymphocyte Syndrome

Class II major histocompatibility complex (MHC) deficiency, also called **bare lymphocyte syndrome,** is a rare heterogeneous group of autosomal recessive diseases in which patients express little or no HLA-DP, HLA-DQ, or HLA-DR on B lymphocytes, macrophages, and dendritic cells and fail to express class II MHC molecules in response to IFN-γ. They express normal or only slightly reduced levels of class I MHC molecules and β_2-microglobulin. Most cases of the bare lymphocyte syndrome are due to mutations in genes encoding proteins that regulate class II MHC transcription. For example, mutations in the constitutively expressed transcription factor RFX5 or the IFN-γ–inducible transcriptional activator CIITA lead to reduced class II MHC expression and a failure of antigen-presenting cells (APCs) to activate $CD4^+$ T lymphocytes. Failure of antigen presentation may result in defective positive selection of T cells in the thymus with a reduction in the number of mature $CD4^+$ T cells or defective activation of cells in the periphery. Affected individuals are deficient in DTH responses and in antibody responses to T cell–dependent protein antigens. The disease appears within the first year of life and is usually fatal unless it is treated by bone marrow transplantation.

Defective Class I MHC Expression

Autosomal recessive class I MHC deficiencies have also been described and are characterized by decreased $CD8^+$ T cell numbers and function. In some cases, the failure to express class I MHC molecules is due to mutations in the gene encoding the TAP-1 or TAP-2 subunit of the TAP (transporter associated with antigen processing) complex, which normally pumps peptides into the endoplasmic reticulum, where they are required for class I MHC assembly (see Chapter 6). These TAP-deficient patients express few cell surface class I MHC molecules, a phenotype similar to TAP gene knockout mice. Such patients suffer mainly from respiratory tract bacterial infections and not viral infections, which is surprising considering that a principal function of $CD8^+$ T cells is defense against viruses.

Immunodeficiency Associated with Other Inherited Diseases

Variable degrees of B and T cell immunodeficiency occur in certain congenital diseases with a wide spectrum of abnormalities involving multiple organ systems. One such disorder is the **Wiskott-Aldrich syndrome,** an X-linked disease characterized by eczema, thrombocytopenia (reduced blood platelets), and susceptibility to bacterial infection. In the initial stages of the disease, lymphocyte numbers are normal, and the principal defect is an inability to produce antibodies in response to T cell–independent polysaccharide antigens, because of which these patients are especially susceptible to infections with encapsulated pyogenic bacteria. The lymphocytes (and platelets) are smaller than normal. With increasing age, the patients show reduced numbers of lymphocytes and more severe immunodeficiency. The defective gene responsible for the Wiskott-Aldrich syndrome encodes a cytoplasmic protein expressed exclusively in bone marrow–derived cells that interacts both with adapter molecules, such as Grb-2 (see Chapter 8), and with small G proteins of the Rho family that regulate the actin cytoskeleton. Expression of many cell surface glycoproteins is also reduced, including the sialic acid–rich glycoprotein called CD43 (or sialophorin), which is normally expressed on lymphocytes, macrophages, neutrophils, and platelets. Cumulatively, these alterations may interfere with trafficking of leukocytes to sites of inflammation.

Another multisystem congenital disease associated with immunodeficiency is **ataxia-telangiectasia.** It is an autosomal recessive disorder characterized by abnormal gait (ataxia), vascular malformations (telangiectases), neurologic deficits, increased incidence of tumors, and immunodeficiency. The immunologic defects are of variable severity and may affect both B and T cells. The most common humoral immune defect is IgA and IgG2 deficiency. The T cell defects, which are usually less pronounced, are associated with thymic hypoplasia. Patients experience upper and lower respiratory tract bacterial infections, multiple autoimmune phenomena, and increasingly frequent cancers with advancing age. The gene responsible for this disorder is located on chromosome 11 and encodes a protein that is related to the enzyme phosphatidylinositol-3 kinase, which was described as participating in T cell activation by antigens (see Chapter 8). The precise function of the ataxia-telangiectasia gene product is unknown, but it may play a role in DNA repair.

Defects in Innate Immunity

Innate immunity constitutes the first line of defense against infectious organisms. Two important mediators of innate immunity are phagocytes and complement, which also participate in the effector phases of adaptive immunity. Therefore, congenital disorders of phagocytes and the complement system result in recurrent infections of varying severity. Complement deficiencies were described in Chapter 14 (see Box 14–2). In this section of the chapter, we discuss some examples of congenital phagocyte disorders (Table 20–4).

Defect in Microbicidal Activities of Phagocytes: Chronic Granulomatous Disease

Chronic granulomatous disease (CGD) is a rare disease, estimated to affect about 1 in 1 million individuals in the United States. About two thirds of cases show an X-linked recessive pattern of inheritance, and the remainder are autosomal recessive. The disease is characterized by recurrent intracellular bacterial and fungal infections, usually from early childhood. Because the infections are not controlled by phagocytes, they stim-

Table 20–4. Congenital Disorders of Innate Immunity

Disease	Functional deficiencies and clinical problems	Mechanisms of defect
Chronic granulomatous disease	Defective production of reactive oxygen intermediates by phagocytes; recurrent intracellular bacterial and fungal infections	Mutations in genes encoding components of the phagocyte oxidase enzyme, most often cytochrome b558
Leukocyte adhesion deficiency-1	Absent or deficient expression of β_2 integrins causing defective leukocyte adhesion-dependent functions; recurrent bacterial and fungal infections	Mutations in gene encoding the β chain (CD18) of β_2 integrins
Leukocyte adhesion deficiency-2	Absent or deficient expression of leukocyte ligands for endothelial E- and P-selectins causing failure of leukocyte migration into tissues; recurrent bacterial and fungal infections	Mutations in gene encoding a GDP-fucose transporter required for synthesis of the sialyl Lewis X component of E- and P-selectin ligands
Chédiak-Higashi syndrome	Defective lysosomal function in neutrophils, macrophages, and dendritic cells; defective granule function in natural killer cells; recurrent infections by pyogenic bacteria	Mutation in a gene of unknown function leading to increased fusion of cytoplasmic granules

ulate chronic cell-mediated immune responses resulting in T cell–mediated macrophage activation and the formation of granulomas composed of activated macrophages. The disease is often fatal, even with aggressive antibiotic therapy.

CGD is caused by mutations in a component of the phagocyte oxidase enzyme, most often the 91-kD membrane protein cytochrome b_{558}, also known as phox (phagocyte oxidase)-91. This mutation results in defective production of superoxide anion, a reactive oxygen intermediate that constitutes a major microbicidal mechanism of phagocytes (see Chapter 12). Defective production of reactive oxygen intermediates results in a failure to kill phagocytosed microbes. The cytokine IFN-γ stimulates the production of superoxide by normal neutrophils, as well as CGD neutrophils, especially in cases in which the phox-91 gene is intact but its transcription is reduced. IFN-γ enhances transcription of the phox-91 gene and also stimulates other components of the phagocyte oxidase enzyme. Once neutrophil superoxide production is restored to about 10% of normal levels, resistance to infection is greatly improved. IFN-γ therapy is now commonly used for the treatment of X-linked CGD.

Leukocyte Adhesion Deficiencies

Leukocyte adhesion deficiency type 1 (LAD-1) is a rare autosomal recessive disorder characterized by recurrent bacterial and fungal infections and impaired wound healing. In these patients, most adhesion-dependent functions of leukocytes are abnormal. These functions include adherence to endothelium, neutrophil aggregation and chemotaxis, phagocytosis, and cytotoxicity mediated by neutrophils, NK cells, and T lymphocytes. The molecular basis of the defect is absent or deficient expression of the β_2 integrins, or the CD11CD18 family of glycoproteins, due to various mutations in the CD18 gene. The β_2 integrins include leukocyte function–associated antigen-1 (LFA-1 or CD11aCD18), Mac-1 (CD11bCD18), and p150,95 (CD11cCD18). These proteins participate in the adhesion of leukocytes to other cells, notably endothelial cells, and the binding of T lymphocytes to APCs (see Chapter 6, Box 6–2).

LAD-2 is another disorder described in a small number of patients that is clinically similar to LAD-1 but is not due to integrin defects. In contrast, LAD-2 results from an absence of sialyl Lewis X, the carbohydrate ligand on neutrophils that is required for binding to E-selectin and P-selectin on cytokine-activated endothelium (see Chapter 6, Box 6–3). This defect is caused by a mutation in a fucose transporter gene leading to an inability to add fucose moieties to carbohydrates that are part of the sialyl Lewis X component of selectin ligands.

Defect in NK Cells and Other Leukocytes: The Chédiak-Higashi Syndrome

The Chédiak-Higashi syndrome is a rare autosomal recessive disorder characterized by recurrent infections by pyogenic bacteria, partial oculocutaneous albinism, and infiltration of various organs by non-neoplastic lymphocytes. The neutrophils, monocytes, and lymphocytes of these patients contain giant cytoplasmic granules. It is thought that this disease is due to a cellular abnormality leading to increased fusion of cytoplasmic granules. This increased granule fusion affects the lysosomes of neutrophils and macrophages (causing reduced resistance to infection), melanocytes (causing albinism), cells of the nervous system (causing nerve defects), and platelets (leading to bleeding disorders). The gene responsible for this disorder has been mapped to chromosome 1 and encodes a widely expressed cytosolic protein. It is not known how defects in the protein encoded by this gene lead to abnormal granule membrane fusion. The giant lysosomes found in neutrophils form during the maturation of these cells from myeloid precursors. Some of these neutrophil precursors die prematurely and cause moderate leukopenia. Surviving neutrophils may contain reduced levels of the lysosomal enzymes that normally function in microbial killing. These cells are also defective in chemotaxis and phagocytosis, further contributing to their deficient microbicidal activity. Defects in the lysosomes of dendritic cells and macrophages may impair antigen processing and presentation. NK cell function in these patients is impaired, probably because of an abnormality in the cytoplasmic granules that store proteins mediating cytolysis. Interestingly, cytolytic T lymphocyte (CTL)–mediated killing is normal.

A mutant mouse strain called the **beige mouse** is an animal model for the Chédiak-Higashi syndrome. This strain is characterized by deficient NK cell function and giant lysosomes in leukocytes. The beige mutation has been mapped to the mouse homologue of the human Chédiak-Higashi gene.

Therapeutic Approaches for Congenital Immunodeficiencies

The current treatment of immunodeficiencies has two aims—to minimize and control infections and to replace the defective or absent components of the immune system by adoptive transfer or transplantation. **Passive immunization** with pooled gamma globulin is enormously valuable for agammaglobulinemic patients and has been lifesaving for many boys with X-linked agammaglobulinemia. **Bone marrow transplantation** is currently the treatment of choice for various immunodeficiency diseases and has been successful in the treatment of SCID with ADA deficiency, Wiskott-Aldrich syndrome, bare lymphocyte syndrome, and LAD. It is most successful with careful T cell depletion from the marrow and HLA matching to prevent graft-versus-host disease (see Chapter 16). Enzyme replacement therapy for ADA and PNP deficiencies has been attempted, with red blood cell transfusions used as a source of the enzymes. This approach has produced temporary clinical improvement in several patients with autosomal SCID. Injection of bovine ADA conjugated to polyethylene glycol to prolong its serum half-life has proved successful in some cases, but the benefits are usually short-lived.

In theory, the therapy of choice for congenital disorders of lymphocytes is to replace the defective gene in self-renewing precursor cells. Gene replacement remains a distant goal for most human immunodeficiencies at present, despite considerable effort. The main obstacles to this type of gene therapy are difficulties in purifying self-renewing stem cells, which are the ideal target for introduction of the replacement gene, and the lack of a method for introducing genes into cells to achieve stable, long-lived, and high-level expression. A small number of patients with X-linked SCID have been successfully treated by transplantation of autologous bone marrow cells engineered to express a normal γ_C chain gene. This is the first disease to be treated by gene therapy, but it is not known how long-lived the gene replacement will be. For unknown reasons, gene therapy has not been as successful in treating patients with autosomal SCID caused by ADA mutations.

Acquired (Secondary) Immunodeficiencies

Deficiencies of the immune system often develop because of abnormalities that are not genetic but acquired during life (Table 20–5). The most important of these abnormalities is HIV infection, and this is described in the next section. Acquired immunodeficiency diseases are caused by two main types of pathogenic mechanisms. First, immunosuppression may occur as a biologic complication of another disease process. Second, so-called iatrogenic immunodeficiencies may develop as complications of therapy for other diseases.

Diseases in which immunodeficiency is a common complicating element include malnutrition, neoplasms, and infections. Protein-calorie malnutrition is extremely common in developing countries and is associated with impaired cellular and humoral immunity to microorganisms. Much of the morbidity and mortality that afflict malnourished people is due to infections. The basis for the immunodeficiency is not well defined, but it is reasonable to assume that the global metabolic disturbances in these individuals, caused by deficient intake of protein, fat, vitamins, and minerals, will adversely affect maturation and function of the cells of the immune system.

Table 20–5. Acquired Immunodeficiencies

Cause	Mechanism
Human immunodeficiency virus infection	Depletion of CD4+ helper T cells
Protein-calorie malnutrition	Metabolic derangements inhibit lymphocyte maturation and function
Irradiation and chemotherapy for cancer	Decreased bone marrow lymphocyte precursors
Cancer metastases to bone marrow	Reduced site of leukocyte development
Removal of spleen	Decreased phagocytosis of microbes

Patients with advanced widespread cancer are often susceptible to infection because of impaired cell-mediated and humoral immune responses to a variety of organisms. Bone marrow tumors, including cancers metastatic to marrow and leukemias that arise in the marrow, may interfere with the growth and development of normal lymphocytes and other leukocytes. In addition, tumors may produce substances that interfere with lymphocyte development or function. An example of malignancy-associated immunodeficiency is the impairment in T cell function commonly observed in patients with a type of lymphoma called Hodgkin's disease. This defect was first characterized as an inability to mount a DTH reaction on intradermal injection of various common antigens to which the patients were previously exposed, such as *Candida* or tetanus toxoid. Other *in vitro* measures of T cell function, such as proliferative responses to polyclonal activators, are also impaired in patients with Hodgkin's disease. Such a generalized deficiency in DTH responses is called **anergy.** The cause of these T cell abnormalities is unknown.

Various types of infections lead to immunosuppression. Viruses other than HIV are known to impair immune responses; examples include the measles virus and human T cell lymphotropic virus 1 (HTLV-1). Both viruses can infect lymphocytes, which may be a basis for their immunosuppressive effects. Like HIV, HTLV-1 is a retrovirus with tropism for $CD4^+$ T cells; however, instead of killing helper T cells, it transforms them and produces an aggressive T cell malignant disease called adult T cell leukemia/lymphoma (ATL). Patients with ATL typically have severe immunosuppression with multiple opportunistic infections. Chronic infections with *Mycobacterium tuberculosis* and various fungi frequently result in anergy to many antigens. Chronic parasitic infections may also lead to immunosuppression. For example, African children with chronic malarial infections have depressed T cell function, which may be important in the pathogenesis of EBV-associated malignant tumors (see Chapter 17, Box 17–2).

Iatrogenic immunosuppression is most often due to drug therapies that either kill or functionally inactivate lymphocytes. Some drugs are given intentionally to immunosuppress patients, either for the treatment of inflammatory diseases or to prevent rejection of tissue allografts. The most commonly used anti-inflammatory and immunosuppressive drugs are corticosteroids and cyclosporine, respectively. Various chemotherapeutic drugs are administered to patients with cancer, and these drugs are usually cytotoxic to both mature and developing lymphocytes as well as to granulocyte and monocyte precursors. Thus, cancer chemotherapy is almost always accompanied by a period of immunosuppression and risk of infection.

Radiation treatment of patients with cancer carries the same risks.

One other form of acquired immunosuppression results from the absence of a spleen caused by surgical removal of the organ after trauma and as treatment of certain hematologic diseases or by infarction in sickle cell disease. Patients without spleens are more susceptible to infection by some organisms, particularly encapsulated bacteria such as *Streptococcus pneumoniae.* This enhanced susceptibility is due to absence of the important function of the spleen in phagocytic clearance of opsonized blood-borne microbes.

Human Immunodeficiency Virus and the Acquired Immunodeficiency Syndrome

AIDS is the disease caused by infection with HIV and is characterized by profound immunosuppression with associated opportunistic infections and malignant tumors, wasting, and central nervous system (CNS) degeneration. HIV infects a variety of cells of the immune system, including CD4-expressing helper T cells, macrophages, and dendritic cells. HIV evolved as a human pathogen very recently relative to most other known human pathogens, and the HIV epidemic was first identified only in the 1980s. However, the degree of morbidity and mortality caused by HIV and the global impact of HIV infection on health care resources and economics are already enormous and continue to grow. HIV has infected 50 to 60 million people and has caused the death of nearly 20 million adults and children. In the year 2001, there were almost 40 million people living with HIV infection and AIDS, of which 70% were in Africa and 15% in Asia. It is estimated that there were 5 million people newly infected with HIV during the year, and 3 million deaths were caused by AIDS. Currently, no prophylactic immunization or cure is known for AIDS, although new therapies are being developed. In this section of the chapter, we describe the molecular and biologic properties of HIV, the nature and possible causes of HIV-induced immunodeficiency, and the clinical and epidemiologic features of HIV-related diseases.

Molecular and Biologic Features of HIV

HIV is a member of the lentivirus family of animal retroviruses. Lentiviruses, including visna virus of sheep and the bovine, feline, and simian immunodeficiency viruses (SIV), are capable of long-term latent infection of cells and short-term cytopathic effects, and they all produce slowly progressive, fatal diseases that include wasting syndromes and CNS degeneration. Two closely related types of HIV, designated HIV-1 and HIV-2, have been identified. HIV-1 is by far the most common cause of AIDS, but HIV-2, which differs in genomic structure and antigenicity, causes a similar clinical syndrome.

HIV Structure and Genes

An infectious HIV particle consists of two identical strands of RNA packaged within a core of viral proteins and surrounded by a phospholipid bilayer envelope derived from the host cell membrane but including virally encoded membrane proteins (Fig. 20–3). The RNA genome of HIV is ~9.2 kb long and has the basic arrangement of nucleic acid sequences characteristic of all known retroviruses (Fig. 20–4). Long terminal repeats (LTRs) at each end of the genome regulate viral integration into the host genome, viral gene expression, and viral replication. The *gag* sequences encode core structural proteins. The *env* sequences encode the envelope glycoproteins gp120 and gp41, which are required for infection of cells. The *pol* sequences encode reverse transcriptase, integrase, and viral protease enzymes required for viral replication. In addition to these typical retrovirus genes, HIV-1 also includes six other regulatory genes, namely, the *tat, rev, vif, nef, vpr,* and *vpu* genes, whose products regulate viral reproduction in various ways. The functions of these genes are summarized in Figure 20–4.

Viral Life Cycle

HIV infection of cells begins when the envelope glycoprotein (Env) of a viral particle binds to both CD4 and a coreceptor that is a member of the chemokine receptor family (Fig. 20–5). The viral particles that initiate infection are usually in the blood, semen, or other body fluids of one individual and are introduced into another individual by sexual contact, needle stick, or transplacental passage. Env is a complex composed of a transmembrane gp41 subunit and an external, noncovalently associated gp120 subunit. These subunits are produced by proteolytic cleavage of a gp160 precursor. The Env complex is expressed as a trimeric structure of three gp120/gp41 pairs. This complex mediates a multistep process of fusion of the virion envelope with the membrane of the target cell (Fig. 20–6). The first step of this process is the binding of gp120 subunits to CD4 molecules, which induces a conformational change that promotes secondary gp120 binding to a chemokine coreceptor. Coreceptor binding induces a conformational change in gp41 that exposes a hydrophobic region, called the fusion peptide, that inserts into the cell membrane and enables the viral membrane to fuse with the target cell membrane. After the virus completes its life cycle in the infected cell (described later), free viral particles are released from one infected cell and bind to an uninfected cell, thus propagating the infection. In addition, gp120 and gp41, which are expressed on the plasma membrane of infected cells before virus is released, can mediate cell-cell fusion with an uninfected CD4- and coreceptor-expressing cell, and HIV genomes can then be passed between the fused cells directly.

The identification of CD4 and chemokine receptors as HIV receptors involved several different experimental approaches and clinical observations.

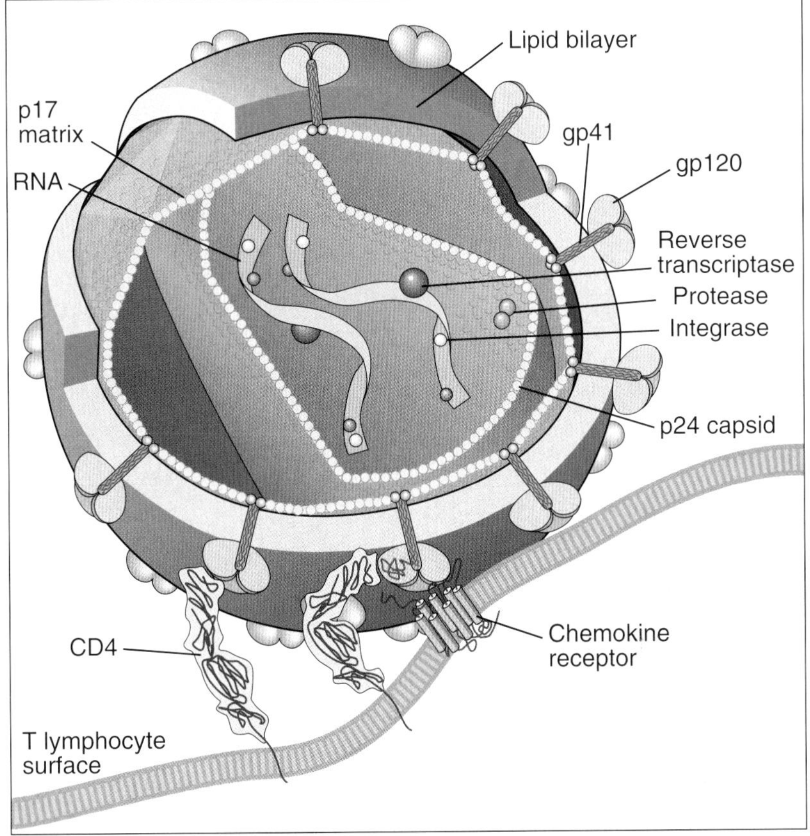

Figure 20–3 Structure of HIV-1.
An HIV-1 virion is shown next to a T cell surface. HIV-1 consists of two identical strands of RNA (the viral genome) and associated enzymes, including reverse transcriptase, integrase, and protease, packaged in a cone-shaped core composed of p24 capsid protein with a surrounding p17 protein matrix, all surrounded by a phospholipid membrane envelope derived from the host cell. Virally encoded membrane proteins (gp41 and gp120) are bound to the envelope. CD4⁻ and chemokine receptors on the host cell surface function as HIV-1 receptors. (Adapted from front cover. The new face of AIDS. Science 272:1841–2102, 1996. © 2000 Terese Winslow.)

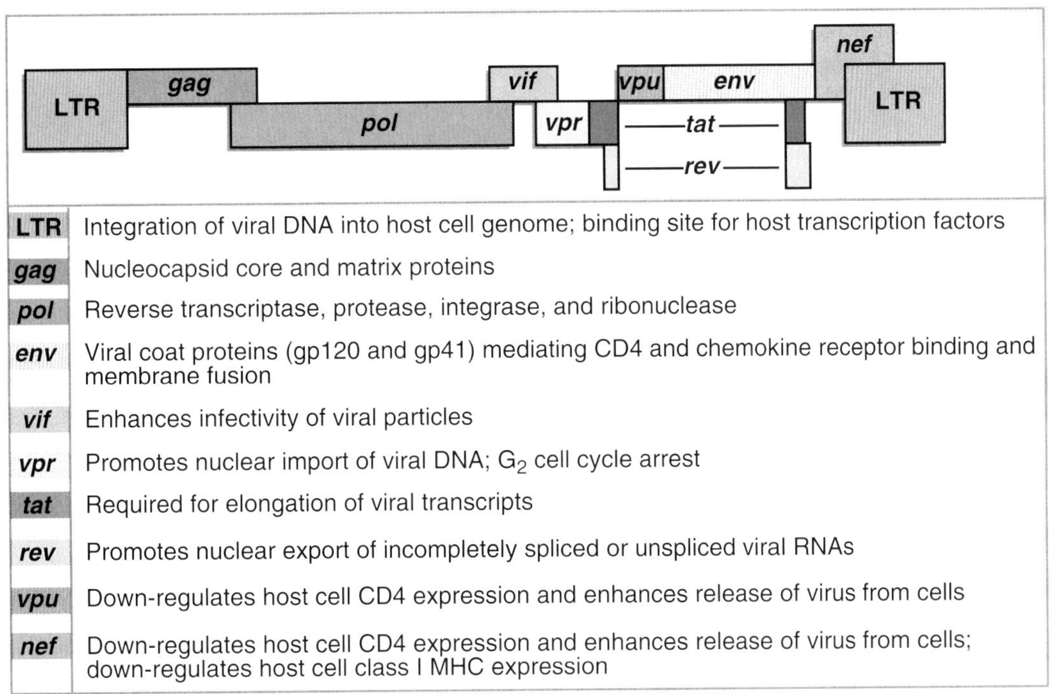

Figure 20–4 HIV-1 genome.
The genes along the linear genome are indicated as differently colored blocks. Some genes use some of the same sequences as other genes, as shown by overlapping blocks, but are read differently by host cell RNA polymerase. Similarly shaded blocks separated by lines indicate genes whose coding sequences are separated in the genome and require RNA splicing to produce functional messenger RNA. LTR, long terminal repeat. (Adapted from Greene W. AIDS and the immune system. Copyright 1993 by Scientific American, Inc. All rights reserved.)

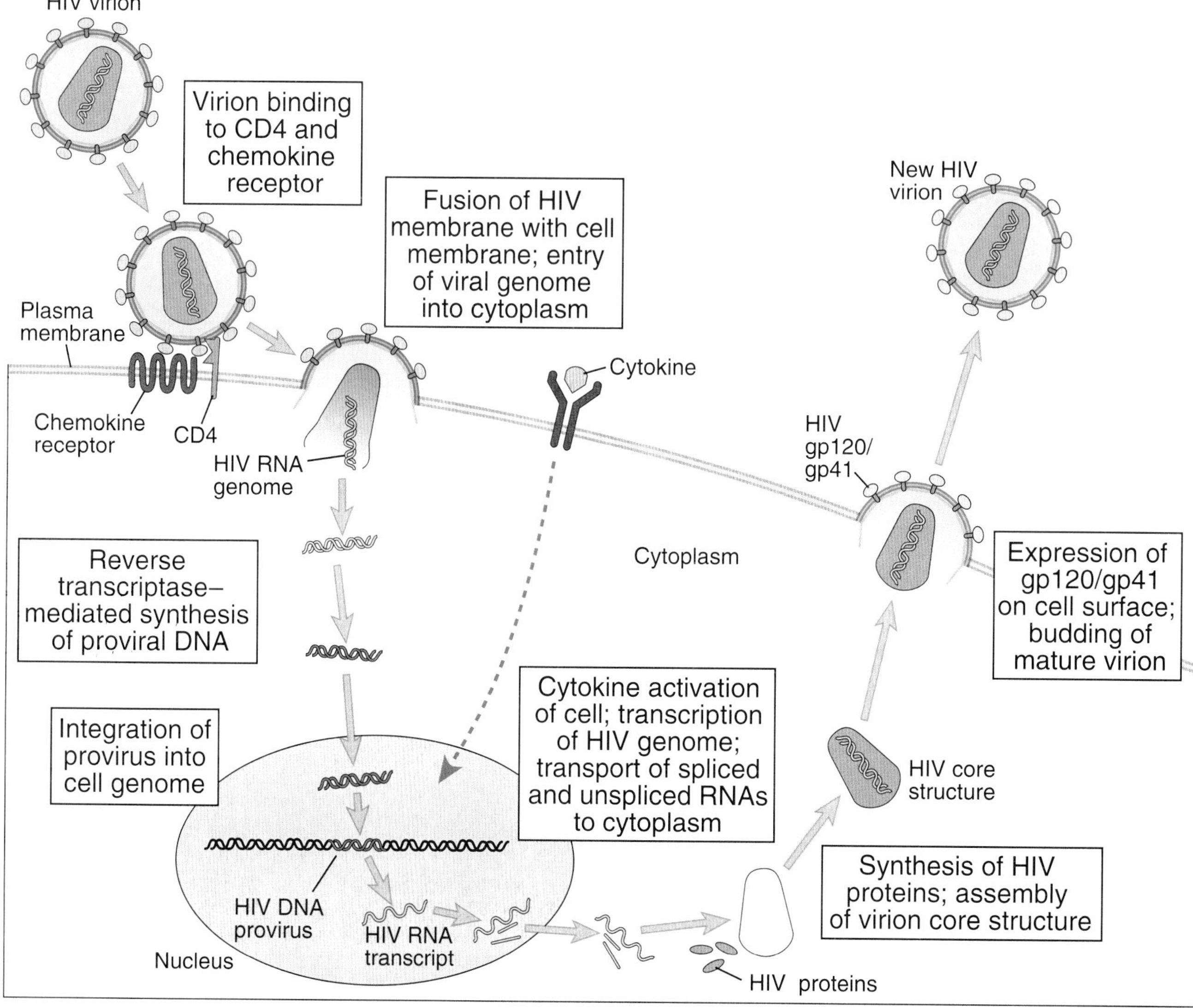

Figure 20–5 HIV life cycle.
The sequential steps in the life cycle of HIV are shown, from initial infection of a host cell to viral replication and release of a new virion. For the sake of clarity, the production and release of only one new virion are shown. An infected cell actually produces many virions, each capable of infecting cells, thereby amplifying the infectious cycle.

- CD4 was first suspected as a viral receptor because of the selective destruction of CD4$^+$ T cells in HIV-infected individuals and the subsequent demonstration that HIV infects CD4$^+$ cells only *in vitro.* Receptor-binding studies using purified recombinant molecules have established that gp120 specifically binds to CD4, and mutational and x-ray crystallographic studies have identified the regions of both molecules that interact physically.

- The requirement for a coreceptor in addition to CD4 in HIV infection was first suspected because expression of recombinant human CD4 in many nonhuman cell lines did not render the cells susceptible to HIV infection but subsequent fusion with human cells did. A second phenomenon indicating a role for cofactors in HIV infection is the existence of different isolates of HIV that have distinct tropisms for different cell populations in a pattern that does not correlate with CD4 expression. All HIV strains can infect and replicate in freshly isolated human CD4$^+$ T cells that are activated *in vitro.* In contrast, some strains will infect primary cultures of human macrophages but not continuous T cell lines (macrophage-tropic, or M-tropic, virus), whereas other strains will infect T cell lines but not macrophages (T-tropic virus). Some virus strains also infect both T cell lines and macrophages (dual-tropic virus). The tropism for macrophages or T cell lines was shown to be related to the ability of the Env proteins to mediate fusion of the virus with the membranes of the two different cell types, and cell-cell fusion experiments indicated that cofactors in addition to CD4 were involved in determining tropism. We now know that the tropism is related to the expression of different chemokine receptors on the macrophage or T cell lines.

- The initial demonstration that a chemokine receptor can act as a cofactor for HIV entry into a cell was

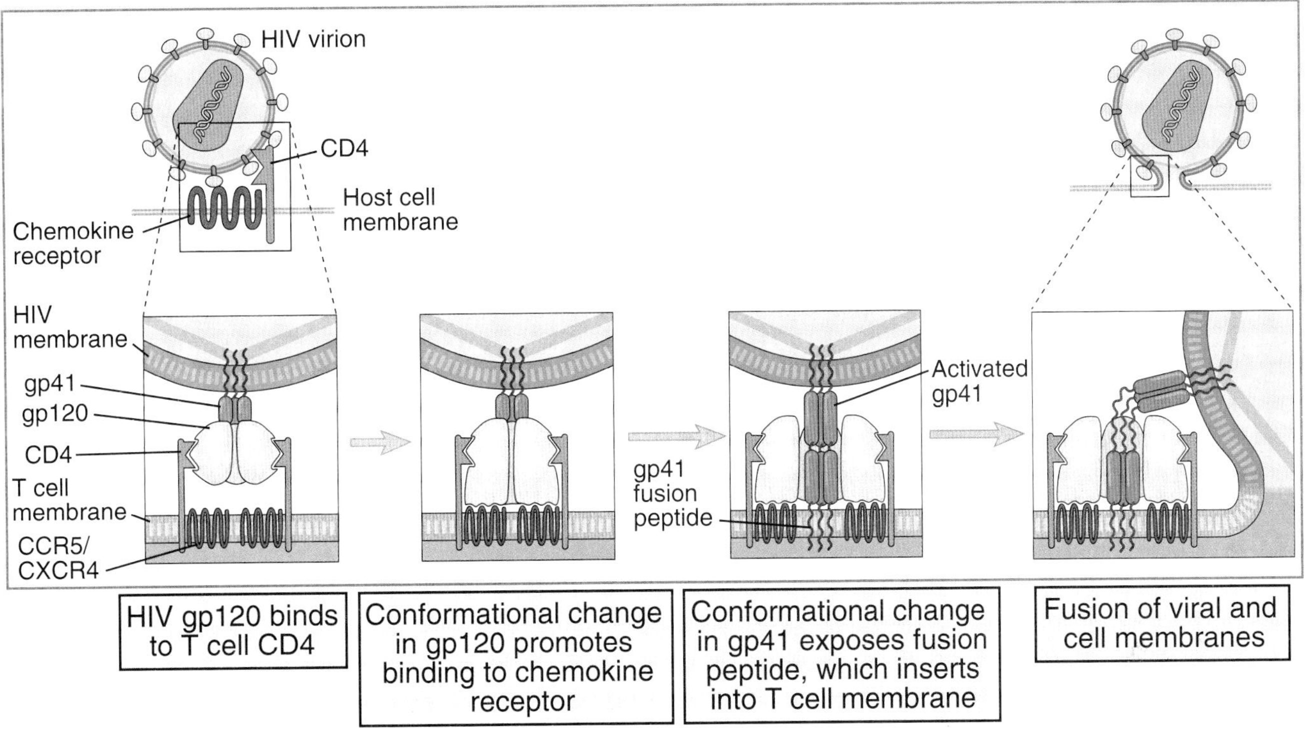

Figure 20–6 Mechanism of HIV entry into a cell.
In the model depicted, sequential conformational changes in gp120 and gp41 are induced by binding to CD4. These changes promote binding of the virus to the coreceptor (a chemokine receptor) and fusion of the HIV-1 and host cell membranes. The fusion peptide of activated gp41 contains hydrophobic amino acid residues that mediate insertion into the host cell plasma membrane.

accomplished by screening human cDNA libraries for the ability to confer infectivity of a human CD4-expressing mouse cell line by a T cell line–tropic HIV strain. A cDNA isolated by this strategy encoded the CXCR4 chemokine receptor, which binds the chemokines SDF-1α and SDF-1β. Concurrent with these studies, investigators discovered that soluble factors released by $CD8^+$ T cells could suppress HIV infection of macrophages by macrophage-tropic virus. These factors were identified as the chemokines RANTES (regulated by activation, normal T cell expressed and secreted), MIP-1α (macrophage inflammatory protein-1α) and MIP-1β, all of which bind to the CCR5 receptor. Transfection of recombinant CCR5 into cell lines that resisted infection by macrophage-tropic virus conferred susceptibly to infection.

More than seven different chemokine receptors have been shown to serve as coreceptors for HIV entry into cells, and several other proteins belonging to the seven-membrane–spanning G protein–coupled receptor family, such as the leukotriene B_4 receptor, can also mediate HIV infection of cells. The specificities of different viral isolates for different coreceptors are based on differences in amino acid sequences of gp120, and mutations in gp120 can thus alter the cell tropism of the virus. Furthermore, in many HIV-infected individuals, there is an evolution from the production of virus that uses CCR5 early in the disease to virus that binds to CXCR4 late in the disease. This switch correlates with a change from the isolation of predominantly macrophage-tropic virus early in disease to the isolation of T cell line–tropic virus late. Currently, HIV variants are described as X4 for CXCR4 binding, R5 for CCR5 binding, or R5X4 for the ability to bind to both chemokine receptors. The importance of CCR5 in HIV infection *in vivo* is supported by the finding that individuals who do not express this receptor because of genetic mutations are resistant to HIV infection.

Once an HIV virion enters a cell, the enzymes within the nucleoprotein complex become active and begin the viral reproductive cycle (see Fig. 20–5). The nucleoprotein core of the virus becomes disrupted, the RNA genome of HIV is transcribed into a double-stranded DNA form by viral reverse transcriptase, and the viral DNA enters the nucleus. The viral integrase also enters the nucleus and catalyzes the integration of viral DNA into the host cell genome. Some evidence shows that the integration event is enhanced by concomitant T cell activation by antigens or bacterial superantigens. The integrated HIV DNA is called the **provirus.** The provirus may remain transcriptionally inactive for months or years, with little or no production of new viral proteins or virions, and in this way HIV infection of an individual cell can be latent.

Transcription of the genes of the integrated DNA provirus is regulated by the LTR upstream of the viral structural genes, and cytokines or other physiologic stimuli to T cells and macrophages enhance viral gene transcription. The LTRs contain polyadenylation signal sequences, the TATA box promoter sequence, and binding sites for two host cell transcription factors, NF-κB and SP1. Initiation of HIV gene transcription in T cells is linked to physiologic activation of the T cell by antigen or cytokines. For example, polyclonal activators of T cells, such as phytohemagglutinin, IL-2, tumor necrosis factor (TNF), and lymphotoxin, stimulate HIV gene expression in infected T cells, and IL-1, IL-3, IL-6, TNF, lymphotoxin, IFN-γ, and granulocyte-macrophage colony-stimulating factor (GM-CSF) stimulate HIV gene expression and viral replication in infected monocytes and macrophages. TCR and cytokine stimulation of HIV gene transcription probably involves the activation of NF-κB and its binding to sequences in the LTR. This phenomenon is significant to the pathogenesis of AIDS because the normal response of a latently infected T cell to a microbe may be the way in which latency is ended and virus production begins. The multiple infections that AIDS patients acquire thus stimulate HIV production and infection of additional cells.

The Tat protein is required for HIV gene expression and acts by enhancing the production of complete viral mRNA transcripts. Even in the presence of optimal signals to initiate transcription, few if any HIV mRNA molecules are actually synthesized because transcription of HIV genes by mammalian RNA polymerase is inefficient and the polymerase complex usually stops before the mRNA is completed. Tat protein binds to the nascent mRNA (not to viral DNA) and increases the "processivity" of RNA polymerase by several hundred-fold, which allows transcription to be completed to produce a functional viral mRNA.

Synthesis of mature, infectious viral particles begins after full-length viral RNA transcripts are produced and the viral genes are expressed as proteins. The mRNAs encoding the various HIV proteins are derived from a single full-genome-length transcript by differential splicing events. HIV gene expression may be divided into an early stage, during which regulatory genes are expressed, and a late stage, during which structural genes are expressed and full-length viral genomes are packaged. The Rev, Tat, and Nef proteins are early gene products encoded by fully spliced mRNAs that are exported from the nucleus and translated into proteins in the cytoplasm soon after infection of a cell. Late genes include *env, gag,* and *pol,* which encode the structural components of the virus and are translated from singly spliced or unspliced RNA. The Rev protein initiates the switch from early to late gene expression by promoting the export of these incompletely spliced late gene RNAs out of the nucleus. The *pol* gene product is a precursor protein that is sequentially cleaved to form reverse transcriptase, protease, ribonuclease, and integrase enzymes. As mentioned before, reverse transcriptase and integrase proteins are required for producing a DNA copy of the viral RNA genome and integrating it as a provirus into the host genome. The *gag* gene encodes a 55-kD protein that is proteolytically cleaved into p24, p17, and p15 polypeptides by the action of the viral protease encoded by the *pol* gene. These polypeptides are the core proteins that are required for assembly of infectious viral particles. The primary product of the *env* gene is a 160-kD glycoprotein (gp160) that is cleaved by cellular proteases within the endoplasmic reticulum into the gp120 and gp41 proteins required for HIV binding to cells, as discussed earlier. Current antiviral drug therapy for HIV disease includes inhibitors of the enzymes reverse transcriptase, protease, and integrase.

After transcription of various viral genes, viral proteins are synthesized in the cytoplasm. Assembly of infectious viral particles then begins by packaging full-length RNA transcripts of the proviral genome within a nucleoprotein complex that includes the *gag* core proteins and the *pol*-encoded enzymes required for the next cycle of integration. This nucleoprotein complex is then enclosed within a membrane envelope and released from the cell by a process of budding from the plasma membrane. The rate of virus production can reach sufficiently high levels to cause cell death, as discussed later.

The Course of HIV Disease

The development of AIDS is related to the ability of HIV to destroy the host immune system and the inability of the host immune response to eradicate HIV infection. We next describe what is known or hypothesized to be the progression of events in HIV disease, including the basis for immunosuppression. We include in this discussion the role of the host's immune response in both aggravating and limiting the pathologic effects of the virus.

Steps in HIV Infection and Pathogenesis

HIV disease begins with acute infection, which is only partly controlled by the adaptive immune response and advances to chronic progressive infection of peripheral lymphoid tissues (Fig. 20–7). The course of HIV disease can be followed by measuring the amount of virus in the patient's plasma and by the blood CD4$^+$ T cell count (Fig. 20–8). Primary infection occurs when HIV virions in the blood, semen, or other body fluids from one individual enter the cells of another individual by the gp120/gp41–cell receptor–mediated fusion events described earlier. Depending on the site of initial exposure to virus, CD4$^+$ T cells and monocytes in the blood or CD4$^+$ T cells and macrophages within mucosal tissues may be the first cells infected. It is likely that dendritic cells in epithelia at sites of virus entry capture the virus and then migrate into the lymph nodes. Dendritic cells express a protein with a mannose-binding lectin domain that may be particularly important in binding the HIV envelope. Thus, dendritic cells may play a key role in the initial dissemination of HIV into lymphoid tissues. Once in lymphoid tissues, dendritic cells may pass HIV on to CD4$^+$ T cells through direct cell-cell contact. Within days after the first exposure to HIV, abundant viral replication can be detected in the lymph nodes. This replication leads to viremia, during which high numbers of HIV particles are present in the patient's blood, accompanied by an

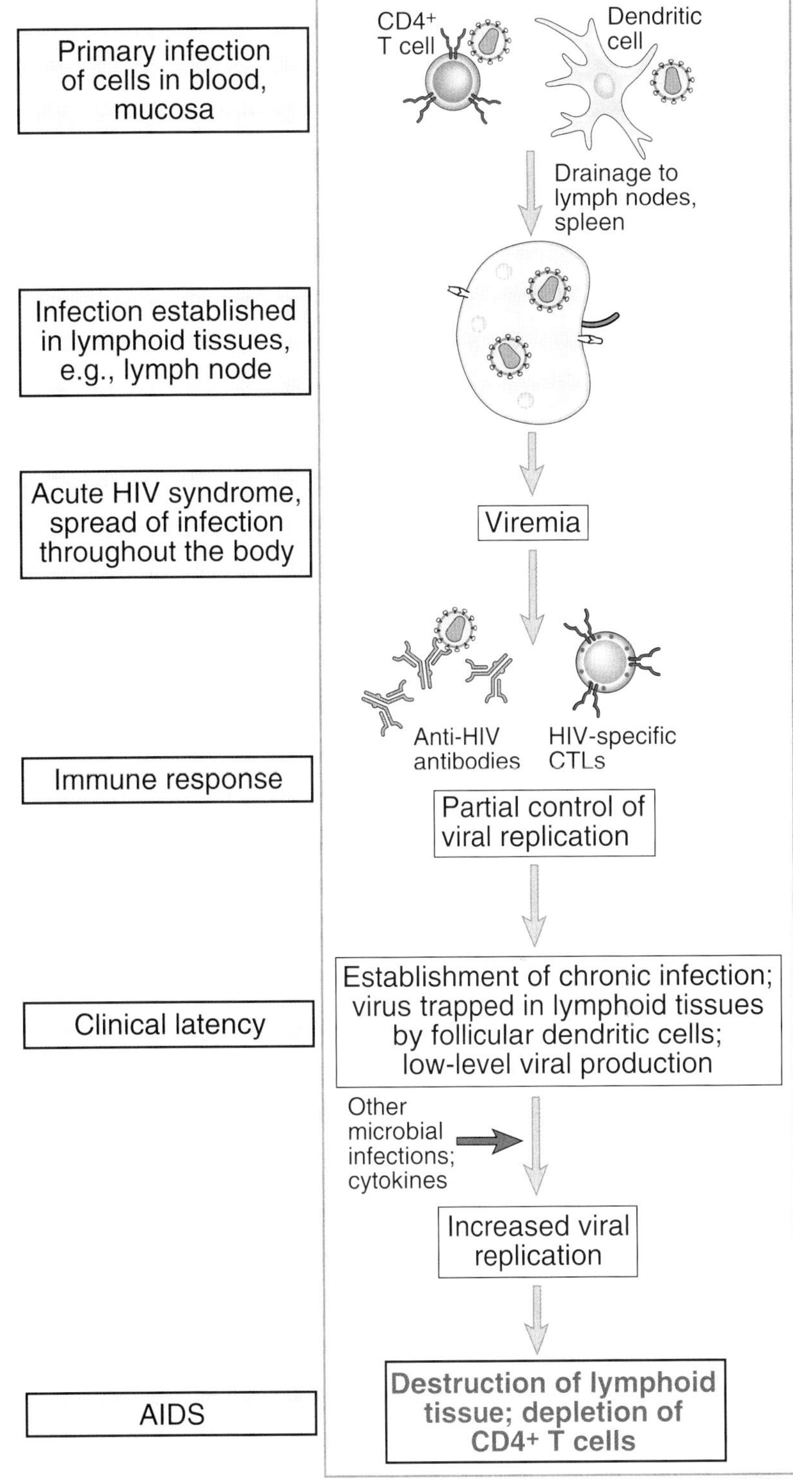

Figure 20–7 Progression of HIV infection. The clinical stages of HIV disease correlate with a progressive spread of HIV from the initial site of infection to lymphoid tissues throughout the body. The immune response of the host temporarily controls acute infection but does not prevent the establishment of chronic infection of cells in lymphoid tissues. Cytokine stimuli induced by other microbes serve to enhance HIV production and progression to AIDS.

acute HIV syndrome that includes a variety of nonspecific signs and symptoms typical of many viral diseases (Table 20–6). The viremia allows the virus to disseminate throughout the body and to infect helper T cells, macrophages, and dendritic cells in peripheral lymphoid tissues. As the HIV infection spreads, the adaptive immune system mounts both humoral and cell-mediated immune responses directed at viral antigens, which we will describe later. These immune responses partially control the infection and viral production, and such control is reflected by a drop in viremia to low but detectable levels by ~12 weeks after the primary exposure (see Fig. 20–8).

After the initial acute infection, a second phase of the disease develops during which lymph nodes and the spleen are sites of continuous HIV replication and

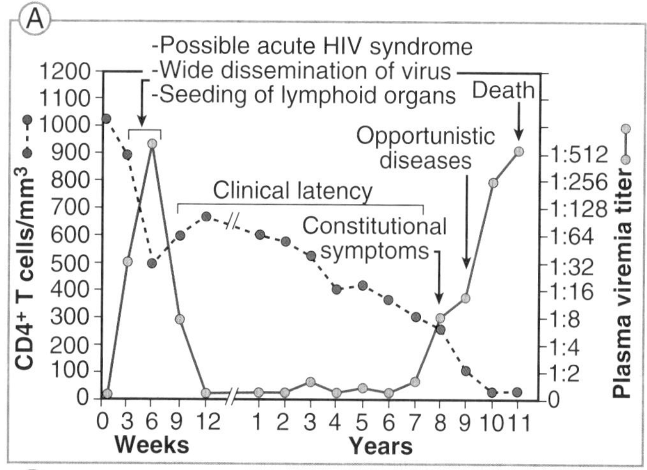

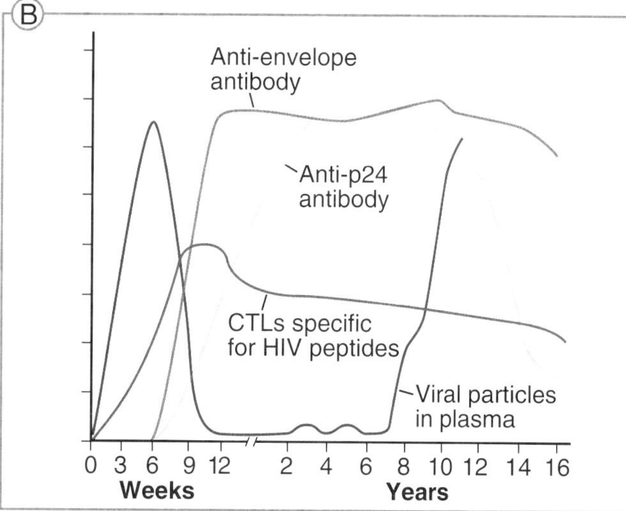

Figure 20–8 Clinical course of HIV disease.

A. Plasma viremia, blood CD4$^+$ T cell counts, and clinical stages of disease. About 12 weeks after infection, blood-borne virus (plasma viremia) is reduced to very low levels (detectable only by sensitive reverse transcriptase–polymerase chain reaction assays) and stays this way for many years. Nonetheless, CD4$^+$ T cell counts steadily decline during this clinical latency period because of active viral replication and T cell infection in lymph nodes. When CD4$^+$ T cell counts drop below a critical level (about 200/mm^3), the risk of infection and other clinical components of AIDS is high. (From Pantaleo G, C Graziosi, and A Fauci. The immunopathogenesis of human immunodeficiency virus infection. New England Journal of Medicine 328:327–335, 1993. Copyright © 1993 Massachusetts Medical Society. All rights reserved.)

B. Immune response to HIV infection. A CTL response to HIV is detectable by 2 to 3 weeks after the initial infection and peaks by 9 to 12 weeks. Marked expansion of virus-specific CD8$^+$ T cell clones occurs during this time, and up to 10% of a patient's CTLs may be HIV specific at 12 weeks. The humoral immune response to HIV peaks at about 12 weeks.

cell destruction (see Fig. 20–7). During this period of the disease, the immune system remains competent at handling most infections with opportunistic microbes, and few or no clinical manifestations of the HIV infection are present. Therefore, this phase of HIV disease is called the clinical latency period. Only low levels of virus are produced during the latent phase, and the majority of peripheral blood T cells do not harbor the virus. However, destruction of CD4$^+$ T cells within lymphoid tissues steadily progresses during the clinically latent period, and the number of circulating blood CD4$^+$ T cells steadily declines (see Fig. 20–8). More than 90% of the body's ~10^{12} T cells are normally found in lymphoid tissues, and it is estimated that HIV destroys up to 1 to 2 × 10^9 CD4$^+$ T cells every day. Early in the course of the disease, the body may continue to make new CD4$^+$ T cells, and therefore CD4$^+$ T cells can be replaced almost as quickly as they are destroyed. At this stage, up to 10% of CD4$^+$ T cells in lymphoid organs may be infected, but the number of circulating CD4$^+$ T cells that are infected at any one time may represent less than 0.1% of the total CD4$^+$ T cells in an individual. Eventually, during a period of years, the continuous cycle of virus infection, T cell death, and new infection leads to a steady decline in the number of CD4$^+$ T cells in the lymphoid tissues and the circulation.

During the chronic progressive phase of HIV disease, the patient becomes susceptible to other infections, and immune responses to these infections may stimulate HIV production and accelerate the destruction of lymphoid tissues. As discussed earlier, HIV gene transcription can be enhanced by stimuli that activate T cells, such as antigens and a variety of cytokines. Cytokines, such as TNF, that are produced by the innate immune system in response to microbial infections are particularly effective in boosting HIV production. Thus, as the immune system attempts to eradicate other microbes, it brings about its own destruction by HIV.

HIV disease progresses to the final and almost invariably lethal phase, called AIDS, when destruction of the peripheral lymphoid tissue is essentially complete and the blood CD4$^+$ T cell count drops below 200 cells/mm^3. HIV viremia may climb dramatically as viral replication in other reservoirs accelerates unchecked. Patients with AIDS suffer from combinations of opportunistic infections, neoplasms, cachexia (HIV wasting syndrome), kidney failure (HIV nephropathy), and CNS degeneration (AIDS encephalopathy) (see Table 20–6). Because CD4$^+$ helper T cells are essential for both cell-mediated and humoral immune responses to various microbes, the loss of these lymphocytes is the main reason that patients with AIDS become suscepti-

Table 20–6. Clinical Features of HIV Infection

Phase of disease	Clinical feature
Acute HIV disease	Fever, headaches, sore throat with pharyngitis, generalized lymphadenopathy, rashes
Clinical latency period	Declining blood CD4+ T cell amount
AIDS	**Opportunistic infections** Protozoa *(Pneumocystis carinii, Cryptosporidium)* Bacteria *(Toxoplasma, Mycobacterium avium, Nocardia, Salmonella)* Fungi *(Candida, Cryptococcus neoformans, Coccidioides immitis, Histoplasma capsulatum)* Viruses (cytomegalovirus, herpes simplex, varicella-zoster) **Tumors** Lymphomas (including EBV-associated B cell lymphomas) Kaposi's sarcoma Cervical carcinoma **Encephalopathy** **Wasting syndrome**

ble to many different types of infections. Furthermore, many of the tumors that arise in patients with AIDS have a viral etiology, and their prevalence in the setting of AIDS reflects an inability of the HIV-infected patient to mount an effective immune response against oncogenic viruses. Most of the opportunistic infections and neoplasms associated with HIV infection do not occur until after the blood CD4$^+$ T cell count drops below 200 cells/mm^3. The mechanisms underlying cachexia and CNS degeneration in AIDS are not well understood. Cachexia is often seen in patients with chronic inflammatory diseases and may reflect a combination of effects of inflammatory cytokines (such as TNF) on appetite and metabolism. The CNS disease in AIDS may be due to neuronal damage by the virus or by shed viral proteins such as gp120 and Tat as well as to the effects of cytokines elaborated by infected microglial cells.

HIV Reservoirs and Viral Turnover

The virus detected in patients' blood is produced mostly by short-lived infected CD4$^+$ T cells and in smaller amounts by other infected cells. New drug therapies have been developed that block all detectable HIV production for several years, as we will discuss later. The reduction in plasma virus levels has been monitored in patients receiving this therapy by sensitive reverse transcriptase–polymerase chain reaction assays for viral genomes (Fig. 20–9). Three phases of decay of plasma viremia have been observed or predicted by mathematical modeling, and these decay curves have been used to surmise the distribution of HIV in different cellular reservoirs. The therapy induces a rapid initial decline in plasma virus levels, with a half-life of less than 1 day. This rapid decline suggests that the virus is produced by short-lived cells, most likely activated CD4$^+$ T cells, which are likely to be major reservoirs and sources of the virus in infected patients. A second decay phase of plasma HIV with a half-life of about 2 weeks brings the amount of plasma virus to below detectable levels in patients receiving drug therapy. This drop may reflect the slower loss of a reservoir of virus in macrophages. A third phase of very slow decay of plasma HIV is predicted on the basis of mathematical models, and it is hypothesized that this pool of virus is present in latently infected memory T cells. Because of the long life span of memory cells, it could take decades for this reservoir of virus to be eliminated even if all new rounds of infection were blocked.

Mechanisms of Immunodeficiency

HIV infection ultimately results in impaired function of both the adaptive and innate immune systems. The most prominent defects are in cell-mediated immunity, and they can be attributed to several mechanisms, including direct cytopathic effects of the virus and indirect effects.

An important cause of the loss of CD4$^+$ T cells in HIV-infected people is the direct cytopathic effects of infection of these cells by HIV. Death of CD4$^+$ T cells is associated with production of virus in infected cells and is a major cause of the decline in the numbers of these cells. Several direct toxic effects of HIV on infected CD4$^+$ cells have been described:

- The process of virus production, with expression of gp41 in the plasma membrane and budding of viral particles, may lead to increased plasma membrane permeability and the influx of lethal amounts of calcium, which induces apoptosis, or osmotic lysis of the cell caused by the influx of water.
- Viral production can interfere with cellular protein synthesis and expression and thereby lead to cell death.
- Unintegrated viral DNA in the cytoplasm of infected cells, or large amounts of nonfunctional viral RNA, may be toxic to the infected cells.
- The plasma membranes of HIV-infected T cells fuse with uninfected CD4$^+$ T cells by virtue of gp120-CD4 interactions, and multinucleated giant cells or syncytia are formed. The process of HIV-induced syncytia formation can be lethal to HIV-infected T cells as well as to uninfected CD4$^+$ T cells that fuse to the infected cells. The phenomenon has largely been observed *in vitro*, and syncytia are rarely seen in the tissues of patients with AIDS.

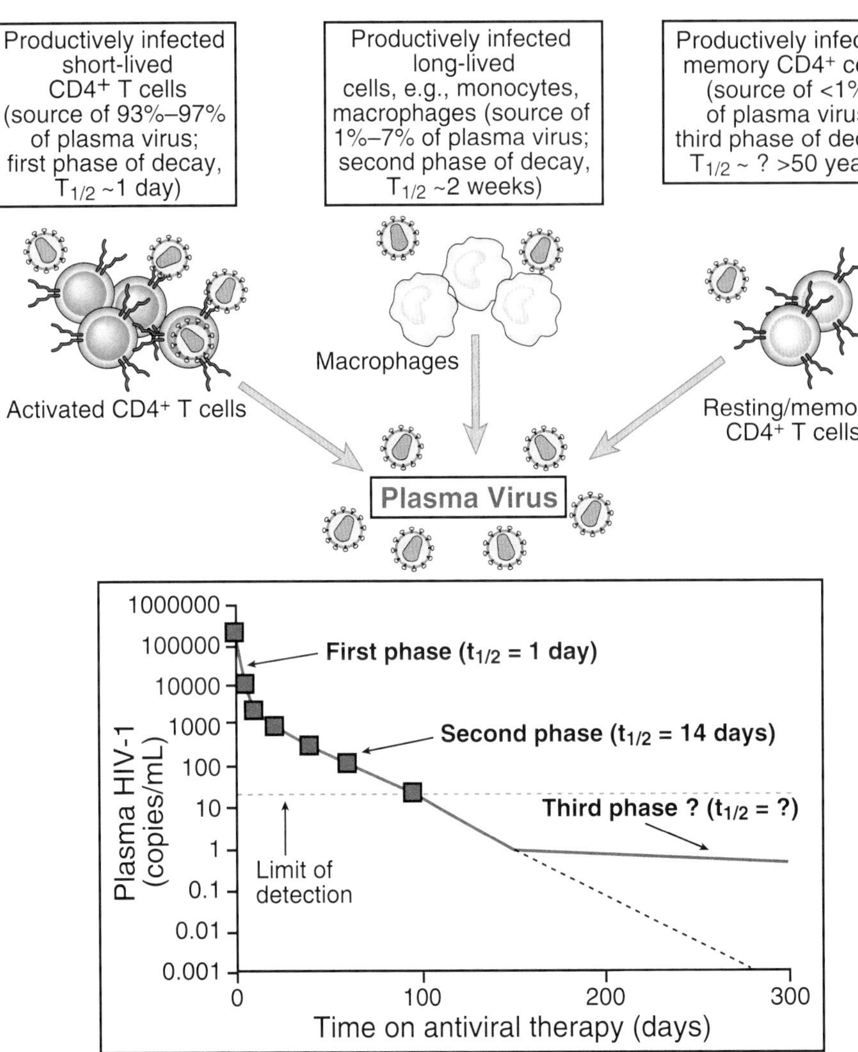

Figure 20–9 Cellular reservoirs of HIV.

Three cellular reservoirs of HIV-1 that contribute to plasma viremia have been identified by mathematical modeling of the decay of plasma HIV-1 mRNA after initiation of highly active antiretroviral therapy. This therapy, which includes combinations of reverse transcriptase and protease inhibitors, can effectively block all new cycles of viral reproduction but will not eliminate provirus from latently infected cells. (Modified from Finzi D, and RF Siliciano. Viral dynamics in HIV-1 infection. Cell 93:665–671, 1998. Copyright 1998, with permission from Elsevier Science.)

Mechanisms in addition to direct lysis of infected CD4⁺ T cells by virus have been proposed for the depletion and loss of function of these cells in HIV-infected individuals. Uninfected cells may be chronically activated by the infections that are common in patients infected with HIV and also by cytokines produced in response to these infections. Activation of the T cells may be followed by apoptosis, often referred to as activation-induced cell death (but not involving death receptors; see Box 10–2, Chapter 10). This pathway of apoptosis of activated lymphocytes may account for the observation that the loss of T cells greatly exceeds the numbers of HIV-infected cells. HIV-specific CTLs are present in many patients with AIDS, and these cells can kill infected $CD4^+$ T cells. In addition, antibodies against HIV envelope proteins may bind to HIV-infected $CD4^+$ T cells and target the cells for antibody-dependent cell-mediated cytotoxicity (ADCC). Binding of gp120 to newly synthesized intracellular CD4 may interfere with normal protein processing in the endoplasmic reticulum and block cell surface expression of CD4, making the cells incapable of responding to antigenic stimulation. Other proposed mechanisms include defective maturation of $CD4^+$ T cells in the thymus. The relative importance of these indirect mechanisms in $CD4^+$ T cell depletion in HIV-infected patients is uncertain and controversial.

Defects in the immune system of HIV-infected individuals are detectable even before significant depletion of $CD4^+$ T cells. These defects include a decrease in memory T cell responses to antigens, poor CTL responses to viral infection, and weak humoral immune responses to antigens even though total serum Ig levels may be elevated. The mechanisms of these defects are not well understood, and many theories based on often controversial data abound. The defects may be a result of the direct effects of HIV infection on $CD4^+$ T cells, including the effects of soluble gp120 released from infected cells binding to uninfected cells. For example, CD4 that has bound gp120 may not be available to interact with class II MHC molecules on APCs, and thus T cell responses to antigens would be inhibited. Alternatively, gp120 binding to CD4 may deliver signals that down-regulate helper T cell function. Some studies have demonstrated that the proportion of IL-2– and IFN-γ–secreting (T_H1) T cells decreases in HIV-infected patients and the proportion of IL-4– and IL-10–secreting (T_H2-like) T cells increases. Postulated mechanisms for this preferential decline of T_H1 cells are that HIV infection inhibits the transcription of T_H1 cytokines and that T_H1 cells are more susceptible than T_H2 cells to the apoptotic effects of HIV gene products (e.g., gp120 or Tat). This altered balance of T_H1 and T_H2 responses may partially explain the susceptibility of HIV-infected individuals to infection by intracellular microbes because IFN-γ activates and IL-4 and IL-10 inhibit macrophage-mediated killing of such microbes.

The Tat protein may play some role in the pathogenesis of immunodeficiency caused by HIV. Within T cells, Tat can interact with a variety of regulatory proteins, such as the p300 coactivator of transcription, and these interactions can interfere with normal T cell functions such as cytokine synthesis. Remarkably, Tat not only enters the nucleus of infected T cells but can also escape across the plasma membrane and enter neighboring cells, thus interfering with activation of uninfected T cells in a paracrine fashion.

Macrophages, dendritic cells, and follicular dendritic cells also play important roles in HIV infection and the progression of immunodeficiency.

- Macrophages express much lower levels of CD4 than helper T lymphocytes do, but they do express CCR5 coreceptors and are susceptible to HIV infection. As noted earlier, some strains of HIV may preferentially infect macrophages on the basis of a predilection for binding to the CCR5 coreceptor over the CXCR4 coreceptor expressed on T cells. However, macrophages are relatively resistant to the cytopathic effects of HIV, possibly because high CD4 expression is required for virus-induced cytotoxicity. Macrophages may also be infected by a gp120/gp41-independent route, such as phagocytosis of other infected cells or Fc receptor–mediated endocytosis of antibody-coated HIV virions. Because macrophages can be infected but are not generally killed by the virus, they may become a reservoir for the virus. In fact, the quantity of macrophage-associated HIV exceeds T cell–associated virus in most tissues from patients with AIDS, including the brain and lung. HIV-infected macrophages may be impaired in antigen presentation functions and cytokine secretion.
- Dendritic cells can also be infected by HIV. Like macrophages, dendritic cells are not directly injured by HIV infection. However, these cells form intimate contact with naive T cells during the course of antigen presentation. It is proposed that dendritic cells infect naive T cells during these encounters and may thus be an important pathway for T cell injury. Infected macrophages may play a similar role.
- Follicular dendritic cells (FDCs) in the germinal centers of lymph nodes and the spleen trap large amounts of HIV on their extended surfaces, in part by Fc receptor–mediated binding of antibody-coated virus. Although FDCs are not efficiently infected, they contribute to the pathogenesis of HIV-associated immunodeficiency in at least two significant ways. First, the FDC surface is a reservoir for HIV that can infect macrophages and $CD4^+$ T cells in the lymph node. Second, the normal functions of FDCs in immune responses are impaired, and they may eventually be destroyed by the virus. Although the mechanisms of HIV-induced death of FDCs are not understood, the net result of loss of the FDC network in the lymph nodes and spleen is a dramatic dissolution of the architecture of the peripheral lymphoid system.

Immune Responses to HIV

Both humoral and cell-mediated immune responses specific for HIV gene products occur in HIV-infected patients. The early response to HIV infection is, in fact, similar in many ways to the immune response to other viruses and serves effectively to clear most of the virus present in the blood and in circulating T cells. Nonetheless, it is clear that these immune responses fail to eradicate all virus, and the infection eventually overwhelms the immune system in most individuals. Despite the poor effectiveness of immune responses to the virus, it is important to characterize them for three reasons. First, the immune responses may be detrimental to the host, for example, by stimulating the uptake of opsonized virus into uninfected cells by Fc receptor–mediated endocytosis or by eradication of $CD4^+$ T cells expressing viral antigens by $CD8^+$ CTLs. Second, antibodies against HIV are diagnostic markers of HIV infection that are widely used for screening purposes. Third, the design of effective vaccines for immunization against HIV requires knowledge of the viral epitopes that are most likely to stimulate protective immunity.

The initial adaptive immune response to HIV infection is characterized by a massive expansion of $CD8^+$ CTLs specific for peptides derived from HIV proteins. As many as 10% or more of circulating $CD8^+$ T cells may be specific for HIV during the early stages of infection. The partial control of HIV infection, reflected by the reduction in viremia and transition to the clinically latent phase, may largely be due to this CTL response (see Fig. 20–8).

Antibody responses to a variety of HIV antigens are detectable within 6 to 9 weeks after infection, but there is little evidence that the antibodies have any beneficial effect in controlling the infection. The most immunogenic HIV molecules that elicit antibody responses appear to be the envelope glycoproteins, and high titers of anti-gp120 and anti-gp41 antibodies are present in most HIV-infected individuals. Other anti-HIV antibodies found frequently in patients' sera include antibodies to p24, reverse transcriptase, and *gag* and *pol* products (see Fig. 20–8). The effect of these antibodies on the clinical course of HIV infection is probably minimal. Interestingly, anti-envelope antibodies are generally poor inhibitors of viral infectivity or cytopathic effects, which supports the hypothesis that the most immunogenic epitopes of the envelope glycoproteins are least important for the functions of these molecules. Low titers of neutralizing antibodies that can inactivate HIV *in vitro* are present in HIV-infected patients, as are antibodies that can mediate ADCC. These antibodies are usually specific for gp120. No correlation has been found between the titers of these antibodies and the clinical course. Standard screening protocols for HIV use immunofluorescence or enzyme-linked immunoassays to detect anti-HIV antibodies in patients' sera. Positive screening test results are often followed by Western blot or radioimmunoassay to detect serum antibodies specific for particular viral proteins.

Mechanisms of Immune Evasion by HIV

The failure of cell-mediated and humoral immune responses to eradicate HIV infection is probably due to several factors. Importantly, because of the depletion and functional inhibition of the $CD4^+$ T cells, the immune responses may be too compromised to eliminate the virus. In addition, several features of HIV may help the virus to evade host immunity.

- ***HIV has an extremely high mutation rate because of error-prone reverse transcription, and in this way it may evade detection by antibodies or T cells generated in response to viral proteins.*** It has been estimated that in an infected person, every possible point mutation in the viral genome occurs every day. A region of the gp120 molecule, called the V3 loop, is one of the most antigenically variable components of the virus; it varies in HIV isolates taken from the same individual at different times. Furthermore, the regions of the V3 loop that are critical for viral entry and therefore are less frequently mutated are not readily exposed to the humoral immune system. It is possible that the host immune response may work as a selective pressure that promotes survival of the most genetically variable viruses.
- ***HIV-infected cells may evade CTLs through down-regulation of class I MHC molecule expression.*** The HIV Nef protein inhibits expression of class I MHC molecules, particularly HLA-A and HLA-B proteins, mainly by promoting internalization of these molecules.
- ***HIV infection may preferentially inhibit cell-mediated immunity.*** We have mentioned previously that in infected individuals, T_H2 cells specific for HIV and other microbes may expand relative to T_H1 cells. Because T_H2 cytokines inhibit cell-mediated immunity, the net result of this imbalance is a form of dysregulation (sometimes called immune deviation) that increases host susceptibility to infection by intracellular microbes, including HIV itself.

Transmission of HIV and Epidemiology of AIDS

The modes of transmission of HIV from one individual to another are the major determinants of the epidemiologic features of AIDS. The virus is transmitted by three major routes:

- Intimate sexual contact is the most frequent mode of transmission, either between heterosexual couples (an increasingly frequent mode of transmission in Africa and Asia) or between homosexual male partners. In sub-Saharan Africa, where the infection rate is the highest in the world (estimated to be about 10,000 new cases every day), more than half the infected individuals are women who acquired the virus by heterosexual transmission.
- Inoculation of a recipient with infected blood or blood products is the second most frequent mode of HIV transmission. Needles shared by intravenous drug abusers account for most cases of this form of transmission. With the advent of routine laboratory screening, transfusion of blood or blood products in a clinical setting accounts for a small portion of HIV infections. Patients infected in this way may then infect other individuals by sexual contact.
- Mother-to-child transmission of HIV accounts for the majority of pediatric cases of AIDS. This type of transmission occurs most frequently *in utero* or during childbirth, although transmission through breast milk is also possible.

Major groups at risk for the development of AIDS in the United States include homosexual or bisexual males, intravenous drug abusers, heterosexual partners of members of other risk groups, and babies born of infected mothers. Health care workers have a small increased risk of infection. In Africa, the majority of HIV infections occur by sexual transmission from one heterosexual partner to another.

Treatment and Prevention of AIDS and Vaccine Development

Active research efforts have been aimed at development of reagents that interfere with the viral life cycle. Treatment of HIV infection and AIDS now includes the administration of three classes of antiviral drugs, used in combination, that target viral molecules for which no human homologues exist. The first type of drug to be widely used consists of nucleoside analogues that inhibit reverse transcriptase activity. These drugs include deoxythymidine nucleoside analogues such as 3′-azido-3′-deoxythymidine (AZT), deoxycytidine nucleoside analogues, and deoxyadenosine analogues. When these drugs are used alone, they are often effective in significantly reducing plasma HIV RNA levels for several months to years. They usually do not halt progression of HIV-induced disease, largely because of the evolution of virus with mutated forms of reverse transcriptase that are resistant to the drugs. More recently, viral protease inhibitors have been developed that block the processing of precursor proteins into mature viral capsid and core proteins. When these protease inhibitors are used alone, mutant viruses resistant to their effects rapidly emerge. However, protease inhibitors are now being used in combination with two different reverse transcriptase inhibitors. This new triple-drug therapy, commonly referred to as HAART (highly active antiretroviral therapy), has proved to be remarkably effective in reducing plasma viral RNA to undetectable levels in most treated patients for up to 3 years. However, no therapy has resulted in sterilization, and resistance to the drugs develops during longer periods of treatment. Furthermore, it could theoretically take decades of effective antiviral drug therapy to eradicate reservoirs of latently infected cells. Other formidable problems associated with these new drug therapies, which will impair their effective use in many parts of the world, include high expense, complicated administration schedules, and serious side effects.

New classes of anti-HIV drugs now in clinical trials include inhibitors of viral entry (chemokine receptor antagonists and inhibitors of viral–cell membrane fusion) and integrase inhibitors that prevent integration of proviral DNA into the host cell DNA.

The individual infections experienced by patients with AIDS are treated with the appropriate prophylaxis, antibiotics, and support measures. More aggressive antibiotic therapy is often required than for similar infections in less compromised hosts.

Efforts at preventing HIV infection are extremely important and potentially effective in controlling the HIV epidemic. In the United States, the routine screening of blood products for evidence of donor HIV infection has already reduced the risk of this mode of transmission to negligible levels. Various public health measures to increase condom use and to reduce the use of contaminated needles by intravenous drug users are now widespread. Perhaps the most effective efforts at prevention are campaigns to increase public awareness of HIV.

The development of an effective vaccine against HIV has become a major priority for biomedical research institutions worldwide. The task has been complicated by the ability of the virus to mutate and vary many of its immunogenic antigens. Furthermore, although we know many of the viral proteins that induce humoral and CTL responses during the natural course of infection, these responses are ineffective in preventing disease. It is likely that an effective vaccine will have to stimulate both humoral and cell-mediated responses to viral antigens that are critical for the viral life cycle. To achieve this goal, several approaches are being tried for HIV vaccine development. Much of the preliminary work has involved SIV infection of macaques, and effective vaccines against SIV have already been developed. This success is encouraging because SIV is molecularly closely related to HIV and causes a disease similar to AIDS in macaques. Various live virus vaccines have been tested in the hope that they will induce strong CTL responses. Such vaccines include nonvirulent recombinant hybrid viruses composed of part SIV and part HIV sequences or viruses that have been attenuated by deletions in one or more parts of the viral genome, such as the *nef* gene. One concern with live virus vaccines is their potential to cause disease if they are not completely attenuated and possibly after recombination *in vivo* with wild-type HIV to produce a pathogenic variant. Another approach that avoids this safety concern but retains efficacy in inducing CTL-mediated immunity is the use of live recombinant non-HIV viral vectors carrying HIV genes. Preliminary trials in human volunteers have already shown that canarypox vaccines expressing several HIV-1 genes can induce strong CTL responses to the HIV antigens. Many DNA vaccines have also been studied; these vaccines are composed of combinations of structural and regulatory genes of SIV or HIV packaged in mammalian DNA expression vectors. Combinations of vaccines, such as initial immunization with a DNA vaccine followed by boosting with a canarypox vector expressing HIV genes, have given some of the most promising results to date. Recombinant protein or peptide subunit vaccines that elicit antibodies are of limited value by themselves because the antibodies often do not neutralize clinical isolates of HIV. It is possible that such vaccines may be useful given with live virus vaccines.

Summary

- Immunodeficiency diseases are caused by congenital or acquired defects in lymphocytes, phagocytes, and other mediators of adaptive and innate immunity. These diseases are associated with an increased susceptibility to infection, the nature and severity of which depend largely on which component of the immune system is abnormal and the extent of the abnormality.
- Defects in lymphocyte development can affect both T and B cells (e.g., X-linked and autosomal forms of SCID), only B cells (e.g., X-linked agammaglobulinemia), or only T cells (e.g., DiGeorge syndrome).
- Defects in lymphocyte activation can affect lymphocyte responses to antigen, antigen presentation (e.g., bare lymphocyte syndrome of TAP deficiency), or T cell–B cell collaboration (X-linked hyper-IgM syndrome).
- Defects in phagocytes include defects in microbial killing (e.g., CGD or Chédiak-Higashi syndrome) and defects in leukocyte migration and adhesion (e.g., LAD).
- Treatment of congenital immunodeficiencies involves transfusions of antibodies, bone marrow or stem cell transplantation, or enzyme replacement. Gene therapy may offer improved treatments in the future.
- Acquired immunodeficiencies are caused by infections, malnutrition, disseminated cancer, and immunosuppressive therapy for transplant rejection or autoimmune diseases.
- AIDS is a severe immunodeficiency caused by infection with HIV. This RNA virus infects $CD4^+$ T lymphocytes, macrophages, and dendritic cells and causes massive dysfunction of the adaptive immune system. Most of the immunodeficiency in AIDS can be ascribed to the depletion of $CD4^+$ T cells.
- HIV enters cells by binding to both the CD4 molecule and a coreceptor of the chemokine receptor family. Once inside the cell, the viral genome is reverse-transcribed into DNA and incorporated into

the cellular genome. Viral gene transcription and viral reproduction are stimulated by signals that normally activate the host cell. Production of virus is accompanied by cell death.

- $CD4^+$ T cell depletion in HIV-infected individuals is due to direct cytopathic effects of the virus, toxic effects of viral products such as shed gp120, and indirect effects such as activation-induced cell death or CTL killing of infected $CD4^+$ cells.
- Several reservoirs of HIV exist in infected individuals, including short-lived activated $CD4^+$ T cells, longer lived macrophages, and very long lived, latently infected resting T cells.
- HIV-induced depletion of $CD4^+$ T cells results in greatly increased susceptibility to infection by a number of opportunistic microorganisms. In addition, HIV-infected patients have an increased incidence of tumors, particularly Kaposi's sarcoma and EBV-associated B cell lymphomas, and encephalopathy frequently develops, the mechanism of which is not fully understood.
- HIV has a high mutation rate, which allows the virus to evade host immune responses as well as drug therapies. Genetic variability also poses a problem for the design of an effective vaccine against HIV. HIV infection can be treated by a combination of inhibitors of viral enzymes.

Selected Readings

Berger EA, PM Murphy, and JM Farber. Chemokine receptors as HIV-1 coreceptors: roles in viral entry, tropism, and disease. Annual Review of Immunology 17:657–700, 1999.

Blankson JN, D Persaud, and RF Siliciano. The problem of viral reservoirs in HIV-1 infection. Annual Review of Medicine 53:557–593, 2002.

Buckley RH. Primary immunodeficiency diseases due to defects in lymphocytes. New England Journal of Medicine 343:1313–1324, 2000.

Cullen BR. HIV-1 auxiliary proteins: making connections in a dying cell. Cell 93:685–692, 1998.

Fischer A. Primary immunodeficiencies: natural mutant models for the study of the immune system. Scandinavian Journal of Immunology 55:238–241, 2002.

Fischer A, S Hacein-Bey, F LeDeist, et al. Gene therapy for human severe combined immunodeficiencies. Immunity 15:1–4, 2001.

Frankel AD, and JAT Young. HIV-1: fifteen proteins and an RNA. Annual Review of Biochemistry 67:1–25, 1998.

Gandhi RT, and BD Walker. Immunologic control of HIV-1. Annual Review of Medicine 53:149–172, 2002.

Greenberg PD, and SR Riddell. Deficient cellular immunity—finding and fixing the defects. Science 285:546–551, 1999.

Grossman Z, M Meier-Schellersheim, AE Sousa, RM Victorino, and WE Paul. $CD4^+$ T-cell depletion in HIV infection: are we closer to understanding the cause? Nature Medicine 8:319–323, 2002.

Haase AT. Population biology of HIV-1 infection: Viral and $CD4^+$ T cell demographics and dynamics in lymphoid tissues. Annual Review of Immunology 17:625–656, 1999.

Hazenberg MD, D Hamann, H Schuitemaker, and F Miedema. T cell depletion in HIV-1 infection: how $CD4^+$ T cells go out of stock. Nature Immunology 1:285–289, 2000.

Kinter A, J Arthos, C Cicala, and AS Fauci. Chemokines, cytokines and HIV: a complex network of interactions that influence HIV pathogenesis. Immunological Reviews 177:88–98, 2000.

LaBranche CC, G Galasso, JP Moore, et al. HIV fusion and its inhibition. Antiviral Research 50:95–115, 2001.

Leonard WJ. Cytokines and immunodeficiency diseases. Nature Reviews Immunology 1:200–208, 2001.

Letvin NL, DH Barouch, and DC Montefiori. Prospects for vaccine protection against HIV-1 infection and AIDS. Annual Review of Immunology 20:73–99, 2002.

Littman DR. Chemokine receptors: keys to AIDS pathogenesis? Cell 29:677–680, 1998.

McMichael AJ, and SL Rowland-Jones. Cellular immune responses to HIV. Nature 410:980–987, 2001.

Meischl C, and D Roos. The molecular basis of chronic granulomatous disease. Springer Seminars in Immunopathology 19:417–434, 1998.

Morra M, D Howie, M Simarro, et al. X-linked lymphoproliferative disease: a progressive immunodeficiency. Annual Review of Immunology 19:657–682, 2001.

Reith W, and B Mach. The bare lymphocyte syndrome and the regulation of MHC expression. Annual Review of Immunology 19:331–373, 2001.

Robinson HL. New hope for an AIDS vaccine. Nature Reviews Immunology 2:239–250, 2002.

Snapper SB, and FS Rosen. The Wiskott-Aldrich syndrome protein (WASP): roles in signaling and cytoskeletal organization. Annual Review of Immunology 17:905–929, 1999.

Spritz RA. Genetic defects in Chédiak-Higashi syndrome and the beige mouse. Journal of Clinical Immunology 18:97–105, 1998.

Sugamura K, H Asao, M Kondo, N Tanaka, N Ishii, K Ohbo, M Nakamura, and T Takeshita. Interleukin-2 receptor gamma chain: its role in multiple cytokine receptor complexes and T cell development in XSCID. Annual Review of Immunology 14:179–206, 1996.

Appendix I

Glossary

αβ T cell receptor (αβ TCR). The most common form of TCR, expressed on both $CD4^+$ and $CD8^+$ T cells. The αβ TCR recognizes peptide antigen bound to an MHC molecule. Both α and β chains contain highly variable (V) regions that together form the antigen-binding site as well as constant (C) regions. TCR V and C regions are structurally homologous to the V and C regions of Ig molecules.

ABO blood group antigens. Glycosphingolipid antigens present on many cell types, including red blood cells. These antigens differ between different individuals, depending on inherited alleles encoding the enzymes required for synthesis of the antigens. The ABO antigens act as alloantigens responsible for blood transfusion reactions and hyperacute rejection of allografts.

Accessory molecule. A lymphocyte cell surface molecule distinct from the antigen receptor complex that mediates adhesive or signaling functions important for activation or migration of the lymphocyte.

Acquired immunodeficiency. A deficiency in the immune system that is acquired after birth, usually because of infection (e.g., AIDS), and that is not related to a genetic defect.

Acquired immunodeficiency syndrome (AIDS). A disease caused by human immunodeficiency virus (HIV) infection that is characterized by depletion of $CD4^+$ T cells leading to a profound defect in cell-mediated immunity. Clinically, AIDS includes opportunistic infections, malignant tumors, wasting, and encephalopathy.

Activation protein-1 (AP-1). A family of DNA-binding transcription factors composed of dimers of two proteins that bind to one another through a shared structural motif called a leucine zipper. The best characterized AP-1 factor is composed of the proteins Fos and Jun. AP-1 is involved in transcriptional regulation of many different genes important in the immune system, such as cytokine genes.

Active immunity. The form of adaptive immunity that is induced by exposure to a foreign antigen and activation of lymphocytes and in which the immunized individual plays an active role in responding to the antigen. This type contrasts with passive immunity, in which an individual receives antibodies or lymphocytes from another individual who was previously actively immunized.

Acute-phase reactants. Proteins, mostly synthesized in the liver, whose plasma concentrations increase shortly after infection as part of the systemic inflammatory response syndrome. Examples include C-reactive protein, fibrinogen, and serum amyloid A protein. Hepatic synthesis of these molecules is up-regulated by inflammatory cytokines, especially IL-6 and TNF. The acute-phase reactants play various roles in the innate immune response to microbes.

Acute-phase response. The increase in plasma concentrations of several proteins, called acute-phase reactants, that occurs as part of the early innate immune response to infections.

Acute rejection. A form of graft rejection involving vascular and parenchymal injury mediated by T cells, macrophages, and antibodies that usually begins after the first week of transplantation. Differentiation of effector T cells and production of antibodies that mediate acute rejection occur in response to the graft, thus the delay in onset.

Adapter protein. Proteins involved in lymphocyte signal transduction pathways by serving as bridge molecules or scaffolds for the recruitment of other signaling molecules. During lymphocyte activation, adapter molecules may be phosphorylated on tyrosine residues to enable them to bind other proteins containing Src homology 2 (SH2) domains. Adapter molecules involved in T cell activation include LAT, SLP-76, and Grb-2.

Adaptive immunity. The form of immunity that is mediated by lymphocytes and stimulated by exposure to infectious agents. In contrast to innate immunity, adaptive immunity is characterized by exquisite specificity for distinct macromolecules and memory, which is the ability to respond more vigorously to repeated exposure to the same microbe. Adaptive immunity is also called specific immunity.

Addressin. Molecules expressed on endothelial cells in different anatomic sites that bind to counter-receptors on lymphocytes called homing receptors and that direct organ-specific lymphocyte homing. Mucosal addressin cell adhesion molecule-1 (MadCAM-1) is an example of an addressin expressed in Peyer's patch in the intestinal wall that binds to the integrin $\alpha_4\beta_7$ on gut-homing T cells.

Adhesion molecule. A cell surface molecule whose function is to promote adhesive interactions with other cells or the extracellular matrix. Leukocytes express various types of adhesion molecules, such as selectins, integrins, and members of the Ig superfamily, and these molecules play crucial roles in cell migration and cellular activation in innate and adaptive immune responses.

Adjuvant. A substance, distinct from antigen, that enhances T cell activation by promoting the accumulation and activation of other leukocytes, called accessory cells, at a site of antigen exposure. Adjuvants enhance accessory cell expression of T cell–activating costimulators and cytokines and may also prolong the expression of peptide-MHC complexes on the surface of APCs.

Adoptive transfer. The process of transferring lymphocytes from one, usually immunized, individual into another individual. Adoptive transfer is used in research to define the role of a particular cell population (e.g., $CD4^+$ T cells) in an immune response. Clinically, adoptive transfer of tumor-reactive T lymphocytes is used in experimental cancer therapy.

Affinity. The strength of the binding between a single binding site of a molecule (e.g., an antibody) and a ligand (e.g., an antigen). The affinity of a molecule X for a ligand Y is represented by the dissociation constant (K_d), which is the concentration of Y that is required to occupy the combining sites of half the X molecules present in a solution. A smaller K_d indicates a stronger or higher affinity interaction, and a lower concentration of ligand is needed to occupy the sites.

Affinity chromatography. A technique used to purify an antigen from a solution by passing it through a column packed with antibody that binds the antigen and is attached to a solid support such as agarose beads.

Affinity maturation. The process that leads to increased affinity of antibodies for a particular protein antigen as a humoral response progresses. Affinity maturation is the result of somatic mutation of Ig genes, followed by selective survival of the B cells producing the highest affinity antibodies.

Allele. One of different forms of a gene present at a particular chromosomal locus. An individual who is heterozygous at a locus has two different alleles, each on a different member of a pair of chromosomes, one inherited from the mother and one from the father. If a particular gene in a population has many different alleles, the gene or locus is said to be polymorphic. The MHC locus is extremely polymorphic.

Allelic exclusion. The exclusive expression of only one of two inherited alleles encoding Ig heavy and light chains and TCR β chains. Allelic exclusion occurs when the protein product of one productively recombined antigen receptor locus on one chromosome blocks rearrangement of the corresponding locus on the other chromosome. This property ensures that all the antigen receptors expressed by one clone of lymphocytes will have the identical antigen specificities. Because the TCR α chain locus does not show allelic exclusion, some T cells do express two different types of TCR.

Allergen. An antigen that elicits an immediate hypersensitivity (allergic) reaction. Allergens are proteins or chemicals bound to proteins that induce IgE antibody responses in atopic individuals.

Allergy. A form of atopy or immediate hypersensitivity disease, often referring to the type of antigen that elicits the disease, such as food allergy, bee sting allergy, and penicillin allergy. All these conditions are related to antigen-induced mast cell or basophil activation.

Alloantibody. An antibody specific for an alloantigen (i.e., an antigen present in some individuals of a species but not in others).

Alloantigen. A cell or tissue antigen that is present in some members of a species and not in others and that is recognized as foreign on an allograft. Alloantigens are usually products of polymorphic genes.

Alloantiserum. The alloantibody-containing serum of an individual who has previously been exposed to one or more alloantigens.

Allogeneic graft. An organ or tissue graft from a donor who is of the same species but genetically nonidentical to the recipient (also called an allograft).

Alloreactive. Reactive to alloantigens; describes T cells or antibodies from one individual that will recognize antigens on cells or tissues of another genetically nonidentical individual.

Allotype. The property of a group of antibody molecules defined by their sharing a particular allotope; that is, antibodies that share a particular allotope belong to the same allotype. Allotype is also often used synonymously with allotope, which refers to an antigenic determinant found on the antibodies of some individuals but not others.

Altered peptide ligands (APLs). Peptides with altered TCR contact residues that elicit responses different from the responses to native peptide ligands. Altered peptide ligands may be important in the regulation of T cell activation in physiologic, pathologic, or therapeutic situations.

Alternative pathway of complement activation. An antibody-independent pathway of activation of the complement system that occurs when the C3b protein binds to microbial cell surfaces. The alternative pathway is a component of the innate immune system and mediates inflammatory responses to infection as well as direct lysis of microbes.

Anaphylactic shock. Cardiovascular collapse occurring in the setting of a systemic immediate hypersensitivity reaction.

Anaphylatoxins. The C5a, C4a, and C3a complement fragments that are generated during complement activation. The anaphylatoxins bind specific cell surface receptors and promote acute inflammation by stimulating neutrophil chemotaxis and activating mast cells. At high concentrations, anaphylatoxins activate enough mast cells to mimic anaphylaxis.

Anaphylaxis. An extreme systemic form of immediate hypersensitivity in which mast cell or basophil mediators cause bronchial constriction, massive tissue edema, and cardiovascular collapse.

Anchor residues. The amino acid residues of a peptide whose side chains fit into pockets in the peptide-binding cleft of an MHC molecule. The side chains bind to complementary amino acids in the MHC molecule and therefore serve to anchor the peptide in the cleft of the MHC molecule.

Anergy. A state of unresponsiveness to antigenic stimulation. Clinically, anergy describes the lack of T cell–dependent cutaneous delayed-type hypersensitivity reactions to common antigens. Lymphocyte anergy (also called clonal anergy) is the failure of clones of T or B cells to react to antigen and may be a mechanism of maintaining immunologic tolerance to self.

Angiogenesis. New blood vessel formation regulated by a variety of protein factors elaborated by cells of the innate and adaptive immune systems and often accompanying chronic inflammation.

Antagonist peptide. Variant peptide ligands of a TCR in which one or two TCR contact residues have been changed and in which negative signals are delivered to specific T cells that inhibit responses to native peptides.

Antibody. A type of glycoprotein molecule, also called immunoglobulin (Ig), produced by B lymphocytes that binds antigens, often with a high degree of specificity and affinity. The basic structural unit of an antibody is composed of two identical heavy chains and two identical light chains. N-terminal variable regions of the heavy and light chains form the antigen-binding sites, whereas the C-terminal constant regions of the heavy chains functionally interact with other molecules in the immune system. Every individual has millions of different antibodies, each with a unique antigen-binding site. Secreted antibodies perform various effector functions, including neutralizing antigens, activating complement, and promoting leukocyte-dependent destruction of microbes.

Antibody-dependent cell-mediated cytotoxicity (ADCC). A process by which NK cells are targeted to IgG-coated cells, resulting in lysis of the antibody-coated cells. A specific receptor for the constant region of IgG, called FcγRIII (CD16), is expressed on the NK cell membrane and mediates binding to the IgG.

Antibody feedback. The down-regulation of antibody production by secreted IgG antibodies that occurs when antigen-antibody complexes simultaneously engage B cell membrane Ig and Fcγ receptors (FcγRII). Under these conditions, the cytoplasmic tails of the Fcγ receptors transduce inhibitory signals inside the B cell.

Antibody repertoire. The collection of different antibody specificities expressed in an individual.

Antibody-secreting cell. A B lymphocyte that has undergone differentiation and produces the secretory form of Ig. Antibody-secreting cells are produced in response to antigen and reside in the spleen and lymph nodes as well as in the bone marrow.

Antigen. A molecule that binds to an antibody or a TCR. Antigens that bind to antibodies include all classes of molecules. TCRs bind only peptide fragments of proteins complexed with MHC molecules; both the peptide ligand and the native protein from which it is derived are called T cell antigens.

Antigen presentation. The display of peptides bound by MHC molecules on the surface of an APC that permits specific recognition by TCRs and activation of T cells.

Antigen processing. The intracellular conversion of protein antigens derived from the extracellular space or the cytosol into peptides and loading of these peptides onto MHC molecules for display to T lymphocytes.

Antigen-presenting cell (APC). A cell that displays peptide fragments of protein antigens, in association with MHC molecules, on its surface and activates antigen-specific T cells. In addition to displaying peptide-MHC complexes, APCs must also express costimulatory molecules to activate T lymphocytes optimally.

Antiserum. Serum from an individual previously immunized against an antigen that contains antibody specific for that antigen.

Apoptosis. A process of cell death characterized by DNA cleavage, nuclear condensation and fragmentation, and plasma membrane blebbing that leads to phagocytosis of the cell without inducing an inflammatory response. This type of cell death is important in lymphocyte development, regulation of lymphocyte responses to foreign antigens, and maintenance of tolerance to self antigens.

Arthus reaction. A localized form of experimental immune complex–mediated vasculitis induced by injection of an antigen subcutaneously into a previously immunized animal or into an animal that has been given intravenous antibody specific for the antigen. Circulating antibodies bind to the injected antigen and form immune complexes that are deposited in the walls of small arteries at the injection site and give rise to a local cutaneous vasculitis with necrosis.

Atopy. The propensity of an individual to produce IgE antibodies in response to various environmental antigens and to develop strong immediate hypersensitivity (allergic) responses. People who have allergies to environmental antigens, such as pollen or house dust, are said to be atopic.

Autoantibody. An antibody produced in an individual that is specific for a self antigen. Autoantibodies can cause damage to cells and tissues and are produced in excess in systemic autoimmune diseases, such as systemic lupus erythematosus.

Autocrine factor. A molecule that acts on the same cell that produces the factor. For example, IL-2 is an autocrine T cell growth factor that stimulates mitotic activity of the T cell that produces it.

Autoimmune disease. A disease caused by a breakdown of self-tolerance such that the adaptive immune system responds to self antigens and mediates cell and tissue damage. Autoimmune diseases can be organ specific (e.g., thyroiditis or diabetes) or systemic (e.g., systemic lupus erythematosus).

Autoimmunity. The state of adaptive immune system responsiveness to self antigens that occurs when mechanisms of self-tolerance fail.

Autologous graft. A tissue or organ graft in which the donor and recipient are the same individual. Autologous bone marrow and skin grafts are commonly performed in clinical medicine.

Avidity. The overall strength of interaction between two molecules, such as an antibody and antigen. Avidity depends on both the affinity and the valency of interactions. Therefore, the avidity of a pentameric IgM antibody, with 10 antigen-binding sites, for a multivalent antigen may be much greater than the avidity of a dimeric IgG molecule for the same antigen. Avidity can be used to describe the strength of cell-cell interactions, which are mediated by many binding interactions between cell surface molecules.

B cell tyrosine kinase (Btk). A tyrosine kinase of the Src family that plays an essential role in B cell maturation. Mutations in the gene encoding Btk cause X-linked agammaglobulinemia, a disease characterized by failure of B cells to mature beyond the pre-B cell stage.

B lymphocyte. The only cell type capable of producing antibody molecules and therefore the central cellular component of humoral immune responses. B lymphocytes, or B cells, develop in the bone marrow, and mature B cells are found mainly in lymphoid follicles in secondary lymphoid tissues, in bone marrow, and in low numbers in the circulation.

B lymphocyte antigen receptor (BCR) complex. A multiprotein complex expressed on the surface of B lymphocytes that recognizes antigen and transduces activating signals into the cell. The BCR includes membrane Ig, which is responsible for binding antigen, and Igα and Igβ proteins, which initiate signaling events.

Bare lymphocyte syndrome. An immunodeficiency disease characterized by a lack of class II MHC molecule expression that leads to defects in antigen presentation and cell-mediated immunity. The disease is caused by mutations in genes encoding factors that regulate class II MHC gene transcription.

Basophil. A type of bone marrow–derived, circulating granulocyte with structural and functional similarities to mast cells that has granules containing many of the same inflammatory mediators as mast cells and expresses a high-affinity Fc receptor for IgE. Basophils that are recruited into tissue sites where antigen is present may contribute to immediate hypersensitivity reactions.

Biogenic amines. Low molecular weight, nonlipid compounds, such as histamine, that share the structural feature of an amine group, are stored in and released from the cytoplasmic granules of mast cells, and mediate many of the biologic effects of immediate hypersensitivity (allergic) reactions. (Biogenic amines are sometimes called vasoactive amines.)

Biologic response modifiers. Molecules, such as cytokines, used clinically as modulators of inflammation, immunity, and hematopoiesis.

Bone marrow. The central cavity of bone that is the site of generation of all circulating blood cells in adults, including immature lymphocytes, and the site of B cell maturation.

Bone marrow transplantation. The transplantation of bone marrow, including stem cells that give rise to all mature blood cells and lymphocytes; it is performed clinically to treat hematopoietic or lymphopoietic disorders and malignant diseases and is also used in various immunologic experiments in animals.

Bronchial asthma. An inflammatory disease usually caused by repeated immediate hypersensitivity reactions in the lung that leads to intermittent and reversible airway obstruction, chronic bronchial inflammation with eosinophils, and bronchial smooth muscle cell hypertrophy and hyperreactivity.

Burkitt's lymphoma. A malignant B cell tumor that is defined by histologic features but almost always carries a reciprocal chromosomal translocation involving Ig gene loci and the cellular *myc* gene on chromosome 8. Many cases of Burkitt's lymphoma are associated with Epstein-Barr virus infection.

C (constant region) gene segments. The DNA sequences in the Ig and TCR gene loci that encode the nonvariable portions of Ig heavy and light chains and TCR α, β, γ, and δ chains.

C1. A serum complement system protein composed of several polypeptide chains that initiates the classical pathway of complement activation by attaching to the Fc portions of IgG or IgM antibody that has bound antigen.

C1 inhibitor (C1 INH). A plasma protein inhibitor of the classical pathway of complement activation. C1 INH is a serine protease inhibitor (serpin) that mimics the normal substrates of the C1r and C1s components of C1. A genetic deficiency in C1 INH causes the disease hereditary angioneurotic edema.

C3. The central and most abundant complement system protein; it is involved in both the classical and alternative pathway cascades. C3 is proteolytically cleaved during complement activation to generate a C3b fragment, which covalently attaches to cell or microbial surfaces, and a C3a fragment, which has various proinflammatory activities.

C3 convertase. A multiprotein enzyme complex generated by the early steps of either the classical or alternative pathway of complement activation. C3 convertase cleaves C3, which gives rise to two proteolytic products called C3a and C3b.

C5 convertase. A multiprotein enzyme complex generated by C3b binding to C3 convertase. C5 convertase cleaves C5 and initiates the late steps of complement activation leading to formation of the membrane attack complex and lysis of cells.

Calcineurin. A cytoplasmic serine/threonine phosphatase that dephosphorylates and thereby activates the transcription factor NFAT. Calcineurin is activated by calcium signals generated through TCR signaling in response to antigen recognition, and the immunosuppressive drugs cyclosporine and FK-506 work by blocking calcineurin activity.

Carcinoembryonic antigen (CEA, CD66). A highly glycosylated membrane protein; increased expression of CEA in many carcinomas of the colon, pancreas, stomach, and breast results in a rise in serum levels. The level of serum CEA is used to monitor the persistence or recurrence of metastatic carcinoma after treatment. Because CEA expression is normally high in many tissues during fetal life but is suppressed in adults except in tumor cells, it is called an oncofetal tumor antigen.

Caspases. Intracellular proteases with cysteines in their active sites that cleave substrates at the C-terminal sides of aspartic acid residues and are components of enzymatic cascades that cause apoptotic death of cells. Lymphocyte caspases may be activated by two pathways; one is associated with mitochondrial permeability changes in growth factor–deprived cells, and the other is associated with signals from death receptors in the plasma membrane.

Cathepsins. Thiol and aspartyl proteases with broad substrate specificities. The most abundant proteases of endosomes in APCs, cathepsins probably play an important role in generating peptide fragments from exogenous protein antigens that bind to class II MHC molecules.

CD molecules. Cell surface molecules expressed on various cell types in the immune system that are designated by the "cluster of differentiation" or CD number. See Appendix II for a list of CD molecules.

Cell-mediated immunity (CMI). The form of adaptive immunity that is mediated by T lymphocytes and serves as the defense mechanism against microbes that survive within phagocytes or infect nonphagocytic cells. CMI responses include $CD4^+$ T cell–mediated activation of macrophages that have phagocytosed microbes and $CD8^+$ CTL killing of infected cells.

Central tolerance. A form of self-tolerance induced in generative (central) lymphoid organs as a consequence of immature self-reactive lymphocytes recognizing self antigens and subsequently leading to their death or inactivation. Central tolerance prevents the emergence of lymphocytes with high-affinity receptors for the ubiquitous self antigens that are likely to be present in the bone marrow or thymus.

Chédiak-Higashi syndrome. A rare autosomal recessive immunodeficiency disease caused by a defect in the cytoplasmic granules of various cell types that affects the lysosomes of neutrophils and macrophages as well as the granules of CTLs and NK cells. Patients show reduced resistance to infection with pyogenic bacteria.

Chemokine receptors. Cell surface receptors for chemokines that transduce signals stimulating the migration of leukocytes. These receptors are members of the seven-transmembrane α-helical, G protein–linked family of receptors.

Chemokines. A large family of structurally homologous, low molecular weight cytokines that stimulate leukocyte movement and regulate the migration of leukocytes from the blood to tissues.

Chemotaxis. Movement of a cell directed by a chemical concentration gradient. The movement of lymphocytes, polymorphonuclear leukocytes, monocytes, and other leukocytes into various tissues is often directed by gradients of low molecular weight cytokines called chemokines.

Chromosomal translocation. A chromosomal abnormality in which a segment of one chromosome is transferred to another. Many malignant diseases of lymphocytes are associated with chromosomal translocations involving an Ig or TCR locus and a chromosomal segment containing a cellular oncogene.

Chronic granulomatous disease. A rare inherited immunodeficiency disease caused by a defect in the gene encoding a component of the phagocyte oxidase enzyme that is needed for microbial killing by polymorphonuclear leukocytes and macrophages. The disease is characterized by recurrent intracellular bacterial and fungal infections, often accompanied by chronic cell-mediated immune responses and the formation of granulomas.

Chronic rejection. A form of allograft rejection characterized by fibrosis with loss of normal organ structures occurring during a prolonged period. In many cases, the major pathologic event in chronic rejection is graft arterial occlusion, which is caused by proliferation of intimal smooth muscle cells and is called graft arteriosclerosis.

c-Kit ligand (stem cell factor). A protein required for hematopoiesis, early steps in T cell development in the thymus, and mast cell development. c-Kit ligand is produced in membrane-bound and soluble forms by stromal cells in the bone marrow and thymus and binds to the c-Kit tyrosine kinase membrane receptor on pluripotent stem cells.

Class I major histocompatibility complex (MHC) molecule. One of two forms of polymorphic, heterodimeric membrane proteins that bind and display peptide fragments of protein antigens on the surface of APCs for recognition by T lymphocytes. Class I MHC molecules usually display peptides derived from the cytoplasm of the cell.

Class II–associated invariant chain peptide (CLIP). A peptide remnant of the invariant chain that sits in the class II MHC peptide-binding cleft and is removed by action of the HLA-DM molecule before the cleft becomes accessible to peptides produced from extracellular protein antigens.

Class II major histocompatibility complex (MHC) molecule. One of two forms of polymorphic, heterodimeric membrane proteins that bind and display peptide fragments of protein antigens on the surface of APCs for recognition by T lymphocytes. Class II MHC molecules usually display peptides derived from extracellular proteins that are internalized into phagocytic or endocytic vesicles.

Class II vesicle (CIIV). A membrane-bound organelle identified in murine B cells that is important in the class II MHC pathway of antigen presentation. The CIIV is similar to the MHC class II compartment (MIIC) identified in other cells and contains all the components required for the formation of complexes of peptide antigens and class II MHC molecules, including the enzymes that degrade protein antigens, class II molecules, invariant chain, and HLA-DM.

Classical pathway of complement activation. The pathway of activation of the complement system that is initiated by binding of antigen-antibody complexes to the C1 molecule and induces a proteolytic cascade involving multiple other complement proteins. The classical pathway is an effector arm of the humoral immune system that generates inflammatory mediators, opsonins for phagocytosis of antigens, and lytic complexes that destroy cells.

Clonal anergy. A state of antigen unresponsiveness of a clone of T lymphocytes experimentally induced by recognition of antigen in the absence of additional signals (costimulatory signals) required for functional activation. Clonal anergy is considered a model for one mechanism of tolerance to self antigens and may be applicable to B lymphocytes as well.

Clonal deletion. A mechanism of lymphocyte tolerance in which an immature T cell in the thymus or an immature B cell in the bone marrow undergoes apoptotic death as a consequence of recognizing an abundant antigen in the generative organ.

Clonal expansion. The increase in number of lymphocytes specific for an antigen that results from antigen stimulation and proliferation of naive T cells. Clonal expansion occurs in lymphoid tissues and is required to generate enough antigen-specific effector lymphocytes from rare naive precursors to eradicate infections.

Clonal ignorance. A form of lymphocyte unresponsiveness in which self antigens are ignored by the immune system even though lymphocytes specific for those antigens remain viable and functional.

Clonal selection hypothesis. A fundamental tenet of the immune system (no longer a hypothesis) stating that every individual possesses numerous clonally derived lymphocytes, each clone having arisen from a single precursor and being capable of recognizing and responding to a distinct antigenic determinant. When an antigen enters, it selects a specific preexisting clone and activates it.

c-*myc*. A cellular proto-oncogene that encodes a nuclear factor involved in cell cycle regulation. Translocations of the c-*myc* gene into Ig gene loci are associated with B cell malignant neoplasms.

Collectins. A family of proteins, including mannose-binding lectin, that are characterized by a collagen-like domain and a lectin (i.e., carbohydrate-binding) domain. Collectins play a role in the innate immune system by acting as microbial pattern recognition receptors, and they may activate the complement system by binding to C1q.

Colony-stimulating factors (CSFs). Cytokines that promote the expansion and differentiation of bone marrow progenitor cells. CSFs are essential for the maturation of red blood cells, granulocytes, monocytes, and lymphocytes. Examples of CSFs are granulocyte-monocyte colony-stimulating factor (GM-CSF), c-Kit ligand, IL-3, and IL-7.

Combinatorial diversity. Combinatorial diversity describes the many different combinations of variable, diversity, and joining segments that are possible as a result of somatic recombination of DNA in the Ig and TCR loci during B cell or T cell development. Combinatorial diversity is one mechanism for the generation of large numbers of different antigen receptor genes from a limited number of DNA gene segments.

Complement. A system of serum and cell surface proteins that interact with one another and with other molecules of the immune system to generate important effectors of innate and adaptive immune responses. The classical and alternative pathways of the complement system are activated by antigen-antibody complexes or microbial surfaces, respectively, and consist of a cascade of proteolytic enzymes that generate inflammatory mediators and opsonins. Both pathways lead to the formation of a common terminal cell lytic complex that is inserted in cell membranes.

Complement receptor type 1 (CR1). A high-affinity receptor for the C3b and C4b fragments of complement. Phagocytes use CR1 to mediate internalization of C3b- or C4b-coated particles. CR1 on erythrocytes serves in the clearance of immune complexes from the circulation. CR1 is also a regulator of complement activation.

Complement receptor type 2 (CR2). A receptor expressed on B cells and follicular dendritic cells that binds proteolytic fragments of the C3 complement protein, including C3d, C3dg, and iC3b. CR2 functions to stimulate humoral immune responses by enhancing B cell activation by antigen and by promoting the trapping of antigen-antibody complexes in germinal centers. CR2 is also the receptor for Epstein-Barr virus.

Complementarity-determining region (CDR). Short segments of Ig and TCR proteins that contain most of the sequence differences among different antibodies or TCRs and that make contact with antigen. Three CDRs are present in the variable domain of each antigen receptor polypeptide chain and six CDRs in an intact Ig or TCR molecule. These hypervariable segments assume loop structures that together form a surface that is complementary to the three-dimensional structure of the bound antigen.

Congenic mouse strains. Inbred mouse strains that are identical to one another at every genetic locus except the one for which they are selected to differ; such strains are created by repetitive back-crossbreeding and selection for a particular trait. Congenic strains that differ from one another only at a particular MHC allele have been useful in defining the function of MHC molecules.

Constant (C) region. The portion of Ig or TCR polypeptide chains that does not vary in sequence among different clones and is not involved in antigen binding.

Contact sensitivity. The propensity for a T cell–mediated, delayed-type hypersensitivity reaction to develop in the skin on contact with a particular chemical agent. Chemicals that elicit contact hypersensitivity bind to and modify self proteins or molecules on the surfaces of APCs, which are then recognized by $CD4^+$ or $CD8^+$ T cells.

Coreceptor. A lymphocyte surface receptor that binds to an antigen complex at the same time that membrane Ig or TCR binds the antigen and delivers signals required for optimal lymphocyte activation. CD4 and CD8 are T cell coreceptors that bind nonpolymorphic parts of an MHC molecule concurrently with the TCR binding to polymorphic residues and the bound peptide. CR2 is a coreceptor on B cells that binds to complement-opsonized antigens at the same time that membrane Ig binds another part of the antigen.

Costimulator. A molecule on the surface of or secreted by an APC that provides a stimulus (or second signal) required for the activation of naive T cells, in addition to antigen. The best defined costimulators are the B7 molecules on professional APCs that bind to the CD28 molecule on T cells.

CpG nucleotides. Unmethylated cytidine-guanine sequences found in bacterial DNA that have adjuvant properties in the mammalian immune system and may be important to the efficacy of DNA vaccines.

C-reactive protein (CRP). A member of the pentraxin family of plasma proteins involved in innate immune responses to bacterial infections. CRP is an acute-phase reactant, and it binds to the capsule of pneumococcal bacteria. CRP also binds to C1q and may thereby activate complement or act as an opsonin by interacting with phagocyte C1q receptors.

Crossmatching. A screening test performed to minimize the chance of graft rejection in which a patient in need of an allograft is tested for the presence of preformed antibodies against donor cell surface antigens (usually MHC antigens). The test involves mixing the recipient serum with leukocytes from potential donors, adding complement, and observing whether cell lysis occurs.

Cross-priming. A mechanism by which a professional APC activates (or primes) a naive $CD8^+$ CTL specific for the antigens of a third cell (e.g., a virus-infected or tumor cell). Cross-priming occurs, for example, when an infected (often apoptotic) cell is ingested by a professional APC and the microbial antigens are processed and presented in association with class I MHC molecules, just like any other phagocytosed antigen. The professional APC also provides costimulation for the T cells. Also called **cross-presentation**.

Cutaneous immune system. The components of the innate and adaptive immune system found in the skin that function together in a specialized way to detect and respond to environmental antigens. Components of the cutaneous immune system include keratinocytes, Langerhans cells, intraepithelial lymphocytes, and dermal lymphocytes.

Cyclosporine. An immunosuppressive drug used to prevent allograft rejection that functions by blocking T cell cytokine gene transcription. Cyclosporine (also called cyclosporin A) binds to a cytosolic protein called cyclophilin, and cyclosporine-cyclophilin complexes bind to and inhibit calcineurin, thereby inhibiting activation and nuclear translocation of the transcription factor NFAT.

Cytokines. Proteins produced by many different cell types that mediate inflammatory and immune reactions. Cytokines are principal mediators of communication between cells of the immune system.

Cytolytic (or cytotoxic) T lymphocyte (CTL). A type of T lymphocyte whose major effector function is to recognize and kill host cells infected with viruses or other intracellular microbes. CTLs usually express CD8 and recognize microbial peptides displayed by class I MHC molecules. CTL killing of infected cells involves the release of cytoplasmic granules whose contents include membrane pore-forming proteins and enzymes.

Cytopathic effect of viruses. Harmful effects of viruses on host cells that are caused by any of a variety of biochemical or molecular mechanisms and are independent of the host immune response to the virus. Some viruses have little cytopathic effect but still cause disease because the immune system recognizes and destroys the infected cells.

Defensins. Cysteine-rich peptides present in the skin and in neutrophil granules that act as broad-spectrum antibiotics to kill a wide variety of bacteria and fungi. The synthesis of defensins is increased in response to inflammatory cytokines such as IL-1 and TNF.

Delayed-type hypersensitivity (DTH). An immune reaction in which T cell–dependent macrophage activation and inflammation cause tissue injury. A DTH reaction to the subcutaneous injection of antigen is often used as an assay for cell-mediated immunity (e.g., the purified protein derivative skin test for immunity to *Mycobacterium tuberculosis*). DTH is a frequent accompaniment of protective cell-mediated immunity against microbes.

Delayed xenograft rejection. A frequent form of rejection of xenografts that occurs within 2 to 3 days of transplantation and is characterized by intravascular thrombosis and fibrinoid necrosis of vessel walls. Delayed xenograft rejection is likely to be caused by antibody- and cytokine-mediated endothelial activation and damage.

Dendritic cells. Bone marrow–derived immune accessory cells found in epithelial and lymphoid tissues that are morphologically characterized by thin membranous projections. Dendritic cells function as APCs for naive T lymphocytes and are important for initiation of adaptive immune responses to protein antigen.

Desensitization. A method of treating immediate hypersensitivity disease (allergies) that involves repetitive administration of low doses of an antigen to which individuals are allergic. This process often prevents severe allergic reactions on subsequent environmental exposure to the antigen, but the mechanisms are not well understood.

Determinant. The specific portion of a macromolecular antigen to which an antibody binds. In the case of a protein antigen recognized by a T cell, the determinant is the peptide portion that binds to an MHC molecule for recognition by the TCR. Synonymous with **epitope**.

Determinant selection model. A model to explain MHC-linked immune responses that was proposed before the demonstration of peptide-MHC molecule binding. The model states that the products of MHC genes in each individual select which determinants of protein antigens will be immunogenic in that individual.

Diacylglycerol (DAG). A membrane-bound signaling molecule generated by phospholipase C (PLCγ1)–mediated hydrolysis of the plasma membrane phospholipid phosphatidylinositol 4,5-bisphosphate (PIP_2) during antigen activation of lymphocytes. The main function of DAG is to activate an enzyme called protein kinase C that participates in the generation of active transcription factors.

DiGeorge syndrome. A selective T cell deficiency caused by a congenital malformation that results in defective development of the thymus, parathyroid glands, and other structures that arise from the third and fourth pharyngeal pouches.

Direct antigen presentation (or direct allorecognition). Presentation of cell surface allogeneic MHC molecules by graft cells to a graft recipient's T cells that leads to T cell activation, with no requirement for processing. Direct recognition of foreign MHC molecules is a cross-reaction in which a normal TCR that recognizes a self MHC molecule plus foreign peptide cross-reacts with an allogeneic MHC molecule plus peptide. Direct presentation is partly responsible for strong T cell responses to allografts.

Diversity. The existence of a large number of lymphocytes with different antigenic specificities in any individual (i.e., the lymphocyte repertoire is large and diverse). Diversity is a fundamental property of the adaptive immune system and is the result of variability in the structures of the antigen-binding sites of lymphocyte receptors for antigens (antibodies and TCRs).

Diversity (D) segments. Short coding sequences between the variable (V) and constant (C) gene segments in the Ig heavy chain and TCR β and γ loci that together with J segments are somatically recombined with V segments during lymphocyte development. The resulting recombined VDJ DNA codes for the carboxyl terminal ends of the antigen receptor V regions, including the third hypervariable (CDR) regions. Random use of D segments contributes to the diversity of the antigen receptor repertoire.

DNA vaccine. A vaccine composed of a bacterial plasmid containing a complementary DNA encoding a protein antigen. DNA vaccines presumably work because professional APCs are transfected *in vivo* by the plasmid and express immunogenic peptides that elicit specific responses. Furthermore, the plasmid DNA contains CpG nucleotides that act as potent adjuvants. DNA vaccines may elicit strong CTL responses.

Double-negative thymocyte. A subset of developing T cells (thymocytes) in the thymus that express neither CD4 nor CD8. Most double-negative thymocytes are at an early developmental stage and do not express antigen receptors. They will later express both CD4 and CD8 during the intermediate double-positive stage before further maturation to single-positive T cells expressing only CD4 or CD8.

Double-positive thymocyte. A subset of developing T cells (thymocytes) in the thymus at an intermediate developmental stage that express both CD4 and CD8. Double-positive thymocytes also express TCRs and are subject to selection processes, the survivors of which mature to single-positive T cells expressing only CD4 or CD8.

Ectoparasite. Parasites that live on the surface of an animal, such as ticks and mites. Both the innate and adaptive immune systems may play a role in protection against ectoparasites, often by destroying the larval stages of these organisms.

Effector cells. The cells that perform effector functions during an immune response, such as secreting cytokines (e.g., helper T cells), killing microbes (e.g., macrophages), killing microbe-infected host cells (e.g., CTLs), or secreting antibodies (e.g., differentiated B cells).

Effector phase. The phase of an immune response, after the recognition and activation phases, in which a foreign antigen is actually destroyed or inactivated. For example, in a humoral immune response, the effector phase may be characterized by antibody-dependent complement activation and phagocytosis of antibody- and complement-opsonized bacteria.

Endosome. An intracellular membrane-bound vesicle into which extracellular proteins are internalized during antigen processing. Endosomes have an acidic pH and contain proteolytic enzymes that degrade proteins into peptides that bind to class II MHC molecules. A subset of class II MHC–rich endosomes, called MIIC, play a special role in antigen processing and presentation by the class II pathway.

Endotoxin. A component of the cell wall of gram-negative bacteria, also called **lipopolysaccharide** (LPS), that is released from dying bacteria and stimulates many innate immune responses, including the secretion of cytokines, induction of microbicidal activities of macrophages, and expression of leukocyte adhesion molecules on endothelium. Endotoxin contains both lipid components and carbohydrate (polysaccharide) moieties.

Enhancer. A regulatory nucleotide sequence in a gene that is located either upstream or downstream of the promoter, binds transcription factors, and increases the activity of the promoter. In cells of the immune system, enhancers are responsible for integrating cell surface signals that lead to induced transcription of genes encoding many of the effector proteins of an immune response, such as cytokines.

Envelope glycoprotein (Env). A membrane glycoprotein encoded by a retrovirus that is expressed on the plasma membrane of infected cells and on the host cell–derived membrane coat of viral particles. Env proteins are often required for viral infectivity. The Env proteins of HIV include gp41 and gp120, which bind to CD4 and chemokine receptors, respectively, on human T cells and mediate fusion of the viral and T cell membranes.

Enzyme-linked immunosorbent assay (ELISA). A method of quantifying an antigen immobilized on a solid surface by use of a specific antibody with a covalently coupled enzyme. The amount of antibody that binds the antigen is proportional to the amount of antigen present and is determined by spectrophotometrically measuring the conversion of a clear substrate to a colored product by the coupled enzyme.

Eosinophil. A bone marrow–derived granulocyte that is abundant in the inflammatory infiltrates of immediate hypersensitivity late-phase reactions and that contributes to many of the pathologic processes in allergic diseases. Eosinophils are important in defense against extracellular parasites, including helminths.

Epitope. The specific portion of a macromolecular antigen to which an antibody binds. In the case of a protein antigen recognized by a T cell, an epitope is the peptide portion that binds to an MHC molecule for recognition by the TCR. Synonymous with **determinant**.

Epstein-Barr virus (EBV). A double-stranded DNA virus of the herpesvirus family that is the etiologic agent of infectious mononucleosis and is associated with some B cell malignant tumors and nasopharyngeal carcinoma. EBV infects B lymphocytes and some epithelial cells by specifically binding to CR2 (CD21).

Equilibrium dialysis. A method of determining the affinity of interaction between a macromolecule such as an antibody and a small ligand such as a hapten. A solution of the macromolecule, at a defined concentration, is confined within a semipermeable membrane and immersed in a solution containing the small ligand. The membrane does not permit the macromolecule to pass through, but the small ligand can pass across the membrane freely. The concentration of the small ligand in solution at equilibrium is used to calculate the affinity of binding to the macromolecule.

Experimental autoimmune encephalomyelitis. An animal model of autoimmune demyelinating disease of the central nervous system (e.g., multiple sclerosis) that is induced in rodents by immunization with components of the myelin sheath (e.g., myelin basic protein) of nerves, mixed with an adjuvant. The disease is mediated in large part by cytokine-secreting $CD4^+$ T cells specific for the myelin sheath proteins.

Extravasation. Escape of the fluid and cellular components of blood from a blood vessel into tissues.

Fab (fragment, antigen-binding). A proteolytic fragment of an IgG antibody molecule that includes one complete light chain paired with one heavy chain fragment containing the variable domain and only the first constant domain. Fab fragment retains the ability to monovalently bind an antigen but cannot interact with IgG Fc receptors on cells or with complement. Therefore, Fab preparations are used in research and therapeutic applications when antigen binding is desired without activation of effector functions. (Fab′ fragment retains the hinge region of the heavy chain.)

$F(ab')_2$ fragment. A proteolytic fragment of an IgG molecule that includes two complete light chains but only the variable domain, first constant domain, and hinge region of the two heavy chains. $F(ab')_2$ fragments retain the entire bivalent antigen-binding region of an intact IgG molecule but cannot bind complement or IgG Fc receptors. They are used in research and therapeutic applications when antigen binding is desired without antibody effector functions.

Fas (CD95). A member of the TNF receptor family that is expressed on the surface of T cells and many other cell types and initiates a signaling cascade leading to apoptotic death of the cell. The death pathway is initiated when Fas binds to Fas ligand expressed on activated T cells. Fas-mediated killing of T cells, called activation-induced cell death, is important for the maintenance of self-tolerance. Mutations in the Fas gene cause systemic autoimmune disease.

Fas ligand (CD95 ligand). A membrane protein that is a member of the TNF family of proteins expressed on activated T cells. Fas ligand binds to Fas, thereby stimulating a signaling pathway leading to apoptotic cell death of the Fas-expressing cell. Mutations in the Fas ligand gene cause systemic autoimmune disease in mice.

Fc (fragment, crystalline). A proteolytic fragment of IgG that contains only the disulfide-linked carboxyl terminal regions of the two heavy chains. Fc is also used to describe the corresponding region of an intact Ig molecule that mediates effector functions by binding to cell surface receptors or the C1q complement protein. (Fc fragments are so named because they tend to crystallize out of solution.)

Fc receptor. A cell surface receptor specific for the carboxyl terminal constant region of an Ig molecule. Fc receptors are typically multichain protein complexes that include signaling components and Ig-binding components. Several types of Fc receptors exist, including those specific for different IgG isotypes, IgE, and IgA. Fc receptors mediate many of the cell-dependent effector functions of antibodies, including phagocytosis of antibody-bound antigens, antigen-induced activation of mast cells, and targeting and activation of NK cells.

FcεRI. A high-affinity receptor for the carboxyl terminal constant region of IgE molecules that is expressed on mast cells and basophils. FcεRI molecules on mast cells are usually occupied by IgE, and antigen-induced cross-linking of these IgE-FcεRI complexes activates the mast cell and initiates immediate hypersensitivity reactions.

Fcγ receptor (FcγR). A specific cell surface receptor for the carboxyl terminal constant region of IgG molecules. There are several different types of Fcγ receptors, including a high-affinity FcγRI that mediates phagocytosis by macrophages and neutrophils, a low-affinity FcγRIIB that transduces inhibitory signals in B cells, and a low-affinity FcγRIIIA that mediates targeting and activation of NK cells.

First-set rejection. Allograft rejection in an individual who has not previously received a graft or otherwise been exposed to tissue alloantigens from the same donor. First-set rejection usually takes about 7 to 10 days.

FK-506. An immunosuppressive drug used to prevent allograft rejection that functions by blocking T cell cytokine gene transcription, similar to cyclosporine. FK-506 binds to a cytosolic protein called FK-506–binding protein, and the resulting complex binds to calcineurin, thereby inhibiting activation and nuclear translocation of the transcription factor NFAT.

Flow cytometry. A method of analysis of the phenotype of cell populations requiring a specialized instrument (flow cytometer) that can detect fluorescence on individual cells in a suspension and thereby determine the number of cells expressing the molecule to which a fluorescent probe binds. Suspensions of cells are incubated with fluorescently labeled antibodies or other probes, and the amount of probe bound by each cell in the population is measured by passing the cells one at a time through a fluorimeter with a laser-generated incident beam.

Fluorescence-activated cell sorter (FACS). An adaptation of the flow cytometer that is used for the purification of cells from a mixed population according to which and how much fluorescent probe the cells bind. Cells are first stained with fluorescently labeled probe, such as an antibody specific for a surface antigen of a cell population. The cells are then passed one at a time through a fluorimeter with a laser-generated incident beam and are differentially deflected by electromagnetic fields whose strength and direction are varied according to the measured intensity of the fluorescence signal.

Follicle. See **Lymphoid follicle.**

Follicular dendritic cells. Cells found in lymphoid follicles that express complement receptors, Fc receptors, and CD40 ligand and have long cytoplasmic processes that form a meshwork integral to the architecture of a lymphoid follicle. Follicular dendritic cells display antigens on their surface for B cell recognition and are involved in the activation and selection of B cells expressing high-affinity membrane Ig during the process of affinity maturation.

***N*-Formylmethionine.** An amino acid that initiates all bacterial proteins and no mammalian proteins (except those synthesized within mitochondria) and serves as a signal to the innate immune system of infection. Specific receptors for *N*-formylmethionine–containing peptides are expressed on neutrophils and mediate activation of the neutrophils.

G protein–coupled receptor family. A diverse family of receptors for hormones, lipid inflammatory mediators, and chemokines that use associated trimeric G proteins for intracellular signaling.

G proteins. Proteins that bind guanyl nucleotides and act as exchange molecules by catalyzing the replacement of bound guanosine diphosphate (GDP) by guanosine triphosphate (GTP). G proteins with bound GTP can activate a variety of cellular enzymes in different signaling cascades. Trimeric GTP-binding proteins are associated with the cytoplasmic portions of many cell surface receptors, such as chemokine receptors. Other small soluble G proteins, such as Ras and Rac, are recruited into signaling pathways by adapter proteins.

γδ T cell receptor (γδ TCR). A form of TCR that is distinct from the more common αβ TCR and is expressed on a subset of T cells found mostly in epithelial barrier tissues. Although structurally similar to the αβ TCR, the forms of antigen recognized by γδ TCRs are poorly understood; they do not recognize peptide complexes bound to polymorphic MHC molecules.

Generative lymphoid organ. Organs in which lymphocytes develop from immature precursors. The bone marrow and thymus are the major generative lymphoid organs in which B cells and T cells develop, respectively.

Germinal center. A lightly staining region within a lymphoid follicle in spleen, lymph node, or mucosal lymphoid tissue that forms during T cell–dependent humoral immune responses and is the site of B cell affinity maturation.

Germline organization. The inherited arrangement of variable, diversity, joining, and constant region gene segments of the antigen receptor loci in nonlymphoid cells or in immature lymphocytes. In developing B or T lymphocytes, the germline organization is modified by somatic recombination to form functional Ig or TCR genes.

Glomerulonephritis. Inflammation of the renal glomeruli, often initiated by immunopathologic mechanisms such as deposition of circulating antigen-antibody complexes in the glomerular basement membrane or binding of antibodies to antigens expressed in the glomerulus. The antibodies can activate complement and phagocytes, and the resulting inflammatory response can lead to renal failure.

Graft. A tissue or organ that is removed from one site and placed in another site, usually in a different individual.

Graft arteriosclerosis. Occlusion of graft arteries caused by proliferation of intimal smooth muscle cells. This process is evident within 6 months to a year after transplantation and is responsible for chronic rejection of vascularized organ grafts. The mechanism is likely to be a result of a chronic immune response to vessel wall alloantigens. Graft arteriosclerosis is also called accelerated arteriosclerosis.

Graft rejection. A specific immune response to an organ or tissue graft that leads to inflammation, damage, and possibly graft failure.

Graft-versus-host disease. A disease occurring in bone marrow transplant recipients that is caused by the reaction of mature T cells in the marrow graft with alloantigens on host cells. The disease most often affects the skin, liver, and intestines.

Granulocyte colony-stimulating factor (G-CSF). A cytokine made by activated T cells, macrophages, and endothelial cells at sites of infection that acts on bone marrow to increase the production of and mobilize neutrophils to replace those consumed in inflammatory reactions.

Granulocyte-monocyte colony-stimulating factor (GM-CSF). A cytokine made by activated T cells, macrophages, endothelial cells, and stromal fibroblasts that acts on bone marrow to increase the production of neutrophils and monocytes. GM-CSF is also a macrophage-activating factor and promotes the differentiation of Langerhans cells into mature dendritic cells.

Granuloma. A nodule of inflammatory tissue composed of clusters of activated macrophages and T lymphocytes, often with associated necrosis and fibrosis. Granulomatous inflammation is a form of chronic delayed-type hypersensitivity, often in response to persistent microbes, such as *Mycobacterium tuberculosis* and some fungi, or in response to particulate antigens that are not readily phagocytosed.

Granzyme. A serine protease enzyme found in the granules of CTLs and NK cells that is released by exocytosis, enters target cells mainly through perforin-created membrane "holes," and proteolytically cleaves and activates caspases, which in turn cleave several substrates and induce target cell apoptosis.

H-2 molecule. An MHC molecule in the mouse. The mouse MHC was originally called the H-2 locus.

Haplotype. The set of MHC alleles inherited from one parent and therefore on one chromosome.

Hapten. A small chemical that can bind to an antibody but must be attached to a macromolecule (carrier) to stimulate an adaptive immune response specific for that chemical. For example, immunization with dinitrophenol (DNP) alone will not stimulate an anti-DNP antibody response, but immunization with a protein with covalently bonded DNP hapten will.

Heavy chain class (isotype) switching. The process by which a B lymphocyte changes the class, or isotype, of the antibodies that it produces, from IgM to IgG, IgE, or IgA, without changing the antigen specificity of the antibody. Heavy chain class switching is regulated by helper T cell cytokines and CD40 ligand and involves recombination of B cell VDJ segments with downstream heavy chain gene segments.

Helminth. A parasitic worm. Helminthic infections often elicit T_H2-regulated immune responses characterized by eosinophil-rich inflammatory infiltrates and IgE production.

Helper T cells. The functional subset of T lymphocytes whose main effector functions are to activate macrophages in cell-mediated immune responses and to promote B cell antibody production in humoral immune responses. These effector functions are mediated by secreted cytokines and by T cell CD40 ligand binding to macrophage or B cell CD40. Most helper T cells express the CD4 molecule.

Hematopoiesis. The development of mature blood cells, including erythrocytes, leukocytes, and platelets, from pluripotent stem cells in the bone marrow and fetal liver. Hematopoiesis is regulated by several different cytokine growth factors produced by bone marrow stromal cells, T cells, and other cell types.

Hematopoietic stem cell. An undifferentiated bone marrow cell that divides continuously and gives rise to additional stem cells and cells of multiple different lineages. A hematopoietic stem cell in the bone marrow will give rise to cells of the lymphoid, myeloid, and erythrocytic lineage.

High endothelial venule (HEV). Specialized venules that are the sites of lymphocyte extravasation from the blood into the stroma of a peripheral lymph node or mucosal lymphoid tissue. HEVs are lined by plump endothelial cells that protrude into the vessel lumen and express unique adhesion molecules involved in binding naive T cells.

Highly active antiretroviral therapy (HAART). Combination chemotherapy for HIV infection consisting of reverse transcriptase inhibitors and a viral protease inhibitor. HAART can reduce plasma virus titers to below detectable levels for more than 1 year and slow the progression of HIV disease.

Hinge region. A region of Ig heavy chains between the first two constant domains that can assume multiple conformations, thereby imparting flexibility in the orientation of the two antigen-binding sites. Because of the hinge region, an antibody molecule can simultaneously bind two epitopes that are anywhere within a range of distances from one another.

Histamine. A biogenic amine stored in the granules of mast cells that is one of the important mediators of immediate hypersensitivity. Histamine binds to specific receptors in various tissues and causes increased vascular permeability and contraction of bronchial and intestinal smooth muscle.

HLA. See **Human leukocyte antigens.**

HLA-DM. A peptide exchange molecule that plays a critical role in the class II MHC pathway of antigen presentation. HLA-DM is found in the specialized MIIC endosomal compartment and facilitates removal of the invariant chain–derived CLIP peptide and the binding of other peptides to class II MHC molecules. HLA-DM is encoded by a gene in the MHC and is structurally similar to class II MHC molecules, but it is not polymorphic.

Homeostasis. In the adaptive immune system, the maintenance of a constant number and diverse repertoire of lymphocytes, despite the emergence of new lymphocytes and tremendous expansion of individual clones that may occur during responses to immunogenic antigens. Homeostasis is achieved by several regulated pathways of lymphocyte death and inactivation.

Homing receptor. Adhesion molecules expressed on the surface of lymphocytes that are responsible for the different pathways of lymphocyte recirculation and tissue homing. Homing receptors bind to ligands (addressins) expressed on endothelial cells in particular vascular beds.

Human immunodeficiency virus (HIV). The etiologic agent of AIDS. HIV is a retrovirus that infects a variety of cell types, including CD4-expressing helper T cells, macrophages, and dendritic cells, and causes chronic progressive destruction of the immune system.

Human leukocyte antigens (HLA). MHC molecules expressed on the surface of human cells. Human MHC molecules were first identified as alloantigens on the surface of white blood cells (leukocytes) that bound serum antibodies from individuals previously exposed to other individuals' cells (e.g., mothers or transfusion recipients).

Humanized antibody. A monoclonal antibody encoded by a recombinant hybrid gene and composed of the antigen-binding sites from a murine monoclonal antibody and the constant region of a human antibody. Humanized antibodies are less likely than mouse monoclonal antibodies to induce an anti-antibody response in humans; they are used clinically in the treatment of tumors and transplant rejection.

Humoral immunity. The type of adaptive immune response mediated by antibodies produced by B lymphocytes. Humoral immunity is the principal defense mechanism against extracellular microbes and their toxins.

Hybridoma. A cell line derived by cell fusion, or somatic cell hybridization, between a normal lymphocyte and an immortalized lymphocyte tumor line. B cell hybridomas created by fusion of normal B cells of defined antigen specificity with a myeloma cell line are used to produce monoclonal antibodies. T cell hybridomas created by fusion of a normal T cell of defined specificity with a T cell tumor line are commonly used in research.

Hyperacute rejection. A form of allograft or xenograft rejection that begins within minutes to hours after transplantation and that is characterized by thrombotic occlusion of the graft vessels. Hyperacute rejection is mediated by preexisting antibodies in the host circulation that bind to donor endothelial antigens, such as blood group antigens or MHC molecules, and activate the complement system.

Hypersensitivity diseases. Disorders caused by immune responses. Hypersensitivity diseases include autoimmune diseases, in which immune responses are directed against self antigens, and diseases that result from uncontrolled or excessive responses against foreign antigens, such as microbes and allergens. The tissue damage that occurs in hypersensitivity diseases is due to the same effector mechanisms used by the immune system to protect against microbes.

Hypervariable loop (hypervariable region). Short segments of about 10 amino acid residues within the variable regions of antibody or TCR proteins that form loop structures that contact antigen. Three hypervariable loops, also called CDRs, are present in each antibody heavy chain and light chain and in each TCR chain. Most of the variability between different antibodies or TCRs is located within these loops.

Idiotype. The property of a group of antibodies or TCRs defined by their sharing a particular idiotope; that is, antibodies that share a particular idiotope belong to the same idiotype. Idiotype is also used to describe the collection of idiotopes expressed by an Ig molecule, and it is often used synonymously with idiotope.

Idiotypic network. A network of complementary interactions involving idiotypes and anti-idiotypic antibodies (or T cells) that, according to the network hypothesis, reach a steady state at which the immune system is at homeostasis. Theoretically, when one or a few clones of lymphocytes respond to a foreign antigen, their idiotypes are expanded and anti-idiotype responses are triggered that function to shut off the antigen-specific response.

Igα and Igβ. Proteins that are required for surface expression and signaling functions of membrane Ig on B cells. Igα and Igβ pairs are disulfide linked to one another, noncovalently associated with the cytoplasmic tail of membrane Ig, and form the BCR complex. The cytoplasmic domains of Igα and Igβ contain ITAMs that are involved in early signaling events during antigen-induced B cell activation.

IL-1 receptor antagonist (IL-1ra). A natural inhibitor of IL-1 produced by mononuclear phagocytes that is structurally homologous to IL-1 and binds to the same receptors but is biologically inactive. Attempts to use IL-1 inhibitors to reduce inflammation in diseases such as rheumatoid arthritis are ongoing.

Immature B lymphocyte. A membrane IgM^+, IgD^- B cell, recently derived from marrow precursors, that does not proliferate or differentiate in response to antigens but rather may undergo apoptotic death or become functionally unresponsive. This property is important for the negative selection of B cells that are specific for self antigens present in the bone marrow.

Immediate hypersensitivity. The type of immune reaction responsible for allergic diseases and dependent on IgE plus antigen-mediated stimulation of tissue mast cells and basophils. The mast cells and basophils release mediators that cause increased vascular permeability, vasodilation, bronchial and visceral smooth muscle contraction, and local inflammation.

Immune complex. A multimolecular complex of antibody molecules with bound antigen. Because each antibody molecule has a minimum of two antigen-binding sites and many antigens are mutivalent, immune complexes can vary greatly in size. Immune complexes activate effector mechanisms of humoral immunity, such as the classical complement pathway and Fc receptor–mediated phagocyte activation. Deposition of circulating immune complexes in blood vessel walls or renal glomeruli can lead to inflammation and disease.

Immune complex disease. An inflammatory disease caused by the deposition of antigen-antibody complexes in blood vessel walls resulting in local complement activation and phagocyte recruitment. Immune complexes may form because of overproduction of antibodies to microbial antigens or as a result of autoantibody production in the setting of an autoimmune disease such as systemic lupus erythematosus. Immune complex deposition in the specialized capillary basement membranes of renal glomeruli can cause glomerulonephritis and impair renal function. Systemic deposition of immune complexes in arterial walls can cause thrombosis and ischemic damage to various organs.

Immune deviation. The conversion of a T cell response associated with one set of cytokines, such as T_H1 cytokines that stimulate cell-mediated immunity, to a response associated with other cytokines, such as T_H2 cytokines that stimulate the production of selected antibody isotypes.

Immune inflammation. Inflammation that is a result of an adaptive immune response to antigen. The cellular infiltrate at the inflammatory site may include cells of the innate immune system such as neutrophils and macrophages, which are recruited as a result of the actions of T cell cytokines.

Immune response. A collective and coordinated response to the introduction of foreign substances in an individual mediated by the cells and molecules of the immune system.

Immune response (Ir) genes. Originally defined as genes in inbred strains of rodents that were inherited in a dominant mendelian manner and that controlled the ability of the animals to make antibodies against simple synthetic polypeptides. We now know that Ir genes are polymorphic MHC genes that encode peptide-binding molecules required for the activation of T lymphocytes and are therefore also required for helper T cell–dependent B cell (antibody) responses to protein antigens.

Immune surveillance. The concept that a physiologic function of the immune system is to recognize and destroy clones of transformed cells before they grow into tumors and to kill tumors after they are formed. The term *immune surveillance* is sometimes used in a general sense to describe the function of T lymphocytes to detect and destroy any cell, not necessarily a tumor cell, that is expressing foreign (e.g., microbial) antigens.

Immune system. The molecules, cells, tissues, and organs that collectively function to provide immunity, or protection, against foreign organisms.

Immunity. Protection against disease, usually infectious disease, mediated by a collection of molecules, cells, and tissues collectively called the immune system. In a broader sense, immunity refers to the ability to respond to foreign substances, including microbes or molecules.

Immunoblot. An analytical technique in which antibodies are used to detect the presence of an antigen bound to (i.e., blotted on) a solid matrix such as filter paper (also known as a Western blot).

Immunodominant epitope. A linear amino acid sequence of a multideterminant protein antigen for which most of the responding T cells in any individual are specific. Immunodominant epitopes correspond to the peptides proteolytically generated within APCs that bind most avidly to MHC molecules and are most likely to stimulate T cells.

Immunofluorescence. A technique in which a molecule is detected by use of an antibody labeled with a fluorescent probe. For example, in immunofluorescence microscopy, cells that express a particular surface antigen can be stained with a fluorescein-conjugated antibody specific for the antigen and then visualized with a fluorescent microscope.

Immunogen. An antigen that induces an immune response. Not all antigens are immunogens. For example, small molecular weight compounds may not stimulate an immune response unless they are linked to macromolecules.

Immunoglobulin domain. A three-dimensional globular structural motif found in many proteins in the immune system, including Igs, TCRs, and MHC molecules. Ig domains are about 110 amino acid residues in length, include an internal disulfide bond, and contain two layers of β-pleated sheet, each layer composed of three to five strands of antiparallel polypeptide chain. Ig domains are classified as V-like or C-like on the basis of closest homology to either the Ig V or C domains.

Immunoglobulin superfamily. A large family of proteins that contain a globular structural motif called an Ig domain, or Ig fold, originally described in antibodies. Many proteins of importance in the immune system, including antibodies, TCRs, MHC molecules, CD4, and CD8, are members of this superfamily.

Immunoglobulin (Ig). Synonymous with antibody (see **Antibody**).

Immunoglobulin heavy chain. One of two types of polypeptide chains in an antibody molecule. The basic structural unit of an antibody includes two identical, disulfide-linked heavy chains and two identical light chains. Each heavy chain is composed of a variable (V) Ig domain and three or four constant (C) Ig domains. The different antibody isotypes, including IgM, IgD, IgG, IgA, and IgE, are distinguished by structural differences in their heavy chain constant regions. The heavy chain constant regions also mediate effector functions, such as complement activation or engagement of phagocytes.

Immunoglobulin light chain. One of two types of polypeptide chains in an antibody molecule. The basic structural unit of an antibody includes two identical light chains, each disulfide linked to one of two identical heavy chains. Each light chain is composed of one variable (V) Ig domain and one constant (C) Ig domain. There are two light chain isotypes, called κ and λ, both functionally identical. About 60% of human antibodies have κ light chains and 40% have λ light chains.

Immunohistochemistry. A technique to detect the presence of an antigen in histologic tissue sections by use of an enzyme-coupled antibody that is specific for the antigen. The enzyme converts a colorless substrate to a colored insoluble substance that precipitates at the site where the antibody and thus the antigen are localized. The position of the colored precipitate, and therefore the antigen, in the tissue section is observed by conventional light microscopy. Immunohistochemistry is a routine technique in diagnostic pathology and various fields of research.

Immunologic tolerance. See **Tolerance.**

Immunologically privileged site. A site in the body that is inaccessible to or constitutively suppresses immune responses. The anterior chamber of the eye, the testes, and the brain are examples of immunologically privileged sites.

Immunoperoxidase technique. A common immunohistochemical technique in which a horseradish peroxidase–coupled antibody is used to identify the presence of an antigen in a tissue section. The peroxidase enzyme converts a colorless substrate to an insoluble brown product that is observable by light microscopy.

Immunoprecipitation. A technique for the isolation of a molecule from a solution by binding it to an antibody and then rendering the antigen-antibody complex insoluble, either by precipitation with a second anti-antibody or by coupling the first antibody to an insoluble particle or bead.

Immunoreceptor tyrosine-based activation motif (ITAM). A conserved motif composed of two copies of the sequence tyrosine-X-X-leucine (where X is an unspecified amino acid) found in the cytoplasmic tails of various membrane proteins in the immune system that are involved in signal transduction. ITAMS are present in the ζ and CD3 proteins of the TCR complex, in Igα and Igβ proteins in the BCR complex, and in several Ig Fc receptors. When these receptors bind their ligands, the tyrosine residues of the ITAMs become phosphorylated and form docking sites for other molecules involved in propagating cell-activating signal transduction pathways.

Immunoreceptor tyrosine-based inhibition motif (ITIM). A six–amino acid (isoleucine-X-tyrosine-X-X-leucine) motif found in the cytoplasmic tails of various inhibitory receptors in the immune system, including FcγRIIB on B cells and killer cell Ig-like receptors (KIR) on NK cells. When these receptors bind their ligands, the ITIMs become phosphorylated on their tyrosine residue and form a docking site for protein tyrosine phosphatases, which in turn function to inhibit other signal transduction pathways.

Immunosuppression. Inhibition of one or more components of the adaptive or innate immune system as a result of an underlying disease or intentionally induced by drugs for the purpose of preventing or treating graft rejection or autoimmune disease. A commonly used immunosuppressive drug is cyclosporine, which blocks T cell cytokine production.

Immunotherapy. The treatment of a disease with therapeutic agents that promote or inhibit immune responses. Cancer immunotherapy, for example, involves promoting active immune responses to tumor antigens or administering anti-tumor antibodies or T cells to establish passive immunity.

Immunotoxins. Reagents that may be used in the treatment of cancer and consist of covalent conjugates of a potent cellular toxin, such as ricin or diphtheria toxin, with antibodies specific for antigens expressed on the surface of tumor cells. It is hoped that such reagents can specifically target and kill tumor cells without damaging normal cells, but safe and effective immunotoxins have yet to be developed.

Inbred mouse strain. A strain of mice created by repetitive mating of siblings that is characterized by homozygosity at every genetic locus. Every mouse of an inbred strain is genetically identical (syngeneic) to every other mouse of the same strain.

Indirect antigen presentation (or indirect allorecognition). In transplantation immunology, a pathway of presentation of donor (allogeneic) MHC molecules by recipient APCs that involves the same mechanisms used to present microbial proteins. The allogeneic MHC proteins are processed by recipient professional APCs, and peptides derived from the allogeneic MHC molecules are presented, in association with recipient (self) MHC molecules, to host T cells. In contrast to indirect antigen presentation, direct antigen presentation involves recipient T cell recognition of unprocessed allogeneic MHC molecules on the surface of graft cells.

Inflammation. A complex reaction of the innate immune system in vascularized tissues that involves the accumulation and activation of leukocytes and plasma proteins at a site of infection, toxin exposure, or cell injury. Inflammation is initiated by changes in blood vessels that promote leukocyte recruitment. Local adaptive immune responses can promote inflammation. Although inflammation serves a protective function in controlling infections and promoting tissue repair, it can also cause tissue damage and disease.

Inflammatory bowel disease (IBD). A group of disorders, including ulcerative colitis and Crohn's disease, characterized by chronic inflammation in the gastrointestinal tract. The etiology of IBD is not known, but some evidence indicates that immune mechanisms may be involved. IBD develops in gene knockout mice lacking IL-2, IL-10, or the TCR α chain.

Innate immunity. Protection against infection that relies on mechanisms that exist before infection, are capable of a rapid response to microbes, and react in essentially the same way to repeated infections. The innate immune system includes epithelial barriers, phagocytic cells (neutrophils, macrophages), NK cells, the complement system, and cytokines, largely made by mononuclear phagocytes, that regulate and coordinate many of the activities of the cells of innate immunity.

Inositol 1,4,5-triphosphate (IP_3). A cytoplasmic signaling molecule generated by phospholipase C (PLCγ1)–mediated hydrolysis of the plasma membrane phospholipid PIP_2 during antigen activation of lymphocytes. The main function of IP_3 is to stimulate the release of intracellular stores of calcium from membrane-bound compartments such as the endoplasmic reticulum.

Insulin-dependent diabetes mellitus. A disease characterized by a lack of insulin that leads to various metabolic and vascular abnormalities. The insulin deficiency results from autoimmune destruction of the insulin-producing β cells of the islets of Langerhans in the pancreas, usually during childhood. $CD4^+$ and $CD8^+$ T cells, antibodies, and cytokines have been implicated in the islet cell damage. Also called type 1 diabetes mellitus.

Integrins. Heterodimeric cell surface proteins whose major functions are to mediate the adhesion of leukocytes to other leukocytes, endothelial cells, and extracellular matrix proteins. Integrins are important for T cell interactions with APCs and for migration of leukocytes from blood into tissues. The ligand-binding affinity of the integrins can be regulated by various stimuli, and the cytoplasmic domains of integrins bind to the cytoskeleton. There are two main subfamilies of integrins; the members of each family express a conserved β chain (β_1, or CD29, and β_2, or CD18) associated with different α chains. VLA-4 (very late activation protein-4) is a β_1 integrin expressed on T cells, and LFA-1 (leukocyte function–associated antigen-1) is a β_2 integrin expressed on T cells and phagocytes.

Interferon-γ (IFN-γ). A cytokine produced by T lymphocytes and NK cells whose principal function is to activate macrophages in both innate immune responses and adaptive cell-mediated immune responses. (IFN-γ is also called immune or type II interferon.)

Interleukin (IL). Another name for a cytokine originally used to describe a cytokine made by leukocytes that acts on leukocytes. The term is now generally used with a numerical suffix to designate a structurally defined cytokine regardless of its source or target.

Interleukin-1 (IL-1). A cytokine produced mainly by activated mononuclear phagocytes whose principal function is to mediate host inflammatory responses in innate immunity. The two forms of IL-1 (α and β) bind to the same receptors and have identical biologic effects, including induction of endothelial cell adhesion molecules, stimulation of chemokine production by endothelial cells and macrophages, stimulation of the synthesis of acute-phase reactants by the liver, and fever.

Interleukin-2 (IL-2). A cytokine produced by antigen-activated T cells that acts in an autocrine manner to stimulate T cell proliferation and also potentiates the apoptotic cell death of antigen-activated T cells. Thus, IL-2 is required for both the induction and self-regulation of T cell–mediated immune responses. IL-2 also stimulates the proliferation and effector functions of NK cells and B cells.

Interleukin-3 (IL-3). A cytokine produced by $CD4^+$ T cells that promotes the expansion of immature marrow progenitors of all known mature blood cell types. IL-3 is also known as multilineage colony-stimulating factor.

Interleukin-4 (IL-4). A cytokine produced mainly by the T_H2 subset of $CD4^+$ helper T cells whose functions include induction of differentiation of T_H2 cells from naive $CD4^+$ precursors, stimulation of IgE production by B cells, and suppression of IFN-γ–dependent macrophage functions.

Interleukin-5 (IL-5). A cytokine produced by $CD4^+$ T_H2 cells and activated mast cells that stimulates the growth and differentiation of eosinophils and activates mature eosinophils.

Interleukin-6 (IL-6). A cytokine produced by many cell types, including activated mononuclear phagocytes, endothelial cells, and fibroblasts, that functions in both innate and adaptive immunity. IL-6 stimulates the synthesis of acute-phase proteins by hepatocytes as well as the growth of antibody-producing B lymphocytes.

Interleukin-7 (IL-7). A cytokine secreted by bone marrow stromal cells that stimulates survival and expansion of immature, but lineage-committed, precursors of B and T lymphocytes.

Interleukin-10 (IL-10). A cytokine produced by activated macrophages and some helper T cells whose major function is to inhibit activated macrophages and therefore to maintain homeostatic control of innate and cell-mediated immune reactions.

Interleukin-12 (IL-12). A cytokine produced by mononuclear phagocytes and dendritic cells that serves as a mediator of the innate immune response to intracellular microbes and is a key inducer of cell-mediated immune responses to these microbes. IL-12 activates NK cells, promotes IFN-γ production by NK cells and T cells, enhances the cytolytic activity of NK cells and CTLs, and promotes the development of T_H1 cells.

Interleukin-15 (IL-15). A cytokine produced by mononuclear phagocytes and other cells in response to viral infections whose principal function is to stimulate the proliferation of NK cells. It is structurally similar to IL-2.

Interleukin-18 (IL-18). A cytokine produced by macrophages in response to LPS and other microbial products that functions together with IL-12 as an inducer of cell-mediated immunity. IL-18 synergizes with IL-12 in stimulating the production of IFN-γ by NK cells and T cells. IL-18 is structurally homologous to but functionally different from IL-1.

Intracellular bacterium. A bacterium that survives or replicates within cells, usually in endosomes. The principal defense against intracellular bacteria, such as *Mycobacterium tuberculosis,* is cell-mediated immunity.

Intraepidermal lymphocytes. T lymphocytes found within the epidermal layer of the skin. In the mouse, most of the intraepidermal T cells express the γδ form of TCR (see **Intraepithelial T lymphocytes**).

Intraepithelial T lymphocytes. T lymphocytes present in the epidermis of the skin and in mucosal epithelia that typically express a limited diversity of antigen receptors. Some of these lymphocytes may recognize microbial products, such as glycolipids, associated with nonpolymorphic class I MHC–like molecules. Intraepithelial T lymphocytes may be considered effector cells of innate immunity and function in host defense by secreting cytokines and activating phagocytes and by killing infected cells.

Invariant chain (I_i). A nonpolymorphic protein that binds to newly synthesized class II MHC molecules in the endoplasmic reticulum. The invariant chain prevents loading of the class II MHC peptide-binding cleft with peptides present in the endoplasmic reticulum, and such peptides are left to associate with class I molecules. The invariant chain also promotes folding and assembly of class II molecules and directs newly formed class II molecules to the specialized endosomal MIIC compartment, where peptide loading takes place.

Isotype. One of five types of antibodies, determined by which of five different forms of heavy chain are present. Antibody isotypes include IgM, IgD, IgG, IgA, and IgE, and each isotype performs a different set of effector functions. Additional structural variations characterize distinct subtypes of IgG and IgA.

J chain. A small polypeptide that is disulfide bonded to the tail pieces of multimeric IgM and IgA antibodies.

JAK/STAT signaling pathway. A signaling pathway initiated by cytokine binding to type I and type II cytokine receptors. This pathway sequentially involves activation of receptor-associated Janus kinase (JAK) tyrosine kinases, JAK-mediated tyrosine phosphorylation of the cytoplasmic tails of cytokine receptors, docking of signal transducers and activators of transcription (STATs) to the phosphorylated receptor chains, JAK-mediated tyrosine phosphorylation of the associated STATs, dimerization and nuclear translocation of the STATs, and STAT binding to regulatory regions of target genes causing transcriptional activation of those genes.

Janus kinases (JAK kinases). A family of tyrosine kinases that associate with the cytoplasmic tails of several different cytokine receptors, including the receptors for IL-2, IL-4, IFN-γ, IL-12, and others. In response to cytokine binding and receptor dimerization, JAKs phosphorylate the cytokine receptors to permit the binding of STATs, and then the JAKs phosphorylate and thereby activate the STATs. Different JAK kinases associate with different cytokine receptors.

Joining (J) segments. Short coding sequences, between the variable (V) and constant (C) gene segments in all the Ig and TCR loci, that together with D segments are somatically recombined with V segments during lymphocyte development. The resulting recombined VDJ DNA codes for the carboxyl terminal ends of the antigen receptor V regions, including the third hypervariable (CDR) regions. Random use of different

J segments contributes to the diversity of the antigen receptor repertoire.

Junctional diversity. The diversity in antibody and TCR repertoires that is attributed to the random addition or removal of nucleotide sequences at junctions between V, D, and J gene segments.

Kaposi's sarcoma. A malignant tumor of vascular cells that frequently arises in patients with AIDS. Kaposi's sarcoma is associated with infection by the Kaposi's sarcoma–associated herpesvirus (human herpesvirus 8).

Killer Ig-like receptors (KIRs). Ig superfamily receptors expressed by NK cells that recognize different alleles of HLA-A, HLA-B, and HLA-C molecules. Some KIRs have signaling components with ITIMS in their cytoplasmic tails, and these deliver inhibitory signals to inactivate the NK cells. Some members of the KIR family have short cytoplasmic tails without ITIMs, and these function as activating receptors.

Knockout mouse. A mouse with a targeted disruption of one or more genes that is created by homologous recombination techniques. Knockout mice lacking functional genes encoding cytokines, cell surface receptors, signaling molecules, and transcription factors have provided extensive information about the roles of these molecules in the immune system.

Langerhans cells. Immature dendritic cells found as a continuous meshwork in the epidermal layer of the skin whose major function is to trap and transport protein antigens to draining lymph nodes. During their migration to the lymph nodes, Langerhans cells mature into lymph node dendritic cells, which can efficiently present antigen to naive T cells.

Large granular lymphocyte. Another name for an NK cell based on the morphologic appearance of this cell type in the blood.

Late-phase reaction. A component of the immediate hypersensitivity reaction that ensues 2 to 4 hours after mast cell and basophil degranulation and that is characterized by an inflammatory infiltrate of eosinophils, basophils, neutrophils, and lymphocytes. Repeated bouts of this late-phase inflammatory reaction can cause tissue damage.

Lck. An Src family nonreceptor tyrosine kinase that noncovalently associates with the cytoplasmic tails of CD4 and CD8 molecules in T cells and is involved in the early signaling events of antigen-induced T cell activation. Lck mediates tyrosine phosphorylation of the cytoplasmic tails of CD3 and ζ proteins of the TCR complex.

Lectin pathway of complement activation. A pathway of complement activation triggered, in the absence of antibody, by the binding of microbial polysaccharides to circulating lectins such as MBL. MBL is structurally similar to C1q and activates the C1r–C1s enzyme complex (like C1q) or activates another serine esterase, called mannose-binding protein–associated serine esterase. The remaining steps of the lectin pathway, beginning with cleavage of C4, are the same as the classical pathway.

Leishmania. An obligate intracellular protozoan parasite that infects macrophages and can cause a chronic inflammatory disease involving many tissues. *Leishmania* infection in mice has served as a model system for study of the effector functions of several cytokines and the helper T cell subsets that produce them. T_H1 responses to *Leishmania major* and associated IFN-γ production control infection, whereas T_H2 responses with IL-4 production lead to disseminated lethal disease.

Lethal hit. A term used to describe the events that result in irreversible damage to a target cell when a CTL binds to it. The lethal hit includes CTL granule exocytosis, perforin polymerization in the target cell membrane, and entry of calcium ions and apoptosis-inducing enzymes (granzymes) into the target cell cytoplasm.

Leukemia. A malignant disease of bone marrow precursors of blood cells in which large numbers of leukemic cells usually occupy the bone marrow and often circulate in the blood stream. Lymphocytic leukemias are derived from B or T cell precursors, myelogenous leukemias are derived from granulocyte or monocyte precursors, and erythroid leukemias are derived from red blood cell precursors.

Leukocyte adhesion deficiency (LAD). One of a rare group of immunodeficiency diseases with infectious complications that is caused by defective expression of the leukocyte adhesion molecules required for tissue recruitment of phagocytes and lymphocytes. LAD-1 is due to mutations in the gene encoding the CD18 protein, which is part of β_2 integrins. LAD-2 is caused by mutations in a gene that encodes a fucose transporter involved in the synthesis of leukocyte ligands for endothelial selectins.

Leukotrienes. A class of arachidonic acid–derived lipid inflammatory mediators produced by the lipoxygenase pathway in many cell types. Mast cells make abundant leukotriene C_4 (LTC_4) and its degradation products LTD_4 and LTE_4, which bind to specific receptors on smooth muscle cells and cause prolonged bronchoconstriction. Leukotrienes contribute to the pathologic processes of bronchial asthma. Collectively, LTC_4, LTD_4, and LTE_4 constitute what was once called slow-reacting substance of anaphylaxis.

Lipopolysaccharide. Synonymous with **endotoxin**.

Live viral vaccine. A vaccine composed of a live but nonpathogenic (attenuated) form of a virus. Attenuated viruses carry mutations that interfere with the viral life cycle or pathogenesis. Because live virus vaccines actually infect the recipient cells, they can effectively stimulate immune responses, such as the CTL response, that are optimal for protecting against wild-type viral infection. A commonly used live virus vaccine is the Sabin poliovirus vaccine, and there is much interest in development of an attenuated live virus vaccine to protect against HIV infection.

LMP-2 and LMP-7. Two catalytic subunits of the proteasome, the organelle that degrades cytosolic proteins into peptides in the class I MHC pathway of antigen presentation. LMP-2 and LMP-7 are encoded by genes in the MHC, are up-regulated by IFN-γ, and are particularly important for generating class I MHC–binding peptides.

Lymph node. Small nodular, encapsulated aggregates of lymphocyte-rich tissue situated along lymphatic channels throughout the body where adaptive immune responses to lymph-borne antigens are initiated.

Lymphatic system. A system of vessels throughout the body that collects tissue fluid called lymph, originally derived from the blood, and returns it, through the thoracic duct, to the circulation. Lymph nodes are interspersed along these vessels and trap and retain antigens present in the lymph.

Lymphocyte homing. The directed migration of subsets of circulating lymphocytes into particular tissue sites. Lymphocyte homing is regulated by the selective expression of adhesion molecules, called homing receptors, on the lymphocytes and the tissue-specific expression of endothelial ligands for these homing receptors, called addressins, in different vascular beds. For example, some T lymphocytes preferentially home to intestinal lymphoid tissue (e.g., Peyer's patches), and this directed migration is regulated by binding of the VLA-4 integrin on the T cells to the MadCAM addressin on Peyer's patch endothelium.

Lymphocyte maturation. The process by which pluripotent bone marrow precursor cells develop into mature, antigen receptor–expressing naive B or T lymphocytes that populate peripheral lymphoid tissues. This process takes place in the specialized environments of the bone marrow (for B cells) and the thymus (for T cells).

Lymphocyte migration. The movement of lymphocytes from the blood stream into peripheral tissues.

Lymphocyte recirculation. The continuous movement of lymphocytes through the blood stream and lymphatics, between the lymph nodes or spleen, and, if activated, to peripheral inflammatory sites.

Lymphocyte repertoire. The complete collection of antigen receptors and therefore antigen specificities expressed by the B and T lymphocytes of an individual.

Lymphoid follicle. A B cell–rich region of a lymph node or the spleen that is the site of antigen-induced B cell proliferation and differentiation. In T cell–dependent B cell responses to protein antigens, a germinal center forms within the follicles.

Lymphokine. An old name for a cytokine (soluble protein mediator of immune responses) produced by lymphocytes.

Lymphokine-activated killer (LAK) cell. NK cells with enhanced cytolytic activity for tumor cells as a result of exposure to high doses of IL-2. LAK cells generated *in vitro* have been adoptively transferred back into patients with cancer to treat their tumors.

Lymphoma. A malignant tumor of B or T lymphocytes usually arising in and spreading between lymphoid tissues but that may spread to other tissues. Lymphomas often express phenotypic characteristics of the normal lymphocytes from which they were derived.

Lymphotoxin (LT, TNF-β). A cytokine produced by T cells that is homologous to and binds to the same receptors as TNF. Like TNF, LT has proinflammatory effects, including endothelial and neutrophil activation. LT is also critical for the normal development of lymphoid organs.

Lysosome. A membrane-bound, acidic organelle abundant in phagocytic cells that contains proteolytic enzymes that degrade proteins derived both from the extracellular environment and from within the cell. Lysosomes are involved in the class II MHC pathway of antigen processing.

M cells. Specialized epithelial cells overlying Peyer's patches in the gut that play a role in delivering antigens to Peyer's patches.

Macrophage. A tissue-based phagocytic cell derived from blood monocytes that plays important roles in innate and adaptive immune responses. Macrophages are activated by microbial products such as endotoxin and by T cell cytokines such as IFN-γ. Activated macrophages phagocytose and kill microorganisms, secrete proinflammatory cytokines, and present antigens to helper T cells. Macrophages may assume different morphologic forms in different tissues, including the microglia of the central nervous system, Kupffer cells in the liver, alveolar macrophages in the lung, and osteoclasts in bone.

Major histocompatibility complex (MHC). A large genetic locus (on human chromosome 6 and mouse chromosome 17) that includes the highly polymorphic genes encoding the peptide-binding molecules recognized by T lymphocytes. The MHC locus also includes genes encoding cytokines, molecules involved in antigen processing, and complement proteins.

Major histocompatibility complex (MHC) molecule. A heterodimeric membrane protein encoded in the MHC locus that serves as a peptide display molecule for recognition by T lymphocytes. Two structurally distinct types of MHC molecules exist. Class I MHC molecules are present on most nucleated cells, bind peptides derived from cytosolic proteins, and are recognized by $CD8^+$ T cells. Class II MHC molecules are restricted largely to professional APCs, bind peptides derived from endocytosed proteins, and are recognized by $CD4^+$ T cells.

Mannose receptor. A carbohydrate-binding receptor (lectin) expressed by macrophages that binds mannose and fucose residues on microbial cell walls and mediates phagocytosis of the organisms.

Mannose-binding lectin (MBL). A plasma protein that binds to mannose residues on bacterial cell walls and acts as an opsonin by promoting phagocytosis of the bacterium by macrophages. Macrophages express a surface receptor for C1q that can also bind MBL and mediate uptake of the opsonized organisms.

Marginal zone. A peripheral region of splenic lymphoid follicles containing macrophages that are particularly efficient at trapping polysaccharide antigens. Such antigens may persist for prolonged periods on the surfaces of marginal zone macrophages, where they are recognized by specific B cells, or they may be transported into follicles.

Mast cell. The major effector cell of immediate hypersensitivity (allergic) reactions. Mast cells are derived from the marrow, reside in most tissues adjacent to blood vessels, express a high-affinity Fc receptor for IgE, and contain numerous mediator-filled granules. Antigen-induced cross-linking of IgE bound to the mast cell Fc receptors causes release of their granule contents as well as new synthesis and secretion of other mediators, leading to an immediate hypersensitivity reaction.

Mature B cell. IgM- and IgD-expressing, functionally competent naive B cells that represent the final stage of B cell maturation in the bone marrow and that populate peripheral lymphoid organs.

Membrane attack complex (MAC). A lytic complex of the terminal components of the complement cascade, including multiple copies of C9, that forms in the membranes of target cells. The MAC causes lethal ionic and osmotic changes in cells.

Memory. The property of the adaptive immune system to respond more rapidly, with greater magnitude, and more effectively to a repeated exposure to an antigen, compared with the response to the first exposure.

Memory lymphocytes. B or T lymphocytes that mediate rapid and enhanced (i.e., memory or recall) responses to second and subsequent exposures to antigens. Memory B and T cells are produced by antigen stimulation of naive lymphocytes and survive in a functionally quiescent state for many years after the antigen is eliminated.

MHC class II (MIIC) compartment. A subset of endosomes (membrane-bound vesicles involved in cell trafficking pathways) found in macrophages and human B cells that are important in the class II MHC pathway of antigen presentation. The MIIC contains all the components required for formation of peptide–class II MHC molecule complexes, including the enzymes that degrade protein antigens, class II molecules, invariant chain, and HLA-DM.

MHC restriction. The characteristic of T lymphocytes that they recognize a foreign peptide antigen only when it is bound to a particular allelic form of an MHC molecule.

MHC-tetramer. A reagent used to identify and enumerate T cells that specifically recognize a particular MHC-peptide complex. The reagent consists of four recombinant, biotinylated MHC molecules (usually class I) bound to a fluorochrome-labeled avidin molecule and loaded with a peptide. T cells that bind the MHC-tetramer can be detected by flow cytometry.

β_2-Microglobulin. The light chain of a class I MHC molecule. β_2-Microglobulin is an extracellular protein encoded by a nonpolymorphic gene outside the MHC, is structurally homologous to an Ig domain, and is invariant among all class I molecules.

Mitogen-activated protein (MAP) kinase cascade. A signal transduction cascade initiated by the active form of the Ras protein and involving the sequential activation of three serine/threonine kinases, the last one being MAP kinase. MAP kinase in turn phosphorylates and activates other enzymes or transcription factors. The MAP kinase pathway is one of several signal pathways activated by antigen binding to the TCR.

Mixed leukocyte reaction (MLR). An *in vitro* reaction of alloreactive T cells from one individual against MHC antigens on blood cells from another individual. The MLR involves proliferation of and cytokine secretion by both $CD4^+$ and $CD8^+$ T cells and is used as a screening test to assess the compatibility of a potential graft recipient with a potential donor.

Molecular mimicry. A postulated mechanism of autoimmunity triggered by infection with a microbe containing antigens that cross-react with self antigens. Immune responses to the microbe result in reactions against self tissues.

Monoclonal antibody. An antibody that is specific for one antigen and is produced by a B cell hybridoma (a cell line derived by the fusion of a single normal B cell and an immortal B cell tumor line). Monoclonal antibodies are widely used in research and clinical diagnosis and therapy.

Monocyte. A type of bone marrow–derived circulating blood cell that is the precursor of tissue macrophages. Monocytes are actively recruited into inflammatory sites, where they differentiate into macrophages.

Monocyte colony-stimulating factor (M-CSF). A cytokine made by activated T cells, macrophages, endothelial cells, and stromal fibroblasts that stimulates the production of monocytes from bone marrow precursor cells.

Monokine. An old name for a cytokine produced by mononuclear phagocytes.

Mononuclear phagocytes. Cells with a common bone marrow lineage whose primary function is phagocytosis. These cells function as accessory cells in the recognition and activation phases of adaptive immune responses and as effector cells in innate and adaptive immunity. Mononuclear phagocytes circulate in the blood in an incompletely differentiated form called monocytes, and once they settle in tissues, they mature into macrophages.

Mucosa-associated lymphoid tissue. Lymphocytes and accessory cells within the mucosa of the gastrointestinal and respiratory tracts that are sites of adaptive immune responses to environmental antigens. Mucosa-associated lymphoid tissues include intraepithelial lymphocytes, mainly T cells, and organized collections of lymphocytes, often rich in B cells, below mucosal epithelia, such as Peyer's patches in the gut or pharyngeal tonsils.

Mucosal immune system. A part of the immune system that responds to and protects against microbes that enter the body through mucosal surfaces, such as the gastrointestinal and respiratory tracts. The mucosal immune system is composed of mucosa-associated lymphoid tissues, which are collections of lymphocytes and accessory cells in the epithelia and lamina propria of mucosal surfaces.

Multiple myeloma. A malignant tumor of antibody-producing B cells that often secretes Igs or parts of Ig molecules. The monoclonal antibodies produced by multiple myelomas were critical for early biochemical analyses of antibody structure.

Mycobacterium. A genus of aerobic bacteria, many species of which can survive within phagocytes and cause disease. The principal host defense against mycobacteria such as *M. tuberculosis* is cell-mediated immunity.

N nucleotides. The name given to nucleotides randomly added to the junctions between V, D, and J gene segments in Ig or TCR genes during lymphocyte development. The addition of up to 20 of these nucleotides, which is mediated by the enzyme terminal deoxyribonucleotidyl transferase, contributes to the diversity of the antibody and TCR repertoires.

Naive lymphocyte. A mature B or T lymphocyte that has not previously encountered antigen, nor is it the progeny of an antigen-stimulated mature lymphocyte. When naive lymphocytes are stimulated by antigen, they differentiate into effector lymphocytes, such as antibody-secreting B cells or helper T cells and CTLs. Naive lymphocytes have surface markers and recirculation patterns that are distinct from those of previously activated lymphocytes. ("Naive" also refers to an unimmunized individual.)

Natural antibodies. IgM antibodies, largely produced by B-1 cells, specific for bacteria that are common in the environment and gastrointestinal tract. Normal individuals contain natural antibodies without any evidence of infection, and these antibodies serve as a preformed defense mechanism against microbes that succeed in penetrating epithelial barriers. Some of these antibodies cross-react with ABO blood group antigens and are responsible for transfusion reactions.

Natural killer (NK) cells. A subset of bone marrow–derived lymphocytes, distinct from B or T cells, that function in innate immune responses to kill microbe-infected cells by direct lytic mechanisms and by secreting IFN-γ. NK cells do not express clonally distributed antigen receptors like Ig receptors or TCRs, and their activation is regulated by a combination of cell surface stimulatory and inhibitory receptors, the latter recognizing self MHC molecules.

Negative selection. The process by which developing lymphocytes that express self-reactive antigen receptors are eliminated, thereby contributing to the maintenance of self-tolerance. Negative selection of developing T lymphocytes (thymocytes) is best understood and involves high-avidity binding of a thymocyte to self MHC molecules with bound peptides on thymic APCs leading to apoptotic death of the thymocyte.

Neonatal Fc receptor (FcRn). An IgG-specific Fc receptor that mediates the transport of maternal IgG across the placenta and the neonatal intestinal epithelium. FcRn resembles a class I MHC molecule. An adult form of this receptor functions to protect plasma IgG antibodies from catabolism.

Neonatal immunity. Passive humoral immunity to infections in mammals in the first months of life, before full development of the immune system. Neonatal immunity is mediated by maternally produced antibodies transported across the placenta into the fetal circulation before birth or derived from ingested milk and transported across the gut epithelium.

Neutrophil (also polymorphonuclear leukocyte, PMN). A phagocytic cell characterized by a segmented lobular nucleus and cytoplasmic granules filled with degradative enzymes. PMNs are the most abundant type of circulating white blood cells and are the major cell type mediating acute inflammatory responses to bacterial infections.

Nitric oxide. A biologic effector molecule with a broad range of activities that in macrophages functions as a potent microbicidal agent to kill ingested organisms.

Nitric oxide synthase. A member of a family of enzymes that synthesize the vasoactive and microbicidal compound nitric oxide from L-arginine. Macrophages express an inducible form of this enzyme on activation by various microbial or cytokine stimuli.

Nuclear factor κB (NF-κB). A family of transcription factors composed of homodimers or heterodimers of proteins homologous to the c-Rel protein. NF-κB proteins are important in the transcription of many genes in both innate and adaptive immune responses.

Nuclear factor of activated T cells (NFAT). A transcription factor required for the expression of IL-2, IL-4, TNF, and other cytokine genes. The four different NFATs are each encoded by separate genes; NFATp and NFATc are found in T cells. Cytoplasmic NFAT is activated by calcium/calmodulin-dependent, calcineurin-mediated dephosphorylation that permits NFAT to translocate into the nucleus and bind to consensus binding sequences in the regulatory regions of IL-2, IL-4, and other cytokine genes, usually in association with other transcription factors such as AP-1.

Nude mouse. A strain of mice that lacks development of the thymus, and therefore T lymphocytes, as well as hair follicles. Nude mice have been used experimentally to define the role of T lymphocytes in immunity and disease.

Oncofetal antigen. Proteins that are expressed at high levels on some types of cancer cells and in normal developing (fetal) but not adult tissues. Antibodies specific for these proteins are often used in histopathologic identification of tumors or to monitor the progression of tumor growth in patients. CEA (CD66) and alpha-fetoprotein are two oncofetal antigens commonly expressed by certain carcinomas.

Opsonin. A macromolecule that becomes attached to the surface of a microbe and can be recognized by surface receptors of neutrophils and macrophages and that increases the efficiency of phagocytosis of the microbe. Opsonins include IgG antibodies, which are recognized by the Fcγ receptor on phagocytes, and fragments of complement proteins, which are recognized by CR1 (CD35) and by the leukocyte integrin Mac-1.

Opsonization. The process of attaching opsonins, such as IgG or complement fragments, to microbial surfaces to target the microbes for phagocytosis.

Oral tolerance. The suppression of systemic humoral and cell-mediated immune responses to an antigen after the oral administration of that antigen as a result of anergy of antigen-specific T cells or the production of immunosuppressive cytokines such as transforming growth factor-β. Oral tolerance is a possible mechanism for preventing immune responses to food antigens and to bacteria that normally reside as commensals in the intestinal lumen.

P nucleotides. Short inverted repeat nucleotide sequences in the VDJ junctions of rearranged Ig and

TCR genes that are generated by RAG-1– and RAG-2–mediated asymmetric cleavage of hairpin DNA intermediates during somatic recombination events. P nucleotides contribute to the junctional diversity of antigen receptors.

Paracrine factor. A molecule that acts on cells in proximity to the cell that produces the factor. Most cytokines act in a paracrine fashion.

Partial agonist. A variant peptide ligand of a TCR that induces only a subset of the functional responses by the T cell or responses entirely different from responses to the unaltered (native) peptide. For instance, a partial agonist may stimulate production of only some of the many cytokines that are induced by the native peptide or quantitatively smaller responses. Partial agonist peptides are usually synthetic peptides in which one or two TCR contact residues have been changed; they are also called APLs.

Passive immunity. The form of immunity to an antigen that is established in one individual by transfer of antibodies or lymphocytes from another individual who is immune to that antigen. The recipient of such a transfer can become immune to the antigen without ever having been exposed to or having responded to the antigen. An example of passive immunity is the transfer of human sera containing antibodies specific for certain microbial toxins or snake venom to a previously unimmunized individual.

Pathogenicity. The ability of a microorganism to cause disease. Multiple mechanisms may contribute to pathogenicity, including production of toxins, stimulation of host inflammatory responses, and perturbation of host cell metabolism.

Pattern recognition receptors. Receptors of the innate immune system that recognize frequently encountered structures called molecular patterns produced by microorganisms and that facilitate innate immune responses against the microorganisms. Examples of pattern recognition receptors include CD14 receptors on macrophages, which bind bacterial endotoxin leading to macrophage activation, and the mannose receptor on phagocytes, which binds microbial glycoproteins or glycolipids.

Pentraxins. A family of plasma proteins that contain five identical globular subunits; includes the acute-phase reactant C-reactive protein.

Peptide-binding cleft. The portion of an MHC molecule that binds peptides for display to T cells. The cleft is composed of paired α-helices resting on a floor made up of an eight-stranded β-pleated sheet. The polymorphic residues, which are the amino acids that vary among different MHC alleles, are located in and around this cleft.

Perforin. A pore-forming protein, homologous to the C9 complement protein, that is present as a monomer in the granules of CTLs and NK cells. When perforin monomers are released from the granules of activated CTLs or NK cells, they undergo polymerization in the lipid bilayer of the target cell plasma membrane and form a large aqueous channel. This channel can cause osmotic lysis of the target cell and serve as a channel for the influx of enzymes derived from the CTL granules.

Periarteriolar lymphoid sheath (PALS). A cuff of lymphocytes surrounding small arterioles in the spleen, adjacent to lymphoid follicles. A PALS contains mainly T lymphocytes, about two thirds of which are $CD4^+$ and one third $CD8^+$. In humoral immune responses to protein antigens, B lymphocytes are activated at the interface between the PALS and follicles and then migrate into the follicles to form germinal centers.

Peripheral lymphoid organs and tissues. Organized collections of lymphocytes and accessory cells, including the spleen, lymph nodes, and mucosa-associated lymphoid tissues, in which adaptive immune responses are initiated.

Peripheral tolerance. Physiologic unresponsiveness to self antigens that are present in peripheral tissues and not usually in the generative lymphoid organs. Peripheral tolerance is induced by the recognition of antigens without adequate levels of the costimulators required for lymphocyte activation or by persistent and repeated stimulation by these self antigens.

Peyer's patches. Organized lymphoid tissue in the lamina propria of the small intestine in which immune responses to ingested antigens may be initiated. Peyer's patches are composed mostly of B cells, with smaller numbers of T cells and accessory cells, all arranged in follicles similar to those found in lymph nodes, often with germinal centers.

Phagocytosis. The process by which certain cells of the innate immune system, including macrophages and neutrophils, engulf large particles (>0.5 µm in diameter) such as intact microbes. The cell surrounds the particle with extensions of its plasma membrane by an energy- and cytoskeleton-dependent process; this process results in the formation of an intracellular vesicle called a phagosome, which contains the ingested particle.

Phagosome. A membrane-bound intracellular vesicle that contains microbes or particulate material from the extracellular environment. Phagosomes are formed during the process of phagocytosis, and fusion with other vesicular structures such as lysosomes leads to enzymatic degradation of the ingested material.

Phosphatase (protein phosphatase). An enzyme that removes phosphate groups from the side chains of certain amino acid residues of proteins. Protein phosphatases in lymphocytes, such as CD45 or calcineurin, regulate the activity of various signal transduction molecules and transcription factors. Some protein phosphatases may be specific for phosphotyrosine residues and others for phosphoserine and phosphothreonine residues.

Phospholipase Cγ (PLCγ). An enzyme that catalyzes hydrolysis of the plasma membrane phospholipid PIP_2 to generate two signaling molecules, IP_3 and DAG. PLCγ becomes activated in lymphocytes by antigen binding to the antigen receptor.

Phytohemagglutinin (PHA). A carbohydrate-binding protein, or lectin, produced by plants that cross-links human T cell surface molecules, including the T cell receptor, thereby inducing polyclonal activation and agglutination of T cells. PHA is frequently used in experimental immunology to study T cell activation. In clinical medicine, PHA is used to assess whether a patient's T cells are functional or to induce T cell mitosis for the purpose of generating karyotypic data.

Plasma cell. A terminally differentiated antibody-secreting B lymphocyte with a characteristic histologic appearance, including an oval shape, eccentric nucleus, and perinuclear halo.

Platelet-activating factor (PAF). A lipid mediator derived from membrane phospholipids in several cell types, including mast cells and endothelial cells. PAF can cause bronchoconstriction and vascular dilatation and leak and may be an important mediator in asthma.

Polyclonal activators. Agents that are capable of activating many clones of lymphocytes, regardless of their antigen specificities. Examples of polyclonal activators include anti-IgM antibodies for B cells and anti-CD3 antibodies, bacterial superantigens, and PHA for T cells.

Poly-Ig receptor. An Fc receptor expressed by mucosal epithelial cells that mediates the transport of IgA and IgM through the epithelial cells into the intestinal lumen.

Polymerase chain reaction (PCR). A rapid method of copying and amplifying specific DNA sequences up to about 1 kb in length that is widely used as a preparative and analytical technique in all branches of molecular biology. The method relies on the use of short oligonucleotide primers complementary to the sequences at the ends of the DNA to be amplified and involves repetitive cycles of melting, annealing, and synthesis of DNA.

Polymorphism. The existence of two or more alternative forms, or variants, of a gene that are present at stable frequencies in a population. Each common variant of a polymorphic gene is called an allele, and one individual may carry two different alleles of a gene, each inherited from a different parent. The MHC genes are the most polymorphic genes in the mammalian genome.

Polyvalency. The presence of multiple identical copies of an epitope on a single antigen molecule, cell surface, or particle. Polyvalent antigens, such as bacterial capsular polysaccharides, are often capable of activating B lymphocytes independent of helper T cells.

Positive selection. The process by which developing T cells in the thymus (thymocytes) whose TCRs bind to self MHC molecules are rescued from programmed cell death, whereas thymocytes whose receptors do not recognize self MHC molecules die by default. Positive selection ensures that mature T cells are self MHC restricted and that $CD8^+$ T cells are specific for complexes of peptides with class I MHC molecules and $CD4^+$ T cells for complexes of peptides with class II MHC molecules.

Pre-B cell. A developing B cell present only in hematopoietic tissues that is at a maturational stage characterized by expression of cytoplasmic Ig μ heavy chains and surrogate light chains but not Ig light chains. Pre-B cell receptors composed of μ chains and surrogate light chains deliver signals that stimulate further maturation of the pre-B cell into an immature B cell.

Pre-B cell receptor. A receptor expressed on maturing B lymphocytes at the pre-B cell stage that is composed of an Ig μ heavy chain and an invariant surrogate light chain. The surrogate light chain is composed of two proteins, including the λ5 protein, which is homologous to the λ light chain C domain, and the V pre-B protein, which is homologous to a V domain. The pre-B cell receptor associates with the Igα and Igβ signal transduction proteins to form the pre-B cell receptor complex. Pre-B cell receptors are required for stimulating the proliferation and continued maturation of the developing B cell. It is not known whether the pre-B cell receptor binds a specific ligand.

Pre-cytolytic T lymphocyte (pre-CTL). A mature, naive $CD8^+$ T lymphocyte that cannot perform effector functions but, on activation by antigen and costimulators, will differentiate into a CTL capable of lysing target cells and secreting cytokines.

Pre-T cell. A developing T lymphocyte in the thymus at a maturational stage characterized by expression of the TCR β chain, but not the α chain or CD4 or CD8. In pre-T cells, the TCR β chain is found on the cell surface as part of the pre-T cell receptor.

Pre-T cell receptor. A receptor expressed on the surface of pre-T cells that is composed of the TCR β chain and an invariant pre-Tα protein. This receptor associates with CD3 and ζ molecules to form the pre-T cell receptor complex. The function of this complex is similar to that of the pre-B cell receptor in B cell development, namely, the delivery of signals that stimulate further proliferation, antigen receptor gene rearrangements, and other maturational events. It is not known whether the pre-T cell receptor binds a specific ligand.

Pre-Tα. An invariant transmembrane protein with a single extracellular Ig-like domain that associates with TCR β chain in pre-T cells to form the pre-T cell receptor.

Primary immune response. An adaptive immune response that occurs after the first exposure of an individual to a foreign antigen. Primary responses are characterized by relatively slow kinetics and small magnitude compared with the responses after a second or subsequent exposure.

Primary immunodeficiency. A genetic defect in which an inherited deficiency in some aspect of the innate or adaptive immune system leads to an increased susceptibility to infections. Primary immunodeficiency is frequently manifested early in infancy and childhood but is sometimes clinically detected later in life.

Pro-B cell. A developing B cell in the bone marrow that is the earliest cell committed to the B lymphocyte lineage. Pro-B cells do not produce Ig, but they can be distinguished from other immature cells by the expression of B lineage–restricted surface molecules such as CD19 and CD10.

Professional antigen-presenting cells (professional APCs). APCs for naive helper T lymphocytes, used to refer to dendritic cells, mononuclear phagocytes, and B lymphocytes, all of which are capable of expressing class II MHC molecules and costimulators. The most important professional APCs for initiating primary T cell responses are dendritic cells.

Programmed cell death. A pathway of cell death by apoptosis that occurs in lymphocytes deprived of necessary survival stimuli, such as growth factors or co-stimulators. Programmed cell death, also called death by neglect or passive cell death, is characterized by the release of mitochondrial cytochrome *c* into the cytoplasm, activation of caspase-9, and initiation of the apoptotic pathway.

Promoter. A DNA sequence immediately 5′ to the transcription start site of a gene where the proteins that initiate transcription bind. The term *promoter* is often used to mean the entire 5′ regulatory region of a gene, including enhancers, which are additional sequences that bind transcription factors and interact with the basal transcription complex to increase the rate of transcriptional initiation. Other enhancers may be located at a significant distance from the promoter, either 5′ of the gene, in introns, or 3′ of the gene.

Prostaglandins. A class of lipid inflammatory mediators derived from arachidonic acid in many cell types through the cyclooxygenase pathway. Activated mast cells make prostaglandin D_2 (PGD_2), which binds to receptors on smooth muscle cells and acts as a vasodilator and a bronchoconstrictor. PGD_2 also promotes neutrophil chemotaxis and accumulation at inflammatory sites.

Pro-T cell. A developing T cell in the thymic cortex that is a recent arrival from the bone marrow and does not express TCRs, CD3, ζ chains, or CD4 or CD8 molecules. Pro-T cells are also called double-negative thymocytes.

Protease. An enzyme that cleaves peptide bonds and thereby breaks proteins down into peptides. Different kinds of proteases have different specificities for bonds between particular amino acid residues. Proteases inside phagocytes are important for killing ingested microbes during innate immune responses, and proteases released from phagocytes at inflammatory sites can cause tissue damage. Proteases in APCs are critical for generating peptide fragments of protein antigens that bind to MHC molecules during T cell–mediated immune responses.

Proteasome. A large multiprotein enzyme complex with a broad range of proteolytic activity that is found in the cytoplasm of most cells and generates from cytosolic proteins the peptides that bind to class I MHC molecules. Proteins are targeted for proteasomal degradation by covalent linkage of ubiquitin molecules.

Protein kinase C (PKC). Any of several isoforms of an enzyme that mediates the phosphorylation of serine and threonine residues in many different protein substrates and thereby serves to propagate various signal transduction pathways leading to transcription factor activation. In T and B lymphocytes, PKC is activated by DAG, which is generated in response to antigen receptor ligation.

Protein tyrosine kinases (PTKs). Enzymes that mediate the phosphorylation of tyrosine residues in proteins and thereby promote phosphotyrosine-dependent protein-protein interactions. PTKs are involved in numerous signal transduction pathways in cells of the immune system.

Protozoa. Single-celled eukaryotic organisms, many of which are human parasites and cause diseases. Examples of pathogenic protozoa include *Entamoeba histolytica,* which causes amebic dysentery; *Plasmodium,* which causes malaria; and *Leishmania,* which causes leishmaniasis. Protozoa stimulate both innate and adaptive immune responses. It has proved difficult to develop effective vaccines against many of these organisms.

Provirus. A DNA copy of the genome of a retrovirus that is integrated into the host cell genome and from which viral genes are transcribed and the viral genome is reproduced. HIV proviruses can remain inactive for long periods and thereby represent a latent form of HIV infection that is not accessible to immune defense.

Purified antigen (subunit) vaccine. A vaccine composed of purified antigens or subunits of microbes. Examples of this type of vaccine include diphtheria and tetanus toxoids, pneumococcus and *Haemophilus influenzae* polysaccharide vaccines, and purified polypeptide vaccines against hepatitis B and influenza virus. Purified antigen vaccines may stimulate antibody and helper T cell responses, but they do not generate CTL responses.

Pyogenic bacteria. Bacteria, such as the gram-positive staphylococci and streptococci, that induce inflammatory responses rich in polymorphonuclear leukocytes (giving rise to pus). Antibody responses to these bacteria greatly enhance the efficacy of innate immune effector mechanisms to clear infections.

Rac. A small guanine nucleotide–binding protein that is activated by the GDP-GTP exchange factor Vav during the early events of T cell activation. GTP•Rac triggers a three-step protein kinase cascade that culminates in activation of the stress-activated protein (SAP) kinase, c-Jun N-terminal kinase (JNK), and p38 kinase, which are similar to the MAP kinases.

Radioimmunoassay. A highly sensitive and specific immunologic method of quantifying the concentration of an antigen in a solution that relies on a radioactively labeled antibody specific for the antigen. Usually, two antibodies specific for the antigen are used. The first antibody is unlabeled but attached to a solid support, where it binds and immobilizes the antigen whose concentration is being determined. The amount of the second, labeled antibody that binds to the immobilized antigen, as determined by radioactive decay detectors, is proportional to the concentration of antigen in the test solution.

Ras. A member of a family of 21-kD guanine nucleotide–binding proteins with intrinsic GTPase activity that are involved in many different signal transduction pathways in diverse cell types. Mutated *ras* genes are associated with neoplastic transformation. In T cell activation, Ras is recruited to the plasma membrane by tyrosine-phosphorylated adapter proteins, where it is activated by GDP-GTP exchange factors.

GTP•Ras then initiates the MAP kinase cascade, which leads to expression of the *fos* gene and assembly of the AP-1 transcription factor.

Reactive oxygen intermediates (ROIs). Highly reactive metabolites of oxygen, including superoxide anion, hydroxyl radical, and hydrogen peroxide, that are produced by activated phagocytes. ROIs are used by the phagocytes to form oxyhalides that damage ingested bacteria. ROIs may also be released from cells and promote inflammatory responses or cause tissue damage.

Reagin. IgE antibody that mediates an immediate hypersensitivity reaction.

Receptor editing. A process by which some immature B cells that recognize self antigens in the bone marrow may be induced to change their Ig specificities. Receptor editing involves reactivation of the RAG genes, additional light chain VJ recombinations, and new Ig light chain production, which allows the cell to express a different Ig receptor that is not self-reactive.

Recombination-activating gene 1 and 2 (*RAG1* and *RAG2*). The genes encoding RAG-1 and RAG-2 proteins, which are the lymphocyte-specific components of V(D)J recombinase and are expressed in developing B and T cells. RAG proteins bind to recombination recognition sequences and are critical for DNA recombination events that form functional Ig and TCR genes. Therefore, RAG proteins are required for expression of antigen receptors and for the maturation of B and T lymphocytes.

Recombination signal sequences. Specific DNA sequences found adjacent to the V, D, and J segments in the antigen receptor loci and recognized by the RAG-1/RAG-2 component of V(D)J recombinase. The recognition sequences consist of a highly conserved stretch of 7 nucleotides, called the heptamer, located adjacent to the V, D, or J coding sequence, followed by a spacer of exactly 12 or 23 nonconserved nucleotides and a highly conserved stretch of 9 nucleotides, called the nonamer.

Red pulp. An anatomic and functional compartment of the spleen composed of vascular sinusoids, scattered among which are large numbers of erythrocytes, macrophages, dendritic cells, sparse lymphocytes, and plasma cells. Red pulp macrophages clear the blood of microbes, other foreign particles, and damaged red blood cells.

Regulatory T cells. A population of T cells that regulates the activation of other T cells and may be necessary to maintain peripheral tolerance to self antigens. Regulatory T cells are $CD4^+$ and express activation markers.

Respiratory burst. The process by which reactive oxygen intermediates such as superoxide anion, hydroxyl radical, and hydrogen peroxide are produced in macrophages and polymorphonuclear leukocytes. The respiratory burst is mediated by the enzyme phagocyte oxidase and is usually triggered by inflammatory mediators, such as LTB_4, PAF, and TNF, or by bacterial products, such as *N*-formylmethionyl peptides.

Reverse transcriptase. An enzyme encoded by retroviruses, such as HIV, that synthesizes a DNA copy of the viral genome from the RNA genomic template. Purified reverse transcriptase is used widely in molecular biology research for purposes of cloning complementary DNAs encoding a gene of interest from messenger RNA. Reverse transcriptase inhibitors are used as drugs to treat HIV-1 infection.

Reverse transcriptase–polymerase chain reaction (RT-PCR). An adaptation of the polymerase chain reaction (PCR) used to amplify a complementary DNA (cDNA) of a gene of interest. In this method, RNA is isolated from a cell expressing the gene, and cDNAs are synthesized by use of the reverse transcriptase enzyme. The cDNA of interest is then amplified by conventional PCR techniques with gene-specific primers.

Rh blood group antigens. A complex system of protein alloantigens expressed on red blood cell membranes that are the cause of transfusion reactions and hemolytic disease of the newborn. The most clinically important Rh antigen is designated D.

Rheumatoid arthritis. An autoimmune disease characterized primarily by inflammatory damage to joints and sometimes inflammation of blood vessels, lungs, and other tissues. $CD4^+$ T cells, activated B lymphocytes, and plasma cells are found in the inflamed joint lining (synovium), and numerous proinflammatory cytokines, including IL-1 and TNF, are present in the synovial (joint) fluid.

RNase protection assay. A sensitive method of detecting and quantifying messenger RNA (mRNA) copies of particular genes based on hybridization of the mRNA to radiolabeled RNA probes and digestion of unhybridized RNA with the enzyme RNase. The double-stranded RNA duplexes created during the hybridization reaction resist degradation by RNase and are of a particular size determined by the length of the probe. They can be separated by gel electrophoresis and are detected and quantitated by radioautography.

Scavenger receptors. A family of cell surface receptors expressed on macrophages, originally defined as receptors that mediate endocytosis of oxidized or acetylated low-density lipoprotein particles but that also bind and mediate the phagocytosis of a variety of microbes.

SCID mouse. A mouse strain in which B and T cells are absent because of an early block in maturation from bone marrow precursors. SCID mice carry a mutation in a component of the enzyme DNA-dependent protein kinase, which is required for double-stranded DNA break repair. Deficiency of this enzyme results in abnormal joining of Ig and TCR gene segments during recombination and therefore failure to express antigen receptors.

Secondary immune response. An adaptive immune response that occurs on second exposure to an antigen. A secondary response is characterized by more rapid kinetics and greater magnitude relative to the primary immune response, which occurs on first exposure.

Second-set rejection. Allograft rejection in an individual who has previously been sensitized to the donor's tissue alloantigens by having received another graft or transfusion from that donor. In contrast to first-set rejection, which occurs in an individual who has not previously been sensitized to the donor alloantigens, second-set rejection is rapid and occurs in 2 to 3 days as a result of immunologic memory.

Secretory component. The proteolytically cleaved portion of the extracellular domain of the poly-Ig receptor that remains bound to an IgA molecule in mucosal secretions.

Selectin. Any one of three separate but closely related carbohydrate-binding proteins that mediate adhesion of leukocytes to endothelial cells. Each of the selectin molecules is a single-chain transmembrane glycoprotein with a similar modular structure, including an extracellular calcium-dependent lectin domain. The selectins include L-selectin (CD62L), expressed on leukocytes; P-selectin (CD62P), expressed on platelets and activated endothelium; and E-selectin (CD62E), expressed on activated endothelium.

Selective immunoglobulin deficiency. Immunodeficiencies characterized by a lack of only one or a few Ig classes or subclasses. Selective IgA deficiency is the most common selective Ig deficiency, followed by IgG3 and IgG2 deficiencies. Patients with these disorders may be at increased risk for bacterial infections, but many are normal.

Self MHC restriction. The limitation (or restriction) of antigens that can be recognized by an individual's T cells to complexes of peptides bound to major histocompatibility complex (MHC) molecules that were present in the thymus during T cell maturation (i.e., self MHC molecules). The T cell repertoire is self MHC restricted as a result of the process of positive selection.

Self-tolerance. Unresponsiveness of the adaptive immune system to self antigens, largely as a result of inactivation or death of self-reactive lymphocytes induced by exposure to those self antigens. Self-tolerance is a cardinal feature of the normal immune system, and failure of self-tolerance leads to autoimmune diseases.

Septic shock. An often lethal complication of severe gram-negative bacterial infection with spread to the blood stream (sepsis) that is characterized by vascular collapse, disseminated intravascular coagulation, and metabolic disturbances. This syndrome is due to the effects of bacterial LPS and cytokines, including TNF, IL-12, and IL-1. Septic shock is also called endotoxin shock.

Seroconversion. The production of detectable antibodies in the serum specific for a microorganism during the course of an infection or in response to immunization.

Serology. The study of blood (serum) antibodies and their reactions with antigens. The term *serology* is often used to refer to the diagnosis of infectious diseases by detection of microbe-specific antibodies in the serum.

Serotype. An antigenically distinct subset of a species of an infectious organism that is distinguished from other subsets by serologic (i.e., serum antibody) tests. Humoral immune responses to one serotype of microbes (e.g., influenza virus) may not be protective against another serotype.

Serum. The cell-free fluid that remains when blood or plasma forms a clot. Blood antibodies are found in the serum fraction.

Serum amyloid A (SAA). An acute-phase protein whose serum concentration rises significantly in the setting of infection and inflammation, mainly because of IL-1– and TNF-induced synthesis by the liver. SAA activates leukocyte chemotaxis, phagocytosis, and adhesion to endothelial cells.

Serum sickness. A disease caused by the injection of large doses of a protein antigen into the blood and characterized by the deposition of antigen-antibody (immune) complexes in blood vessel walls, especially in the kidneys and joints. Immune complex deposition leads to complement fixation and leukocyte recruitment and subsequently to glomerulonephritis and arthritis. Serum sickness was originally described as a disorder that occurred in patients receiving injections of serum containing antitoxin antibodies to prevent diphtheria.

Severe combined immunodeficiency (SCID). Immunodeficiency diseases in which both B and T lymphocytes do not develop or do not function properly, and therefore both humoral and cell-mediated immunity are impaired. Children with SCID usually have infections during the first year of life and succumb to these infections unless the immunodeficiency is treated. SCID has several different genetic causes.

Shwartzman reaction. An experimental model of the pathologic effects of bacterial LPS and TNF in which two intravenous injections of LPS are administered to a rabbit 24 hours apart. After the second injection, the rabbit suffers disseminated intravascular coagulation and neutrophil and platelet plugging of small blood vessels.

Signal transducer and activator of transcription (STAT). A member of a family of proteins that function as signaling molecules and transcription factors in response to binding of cytokines to type I and type II cytokine receptors. STATs are present as inactive monomers in the cytoplasm of cells and are recruited to the cytoplasmic tails of cross-linked cytokine receptors, where they are tyrosine phosphorylated by JAKs. The phosphorylated STAT proteins dimerize and move to the nucleus, where they bind to specific sequences in the promoter regions of various genes and stimulate their transcription. Different STATs are activated by different cytokines.

Simian immunodeficiency virus. A lentivirus closely related to HIV-1 that causes disease similar to AIDS in monkeys.

Single-positive thymocyte. A maturing T cell precursor in the thymus that expresses CD4 or CD8 molecules but not both. Single-positive thymocytes are found mainly in the medulla and have matured from the double-positive stage, during which thymocytes express both CD4 and CD8 molecules.

Smallpox. A disease caused by variola virus. Smallpox was the first infectious disease shown to be preventable by vaccination and the first disease to be completely eradicated by a worldwide vaccination program.

Somatic hypermutation. High-frequency point mutations in Ig heavy and light chains that occur in germinal center B cells. Mutations that result in increased affinity of antibodies for antigen impart a selective survival advantage to the B cells producing those antibodies and lead to affinity maturation of a humoral immune response.

Somatic recombination. The process of DNA recombination by which the functional genes encoding the variable regions of antigen receptors are formed during lymphocyte development. A relatively limited set of inherited, or germline, DNA sequences that are initially separated from one another are brought together by enzymatic deletion of intervening sequences and religation. This process occurs only in developing B or T lymphocytes. This process is sometimes referred to as somatic rearrangement.

Southern blot. A technique used to determine the organization of genomic DNA around a particular gene. The DNA is cut into fragments by restriction endonucleases, different-sized fragments are electrophoretically separated in a gel, and the DNA is then immobilized (blotted) onto a sheet of nitrocellulose or nylon. The position and therefore the size of a particular DNA fragment can then be detected by use of a radioactively labeled DNA probe with a homologous sequence. (See Appendix III for a detailed description.)

Specificity. A cardinal feature of the adaptive immune system, namely, that immune responses are directed toward and able to distinguish between distinct antigens or small parts of macromolecular antigens. This fine specificity is attributed to lymphocyte antigen receptors that may bind to one molecule but not to another with only minor structural differences from the first.

Spleen. A secondary lymphoid organ in the left upper quadrant of the abdomen. The spleen is the major site of adaptive immune responses to blood-borne antigens. The red pulp of the spleen is composed of blood-filled vascular sinusoids lined by active phagocytes that ingest opsonized antigens and damaged red blood cells. The white pulp of the spleen contains lymphocytes and lymphoid follicles where B cells are activated.

Src homology 2 (SH2) domain. A three-dimensional domain structure of about 100 amino acid residues present in many signaling proteins that permits specific noncovalent interactions with other proteins by binding to phosphotyrosines. Each SH2 domain has a unique binding specificity that is determined by the amino acid residues adjacent to the phosphotyrosine on the target protein. Several proteins involved in early signaling events in T and B lymphocytes interact with one another through SH2 domains.

Src homology 3 (SH3) domain. A three-dimensional domain structure of about 60 amino acid residues present in many signaling proteins that mediates protein-protein binding. SH3 domains bind to proline residues and function cooperatively with the SH2 domains of the same protein. For instance, Sos, the guanine nucleotide exchange factor for Ras, contains both SH2 and SH3 domains, and both are involved in Sos binding to the adapter protein Grb-2.

Stem cell. An undifferentiated cell that divides continuously and gives rise to additional stem cells and to cells of multiple different lineages. For example, all blood cells arise from a common hematopoietic stem cell.

Superantigens. Proteins that bind to and activate all the T cells in an individual that express a particular set or family of V_β TCR genes. Superantigens are presented to T cells by binding to nonpolymorphic regions of class II MHC molecules on APCs, and they interact with conserved regions of TCR V_β domains. Several staphylococcal enterotoxins are superantigens. Their importance lies in their ability to activate many T cells, which results in large amounts of cytokine production and a clinical syndrome that is similar to septic shock.

Suppressor T cell. T cells that block the activation and function of other effector T lymphocytes. Suppressor function may be attributed to a still poorly defined population of T cells currently called **regulatory T cells.**

Surrogate light chain. A complex of two nonvariable proteins that associate with Ig μ heavy chains in pre-B cells to form the pre-B cell receptor. The two surrogate light chain proteins include V pre-B protein, which is homologous to a light chain V domain, and λ5, which is covalently attached to the μ heavy chain by a disulfide bond.

Switch recombination. The molecular mechanism underlying Ig isotype switching in which a rearranged VDJ gene segment in an antibody-producing B cell recombines with a downstream C gene and the intervening C gene is deleted. DNA recombination events in switch recombination are triggered by CD40 and cytokines and involve nucleotide sequences called switch regions located in the introns at the 5′ end of each C_H locus.

Syngeneic. Genetically identical. All animals of an inbred strain and monozygotic twins are syngeneic.

Syngeneic graft. A graft from a donor who is genetically identical to the recipient. Syngeneic grafts are not rejected.

Synthetic vaccine. Vaccines composed of recombinant DNA–derived antigens. Synthetic vaccines for hepatitis B virus and herpes simplex virus are now in use.

Systemic inflammatory response syndrome (SIRS). The systemic changes observed in patients who have disseminated bacterial infections. In its mild form, SIRS consists of neutrophilia, fever, and a rise in acute-phase reactants in the plasma. These changes are stimulated by bacterial products such as LPS and are mediated by cytokines of the innate immune system. In severe cases, SIRS may include disseminated intravascular coagulation, adult respiratory distress syndrome, and septic shock.

Systemic lupus erythematosus (SLE). A chronic systemic autoimmune disease that affects predominantly women and is characterized by rashes, arthritis, glomerulonephritis, hemolytic anemia, thrombocytopenia, and central nervous system involvement. Many different autoantibodies are found in patients with SLE, particularly anti-DNA antibodies. Many of the manifestations of SLE are due to the formation of immune complexes composed of autoantibodies and their specific antigens, with deposition of these complexes in small blood vessels in various tissues. The underlying mechanism for the breakdown of self-tolerance in SLE is not understood.

T cell receptor (TCR). The clonally distributed antigen receptor on $CD4^+$ and $CD8^+$ T lymphocytes that recognizes complexes of foreign peptides bound to self MHC molecules on the surface of APCs. The most common form of TCR is composed of a heterodimer of two disulfide-linked transmembrane polypeptide chains, designated α and β, each containing one N-terminal Ig-like variable (V) domain, one Ig-like constant (C) domain, a hydrophobic transmembrane region, and a short cytoplasmic region. (Another less common type of TCR, composed of γ and δ chains, is found on a small subset of T cells and recognizes different forms of antigen.)

T cell receptor complex. A multiprotein plasma membrane complex on T lymphocytes that is composed of the highly variable, antigen-binding TCR heterodimer and the invariant signaling proteins CD3 δ, ε, and γ and the ζ chain.

T lymphocyte. The cell type that mediates cell-mediated immune responses in the adaptive immune system. T lymphocytes mature in the thymus, circulate in the blood, populate secondary lymphoid tissues, and are recruited to peripheral sites of antigen exposure. They express antigen receptors (TCRs) that recognize peptide fragments of foreign proteins bound to self MHC molecules. Functional subsets of T lymphocytes include $CD4^+$ helper T cells and $CD8^+$ CTLs.

T-dependent antigen. An antigen that requires both B cells and helper T cells to stimulate an antibody response. T-dependent antigens are protein antigens that contain some epitopes recognized by T cells and other epitopes recognized by B cells. Helper T cells produce cytokines and cell surface molecules that stimulate B cell growth and differentiation into antibody-secreting cells. Humoral immune responses to T-dependent antigens are characterized by isotype switching, affinity maturation, and memory.

T_H1 cells. A functional subset of helper T cells that secrete a particular set of cytokines, including IFN-γ, and whose principal function is to stimulate phagocyte-mediated defense against infections, especially with intracellular microbes.

T_H2 cells. A functional subset of helper T cells that secrete a particular set of cytokines, including IL-4 and IL-5, and whose principal functions are to stimulate IgE and eosinophil/mast cell–mediated immune reactions and to down-regulate T_H1 responses.

Thymic epithelial cells. Epithelial cells abundant in the cortical and medullary stroma of the thymus that play a critical role in T cell development. Thymic epithelial cells secrete factors, such as IL-7, that are required for the early stages of T cell development. In the process of positive selection, maturing T cells must recognize self peptides bound to MHC molecules on the surface of thymic epithelial cells to be rescued from programmed cell death.

Thymocyte. A precursor of a mature T lymphocyte present in the thymus.

Thymus. A bilobed organ situated in the anterior mediastinum that is the site of maturation of T lymphocytes from bone marrow–derived precursors. Thymic tissue is divided into an outer cortex and an inner medulla and contains stromal thymic epithelial cells, macrophages, dendritic cells, and numerous T cell precursors (thymocytes) at various stages of maturation.

T-independent antigen. Nonprotein antigens, such as polysaccharides and lipids, that can stimulate antibody responses without a requirement for antigen-specific helper T lymphocytes. T-independent antigens usually contain multiple identical epitopes that can cross-link membrane Ig on B cells and thereby activate the cells. Humoral immune responses to T-independent antigens show relatively little heavy chain isotype switching or affinity maturation, two processes that require signals from helper T cells.

Tissue typing. The determination of the particular MHC alleles expressed by an individual for the purpose of matching allograft donors and recipients. Tissue typing, also called HLA typing, is usually done by testing whether sera known to be reactive with certain MHC gene products mediate complement-dependent lysis of an individual's lymphocytes. PCR techniques are now also used to determine whether an individual carries a particular MHC allele.

TNF receptor–associated factors (TRAFs). A family of adapter molecules that interact with the cytoplasmic domains of various receptors in the TNF receptor family, including TNF-RII, lymphotoxin (LT)–β receptor, and CD40. Each of these receptors contains a cytoplasmic motif that binds different TRAFs, which in turn engage other signaling molecules leading to activation of the transcription factors AP-1 and NF-κB. A transforming gene product of Epstein-Barr virus encodes a protein with a domain that binds TRAFs, and therefore infection by the virus mimics TNF- or CD40-induced signals.

Tolerance. Unresponsiveness of the adaptive immune system to antigens, as a result of inactivation or death of antigen-specific lymphocytes, induced by exposure to the antigens. Tolerance to self antigens is a normal feature of the adaptive immune system, but tolerance to foreign antigens may be induced under certain conditions of antigen exposure.

Tolerogen. An antigen that induces immunologic tolerance, in contrast to an immunogen, which induces an immune response. Many antigens can be either tolerogens or immunogens, depending on how they are administered. Tolerogenic forms of antigens include large doses of the proteins administered without adjuvants, APLs, and orally administered antigens.

Toll-like receptors. Cell surface molecules on phagocytes and other cell types that are involved in recognition of microbial structures, such as endotoxin, and the generation of signals that lead to the activation of innate immune responses. Toll-like receptors share structural homology and signal transduction pathways with the type I IL-1 receptor.

Toxic shock syndrome. An acute illness characterized by shock, skin exfoliation, conjunctivitis, and diarrhea that is associated with tampon use and caused by a *Staphylococcus aureus* superantigen.

Transforming growth factor-β (TGF-β). A cytokine produced by activated T cells, mononuclear phagocytes, and other cells whose principal actions are to inhibit the proliferation and differentiation of T cells, to inhibit the activation of macrophages, and to counteract the effects of proinflammatory cytokines.

Transfusion. Transplantation of circulating blood cells, platelets, or plasma from one individual to another. Transfusions are performed to treat blood loss from hemorrhage or to treat a deficiency in one or more blood cell types resulting from inadequate production or excess destruction.

Transfusion reactions. An immunologic reaction against transfused blood products, usually mediated by preformed antibodies in the recipient that bind to donor blood cell antigens, such as ABO blood group antigens or histocompatibility antigens. Transfusion reactions can lead to intravascular lysis of red blood cells and, in severe cases, kidney damage, fever, shock, and disseminated intravascular coagulation.

Transgenic mouse. A mouse that expresses an exogenous gene that has been introduced into the genome by injection of a specific DNA sequence into the pronuclei of fertilized mouse eggs. Transgenes insert randomly at chromosomal break points and are subsequently inherited as simple mendelian traits. By the design of transgenes with tissue-specific regulatory sequences, mice can be produced that express a particular gene only in certain tissues. Transgenic mice are used extensively in immunology research to study the functions of various cytokines, cell surface molecules, and intracellular signaling molecules.

Transplantation. The process of transferring cells, tissues, or organs (i.e., grafts) from one individual to another or from one site to another in the same individual. Transplantation is used to treat a variety of diseases in which there is a functional disorder of a tissue or organ. The major barrier to successful transplantation between individuals is immunologic reaction (rejection) to the transplanted graft.

Transporter associated with antigen processing (TAP). An adenosine triphosphate (ATP)–dependent peptide transporter that mediates the active transport of peptides from the cytosol to the site of assembly of class I MHC molecules inside the endoplasmic reticulum. TAP is a heterodimeric molecule composed of TAP-1 and TAP-2 polypeptides, both encoded by genes in the MHC. Because peptides are required for stable assembly of class I MHC molecules, TAP-deficient animals express few cell surface class I MHC molecules, which results in diminished development and activation of $CD8^+$ T cells.

Tumor immunity. Protection against the development of tumors by the immune system. Although immune responses to naturally occurring tumors can frequently be demonstrated, true immunity may occur only in the case of a subset of these tumors that express immunogenic antigens (e.g., tumors that are caused by oncogenic viruses and therefore express viral antigens). Research efforts are under way to enhance weak immune responses to other tumors by a variety of approaches.

Tumor-infiltrating lymphocytes (TILs). Lymphocytes isolated from the inflammatory infiltrates present in and around surgical resection samples of solid tumors that are enriched with tumor-specific CTLs and NK cells. In an experimental mode of cancer treatment, TILs are grown *in vitro* in the presence of high doses of IL-2 and are then adoptively transferred back into patients with the tumor.

Tumor necrosis factor (TNF). A cytokine produced mainly by activated mononuclear phagocytes that functions to stimulate the recruitment of neutrophils and monocytes to sites of infection and to activate these cells to eradicate microbes. TNF stimulates vascular endothelial cells to express new adhesion molecules, induces macrophages and endothelial cells to secrete chemokines, and promotes apoptosis of target cells. In severe infections, TNF is produced in large amounts and has systemic effects, including induction of fever, synthesis of acute-phase proteins by the liver, and cachexia. The production of large amounts of TNF can cause intravascular thrombosis and shock. (TNF-β, or lymphotoxin, is a closely related cytokine with biologic effects identical to those of TNF-α but is produced by T cells.)

Tumor necrosis factor (TNF) receptors. Cell surface receptors for TNF-α and TNF-β (LT), present on most cell types. There are two distinct TNF receptors, TNF-RI and TNF-RII, but most biologic effects of TNF are mediated by TNF-RI. TNF receptors are members of a family of homologous receptors with cysteine-rich extracellular motifs that include Fas and CD40.

Tumor-specific antigen. An antigen whose expression is restricted to a particular tumor and is not expressed by normal cells. Tumor-specific antigens may serve as target antigens for antitumor immune responses.

Tumor-specific transplantation antigen (TSTA). An antigen expressed on experimental animal tumor cells that can be detected by induction of immunologic rejection of tumor transplants. TSTAs were originally defined on chemically induced rodent sarcomas and shown to stimulate CTL-mediated rejection of transplanted tumors.

Two-signal hypothesis. A now proven hypothesis that states that the activation of lymphocytes requires two distinct signals, the first being antigen and the second either microbial products or components of innate immune responses to microbes. The requirement for antigen (so-called signal 1) ensures that the ensuing immune response is specific. The requirement for additional stimuli triggered by microbes or innate immune reactions (signal 2) ensures that immune responses are induced when they are needed, that is, against microbes and other noxious substances and not against harmless substances, including self antigens. Signal 2 is referred to as costimulation and is often mediated by membrane molecules on professional APCs, such as B7 proteins.

Type I cytokine receptors. A family of cytokine receptors, also called hemopoietin receptors, that contain conserved structural motifs in their extracellular domains and bind cytokines that fold into four α-helical strands, including growth hormone, IL-2, IL-3, IL-4, IL-5, IL-6, IL-7, IL-9, IL-11, IL-13, IL-15, GM-CSF, and G-CSF. Some of these receptors consist of a ligand-binding chain and one or more signal-transducing chains, and all of these chains have the same structural motifs. Type I cytokine receptors are dimerized on binding their cytokine ligands, and they signal through JAK/STAT pathways.

Type I interferons (IFN-α, IFN-β). A family of cytokines, including several structurally related IFN-α proteins and a single IFN-β protein, all of which have potent antiviral actions. The major source of IFN-α is mononuclear phagocytes; IFN-β is produced by many cells, including fibroblasts. Both IFN-α and IFN-β bind to the same cell surface receptor and induce similar biologic responses. Type I IFNs inhibit viral replication, increase the lytic potential of NK cells, increase expression of class I MHC molecules on virus-infected cells, and stimulate the development of T_H1 cells, especially in humans.

Ubiquitination. Covalent linkage of several copies of a small polypeptide called ubiquitin to a protein. Ubiquitination serves to target the protein for proteolytic degradation by proteasomes, a critical step in the class I MHC pathway of antigen processing and presentation.

Urticaria. Localized transient swelling and redness of the skin caused by leakage of fluid and plasma proteins from small vessels into the dermis during an immediate hypersensitivity reaction.

V gene segments. A DNA sequence that encodes the variable domain of an Ig heavy chain or light chain or a TCR α, β, γ, or δ chain. Each antigen receptor locus contains many different V gene segments, any one of which may recombine with downstream D or J segments during lymphocyte maturation to form functional antigen receptor genes.

V(D)J recombinase. A collection of enzymes that together mediate the somatic recombination events that form functional antigen receptor genes in developing B and T lymphocytes. Some of the enzymes, such as RAG-1 and RAG-2, are found only in developing lymphocytes, and others are ubiquitous DNA repair enzymes.

Vaccine. A preparation of microbial antigen, often combined with adjuvants, that is administered to individuals to induce protective immunity against microbial infections. The antigen may be in the form of live but avirulent microorganisms, killed microorganisms, purified macromolecular components of a microorganism, or a plasmid that contains a complementary DNA encoding a microbial antigen.

Variable region. The extracellular, N-terminal region of an Ig heavy or light chain or a TCR α, β, γ, or δ chain that contains variable amino acid sequences that differ between every clone of lymphocytes and that are responsible for the specificity for antigen. The antigen-binding variable sequences are localized to extended loop structures or hypervariable segments.

Virus. A primitive obligate intracellular parasitic organism or infectious particle that consists of a simple nucleic acid genome packaged in a protein capsid, sometimes surrounded by a membrane envelope. Many pathogenic animal viruses cause a wide range of diseases. Humoral immune responses to viruses can be effective in blocking infection of cells, and NK cells and CTLs are necessary to kill cells already infected.

Western blot. An immunologic technique to determine the presence of a protein in a biologic sample. The method involves separation of proteins in the sample by electrophoresis, transfer of the protein array from the electrophoresis gel to a support membrane by capillary action (blotting), and finally detection of the protein by binding of an enzymatically or radioactively labeled antibody specific for that protein.

Wheal and flare reaction. Local swelling and redness in the skin at a site of an immediate hypersensitivity reaction. The wheal reflects increased vascular permeability and the flare results from increased local blood flow, both changes resulting from mediators such as histamine released from activated dermal mast cells.

White pulp. The part of the spleen that is composed predominantly of lymphocytes, arranged in periarteriolar lymphoid sheaths, and follicles and other leukocytes. The remainder of the spleen contains sinusoids lined with phagocytic cells and filled with blood, called the **red pulp.**

Wiskott-Aldrich syndrome. An X-linked disease characterized by eczema, thrombocytopenia (reduced blood platelets), and immunodeficiency manifested as susceptibility to bacterial infections. The defective gene encodes a cytosolic protein involved in signaling cascades and regulation of the actin cytoskeleton.

Xenoantigen. An antigen on a graft from another species.

Xenogeneic graft (xenograft). An organ or tissue graft derived from a species different from the recipient. Transplantation of xenogeneic grafts (e.g., from a pig) to humans is not yet practical because of special problems related to immunologic rejection.

Xenoreactive. Describing a T cell or antibody that recognizes and responds to an antigen on a graft from another species (a xenoantigen). The T cell may recognize an intact xenogeneic MHC molecule or a peptide derived from a xenogeneic protein bound to a self MHC molecule.

X-linked agammaglobulinemia. An immunodeficiency disease, also called Bruton's agammaglobulinemia, characterized by a block in early B cell maturation and absence of serum Ig. Patients suffer from pyogenic bacterial infections. The disease is caused by mutations or deletions in the gene encoding Btk, an enzyme involved in signal transduction in developing B cells.

X-linked hyper-IgM syndrome. A rare immunodeficiency disease caused by mutations in the CD40 ligand gene and characterized by failure of B cell heavy chain isotype switching and cell-mediated immunity. Patients suffer from both pyogenic bacterial and protozoal infections.

Zeta-associated protein of 70 kD (ZAP-70). An Src family cytoplasmic protein tyrosine kinase that is critical for early signaling steps in antigen-induced T cell activation. ZAP-70 binds to phosphorylated tyrosines in the cytoplasmic tails of the ζ chain of the TCR complex and in turn phosphorylates adapter proteins that recruit other components of the signaling cascade.

ζ Chain. A transmembrane protein expressed in T cells as part of the TCR complex that contains ITAMs in its cytoplasmic tail and binds the ZAP-70 protein tyrosine kinase during T cell activation.

Appendix **II**

Principal Features of CD Molecules

CD designation	Common synonyms	Molecular structure, Family	Main cellular expression	Known or proposed functions
CD1a*	R4	49 kD; class I MHC family; β_2 microglobulin associated	Thymocytes, dendritic cells (including Langerhans cells)	Presentation of nonpeptide (lipid and glycolipid) antigens to some T cells
CD1b	—	45 kD; class I MHC family; β_2 microglobulin associated	Same as CD1a	Same as CD1a
CD1c	—	43 kD; class I MHC family; β_2 microglobulin associated	Thymocytes, dendritic cells (including Langerhans cells), some B cells	Same as CD1a
CD1d	—	43 kD; class I MHC family; β_2 microglobulin associated	Thymocytes, dendritic cells (including Langerhans cells), intestinal epithelial cells	Same as CD1a
CD2	T11; LFA-2; sheep red blood cell receptor	50 kD; Ig superfamily; CD2/CD48/CD58 family	T cells, thymocytes, NK cells	Adhesion molecule (binds CD58); T cell activation; CTL- and NK cell–mediated lysis
CD3γ	T3; Leu-4	25–28 kD; associated with CD3δ and CD3ε in TCR complex; Ig superfamily; ITAM in cytoplasmic tail	T cells, thymocytes	Cell surface expression of and signal transduction by the T cell antigen receptor
CD3δ	T3; Leu-4	20 kD; associated with CD3δ and CD3ε in TCR complex; Ig superfamily; ITAM in cytoplasmic tail	T cells, thymocytes	Cell surface expression of and signal transduction by the T cell antigen receptor
CD3ε	T3; Leu-4	20 kD; associated with CD3δ and CD3ε in TCR complex; Ig superfamily; ITAM in cytoplasmic tail	T cells, thymocytes	Required for cell surface expression of and signal transduction by the T cell antigen receptor
CD4	T4; Leu-3; L3T4	55 kD; Ig superfamily	Class II MHC–restricted T cells, thymocyte subsets, monocytes, and macrophages	Signaling and adhesion coreceptor in class II MHC–restricted antigen-induced T cell activation (binds to class II MHC molecules); thymocyte development; primary receptor for HIV retroviruses
CD5	T1; Ly-1	67 kD; scavenger receptor family	T cells, thymocytes, B cell subset	Signaling molecule; binds CD72
CD6	T12	100–130 kD; scavenger receptor family	T cells, thymocytes, subset of B cells	Adhesion of developing thymocytes with thymic epithelial cells; role in T cell activation

CD designation	Common synonyms	Molecular structure, Family	Main cellular expression	Known or proposed functions
CD7	—	40 kD	Hematopoietic stem cells, thymocytes, subset of T cells	Signaling
CD8α	T8; Leu-2; Lyt2	34 kD; expressed as homodimer or hetero-dimer with CD8β; Ig superfamily	Class I MHC–restricted T cells, thymocyte subsets	Signaling and adhesion coreceptor in class I MHC–restricted antigen-induced T cell activation (binds to class I MHC molecules); thymocyte development
CD8β	T8; Leu-2; Lyt2	34 kD; expressed as heterodimer with CD8α; Ig superfamily	Same as CD8α	Same as CD8α
CD9	DRAP-27; MRP-1	24 kD; tetraspan (TM4SF) family	Platelets, pre-B and immature B cells, activated and differentiating B cells, activated T cells, eosinophils, basophils, endothelial cells, brain and peripheral nerves, vascular smooth muscle cells, cardiac muscle cells, epithelial cells	Role in platelet activation; cell adhesion and migration
CD10	Common acute lymphoblastic leukemia antigen (CALLA); neutral endopeptidase. metalloendopeptidase; enkephalinase	100 kD	Immature and some mature B cells; lymphoid progenitors, granulocytes	Metalloproteinase
CD11a	LFA-1 α chain; α_L integrin subunit	180 kD; noncovalently linked to CD18 to form LFA-1 integrin	Leukocytes	Cell:cell adhesion; binds to ICAM-1 (CD54), ICAM-2 (CD102), and ICAM-3 (CD50)
CD11b	Mac-1; Mo1; CR3 (iC3b receptor); αM integrin chain	165 kD; noncovalently linked to CD18 to form Mac-1 integrin	Granulocytes, monocytes/ macrophages, NK cells	Phagocytosis of iC3b-coated particles; neutrophil and monocyte adhesion to endothelium (binds CD54) and extracellular matrix proteins
CD11c	p150,95; CR4 α chain; α_X integrin chain	145 kD; noncovalently linked to CD18 to form p150,95 integrin	Monocytes/macrophages, granulocytes, NK cells	Similar functions to CD11b; major CD11CD18 integrin on macrophages
CDw12†	p90–120	90–120 kD	Monocytes, granulocytes, NK cells	Phosphoprotein; no known function
CD13	Aminopeptidase N	150 kD; peptidase M1 family	Monocytes, granulocytes, endothelial cells	Aminopeptidase involved in trimming peptides bound to class II molecules and cleaving MIP-1 chemokine to alter target cell specificity; coronavirus receptor
CD14	Mo2; LPS receptor	53 kD; PI linked	Monocytes, macrophages, granulocytes, soluble form in serum	Binds complex of LPS and LPS-binding protein; required for LPS-induced macrophage activation
CD15	Lewis^x (Le^x)	Trisaccharide (poly-*N*-acetyllactosamine) present on several membrane glycoproteins and glycolipids	Granulocytes, monocytes	See CD15s
CD15s	Sialyl Lewis X (sLex)	Poly-*N*-acetyllactosamine; terminal tetrasaccharide on several cell surface glycoproteins	Leukocytes, endothelium	Leukocyte adhesion to endothelial cells; ligand for CD62E, P (selectins)
CD16a	FcγRIIIA	50–70 kD; Ig superfamily	NK cells, macrophages, mast cells	Immune complex–induced cellular activation; antibody-dependent cellular cytotoxicity
CD16b	FcγRIIIB	50 kD; PI linked; Ig superfamily	Neutrophils	Synergy with FcγRII in immune complex–mediated neutrophil activation
CDw17	Lactosylceramide	Lactosyl disaccharide group of the glycosphingolipid lactosylceramide	Monocytes, granulocytes, platelets, subset of B cells	? Phagocytosis of bacteria

CD designation	Common synonyms	Molecular structure, Family	Main cellular expression	Known or proposed functions
CD18	β chain of LFA-1 family; β_2 integrin subunit	95 kD; noncovalently linked to CD11a, CD11b, or CD11c to form β_2 integrins	Leukocytes	See CD11a, CD11b, CD11c
CD19	B4	95 kD; Ig superfamily	Most B cells	B cell activation; forms a coreceptor complex with CD21 and CD81, which delivers signals that synergize with signals from B cell antigen receptor complex
CD20	B1	35–37 kD ; tetraspan (TM4SF) family	Most or all B cells	? Role in B cell activation or regulation; calcium ion channel
CD21	CR2; C3d receptor; B2	145 kD; regulators of complement activation family	Mature B cells, follicular dendritic cells	Receptor for complement fragment C3d; forms a coreceptor complex with CD19 and CD81, which delivers activating signals in B cells; Epstein-Barr virus receptor
CD22	BL-CAM; Lyb8	130–140 kD; ITIM in cytoplasmic tail; Ig superfamily	B cells	Regulation of B cell activation, cross-regulation with CD19
CD23	FcεRIIb; low-affinity IgE receptor	45 kD; C-type lectin	Activated B cells, monocytes, macrophages	Low-affinity Fcε receptor, induced by IL-4; ? regulation of IgE synthesis; ? triggering of monocyte cytokine release
CD24	Heat-stable antigen (HSA)	35–45 kD; PI linked	B cells, granulocytes	?
CD25	IL-2 receptor α chain; TAC; p55	55 kD; regulators of complement activation family; noncovalently associates with IL-2Rβ (CD122) and IL-2Rγ (CD132) chains to form high-affinity IL-2 receptor	Activated T and B cells, activated macrophages	Binds IL-2; subunit of IL-2R
CD26	Adenosine deaminase–binding protein; dipeptidyl-peptidase IV	110 kD; type II transmembrane molecule	Activated T and B cells, macrophages, NK cells	Serine peptidase; ? signaling in T cells
CD27	—	Homodimer of 55 kD chains; TNF-R family	Most T cells, medullary thymocytes, memory B cells, NK cells	Binds CD70; mediates costimulatory signals for T and B cell activation; involved in murine T cell development
CD28	Tp44	Homodimer of 44-kD chains; Ig superfamily	T cells (most CD4, some CD8 cells)	T cell receptor for costimulator molecules CD80 (B7-1) and CD86 (B7-2)
CD29	β chain of VLA antigens; β_1 integrin subunit; platelet GPIIa	130 kD; noncovalently linked with CD49a-d chains to form VLA (β_1) integrins	Leukocytes	Leukocyte adhesion to extracellular matrix proteins and endothelium (see CD49)
CD30	Ki-1	120 kD; TNF-R family	Activated T and B cells, NK cells, monocytes, Reed-Sternberg cells in Hodgkin's disease	Role in activation-induced cell death of $CD8^+$ T cells; binds to CD153 (CD30L) on neutrophils, activated T cells, and macrophages
CD31	PECAM-1; platelet GPIIa	130–140 kD; Ig superfamily	Platelets, monocytes, granulocytes, B cells, endothelial cells	Adhesion molecule involved in the leukocyte diapedesis
CD32	FcγRIIA; FcγRIIB; FcγRIIC	40 kD; Ig superfamily; A, B, and C forms; ITIM in cytoplasmic tail of B form, ITAM in cytoplasmic tail of A and C forms	Macrophages, granulocytes, B cells, eosinophils, platelets	Fc receptor for aggregated IgG; binds C-reactive protein; role in phagocytosis, ADCC; acts as inhibitory receptor that terminates activation signals initiated by the B cell antigen receptor
CD33	Sialoadhesin; sialic acid–dependent cytoadhesion molecule	67 kD; Ig superfamily; sialic acid–binding Ig-like lectin family; ITIMs in cytoplasmic tail	Monocytes, myeloid progenitor cells	Binds sialic acid; ? regulation of signaling in myeloid cells

CD designation	Common synonyms	Molecular structure, Family	Main cellular expression	Known or proposed functions
CD34	gp105–120	116 kD; sialomucin	Precursors of hematopoietic cells, endothelial cells in high endothelial venules	Cell-cell adhesion; binds CD62L (L-selectin)
CD35	CR1; C3b receptor	190–285 kD (four products of polymorphic alleles); regulators of complement activation family	Granulocytes, monocytes, erythrocytes, B cells, follicular dendritic cells	Binds C3b and C4b; promotes phagocytosis of C3b- or C4b-coated particles and immune complexes; regulates complement activation
CD36	Platelet GPIIIb; GPIV	85–90 kD	Platelets, mature monocytes and macrophages, microvascular endothelial cells	Scavenger receptor for oxidized low-density lipoprotein; platelet adhesion; phagocytosis of apoptotic cells
CD37	—	Composed of two or three 40 to 52 kD chains; tetraspan (TM4SF) family	B cells, some T cells and myeloid cells	Forms complexes in membrane with CD53, CD81, CD82, and MHC class II molecules; ? signal transduction
CD38	T10	45 kD	Early and activated B cells, plasma cells, activated T cells	Ectoenzyme with NAD glycohydrolase, ADP ribosyl cyclase, and cyclic ADP ribose hydrolase activities
CD39	ENTPD1: ectonucleoside triphosphate diphosphohydrolase 1	78 kD; ecto-apyrase gene family	Activated B cells, activated NK cells, some T cells, endothelial cells	Ectoenzyme with ADPase and ATPase activities; regulation of platelet aggregation and thrombosis
CD40	—	Homodimer of 44 to 48 kD chains; TNF-R family	B cells, macrophages, dendritic cells, endothelial cells	Binds CD154 (CD40 ligand); role in T cell–dependent B cell, macrophage, dendritic cell, and endothelial cell activation
CD41	Glycoprotein IIb (GPIIb); α_{IIb} integrin chain	Heterodimer of GPIIba (120 kD) and GPIIbb (23 kD); noncovalently linked with GPIIIa (CD61) to form GPIIb/IIIa integrin	Platelets, megakaryocytes	Platelet aggregation and activation; binds fibrinogen, fibronectin (recognizes RGD sequence)
CD42a	Platelet GPIX	22 kD; forms complex with CD42b, c, and d	Platelets, megakaryocytes	Platelet adhesion; binds von Willebrand factor, thrombin
CD42b	Platelet GPIbα	145 kD; disulfide linked with CD42c and forms complex with CD42a and d; mucin	See CD42a	See CD42a
CD42c	Platelet GPIbβ	25 kD; disulfide linked with CD42b and foms complex with CD42a and d	See CD42a	See CD42a
CD42d	Platelet GPV	82 kD; forms complex with CD42a, b, and c	See CD42a	See CD42a
CD43	Sialophorin; leukosialin	95–135 kD; sialomucin	Leukocytes (except circulating B cells)	Adhesive and anti-adhesive functions
CD44	Pgp-1; Hermes	80 to >100 kD, highly glycosylated; cartilage link protein family	Leukocytes, erythrocytes	Binds hyaluronan; involved in leukocyte adhesion to endothelial cells and extracellular matrix; leukocyte aggregation
CD45	Leukocyte common antigen (LCA); T200; B220	Multiple isoforms, 180–220 kD (see CD45R); protein tyrosine phosphatase receptor family; fibronectin type III family	Hematopoietic cells	Tyrosine phosphatase plays critical role in T and B cell antigen receptor–mediated signaling
CD45R	Forms of CD45 with restricted cellular expression	CD45RO: 180 kD CD45RA: 220 kD CD45RB: 190, 205, and 220 kD isoforms	CD45RO: memory T cells, subset of B cells, monocytes, macrophages CD45RA: naive T cells, B cells, monocytes CD45RB: B cells, subset of T cells	See CD45
CD46	Membrane cofactor protein (MCP)	52–58 kD; regulators of complement activation family	Leukocytes, epithelial cells, fibroblasts	Regulation of complement activation

CD designation	Common synonyms	Molecular structure, Family	Main cellular expression	Known or proposed functions
CD47R	Rh-associated protein; integrin-associated protein (IAP); CDw149	45–60 kD; Ig superfamily	Broad	Thrombospondin receptor; adhesion
CD48	BCM1; Blast-1; Hu; Lym3; OX-45	45 kD; PI linked; Ig superfamily; CD2/CD48/CD58 family	Leukocytes	Ligand for CD244; mouse receptor for CD2; ? role in leukocyte adhesion and signaling
CD49a	α_1 integrin subunit	210 kD; noncovalently linked to CD29 to form VLA-1 (β_1 integrin)	Activated T cells, monocytes	Leukocyte adhesion to extracellular matrix; binds collagens, laminin
CD49b	α_2 integrin subunit; platelet GPIa	170 kD; noncovalently linked to CD29 to form VLA-2 (β_1 integrin)	Platelets, activated T cells, monocytes, some B cells	Leukocyte adhesion to extracellular matrix; binds collagen, laminin
CD49c	α_3 integrin subunit	Dimer of 130 and 25 kD chains; noncovalently linked to CD29 to form VLA-3 (β_1 integrin)	T cells, some B cells, monocytes	Leukocyte adhesion to extracellular matrix; binds fibronectin, collagens, laminin
CD49d	α_4 integrin subunit	150 kD; noncovalently linked to CD29 to form VLA-4 ($\alpha_4\beta_1$) integrin or to β_7 to form $\alpha_7\beta_7$ integrin	T cells, monocytes, B cells	Leukocyte adhesion to endothelium and extracellular matrix; binds to VCAM-1 and MAdCAM-1; binds fibronectin and collagens
CD49e	α_5 integrin subunit	Heterodimer of 135 and 25 kD chains; noncovalently linked to CD29 to form VLA-5 (β_1 integrin)	T cells, few B cells and monocytes	Adhesion to extracellular matrix; binds fibronectin
CD49f	α_6 integrin subunit	Heterodimer of 125 and 25 kD chains; noncovalently linked to CD29 to form VLA-6 ($\beta 1$ integrin)	Platelets, megakaryocytes, activated T cells, monocytes	Adhesion to extracellular matrix; binds fibronectin
CD50	ICAM-3	110–140 kD; Ig superfamily	Leukocytes, some endothelium	Adhesion; binds CD11aCD18
CD51	α_V integrin subunit; vitronectin receptor α chain	Heterodimer of 125 and 24 kD chains; noncovalently associates with CD61 to form vitronectin receptor integrin	Platelets, megakaryocytes	Adhesion: receptor for vitronectin, fibrinogen, von Willebrand factor (binds RGD sequence)
CD52	—	25–29 kD	Thymocytes, lymphocytes, monocytes, macrophages, male genital tract epithelial cells	Function unknown; anti-CD52 antibodies used to treat lymphoid malignant tumors
CD53	OX44	32–42 kD; tetraspan (TM4SF) family	Hematopoietic cells	? Signaling
CD54	ICAM-1	75–114 kD; Ig superfamily	Endothelial cells, T cells, B cells, monocytes, endothelial cells (cytokine inducible)	Cell-cell adhesion; ligand for CD11aCD18 (LFA-1) and CD11bCD18 (Mac-1); receptor for rhinovirus
CD55	Decay-accelerating factor (DAF)	55–70 kD; PI linked; regulators of complement activation family	Broad	Regulation of complement activation; binds C3b, C4b
CD56	Leu-19; NKH1	175–220 kD; isoform of neural cell adhesion molecule (N-CAM); Ig superfamily	NK cells, subset of T and B cells, brain	Homotypic adhesion
CD57	HNK-1; Leu-7	Carbohydrate epitope on many cell surface glycoproteins and glycolipids	NK cells, subset of T cells, monocytes	? Adhesion

CD designation	Common synonyms	Molecular structure, Family	Main cellular expression	Known or proposed functions
CD58	Lymphocyte function–associated antigen-3 (LFA-3)	40–70 kD; PI linked or integral membrane protein; CD2/CD48/CD58 family	Broad	Leukocyte adhesion; T cell costimulation; binds CD2
CD59	Membrane inhibitor of reactive lysis (MIRL)	18–20 kD; PI linked; Ly-6 superfamily	Broad	Binds C9; inhibits formation of complement membrane attack complex
CDw60	GD3	120 kD; 9-*O*-acetylated disialosyl group predominantly found on ganglioside D3	Subset of T cells, platelets, thymic epithelium, activated keratinocytes	Unknown
CD61	β_3 integrin subunit; vitronectin receptor β chain; GPIIIa component of GPIIb/GPIIIa integrin	110 kD; noncovalently linked to CD51 to form vitronectin receptor (integrin); non-covalently linked to CD41 to form GPIIb/GPIIIa (integrin)	Platelets, megakaryocytes, endothelial cells, leukocytes	See CD51, CD41
CD62E	E-selectin; ELAM-1	115 kD; selectin family	Endothelial cells	Leukocyte-endothelial adhesion
CD62L	L-selectin; LAM-1; MEL-14	74–95 kD; selectin family	B cells, T cells, monocytes, granulocytes, some NK cells	Leukocyte-endothelial adhesion; homing of naive T cells to peripheral lymph nodes
CD62P	P-selectin; gmp140; PADGEM	120 kD; selectin family	Platelets, endothelial cells; (present in granules, translocated to cell surface upon activation)	Leukocyte adhesion to endothelium, platelets; binds CD162 (PSGL-1)
CD63	Granulophysin; lysosome-associated membrane protein 3 (LAMP-3)	40–60 kD; tetraspan (TM4SF) family	Activated platelets, endothelial cells, neutrophils, monocytes, macrophages	Unknown
CD64	FcγRI	75 kD; Ig superfamily; non-covalently associated with the common FcRγ chain	Monocytes, macrophages, activated neutrophils	High-affinity Fcγ receptor; role in phagocytosis, ADCC, macrophage activation
CD65	Ceramide-dodecasaccharide; VIM-2	Carbohydrate epitope on ceramide glycolipid	Granulocytes	Unknown
CD66a	NCA-160 biliary glycoprotein (BGP)	140–180 kD; Ig superfamily; carcinoembryonic antigen (CEA) family	Granulocytes, epithelial cells	Unknown; receptor for *Neisseria gonorrhoeae* and *Neisseria meningitidis*
CD66b	CD67; CGM6; NCA-95	95–100 kD; Ig superfamily; carcinoembryonic antigen (CEA) family	Granulocytes	? Role in cell-cell adhesion; ? role in signaling
CD66c	NCA	90 kD; Ig superfamily; carcinoembryonic antigen (CEA) family	Granulocytes, epithelial cells	? Role in cell-cell adhesion; ? regulates integrin activity
CD66d	CGM1	35 kD; Ig superfamily; carcinoembryonic antigen (CEA) family	Granulocytes	? Role in cell-cell adhesion; ? regulates integrin activity
CD66e	Carcinoembryonic antigen (CEA)	180–220 kD; Ig superfamily; carcinoembryonic antigen (CEA) family	Colonic and other epithelial cells	? Adhesion; clinical marker of carcinoma burden
CD66f	Pregnancy-specific glycoprotein (PSG)	54–72 kD; Ig superfamily; carcinoembryonic antigen (CEA) family	Placental syncytiotrophoblasts, fetal liver	Unknown
CD68	Macrosialin	110 kD; mucin; lysosome-associated membrane protein (LAMP) family; scavenger receptor family	Monocytes, macrophages, dendritic cells, granulocytes, activated T cells, subset of B cells, intracellular protein, weak surface expression	Unknown

CD designation	Common synonyms	Molecular structure, Family	Main cellular expression	Known or proposed functions
CD69	Activation inducer molecule (AIM)	Homodimer of 28 to 32 kD chains; C-type lectin	Activated leukocytes including T cells, B cells, NK cells, neutrophils, basophils, eosinophils, platelets, Langerhans cells	Signaling in different cell types
CD70	Ki-24	75–170 kD; TNF family	Activated T and B cells, macrophages	Binds CD27; provides costimulatory signals for T and B cell activation
CD71	T9; transferrin receptor	Homodimer of 95-kD chains	Activated T and B cells, macrophages, proliferating cells	Receptor for transferrin; role in iron metabolism, cell growth
CD72	Lyb-2 (mouse)	Homodimer of 39 to 43 kD chains; C-type lectin	B cells	Ligand for CD5; ? role in T cell–B cell interactions
CD73	Ecto-5'-nucleotidase	69–70 kD; PI linked	Subsets of T and B cells, germinal center follicular dendritic cells	Ecto-5'-nucleotidase; signaling in T cells
CD74	Class II MHC invariant (γ) chain; I_i	33–35 and 41 kD isoforms	B cells, monocytes, macrophage, other class II MHC–expressing cells	Associates with and directs intracellular sorting of newly synthesized class II MHC molecules
CD75	Lactosamines	Carbohydrate epitope		Unknown
CD75s	—	Carbohydrate epitope; sialoglycan	Mature B cells, subset of T cells	Cell adhesion; binds CD22
CD77	Pk blood group antigen; Burkitt's lymphoma antigen (BLA); ceramide trihexoside (CTH); globotriaosylceramide (Gb3)	Carbohydrate epitope	Germinal center B cells	Unknown; ? induces apoptosis
CD79a	Igα, MB1	32–33 kD; forms dimer with CD79b; Ig superfamily; ITAM in cytoplasmic tail	Mature B cells	Required for cell surface expression of and signal transduction by the B cell antigen receptor complex
CD79b	Igβ, B29	37–39 kD; forms dimer with CD79a; Ig superfamily; ITAM in cytoplasmic tail	Mature B cells	Required for cell surface expression of and signal transduction by the B cell antigen receptor complex
CD80	B7-1; BB1	60 kD; Ig superfamily	Dendritic cells, activated B cells and macrophages	Costimulator for T lymphocyte activation; ligand for CD28 and CD152 (CTLA-4)
CD81	Target for antiproliferative antigen-1 (TAPA-1)	26 kD; tetraspan (TM4SF) family	Hematopoietic cells, endothelium, epithelial cells	B cell activation; forms a coreceptor complex with CD19 and CD21, which delivers signals that synergize with signals from B cell antigen receptor complex
CD82	4F9; C33; IA4; KAI1; R2	45–90 kD; tetraspan (TM4SF) family	Broad	? Signal transduction
CD83	HB15	43 kD; Ig superfamily	Dendritic cells, Langerhans cells, germinal center B cells	Unknown
CD84	—	68–80 kD; Ig superfamily; CD2/CD48/CD58 family	Monocytes, macrophages, subset of T cells, mature B cells, platelets	Unknown
CD85	—	110 kD; Ig superfamily	B cells, plasma cells, monocytes, T cell subset	? Signaling
CD86	B7-2	80 kD; Ig superfamily	B cells, monocytes, dendritic cells; some T cells	Costimulator for T lymphocyte activation; ligand for CD28 and CD152 (CTLA-4)
CD87	Urokinase plasminogen activator receptor (uPAR)	35–59 kD; PI linked	T cells, NK cells, monocytes, neutrophils, endothelial cells	Receptor for urokinase plasminogen activator; role in inflammatory cell adhesion and migration

CD designation	Common synonyms	Molecular structure, Family	Main cellular expression	Known or proposed functions
CD88	C5a receptor	43 kD; G protein–coupled, 7-membrane–spanning receptor family	Granulocytes, dendritic cells, mast cells	Receptor for C5a complement fragment; role in complement-induced inflammation
CD89	Fcα receptor (FcαR)	45–100 kD; Ig superfamily; noncovalently associated with the common FcR γ chain	Granulocytes, monocytes, macrophages, T cells, NK cells	Binds IgA; mediates IgA-dependent cellular cytotoxicity
CD90	Thy-1	25–35 kD; PI linked; Ig superfamily	Thymocytes, peripheral T cells (mice), neurons (all species)	Marker for T cells; ? role in T cell activation
CD91	α2-macroglobulin receptor; low-density lipoprotein receptor–related protein (LRP)	600 kD; LDL receptor family	Macrophages and monocytes	Binds low-density lipoproteins
CD92	CTL1	70 kD	Monocytes, granulocytes, endothelium	Unknown
CDw93	—	110 kD; sialoglycoprotein	Neutrophils, monocytes, endothelial cells	Unknown
CD94	Kp43; KIR	30 kD; C-type lectin; on NK cells, covalently assembles with other C-type lectin molecules (NKG2)	NK cells; subset of $CD8^+$ T cells	CD94/NKG2 complex functions as an NK cell killer inhibitory receptor; binds HLA-E class I MHC molecules
CD95	Fas antigen, APO-1	Homotrimer of 45 kD chains; TNF receptor family	Multiple cell types	Binds Fas ligand; mediates signals leading to activation-induced cell death
CD96	T cell activation increased late expression (TACTILE)	160, 180, 240 kD forms; Ig superfamily; mucin	T cells	Unknown
CD97	BL-KDD/F12	74, 80, 89 kD forms; G protein–coupled receptor family	Broad	Unknown
CD98	4F2; FRP-1	Heterodimer of 40 and 80-kD subunits	Broad	? Amino acid transporter
CD99	E2; MIC2	32 kD	Broad	Unknown
CD100	SEMA4D	120 kD; Ig superfamily; semaphorin	Hematopoietic cells	? Signaling
CD101	P126; V7	Homodimer of 120 kD chains; Ig superfamily	Granulocytes, monocytes, dendritic cells, activated T cells	? Inhibitory signaling in T cells
CD102	ICAM-2	55–65 kD; Ig superfamily	Endothelial cells, monocytes, some lymphocytes	Ligand for CD11aCD18 (LFA-1); cell-cell adhesion
CD103	HML-1; α_E integrin subunit	Dimer of 150 and 25 kD subunits; noncovalently linked to β_7 integrin subunit to form $\alpha_E\beta_7$ integrin	Intraepithelial lymphocytes, other cell types	Role in T cell homing to mucosa; binds E-cadherin
CD104	β_4 integrin subunit	205–220 kD; noncovalently linked to CD49f (α_6) integrin subunit to form to $\alpha_6\beta_4$ integrin	Thymocytes, epithelial cells	Adhesion; binds laminin
CD105	Endoglin	Homodimer of 90-kD subunits	Endothelial cells, activated macrophages	Binds TGF-β; modulates cellular responses to TGF-β
CD106	Vascular cell adhesion molecule-1 (VCAM-1); INCAM-110	100–110 kD; Ig superfamily	Endothelial cells, macrophages, follicular dendritic cells, marrow stromal cells	Adhesion; receptor for CD49dCD29 (VLA-4) integrin; role in lymphocyte trafficking, activation; role in hematopoiesis
CD107a	Lysosome-associated membrane-protein 1 (LAMP-1)	110–120 kD	Activated platelets, activated T cells, activated endothelium, activated neutrophils	Lysosomal protein translocated to cell surface after activation; ? adhesion

CD designation	Common synonyms	Molecular structure, Family	Main cellular expression	Known or proposed functions
CD107b	Lysosome-associated membrane protein 2 (LAMP-2)	120 kD	Activated platelets, activated T cells, activated endothelium, activated neutrophils	Lysosomal protein translocated to cell surface after activation; ? adhesion
CD108	John-Milton-Hagen (JMH) human blood group antigen	76 kD; PI linked	Erythrocytes, lymphocytes	Unknown
CD109	8A3; E123	170 kD; PI linked	Endothelial cells, activated platelets, activated T lymphocytes	Unknown
CD110	MPL; TPO-R; C-MPL	85–92 kD; hematopoietin receptor family	Hematopoietic cells	Thrombopoietin receptor; megakaryocyte differentiation
CD111	PVRL1; PRR1; HevC; nectin-l	75 kD; Ig superfamily; poliovirus receptor family	Hemopoietic cells; epithelial cells; neurons	Adhesion molecule; herpesvirus receptor
CD112	PVR2; HveB; nectin-2	64–72 kD Ig superfamily; poliovirus receptor family	Hematopoietic cells	Adhesion; herpesvirus receptor
CD114	Granulocyte colony-stimulating factor (G-CSF) receptor	150 kD; Ig superfamily; type I cytokine receptor family	Granulocytes, monocytes, platelets, endothelial cells, hematopoietic cells	Binds and mediates biologic effects of G-CSF
CD115	Macrophage colony-stimulating factor receptor (M-CSFR); CSF-1R	150 kD; Ig superfamily; tyrosine kinase receptor family	Monocytes, macrophages, hematopoietic cells	Binds and mediates biologic effects of M-CSF
CD116	Granulocyte-monocyte colony-stimulating factor receptor (GM-CSFR) α chain	80 kD; interacts with the common β subunit (CDw131) of the GM-CSF, IL-3, and IL-5 receptors; type I cytokine receptor family	Myeloid cells and their hematopoietic precursors	Binds and mediates biologic effects of GM-CSF
CD117	c-Kit, stem cell factor receptor	145 kD; Ig superfamily; tyrosine kinase receptor family	Hematopoietic stem and progenitor cells, tissue mast cells	Binds and mediates biologic effects of c-Kit ligand (stem cell factor)
CD118	Interferon (IFN)-α, β receptor	Type II cytokine receptor family	Broad	Binds and mediates biologic effects of IFN-α/β
CD119	Interferon (IFN)-γ receptor	90–100 kD;	Macrophages, monocytes, dendritic cells, B cells, T cells, endothelium, epithelial cells	Binds and mediates biologic effects of IFN-γ
CD120a	55 kD tumor necrosis factor (TNF) receptor; TNF-RI	Homotrimer of 55 kD chains; TNF-R family	Broad	Binds and mediates most biologic effects of TNF-α and TNF-β
CD120b	75 kD tumor necrosis factor (TNF) receptor; TNF-RII	Homotrimer of 75 kD chains; TNF-R family	Broad	Binds and mediates some biologic effects of TNF-α and TNF-β
CD121a	Type 1 IL-1 receptor	80 kD; Ig superfamily	Broad	Binds and mediates biologic effects of IL-1α and IL-1β
CD121b	Type 2 IL-1 receptor	60–70 kD; Ig superfamily	B cells	Decoy receptor that binds IL-1α and IL-1β but does not mediate biologic effects
CD122	IL-2 receptor β chain	70–75 kD; type I cytokine receptor family; associates with CD25 and CD132 to form high-affinity IL-2R	T cells, B cells, NK cells, monocytes, macrophages	Signaling and binding component of IL-2 and IL-15 receptors; critical for mediating biologic effects of IL-2 and IL-15 on T cells and NK cells
CD123	IL-3 receptor α chain	70 kD; type I cytokine receptor family; associates with the common CD131 signaling chain	Monocytes, macrophages, megakaryocytes, bone hematopoietic precursor cells	Binds IL-3 and in association with CD131, mediates biologic effects of IL-3
CDw124	IL-4 receptor α chain	140 kD; type I cytokine receptor family; associates with CD132 to form functional IL-4 receptor	B cells, T cell, endothelium, hematopoietic precursor cells	Cytokine binding subunit of IL-4 receptor; also subunit of IL-13 receptor
CD125	IL-5 receptor α chain	60 kD; type I cytokine receptor family; associates with CDw131 to form functional IL-5 receptor	Eosinophils, activated B cells, basophils	Binds IL-5 and in association with CDw131 mediates biologic effects of IL-5

CD designation	Common synonyms	Molecular structure, Family	Main cellular expression	Known or proposed functions
CD126	IL-6 receptor α chain	80 kD; type I cytokine receptor family; Ig superfamily; associates with CDw130 to form functional IL-6 receptor	Activated B cells, plasma cells, other leukocytes	Binds IL-6 and in association with CDw130 mediates biologic effects of IL-6
CD127	IL-7 receptor α chain	65–70/90 kD; type I cytokine receptor family; associates with CD132 to form functional IL-7 receptor	Lymphocyte precursors in bone marrow, T cells	Binds IL-7 and in association with CD132 mediates biologic effects of IL-7
CDw128a	CXCR1; IL-8 receptor α	58–67; G protein–coupled, 7-membrane–spanning receptor family	Neutrophils, basophils, mast cells, T cell subsets	Binds and mediates biologic effects of IL-8
CDw128b	CXCR2;IL-8 receptor β	G protein–coupled, 7-membrane–spanning receptor family	Neutrophils, mast cells	Binds and mediates biologic effects of IL-8
CD129	Unassigned			
CD130	IL-6 receptor β chain (IL-6Rβ); IL-11 receptor β chain (IL-11Rβ); oncostatin M receptor β chain (OSMRβ); leukemia inhibitory factor receptor β (LIFRβ); gp130	130–140 kD; Ig superfamily; type I cytokine receptor family; associates with ligand binding chains of IL-6 (CD126), IL-11, oncostatin M, and leukemia inhibitory factor receptors	Broad	Signaling functions of receptors for IL-6, IL-11, oncostatin M, and LIF
CD131	Common β subunit of IL-3 receptor (IL-3R), IL-5 receptor (IL-5R), and granulocyte-monocyte colony-stimulating factor receptor (GM-CSFR)	120–140 kD; Ig superfamily; type I cytokine receptor family; associates with α chains of IL-3R (CD123), IL-5R (CD125), and GM-CSFR (CD116)	Myeloid cells and their progenitors, early B cells	Signaling functions of receptors for IL-3, IL-5, and GM-CSF
CD132	Common γ chain (γc) of IL-2 receptor (IL-2R), IL-4 receptor (IL-4R), IL-7 receptor (IL-7R), IL-9 receptor (IL-9R), and interleukin-15 receptor (IL-15R)	64 kD; Ig superfamily; type I cytokine receptor family; associates with other chains of IL-2R (CD25, CD122), IL-4R (CD124), IL-7R (CD127), IL-9R, and IL-15R (IL-15Rα, CD122)	T cells, B cells, NK cells, monocytes, macrophages, neutrophils	Some of the signaling functions of receptors for IL-2, IL-4, IL-7, IL-9, and IL-15
CD133	PROML1; AC133; hematopoietic stem cell antigen	120 kD; pentaspan transmembrane glycoprotein family	Various stem cells	Unknown
CD134	OX40	50 kD; TNF receptor family	Activated T cells	Costimulatory signaling in T cells; binds OX40 ligand
CD135	FMS-like tyrosine kinase 3 (Flt-3); Flk-2; STK-1	130 kD; tyrosine kinase receptor family	Myeloid and B cell progenitor cells	Growth factor receptor involved in hematopoiesis; binds Flt-3
CDw136	Macrophage-stimulating protein receptor (MSP receptor); Ron	Heterodimer of 150 kD and 40 kD chains; tyrosine kinase receptor family	Epithelial cells from various tissues	Role in cell migration and growth; binds incompletely characterized growth factors— macrophage stimulating protein (MSP) and hepatocyte growth factor-like (HGFL)
CDw137	4-1BB, induced by lymphocyte activation (ILA)	85 kD; TNF-receptor family	T lymphocytes, B lymphocytes, monocytes, epithelial cells	Costimulation of T cells; binds an incompletely characterized ligand on B cells and macrophages
CD138	Syndecan-1	Heparan sulfate proteoglycan	B cells	Unknown
CD139		209, 228 kD	B lymphocytes, monocytes, granulocytes	Unknown

CD designation	Common synonyms	Molecular structure, Family	Main cellular expression	Known or proposed functions
CD140a	Platelet-derived growth factor receptor A (PDGFR A)	180 kD; tyrosine kinase receptor family; associates with β chain of PDGFR	Broad	In association with CD140b, binds and mediates biologic effects of PDGF
CD140b	Platelet-derived growth factor receptor B (PDGFR b)	180 kD; tyrosine kinase receptor family; associates with α chain of PDGFR	Broad	In association with CD140a, binds and mediates biologic effects of PDGF
CD141	Fetomodulin; thrombomodulin (TM)	75 kD, 105 kD; C-type lectin	Endothelium	Regulation of coagulation
CD142	Coagulation factor III; thromboplastin; tissue factor (TF)	Coagulation factor III; thromboplastin; tissue factor (TF)	Epithelial cells and stromal cells in various tissues, activated endothelial cells	Binds factor VIIa to form an enzyme that initiates the blood clotting cascade; regulates factor VIIa serine protease activity
CD143	Angiotensin-converting enzyme (ACE)	170–180 kD	Endothelial cells, epithelial cells, neurons, activated macrophages, some T cells	Peptidyl-dipeptide hydrolase involved in metabolism of vasoactive peptides angiotensin II and bradykinin
CD144	Cadherin-5; VE-cadherin	139,135 kD; cadherin family	Endothelial cells	Organizes adherent junction in endothelial cells, which control cell-cell adhesion, permeability, and migration
CD146	A32; MCAM, MUC18, Mel-CAM, S-endo	118, 139 kD; Ig superfamily	Endothelium, smooth muscle, subpopulation of activated T cells	? Cell junction adhesion molecule
CD147	5A11; basigin; CE9; HT7; M6; neurothelin;OX-47	55–65 kD; Ig superfamily	Leukocytes, red blood cells, platelets, endothelial cells	? Adhesion
CD148	HPTP-η	240–260 kD; protein tyrosine phosphatase	Granulocytes, monocytes, T cells, dendritic cells, platelets, fibroblasts, nerve cells	Unknown
CD150	Signaling lymphocyte activation molecule (SLAM); IPO-3	75–95 kD; Ig superfamily	Thymocytes, activated lymphocytes, dendritic cells, endothelial cells	Regulation of B cell–T cell interactions and proliferative signals in B lymphocytes; binds itself as a self ligand
CD151	PETA-3; SFA-1	32 kD; tetraspan (TM4SF) family	Platelets, megakaryocytes, hematopoietic cells, epithelial cells, endothelium	? Adhesion, platelet aggregation
CD152	Cytotoxic T lymphocyte–associated protein-4 (CTLA-4)	33, 50 kD; Ig superfamily	Activated T lymphocytes	Inhibitory signaling in T cells; binds CD80 (B7-1) and CD86 (B7-2) on antigen-presenting cells
CD153	CD30 ligand (CD30L)	40 kD; TNF family	Activated T cells, resting B cells, granulocytes, thymocytes	Role in activation-induced cell death of $CD8^+$ T cells; binds to CD30
CD154	CD40 ligand (CD40L); T-BAM; TNF-related activation protein (TRAP); gp39	Homotrimer of 32 to 39 kD chains; TNF receptor family	Activated $CD4^+$ T cells	Activates B cells, macrophages, and endothelial cells; ligand for CD40
CD155	Poliovirus receptor	80–90 kD; Ig superfamily	Broad	Unknown function; used by poliovirus to infect cells
CD156a	ADAM8; MS2	69 kD; metalloprotease family; disintegrin family	Neutrophils, monocytes	? Role in leukocyte extravasation
CD156b	ADAM17: tumor necrosis factor α converting enzyme (TACE)	100–120 kD; disintegrin and metalloprotease families	Broad	Proteolysis and release of active forms of TNF and TGFα
CD157	BP-3/IF-7; BST-1; Mo5	42–45 , 50 kD; PI linked	Granulocytes, monocytes, B and T cell progenitor cells, bone marrow stromal cells	ADP ribosyl cyclase and cyclic ADP ribose hydrolase activities; ? role in lymphocyte development

CD designation	Common synonyms	Molecular structure, Family	Main cellular expression	Known or proposed functions
CD158	Killer Ig-like receptor (KIR)	50, 58 kD; Ig superfamily; ITIMS in cytoplasmic tail or ITAM	NK cells	Inhibition or activation of NK cells upon interaction with the appropriate class I HLA-C alleles
CD159a	NKG2A; NKG2B; KLRC1	C-type lectin	NK cells	Inhibition or activation of NK cells upon interaction with the appropriate HLA-C alleles
CD160	BY55 antigen; NK1; NK28	80 kD homodimer; Ig superfamily	NK cells; cytolytic T lymphocytes	Binds class I MHC–like molecules; regulation of NK cell activation
CD161	NKR-P1A; KLRB1	Homodimer of 40 kD chains; C-type lectin	NK cells, subset of T cells	Role in NK cell activation
CD162	PSGL-1	Homodimer of 120 kD chains; sialomucin	T cells, monocytes, granulocytes, some B cells	Ligand for selectins (CD62E, CD62P, CD62L); adhesion of leukocytes to endothelium
CD163	GHI/61; M130	130 kD; scavenger receptor cysteine-rich family	Monocytes, macrophages	Unknown
CD164	MUC-24; multiglycosylated core protein 24 (MGC-24v)	80–90 kD; sialomucin	Hematopoietic progenitor cells	? Adhesion of hematopoietic cells to bone marrow stroma
CD165	AD2; gp37	37, 42 kD	Mature lymphocytes, thymocytes, thymic epithelial cells, monocytes, platelets, CNS neurons	? Adhesion between thymocytes and thymic epithelial cells
CD166	BEN; DM-GRASP; KG-CAM; SC-1; activated leukocyte cell adhesion molecule (ALCAM)	100–105 kD; Ig superfamily	Activated T cells, activated monocytes, epithelium, neurons, fibroblasts	Binds CD6; unknown function
CD167a	DDR1; trkE; cak; eddr1	62 kD tyrosine kinase receptor family	Normal and transformed epithelial cells	Binds collagen
CD168	HMMR; IHABP; RHAMM	88, 84, 80 kD	Thymocytes, hematopoietic progenitors, malignant B cells, monocytes	Binds hyaluronan; stimulates cellular motility
CD169	Sialoadhesin; siglec-1	180 kD; Ig superfamily; sialic acid–binding Ig-like lectin (siglec) family	Macrophages	Binds sialylated ligands; cell-cell and cell-matrix adhesion
CD170	Siglec-5; OBBP2, CD33L2	70 kD homodimer; Ig superfamily; sialic acid binding–Ig-like lectin (siglec) family	Neutrophils, monocytes, macrophages	Binds sialylated ligands; cell-cell and cell-matrix adhesion
CD171	L1; L1CAM; N-CAM L1	140–220 kD depending on cell type; Ig superfamily	Neurons, Schwann cells, epithelial cells, CD4$^+$ T cells, myelomonocytic cells	Cell adhesion molecule required for normal neurohistogenesis
CD172a	SIRP, MYD-1, SHPS1, SHPS-1, protein tyrosine phosphatase, nonreceptor type substrate 1	Ig superfamily, signal-regulatory-protein (SIRP) family; ITIM in cytoplasmic tail	Neutrophils, monocytes	Inhibitory receptor
CD173	Blood group H type 2	Carbohydrate epitope	Broad	Blood group antigen
CD174	Lewis y	Carbohydrate epitope	Broad	Blood group antigen
CD175	Tn	Carbohydrate epitope	Broad	Blood group antigen
CD175s	Sialyl-Tn	Carbohydrate epitope	Broad	Blood group antigen
CD176	TF	Carbohydrate epitope	Broad	Blood group antigen

CD designation	Common synonyms	Molecular structure, Family	Main cellular expression	Known or proposed functions
CD177	NB1; HNA-2a	64–68 kD	Neutrophils	Unknown
CD178	FasL; CD95L; APO-1; TNFSF6; APT1LG1;	40 kD; forms homotrimers; TNF family	Activated T cells, NK cells, tumor cells, retinal cells, endothelial cells; broadly inducible	Binds CD95 (Fas); induces apoptosis via Fas pathway
CD179a	VpreB; VPREB1; IGVPB; Igι	16–18 kD; Ig superfamily	Pro B and early pre B cells	Associates noncovalently with CD179b to form surrogate light chain component of pre-B cell receptor required for B cell development
CD179b	IGLL1; lambda5; Igomega; IGVPB; 14.1 chain	22 kD; Ig superfamily	ProB and early preB cells	Associates non-covalently with CD179a to form surrogate light chain component of pre-B-cell receptor required for B cell development
CD180	LY64; RP105	95–105 kD; Toll-like receptor (TLR) family	B cells, monocytes, dendritic cells	Associates with MD-1 to form RP105/MD-1 complex, which works with TLR-4 in LPS-induced signaling
CD183	CXCR3; GPR9; CKR-L2; IP10-R; Mig-R	40 kD; CXCR chemokine receptor family	T cells, subsets of B cells and NK cells	Cell surface receptor for chemokines, including IP10, Mig, and I-TAC
CD184	CXCR4; fusin; LESTR; NPY3R; HM89; FB22	40 kD; CXCR chemokine receptor family	Broadly expressed on blood and tissue cells	Cell surface receptor for chemokine SDF1; cofactor for T cell–tropic HIV entry into cells
CD195	L1; L1CAM; N-CAM L1	40 kD; CCR chemokine receptor family	T cells and macrophages	Cell surface receptor for chemokines MCP-2, MIP-1α, MIP-1β, and RANTES; cofactor for macrophage-tropic HIV entry into cells
CDw197	CCR7; CMKBR7; BLR2; EBI1	40 kD; CCR chemokine receptor family	T cells, dendritic cells	Cell surface receptor for chemokines ELC and SLC
CD200	OX-2	41 or 47 kD; Ig superfamily	B cells, CNS neurons, microglial cells	Unknown
CD201	EPC R; CCCA; CCD41; bA42O4.2	49 kD; CD1 MHC family	Endothelial cells	Binds protein C and mediates endothelial cell activation
CD202b	Tie2; tek	145 kD; Ig superfamily; receptor tyrosine kinase family	Endothelial cells, early hematopoietic cells	Role in vascular maturation and remodeling
CD203c	NPP3; PDNP3; PD-Iβ; B10; gp130RB13-6; ENPP3	270 kD; type II transmembrane molecule; ectonucleotide enzyme family	Basophils, mast cells	Ectoenzyme that cleaves phosphodiester and phosphosulfate bonds, including deoxynucleotides, nucleotide sugars, and NAD
CD204	Macrophage scavenger receptor 1; MSR1	220 kD; scavenger receptor family; collagen-like domain	Myeloid cells	Role in cellular internalization of oxidized low-density lipoproteins and many other molecules
CD205	DEC205; LY75; GP200-MR6	205 kD; mannose receptor family	Dendritic cells, B cells	Putative role in antigen uptake
CD206	Macrophage mannose receptor (MMR); MRC1	162 kD; mannose receptor family; C-type lectin family	Macrophages, immature dendritic cells	Binds high-mannose oligosaccharides on microbes; pattern recognition receptor of innate immune system
CD207	Langerin	40 kD; mannose receptor family; C-type lectin family	Langerhans cells	Antigen capture and routing to nonclassical antigen-processing pathway
CD208	Lysosome-associated membrane protein 3; DC-LAMP; TSC403	70–90 kD; lysosome-associated membrane protein (LAMP) family	Dendritic cells	Role in transfer of peptide-MHC class II molecules to the surface of dendritic cells

CD designation	Common synonyms	Molecular structure, Family	Main cellular expression	Known or proposed functions
CD209	Dendritic cell–specific ICAM3-grabbing nonintegrin (DCSIGN)	44 kD; mannose receptor family; C-type lectin	Dendritic cells	Binds ICAM-3 and high-mannose oligosaccharides; cell adhesion receptor mediating dendritic cell migration and T cell activation; HIV receptor
CDw210	IL-10 receptor α; IL10R	90–110 kD; type II cytokine receptor family	Hematopoietic cells	Subunit of IL-10 receptor; associates with IL-10Rβ
CD212	IL-12 receptor β1; IL12RB	Hematopoietin receptor superfamily	Hematopoietic cells	Subunit of the IL-12 receptor complex; associates with IL-10Rβ2
CD213a1	IL-13 receptor α1; IL-13Rα1; IL13RA1; IL13RA	65 kD; Ig superfamily	Broad	Subunit of IL-13 and IL-4 receptor complexes
CD213a2	IL-13 receptor α2; IL-13Rα2; IL-13R; IL13BP	56 kD; hematopoietin receptor superfamily	Broad	High-affinity, nonsignaling IL-13 decoy receptor
CDw217	IL-17 receptor; HIL-17R; VDw217; AW538159	120 kD; cytokine receptor	Hematopoietic cells	Binds and mediates biologic effects of IL-17
CD220	Insulin receptor; INSR	135 kD (α) and 90 kD (β) subunits; tyrosine kinase receptor family	Broad	Binds and mediates many biologic effects of insulin
CD221	Insulin-like growth factor 1 receptor; IGFR1; JTK13	80 kD (α) and 71 kD (β) subunits; tyrosine kinase receptor family	Broad	Binds insulin and IGF and induces DNA synthesis and differentiation; delivers cell survival signals
CD222	Insulin-like growth factor 2 receptor; IGF2R; IGFIIR; mannose-6 phosphate receptor; M6P-R; CIMPR; CI-MPR	250 kD; lectin	Broad	Internalization of IGF-II; internalization and sorting of lysosomal enzymes and other M6P-containing proteins
CD223	Lymphocyte activation gene 3; LAG3	Ig superfamily; CD4 related	Activated T cells and NK cells	Binds class II MHC; unknown function
CD224	γ Glutamyl transpeptidase; GGT, GGT1; EC2.3.2.2	62–68 kD and 22 kD subunits; ectoenzyme, peptidase family T3	Renal tubular cells, pancreas, epididymis, seminal vesicles, vascular endothelium, macrophages, activated T cells, subset of B cells	Role in γ glutamyl cycle involving the degradation and neosynthesis of glutathione
CD225	Interferon-induced transmembrane protein 1; LEU13	17 kD	Leukocytes, endothelial cells	Component of a multimeric complex involved in the transduction of antiproliferative and homotypic adhesion signals
CD226	DNAM-1; PTA1; TLiSA1	65 kD; Ig superfamily	T cells, NK cells, platelets, monocytes, subset of B cells, thymocytes, activated endothelial cells	Mediates cellular adhesion and activation; ligand unknown
CD227	MUC1; episialin; PUM; PEM; EMA; DF3 antigen; H23 antigen	300–700 kD; mucin	Glandular and ductal epithelial cells, human adenocarcinoma, activated T cells, activated monocytes, activated dendritic cells, some B cells	Cell-cell and cell-matrix adhesion; signal transduction; target for immunotherapy of tumors
CD228	Melanotransferrin; melanoma-associated antigen p97; MTF1; MAP97	97 kD; transferrin superfamily	Melanomas	Iron transport functions
CD229	Ly9	100, 120 kD; Ig superfamily; CD2/CD48/CD58 family	B cells, T cells, thymocytes	Putative adhesion functions
CD230	Prion protein (p27-30); CJD, PrP, PRIP, PrPc	27–30 kD; prion family; neuronal sialoglycoprotein	Broad	Cellular protein of unknown function; structural isoform is the transmissible agent causing spongiform encephalopathies

CD designation	Common synonyms	Molecular structure, Family	Main cellular expression	Known or proposed functions
CD231	TM4SF2; A15; TALLA-1; MXS1; CCG-B7; TALLA	150 kD; tetraspan (TM4SF) family	Neurons, neuroblastoma cells, T cell acute lymphoblastic leukemic cells	Unknown
CD232	Plexin C1; PLXN-C1; semaphorin receptor; VESPR	200 kD; plexin family	Neurons	Receptor for virally encoded semaphorins; regulation of cell dissociation and repulsion
CD233	Band 3; erythrocyte membrane protein band 3; AE1; SLC4A1; Diego blood group; EPB3	95–110 kD; anion exchanger family	Erythrocytes, renal tubular epithelial cells	Anion exchanger; attachment site for underlying cytoskeleton
CD234	Fy-glycoprotein; Duffy antigen; duffy antigen receptor for chemokines	35 kD; chemokine receptor family	Erythrocytes; endothelial cells	Bears the Duffy blood group antigens; nonspecific nonsignaling receptor for various chemokines; *Plasmodium vivax* and *Plasmodium knowlesi* receptor
CD235a	Glycophorin A; MN; GPA; MNS	31 kD; glycophorin A family; sialoglycoprotein	Erythrocytes	Prevention of red cell aggregation in the circulation; bears the antigenic determinants for the MN and Ss blood groups
CD235b	Glycophorin B; SS; MNS	24 kD; glycophorin A family; sialoglycoprotein	Erythrocytes	Bears the antigenic determinants for the MN and Ss blood groups
CD236	Glycophorin C/D	24 kD; sialoglycoprotein	Erythrocytes	Mutated form of glycophorin D bears Webb and Dutch blood group antigens; *Plasmodium falciparum* receptor
CD236R	Glycophorin C; GYPC; Gerbich blood group	32 kD; sialoglycoprotein	Erythrocytes	Bears the Gerbich blood group antigens; role in maintenance of the erythrocyte shape
CD238	Kell	93 kD; zinc metalloglycoproteins family	Erythrocytes	Bears the Kell blood group antigens
CD239	B cell adhesion molecule; B-CAM; Lutheran blood group; Auberger blood group	78–85 kD; Ig superfamily	Broad	Bears the Lutheran blood group antigens
CD240CE	Rhesus blood group; CcEe antigens; Rh30CE	30 kD	Erythrocytes	Rh Cc and Ee blood group antigens; associate with Rh50, CD47 and glycophorin B to form the Rh antigen; membrane transport function
CD240D	Rh30D; Rh protein, D antigen	30 kD	Erythrocytes	Major antigen of the Rh system; associates with Rh50, CD47, and glycophorin B to form the RhD group; membrane transport function
CD241	Rhesus blood group–associated glycoprotein RhAg; RH50A	50 kD	Erythrocytes	Role in transport of Rh antigen to cell surface of red blood cells
CD242	ICAM-4; Landsteiner-Wiener blood group	42 kD; ICAM family	Erythrocytes	Adhesion molecule; binds LFA-1; bears Landsteiner-Wiener blood group antigen
CD243	Multidrug resistance-1; MDR-1; P glycoprotein 1; P-GP, PGY1, ABC20, GP170	1170 kD; ATP-binding cassette (ABC) transporter family; MDR/TAP subfamily	Broad	ATP-dependent efflux pump for xenobiotic hydrophobic compounds (e.g., drugs); transporter in the blood-brain barrier
CD244	2B4; NAIL; p38	70 kD; Ig superfamily; CD2/CD48/CD58 family	NK cells, ~50% of $CD8^+$ T cells, $\gamma\delta$ T cells, subset of $CD4^+$ T cells, monocytes, basophils	High-affinity receptor for CD48; modulates various functions of NK cells

CD designation	Common synonyms	Molecular structure, Family	Main cellular expression	Known or proposed functions
CD245	p220/240; NPAT	220/240 kD	T cells	Cell cycle regulation
CD246	Anaplastic lymphoma kinase; Ki-1	177 kD; tyrosine kinase receptor family; insulin receptor subfamily	Brain, anaplastic lymphomas	Unknown; fusion protein with nucleolar phosphoprotein nucleophosmin (NPM) found in anaplastic lymphomas
CD247	Zeta chain; TCRζ	21–23 kD; ITAMs in cytoplasmic tail	T cells, NK cells	Signaling chain of TCR and NK cell–activating receptors

The complete listing of CD molecules is published in Mason D (ed). Leucocyte Typing VII. Oxford University Press, Oxford, 2002.

Current CD molecule information is also available in Shaw S, L Turni, and K Katz (eds). Protein Reviews on the Web: An International WWW Resource/Journal. http://www.ncbi.nlm.nih.gov/prow/

Additional details of the individual CD molecules may be found in Barclay AN, ML Birkeland, MH Brown, AD Beyers, SJ Davis, C Somoza, and AF Williams (eds). The Leukocyte Antigen Facts book, 2nd ed. Academic Press, New York, 1997.

*The small letters affixed to some CD numbers refer to complex CD molecules that are encoded by multiple genes or that belong to families of structurally related proteins. For instance, CD1a, CD1b, and CD1c are structurally related, but distinct forms of a β_2-microglobulin–associated nonpolymorphic protein.

†Antibodies that have been submitted recently or whose reactivity has not been fully confirmed are said to identify putative CD molecules, indicated with a "w" (for "workshop") designation.

Abbreviations: ADCC, antibody-dependent cell-mediated cytotoxicity; ADP, adenosine diphosphate; ATP, adenosine triphosphate; CEA, carcinoembryonic antigen; CR1 type 1 complement receptor; CTL, cytolytic T lymphocyte; ELAM, endothelial cell leukocyte adhesion molecule; GMP, granule membrane protein; GP, glycoprotein; HIV, human immunodeficiency virus; ICAM, intercellular adhesion molecule; IFN, interferon; Ig, immunoglobulin; IL, interleukin; kD, kilodalton; ITAM, immunoreceptor tyrosine-based activation motif; ITIM, immunoreceptor tyrosine-based inhibition motif; LAMP, lysosomal membrane-associated glycoprotein; LFA, lymphocyte function-associated antigen; LPS, lipopolysaccharide; MAC membrane attack complex; MadCAM, mucosal addressin cell adhesion molecule; MHC, major histocompatibility complex; NAD, nicotinamide adenine dinucleotide; NK, natural killer; PECAM, platelet endothelial cell adhesion molecule; PI, phosphatidylinositol; TAC, T cell activation antigen; TCR, T cell receptor; TGF, transforming growth factor; TNF, tumor necrosis factor; VCAM, vascular cell adhesion molecule; VLA, very late activation

Appendix **III**

Laboratory Techniques Commonly Used in Immunology

Many laboratory techniques that are routine in research and clinical settings are based on the use of antibodies. In addition, many of the techniques of modern molecular biology have provided invaluable information about the immune system. We have mentioned these techniques often throughout the book. In this appendix, we describe the principles underlying some of the most commonly used laboratory methods in immunology. Details of how to carry out various assays may be found in laboratory manuals.

Laboratory Methods Using Antibodies

The exquisite specificity of antibodies for particular antigens makes antibodies valuable reagents for detecting, purifying, and quantitating antigens. Because antibodies can be produced against virtually any type of macromolecule and small chemical, antibody-based techniques may be used to study virtually any type of molecule in solution or in cells. The method for producing monoclonal antibodies (see Chapter 3, Box 3–1) has greatly increased our ability to generate antibodies of almost any desired specificity. Historically, many of the uses of antibody depended on the ability of antibody and specific antigen to form large immune complexes, either in solution or in gels, that could be detected by various optical methods. These methods were of great importance in early studies but have now almost entirely been replaced by simpler methods based on immobilized antibodies or antigens.

Quantitation of Antigen by Immunoassays

Immunologic methods of quantifying antigen concentration provide exquisite sensitivity and specificity and have become standard techniques for both research and clinical applications. All modern immunochemical methods of quantitation are based on having a pure antigen or antibody whose quantity can be measured by an indicator molecule. When the indicator molecule is labeled with a radioisotope, as first introduced by Rosalyn Yalow and colleagues, it may be quantified by instruments that detect radioactive decay events; the assay is called a **radioimmunoassay (RIA).** When the indicator molecule is covalently coupled to an enzyme, it may be quantified by determining with a spectrophotometer the rate at which the enzyme converts a clear substrate to a colored product; the assay is called an **enzyme-linked immunosorbent assay (ELISA).** Several variations of RIA and ELISA exist, but the most commonly used version is the sandwich assay (Fig. A–1). The sandwich assay uses two different antibodies reactive with different epitopes on the antigen whose concentration needs to be determined. A fixed quantity of one antibody is attached to a series of replicate solid supports, such as plastic microtiter wells. Test solutions containing antigen at an unknown concentration or a series of standard solutions with known concentrations of antigen are added to the wells and allowed to bind. Unbound antigen is removed by washing, and the second antibody, which is enzyme linked or radiolabeled, is allowed to bind. The antigen serves as a bridge, so the more antigen in the test or standard solutions, the more enzyme-linked or radiolabeled second antibody will bind. The results from the standard solutions are used to construct a binding curve for second antibody as a function of antigen concentration, from which the quantities of antigen in the test solutions may be inferred. When this test is performed with two monoclonal antibodies, it is essential that these antibodies see nonoverlapping determinants on the antigen; otherwise, the second antibody cannot bind.

In an important clinical variant of immunobinding assays, samples from patients may be tested for the presence of antibodies that are specific for a microbial antigen (e.g., antibodies reactive with proteins from

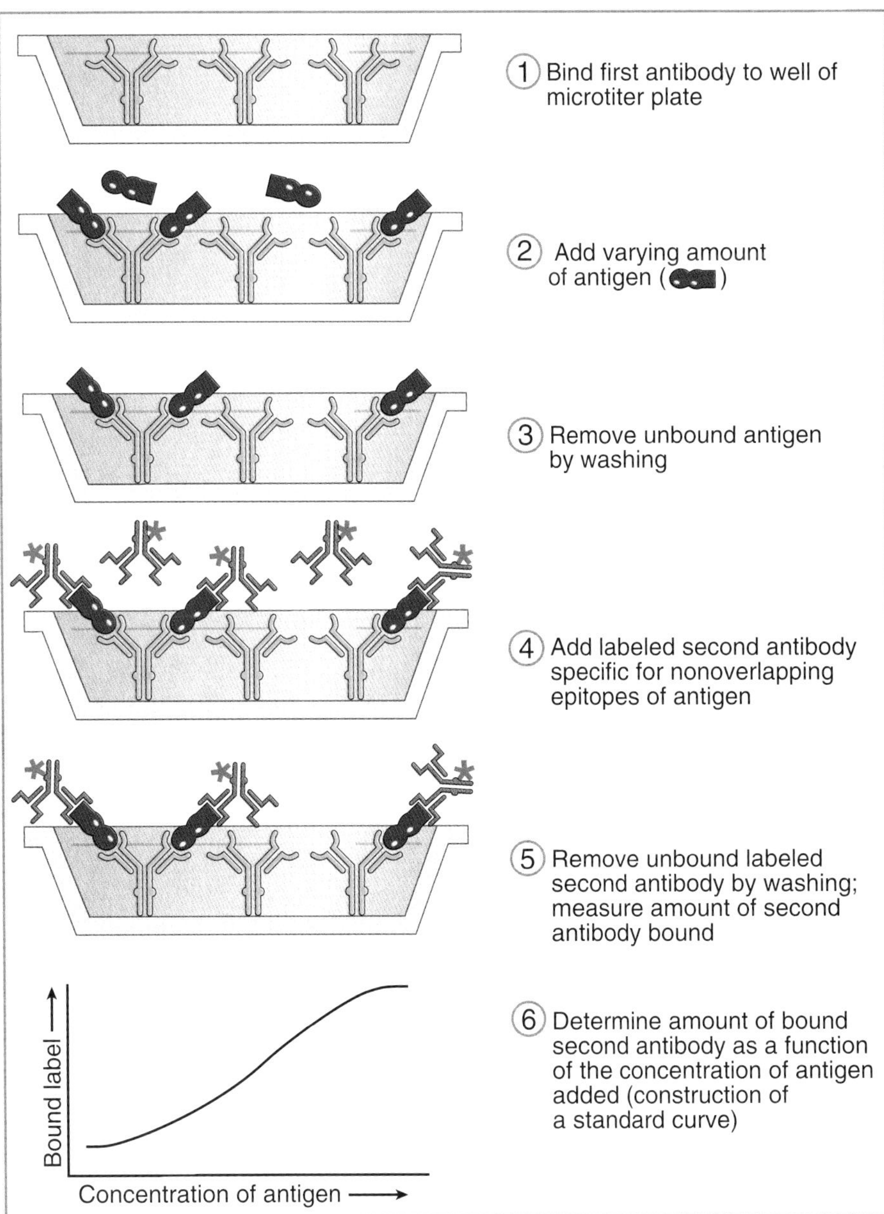

Figure A–1 Sandwich enzyme-linked immunosorbent assay or radioimmunoassay.
A fixed amount of one immobilized antibody is used to capture an antigen. The binding of a second, labeled antibody that recognizes a nonoverlapping determinant on the antigen will increase as the concentration of antigen increases and thus allow quantification of the antigen.

human immunodeficiency virus [HIV] or hepatitis B virus) as indicators of infection. In this case, a saturating quantity of antigen is added to replicate wells containing plate-bound antibody, or the antigen is attached directly to the plate, and serial dilutions of the patient's serum are then allowed to bind. The amount of the patient's antibody bound to the immobilized antigen is determined by use of an enzyme-linked or radiolabeled second antihuman immunoglobulin (Ig) antibody.

Purification and Identification of Proteins

Antibodies can be used to purify proteins from solutions and to identify and characterize proteins. Two commonly used methods to purify proteins are immunoprecipitation and affinity chromatography. Western blotting is a widely used technique to determine the presence and size of a protein in a biologic sample.

Immunoprecipitation and Affinity Chromatography

Immunoprecipitation is a technique in which an antibody specific for one protein antigen in a mixture of proteins is used to isolate the specific antigen from the mixture (Fig. A–2A). In most modern procedures, the antibody is attached to a solid-phase particle (e.g., an agarose bead) either by direct chemical coupling or indirectly. Indirect coupling may be achieved by means of an attached anti-antibody, such as rabbit antimouse Ig antibody, or by means of some other protein with specific affinity for the Fc portion of Ig molecules, such as protein A or protein G from staphylococcal bacteria. After the antibody-coated beads are incubated with the solution of antigen, unbound molecules are separated from the bead-antibody-antigen complex by washing. Specific antigen is then released (eluted) from the antibody by changing the pH or by other solvent conditions that reduce the affinity of binding. The purified antigen can then be analyzed by conventional chemical techniques. Alternatively, a small amount of radiolabeled protein can be purified and the characteristics of the macromolecule inferred from the behavior of the radioactive label in analytical separation techniques, such as sodium dodecyl sulfate–polyacrylamide gel electrophoresis (SDS-PAGE) or isoelectric focusing.

Affinity chromatography, like immunoprecipitation, uses antibodies attached to an insoluble support to remove and thereby purify antigens from a solution (Fig. A–2B). Antibodies specific for the desired antigen are attached to a solid support, such as agarose beads packed into a column, either by direct coupling or indirectly, as described for immunoprecipitation. A complex mixture of antigens is passed through the beads to allow the antigen that is recognized by the antibody to bind. Unbound molecules are washed away, and the bound antigen is eluted by changing the pH or by exposure to a chemical that breaks the antigen-antibody bonds. The same method may be used to purify antibodies from culture supernatants or natural fluids, such as serum, by first attaching the antigen to beads and passing the supernatants or serum through.

Western Blotting

Western blotting (Fig. A–3) is used to determine the relative quantity and the molecular weight of a protein within a mixture of proteins or other molecules. The mixture is first subjected to analytical separation, typically by SDS-PAGE, so that the final positions of different proteins in the gel are a function of their molecular size. The array of separated proteins is then transferred from the separating polyacrylamide gel to a support membrane by capillary action (blotting) or by electrophoresis such that the membrane acquires a replica of the array of separated macromolecules present in the gel. SDS is displaced from the protein during the transfer process, and native antigenic determinants are often regained as the protein refolds. The position of the protein antigen on the membrane can then be detected by binding of labeled antibody specific for that protein, thus providing information about antigen size and quantity. If radiolabeled antibody probes are used, the proteins on the blot are visualized by autoradiographic exposure of film. More recently, antibody probes are labeled with enzymes that generate chemiluminescent signals and leave images on photographic film. The sensitivity and specificity of this technique can be increased by starting with immunoprecipitated proteins instead of crude protein mixtures. This sequential technique is especially useful for detecting protein-protein interactions. For example, the physical association of two different proteins in the membrane of a lymphocyte can be established by immunoprecipitating a membrane extract by use of an antibody specific for one of the proteins and probing a Western blot of the immunoprecipitate by use of a labeled antibody specific for the second protein that may have been co-immunoprecipitated along with the first protein. A variation of the Western blot technique is routinely used to detect the presence of anti-HIV antibodies in patients' sera. In this case, a defined mixture of HIV proteins is separated by SDS-PAGE and blotted onto a membrane, and the membrane is incubated with dilutions of the test serum. The blot is then probed with a second labeled antihuman Ig to detect the presence of HIV-specific antibodies that were in the serum and bound to the HIV proteins.

The technique of transferring proteins from a gel to a membrane is called Western blotting as a biochemist's joke. Southern is the last name of the scientist who first blotted DNA from a separating gel to a membrane, a technique since called Southern blotting. By analogy, Northern blotting was applied to the technique of transferring RNA from a gel to a membrane, and Western blotting was applied to protein transfer. A more detailed description of Southern and Northern blotting is presented later.

Labeling and Detection of Antigens in Cells and Tissues

Antibodies specific for antigens expressed on or in particular cell types are commonly used to identify these cells in tissues or cell suspensions and to separate these

(A) **Immunoprecipitation**

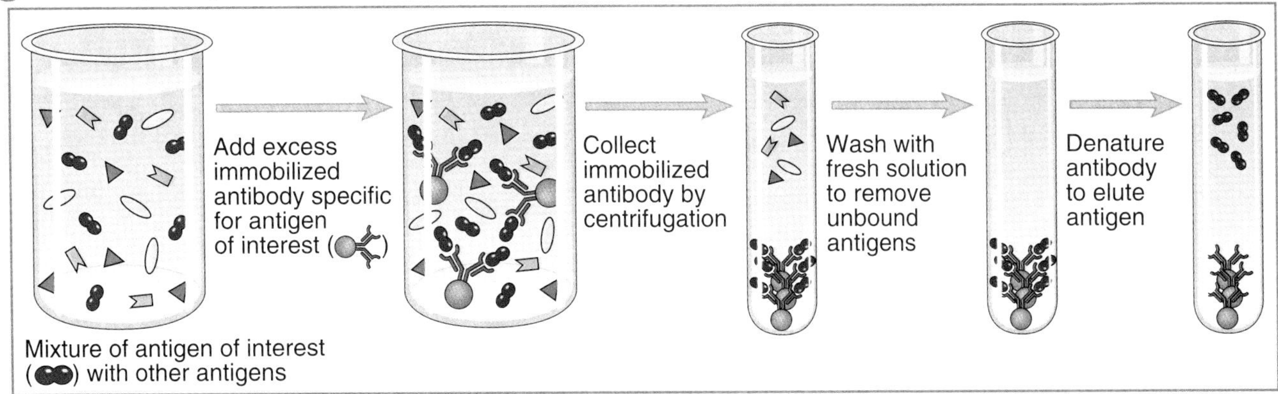

(B) **Affinity chromatography**

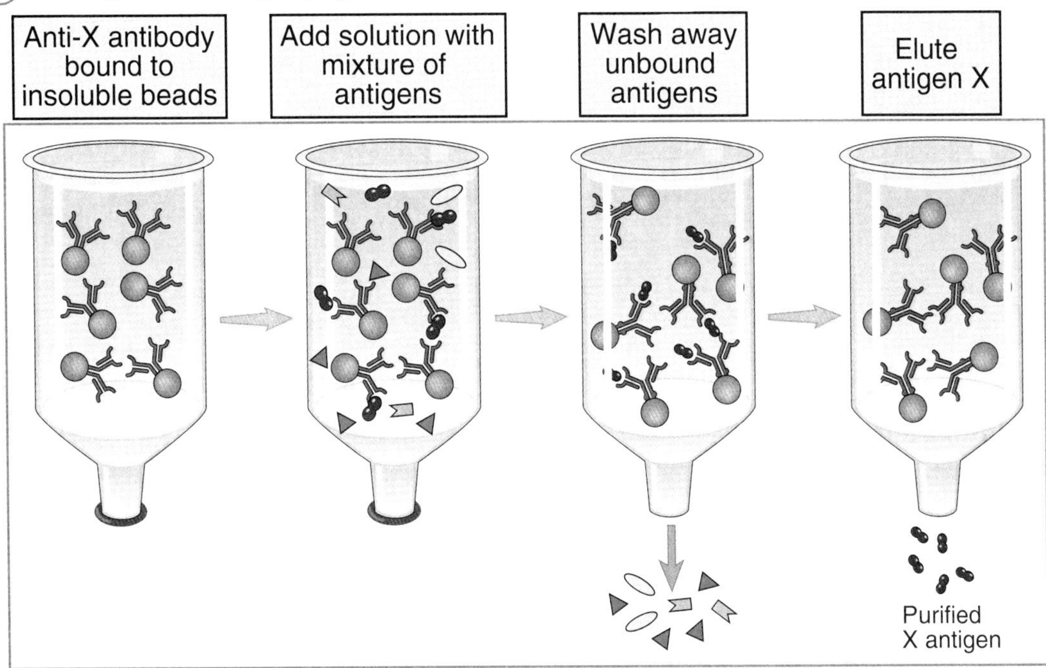

Figure A–2 Isolation of an antigen by immunoprecipitation or affinity chromatography.

A. A particular antigen can be purified from a mixture of antigens in serum or other solutions by adding antibodies specific to the antigen, which are bound to insoluble beads. Unbound antigens are then washed away, and the desired antigen is recovered by changing the pH or ionic strength of the solution so that the affinity of antibody-antigen binding is lowered. Immunoprecipitation can be used as a means of purification, as a means of quantification, or as a means of identification of an antigen. Antigens purified by immunoprecipitation are often analyzed by sodium dodecyl sulfate–polyacrylamide gel electrophoresis.

B. Affinity chromatography is based on the same principle as immunoprecipitation, except that the antibody is fixed to an insoluble matrix or gel, usually in a column. The method is often used to isolate soluble antigens (shown) or antibodies specific for an immobilized antigen.

cells from mixed populations. In these methods, the antibody can be radiolabeled, enzyme linked, or, most commonly, fluorescently labeled, and a detection system is used that can identify the bound antibody.

Flow Cytometry and Fluorescence-Activated Cell Sorting

The tissue lineage, maturation stage, or activation status of a cell can often be determined by analyzing the cell surface or intracellular expression of different molecules. This technique is commonly done by staining the cell with fluorescently labeled probes that are specific for those molecules and measuring the quantity of fluorescence emitted by the cell (Fig. A–4). The flow cytometer is a specialized instrument that can detect fluorescence on individual cells in a suspension and thereby determine the number of cells expressing the molecule to which a fluorescent probe binds. Suspensions of cells are incubated with fluorescently

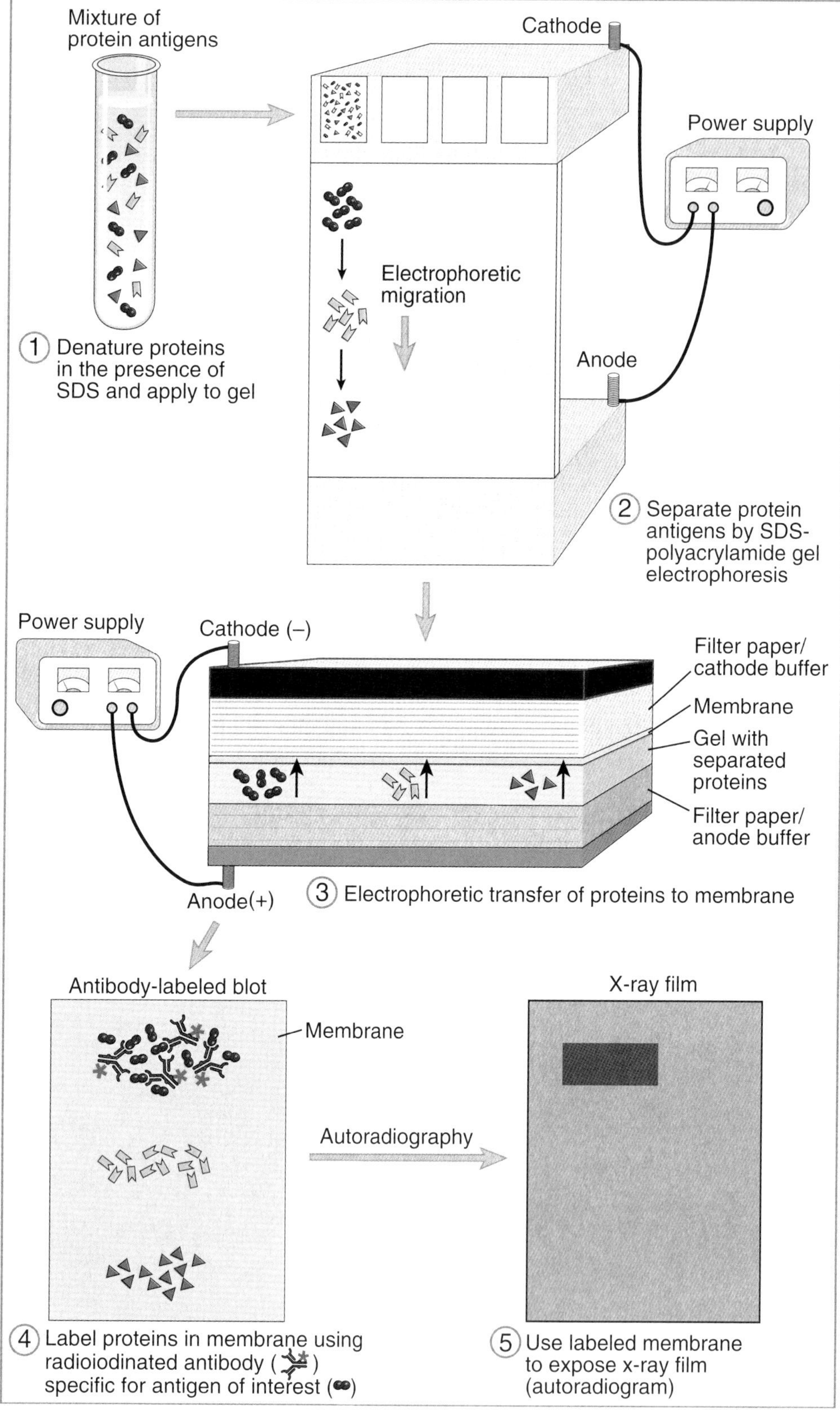

Figure A–3 Characterization of antigens by Western blotting.

Protein antigens, separated by sodium dodecyl sulfate (SDS)–polyacrylamide gel electrophoresis and transferred to a membrane, can be labeled with radioactive or (not shown) enzyme-coupled antibodies. Analysis of an antigen by Western blotting provides information similar to that obtained from immunoprecipitation followed by polyacrylamide gel electrophoresis. Some antibodies work only in one or the other technique.

labeled probes, and the amount of probe bound by each cell in the population is measured by passing the cells one at a time through a fluorimeter with a laser-generated incident beam. The relative amounts of a particular molecule on different cell populations can be compared by staining each population with the same probe and determining the amount of fluorescence emitted. In preparation for flow cytometric analysis, cell suspensions are stained with the fluorescent probes of choice. Most often, these probes are

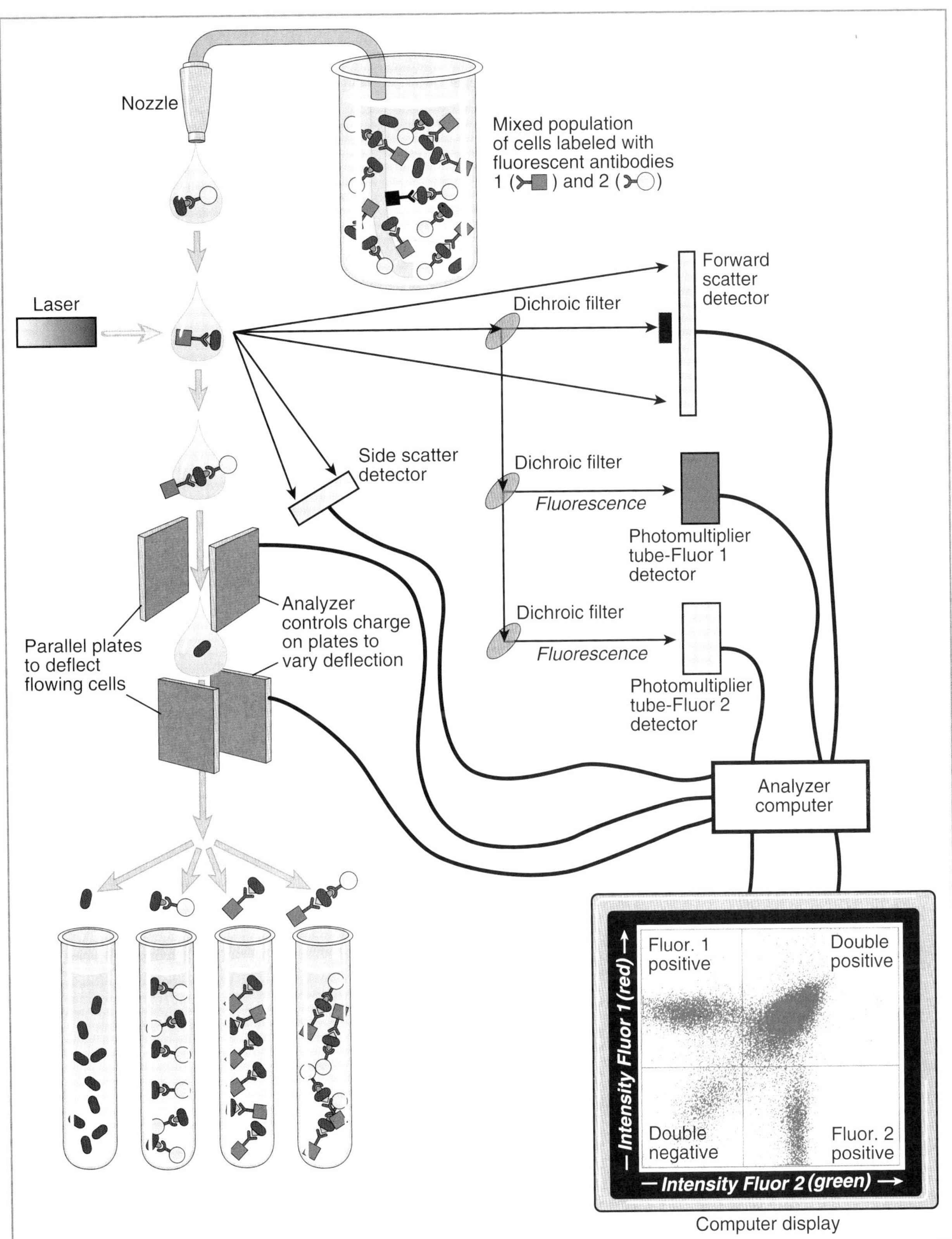

Figure A–4 Principle of flow cytometry and fluorescence-activated cell sorting. The incident laser beam is of a designated wavelength, and the light that emerges from the sample is analyzed for forward and side scatter as well as fluorescent light of two or more wavelengths that depend on the fluorochrome labels attached to the antibodies. The separation depicted here is based on two antigenic markers (two-color sorting). Modern instruments can routinely analyze and separate cell populations on the basis of three or more different colored probes.

fluorochrome-labeled antibodies specific for a cell surface molecule. Alternatively, cytoplasmic molecules can be stained by temporarily permeabilizing cells and permitting the labeled antibodies to enter through the plasma membrane. In addition to antibodies, various fluorescent indicators of cytoplasmic ion concentrations and reduction-oxidation potential can also be detected by flow cytometry. Cell cycle studies can be performed by flow cytometric analysis of cells stained with fluorescent DNA-binding probes such as propidium iodide. Modern flow cytometers can routinely detect three or more different-colored fluorescent signals, each attached to a different antibody or other probe. This technique permits simultaneous analysis of the expression of many different combinations of molecules by a cell. In addition to detecting fluorescent signals, flow cytometers also measure the forward and side light-scattering properties of cells, which reflect cell size and internal complexity, respectively. This information is often used to distinguish different cell types. For example, compared with lymphocytes, neutrophils cause greater side scatter because of their cytoplasmic granules, and monocytes cause greater forward scatter because of their size.

A fluorescence-activated cell sorter (FACS) is an adaptation of the flow cytometer that allows one to separate cell populations according to which and how much fluorescent probe they bind. This technique is accomplished by differentially deflecting the cells with electromagnetic fields whose strength and direction are varied according to the measured intensity of the fluorescence signal. A more rapid but less rigorous separation can be accomplished without a FACS by allowing cells to attach to antibodies bound to plates (panning) or to magnetic beads that can be pulled out of solution by a strong magnet.

Immunofluorescence and Immunohistochemistry

Antibodies can be used to identify the anatomic distribution of an antigen within a tissue or within compartments of a cell. To do so, the tissue or cell is incubated with an antibody that is labeled with a fluorochrome or enzyme, and the position of the label, determined with a suitable microscope, is used to infer the position of the antigen. In the earliest version of this method, called immunofluorescence, the antibody was labeled with a fluorescent dye and allowed to bind to a monolayer of cells or to a frozen section of a tissue. The stained cells or tissues were examined with a fluorescence microscope to locate the antibody. Although sensitive, the fluorescence microscope is not an ideal tool for identifying the detailed structures of the cell or tissue because of a low signal-to-noise ratio. This problem has been overcome by new technologies including confocal microscopy, which uses optical sectioning technology to filter out unfocused fluorescent light, and two-photon microscopy, which prevents out-of-focus light from forming. Alternatively, antibodies may be coupled to enzymes that convert colorless substrates to colored insoluble substances that precipitate at the position of the enzyme. A conventional light microscope may then be used to localize the antibody in a stained cell or tissue. The most common variant of this method uses the enzyme horseradish peroxidase, and the method is commonly referred to as the immunoperoxidase technique. Another commonly used enzyme is alkaline phosphatase. Different antibodies coupled to different enzymes may be used in conjunction to produce simultaneous two-color localizations of different antigens. In other variations, antibody can be coupled to an electron-dense probe such as colloidal gold, and the location of antibody can be determined subcellularly by means of an electron microscope, a technique called immunoelectron microscopy. Different-sized gold particles have been used for simultaneous localization of different antigens at the ultrastructural level.

In all immunomicroscopic methods, signals may be enhanced by use of sandwich techniques. For example, instead of attaching horseradish peroxidase to a specific mouse antibody directed against the antigen of interest, it can be attached to a second anti-antibody (e.g., rabbit antimouse Ig antibody) that is used to bind to the first, unlabeled antibody. When the label is attached directly to the specific, primary antibody, the method is referred to as direct; when the label is attached to a secondary or even tertiary antibody, the method is indirect. In some cases, molecules other than antibody can be used in indirect methods. For example, staphylococcal protein A, which binds to IgG, or avidin, which binds to primary antibodies labeled with biotin, can be coupled to fluorochromes or enzymes.

Measurement of Antigen-Antibody Interactions

In many situations, it is important to know the affinity of an antibody for an antigen. For example, the usefulness of a monoclonal antibody as an experimental or therapeutic reagent depends on its affinity. Antibody affinities for antigen can be measured directly for small antigens (e.g., haptens) by a method called **equilibrium dialysis** (Fig. A–5). In this method, a solution of antibody is confined within a "semipermeable" membrane of porous cellulose and immersed in a solution containing the antigen. (Semipermeable in this context means that small molecules, such as antigen, can pass freely through the membrane pores but that macromolecules, such as antibody, cannot.) If no antibody is present within the membrane-bound compartment, the antigen in the bathing solution enters until the concentration of antigen within the membrane-bound compartment becomes exactly the same as that outside. Another way to view the system is that at dynamic equilibrium, antigen enters and leaves the membrane-bound compartment at exactly the same rate. However, when antibody is present inside the membrane, the net amount of antigen inside the membrane at equilibrium increases by the quantity that is bound to antibody. This phenomenon occurs because only unbound antigen can diffuse across the membrane, and at equilibrium,

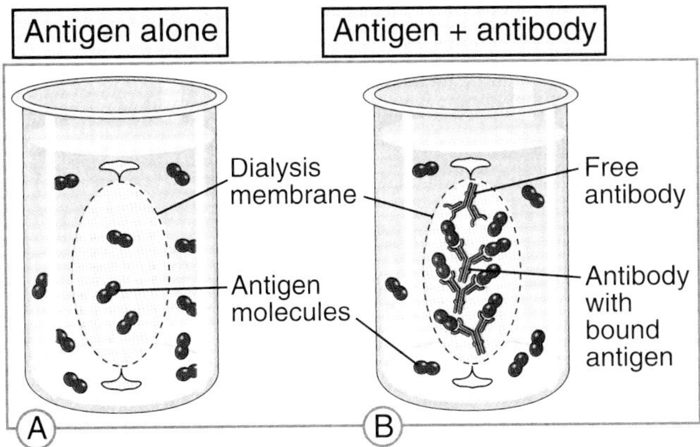

Figure A–5 Analysis of antigen-antibody binding by equilibrium dialysis.

In the presence of antibody (B), the amount of antigen within the dialysis membrane is increased compared with the absence of antibody (A). As described in the text, this difference, caused by antibody binding of antigen, can be used to measure the affinity of the antibody for the antigen. This experiment can be performed only when the antigen is a small molecule (e.g., a hapten) capable of freely crossing the dialysis membrane.

it is the unbound concentration of antigen that must be identical inside and outside the membrane. The extent of the increase in antigen inside the membrane depends on the antigen concentration, on the antibody concentration, and on the dissociation constant (K_d) of the binding interaction. By measuring the antigen and antibody concentrations, by spectroscopy or by other means, K_d can be calculated.

An alternative way to determine K_d is by measuring the rates of antigen-antibody complex formation and dissociation. These rates depend, in part, on the concentrations of antibody and antigen and on the affinity of the interaction. All parameters except the concentrations can be summarized as rate constants, and both the **on-rate constant** (K_{on}) and the **off-rate constant** (K_{off}) can be calculated experimentally by determining the concentrations and the actual rates of association or dissociation, respectively. The ratio of K_{off}/K_{on} allows one to cancel out all the parameters not related to affinity and is exactly equal to the dissociation constant K_d. Thus, one can measure K_d at equilibrium by equilibrium dialysis or calculate K_d from rate constants measured under nonequilibrium conditions.

Analysis of Gene Structure and Expression

Many of the advances in immunology during the last two decades have been a direct result of the advent of powerful techniques for characterizing the structure and expression of genes, synthesizing genes at will, and manipulating genes in cells and animals. In the following section, we outline some of the molecular genetic techniques that are widely used to study the immune system.

Southern Blot Hybridization

Southern blot hybridization, introduced by E. M. Southern, is used to characterize the organization of DNA surrounding a specific nucleic acid sequence, such as a particular gene. In a typical experiment, genomic DNA is chemically extracted from the nuclei of isolated cells or from whole tissues. At this point, the DNA will be present in extremely long segments and must be broken down into small fragments for analysis. This digestion is accomplished by enzymatic cleavage with restriction endonucleases, which cleave double-stranded DNA only at positions of particular symmetric nucleotide sequences, usually about 6 bp in length. Such sequences are called restriction sites and are present at the same positions in every cell, barring somatic mutation or DNA rearrangement. Complete digestion with a particular enzyme leads to cleavage of the genomic DNA, which gives rise to an array of DNA fragments ranging from about 0.5 to 10 kb in size. Different restriction endonucleases produce different arrays of restriction fragments, but each enzyme generally produces the same fragments from the DNA of every cell from an individual. Such is not the case, of course, when one examines genes that rearrange in different ways in different clones of cells, such as the Ig and T cell receptor genes.

To analyze the fragments, the digested DNA is separated according to size by electrophoresis in an agarose gel. The separated fragments are transferred by capillary action (blotting) from the gel to a membrane of nitrocellulose or nylon. Each fragment is then attached in place to the membrane by heating or ultraviolet irradiation. The net result is that the array of fragments is arranged by size on the membrane. Any particular nucleic acid sequence, such as a gene of interest, will be present on one or a few unique-sized fragments, depending only on the choice of restriction endonuclease and the distances between the relevant restriction sites that flank the gene or are located within the gene. The analysis is completed by ascertaining the size of the restriction fragment that contains the gene of interest, which is accomplished by nucleic acid hybridization. Double-stranded DNA can be "melted" into single-stranded DNA by changing the temperature and solvent conditions. When the temperature is lowered, single-stranded DNA will reanneal to form double-stranded DNA. The rate at which reannealing of a sequence occurs is determined by the concentration of DNA containing complementary nucleic acid sequences present in the system. In the Southern blot hybridization technique, the DNA on the membrane is melted and then allowed to reanneal in the presence of a solution containing a large excess of single-stranded DNA (probe) with a sequence complementary to the gene of interest. The probe is typically labeled with radioactive phosphorus (e.g., ^{32}P). It preferentially anneals only to the melted DNA on the membrane that contains the complementary sequence. After excess probe is removed by washing, the location of the bound probe is determined by autoradiography and compared with the positions of DNA fragments of known size.

Restriction sites are generally located at the same positions in the genomes of all individuals of a species. On occasion, this generalization is not true, and a particular restriction site is present only in or near some allelic forms of a gene. This variability in the presence of a particular restriction site leads to variability in the length of the restriction fragment that is detected by Southern blot hybridization if a probe is used that hybridizes near the variable restriction site. The length of the fragment is inherited as a mendelian allele, and its variation among individuals is described as a restriction fragment length polymorphism (RFLP). Southern blotting for RFLPs is now commonly used to study the inheritance of nearby (linked) genes.

Northern Blot Hybridization and RNase Protection Assay

Nucleic acid electrophoresis, blotting, and hybridization with DNA probes have also been used to analyze messenger RNA (mRNA) molecules. In this case, mRNA is isolated from the cell of interest and subjected to electrophoresis without digestion; mRNA is already single stranded, and the gel electrophoresis is run under denaturing conditions to prevent internal hybridization. The position of probe binding can indicate the size of the mRNA (rather than the size of a restriction fragment of DNA), and the extent of probe binding correlates with the abundance of mRNA present in the cell. This technique for RNA analysis is now universally referred to as Northern blotting to contrast it with Southern blotting for analysis of DNA.

A more sensitive technique for the detection of mRNA transcribed from defined genes is the RNase protection assay. In this technique, cellular RNA is hybridized with an excess of a radioactively labeled RNA probe of defined length that is complementary to part of the sequence of a gene of interest. RNase is then added to the RNA mixture to digest only single-stranded RNA. The binding of the RNA probe to mRNA from the cell forms double-stranded RNA duplexes that are protected from digestion by the RNase. After digestion of single-stranded cellular and unhybridized probe RNA, the radioactively labeled RNA duplexes are separated by PAGE and visualized by autoradiography. The predicted position of the radioactive band on the gel, corresponding to a particular mRNA, will be determined by the length of the RNA probe, and the intensity of the band will correspond to the amount of the specific mRNA in the original sample. Multiple RNA probes of different lengths, each complementary to a different gene, are commonly used to detect the presence and quantity of several different mRNAs in a sample simultaneously. For example, the relative amounts of multiple cytokine gene mRNAs made by a helper T cell population can be determined in one RNase protection assay.

Polymerase Chain Reaction

The polymerase chain reaction (PCR) is a rapid and simple method for copying and amplifying specific DNA sequences up to about 1 kb in length. PCR is widely used as a preparative and analytical technique in all branches of molecular biology. To use this method, it is necessary to know the sequence of a short region of DNA on each end of the larger sequence that is to be copied; these short sequences are used to specify oligonucleotide primers. The method consists of repetitive cycles of DNA melting, DNA annealing, and DNA synthesis (Fig. A–6). Double-stranded DNA containing the sequence to be copied and amplified is mixed with a large molar excess of two single-stranded DNA oligonucleotides (the primers). The first primer is identical to the 5′ end of the sense strand of the DNA to be copied, and the second primer is identical to the antisense strand at the 3′ end of the sequence. (Because double-stranded DNA is antiparallel, the second primer is also the inverted complement of the sense strand.) The PCR reaction is initiated by melting the double-stranded DNA at high temperature and cooling the mixture to allow DNA annealing. During annealing, the first primer (present in large molar excess) will hybridize to the 3′ end of the antisense strand, and the second primer (also present in large molar excess) will hybridize to the 3′ end of the sense strand. The annealed mixture is incubated with DNA polymerase I and all four deoxynucleotide triphosphates (A, T, G, and C) to allow new DNA to be synthesized. DNA polymerase I will extend the 3′ end of each bound primer to synthesize the complement of the single-stranded DNA templates. Specifically, the original sense strand is used as a template to make a new antisense strand, and the original antisense strand is used as a template to make a new sense strand. This ends cycle 1. Cycle 2 is initiated when the reaction mixture is remelted and then allowed to reanneal with the primers. In the DNA synthetic step of the second cycle, each strand synthesized in the first cycle serves as an additional template after having hybridized with the appropriate primers. (It follows that the number of templates in the reaction doubles with each cycle, hence the name "chain reaction.") The second cycle is completed when DNA polymerase I extends the primers to synthesize the complement of the templates. PCR reactions can be conducted for 20 or more cycles, with the sequence flanked by the primers doubled at each step. These reactions are routinely automated by temperature-controlled cyclers to regulate melting, annealing, and DNA synthesis and with a DNA polymerase I enzyme isolated from thermostable bacteria that can withstand the temperatures used for melting of DNA.

PCR has many uses. For example, by choosing suitable primers, exon 2 of an unknown HLA-DR β allele (i.e., the exon that encodes the polymorphic β1 protein domain) can be amplified, the amplified DNA ligated into a suitable vector, and the DNA sequence determined without ever isolating the original gene from genomic DNA. This objective was the original purpose

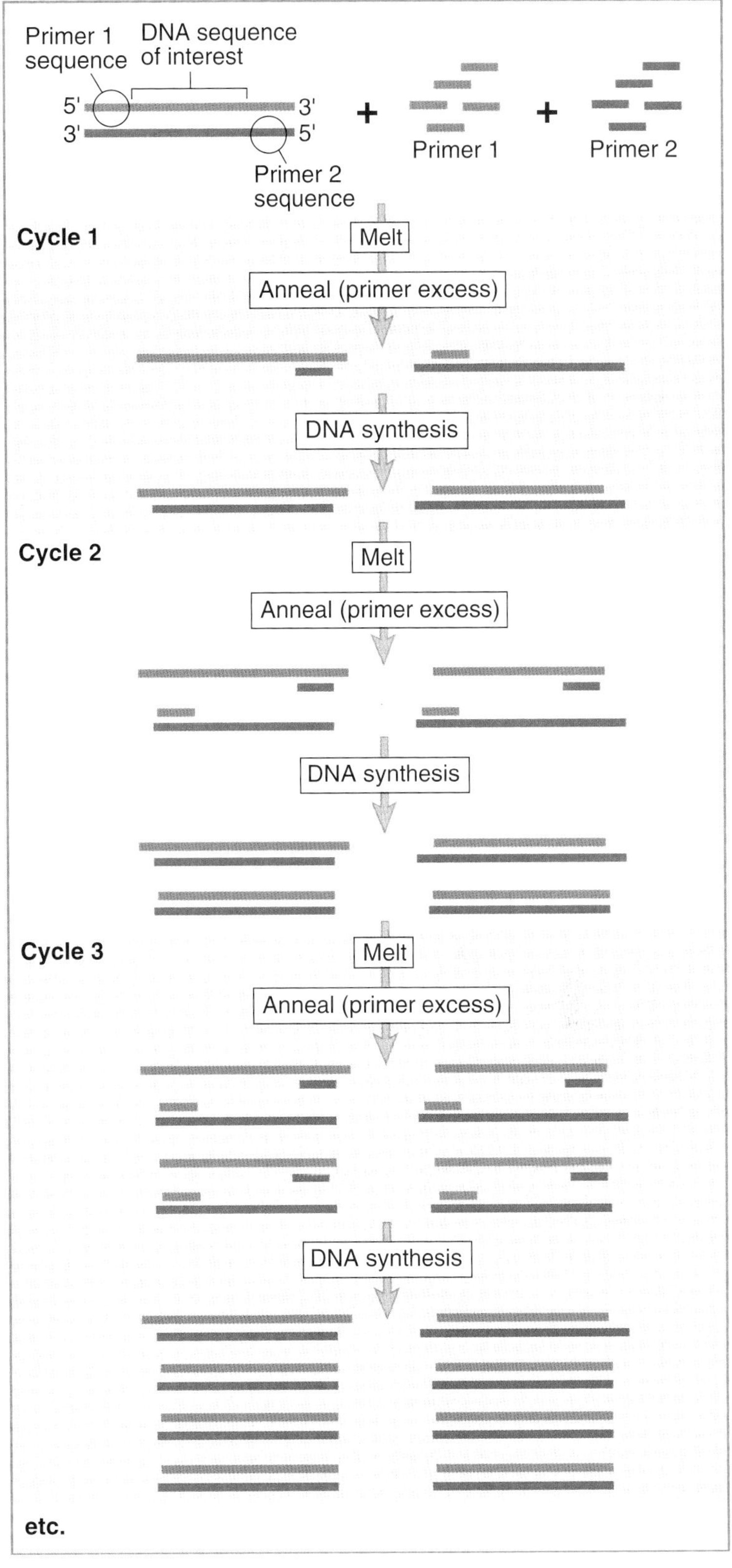

Figure A–6 Polymerase chain reaction. This technique is used to amplify the number of copies of a specific sequence of DNA for either preparative or analytical purposes.

for which PCR was invented. PCR is also widely used for the cloning of known genes or genes related to known genes (e.g., by choosing primers from highly conserved regions of a gene family). PCR can be used to detect or, in some cases, even to quantify the presence of particular DNA sequences in a sample (e.g., the presence of viral sequences in a clinical specimen). Because PCR can amplify DNA only when the two primers are near each other (i.e., within about 1 kb), the technique is useful to detect a specific gene recombination event by choosing primers complementary to sequences that are near one another only in the rearranged DNA. This approach is used to detect antigen receptor gene recombination events and chromosomal translocations. In the reverse transcriptase–PCR (RT-PCR) method, mRNA transcripts of a particular gene are detected by first using reverse transcriptase to make a complementary DNA copy of the mRNA before PCR amplification. Relative quantification of RNA between samples can be achieved by an adaptation of RT-PCR called real-time RT-PCR, in which fluorescent probes are used to follow the accumulation of amplified product during each PCR cycle (i.e., in real time) as opposed to the end point detection by conventional quantitative PCR methods.

Transgenic Mice and Targeted Gene Knockouts

Two important methods for studying the functional effects of specific gene products *in vivo* are the creation of transgenic mice that overexpress a particular gene in a defined tissue and the creation of gene knockout mice, in which a targeted disruption is used to ablate the function of a particular gene. Both techniques have been widely used to analyze many biologic phenomena, including the maturation, activation, and tolerance of lymphocytes.

To create transgenic mice, foreign DNA sequences, called transgenes, are introduced into the pronuclei of fertilized mouse eggs, and the eggs are implanted into the oviducts of pseudopregnant females. Usually, if a few hundred copies of a gene are injected into pronuclei, about 25% of the mice that are born are transgenic. One to 50 copies of the transgene insert in tandem into a random site of breakage in a chromosome and are subsequently inherited as a simple mendelian trait. Because integration usually occurs before DNA replication, most (about 75%) of the transgenic pups carry the transgene in all their cells, including germ cells. In most cases, integration of the foreign DNA does not disrupt endogenous gene function. Also, each founder mouse carrying the transgene is a heterozygote, from which homozygous lines can be bred.

The great value of transgenic technology is that it can be used to express genes in particular tissues by attaching coding sequences of the gene to regulatory sequences that normally drive the expression of genes selectively in that tissue. For instance, lymphoid promoters and enhancers can be used to overexpress genes, such as rearranged antigen receptor genes, in lymphocytes, and the insulin promoter can be used to express genes in the β cells of pancreatic islets. Examples of the utility of these methods for studying the immune system are mentioned in many chapters of this book. Transgenes can also be expressed under the control of promoter elements that respond to drugs or hormones, such as tetracycline or estrogens. In these cases, transcription of the transgene can be controlled at will by administration of the inducing agent.

A powerful method for developing animal models of single-gene disorders, and the most definitive way of

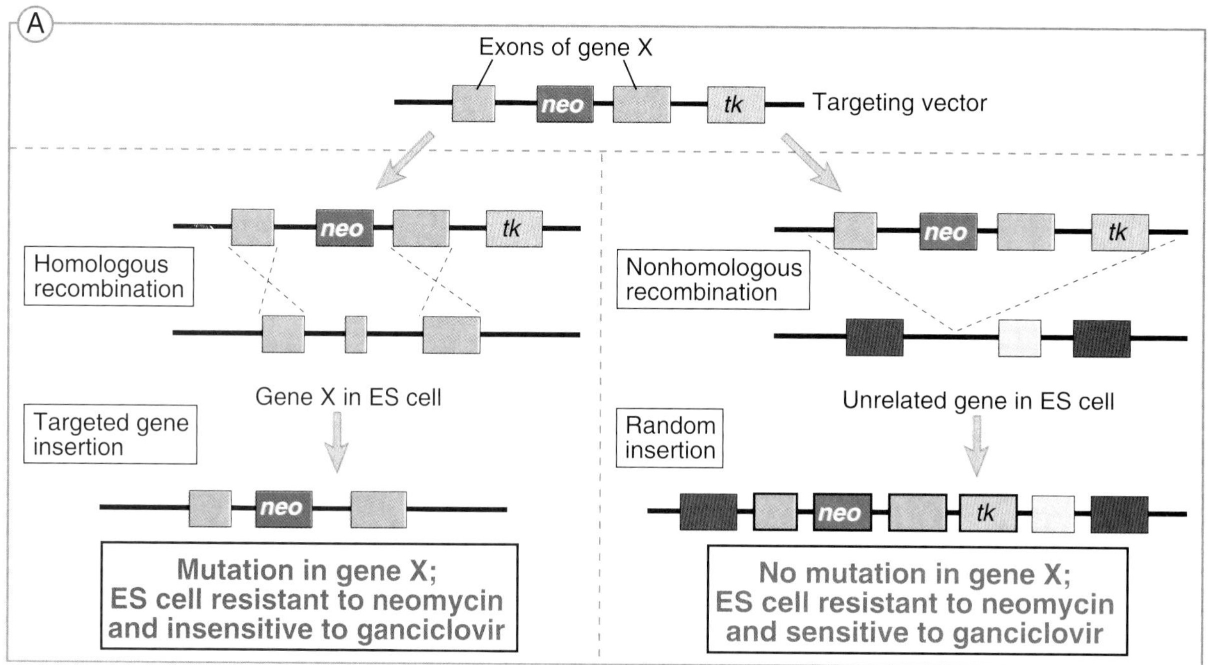

Figure A–7 Generation of gene knockout.
A. The disruption of gene X in an embryonic stem (ES) cell is accomplished by homologous recombination. A population of ES cells is transfected with a targeting vector that contains sequences homologous to two exons of gene X flanking a neomycin resistance gene (*neo*). The *neo* replaces or disrupts one of the exons of gene X on homologous recombination. The thymidine kinase gene (*tk*) in the vector will be inserted into the genome only if random, nonhomologous recombination occurs.

Figure A–7 (*Continued*)
B. The ES cells that were transfected by the targeting vector are selected by neomycin and ganciclovir so that only those cells with targeted insertion (homologous recombination) survive. These cells are then injected into a blastocyst, which is then implanted into the uterus of a pseudopregnant mouse. A chimeric mouse will develop in which some of the tissues are derived from the ES cell carrying the targeted mutation in gene X. These chimeric mice are identified by a mixed-color coat, including the color of the mouse strain from which the ES cells were derived and the color of the mouse strain from which the blastocyst was derived. If the mutation is present in germ cells, it can be propagated by further breeding.

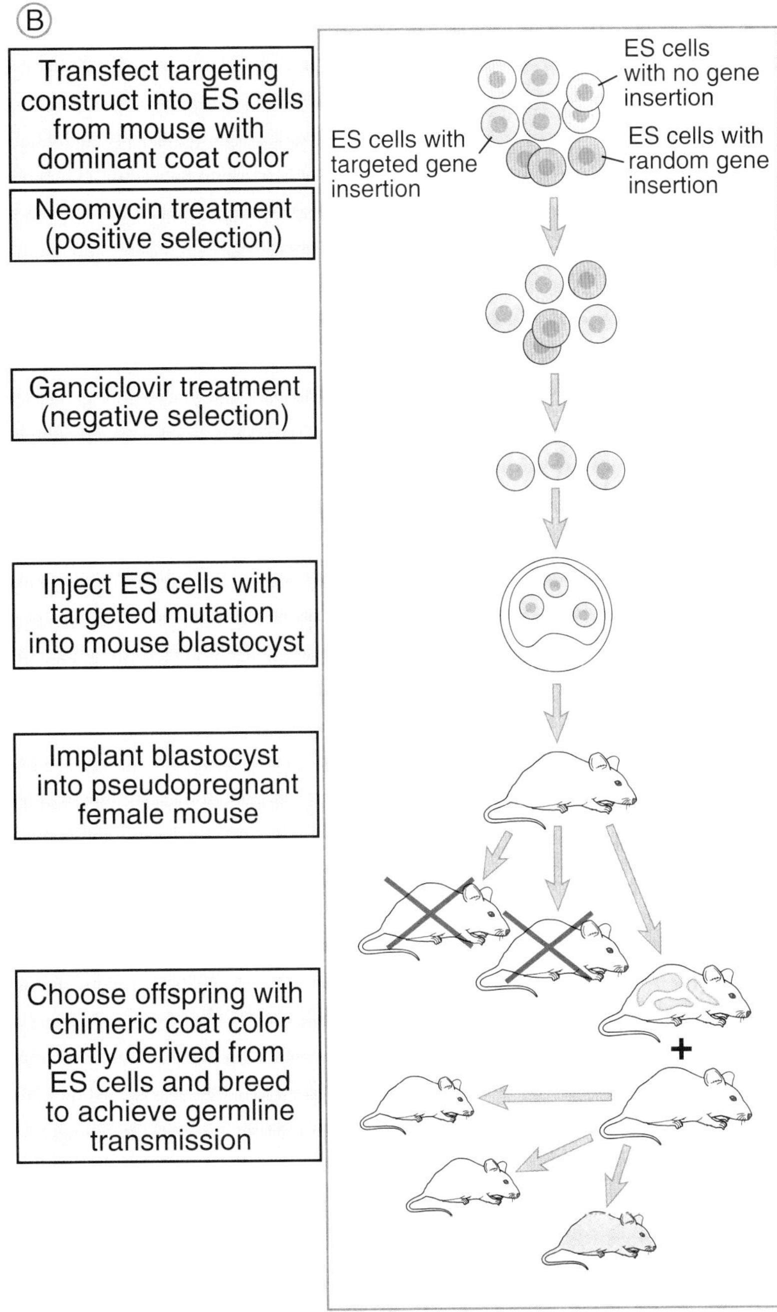

establishing the obligatory function of a gene *in vivo*, is the creation of knockout mice by targeted mutation or disruption of the gene. This technique relies on the phenomenon of homologous recombination. If an exogenous gene is inserted into a cell, for instance, by electroporation, it can integrate randomly into the cell's genome. However, if the gene contains sequences that are homologous to an endogenous gene, it will preferentially recombine with and replace endogenous sequences. To select for cells that have undergone homologous recombination, a drug-based selection strategy is used. The fragment of homologous DNA to be inserted into a cell is placed in a vector typically containing a neomycin resistance gene and a viral thymidine kinase (*tk*) gene (Fig. A–7A). This targeting vector is constructed in such a way that the neomycin resistance gene is always inserted into the chromosomal DNA, but the *tk* gene is lost whenever homologous recombination (as opposed to random insertion) occurs. The vector is introduced into cells, and the cells are grown in neomycin and ganciclovir, a drug that is metabolized by thymidine kinase to generate a lethal product. Cells in which the gene is integrated randomly will be resistant to neomycin but will be killed by ganciclovir, whereas cells in which homologous recombination has occurred will be resistant to both drugs because the *tk* gene will not be incorporated. This positive-negative selection ensures that the inserted gene in surviving cells has undergone homologous recombination with endogenous sequences. The presence of the inserted DNA in the middle of an endogenous gene usually disrupts the coding sequences and ablates expression or function of that gene. In addition, targeting vectors can be designed such that homologous recombination will lead to the deletion of one or more exons of the endogenous gene.

To generate a mouse carrying a targeted gene disruption or mutation, a targeting vector is used to first disrupt the gene in a murine embryonic stem (ES) cell line. ES cells are pluripotent cells derived from mouse embryos that can be propagated and induced to differentiate in culture or that can be incorporated into a mouse blastocyst, which may be implanted in a pseudopregnant mother and carried to term. Importantly, the progeny of the ES cells develop normally into mature tissues that will express the exogenous genes that have been transfected into the ES cells. Thus, the targeting vector designed to disrupt a particular gene is inserted into ES cells, and colonies in which homologous recombination has occurred (on one chromosome) are selected with drugs, as described before (Fig. A–7B). The presence of the desired recombination is verified by analysis of DNA with techniques such as Southern blot hybridization or PCR. The selected ES cells are injected into blastocysts, which are implanted into pseudopregnant females. Mice that develop will be chimeric for a heterozygous disruption or mutation, that is, some of the tissues will be derived from the ES cells and others from the remainder of the normal blastocyst. The germ cells are also usually chimeric, but because these cells are haploid, only some will contain the chromosome copy with the disrupted (mutated) gene. If chimeric mice are mated with normal (wild-type) animals and either sperm or eggs containing the chromosome with the mutation fuse with the wild-type partner, all cells in the offspring derived from such a zygote will be heterozygous for the mutation (so-called germline transmission). Such heterozygous mice can be mated to yield animals that will be homozygous for the mutation with a frequency that is predictable by simple mendelian segregation. Such knockout mice are deficient in expression of the targeted gene.

Homologous recombination can also be used to replace a normal gene sequence with another gene, thereby creating a knock-in mouse strain. In a sense, knock-in mice are mice carrying a transgene at a defined site in the genome rather than in a random site as in conventional transgenic mice. This strategy is used when it is desirable to have the expression of the transgene regulated by certain endogenous DNA sequences, such as a particular enhancer or promoter region. In this case, the targeting vector contains an exogenous gene encoding a desired product as well as sequences homologous to an endogenous gene that are needed to target the site of recombination.

Although the conventional gene-targeting strategy has proved to be of great usefulness in immunology research, the approach has some potentially significant drawbacks. First, the mutation of one gene during development may be compensated for by altered expression of other gene products, and therefore the function of the targeted gene may be obscured. Second, in a conventional gene knockout mouse, the importance of a gene in only one tissue or at only one time during development cannot be easily assessed. Third, a functional selection marker gene, such as the neomycin resistance gene, is permanently introduced into the animal genome, and this alteration may have unpredictable results on the phenotype of the animal. An important refinement of gene knockout technology that can overcome many of these drawbacks takes advantage of the bacteriophage-derived Cre/*loxP* recombination system. The Cre enzyme is a DNA recombinase that recognizes a 34-bp sequence motif called *loxP*, and the enzyme mediates the deletion of gene segments flanked by two *loxP* sites in the same orientation. To generate mice with *loxP*-tagged genes, targeting vectors are constructed with one *loxP* site flanking the neomycin resistance gene at one end and a second *loxP* site flanking the sequences homologous to the target at the other end. These vectors are transfected into ES cells, and mice carrying the *loxP*-flanked but still functional target gene are generated as described for conventional knockout mice. A second strain of mice carrying a *cre* transgene is then bred with the strain carrying the *loxP*-flanked target gene. In the offspring, expression of Cre recombinase will mediate deletion of the target gene. Both the normal gene sequences and the neomycin resistance gene will be deleted. Importantly, expression of the *cre* gene, and therefore deletion of the targeted gene, can be restricted to certain tissues or specified times by the use of *cre* transgene constructs with different promoters. For example, selective deletion of a gene only in helper T cells can be accomplished by using a *cre* transgenic mouse in which *cre* is driven by a CD4 promoter. Alternatively, a steroid-inducible promoter can be used so that Cre expression and subsequent gene deletion only occur after mice are given a dose of dexamethasone. Many other variations on this technology have been devised to create conditional mutants. Cre/*loxP* technology can also be used to create knock-in mice. In this case, *loxP* sites are placed in the targeting vector to flank the neomycin resistance gene and the homologous sequences, but they do not flank the replacement (knock-in) gene sequences. Therefore, after *cre*-mediated deletion, the exogenous gene remains in the genome at the targeted site.

Index

Note: Page numbers followed by the letter f refer to figures and those followed by t refer to tables. Page numbers followed by the letter b indicate boxed material.

C

E

F

N

O

P

T

U

V

W

X

Z